THE AMERICAN MEDICAL ASSOCIATION

GUIDE TO PRESCRIPTION AND OVER-THE-COUNTER DRUGS

Reader's Digest Fund for the Blind is publisher of the Large-Type Edition of *Reader's Digest.* For subscription information about this magazine, please contact Reader's Digest Fund for the Blind, Inc., Dept. 250, Pleasantville, N.Y. 10570.

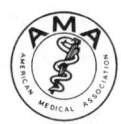

THE AMERICAN MEDICAL ASSOCIATION

GUIDE TO PRESCRIPTION AND OVER-THE-COUNTER DRUGS

EDITOR
Charles B. Clayman, MD

Published by The Reader's Digest Association, Inc.,
with permission of Random House, Inc.

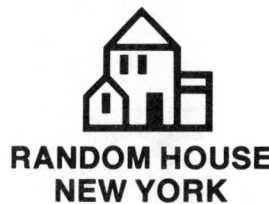

RANDOM HOUSE
NEW YORK

THE AMERICAN MEDICAL ASSOCIATION

James H. Sammons, MD, Executive Vice President
John T. Baker Vice President, Publishing
Frank D. Campion Director, Consumer Book Program
Heidi Hough Managing Editor
James Ferris Editor
Brenda A. Clark Staff Assistant

CONSULTANTS

Charles B. Clayman, MD, Editor

John C. Ballin, PhD
Donald R. Bennett, MD, PhD
Joaquin Chang, BS
Joseph Cranston, Jr., PhD
Sanford C. Dishman, RPh
William R. Felts, MD
Seymour Goren, MD
Gary L. Hubler, RPh
Paul A. Greenberger, MD
Patrick L. Israel, MD
Kenneth F. Lampe, PhD
Fred Levit, MD
Gary S. Lissner, MD

Arline M. McDonald, PhD
Ronald M. Meyer, MD
Carole M. Meyers, MD
Vincent T. Miller, MD
E. Dennis Murphy, MD
Tom E. Nesbitt, MD
Norbert P. Rapoza, PhD
Tor Shwayder, MD
Irwin M.Siegel, MD
Joseph H. Skom, MD
E. M. Steindler, MS
Neil J. Stone, MD
Bonnie B. Wilford

DORLING KINDERSLEY

Senior Editor
Cathy Meeus

Art Editor
Chez Picthall

Editors
Christiane Gunzi, Terence Monaighan, Penny Gray,
Marian Broderick, David Bennett,
Deirdre Clark, Gail Lawther

Additional editorial assistance from
Casey Horton, Jillian Somerscales, Joanna Thomas

Designers
Richard Czapnik, Debra Lee, Gail Jones,
Sandra Schneider

Additional design assistance from
Tracy Timson, Peter Cross, Anne Cuthbert

Editorial Director Amy Carroll

Edited and designed by Dorling Kindersley Limited.

Copyright © 1988 by Dorling Kindersley Limited.
and the American Medical Association

All rights reserved under international and Pan-
American Copyright Conventions. Published in the
United States by Random House, Inc., New York.

Library of Congress Cataloging-in-Publication Data

Main entry under title:

The American Medical Association guide to
prescription and over-the-counter drugs.

Includes index.
1. Drugs – Handbooks, manuals, etc.
2. Drugs, Non-prescription – Handbooks, manuals, etc.
I. American Medical Association.

RM301.12.A44 1988 615'.1 87–43202
ISBN 0–394–56949–0

Manufactured in the United States of America

Computerset by The Setting Studio, Newcastle, England
Reproduction by Llovet SPA, Barcelona, Spain

PREFACE

Those of us over 55 years old can scarcely remember – and those of us under 55 have never known – how relatively powerless medicine really was in the years before World War II. The physician then had only a handful of medicines available to fight disease. But starting with the development of the sulfa drugs in the late 1930s, a parade of new, seemingly miraculous drugs began to transform medicine. First there was penicillin, then streptomycin and cortisone, followed by many others. The ever-growing array of new drugs has enormously expanded the physician's ability to cure or alleviate conditions once considered hopeless.

Simultaneously, the public's desire for authoritative knowledge about the new medicines has grown. To help satisfy that curiosity, to enable a sick person to better understand his or her treatment, to warn people about the harm many drugs can do, we are delighted to add this book to the American Medical Association's Home Health Library.

Developed by the successful British publishing firm Dorling Kindersley, Limited, the concept of this Guide places a strong emphasis on graphics. The factual material has come from many sources – from pharmacologists and pharmacists here and in England, from *Drug Evaluations*, 6th edition, a reference work by the American Medical Association Department of Drugs, and from many US physician specialists active in clinical practice and academic medicine.

Although this Guide lists thousands of medical or medically related substances in the index, it has been impossible to give them equal attention. In the process of selecting, various criteria have been applied. These include medical judgments as to a drug's clinical value and frequency of medically recommended use, based on data from the independent National Drug and Therapeutic Index. Nevertheless, many less commonly used drugs have been included to emphasize the diversity and versatility of modern pharmacology.

Ultimately, the final selections reflect the judgment of the medical editor of this book, Charles B. Clayman, MD. A board-certified internist, he served for several years on the staff of the Department of Drugs of the American Medical Association. Until recently, he divided his time between private medical practice and teaching, with the rank of associate professor of medicine, at the Northwestern University Medical School. Since 1977 he has been a contributing editor of the *Journal of the American Medical Association*.

James H. Sammons, MD
Executive Vice President, American Medical Association

CONTENTS

4 A–Z OF DRUGS

5 GLOSSARY AND INDEX

DRUG POISONING EMERGENCY GUIDE 590

INTRODUCTION

The American Medical Association Guide to Prescription and Over-the-Counter Drugs has been planned and written to provide clear information and practical advice on drugs and medicines in a way that can be readily understood by a non-medical reader. The text reflects current medical knowledge and standard medical practice in the US. It is intended to complement and reinforce the advice of your physician.

How the book is structured

The book is divided into five parts. The first part, Understanding and Using Drugs, provides a general introduction to the effects of drugs and gives general advice on practical questions such as the administration and storage of drugs. The second part, the Drug Finder Index, provides the means of locating information on specific drugs. Part 3, Major Drug Groups, will help you to understand

the uses and mechanisms of action of the principal classes of drugs. Part 4, the A – Z of Drugs, consists of detailed profiles of all commonly prescribed drugs, and also includes special profiles on vitamins and minerals, drugs of abuse and food additives. Part 5 contains a glossary of drug-related terms and a general index.

Finding your way into the book

The information you require, whether on the specific characteristics of an individual drug or on the general effects and uses of a group of drugs, can be easily obtained without prior knowledge of the medical names of drugs or drug classification through one of the two indexes: the Drug Finder Index or the General Index. The diagram on the facing page shows how you can access information throughout the book on the subject concerning you from each of these starting points.

1 UNDERSTANDING AND USING DRUGS

The introductory part of the book, Understanding and Using Drugs, gives a grounding in the fundamental principles underlying the medical use of drugs. Covering such topics as the classification of drugs, mechanisms of action

and the proper use of medications, it provides valuable background information that backs up the more detailed descriptions and advice given in Parts 3 and 4. Read this section before seeking further specific information.

2 DRUG FINDER INDEX

This is composed of two elements. The Color Identification Guide contains photographs of over 250 brand-name tablets and capsules to help you identify medications. The Index of Generic and Brand-Name Drugs helps you to find information on specific drugs.

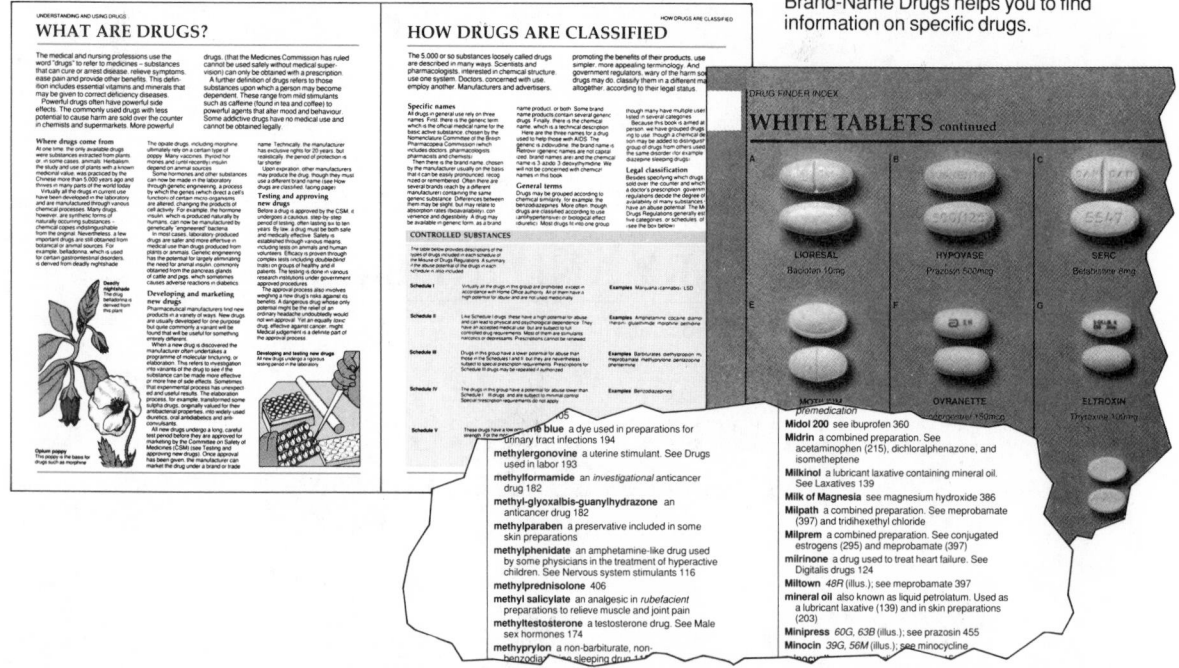

Finding your information

Whether you start by looking up an individual drug or a group of drugs, you will be led by cross-references to relevant information in all parts of the book.

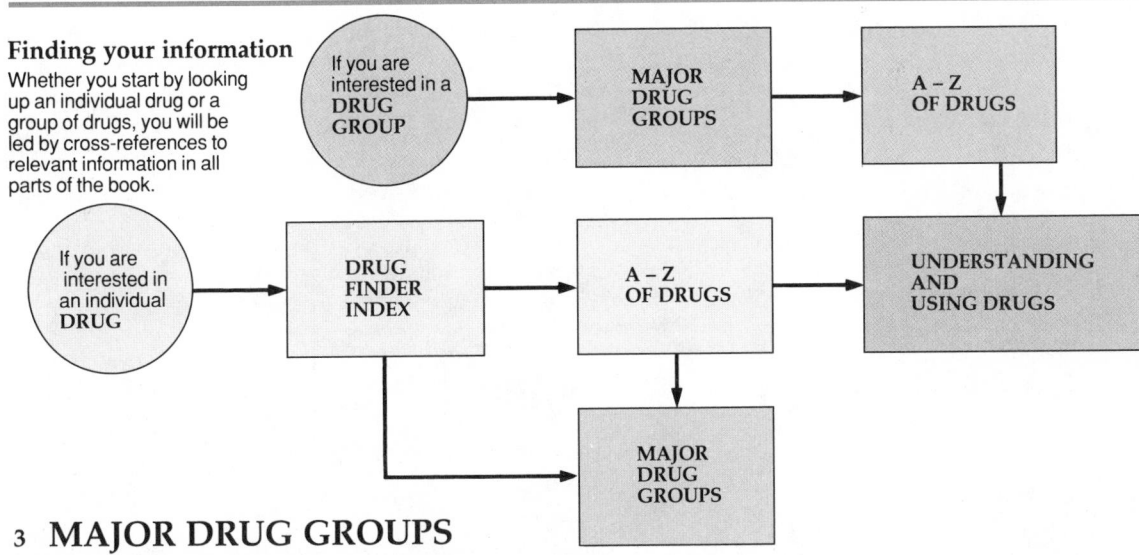

If you are interested in a **DRUG GROUP** → **MAJOR DRUG GROUPS** → **A – Z OF DRUGS**

If you are interested in an individual **DRUG** → **DRUG FINDER INDEX** → **A – Z OF DRUGS** → **UNDERSTANDING AND USING DRUGS**

MAJOR DRUG GROUPS

3 MAJOR DRUG GROUPS

Subdivided into sections dealing with each body system (for example, heart and circulation) or major disease grouping (for example, malignant and immune disease), this part of the book contains descriptions of the principal classes of drugs. Information is given on the uses, actions, effects and risks associated with each group of drugs and is backed up by helpful illustrations and diagrams. Individual drugs in each group are listed to allow cross-reference to Part 4.

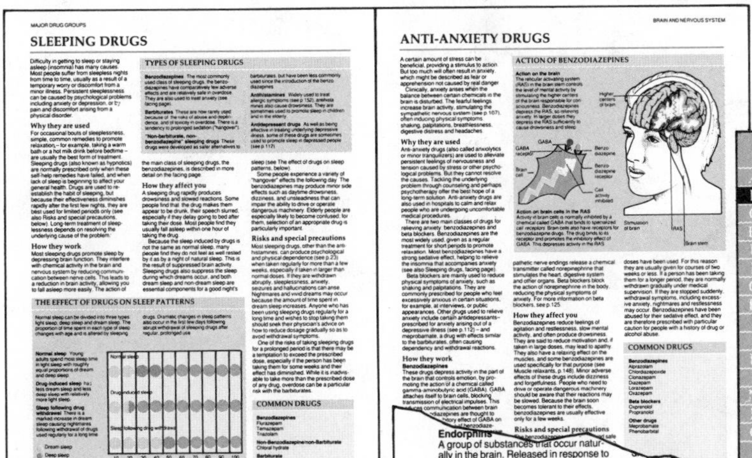

4 A – Z OF DRUGS

This part contains descriptions of individual drugs. The main listing includes 320 profiles of generic drugs written to a standard format to help you find specific information quickly and easily. Cross-references to the relevant major drug groups are provided. Supplementary sections profile vitamins and minerals, drugs of abuse and food additives.

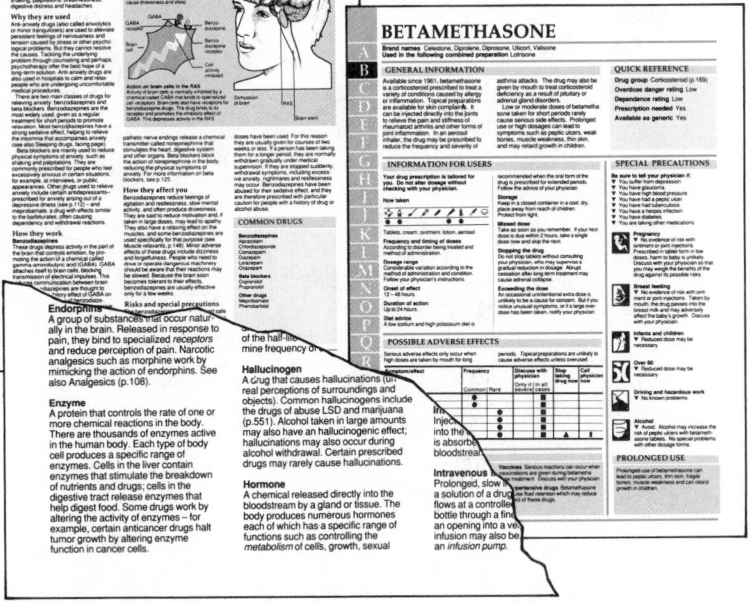

5 GLOSSARY AND INDEX

The glossary explains technical words, printed in italics in the text. The index enables you to look up references throughout the book.

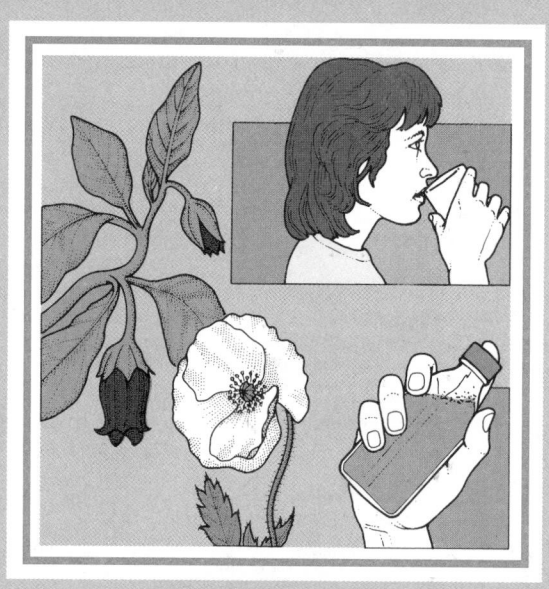

PART

1

UNDERSTANDING AND USING DRUGS

WHAT ARE DRUGS?

In the broadest sense, and that used in most sections of this book, the word "drugs" refers to medicines – substances that can cure or arrest disease, relieve symptoms, ease pain and provide a range of other benefits. That definition includes the vitamins and minerals essential to health that may be given to correct deficiency diseases.

The power of individual drugs varies. The commonly used drugs with less potential to cause harm are sold over the counter in drugstores and supermarkets. More powerful drugs, ones that the US Food and Drug Administration has ruled cannot be used safely without medical supervision, require a physician's prescription.

A further definition of drugs refers to those substances upon which a person may become dependent. These range from mild stimulants such as caffeine (in coffee) to potent agents that alter mood and behavior. Certain of the latter have no medical use and cannot be obtained legally.

Where drugs come from

At one time, drugs were substances extracted from plants, or in some cases, animals. Herbalism, the study and use of plants with presumed medicinal value, was practiced by the Chinese more than 5,000 years ago and thrives in many parts of the world today.

Virtually all the drugs in current use in the US today have been developed in the laboratory and are manufactured through various chemical processes. Many drugs, however, are synthetic forms of naturally occurring substances – chemical copies indistinguishable from the original. Nevertheless, a few important drugs are still obtained from botanical or animal sources. Belladonna, which is used for certain gastrointestinal disorders, is derived from deadly nightshade. The opiate drugs, including morphine, ultimately rely on a certain type of poppy. Many vaccines and thyroid hormones depend on animal sources.

Many hormones and other substances can now be made in the laboratory through genetic engineering, a process by which the genes (which direct a cell's function) of certain microorganisms are altered, changing the products of cell activity. For example, the hormone insulin, which is produced naturally by humans, can now be manufactured by genetically "engineered" bacteria.

In most cases, laboratory-produced drugs are safer and more effective in medical use than drugs produced from plants or animals. Genetic engineering has the potential for largely eliminating the need for animal insulin, commonly obtained from the pancreas glands of cattle and pigs, which sometimes causes adverse reactions in diabetics.

Developing and marketing new drugs

Constantly on the lookout for new products, pharmaceutical manufacturers find them in a variety of ways. Sometimes, after a drug developed for one purpose proves ineffective, a variant will be found that will be useful for something entirely different. When a new drug is discovered, the manufacturer often undertakes a program of molecular tinkering (called elaboration), varying the molecular structure to see if the substance can be made more effective or more free of side effects. Sometimes that experimental process has serendipitous results. The elaboration process, for example, transformed some sulfa drugs, originally valued for their antibacterial properties, into widely used diuretics, oral antidiabetics, and anticonvulsants.

All new drugs undergo a long, careful test period before they are approved for marketing by the US Food and Drug Administration (FDA). (See Testing and approving new drugs, below.) Once approval has been given, the manufacturer can market the drug under a brand name, or trademark. Technically, the manufacturer has exclusive rights for 17 years; but realistically, the period of protection is far shorter.

Upon expiration, other manufacturers may produce the drug, though they must use a different brand name (see How drugs are classified, facing page).

Testing and approving new drugs

Before a drug is approved by the FDA, it undergoes a cautious, step-by-step period of testing, often lasting six to ten years. By federal law, a drug must be both safe and medically effective. Safety is established through various means, including tests on animals and human volunteers. Efficacy is proven through complex tests (including *double-blind* trials) on groups of healthy and ill patients. The testing is done in various research institutions under FDA-approved procedures.

The approval process also involves weighing a new drug's risks against its benefits. A dangerous drug whose only potential might be the relief of an ordinary headache undoubtedly would not win approval. Yet an equally *toxic* drug, effective against cancer, might. Medical judgment is a definite part of the approval process.

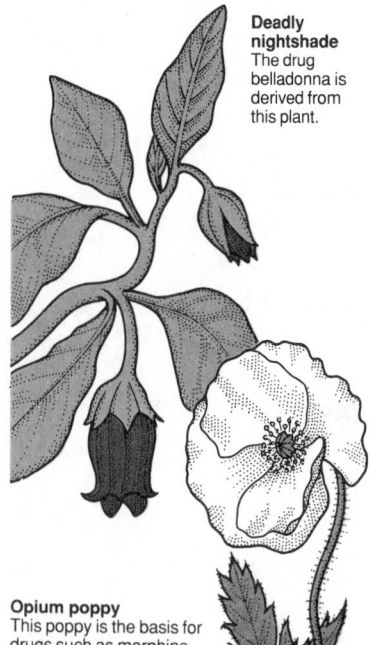

Deadly nightshade
The drug belladonna is derived from this plant.

Opium poppy
This poppy is the basis for drugs such as morphine.

Developing and testing new drugs
All new drugs undergo a rigorous testing period in the laboratory.

HOW DRUGS ARE CLASSIFIED

The 5,000 or so substances loosely called drugs are described in many ways. Scientists and pharmacologists, interested in chemical structure, use one system. Physicians, concerned with use, have another. Manufacturers and advertisers, promoting the benefits of their products, employ simpler, more appealing terminology. And state and federal regulators, wary of the harm some drugs may do, classify them in a different manner altogether, according to their legal status.

Specific names

All drugs in general use rely on three names. The generic term is the official medical name for the basic active substance, chosen by the USAN (US Adopted Name) Council, made up of representatives of the American Medical Association, the US Pharmacopeial Association (physicians and pharmacists) and the American Pharmaceutical Association (pharmacists).

Then there is the brand name, chosen by the manufacturer usually on the basis that it can be easily pronounced, recognized or remembered. Often there are several brands (each by a different manufacturer) containing the same generic substance. Differences between them may be slight, but may relate to absorption rates (bioavailability), convenience and digestibility. A drug may be available in generic form, as a brand name, or both. Some brand names contain several generic substances. Finally, there is the chemical name, which is a technical description.

Here are the three names for a drug used to help those with AIDS. The generic is zidovudine; the brand name is Retrovir (generic names are not capitalized; brand names are); and the chemical name is 3-azido-3-deoxythymidine.

General terms

Drugs may be grouped according to chemical similarity, for example, the benzodiazepines. More often, though, drugs are classified according to use (antihypertensive) or biological effect (diuretic). Most drugs fit into one group, though many have multiple uses and are listed in several categories.

Because this book is aimed at the lay person, we have grouped drugs according to use, though a chemical description may be added to distinguish one group of drugs from others used to treat the same disorder (e.g., benzodiazepine sleeping drugs).

Legal classification

Besides specifying which drugs can be sold over the counter and which require a physician's prescription, state and federal statutes and regulations govern the availability of many substances which have an abuse potential. The controlled substances laws generally establish five categories, or schedules, of drugs (see the table below).

CONTROLLED SUBSTANCES

The table below provides descriptions of the types of drugs usually included in each schedule of controlled substances laws. A summary of regulations concerning prescription renewals is also included. The schedules may vary somewhat from one state to another.

Schedule I	Virtually all the drugs in this group are illegal. All of them have a high potential for abuse and currently do not have an accepted medical use. These drugs are not prescribable.	**Examples** Benzylmorphine, dihydromorphine, heroin, LSD, mescaline, nicocodeine, peyote.
Schedule II	Like Schedule I drugs, these have a high potential for abuse and can lead to serious physical and psychological dependence. Unlike Schedule I drugs, however, they have an accepted medical use. Most of them are stimulants, narcotics or depressants. Prescriptions for them cannot be renewed.	**Examples** Amphetamine, cocaine, codeine, meperidine, morphine, secobarbital.
Schedule III	Drugs in this group have a lower potential for abuse than those in Schedules I and II, but they can nevertheless lead to dependence. Prescriptions for Schedule III drugs can be refilled up to five times in six months if the prescriber authorizes it.	**Examples** Acetaminophen with codeine, aspirin with codeine, methyprylon (sleeping drug), benzphetamine (appetite suppressant), phendimetrazine (appetite suppressant).
Schedule IV	The drugs in this group have a potential for abuse lower than Schedule I – III drugs. The regulations for refilling prescriptions are the same in most states as for Schedule III drugs.	**Examples** Chloral hydrate (sleeping drug), diazepam (anti-anxiety drug, muscle relaxant), ethchlorvynol (sleeping drug), phenobarbital (anticonvulsant), prazepam (anti-anxiety drug).
Schedule V	These drugs have a low potential for abuse. For the most part, they are preparations that contain small amounts of narcotics.	**Examples** (Note: These are all brand-name combination preparations.) Lomotil (antidiarrheal), Parepectolin (antidiarrheal), Cheracol (cough suppressant), Robitussin AC (cough suppressant), Tussi-Organidin liquid (cough suppressant).

HOW DRUGS WORK

Of all the weapons at a physician's disposal, probably none is more effective or more frequently used than the array of drugs developed, for the most part, in the last 50 years. Today, there are drugs that ease the the painful symptoms of disease, drugs that make disorders like hypertension manageable, drugs that soothe inflammation, relieve anxieties and bolster the body's natural defenses.

Before the discovery of the sulfa drugs in 1935, the physician's knowledge of drugs was limited.

At that time, possibly only a dozen or so drugs had clear medical value. That, of course, has changed. Not only is an impressive variety of effective drugs now available; scientific knowledge in the drug field has virtually exploded.

Today's physician understands far better than his predecessors the complex actions of drugs in the body and the effects drugs can have on it, both beneficial and adverse. He can also recognize that some drugs interact harmfully with others, or with certain foods.

DRUG ACTIONS

While the exact workings of some drugs are not fully understood, medical science provides clear knowledge as to what most of them do once they enter or are applied to the human body. Drugs, of course, serve different purposes, sometimes curing a disease, sometimes only alleviating symptoms. Their impact occurs in various parts of the anatomy. But although different drugs act in different ways, their actions generally fall into one of three categories.

Replacing chemicals that are deficient

To function normally, the body requires sufficient levels of certain chemical substances. These include vitamins and minerals, which the body obtains from food. A balanced diet usually supplies what is needed. But when deficiencies occur, various diseases result. Lack of vitamin C causes scurvy, lack of vitamin D leads to rickets, and iron deficiency causes anemia.

Other deficiency diseases arise from a lack of various *hormones*, chemical substances produced by glands which act as internal "messengers." Diabetes mellitus, Addison's disease and hypothyroidism all result from deficiencies of different hormones.

Deficiency diseases are treated with drugs that replace the substances that are missing, or, in the case of some hormone deficiencies, with animal or synthetic replacements.

Interfering with cell function

Many drugs can change the way cells work by stimulating or reducing the normal level of activity. Vaccines, for example, function in this way by increasing the activity of the cells that produce the antibodies that fight invading organisms such as bacteria and viruses. Drugs that act in a similar manner are used in the treatment of a variety of conditions: hormone disorders, blood clotting problems, heart and kidney diseases.

These drugs do their work by altering the transmission system by which messages are sent from one part of the body to another.

A message – to contract a muscle, say – originates in the brain and enters a nerve cell through its receiving end. The message, in the form of an electrical impulse, travels the length of the nerve cell to the sending end. Here a chemical substance called a *neurotransmitter* is released, conducting the message across the tiny gap separating it from an adjacent nerve cell. That process is repeated until the message reaches the appropriate muscle.

Many drugs can alter this process, often by their effect on receptor sites on cells (see the box, left). Some drugs (*agonists*) intensify cell activity, while other drugs (*antagonists*) reduce activity in the cells.

Acting against invading organisms or abnormal cells

Many microorganisms are able to invade the body and cause infection. Some drugs destroy microorganisms, either by preventing their multiplication or by killing them directly. Other drugs treat disease by killing abnormal cells – cancer cells, for example.

RECEPTOR SITES

Many drugs are thought to produce their effects by their action on special sites called *receptors* on the surface of body cells. Natural body chemicals such as *neurotransmitters* bind to these sites, initiating a response in the cell. Cells may have many types of receptors, each of which has an affinity for a different chemical in the body. Drugs may also bind to receptors, either adding to the effect of the body's natural chemicals and enhancing cell response (agonist drugs) or preventing such a chemical from binding to its receptor, and thereby blocking a particular cell response (antagonist drugs).

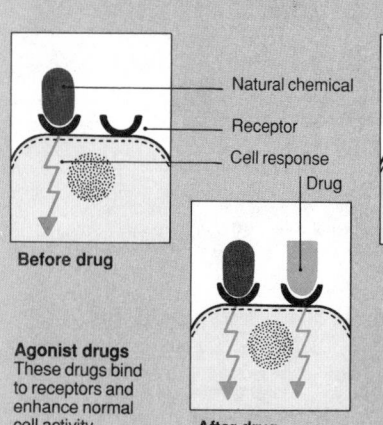

Before drug

Agonist drugs
These drugs bind to receptors and enhance normal cell activity.

After drug

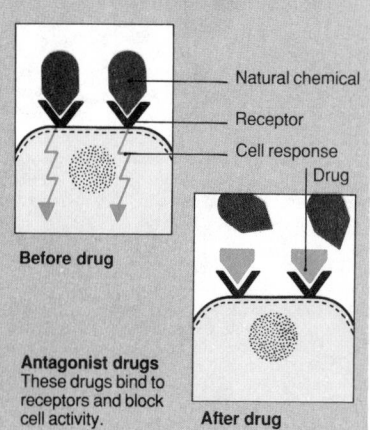

Before drug

Antagonist drugs
These drugs bind to receptors and block cell activity.

After drug

Natural chemical
Receptor
Cell response
Drug

THE EFFECTS OF DRUGS

Before a physician selects a drug to be used in the treatment of a sick person, he or she carefully weighs the benefits and the risks. Obviously, the doctor expects a positive result from the drug, a cure of the condition or at least the relief of symptoms. At the same time, consideration has to be given to the risks, for all drugs are potentially harmful, some of them considerably more so than others.

Reaction time

Some drugs can produce rapid and spectacular relief from the symptoms of disease. Nitroglycerin frequently provides almost immediate relief for the pain of angina; other drugs can quickly alleviate the symptoms of an asthmatic attack. Conversely, some drugs take much longer to produce a response. It may, for example, require several weeks of treatment with an antidepressant drug before a person experiences maximum benefit. This can be worrisome unless the physician has warned of the possibility of a delay in the onset of beneficial effects.

Side effects

The side effects of a drug are the known and frequently experienced, expected reactions to a drug. The old concept of a drug as a "magic bullet" that could be targeted to a specific type of cell is now recognized as inaccurate. Whether a drug is taken by mouth, by injection, or by inhalation, it will be distributed throughout the body, and its effects are unlikely to be restricted to one particular type of tissue or organ.

For example, *anticholinergic* drugs, which are prescribed to relieve spasm in the wall of the intestine, may also affect the eyes, causing blurred vision; the mouth, causing dryness; and the bladder, causing the retention of urine. Such side effects may gradually disappear as the body becomes used to the drug. But if side effects persist, the dose of the drug may have to be

DOSE AND RESPONSE

Not everyone responds in the same way to a drug, and in many cases the dose has to be adjusted to allow for such factors as the age, weight, or general health of the patient.

The dose of any drug should be sufficient to produce a beneficial response but not so great that it will cause excessive adverse effects. If the dose is too low, the drug may not have any effect, either beneficial or adverse; if it is too high, it will not produce any additional benefits and may produce adverse effects. The aim of

drug treatment, therefore, is to achieve a concentration of drug in the blood or tissue that lies somewhere between the minimum effective level and the maximum safe concentration. This is known as the therapeutic range.

For some drugs, such as digitalis drugs, the therapeutic range is quite narrow, so the margin of safety/effectiveness is small. Other drugs, such as penicillin antibiotics, have a much wider therapeutic range.

Wide therapeutic range

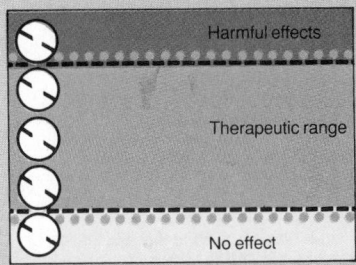

Dosage of drugs with a wide therapeutic range can vary considerably without altering the drug's effects.

Narrow therapeutic range

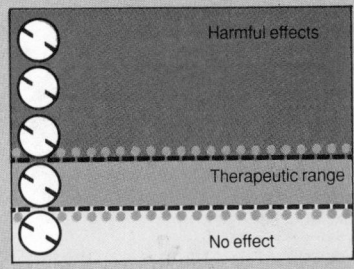

Dosage of drugs with a narrow therapeutic range has to be carefully calculated to achieve the desired effect.

reduced, or the time between doses may have to be increased.

The side effects of certain drugs, especially some anticancer drugs, can often be quite serious. Such drugs are administered because they may be the only agents available for the treatment of a disease that might otherwise prove fatal. However, all drugs, even the mildest, should be regarded as chemicals with a potential for producing serious, *toxic* reactions, especially if they are misused or abused.

Adverse reactions

Adverse reactions are unexpected, unpredictable reactions that are not related to the usual effects of a normal

dose of a drug. Unpredictable drug reactions may be caused by conditions in the patient such as an allergy or a genetic disorder, like the absence of an *enzyme* that usually inactivates the drug. Common adverse reactions of this type include a rash, swelling of the face, or jaundice. They may also be due to interactions with other drugs. Unpredictable drug reactions usually necessitate withdrawal of the drug under medical supervision.

Beneficial vs. adverse effects

In evaluating the risk/benefit ratio of a drug which he or she may prescribe, a physician weighs the therapeutic benefit to the sick person against the possible adverse effects. For example, such side effects as nausea, headache, and diarrhea may result from taking an antibiotic. But they will certainly be considered acceptable risks if the problem is a life-threatening infection requiring immediate treatment. On the other hand, such side effects would be considered unacceptable for an oral contraceptive that is taken over a number of years by a healthy patient.

Because some people are more at risk from adverse drug reactions than others (particularly those with a history of drug allergy), the physician normally checks whether there is any reason why a particular drug should not be given (see Drug treatment in special risk groups, p.20).

PLACEBO RESPONSE

The word placebo – Latin for "I will please" – is used to describe any chemically inert substance given as a substitute for a drug. Any benefit gained from taking a placebo occurs because the person taking it believes that it will produce good results.

New drugs are almost always tested against a placebo preparation in clinical trials as a way to assess the efficacy of a drug before it is marketed. The placebo is made to look identical to the active preparation, and volunteers are not told whether they have been given the active drug or the placebo. Sometimes the physician is also unaware of which preparation an individual has been

given. This is known as a *double-blind* trial. In this way, the purely placebo effect can be eliminated and the effectiveness of the drug determined more realistically.

Sometimes the mere taking of a medicine has a psychological effect that produces a beneficial physical response. This type of placebo response can make an important contribution to the overall effectiveness of a chemically active drug, and is most commonly seen with analgesics, antidepressants and anti-anxiety drugs. Some people, known as placebo responders, are more likely to experience this sort of reaction than the rest of the population.

DRUG INTERACTIONS

When two different drugs are taken together, or when a drug is taken in combination with certain foods or with alcohol, this may produce effects different from those produced when the drug is taken alone. In many cases, this is beneficial, and physicians frequently make use of interactions to increase the effectiveness of a treatment. Very often, more than one drug may be prescribed to treat cancer or high blood pressure (hypertension).

Many interactions, however, are unwanted and may be harmful. They may occur not only between prescription drugs, but also between prescription and over-the-counter drugs. So it is important to read warnings on drug labels and tell your physician if you are taking any drug preparations – both prescription and over-the-counter – that the physician does not know about.

A drug may interact with another drug or with food or alcohol for a number of reasons. The main types of interaction are discussed below.

Altered absorption

Alcohol and some drugs (especially narcotics) slow down the digestive process that empties the stomach contents into the intestine. This may delay the absorption, and therefore the effect, of another drug taken at the same time. Other drugs (for example, metoclopramide, an anti-emetic drug) may speed the rate at which the stomach empties and therefore may increase the rate at which another drug is absorbed and takes effect.

Some drugs also combine with another drug or a food in the intestine to form a compound that is not so readily absorbed. This occurs when tetracycline and iron tablets or antacids are taken together. Milk also reduces the absorption of certain drugs in this way.

Reduced absorption in the intestine

Absorption of drug (A) through the intestinal wall may be reduced if it combines with another drug (B).

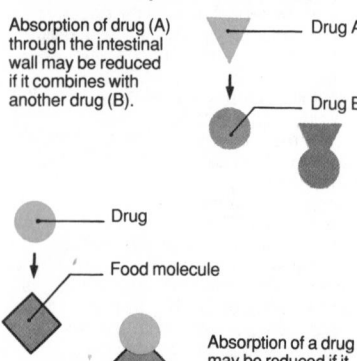

Drug A

Drug B

Drug

Food molecule

Absorption of a drug may be reduced if it combines with a food molecule.

EXAMPLES OF IMPORTANT INTERACTIONS

Adverse interactions between drugs may vary from a simple blocking of a drug's beneficial effect to a serious reaction between two drugs which may be life-threatening. Some of the more threatening adverse interactions occur between the following:

Drugs that depress the central nervous system (sleeping drugs, narcotics, antihistamines and alcohol). The effects of two or more of these drugs in combination may be additive, causing dangerous oversedation.

Drugs that lower blood sugar levels and such drugs as sulfonamides and alcohol. The drug interaction increases the effect of blood sugar-lowering drugs, thus further depressing blood sugar levels.

Oral anticoagulants and other drugs, particularly aspirin and antibiotics. Because these drugs may increase the tendency to bleed, it is essential to check the effects in every case.

Monoamine oxidase inhibitors (MAOIs). There is a large list of drugs and foods which can produce a severe rise in blood pressure when taken with MAOIs. Dangerous drugs include amphetamines and decongestants. Foods that interact include cheese, red wine, beer, and chocolate.

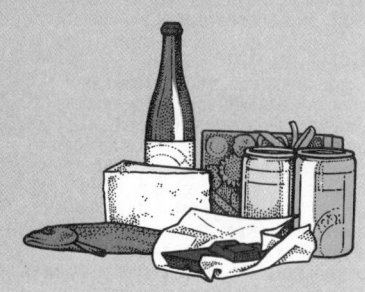

Enzyme effects

Some drugs increase the production of *enzymes* in the liver that break down drugs, while others may inhibit or reduce enzyme production. They therefore affect the rate at which other drugs are activated or inactivated.

Excretion in the urine

A drug may reduce the kidneys' ability to excrete another drug, thereby raising the level of the drug in the blood and increasing its effect.

Receptor effects

Drugs which act on the same *receptors* (p.14) sometimes redouble each other's stimulating effect on the body. Or they may compete with each other in occupying particular receptor sites. Naloxone, for instance, blocks the receptors used by narcotic drugs, thereby helping to reverse the effects of narcotic poisoning.

Similar effects

Drugs that produce similar effects (even though they do not act on the same receptor) may be given together so that a smaller dose of each is required, reducing the side effects of each. This is common practice in the treatment of high blood pressure, in giving anticancer drugs, and also in treating pain. Sometimes two antibiotics may be given simultaneously. Though their effects may be similar, the infecting organisms are less likely to develop resistance.

Reduced protein binding

Some drugs circulate around the body in the bloodstream with a proportion of the drug attached to the proteins of the blood plasma. This means that the amount of the drug attached to plasma proteins is inactive. If another drug is taken, some of the second drug may also attach itself to the plasma proteins and displace the first drug; more of the first drug is then active in the body.

Interaction between protein-bound drugs

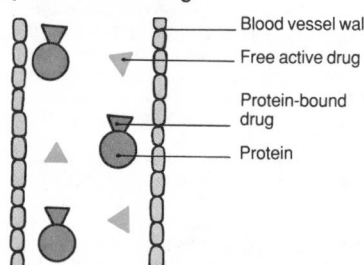

Blood vessel wall

Free active drug

Protein-bound drug

Protein

Protein-bound drug taken alone
Drug molecules that are bound to proteins in the blood are unable to pass into body tissues. Only free drug molecules are active.

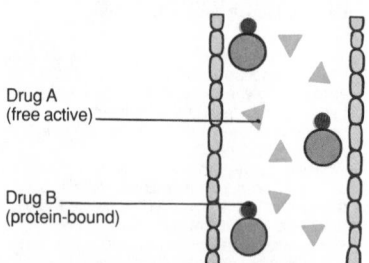

Drug A (free active)

Drug B (protein-bound)

Taken with another protein-bound drug
If a drug (B) with a greater ability to bind with proteins is also taken, the first drug (A) is displaced, increasing the amount of active drug.

METHODS OF ADMINISTRATION

To be effective, the majority of drugs must be absorbed into the bloodstream in order to reach the site where their effects are needed. The method of administering a drug determines the route it takes to get into the bloodstream and the speed at which it is absorbed into the blood.

When a drug is meant to enter the bloodstream it is usually administered in one of the following ways: through the mouth or rectum, by injection, or inhalation. Drugs implanted under the skin or enclosed in a skin patch also enter the bloodstream. These are discussed under Slow-release preparations (p.18).

When it is unnecessary or undesirable for a drug to enter the bloodstream in large amounts, it may be applied *topically* so that its effect is limited mainly to the site of the disorder, such as the surface of the skin or mucous membranes (the membranes of the nose, eyes, ears, mouth, vagina, and rectum). Drugs are administered topically in a variety of preparations, including creams, sprays, drops, and suppositories. Most inhaled drugs also have a local effect.

Very often, a particular drug may be available in different forms. Many drugs are available as tablets and injectable fluid. The choice between a tablet or injection depends on a number of factors, including the severity of the illness, the urgency with which the drug effect is needed, the part of the body requiring treatment, and the patient's general state of health, such as his or her ability to swallow, for example.

The various routes of administration are discussed in greater detail below. For a description of the different forms in which drugs are given, see Drug forms (p.19).

ADMINISTRATION BY MOUTH

Giving drugs by mouth is the most frequently used method of administration. Most drugs that are given by mouth are absorbed into the bloodstream through the walls of the intestine. The speed at which the drug is absorbed and the amount of active drug that is available for use depend on several factors, including the form in which it is given (for example, as a tablet or a liquid) and whether it is taken with food or on an empty stomach. If a drug is taken when the stomach is empty (before meals, for example), it may act more quickly than a drug that is taken when the stomach is full.

Some drugs (like antacids, which neutralize stomach acidity) are taken by mouth to produce a direct effect on the stomach or digestive tract.

Sublingual tablets
Tablets are available which are placed in the mouth but not swallowed. They are absorbed quickly into the bloodstream through the lining of the mouth, which has a rich supply of blood vessels. Both sublingual and buccal tablets act in this way. Sublingual tablets are placed under the tongue; buccal tablets are placed in the pouch between the cheek and teeth.

HOW DRUGS PASS THROUGH THE BODY

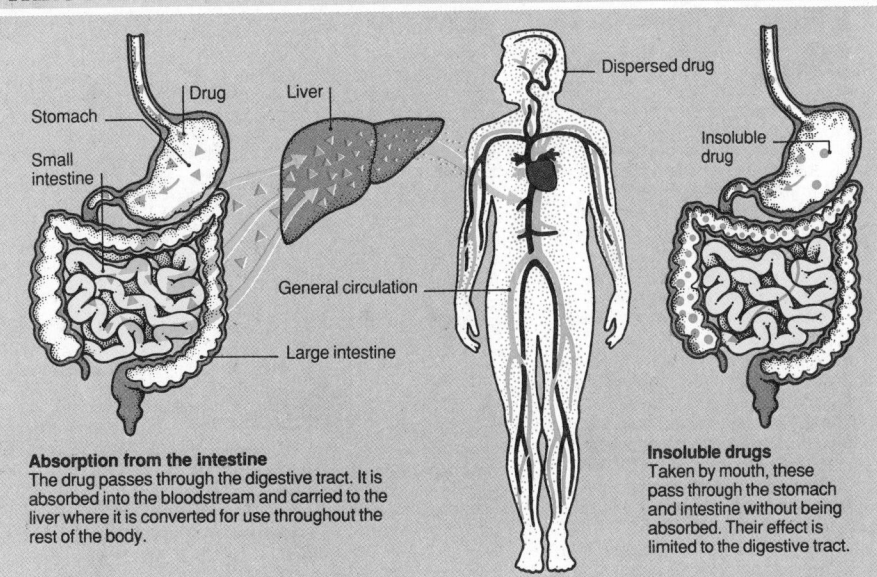

Most drugs taken by mouth reach the bloodstream by absorption through the small intestine wall. Blood vessels supplying the intestine then carry the drug to the liver where it may be broken down into a form that can be used by the body. The drug (or its breakdown product) then enters into the general circulation, which carries it around the body. It may pass back into the intestine before it is reabsorbed into the bloodstream. Some drugs are rapidly excreted via the kidneys; others may build up in fatty tissues in the body.

Certain insoluble drugs cannot be absorbed through the intestine and pass through the digestive tract unchanged. They are useful for treating bowel disorders, but if they are intended to have *systemic* effects elsewhere they must be given by intravenous injection.

Absorption from the intestine
The drug passes through the digestive tract. It is absorbed into the bloodstream and carried to the liver where it is converted for use throughout the rest of the body.

Insoluble drugs
Taken by mouth, these pass through the stomach and intestine without being absorbed. Their effect is limited to the digestive tract.

Labels on diagram: Stomach, Small intestine, Drug, Liver, General circulation, Large intestine, Dispersed drug, Insoluble drug

RECTAL ADMINISTRATION

Drugs intended to have a *systemic* effect may be given in the form of suppositories inserted into the rectum, from whence they are absorbed into the bloodstream. This method may be used to give drugs that might be destroyed by the stomach's digestive juices. It is also sometimes used to administer drugs to people who cannot take medication by mouth, such as those suffering from nausea and vomiting.

Drugs may also be given rectally for local effect, either as suppositories (to relieve hemorrhoids) or as enemas (for ulcerative colitis).

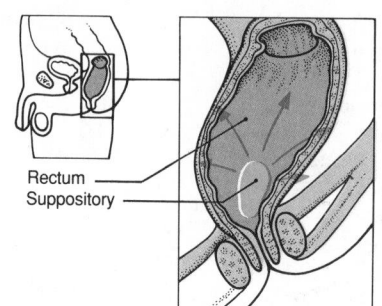

Rectum
Suppository

INHALATION

Drugs may be inhaled to produce a *systemic* effect or a direct local effect on the respiratory tract.

Gases to produce general anesthesia are administered by inhalation and are absorbed into the bloodstream through the lungs, producing a general effect on the body.

Bronchodilators, used to treat certain types of asthma, emphysema and bronchitis, are a common example of drugs administered by inhalation for their direct effect on the respiratory tract, although some of the active drug also reaches the bloodstream.

ADMINISTRATION BY INJECTION

Drugs may be injected into the body to produce a systemic effect. One reason for injecting drugs is the rapid response that follows. Other circumstances which call for injection: a person's intolerance to a drug when taken by mouth; a drug's inability to resist inactivation by stomach acids (insulin is an example); the inability of the drug to pass through the intestinal walls into the bloodstream.

Drug injections may also be given to produce a local effect, as is often done to relieve the pain of arthritis.

The main types of injection – intramuscular, intravenous, and subcutaneous – are described in the illustration (see right). The type of injection depends on the nature of the drug and the condition being treated.

Muscle | Vein | Skin | Fatty tissue

Intramuscular (IM) injection
The drug is injected into a muscle, usually of the thigh, the upper arm or buttock.

Subcutaneous (SQ) injection
The drug is injected directly under the surface of the skin.

Intravenous (IV) injection
The drug is injected directly into a vein and therefore directly into the bloodstream. Drugs given by this route act more quickly than drugs given by other types of injection.

TOPICAL APPLICATION

In treating localized disorders such as skin infections and nasal congestion, it is often preferable when a choice is available to prescribe drugs in a form that has a *topical* rather than a *systemic* effect. The reason is that it is much easier to control the effects of drugs administered locally and to ensure that they produce the maximum benefit with minimum side effects.

Topical preparations are available in a variety of forms, from skin creams, ointments and lotions to vaginal suppositories, nasal sprays, and ear and eye drops. It is important when using topical preparations to follow instructions carefully, avoiding a higher dose than recommended or application for longer than necessary. This will help avoid adverse systemic effects caused by the absorption of larger amounts into the bloodstream.

SLOW-RELEASE PREPARATIONS

A number of disorders can be treated with drug preparations that have been specially formulated to release their active drug slowly over a given period of time. Such preparations may be beneficial when it is inconvenient for a person to visit the physician on a regular basis to receive treatment by injection, or when it is necessary to accurately control the release of small amounts of the drug into the body. Slow release of drugs can be achieved by *depot injections, transdermal patches,* slow-release capsules and tablets, and implants.

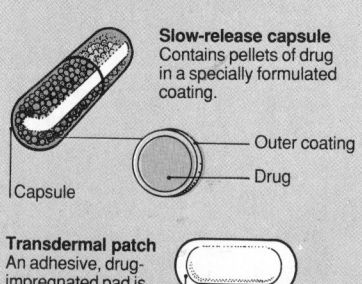

Slow-release capsule
Contains pellets of drug in a specially formulated coating.

Capsule
Outer coating
Drug

Transdermal patch
An adhesive, drug-impregnated pad is placed on the skin. The drug passes slowly into the skin.

Transdermal patch
Skin
Drug

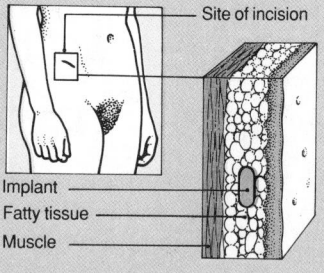

Site of incision

Implant
Fatty tissue
Muscle

Implants
A pellet containing the drug is implanted under the skin in a minor surgical procedure. By this rarely used method, a drug (usually a hormone) is slowly released into the bloodstream.

DRUG FORMS

Most drugs are specially prepared in a form designed for convenience of administration. This helps to ensure that dosages are accurate and that taking the medication is as easy as possible. Inactive ingredients (those with no therapeutic effect) are sometimes added to flavor or color the medicine, or to improve its chemical stability, extending the period during which it is effective.

The more common drug forms are described in detail below.

Tablet

This contains the drug compressed into a solid dosage form, often round in shape. Other ingredients are added to the powder prior to compression, often including an agent to bind the tablet together (see right). In some tablets, the active drug is released slowly after the tablet has been swallowed whole, producing a prolonged (sustained) effect.

Capsule

The drug is contained in a cylindrically shaped gelatin shell that breaks open after the capsule has been swallowed, releasing the drug. Slow-release capsules contain pellets that dissolve in the gastrointestinal tract, releasing the drug slowly (facing page).

Liquids

Some drugs are available in liquid form, the active substance being combined in a solution, suspension or emulsion with other ingredients – solvents, preservatives, and flavoring and coloring agents. Many liquid preparations should be shaken before use to ensure that the active drug is evenly distributed. If it is not, inaccurate dosages will result.

A mixture

A mixture contains one or more drugs, either dissolved to form a solution or suspended in a liquid (often water).

An elixir

An elixir is a solution of a drug, often highly flavored. It usually contains a high proportion of alcohol, plus sugar.

An emulsion

An emulsion is a drug dispersed in oil and water. An emulsifying agent is often included to stabilize the product.

A syrup

A syrup is a concentrated solution of sugar containing the active drug, with flavoring and stabilizing agents added.

Topical skin preparations

These are preparations designed for application to the skin and other surface tissues of the body. Preservatives are usually included to reduce the growth of

WHAT A TABLET CONTAINS

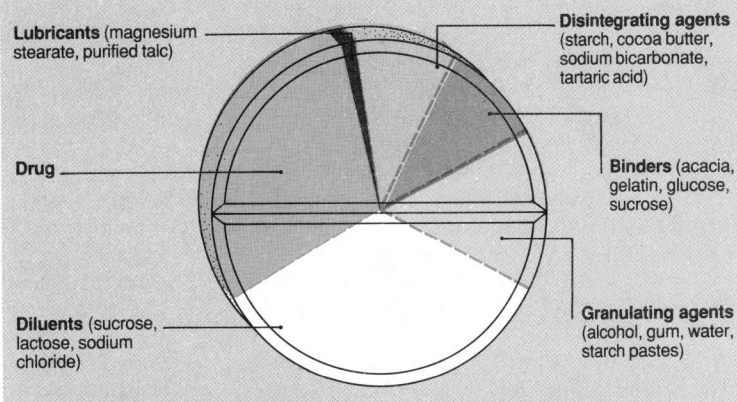

Lubricants (magnesium stearate, purified talc)

Drug

Diluents (sucrose, lactose, sodium chloride)

Disintegrating agents (starch, cocoa butter, sodium bicarbonate, tartaric acid)

Binders (acacia, gelatin, glucose, sucrose)

Granulating agents (alcohol, gum, water, starch pastes)

Diluents add bulk if necessary. Granulating agents and binders enable the ingredient to be formed into a tablet. Lubricants or a sugar coating ensure a smooth surface, and disintegrating agents dissolve the medication. The proportions of each ingredient may vary.

bacteria. The most commonly used types of skin preparations are described below. For a more detailed discussion of the various preparations, see Bases for skin preparations, p.203.

A cream

A cream is a non-greasy preparation used to apply drugs to an area of the body or to cool or moisten the skin. It is less noticeable than an ointment.

An ointment

An ointment is a greasy preparation used to apply drugs to an area of the body, or as a protective agent for dry skin conditions.

A lotion

A lotion is a solution or suspension applied to unbroken skin to cool and dry the area. Some are more suitable for use in hairy areas, since they are not as sticky as creams or ointments.

Injection solutions

Solutions for injections are sterile (germ-free) preparations of a drug dissolved or suspended in a liquid. Other agents (antioxidants) are often added to preserve the stability of the drug or to regulate the acidity or alkalinity of the solution. Most injectable drugs used today are packaged in sterile disposable syringes. This reduces chances of contamination. Certain drugs are still available in multiple-dose vials, and a chemical bactericide is added to prevent the growth of bacteria when the needle is reinserted through the rubber seal. For details on types of injection, see Administration by injection, p.18.

Suppository

A suppository is a solid, bullet-shaped dosage form specially designed for easy insertion into the rectum (rectal suppository) or vagina (vaginal suppository). It contains a drug and an inert (chemically inactive) substance that is often derived from cocoa butter or another type of vegetable oil. The active drug is gradually released in the rectum or vagina as the suppository dissolves at body temperature.

Eye drops

A sterile drug solution (or suspension) dropped behind the eyelid to produce an effect on the eye.

Ear drops

A solution (or suspension) containing a drug introduced into the ear by dropper. Ear drops are usually given to produce an effect on the outer-ear canal.

Nasal drops/spray

A solution of a drug, usually in water, for introduction into the nose to produce a local effect.

Inhalers

Aerosol inhalers contain a solution or suspension of a drug under pressure. A valve mechanism ensures the delivery of the recommended dosage when the inhaler is activated. A mouthpiece fixed to the device facilitates inhalation of the drug as it is released from the canister. The correct technique is important; printed instructions should be followed carefully. Aerosol inhalers are used for respiratory conditions such as asthma (see also p.120).

DRUG TREATMENT IN SPECIAL RISK GROUPS

Different people may respond in different ways to drug treatment. Taking the same drug, one person may suffer adverse effects while another experiences none. However, physicians know that certain groups are always more at risk when they take drugs; the reason is that in those people the body handles drugs differently, or the drug has an atypical effect. Those groups at special risk include infants and children, women who are pregnant or breast-feeding, the elderly and people with long-term medical conditions, especially those who have impaired liver or kidney function.

The reasons that such groups may be more likely to suffer adverse effects are discussed in detail on the following pages. Others who may need special attention include those already taking regular medication who may risk complications when they take another drug. Drug interactions are discussed more fully on p.16.

When physicians prescribe drugs for special risk groups they take extra care to select appropriate medication, adjust dosages and closely monitor the effects of treatment. If you think you may be at special risk, be sure to tell your physician in case he or she is not fully aware of your particular circumstances. Similarly, if you are buying over-the-counter drugs you should ask your physician if you think you may be at risk from any possible adverse effects.

INFANTS AND CHILDREN

Infants and children need a lower dosage of drugs than adults because children have a relatively low body weight. Moreover, because of differences in body composition, as well as the distribution and amount of body fat, and differences in the state of development and function of organs such as the liver and kidneys at different ages, children cannot simply be given a proportion of an adult dose as if they were small adults. Dosages need to be calculated in a more complex way, taking account of both age and weight. Although newborn babies often have to be given very small doses of drugs, older children may need relatively large doses of some drugs.

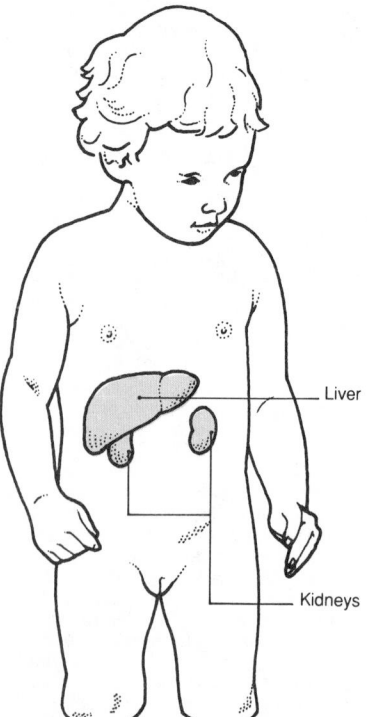

The liver
The liver's enzyme systems are not fully developed when a baby is born. This means that drugs are not broken down as rapidly as in an adult, and may become dangerously concentrated in the baby's body. For this reason, many drugs are not prescribed for babies or are prescribed in very reduced doses. In older children, because the liver is relatively large compared to the rest of the body, some drugs may need to be given in proportionately larger doses.

The kidneys
During the first six months, a baby's kidneys are unable to excrete drugs as efficiently as those of an adult. This, too, may lead to a dangerously high concentration of a drug in the blood. The dose of certain drugs may therefore need to be reduced. Between one and two years of age, kidney function improves, and higher doses of some drugs may then be needed.

Liver

Kidneys

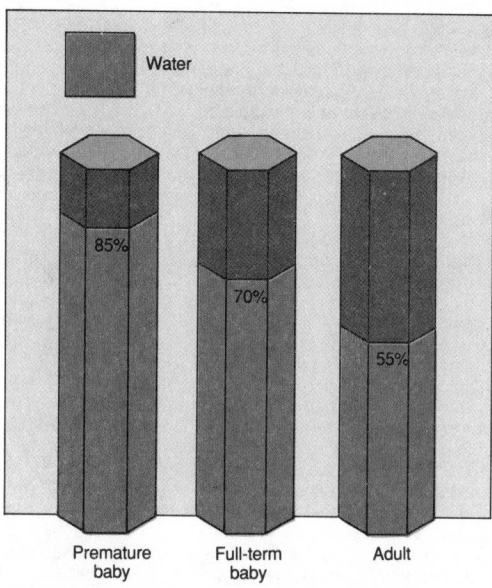

Water

Premature baby — 85%

Full-term baby — 70%

Adult — 55%

Body composition
The proportion of water in the body of a premature baby is about 85 per cent of its body weight, that of a full-term baby is 70 per cent, and that of an adult is only 55 per cent. This means that certain drugs are not as concentrated in an infant's body as in an adult's, and higher doses relative to weight may need to be given initially.

PREGNANT WOMEN

Great care is needed during pregnancy to protect the fetus so that it develops into a healthy baby. Drugs taken by the mother can cross the placenta and enter the baby's bloodstream. With certain drugs, and at particular stages of pregnancy, there is a risk of developmental abnormalities, retarded growth, or post-delivery problems affecting the baby. In addition, some drugs may affect the health of the mother during pregnancy.

Many drugs are known to have adverse effects during pregnancy; others are known to be safe, but in a large number of cases there is no firm evidence to decide on risk or safety. Therefore, the most important rule if you are pregnant or trying to conceive is to consult your physician before taking any prescribed or over-the-counter medication. Drugs such as marijuana, nicotine and alcohol should be avoided. Your physician will balance the potential benefits of drug treatment against any possible risks to decide whether or not a drug should be taken. This is particularly important if you need to take regular medication for a chronic condition such as epilepsy, high blood pressure or diabetes.

Drugs and the stages of pregnancy

Pregnancy is divided into three three-month stages called trimesters. Depending on the trimester in which they are taken, drugs can have different effects on the mother or the fetus or both. Some drugs may be considered safe during one trimester, but not another. Physicians, therefore, often need to change regular medications given during the course of pregnancy.

The trimesters of pregnancy

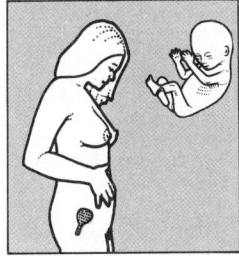

First trimester
During the first three months of pregnancy – the most critical period – drugs may affect the development of fetal organs, leading to congenital malformations. Very severe defects may result in miscarriage.

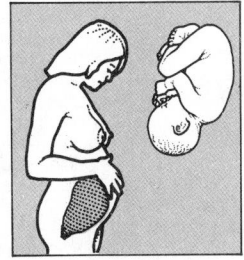

Second trimester
From the fourth through the sixth month some drugs may retard the growth of the fetus. This may also result in a low birthweight.

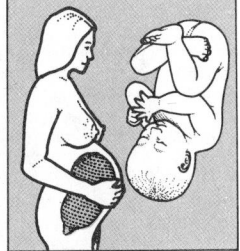

Third trimester
During the last three months of pregnancy, major risks include breathing difficulties in the newborn baby. Some drugs may also affect labor, causing it to be premature, delayed or prolonged.

How drugs cross the placenta

The placenta acts as a filter between the mother's bloodstream and that of the baby. It allows small molecules from nutrients to pass into the baby's blood, while preventing larger particles such as blood cells from doing so. Drug molecules are comparatively small and pass easily through the placental barrier.

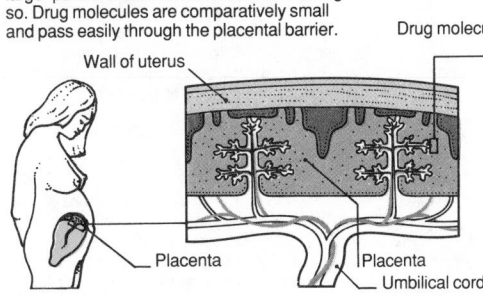

Wall of uterus

Placenta

Placenta
Umbilical cord

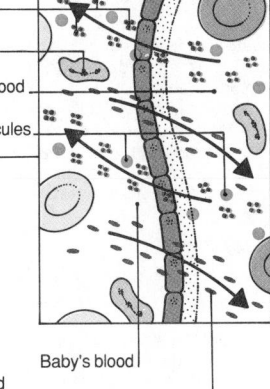

Nutrients

Blood cell

Mother's blood

Drug molecules

Baby's blood

Waste products

BREAST-FEEDING

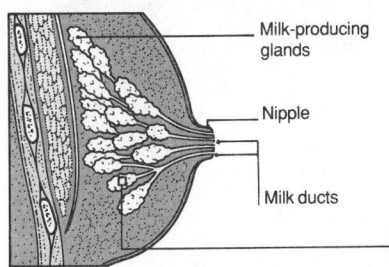

Milk-producing glands

Nipple

Milk ducts

How drugs pass into breast milk
The milk-producing glands in the breast are surrounded by a network of fine blood vessels. Small molecules of substances such as drugs pass from the blood into the milk. Drugs that dissolve easily in fat may pass across in greater concentrations than other drugs.

Just as drugs may cross from the mother's bloodstream into the baby's through the placenta, they may also pass to the baby from the mother's milk.

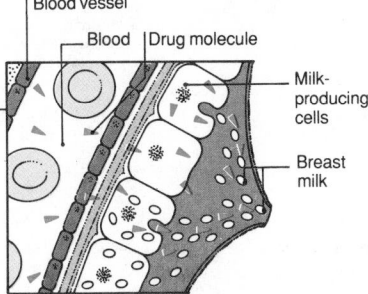

Blood vessel

Blood   Drug molecule

Milk-producing cells

Breast milk

This means that a breast-fed baby will receive small doses of whatever drugs the mother is taking. In many cases this is not a problem, because the amount of drug that passes into the milk is too small to have any significant effect on the baby. However, some drugs can produce unwanted effects on the baby. Antibiotics may sensitize the infant and consequently prevent their use later in life. Sedative drugs may make the baby drowsy and cause feeding problems. Moreover, some drugs may reduce the amount of milk produced by the mother.

Physicians usually advise breast-feeding women to take only essential drugs. When a mother needs to take regular medication while breast-feeding, her baby may also need to be closely monitored for possible adverse effects.

THE ELDERLY

Older people are particularly at risk when taking drugs. This is partly due to the physical changes associated with aging, and partly to the need for some elderly people to take several different drugs at the same time. They may also be at risk because they may be unable to manage their treatment properly, or may lack the information to do so.

Physical changes

Elderly people have a greater risk of accumulating drugs in their bodies because the liver is less efficient at breaking drugs down and the kidneys are less efficient at excreting them. Because of this, in some cases, the normal adult dose will produce side effects, and half a dose may be sufficient to produce a therapeutic effect without the side effects. (See also Kidney and liver disease, below.)

Older people, too, take more drugs than younger people – many take two or more drugs at the same time. Apart from increasing the number of drugs in their systems, taking more than one drug at a time can cause adverse drug interactions (see p.16).

As people grow older some parts of the body, such as the brain and nervous system, become more sensitive to drugs, thus increasing the likelihood of adverse reactions from drugs acting on

those sites. A similar problem may occur due to changes in the body's ratio of body fat. Although allergic reactions (see p.151) are rarely a function of age, changes in the immune system may account for some unexpected reactions.

Accordingly, physicians prescribe more conservatively for older people, especially those with disorders likely to correct themselves in time.

Incorrect use of drugs

Elderly people often suffer harmful effects from their drug treatment because they fail to take their medication regularly or correctly. This may happen because they have been misinformed about how to take it or receive vague instructions. Problems arise sometimes because many elderly people cannot remember whether they have taken the drug and take a double dosage (see Exceeding the dose, p.30). Problems may also occur because the person is confused; this is not necessarily due to senility, but can arise as a result of drug treatment, especially if an elderly person is taking a number of different drugs or a sedative drug.

All prescriptions for the elderly should be especially clearly and fully labeled. Leaflets about the drug and its use are also helpful for the individual or the

Effect of drugs that act on the brain

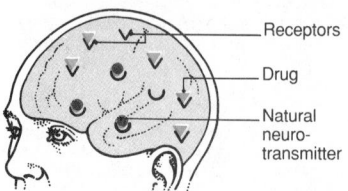

In young people
There are plenty of receptors to take up the drug as well as natural *neurotransmitters*.

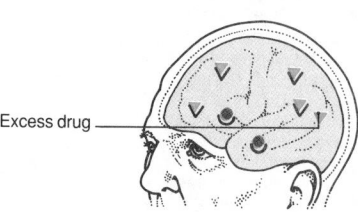

In older brains
There are fewer receptors, so even a reduced drug dose may be excessive.

person taking care of him or her. Where appropriate, special containers with memory aids should be used for dispensing the medication in single doses.

KIDNEY AND LIVER DISEASE

Long-term illnesses affect the way in which people respond to drug treatment. This is especially true of kidney and liver problems. The liver alters the chemical structure of many of the drugs that enter the body (see How drugs pass through the body, p.17) by breaking them down into simpler substances, while the kidneys excrete drugs in the urine. If the effectiveness of the liver or kidneys is curtailed or interfered with by illness, the

effect of drugs on the individual can be marked. In most cases, people with kidney or liver disease will be prescribed a smaller number of drugs and in lower doses. In addition, certain drugs may in rare cases damage the liver or kidneys. A physician may therefore be reluctant to prescribe such a drug to someone with already reduced liver or kidney function to avoid the risk of further damage.

Drugs and kidney disease

People with poor kidney function are at greater risk from drug side effects. There are two reasons for this. First, drugs build up in the system because smaller amounts are excreted in urine. Second, kidney disease can cause protein loss through the urine; that lowers the level of protein in the blood. Some drugs bind to blood proteins, and if there are fewer proteins, a greater proportion of drugs becomes free and active in the body (see Effects of protein loss, left).

Drugs and liver disease

Severe liver diseases such as cirrhosis of the liver and hepatitis affect the way the body breaks down drugs. This can lead to dangerous accumulation of certain drugs in the body. People suffering from these diseases or anything similar should consult their physician before taking any medication (including over-the-counter drugs) or alcohol. Many drugs must be avoided completely since they can cause coma in someone with a damaged or poorly functioning liver.

Effects of protein loss

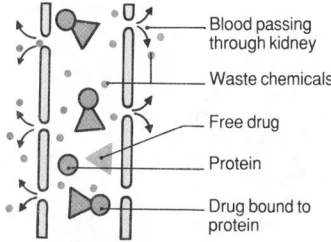

Blood passing through kidney

Waste chemicals

Free drug

Protein

Drug bound to protein

Normal kidney
Some drugs bind to proteins in the blood and are inactive; only free drugs affect the body.

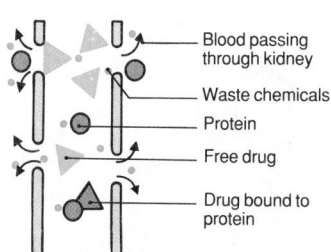

Blood passing through kidney

Waste chemicals

Protein

Free drug

Drug bound to protein

Damaged kidney
Loss of protein increases the amount of active drug, and therefore its overall effect.

DRUG DEPENDENCE

The term "drug dependence" applies far more widely than most people realize. It is usually thought of in association with use of illegal drugs like heroin or with excessive intake of alcohol. But millions of Americans are dependent on other drugs, including stimulants – such as caffeine found in coffee and tea, and nicotine in tobacco – and certain prescription medicines, such as analgesics, sleeping drugs, and tranquilizers (anti-anxiety drugs).

Psychological and physical dependence

Drug dependence, implying a person's inability to control use of a substance with an abuse potential, is of two types. Psychological dependence is an emotional state of craving for a drug whose presence in the body has a desired effect or whose absence has an undesired effect. Physical dependence, which often includes psychological dependence, involves physiological adaptation to a drug or alcohol, charac-terized by severe physical distur-bances – withdrawal symptoms – during a prolonged period of abstinence.

Physical dependence on a drug is further characterized by a developing *tolerance* to the drug's effects; the line between tolerance and lethal dosage is sometimes extremely fine (see Drug tolerance, below).

Drug dependence is now widely preferred to the word addiction, defined as the compulsive use of a substance resulting in physical, psychological or social harm to the user, with continued use despite the harm.

Drugs which cause dependence

Many people who need to take regular medication worry that they may become dependent on their drugs. In fact, only a few groups of drugs produce physical dependence, most of them substances that alter mood or behavior. Such drugs include heroin and the narcotic anal-gesics (morphine, meperidine, and other similar drugs), sleeping drugs and anti-anxiety drugs (benzodiazepines and barbiturates), depressants (alcohol), and nervous system stimulants (amphetamines, cocaine, and nicotine). Consult the drug profile in Part 4 of this book to discover the dependence rating of any drug you are taking.

The use of nicotine in the form of tobacco and the controlled or uncon-trolled use of narcotic analgesics invariably produce physical dependence

DRUG TOLERANCE

Drug tolerance occurs as the body adapts to the actions of a drug. Although people can develop a tolerance to many drugs, it is a dangerous characteristic of virtually all of the drugs of dependence. A person taking them needs larger and larger doses to achieve the original effect; as the dose increases, so do the risks of *toxic* effects and dependence.

The explanation of tolerance, still not fully understood, is highly complex. It stems from one (or both) of two actions. One is the liver increasing its capacity to break down and dispose of the drug, giving lower concen-trations of it in the bloodstream and a shorter duration of action. The other potential action involves adaptation by the cells of the central nervous system, including the brain, to the drug, lowering responsiveness.

Brain tolerance can also lead to cross-tolerance, a person's tolerance to one drug leading to tolerance of similar drugs. For example, the regular drinker who can tol-erate high levels of alcohol (a depressant) can have a sometimes dangerous tolerance to other depressants such as sleeping drugs and anti-anxiety drugs. While cross-tolerance raises problems, it does allow a substance with a less addictive potential to replace the original. The symptoms of alcohol withdrawal can thus be controlled by the anti-anxiety drug diazepam.

Tolerance to some drugs has its benefits. A person can, for example, develop tolerance to the side effects of a drug but remain res-ponsive to its curative powers. Many people taking antidepressants find that side effects such as dry mouth, constipation and blurred vision slowly disappear, with the primary action of the drug continuing.

Increasing tolerance does, however, have its dangers. A person with a developed tolerance tends to increase dosage, some-times to the toxic level.

Dosage and effect in drug tolerance
The chart below shows how some effects (these may be intended or unintended) of a fixed dose of tolerance-producing drugs gradually diminish over a period of time. If after this time the dose is significantly increased, the drug effect is restored. Remember, dosage of prescribed drugs should never be increased except on your physician's instructions.

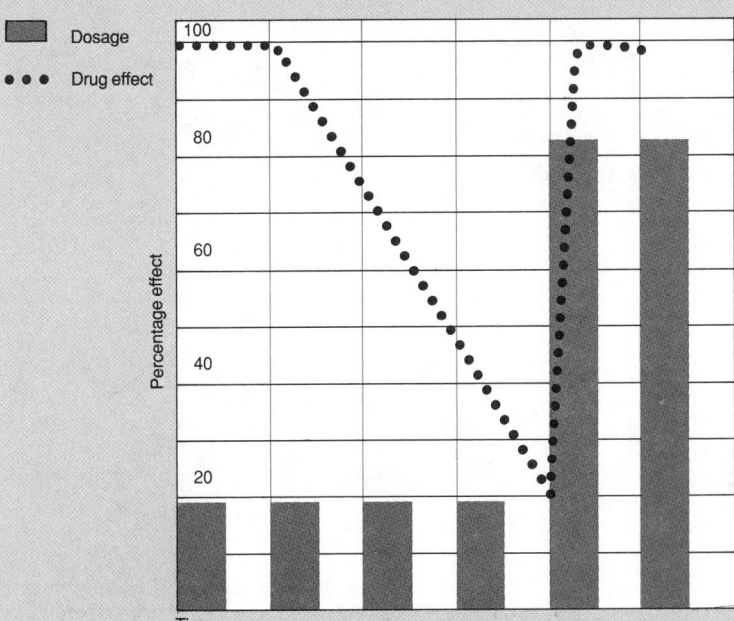

Dosage

Drug effect

DRUG DEPENDENCE continued

if taken regularly over a period of time. However, it is equally true that not all regular users of alcohol become alcoholics. There is much argument over the definition of an alcoholic. The definition preferred by the AMA is: A person who has experienced physical, psychological, social, or occupational impairment due to habitual excessive consumption of alcohol.

Recognizing the dangers of drug dependence

Factors that determine the risk of developing physical dependence include the characteristics of the drug itself, the strength and frequency of doses, and the duration of use. However, the presence of these factors does not always result in dependence. Psychological and physiological factors unique to each individual also enter the equation, and there may be other as yet unknown factors involved. For example, when the use of narcotic analgesics is restricted to the immediate short-term relief of severe pain in a medical setting, long-term dependence is rare. Yet there is a high risk of physical dependence when narcotic analgesics, or other drugs of abuse, are taken for non-medical reasons. There is also risk in some cases of low-dose use when continued over a long period of time for

DRUG ABUSE

The term is defined as any use of drugs that causes physical, psychological, economic, legal, or social harm to the user, or to persons who may be affected by the user's behavior. Drug abuse commonly refers to taking drugs obtained illegally (such as heroin), but may also be used to describe the misuse of drugs generally obtainable legally (nicotine, alcohol), and to drugs obtainable through a physician's prescription only (everything from sleeping drugs and tranquilizers to analgesics and stimulants).

The abuse of prescription drugs deserves more attention than it usually receives. The practice can include the personal use of drugs left over from a previous course of treatment, the sharing with others of drugs prescribed for yourself, the deliberate deception of physicians, the forgery of prescriptions, and the theft of drugs from pharmacies. All of these practices can have dangerous consequences.

Careful attention to the advice in the section on Managing your drug treatment (p.25) will help to avoid inadvertent misuse of drugs. The dangers associated with abuse of individual drugs are discussed under Drugs of abuse (pp.547–554).

Common drugs of abuse
Alcohol
Amphetamines
Amyl nitrite and similar drugs
Cocaine
Heroin
LSD
Marijuana
Meperidine
Mescaline
Nicotine
Phencyclidine
Solvents

chronic pain. No one can say for sure just what leads an individual to drug dependent behavior. A person's physical and psychological make-up are thought to be factors, as well as his social environment, occupational pressures, and outlook on life. Motivation and setting play major roles.

Indiscriminate use of certain prescription drugs has also caused drug

dependence, with the barbiturate sleeping drugs commonly cited. Benzodiazepines, which are much less likely to lead to a single fatal dose, have largely replaced them, though physicians discourage the use of any drug to induce sleep or calm anxiety for more than a few weeks. Appetite suppressants require close supervision. Similarly, amphetamines are now prescribed for fewer conditions than in the past because of the frequency with which they are abused.

Treating drug dependence

When a person is dependent on a drug, the cells in the body have adapted to a new chemical environment. To move someone from that condition to a drug-free state is a complex medical process. But a patient must become completely drug-free before long-term rehabilitation can occur.

The first step, detoxification, can take different forms. In cases of alcohol dependence, abstinence may often be abruptly imposed. With other substances, the drug may be gradually withdrawn, or other safer substances substituted. There are, however, differing schools of thought, and some treatment centers argue for the abrupt cessation method of detoxification for substances besides alcohol.

Withdrawal can be mild or violent, and is occasionally fatal. Expert medical supervision is required. Drugs may be given to provide symptomatic relief.

Once a person is drug-free, rehabilitation measures begin. Drug therapy – such as the use of disulfiram (Antabuse) for alcoholism – psychotherapy, personal counseling and the work of support organizations like Alcoholics Anonymous play an important role.

SYMPTOMS OF WITHDRAWAL

These can range from the mild (sneezing, sweating) to the serious (vomiting, confusion) to the extremely serious (seizures, coma). Alcohol withdrawal may be associated with delirium tremens, very occasionally fatal. Withdrawal from barbiturates can sometimes involve seizures and coma. But under medical guidance, withdrawal symptoms can be

relieved, sometimes with doses of the original drug, or with less addictive substitutes.

Withdrawal symptoms occur because the body has adapted to the action of the drug (see Drug tolerance, p.23). When a drug is continuously present, the body may stop the release of a natural chemical necessary to normal function, like endorphins (below).

Pain and heroin withdrawal

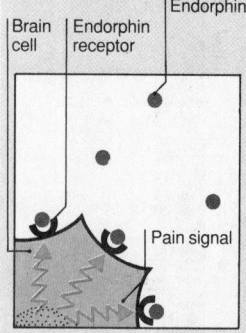

Normal brain
When no drug is present, natural substances called endorphins inhibit the transmission of pain signals.

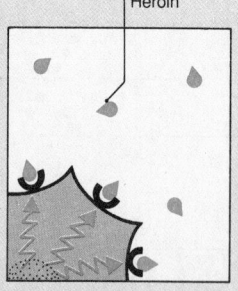

Effect of heroin
Heroin occupies the same receptors in the brain as endorphins and suppresses endorphin production.

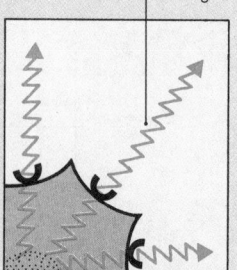

Heroin withdrawal
Abrupt withdrawal of heroin leaves the brain without a buffer to pain signals produced by even minor stimuli.

MANAGING YOUR DRUG TREATMENT

A prescribed drug does not automatically produce a beneficial response. For a drug to have maximum benefit, it must be taken as directed by the physician or manufacturer. It is estimated that two out of every five people for whom a drug is prescribed do not take it properly, if at all. The reasons include failure to understand instructions, fear of adverse reactions, and lack of motivation, often arising after symptoms disappear.

It is your responsibility to take a prescribed drug at the correct time, and in the manner stipulated. To do this, you need to know where to obtain information about the drug (see Questioning your physician, p.26) and to make certain that you understand the instructions.

The following pages describe the practical aspects of drug treatment, from filling a prescription and buying over-the-counter drugs to storing drugs and disposing of old medications safely. Problems caused by mismanaging drug treatment – overdosing, underdosing or stopping the drug altogether – and long-term drug treatment are dealt with on pp. 28 – 30. Information about managing specific drugs is given in Part 4.

OVER-THE-COUNTER DRUGS

Over-the-counter drugs are those for which a prescription is not required. They are sold widely in a variety of outlets (including supermarkets), although some are available only at drugstores.

It is generally accepted that over-the-counter drugs are suitable for self-treatment and are unlikely to produce adverse reactions if taken as directed. But, as with all medicines, they can be harmful if they are misused. The ease with which they can be purchased is no guarantee of their absolute safety. For this reason, when using any over-the-counter medication, the same precautions should be taken as when using a prescription drug.

Using over-the-counter drugs

A number of minor ailments and problems, from coughs and colds to minor cuts and bruises, can be adequately dealt with by using over-the-counter medicines. However, you must be sure to read the directions on the label and follow them carefully, particularly those advising on dosage and on when to see your physician. Most over-the-counter drugs are clearly labeled. They may warn of conditions under which the drug should not be taken, or advise you to consult a physician if symptoms persist.

The pharmacist is usually a good source of information about over-the-counter drugs. He or she cannot make a diagnosis or a decision about therapy, but can tell what is suitable for your complaint. The pharmacist can also tell you when an over-the-counter drug will probably not be effective, and can warn you if self-treatment or prolonged treatment is inadvisable.

It is particularly important to speak to your physician before buying over-the-counter drugs for children. Some conditions, such as diarrhea in young children, should be treated only by a physician. You should also tell your pharmacist about any prescription drugs you are taking.

Buying over-the-counter medications

Various drugs are available over the counter, ranging from cough medicines to eye drops. Your pharmacist can often help you to select the appropriate medication.

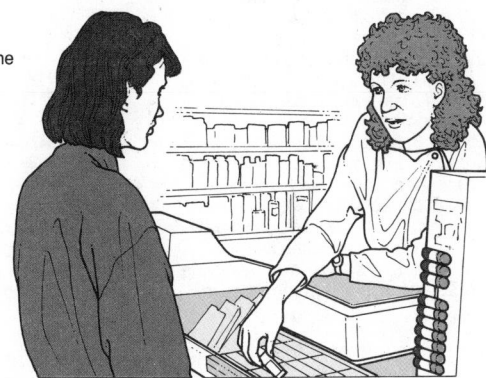

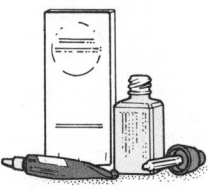

Eye preparations

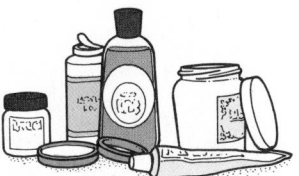

Medicated creams, lotions and powders

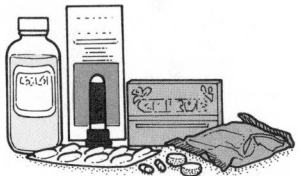

Cough and cold treatments

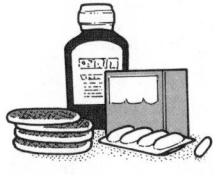

Laxatives

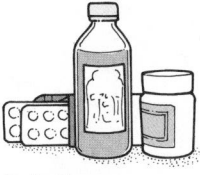

Analgesics

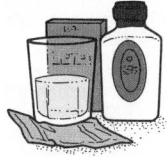

Antacids

PRESCRIPTION DRUGS

Conventional wisdom to the contrary, prescription drugs are not necessarily more potent or effective than over-the-counter drugs. The difference between the two, rather, reflects the policy of the US Food and Drug Administration that all drugs are for over-the-counter sale unless it is impossible to write labeling that will ensure the drug will be used safely without medical supervision.

When a physician prescribes a drug, he or she usually starts treatment at the normal dosage for the disorder being treated. The dosage may later be adjusted (lowered or increased) if the drug is not producing the desired effect or if there are adverse reactions, and the physician may also switch to an alternative drug that may be more effective.

Prescribing generic and brand-name drugs

When writing a prescription for the drug, the physician often has the choice between a generic and a brand-name drug. In some cases, the generic form costs less than the brand-name drug and will produce the same effects. However, since different manufacturers may formulate a drug in different ways – even though the active ingredient is exactly the same – two versions of the same drug do not always produce the same actions or take effect in the same amount of time. Those are factors that a physician must consider before writing a prescription to give you the most effective drug for your disorder/condition. Cost to the patient may be important, but is secondary to medical considerations such as quality and effectiveness.

All states now have laws regarding the substitution of generic drugs for brand-name products. In some, the law is "positive," requiring the pharmacist to substitute a generic product unless the physician has given specific instructions not to substitute. In other states, the law is "negative," forbidding a generic substitution unless the physician authorizes it. Many physicians use a prescription form with a May (or May Not) Substitute box.

Filling your prescription

One of the most important things a pharmacist does is to keep a computerized profile of the drugs taken by regular customers. For that reason, it is highly advisable that you order all your prescription drugs from the same pharmacist or the same pharmacy.

In case you are to take drugs prescribed by more than one physician, or from your dentist in addition to your doctor, the pharmacist's profile calls attention to possible harmful interactions. Physicians do ask if you are taking other medicines, but the profile is a valuable additional safety measure.

A trained and licensed professional, the pharmacist plays a necessary part in the health care system. He or she knows about drug actions, interactions and adverse effects, and is a good source of information about over-the-counter drugs too.

Questioning your physician

Countless surveys unmistakably point to lack of information as the most common reason for drug failure. Responses like "The doctor is too busy to be bothered with a lot of questions" or "The doctor will think I'm stupid if I ask that" recur over and over. Be certain you understand the instructions for a drug before leaving the physician, and don't leave with any questions unanswered.

It is a good idea to make a list of the questions you may want to ask before your visit, and to make a few notes while you are there about what you are told. It is not uncommon to forget some of the instructions your physician gives you during a consultation.

Know what you are taking

Although most of the important information you need will be written on the prescription and on the drug label, you should obtain any additional information as necessary from your physician.

Your physician should tell you the generic or brand name of the drug he or she is prescribing, and exactly what condition or symptom the drug has been prescribed to treat.

As well as knowing the name of the drug prescribed, you should know what dose to take, how often to take it, and whether you should have your prescription refilled. Be certain you understand fully the instructions about how and when to take the drug (see also Taking your medication, facing page). For example, exactly how much is a teaspoon, and does four times a day mean four times during the time you are awake, or four times in twenty-four hours ? Ask your physician how long treatment should last; some drugs cause harmful effects if you abruptly stop taking them, or do not have beneficial effects unless the course is completed.

Risks and special precautions

All drugs have side effects (see The effects of drugs, p.15), and you should know what these are. Ask your physician what the possible adverse reactions of the drug are and what you should do if they occur. Also ask if there are any foods or other drugs you should avoid during treatment and if you can drink alcohol while taking the drug.

Your prescription

Your prescription tells the pharmacist the type and amount of drug to supply, and gives the information that will appear on the container label. Some people like to read prescriptions, to compare instructions written by the physician with those on the label. If there are differences, you may discuss them with the pharmacist.

It is a good idea to ask the pharmacist to include several other facts on the drug label: the name of the drug, the number of tablets or capsules in the container, and how long the drug can be stored.

Patient's name and address

Physician's name and address

Drug name, strength and amount to be dispensed

Special instructions

Physician's signature

Generic substitution instructions

PRESCRIPTION TERMS

ac before meals	**PM** evening
ad lib freely	**po** by mouth
AM morning	**prn** as needed
bid twice a day	**qd** once a day
c with	**qid** four times
cap capsule	a day
cc or **cm** cubic	**s** without
centimeter	**sig ut dict** take as
ext for external use	directed
gtt drops	**stat** at once
h.s. before bedtime	**tab** tablet
mg milligrams	**tid** three times a day
ml milliliter	**top** apply topically
noct at night	**x** times
pc after meals	

TAKING YOUR MEDICATION

Among the most important aspects of managing your drug treatment is knowing how often the drug is to be taken. On an empty stomach? With food? Mixed with something? Specific instructions on such points are given in the individual drug profiles in Part 4.

When to take your drugs

Certain drugs – analgesics and drugs for migraine, for example – are taken only as necessary, as warning symptoms occur. Others are meant to be taken regularly at specified intervals. The prescription or label instructions can be confusing, however. For instance, does three times a day mean three times every eight hours out of 24 – at 8 a.m., 4 p.m. and midnight? Or does it mean take at three equal intervals during waking hours – morning, early afternoon and bedtime? A patient must know just what the precise directions are. Either ask the physician at the time he or she writes the prescription, or phone him or her (or the nurse) later. Try to take your dose at the recommended intervals; taking doses too close together increases the risk of side effects.

The actual time of day that you take a drug is generally flexible, so you can normally schedule your doses to fit your daily routine. This has the additional advantage of making it easier for you to remember to take your drugs. For example, if you are to take the drug three times during the day, it may be most convenient to take the first dose at 7 a.m., the second at 3 p.m. and the third at 11 p.m., while it may be more suitable for another person on the same regimen to take the first dose at 8 a.m., and so on. You must, however, establish

Three times a day ?

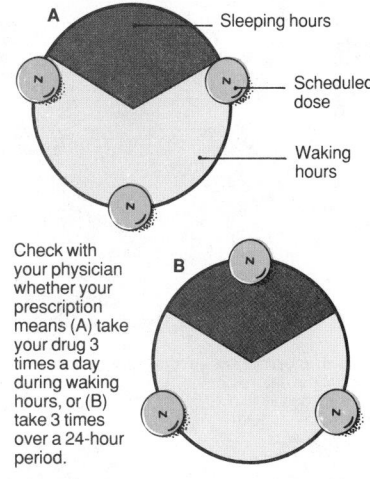

A — Sleeping hours

— Scheduled dose

— Waking hours

Check with your physician whether your prescription means (A) take your drug 3 times a day during waking hours, or (B) take 3 times over a 24-hour period.

TIPS ON TAKING MEDICINES

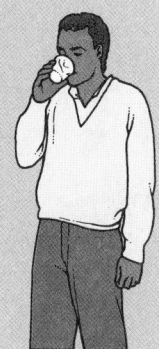

● Whenever possible, take capsules and tablets while standing, or at least when you are in an upright sitting position, and take them with water. If you take them when you are lying down, or without fluid, it is possible for capsules and tablets to become stuck in the esophagus. This can delay the action of the drug and may damage the esophagus.

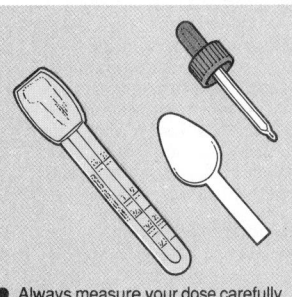

● Always measure your dose carefully, using a 5ml spoon when a teaspoon is specified, or an accurate measure such as a dropper or children's medicine spoon.

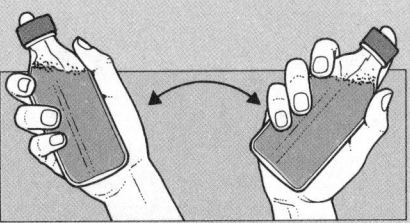

● When taking liquid medicines shake the bottle before measuring each dose, or you may give yourself improper dosages if the active substance has risen to the top or settled at the bottom of the bottle.

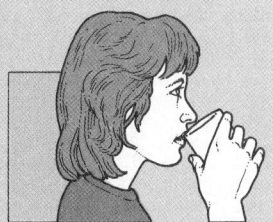

● A drink of cold water taken immediately after an unpleasantly flavored medicine will often hide the taste.

with your pharmacist or your physician whether the drug should be taken with food, in which case you would probably need to take it with your breakfast, lunch, and dinner.

If you are taking several different drugs, ask your physician if they can be taken at the same time, or if they must be taken at different intervals in order to avoid any adverse effects or reduced effectiveness caused by an interaction.

How to take your drugs

If your prescription specifies taking your drug with food – or without food – it is very important to follow this instruction if you are to get the maximum benefit from your treatment. Certain drugs should be taken on an empty stomach (usually one to two hours before eating) so they will be absorbed more quickly into the bloodstream; others should be taken with food to avoid stomach irritation. Similarly, you should comply with any instructions to avoid particular foods. Milk and dairy products may inhibit the absorption of some drugs; fruit juices can break down certain antibacterial drugs in the stomach and thereby decrease their action; alcohol is best avoided with all drugs. (See also Drug interactions, p.16.)

In some cases, when taking diuretics, for example, you may be advised to eat foods rich in potassium. But do not take potassium supplements unless you are advised to do so by your physician (see Potassium, p.540). If you use salt substitutes (all of which contain potassium), remember to tell your physician.

GIVING MEDICINES TO CHILDREN

A number of over-the-counter medicines are specifically prepared for children. Many other medicines have labels that give both adult and children's dosages. For the purposes of drug labeling, anyone 12 years of age or under is considered a child.

When giving over-the-counter medicines to children you should follow the instructions on the label exactly and under no circumstances exceed the dosage recommended for a child. Never give a child even a small proportion of a medicine intended for adult use without the advice of your physician.

Never deceive your child about what you are giving, pretending that tablets are candy or that liquid medicines are soft drinks. Never leave a child's medicine within reach. He or she may be tempted to take an extra dose in order to hasten recovery.

MISSED DOSES

Missing a dose of your medication can be a problem only if you are taking the drug as part of a regular course of treatment. Although missing a drug dose is not uncommon, it is not a cause for concern in most cases. It may sometimes produce a recurrence of symptoms or a change in the action of the drug, so you should know what to do when you have forgotten to take your medication. For advice on individual drugs, consult the drug profile in Part 4.

Additional measures

With some drugs, the timing of doses depends on how long their actions last. When you miss a dose, the amount of drug in your body is lowered, and the effect of the drug may be diminished. You may therefore have to take other steps to avoid unwanted consequences. For example, if you are taking an oral contraceptive containing progesterone only, and forget to take one pill, you should take one as soon as you remember, and for the next 48 hours use another form of contraception.

If you miss more than one dose of any drug you are taking regularly, tell your physician. If you miss even one dose of insulin, consult your physician about how to continue treatment.

If you frequently forget to take your medication you should tell your physician. He or she may be able to simplify your treatment schedule by prescribing a multi-ingredient preparation that contains several drugs in one capsule, or a preparation that releases the drug slowly into the body over a period of time.

REMEMBERING YOUR MEDICATION

If you take several different drugs, it is useful to draw up a chart to remind yourself of when to take each drug. This will also help anyone who looks after you, or a visiting physician unfamiliar with your treatment.

Furosemide (a diuretic to counter fluid retention), two 40mg tablets in the morning (small round tablets).

Spironolactone (another diuretic to counter the potassium loss caused by furosemide), one 50mg tablet in the morning (oval tablets).

The example given here is of a dosage chart made for an older woman suffering from arthritis and a heart condition who has trouble sleeping. Her physician has prescribed the following treatment:

Ibuprofen (for arthritis), three 400mg tablets daily with meals (large round tablets).

Nifedipine (to treat her heart condition), three 10mg capsules a day (one-color capsules).

Temazepam (a sleeping drug), one 20mg capsule at bedtime (two-color capsules).

Dosage chart

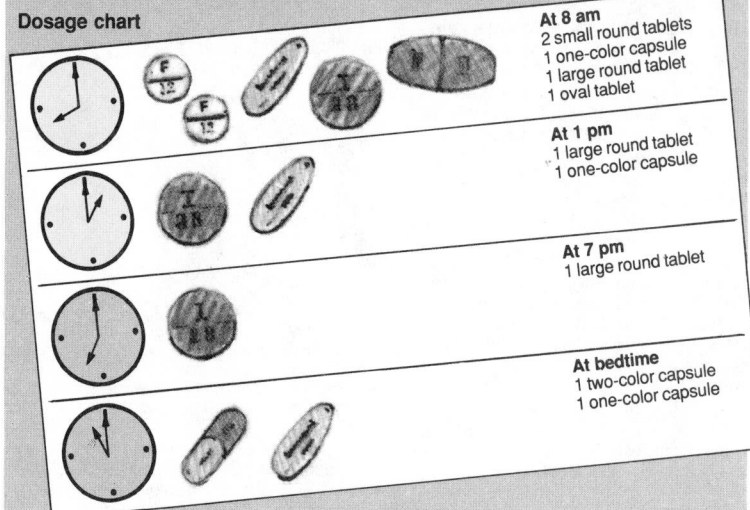

At 8 am
2 small round tablets
1 one-color capsule
1 large round tablet
1 oval tablet

At 1 pm
1 large round tablet
1 one-color capsule

At 7 pm
1 large round tablet

At bedtime
1 two-color capsule
1 one-color capsule

ENDING DRUG TREATMENT

As with missed doses, ending drug treatment too soon can be a problem when you are taking a regular course of drugs. With medication that you take as required, you can stop treatment as soon as you feel better.

Advice on stopping individual drugs is given in the drug profiles in Part 4. Some general guidelines to ending drug treatment are given below.

Risks of stopping too soon

Suddenly stopping drug treatment before completing your course of medication may cause the original condition to recur or lead to other complications, including withdrawal symptoms. Even if you begin to feel better, you still should not stop taking the drug unless your physician advises you to do so. People taking antibiotics often make this mistake. But the disappearance of the

symptoms does not necessarily mean that the infection is cured. The full course of treatment prescribed should always be followed.

Adverse effects

Do not stop taking a drug simply because it produces unpleasant side effects. Many side effects disappear or become bearable after a while. But if they do not, check with your physician who may want to reduce the dosage of the drug gradually or substitute another drug which does not produce the same side effects.

Gradual reduction

While many drugs can be stopped suddenly, others must be reduced gradually to avoid a reaction when treatment ends. This is the case with long-term corticosteroid treatment (see right).

Phased reduction of corticosteroids

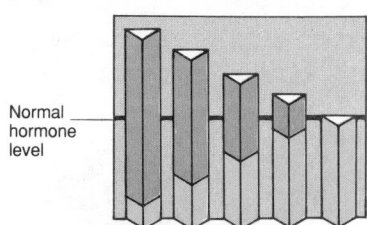

■ Corticosteroid drug

□ Natural adrenal hormone

Normal hormone level

Corticosteroid drugs suppress production in the body of natural adrenal hormones. A phased reduction of the drug dosage allows levels of the natural hormones to revert to normal gradually.

STORING DRUGS

Once you have completed a medically directed course of treatment, you should not keep any unused drugs. But your store of often-needed remedies for headaches, colds, indigestion and so forth does merit some attention. Such drugs should not be used if they show signs of deterioration or if their period of effectiveness has expired (see When to dispose of drugs, right).

How to store drugs

Over-the-counter and prescription drugs should normally be stored in the container in which you purchased them. If you need to put them into other containers, say, special containers designed for the elderly, remember to keep the original container with the label and separate instructions for future reference.

Make certain that caps and lids are replaced and tightly closed after use; loose caps may leak and spill, or hasten deterioration of the drug.

Where to store drugs

The majority of drugs should be stored in a cool, dry place out of direct sunlight, even those in plastic containers or tinted glass. Room temperature is suitable for most drugs, away from sources of direct heat. A few drugs should be stored in the refrigerator. Storage information for individual drugs is given in the drug profiles in Part 4.

All drugs, including cough medicines, iron tablets, and oral contraceptives, should be kept out of the reach of children. If you are in the habit of keeping your medicines where you will see them as a reminder to take them, leave an empty medicine container out instead, and put the medicine itself safely out of reach.

Wall cabinets that can be locked are ideal for storing drugs, as long as the cabinet itself is in a cool, dry place and not, as often happens, in the bathroom, which is frequently warm and humid.

WHEN TO DISPOSE OF DRUGS

Old medications should be flushed down the toilet or returned to the pharmacist, but not put in the garbage. Always dispose of:

● Aspirin and acetaminophen tablets that smell of vinegar.

● Tablets that are chipped, cracked, or discolored, and capsules that have softened, cracked, or stuck together.

● Liquids that have thickened or discolored, or that taste or smell different in any way from the original product.

● Tubes that are cracked, leaky, or hard.

● Ointments and creams that have changed odor, or changed appearance by discoloring, hardening, or separating.

● Any liquid needing refrigeration that has been kept for over two weeks.

● Tablets or capsules over two years old.

LONG-TERM DRUG TREATMENT

Many people may require regular, prolonged, or even lifelong treatment with one or more drugs. People suffering from chronic or recurrent disorders often need lifelong treatment with drugs to control symptoms or prevent complications. Antihypertensive drugs for high blood pressure and insulin or oral antidiabetic drugs for diabetes mellitus are familiar examples. Many other disorders take a long time to cure; people with tuberculosis, for example, usually need at least six months' therapy with antituberculous drugs. Long-term treatment may also be necessary to prevent a condition from occurring, and will have to be taken for as long as the individual is at risk. Antimalarial drugs are a good example.

Possible adverse effects

You may worry that taking a drug for a long period will reduce its effectiveness or that you will become dependent on it. However, *tolerance* develops only with a few drugs; most drugs continue to have the same effect indefinitely. Similarly, taking a drug for more than a few weeks does not normally create dependence.

Changing drug treatment

If you are taking a drug regularly, you will need to know what to do if something else occurs to affect your health. If you wish to become pregnant, for example, you should ask your physician right away if it is preferable to continue on your regular medicine or switch to another less apt to affect your pregnancy. If you contract a new illness, for which an additional drug is prescribed, your regular medication may be altered.

There are a number of other reasons for changing drugs. You may have had an adverse reaction, or an improved preparation may have become available.

Adjusting to long-term treatment

You should establish a daily routine for taking your medication in order to reduce the risk of a missed dose. Usually you should not stop taking your medication, even if there are side effects, without consulting your physician (see Ending drug treatment, p.28). If you become afraid of possible adverse effects from the drug, you should discuss these fears with your physician.

Many people deliberately stop their drugs because they feel well or their symptoms disappear. That can be dangerous, especially with a disease like hypertension which has no noticeable symptoms. Stopping treatment may lead to a recurrence or worsening of a disease. If you are uncertain about why you have to keep taking a drug, ask your physician. Only a few drugs require an alteration in habits. Some drugs should not be taken with alcohol; with one or two drugs you should avoid certain foods. If you require a drug that makes you drowsy, you should not drive a car or operate dangerous equipment.

If you are taking a drug that should not be stopped suddenly or that may interact with other drugs, it is a good idea to carry a warning card or bracelet. Such information might be essential for emergency medical treatment in an accident.

Monitoring treatment

If you are on long-term treatment, you need to visit your physician for periodic checkups. He or she will check your underlying condition and monitor any adverse effects of treatment. Levels of the drug in the blood may be measured. With insulin, in addition to checks with the physician, you need to monitor blood sugar levels each day.

If a drug is known to cause damage to an organ, tests may be done to check the function of the organ. For example, blood and urine tests to check kidney function, or a blood count to check the bone marrow, may be indicated.

Physician checkups
Blood pressure is a concern in the long-term treatment of circulatory disorders.

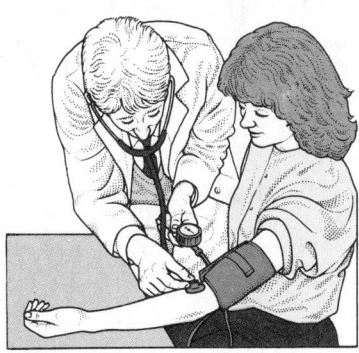

EXCEEDING THE DOSE

Most people associate drug overdoses with attempts at suicide or the fatalities and near fatalities brought on by abuse of street drugs. However, drug overdoses can also occur among people who deliberately or inadvertently exceed the stated dose of a drug that has been prescribed for them by their physician.

A single extra dose of most drugs is unlikely to be a cause for concern, although accidental overdoses can create anxiety in the individual and his or her family, and may cause overdose symptoms which appear in a variety of different forms.

Overdose of some drugs, however, is potentially dangerous even when the dose has been exceeded by only a small amount. Each of the drug profiles in Part 4 of this book gives detailed information on the consequences of exceeding the dose, symptoms to look out for, and what to do. Each drug has been given an overdose danger rating of low, medium or high (described fully on p.212).

Taking an extra dose

People sometimes exceed the stated dose in the mistaken belief that by increasing dosage they will obtain more

Effects of repeated overdose
Repeated overdose of a drug over an extended period may lead to a buildup of high levels of the drug in the body, especially if liver or kidney function is reduced.

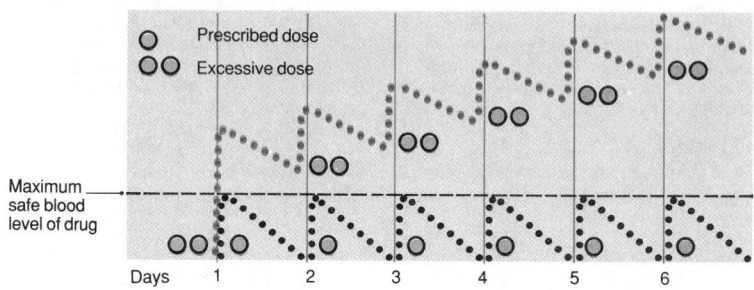

○ Prescribed dose
○○ Excessive dose

Maximum safe blood level of drug

Days 1 2 3 4 5 6

immediate action or a more effective cure. This is a particular risk with *tolerance*-inducing drugs (see Drug dependence, p.23). Others exceed their dose accidentally, by miscalculating the amount or forgetting that the dose has already been taken.

Taking extra doses is often a problem in the elderly, who may repeat their dose through forgetfulness or confusion. This

is a special risk with medicines that cause drowsiness (see also p.22).

In some cases, especially when liver or kidney function is impaired, the drug builds up in the blood because the body cannot break down and excrete the extra dose quickly enough, so that symptoms of poisoning may result (see below left). Symptoms of excessive intake may not be apparent for many days.

When and how to get help

If you are not sure whether you have taken your tablets or medicine, think back and check again. If you honestly cannot remember, assume that you have missed the dose and follow the advice given in the individual drug profiles in Part 4 of this book. If you cannot find your drug there, consult your physician. Make a note to use some system in the future which will help you remember to take your medication.

If you are looking after an elderly person on regular medication who suddenly develops unusual symptoms such as confusion, drowsiness, or unsteadiness, consider the possibility of drug overdose and call the prescribing physician as soon as possible.

Deliberate overdose

While many cases of drug overdose are accidental or the result of a mistaken belief that increasing the dose will enhance the benefits of drug treatment, sometimes an excessive amount of a drug is taken with the intention of causing harm or even as a suicide attempt. Whether or not you think a dangerous amount of a drug has been taken, deliberate overdoses of this kind should always be brought to the attention of your physician. Not only is it necessary to ensure that no physical harm has occurred as a result of the overdose, but the psychological condition of a person who takes such action may indicate the need for additional medical help.

HOW DRUGS ACCUMULATE

In most people, the liver and kidneys are able to cope with an occasional extra dose of a drug. But if they are functioning below normal efficiency, excessive doses may accumulate in the body.

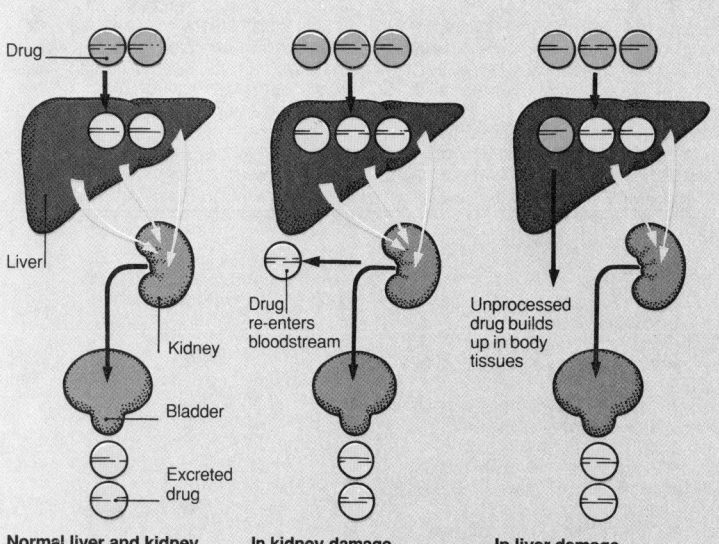

Drug

Liver

Kidney

Bladder

Excreted drug

Drug re-enters bloodstream

Unprocessed drug builds up in body tissues

Normal liver and kidney
Drugs taken by mouth are processed in the liver and later excreted by the kidneys.

In kidney damage
The kidneys cannot eliminate excess drug in the urine; drug levels in the blood may rise.

In liver damage
The liver cannot process the excess drug which may build up in the body tissues.

DOs AND DON'Ts

On this page you will find a summary of the most important practical points concerning the management of your drug treatment. The advice is arranged under general headings, explaining the safest methods of storing drugs and following treatment, whether it is a prescribed medication or an over-the-counter drug. This information is equally applicable whether you are taking medication yourself or supervising the drug treatment of someone in your care.

At the physician's

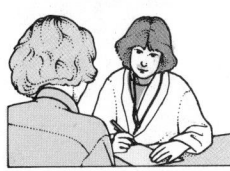

DO
● Tell your physician about any medications you are already taking, both prescription and over-the-counter.
● Tell your physician if you are pregnant, intending to become pregnant, or breast-feeding.
● Tell your physician about any allergic reactions you have experienced to past drug treatments.
● Tell your physician if you have a specific current health problem, such as liver or kidney disease, or if you think you might be at special risk from drug treatment for any other reason.

● Discuss your drug treatment with your physician and make sure you understand the reasons why you have been prescribed a particular drug and what benefits you can expect. People who do not understand the reasons for their treatment often fail to take their medication correctly.

DON'T
▼ Leave your physician's office without a clear understanding of how and when to take your medication.

At the drugstore

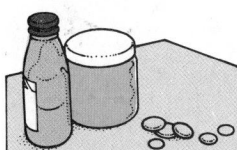

DO
● Ask your pharmacist's advice about over-the-counter drugs if you are not sure what you should buy, or if you think you may react adversely to a drug.
● Try to see the same pharmacist or use the same drugstore to fill your regular prescriptions.
● Be sure you know the name of the drug you have been prescribed, and make sure you always receive the same brand of drug as you had previously if you are refilling a prescription.

● Make sure you understand what is on the drug label.
● Ask the pharmacist to put your medication in a container with an easy-to-remove cap if you have difficulty using child-resistant containers.

DON'T
▼ Send children to the drugstore to get your medication for you.

Giving medicines to children

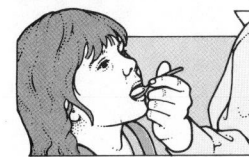

DO
● Check the dose on the label carefully before giving medicines to children.
● Make sure over-the-counter preparations you give to young children for viral infections or fevers of unknown cause do not contain aspirin.

DON'T
▼ Pretend to children that medicinal preparations are candy or soft drinks.
▼ Give any medicines to children under the age of five, except on the advice of your physician.

Taking your medication

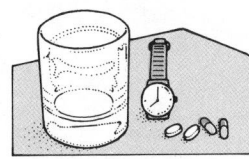

DO
● Make sure that your medication will not make you drowsy or otherwise affect your ability before you drive or perform difficult or dangerous tasks.
● Read the label carefully and do what it says. This is equally important with all types of drugs, creams, and lotions as well as drugs taken by mouth.
● Finish the drug treatment your physician prescribes for you.
● Consult your physician for advice if you experience side effects.

DON'T
▼ Take any prescribed or over-the-counter drugs without first consulting your physician if you are pregnant or trying to conceive.
▼ Offer your medication to other people or take medication that has been prescribed for someone else (even if the symptoms are the same).

Food, drink, and drugs of abuse

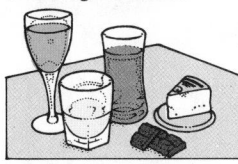

DO
● Check that it is safe to take alcohol with prescribed drugs, and that there are no foods you should avoid.

DON'T
▼ Take medication (except that prescribed by your physician), drugs of abuse, or alcohol if you are pregnant or trying to conceive. They may adversely affect the unborn baby.

Storing medications

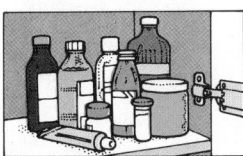

DO
● Take care to store medications in a cool, dry place and protect them from light or refrigerate them, if advised to do so.
● Keep all drugs – including seemingly harmless medications such as cough preparations – locked away out of the reach of children.
● Check your medicine chest regularly in case other members of the family have left their unwanted drugs in it, and to make sure that none of the normal supplies are out of date.

● Keep drugs in their original containers with the original instructions to avoid confusion.

DON'T
▼ Hoard drugs at home. When you have stopped taking a prescribed drug, dispose of it unless it is part of your family first aid kit.

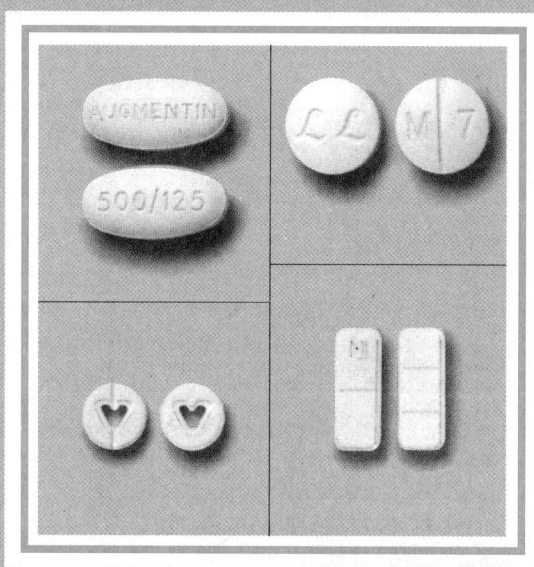

COLOR IDENTIFICATION GUIDE

The following pages contain photographs of brand-name drugs. The guide is divided into two sections – tablets and capsules. These are arranged first according to their color groups, and secondly according to their size. The fact that a particular product is included in no way implies AMA endorsement of that brand over another similar drug.

The products included on these pages represent a selection of the most popular brand names in the United States. Several dosage strengths of some of the more widely prescribed brand names have been included. Each drug is

photographed approximately life-size. Beneath each photograph you will find the name of the tablet or capsule with details of its main generic ingredients and their amounts in grams (g) and milligrams (mg). The drugs are laid out in a grid format. Each entry can be located from the Index of Generic and Brand-Name Drugs by reference to the page number and the letter in the top left-hand corner of each square of the grid.

To locate the photograph of a particular medication, consult the chart, which will direct you to the relevant color section. You will find an example of an entry in the section below.

HOW TO LOCATE YOUR MEDICATION

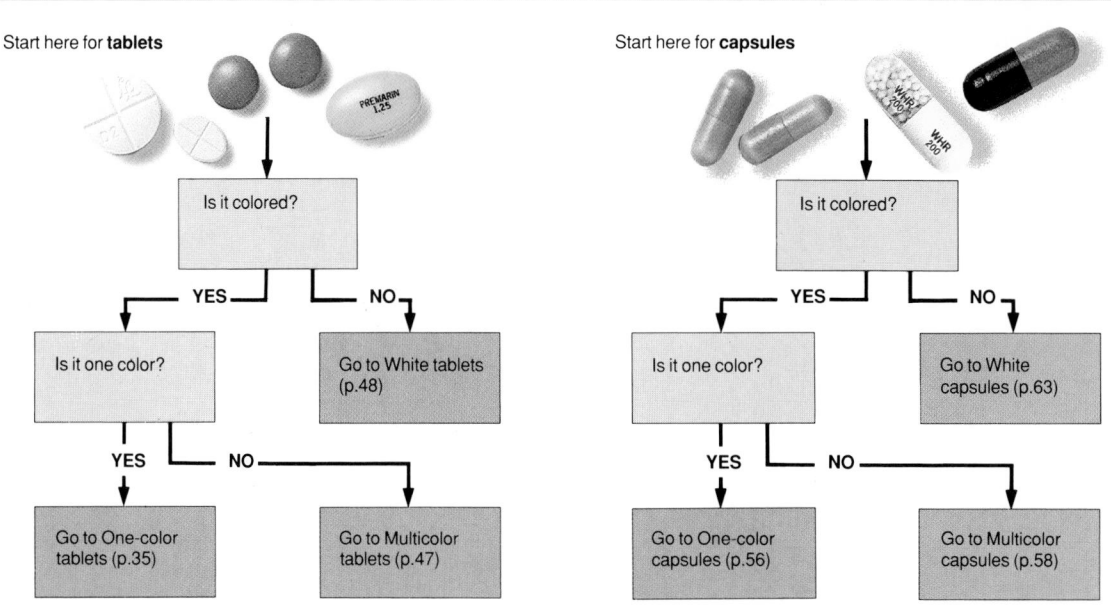

Start here for **tablets**

Is it colored? — YES → Is it one color? — YES → Go to One-color tablets (p.35)

Is it one color? — NO → Go to Multicolor tablets (p.47)

Is it colored? — NO → Go to White tablets (p.48)

Start here for **capsules**

Is it colored? — YES → Is it one color? — YES → Go to One-color capsules (p.56)

Is it one color? — NO → Go to Multicolor capsules (p.58)

Is it colored? — NO → Go to White capsules (p.63)

HOW TO UNDERSTAND THE ENTRIES

This example explains the significance of the text accompanying each photograph that will help you to identify a particular drug.

Identifying marks These are unique to each product, but they may include the name of the manufacturer, brand name of the drug, or a reference number.

Brand name The brand name of the drug.

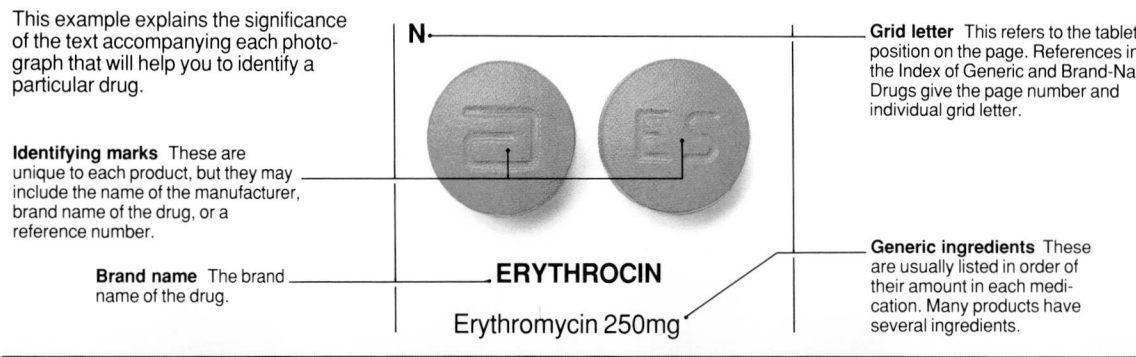

N

ERYTHROCIN

Erythromycin 250mg

Grid letter This refers to the tablet's position on the page. References in the Index of Generic and Brand-Name Drugs give the page number and individual grid letter.

Generic ingredients These are usually listed in order of their amount in each medication. Many products have several ingredients.

ONE-COLOR TABLETS

A

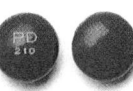

CHOLEDYL

Oxtriphylline 100mg

B

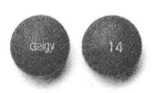

BUTAZOLIDIN

Phenylbutazone 100mg

C

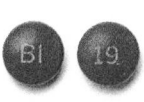

PERSANTINE

Dipyridamole 75mg

D

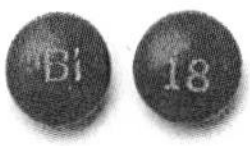

PERSANTINE

Dipyridamole 50mg

E

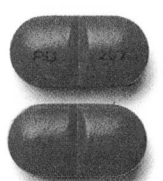

PROCAN SR

Procainamide 100mg

F

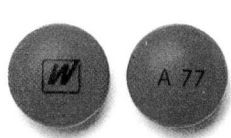

ARALEN

Chloroquine 500mg

G

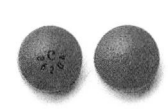

NOLAMINE

Phenylpropanolamine 50mg
Phenindamine 24mg
Chlorpheniramine 4mg

H

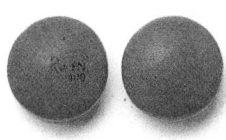

RUFEN

Ibuprofen 400mg

I

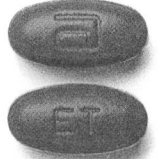

ERYTHROCIN

Erythromycin 500mg

J

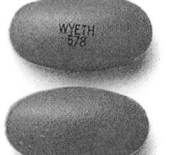

WYAMYCIN S

Erythromycin 500mg

K

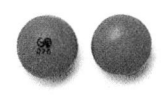

ESTINYL

Ethinyl estradiol 0.05mg

L

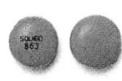

PROLIXIN

Fluphenazine 1mg

M

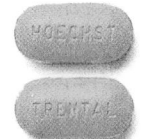

TRENTAL

Pentoxifylline 400mg

N

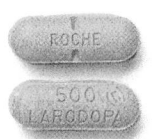

LARODOPA

Levodopa 0.5g

O

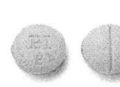

COMBIPRES

Chlorthalidone 15mg
Clonidine 0.1mg

P

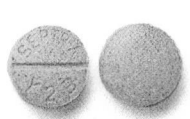

SEPTRA

Sulfamethoxazole 400mg
Trimethoprim 80mg

Q

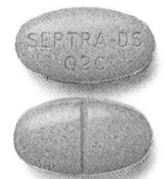

SEPTRA DS

Sulfamethoxazole 800mg
Trimethoprim 160mg

R

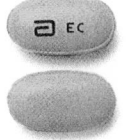

ERYTAB

Erythromycin 250mg

S

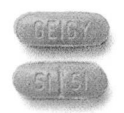

LOPRESSOR

Metoprolol 50mg

T

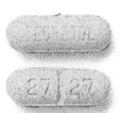

TEGRETOL

Carbamazepine 200mg

ONE-COLOR TABLETS continued

A

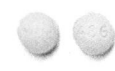

NORDETTE 28
Levonorgestrel 0.15mg
Ethinyl estradiol 0.03mg

B

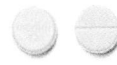

DELTASONE
Prednisolone 2.5mg

C

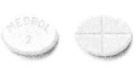

MEDROL
Methylprednisolone 2mg

D

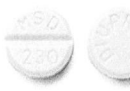

DIUPRES
Chlorothiazide 250mg

E

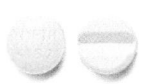

ISORDIL
Isosorbide dinitrate 5mg

F

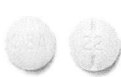

ESIDRIX
Hydrochlorothiazide 25mg

G

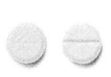

CRYSTODIGIN
Digitoxin 0.1mg

H

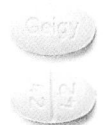

CONSTANT T
Theophylline 200mg

I

ISORDIL (sublingual)
Isosorbide dinitrate 5mg

J

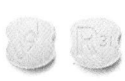

REGROTON
Chlorthalidone 50mg
Reserpine 0.25mg

K

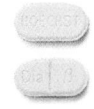

DIABETA
Glyburide 2.5mg

L

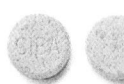

SER-AP-ES
Hydralazine 25mg
Hydrochlorothiazide 15mg
Reserpine 0.1mg

M

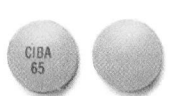

LITHOBID
Lithium carbonate 300mg

N

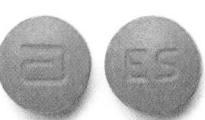

ERYTHROCIN
Erythromycin 250mg

O

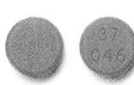

BUTIBEL
Belladonna 15mg
Butabarbital 15mg

P

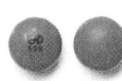

ETRAFON
Amitriptyline 25mg
Perphenazine 2mg

Q

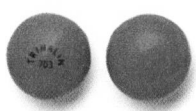

TRINALIN
Pseudoephedrine 120mg
Azatadine 1mg

R

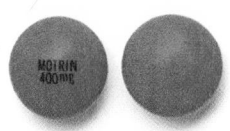

MOTRIN
Ibuprofen 400mg

S

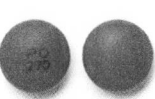

NARDIL
Phenelzine 15mg

T

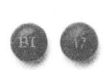

PERSANTINE
Dipyridamole 25mg

A

LUDIOMIL

Maprotiline 50mg

B

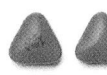

ATARAX

Hydroxyzine 10mg

C

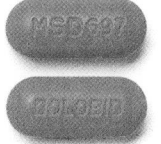

DOLOBID

Diflunisal 500mg

D

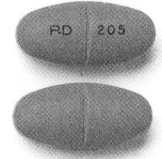

PROCAN SR

Procainamide 750mg

E

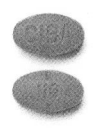

LUDIOMIL

Maprotiline 25mg

F

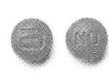

JANIMINE

Imipramine 10mg

G

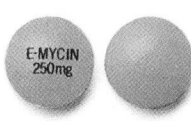

E-MYCIN

Erythromycin 250mg

H

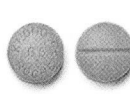

KLONOPIN

Clonazepam 0.5mg

I

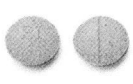

CATAPRES

Clonidine 0.2mg

J

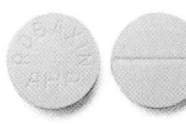

ROBAXIN

Methocarbamol 500mg

K

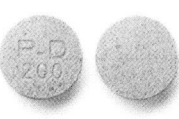

BRONDECON

Oxtriphylline 200mg
Guaifenesin 100mg

L

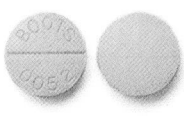

LOPURIN

Allopurinol 300mg

M

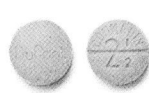

COUMADIN

Warfarin 2.5mg

N

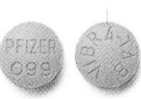

VIBRA-TABS

Doxycycline 100mg

O

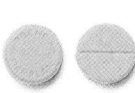

MARPLAN

Isocarboxazid 10mg

P

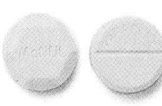

PARAFLEX

Chlorzoxazone 250mg

Q

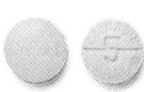

COUMADIN

Warfarin 5mg

R

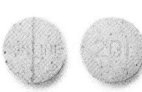

BONINE

Meclizine 25mg

S

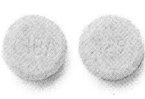

APRESOLINE WITH ESIDRIX

Hydralazine 25mg
Hydrochlorothiazide 15mg

T

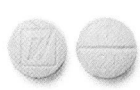

TALWIN NX

Pentazocine 50mg
Naloxone 0.5mg

ONE-COLOR TABLETS continued

A

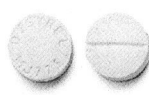

DESYREL

Trazodone 50mg

B

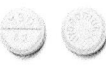

HYDRODIURIL

Hydrochlorothiazide 25mg

C

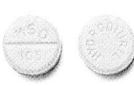

HYDRODIURIL

Hydrochlorothiazide 50mg

D

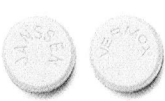

VERMOX

Mebendazole 100mg

E

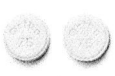

ORTHO-NOVUM 7/7/7

Norethindrone 1mg
Ethinyl estradiol 0.035mg

F

ORTHO-NOVUM 10/11

Norethindrone 1mg
Ethinyl estradiol 0.035mg

G

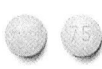

NORDETTE

Levonorgestrel 0.15mg
Ethinyl estradiol 0.03mg

H

PRO-BANTHINE

Propantheline 15mg

I

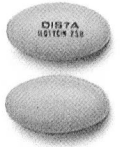

ILOTYCIN

Erythromycin 250mg

J

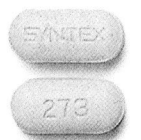

NAPROSYN

Naproxen 375mg

K

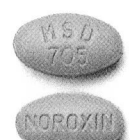

NOROXIN

Norfloxacin 400mg

L

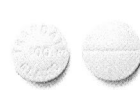

TRANDATE

Labetalol 100mg

M

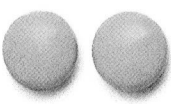

CYCLOSPASMOL

Cyclandelate 100mg

N

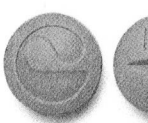

AZULFIDINE

Sulfasalazine 500mg

O

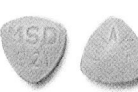

TRIAVIL

Amitriptyline 25mg
Perphenazine 2mg

P

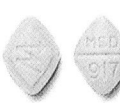

MODURETIC

Amiloride 5mg
Hydrochlorothiazide 50mg

Q

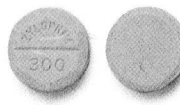

ZYLOPRIM

Allopurinol 300mg

R

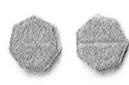

ASENDIN

Amoxapine 50mg

S

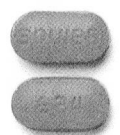

VEETIDS

Penicillin V 250mg

T

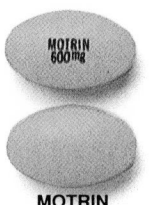

MOTRIN

Ibuprofen 600mg

A

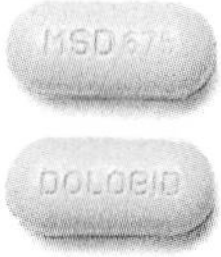

DOLOBID

Diflunisal 250mg

B

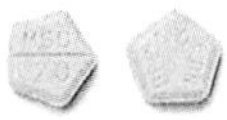

DECADRON

Dexamethasone 0.25mg

C

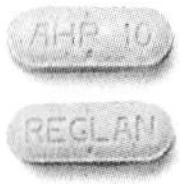

REGLAN

Metoclopramide 10mg

D

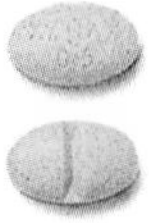

XANAX

Alprazolam 0.5mg

E

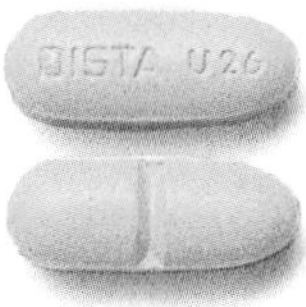

ILOSONE

Erythromycin 500mg

F

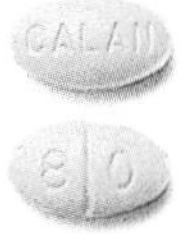

CALAN

Verapamil 80mg

G

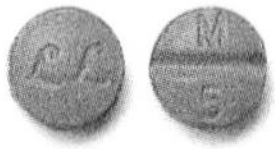

MINOCIN

Minocycline 100mg

H

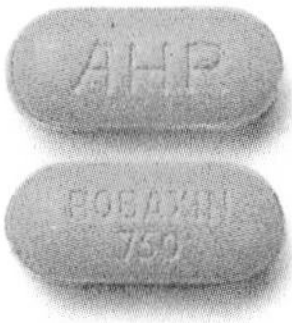

ROBAXIN

Methocarbamol 750mg

I

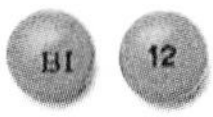

DULCOLAX

Bisacodyl 5mg

J

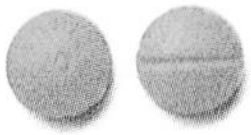

ENDEP

Amitriptyline 10mg

K

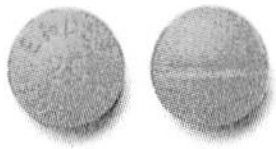

ENDEP

Amitriptyline 25mg

L

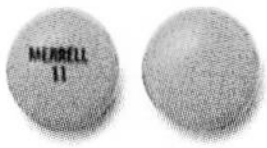

NORPRAMIN

Desipramine 25mg

M

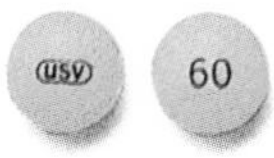

AZOLID

Phenylbutazone 100mg

N

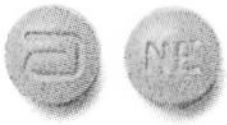

JANIMINE

Imipramine 25mg

O

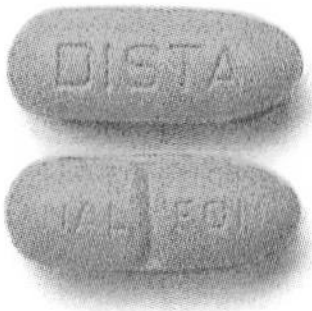

NALFON

Fenoprofen 600mg

P

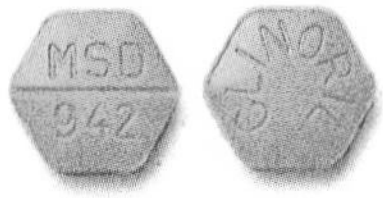

CLINORIL

Sulindac 200mg

Q

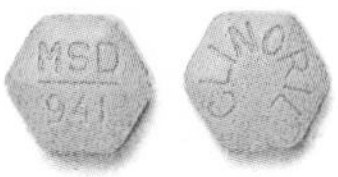

CLINORIL

Sulindac 150mg

R

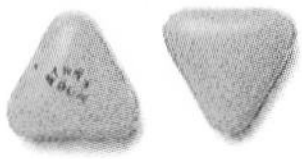

ATARAX

Hydroxyzine 50mg

S

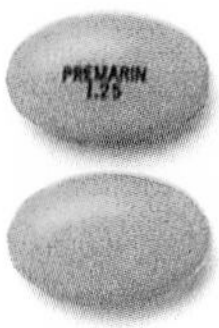

PREMARIN

Conjugated estrogens 1.25mg

T

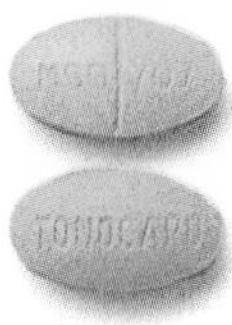

TONOCARD

Tocainide 400mg

ONE-COLOR TABLETS continued

A

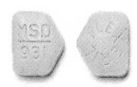

FLEXERIL

Cyclobenzaprine 10mg

B

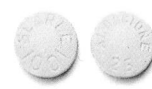

ALDACTONE

Spironolactone 25mg

C

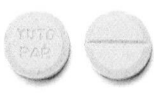

YUTOPAR

Ritodrine 10mg

D

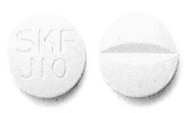

ESKALITH CR

Lithium carbonate 450mg

E

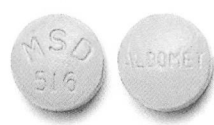

ALDOMET

Methyldopa 500mg

F

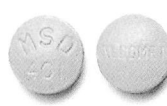

ALDOMET

Methyldopa 250mg

G

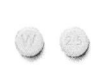

ISORDIL (sublingual)

Isosorbide dinitrate 2.5mg

H

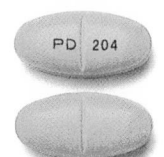

PROCAN SR

Procainamide 500mg

I

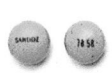

SANSERT

Methysergide 2mg

J

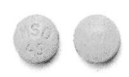

ELAVIL

Amitriptyline 25mg

K

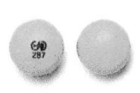

PROLIXIN

Fluphenazine 2.5mg

L

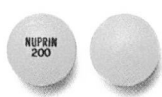

NUPRIN

Ibuprofen 200mg

M

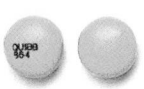

ETRAFON

Amitriptyline 10mg
Perphenazine 2mg

N

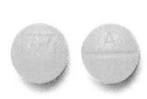

ATABRINE

Quinacrine 100mg

O

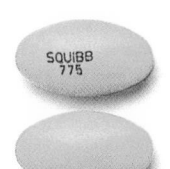

PRONESTYL SR

Procainamide 500mg

P

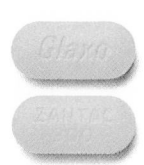

ZANTAC

Ranitidine 300mg

Q

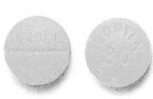

ISOPTIN

Verapamil 80mg

R

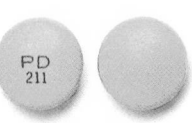

CHOLEDYL

Oxtriphylline 200mg

S

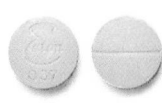

FURADANTIN

Nitrofurantoin 100mg

T

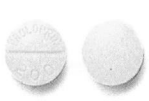

PROLOPRIM

Trimethoprim 200mg

A

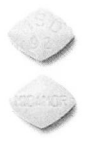

DYMELOR

Acetohexamide 500mg

B

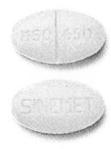

SINEMET

Levodopa 100mg
Carbidopa 25mg

C

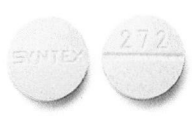

NAPROSYN

Naproxen 250mg

D

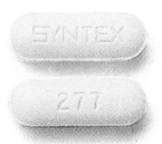

NAPROSYN

Naproxen 500mg

E

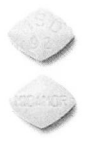

MIDAMOR

Amiloride 5mg

F

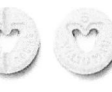

VALIUM

Diazepam 5mg

G

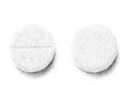

LANOXIN

Digoxin 0.125mg

H

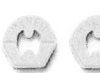

HALDOL

Haloperidol 1mg

I

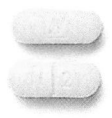

BENEMID

Probenecid 0.5g

J

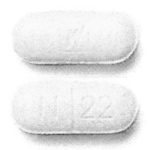

NEGGRAM

Nalidixic acid 500mg

K

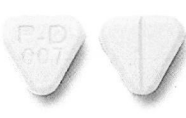

DILANTIN

Phenytoin 50mg

L

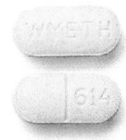

CYCLAPEN W

Cyclacillin 250mg

M

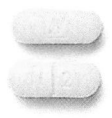

NEGGRAM

Nalidixic acid 250mg

N

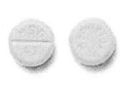

MEPHYTON

Phytonadione 5mg

O

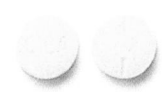

ISMELIN

Guanethidine 10mg

P

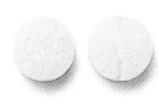

ESIDRIX

Hydrochlorothiazide 50mg

Q

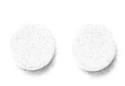

ORTHO-NOVUM 1/50

Norethindrone 1mg
Mestranol 0.05mg

R

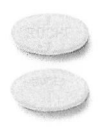

BUMEX

Bumetanide 1mg

S

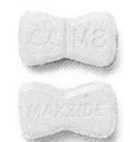

MAXZIDE

Triamterene 75mg
Hydrochlorothiazide 50mg

T

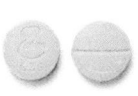

FURADANTIN

Nitrofurantoin 50mg

ONE-COLOR TABLETS continued

A

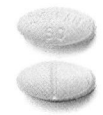

IMURAN

Azathioprine 50mg

B

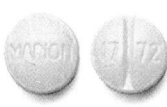

CARDIZEM

Diltiazem 60mg

C

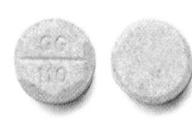

CHLORZOXAZONE WITH APAP

Chlorzoxazone 250mg
with acetaminophen

D

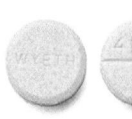

ISORDIL TEMBIDS

Isosorbide dinitrate 40mg

E

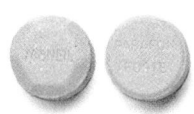

PARAFON FORTE

Acetaminophen 300mg
Chlorzoxazone 250mg

F

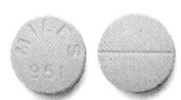

LITHANE

Lithium carbonate 300mg

G

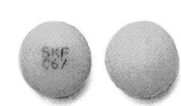

COMPAZINE

Prochlorperazine 10mg

H

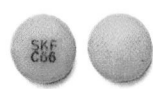

COMPAZINE

Prochlorperazine 5mg

I

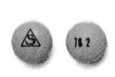

MELLARIL

Thioridazine 10mg

J

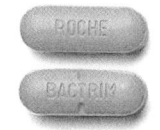

BACTRIM

Sulfamethoxazole 400mg
Trimethoprim 80mg

K

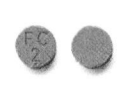

ERGOMAR

Ergotamine 2mg

L

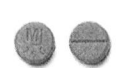

ESTRACE

Estradiol 2mg

M

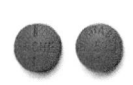

LIBRITABS

Chlordiazepoxide 5mg

N

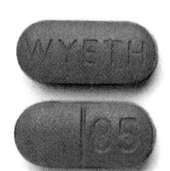

WYGESIC

Acetaminophen 650mg
Propoxyphene 65mg

O

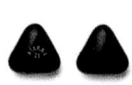

ATARAX

Hydroxyzine 25mg

P

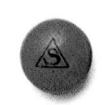

CAFERGOT P – B

Caffeine 100mg Ergotamine 1mg
Pentobarbital 30mg
Belladonna 0.125mg

Q

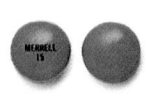

NORPRAMIN

Desipramine 50mg

R

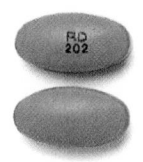

PROCAN-SR

Procainamide 250mg

S

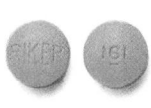

DISIPAL

Orphenadrine 50mg

T

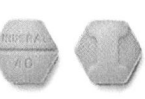

INDERAL

Propranolol 40mg

A

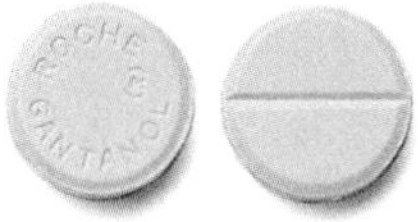

GANTANOL
Sulfamethoxazole 0.5g

B

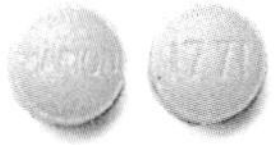

CARDIZEM
Diltiazem 30mg

C

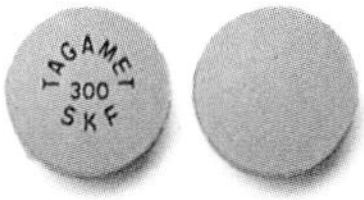

TAGAMET
Cimetidine 300mg

D

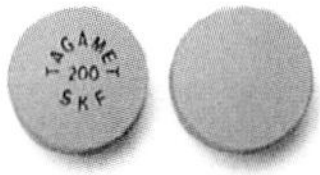

TAGAMET
Cimetidine 200mg

E

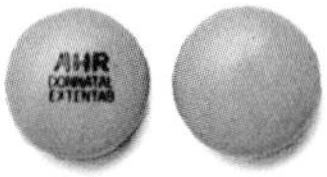

DONNATAL
Phenobarbital 16.2mg
with hyoscyamine, atropine
and scopolamine

F

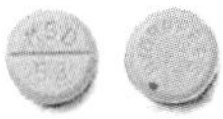

HYDROPRES-25
Hydrochlorothiazide 25mg
Reserpine 0.125mg

G

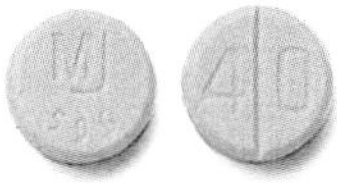

MEGACE
Megestrol 40mg

H

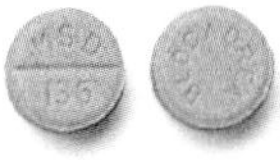

BLOCADREN
Timolol 10mg

I

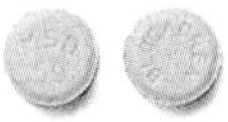

BLOCADREN
Timolol 5mg

J

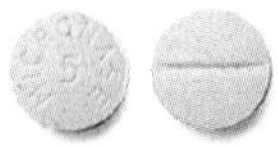

MICRONASE
Glyburide 5mg

K

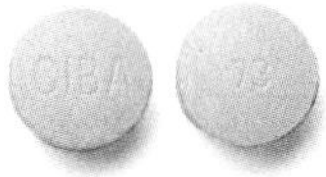

APRESOLINE
Hydralazine 50mg

L

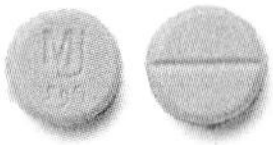

MEGACE
Megestrol 30mg

M

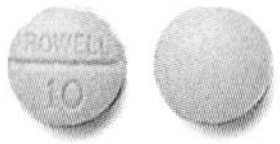

ORASONE
Prednisolone 10mg

N

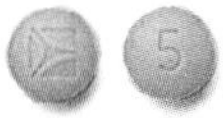

ZAROXOLYN
Metolazone 5mg

O

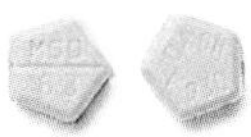

DECADRON
Dexamethasone 0.75mg

P

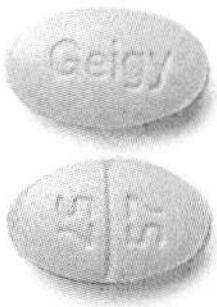

CONSTANT T
Theophylline 300mg

Q

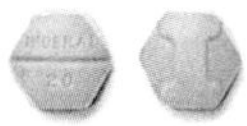

INDERAL
Propranolol 20mg

R

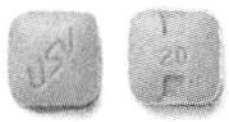

HYGROTON
Chlorthalidone 50mg

S

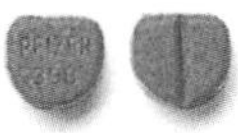

DIABINESE
Chlorpropamide 100mg

T

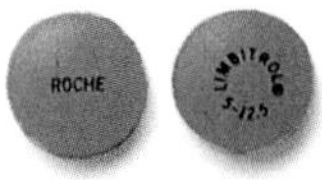

LIMBITROL
Amitriptyline 12.5mg
Chlordiazepoxide 5mg

ONE-COLOR TABLETS continued

A

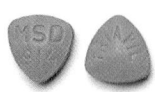

TRIAVIL

Amitriptyline 10mg
Perphenazine 2mg

B

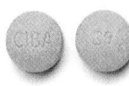

APRESOLINE

Hydralazine 25mg

C

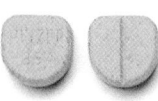

DIABINESE

Chlorpropamide 250mg

D

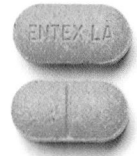

ENTEX LA

Guaifenesin 400mg
Phenylpropanolamine 75mg

E

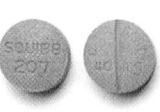

CORGARD

Nadolol 40mg

F

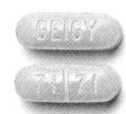

LOPRESSOR

Metoprolol 100mg

G

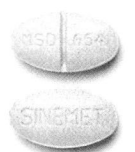

SINEMET

Levodopa 250mg
Carbidopa 25mg

H

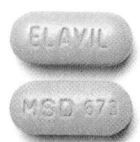

ELAVIL

Amitriptyline 150mg

I

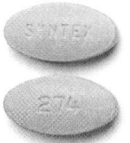

ANAPROX

Naproxen 275mg

J

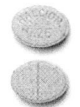

HALCION

Triazolam 0.25mg

K

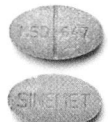

SINEMET

Levodopa 100mg
Carbidopa 10mg

L

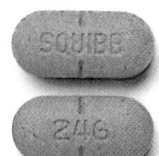

CORGARD

Nadolol 160mg

M

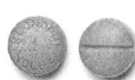

KLONOPIN

Clonazepam 1mg

N

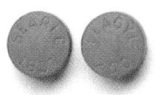

FLAGYL

Metronidazole 250mg

O

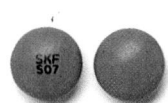

STELAZINE

Trifluoperazine 10mg

P

STELAZINE

Trifluoperazine 5mg

Q

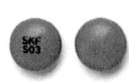

STELAZINE

Trifluoperazine 1mg

R

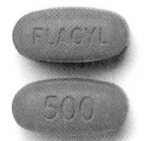

FLAGYL

Metronidazole 500mg

S

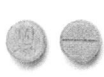

ESTRACE

Estradiol 1mg

T

HALCION

Triazolam 0.125mg

A

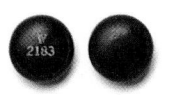

CARAFATE

Sucralfate 1g

B

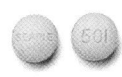

DIULO

Metolazone 2.5mg

C

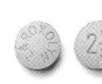

ZAROXOLYN

Metolazone 2.5mg

D

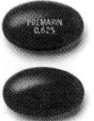

PREMARIN

Conjugated estrogens 0.625mg

E

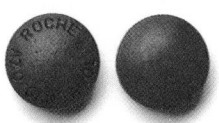

URISED

Atropine 0.03mg
Hyoscyamine 0.03mg and
several antiseptic ingredients

F

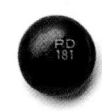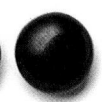

PYRIDIUM

Phenazopyridine 200mg

G

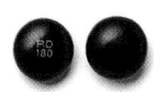

PYRIDIUM

Phenazopyridine 100mg

H

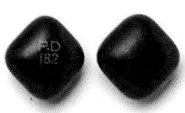

PYRIDIUM PLUS

Phenazopyridine 150mg
Butabarbital 15mg
Hyoscyamine 0.3mg

I

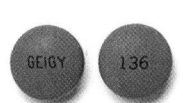

AZO-GANTANOL

Phenazopyridine 100mg
Sulfamethoxazole 0.5mg

J

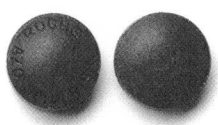

AZO-GANTRISIN

Phenazopyridine 50mg
Sulfisoxazole 0.5mg

K

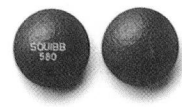

MYCOSTATIN

Nystatin 500,000 units

L

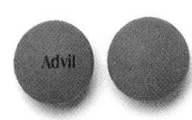

ADVIL

Ibuprofen 200mg

M

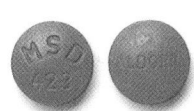

TOFRANIL

Imipramine 50mg

N

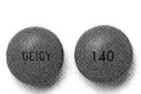

TOFRANIL

Imipramine 25mg

O

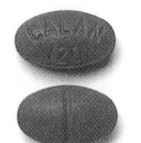

CALAN

Verapamil 120mg

P

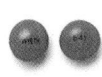

TRIPHASIL

Levonorgestrel 0.05mg
Ethinyl estradiol 0.03mg

Q

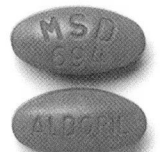

ALDORIL 15

Methyldopa 250mg
Hydrochlorothiazide 15mg

R

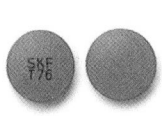

ALDORIL D30

Methyldopa 500mg
Hydrochlorothiazide 30mg

S

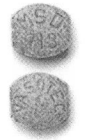

VASOTEC

Enalapril 10mg

T

THORAZINE

Chlorpromazine 50mg

ONE-COLOR TABLETS continued

A

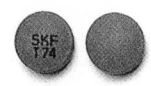

THORAZINE

Chlorpromazine 25mg

B

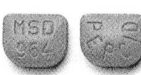

PEPCID

Famotidine 40mg

C

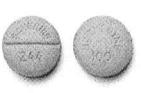

NORMODYNE

Labetalol 100mg

D

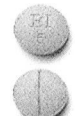

CATAPRES

Clonidine 0.1mg

E

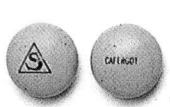

CAFERGOT

Caffeine 100mg
Ergotamine 1mg

F

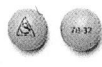

BELLERGAL–S

Phenobarbital 40mg
Ergotamine 0.6mg
Belladonna 0.2mg

G

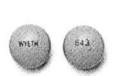

TRIPHASIL

Levonorgestrel 0.05mg
Ethinyl estradiol 0.03mg

H

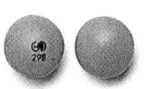

ESTINYL

Ethinyl estradiol 0.02mg

I

MELLARIL

Thioridazine 25mg

J

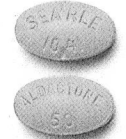

ALDACTONE

Spironolactone 50mg

K

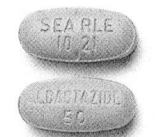

ALDACTAZIDE

Hydrochlorothiazide 50mg
Spironolactone 50mg

L

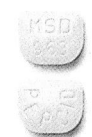

PEPCID

Famotidine 20mg

M

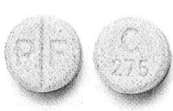

CARDIOQUIN

Quinidine 275mg

N

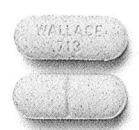

RYNATAN

Phenylephrine 25mg
Pyrilamine 25mg
Chlorpheniramine 8mg

O

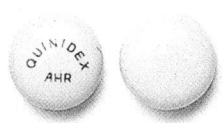

QUINIDEX

Quinidine 300mg

P

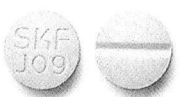

ESKALITH

Lithium carbonate 300mg

Q

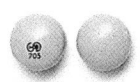

TRILAFON

Perphenazine 2mg

R

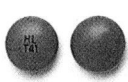

TEMARIL

Trimeprazine 2.5mg

MULTICOLOR TABLETS

A

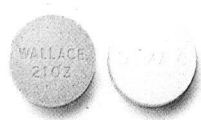

SOMA COMPOUND

Aspirin 325mg
Carisoprodol 200mg

B

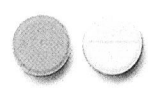

PHENERGAN D

Pseudoephedrine 560mg
Promethazine 6.25mg

C

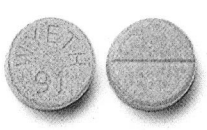

EQUAGESIC

Aspirin 325mg
Meprobamate 200mg

D

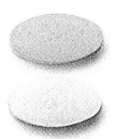

ANTIVERT

Meclizine 25mg

E

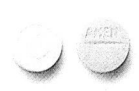

AMEN

Medroxyprogesterone 10mg

F

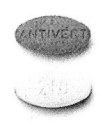

ANTIVERT

Meclizine 12.5mg

G

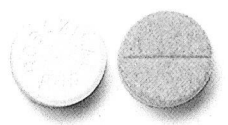

ROBAXISAL

Methocarbamol 400mg
Aspirin 325mg

H

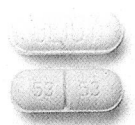

LOPRESSOR HCT

Metoprolol 100mg
Hydrochlorothiazide 25mg

I

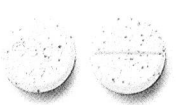

TEGRETOL

Carbamazepine 100mg

J

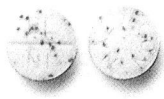

NALDECON

Phenylpropanolamine 40mg
Phenyltoloxamine 15mg with
phenylephrine and chlorpheniramine

K

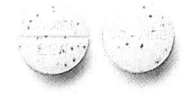

CORZIDE

Nadolol 80mg
Bendroflumethiazide 5mg

L

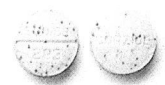

CORZIDE

Nadolol 40mg
Bendroflumethiazide 5mg

M

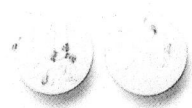

CYTOXAN

Cyclophosphamide 50mg

N

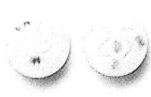

CYTOXAN

Cyclophosphamide 25mg

O

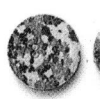

BELLERGAL – S

Phenobarbital 40mg
Ergotamine 0.6mg
Belladonna 0.2mg

P

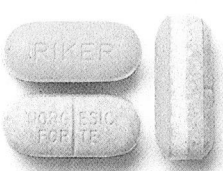

NORGESIC FORTE

Aspirin 385mg
Caffeine 30mg
Orphenadrine 25mg

WHITE TABLETS

A

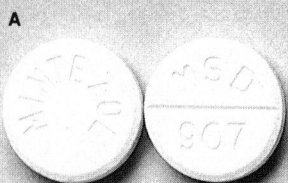

MINTEZOL

Thiabendazole 500mg

B

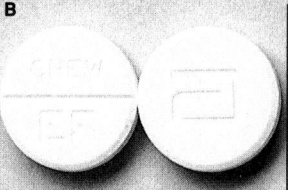

E.E.S.

Erythromycin 200mg

C

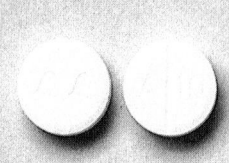

AMICAR

Aminocaproic acid 500mg

D

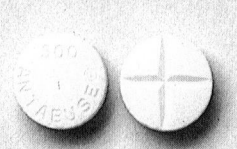

ANTABUSE

Disulfiram 500mg

E

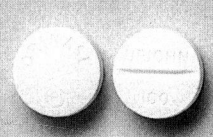

MYAMBUTOL

Ethambutol 400mg

F

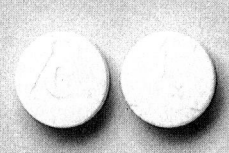

QUINAGLUTE

Quinidine 324mg

G

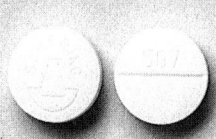

FULVICIN P/G

Griseofulvin 250mg

H

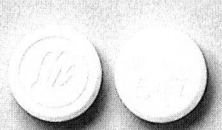

QUINAMM

Quinine 260mg

I

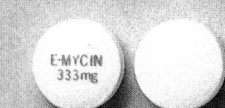

ORINASE

Tolbutamide 0.5mg

J

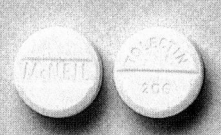

TOLECTIN

Tolmetin 200mg

K

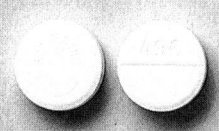

FULVICIN U/F

Griseofulvin 500mg

L

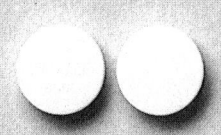

SOMA

Carisoprodol 350mg

M

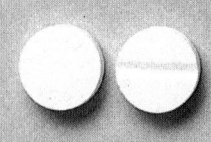

E-MYCIN

Erythromycin 333mg

N

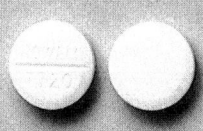

CHENIX

Chenodiol 250mg

O

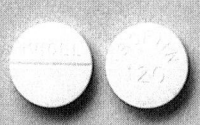

ISOPTIN

Verapamil 120mg

P

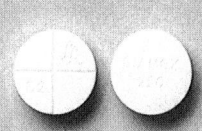

DIAMOX

Acetazolamide 250mg

Q

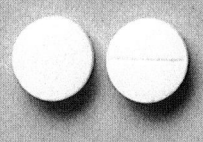

DECONAMINE

Pseudoephedrine 60mg
Chlorpheniramine 4mg

R

MILTOWN

Meprobamate 400mg

S

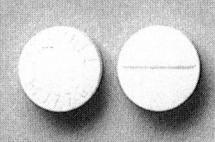

DESYREL

Trazodone 100mg

T

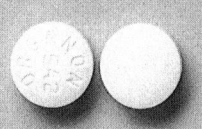

WIGRAINE

Caffeine 100mg
Ergotamine 1mg

A

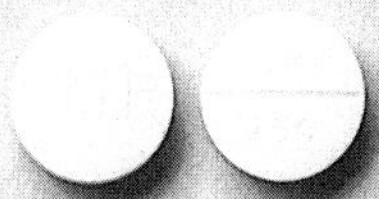

THEOLAIR

Theophylline 250mg

B

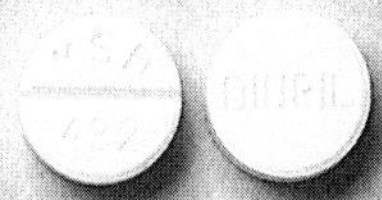

DIURIL

Chlorothiazide 500mg

C

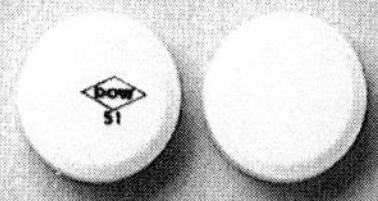

LORELCO

Probucol 250mg

D

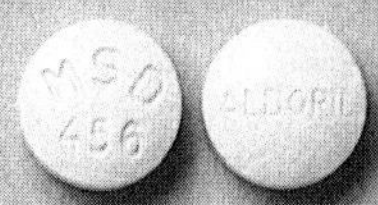

ALDORIL – 25

Methyldopa 250mg
Hydrochlorthiazide 25mg

E

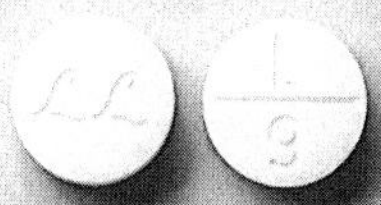

LEDERCILLIN – VK

Penicillin V 500mg

F

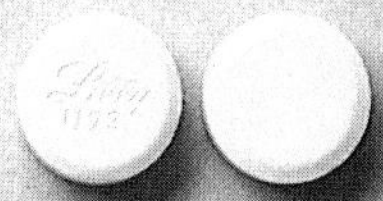

INH

Isoniazid 300mg

G

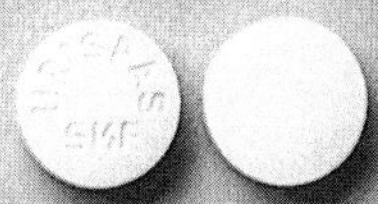

URISPAS

Flavoxate 100mg

H

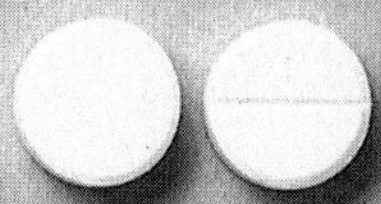

EQUANIL

Meprobamate 400mg

I

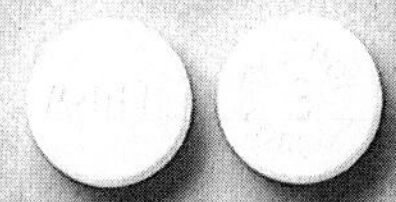

TYLENOL WITH CODEINE

Acetaminophen 300mg
Codeine 30mg

J

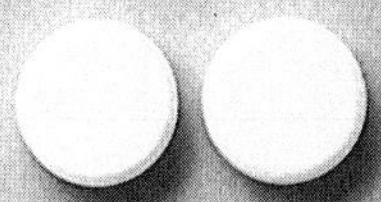

SELDANE

Terfenadine 60mg

K

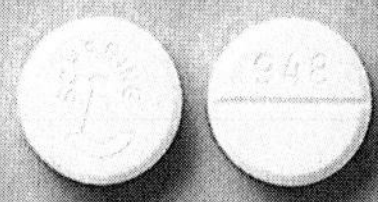

FULVICIN U/F

Griseofulvin 250mg

L

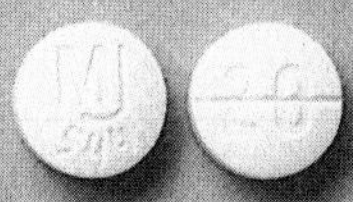

VASODILAN

Isoxsuprine 20mg

M

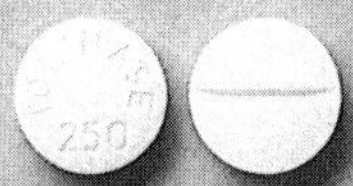

TOLINASE

Tolazamide 250mg

N

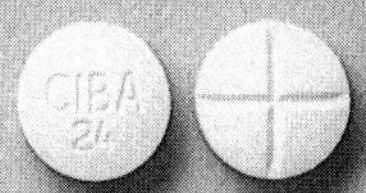

CYTADREN

Aminoglutethimide 250mg

O

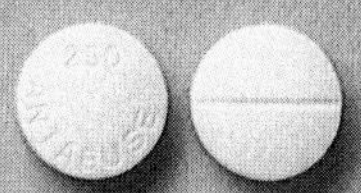

ANTABUSE

Disulfiram 250mg

P

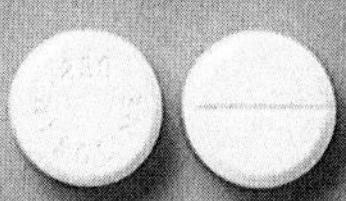

MYSOLINE

Primidone 250mg

Q

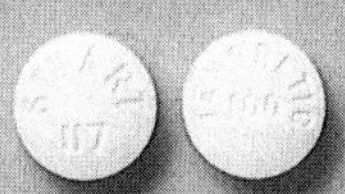

TENORETIC

Atenolol 100mg
Chlorthalidone 25mg

R

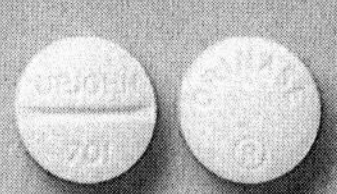

ORINASE

Tolbutamide 250mg

S

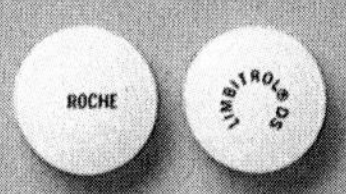

LIMBITROL

Amitriptyline 25mg
Chlordiazepoxide 10mg

T

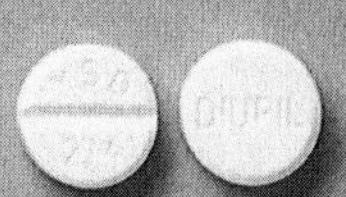

DIURIL

Chlorothiazide 250mg

WHITE TABLETS continued

A

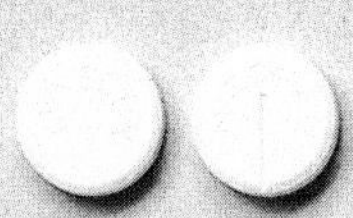

NIZORAL

Ketoconazole 200mg

B

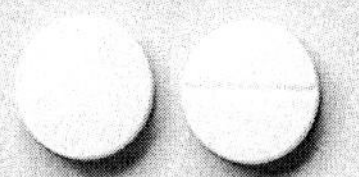

THEO-DUR

Theophylline 100mg

C

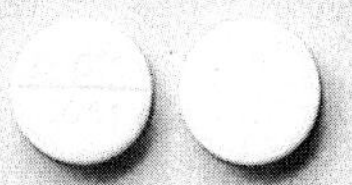

LOPURIN

Allopurinol 100mg

D

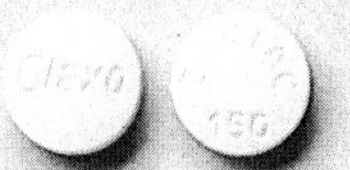

ZANTAC

Ranitidine 150mg

E

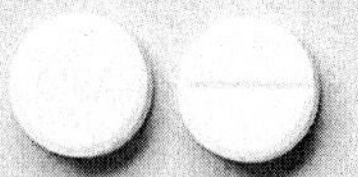

ANTURANE

Sulfinpyrazone 100mg

F

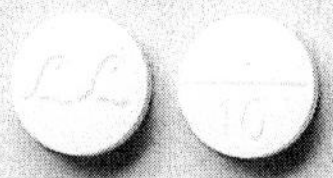

LEDERCILLIN VK

Penicillin V 250mg

G

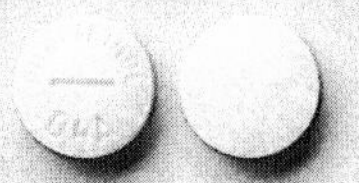

PURINETHOL

Mercaptopurine 50mg

H

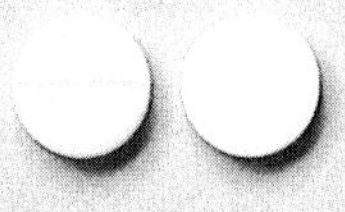

ARTANE

Trihexyphenidyl 5mg

I

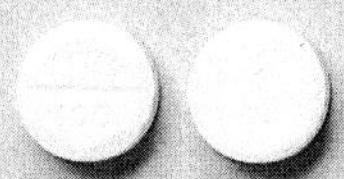

ZYLOPRIM

Allopurinol 100mg

J

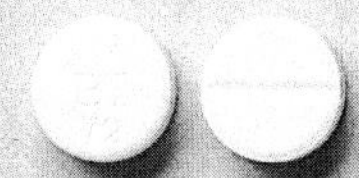

ALUPENT

Metaproterenol 20mg

K

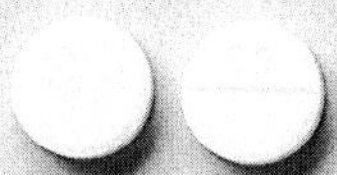

PEN-VEE-K

Penicillin V 250mg

L

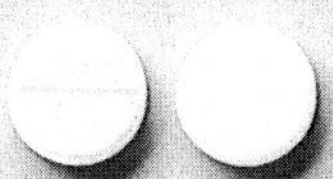

CLOMID

Clomiphene 50mg

M

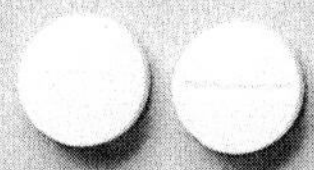

CORTEF

Hydrocortisone 10mg

N

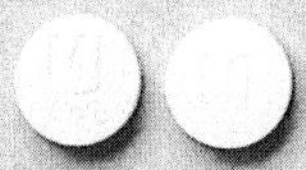

VASODILAN

Isoxsuprine 10mg

O

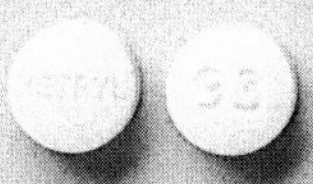

METRYL

Metronidazole 250mg

P

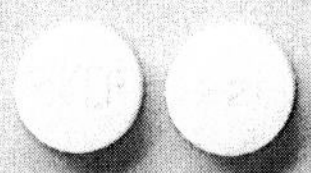

NORFLEX

Orphenadrine 100mg

Q

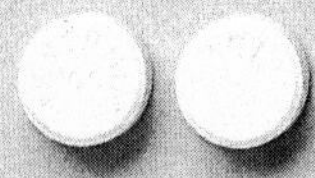

TENORMIN

Atenolol 100mg

R

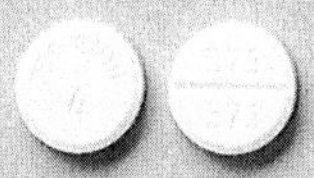

PROVENTIL

Albuterol 4mg

S

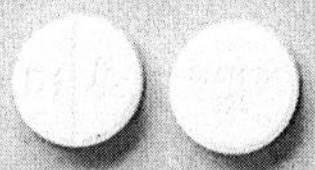

DIAMOX

Acetazolamide 125mg

T

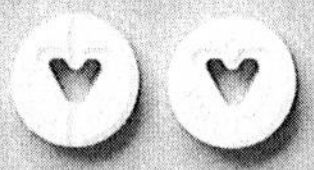

VALIUM

Diazepam 2mg

A

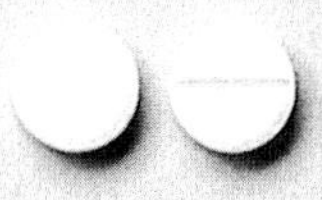

TAPAZOLE

Methimazole 10mg

B

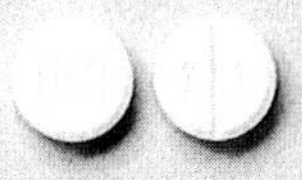

SEROPHENE

Clomiphene 50mg

C

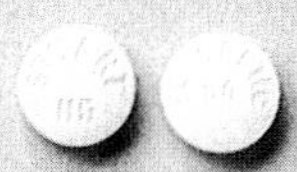

TENORETIC

Atenolol 50mg
Chlorthalidone 25mg

D

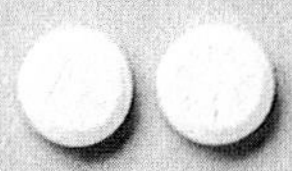

HYDERGINE

Ergoloid mesylates 1mg

E

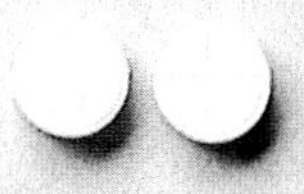

PHENERGAN

Promethazine 25mg

F

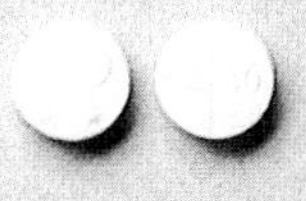

DONNATAL

Phenobarbital 16.2mg with
hyoscyamine, atropine
and scopolamine

G

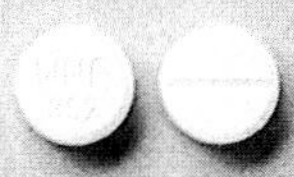

SLO-PHYLLIN

Theophylline 200mg

H

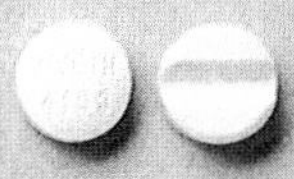

ISORDIL

Isosorbide dinitrate 10mg

I

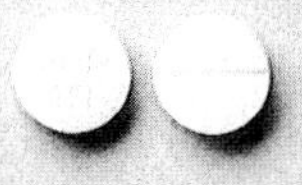

SLO-PHYLLIN

Theophylline 100mg

J

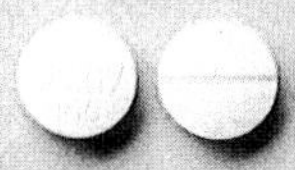

BRETHINE

Terbutaline 5mg

K

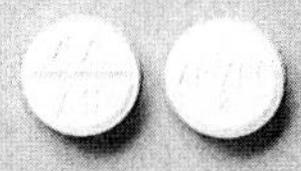

ARTANE

Trihexyphenidyl 2mg

L

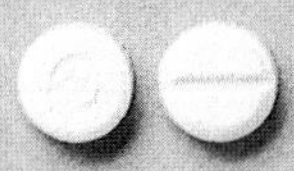

HEXADROL

Dexamethasone 0.75mg

M

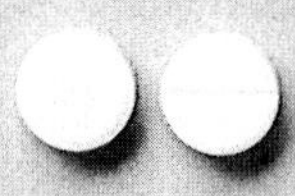

ALUPENT

Metoproterenol 10mg

N

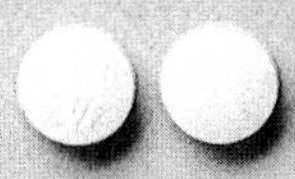

BRICANYL

Terbutaline 2.5mg

O

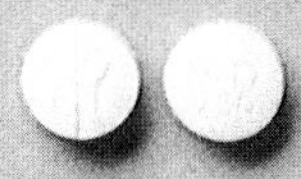

TEDRAL

Theophylline 118mg
Ephedrine 24mg
Phenobarbital 8mg

P

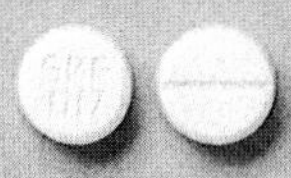

CYTOMEL

Liothyronine 0.05mg

Q

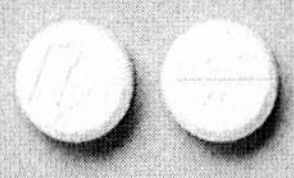

LASIX

Furosemide 40mg

R

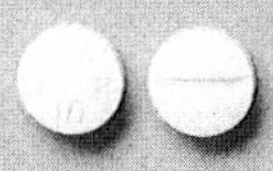

LONITEN

Minoxidil 10mg

S

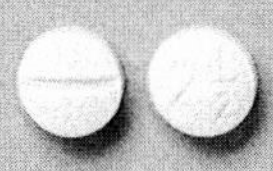

LONITEN

Minoxidil 2.5mg

T

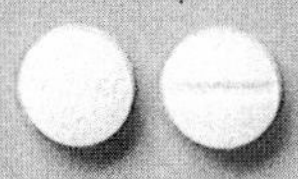

CORTEF

Hydrocortisone 5mg

WHITE TABLETS continued

A

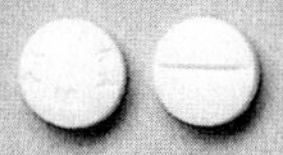

PROVERA

Medroxyprogesterone 10mg

B

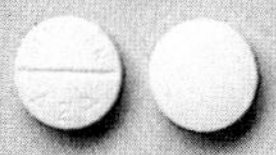

ALKERAN

Melphalan 2mg

C

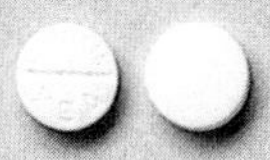

LANOXIN

Digoxin 0.25mg

D

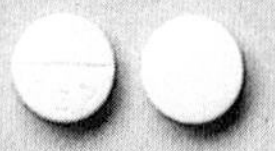

KEMADRIN

Procyclidine 5mg

E

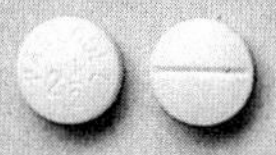

PARLODEL

Bromocriptine 2.5mg

F

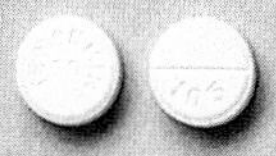

TENORMIN

Atenolol 50mg

G

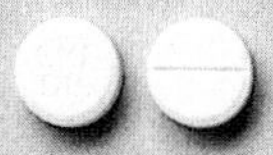

CYTOMEL

Liothyronine 0.025mg

H

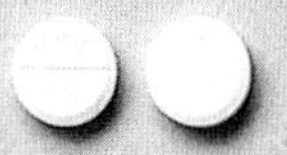

PERIACTIN

Cyproheptadine 4mg

I

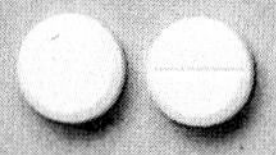

MYSOLINE

Primidone 50mg

J

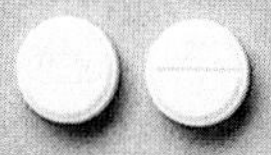

HYGROTON

Chlorthalidone 100mg

K

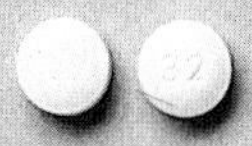

DEMI-REGROTON

Chlorthalidone 25mg
Reserpine 0.125mg

L

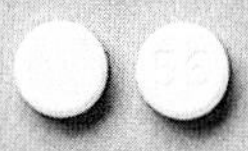

OVRAL

Norgestrel 0.5mg
Ethinyl estradiol 0.05mg

M

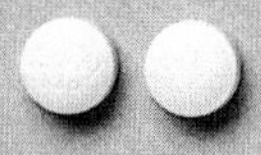

ERGOTRATE MALEATE

Ergonovine 0.2mg

N

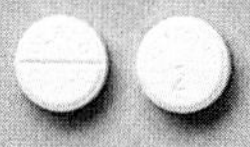

VENTOLIN

Albuterol 2mg

O

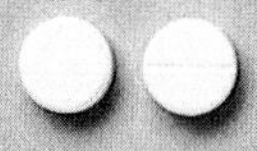

DELTASONE

Prednisolone 5mg

P

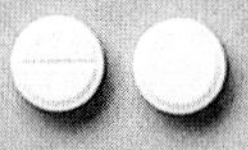

COGENTIN

Benztropine 0.5mg

Q

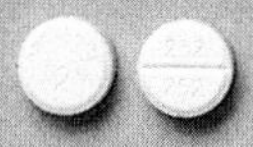

PROVENTIL

Albuterol 2mg

R

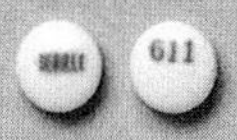

PRO-BANTHINE 7

Propantheline 7.5mg

S

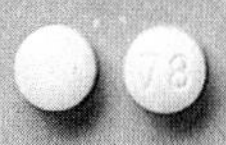

LO/OVRAL

Norgestrel 0.3mg
Ethinyl estradiol 0.03mg

T

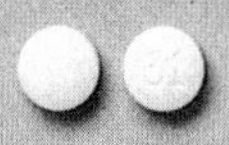

LOMOTIL

Diphenoxylate 2.5mg
Atropine 0.025mg

A

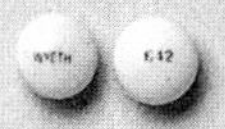

TRIPHASIL

Ethinyl estradiol 0.03mg
Levonorgestrel 0.05mg

B

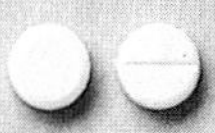

TAPAZOLE

Methimazole 5mg

C

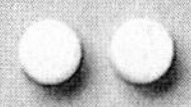

NITROSTAT

Nitroglycerin 0.3mg

D

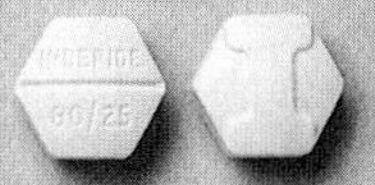

INDERIDE-LA

Propranolol 80mg
Hydrochlorothiazide 50mg

E

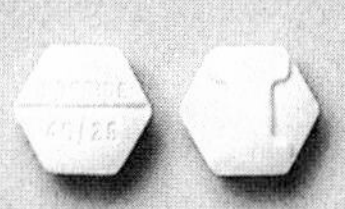

INDERIDE

Propranolol 40mg
Hydrochlorothiazide 25mg

F

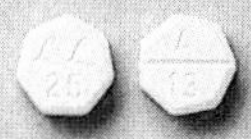

ASENDIN

Amoxapine 25mg

G

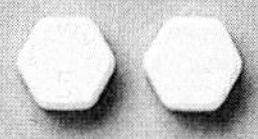

PROVERA

Medroxyprogesterone 5mg

H

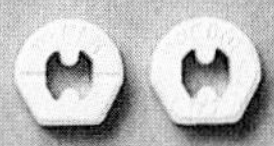

HALDOL

Haloperidol 0.5mg

I

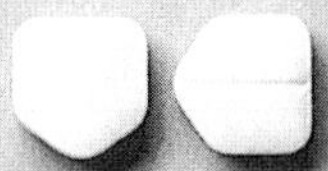

EQUANIL

Meprobamate 200mg

J

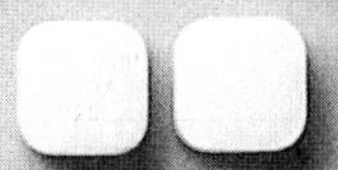

GRISACTIN ULTRA

Griseofulvin 125mg

K

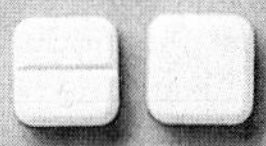

BRICANYL

Terbutaline 5mg

L

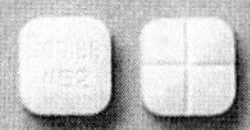

CAPOTEN

Captopril 25mg

M

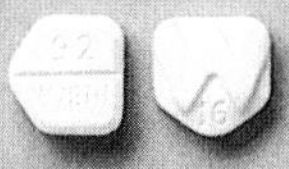

WYTENSIN

Guanabenz 16mg

N

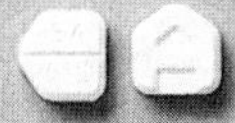

ATIVAN

Lorazepam 1mg

O

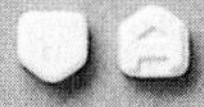

ATIVAN

Lorazepam 0.5mg

P

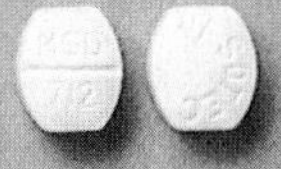

VASOTEC

Enalapril 5mg

Q

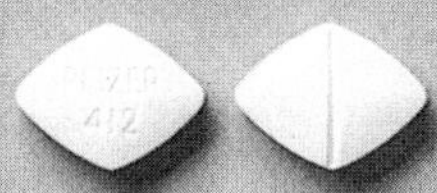

GLUCOTROL

Glipizide 10mg

R

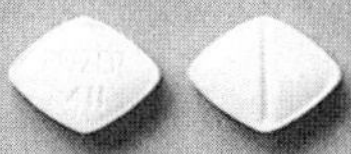

GLUCOTROL

Glipizide 5mg

S

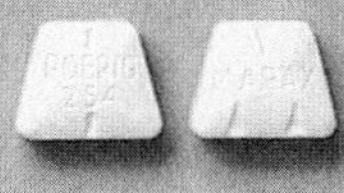

MARAX

Theophylline 130mg
Ephedrine 25mg
Hydroxyzine 10mg

T

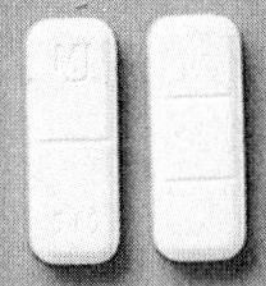

QUIBRON – T SR

Theophylline 300mg

WHITE TABLETS continued

A

DURICEF

Cefadroxil 1g

B

AUGMENTIN

Amoxicillin 500mg
Clavulanate potassium 125mg

C

SMZ-TMP-DS

Sulfamethoxazole 800mg
Trimethoprim 160mg

D

AUGMENTIN

Amoxicillin 250mg
Clavulanate potassium 125mg

E

PENTIDS

Penicillin G 250mg

F

ERYTAB

Erythromycin 333mg

G

V-CILLIN K

Penicillin V 250mg

H

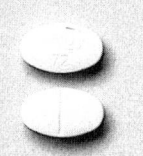

BRETHINE

Terbutaline 2.5mg

I

TRIMPEX

Trimethoprim 100mg

J

THEO-DUR

Theophylline 200mg

K

HYDROCORTONE

Hydrocortisone 20mg

L

HYDROCORTONE

Hydrocortisone 10mg

M

COGENTIN

Benztropine 1mg

N

LIORESAL

Baclofen 10mg

O

HYDERGINE

Ergoloid mesylates 1mg

P

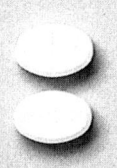

ANAVAR

Oxandrolone 2.5mg

Q

XANAX

Alprazolam 0.25mg

R

MEDROL

Methylprednisolone 4mg

S

LASIX

Furosemide 20mg

T

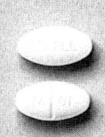

RUFEN

Ibuprofen 600mg

A

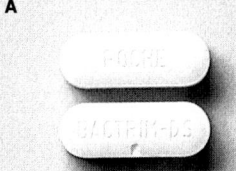

BACTRIM-DS

Sulfamethoxazole 800mg
Trimethoprim 160mg

B

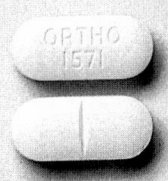

PROTOSTAT

Metronidazole 500mg

C

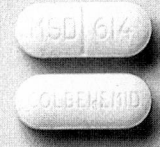

COLBENEMID

Probenecid 0.5mg
Colchicine 0.5mg

D

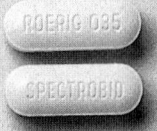

SPECTROBID

Bacampicillin 400mg

E

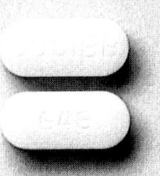

VEETIDS

Penicillin V 500mg

F

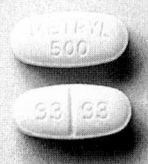

METRYL

Metronidazole 500mg

G

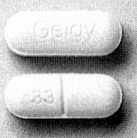

LIORESAL

Baclofen 20mg

H

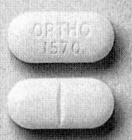

PROTOSTAT

Metronidazole 250mg

I

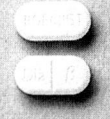

DYMELOR

Acetohexamide 250mg

J

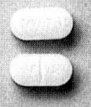

DIABETA

Glyburide 1.25mg

K

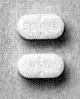

TAVIST-1

Clemastine 1.34mg

L

CAPOTEN

Captopril 12.5mg

ONE-COLOR CAPSULES

A

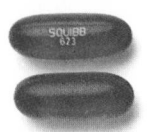

NOCTEC

Chloral hydrate 250mg

B

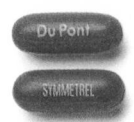

SYMMETREL

Amantadine 100mg

C

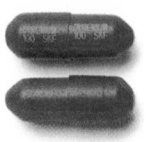

DYRENIUM

Triamterene 100mg

D

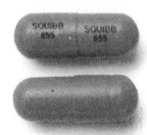

SUMYCIN

Tetracycline 250mg

E

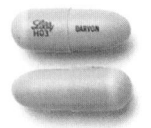

DARVON

Propoxyphene 65mg

F

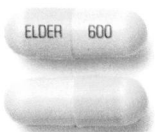

OXSORALEN

Methoxsalen 10mg

G

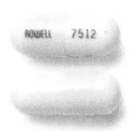

LITHONATE

Lithium carbonate 300mg

H

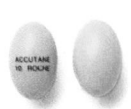

ACCUTANE

Isotretinoin 10mg

I

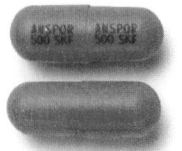

ANSPOR

Cephadrine 500mg

J

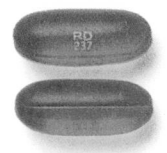

ZARONTIN

Ethosuximide 250mg

K

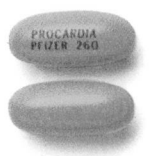

PROCARDIA

Nifedipine 10mg

L

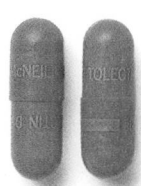

TOLECTIN DS

Tolmetin 400mg

M

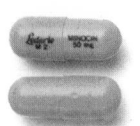

MINOCIN

Minocycline 50mg

N

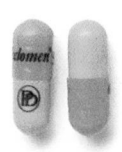

MECLOMEN

Meclofenamate 50mg

O

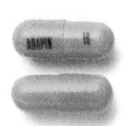

ADAPIN

Doxepin 10mg

P

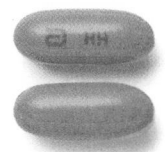

DEPAKENE

Valproic acid 250mg

Q

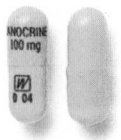

DANOCRINE

Danazol 100mg

R

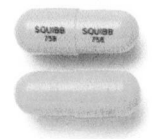

PRONESTYL

Procainamide 250mg

S

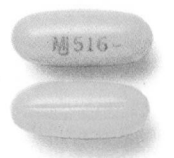

QUIBRON

Theophylline 150mg
Guaifenesin 90mg

T

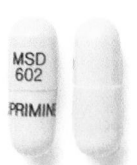

CUPRIMINE

Penicillamine 250mg

A

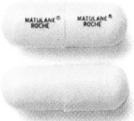

MATULANE

Procarbazine 50mg

B

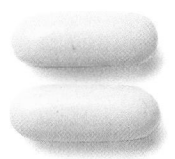

SLO-PHYLLIN GG

Theophylline 150mg
Guaifenesin 90mg

C

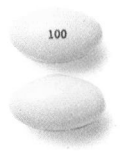

SOMOPHYLLIN T

Theophylline 100mg

D

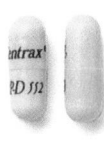

CENTRAX

Prazepam 5mg

E

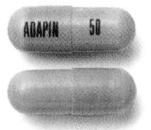

ADAPIN

Doxepin 50mg

F

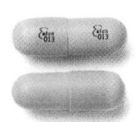

DOPAR

Levodopa 100mg

G

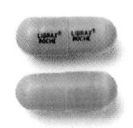

LIBRAX

Chlordiazepoxide 5mg
Clidinium bromide 2.5mg

H

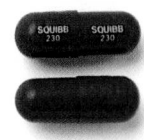

TRIMOX

Amoxicillin 250mg

I

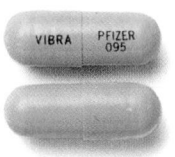

VIBRAMYCIN

Doxycycline 100mg

J

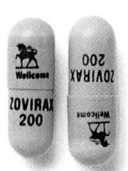

ZOVIRAX

Acyclovir 200mg

K

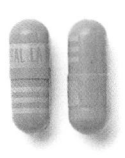

INDERAL-LA

Propranolol 80mg

L

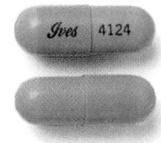

CYCLOSPASMOL

Cyclandelate 200mg

M

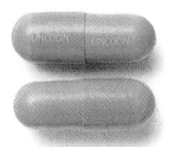

LINCOCIN

Lincomycin 250mg

N

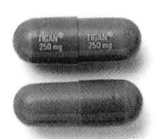

TIGAN

Trimethobenzamide 250mg

O

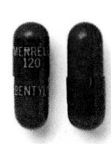

BENTYL

Dicyclomine 10mg

P

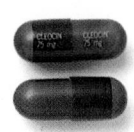

CLEOCIN

Clindamycin 75mg

Q

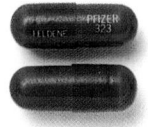

FELDENE

Piroxicam 20mg

R

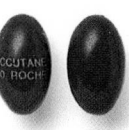

ACCUTANE

Isotretinoin 20mg

S

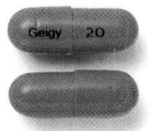

TOFRANIL PM

Imipramine 75mg

T

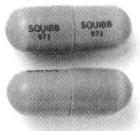

PRINCIPEN

Ampicillin 250mg

MULTICOLOR CAPSULES

A

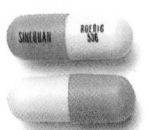

SINEQUAN

Doxepin 50mg

B

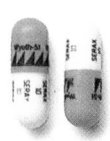

SERAX

Oxazepam 10mg

C

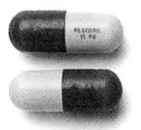

RESTORIL

Temazepam 15mg

D

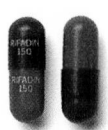

RIFADIN

Rifampin 150mg

E

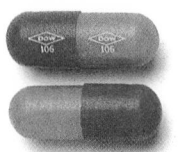

NOVAFED A

Pseudoephedrine 120mg
Chlorpheniramine 8mg

F

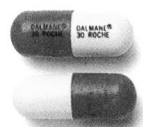

DALMANE

Flurazepam 30mg

G

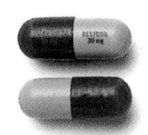

RESTORIL

Temazepam 30mg

H

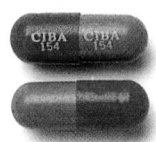

RIMACTANE

Rifampin 300mg

I

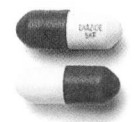

DYAZIDE

Triamterene 50mg
Hydrochlorothiazide 25mg

J

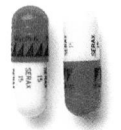

SERAX

Oxazepam 15mg

K

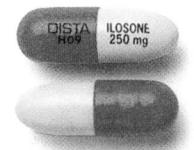

ILOSONE

Erythromycin 250mg

L

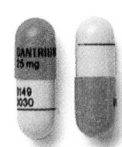

DANTRIUM

Dantrolene 25mg

M

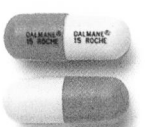

DALMANE

Flurazepam 15mg

N

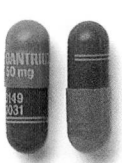

DANTRIUM

Dantrolene 50mg

O

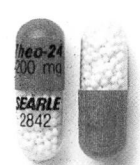

THEO-24

Theophylline 200mg

P

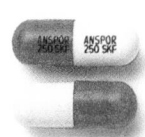

ANSPOR

Cephradine 250mg

Q

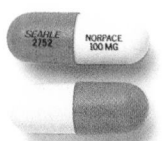

NORPACE

Disopyramide 100mg

R

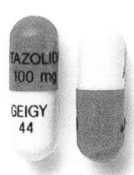

BUTAZOLIDIN

Phenylbutazone 100mg

S

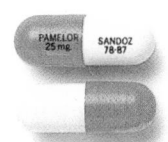

PAMELOR

Nortriptyline 25mg

T

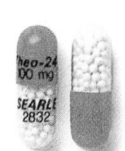

THEO-24

Theophylline 100mg

A

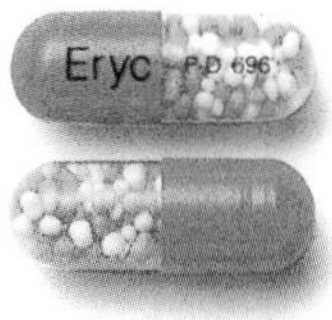

ERYC

Erythromycin 250mg

B

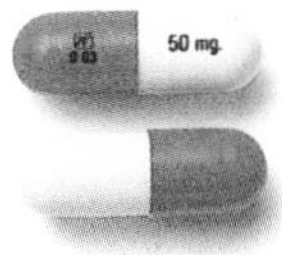

DANOCRINE

Danazol 50mg

C

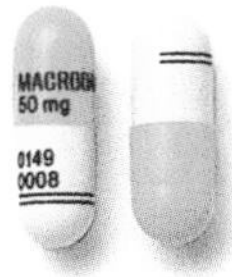

MACRODANTIN

Nitrofurantoin 50mg

D

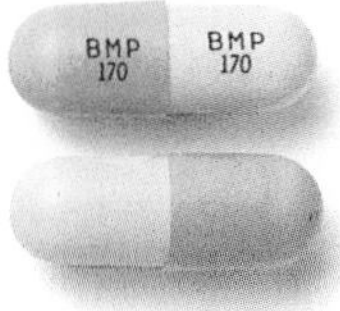

CLOXAPEN

Cloxacillin 500mg

E

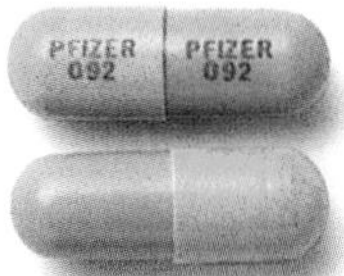

UROBIOTIC

Oxytetracycline 250mg
Sulfamethizole 250mg
Phenazopyridine 50mg

F

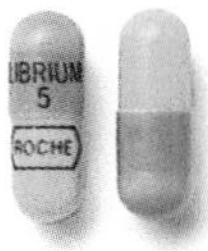

LIBRIUM

Chlordiazepoxide 5mg

G

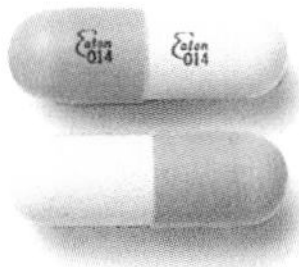

DOPAR

Levodopa 250mg

H

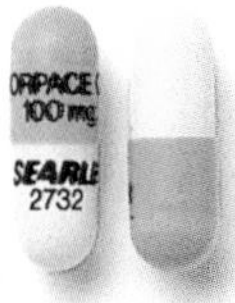

NORPACE CR

Disopyramide 100mg

I

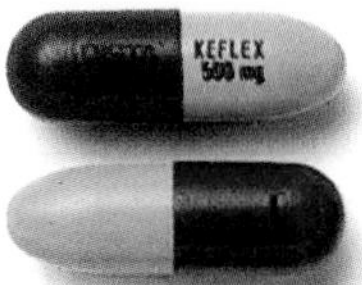

KEFLEX

Cephalexin 500mg

J

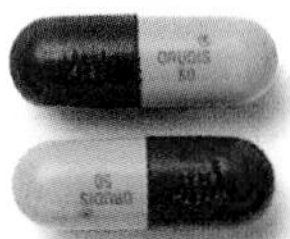

ORUDIS

Ketoprofen 50mg

K

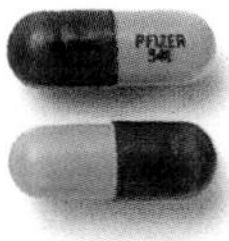

VISTARIL

Hydroxyzine 25mg

L

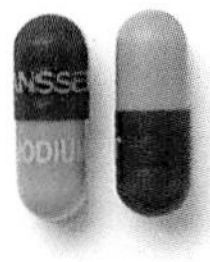

IMODIUM

Loperamide 2mg

M

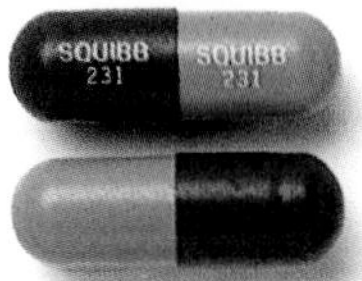

TRIMOX

Amoxicillin 500mg

N

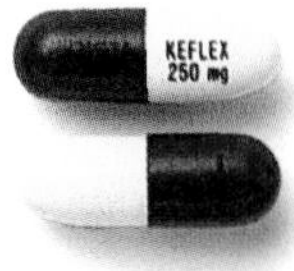

KEFLEX

Cephalexin 250mg

O

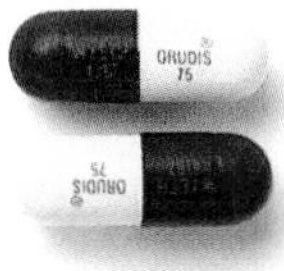

ORUDIS

Ketoprofen 75mg

P

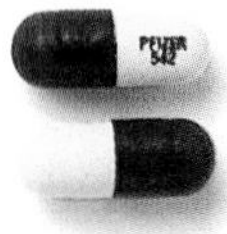

VISTARIL

Hydroxyzine 50mg

Q

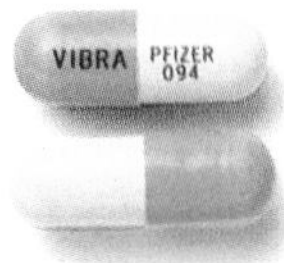

VIBRAMYCIN

Doxycycline 50mg

R

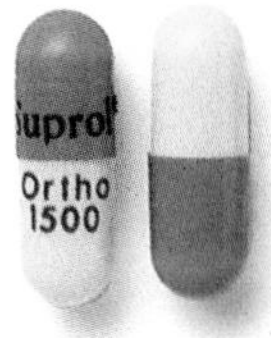

SUPROL

Suprofen 200mg
(withdrawn 1987)

S

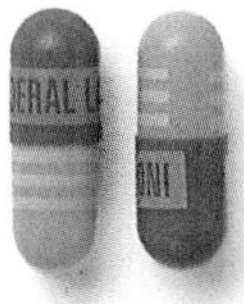

INDERAL–LA

Propranolol 120mg

T

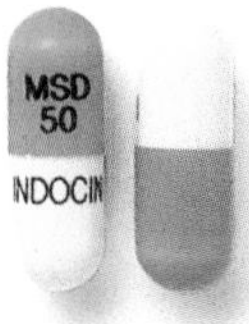

INDOCIN

Indomethacin 50mg

MULTICOLOR CAPSULES continued

A

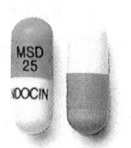

INDOCIN

Indomethacin 25mg

B

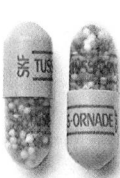

TUSS-ORNADE

Phenylpropanolamine 75mg
Caramiphen 40mg

C

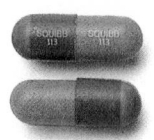

VELOSEF

Cephradine 250mg

D

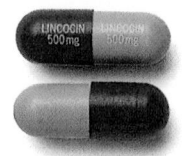

LINCOCIN

Lincomycin 500mg

E

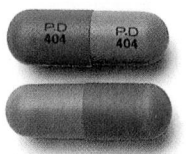

AMCILL

Ampicillin 500mg

F

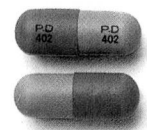

AMCILL

Ampicillin 250mg

G

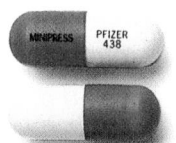

MINIPRESS

Prazosin 5mg

H

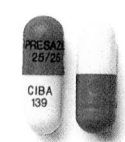

APRESAZIDE

Hydrazaline 25mg
Hydrochlorothiazide 25mg

I

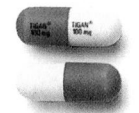

TIGAN

Trimethobenzamide 100mg

J

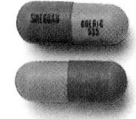

SINEQUAN

Doxepin 25mg

K

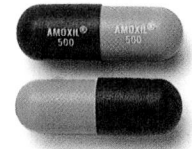

AMOXIL

Amoxicillin 500mg

L

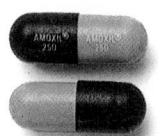

AMOXIL

Amoxicillin 250mg

M

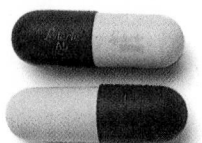

ACHROMYCIN V

Tetracycline 500mg

N

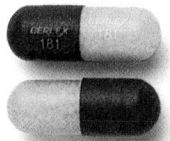

DECONAMINE SR

Pseudoephedrine 60mg
Chlorpheniramine 4mg

O

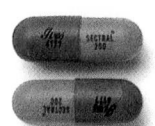

SECTRAL

Acebutolol 200mg

P

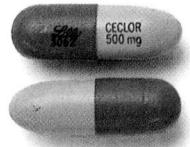

CECLOR

Cefaclor 500mg

Q

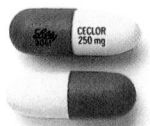

CECLOR

Cefaclor 250mg

R

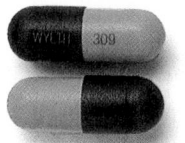

OMNIPEN

Ampicillin 500mg

S

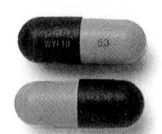

OMNIPEN

Ampicillin 250mg

T

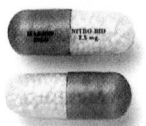

NITRO-BID

Nitroglycerin 2.5mg

A

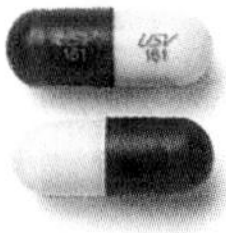

PERTOFRANE

Desipramine 50mg

B

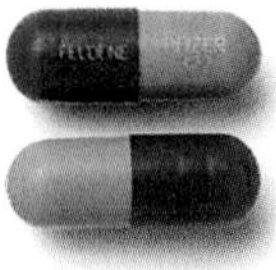

FELDENE

Piroxicam 10mg

C

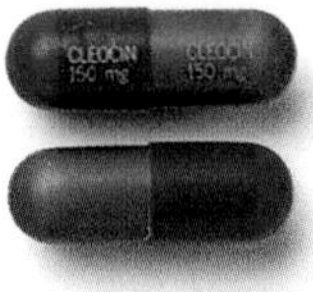

CLEOCIN

Clindamycin 150mg

D

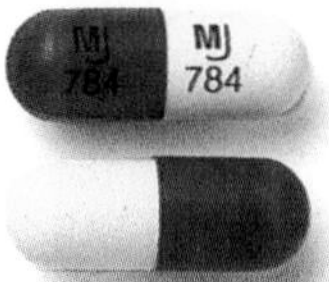

DURICEF

Cefadroxil 500mg

E

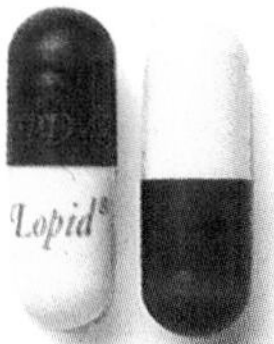

LOPID

Gemfibrozil 300mg

F

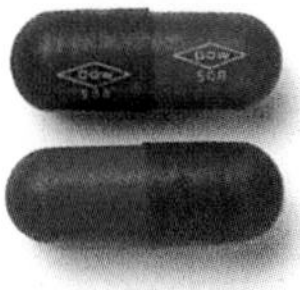

RIFADIN

Rifampin 300mg

G

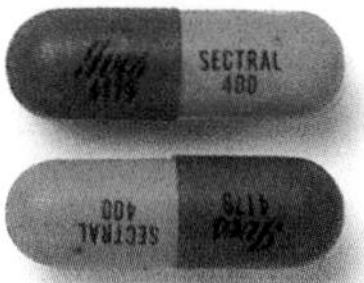

SECTRAL

Acebutolol 400mg

H

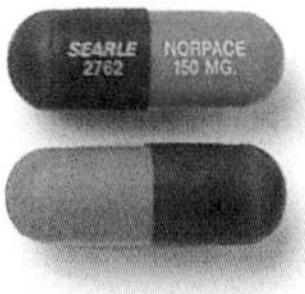

NORPACE

Disopyramide 150mg

I

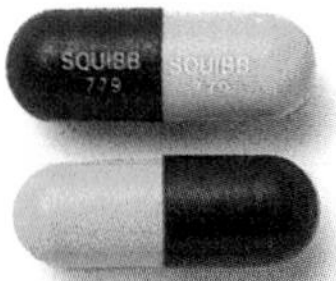

MYSTECLIN-F

Tetracycline 250mg
Amphotericin B 50mg

J

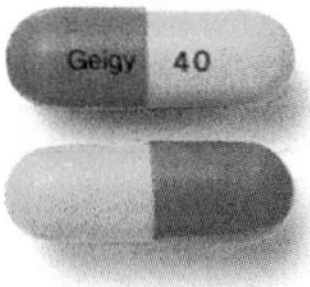

TOFRANIL PM

Imipramine 100mg

K

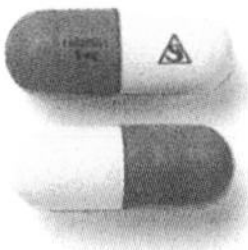

PARLODEL

Bromocriptine 5mg

L

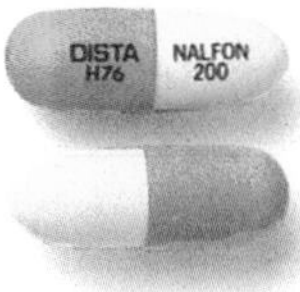

NALFON

Fenoprofen 200mg

M

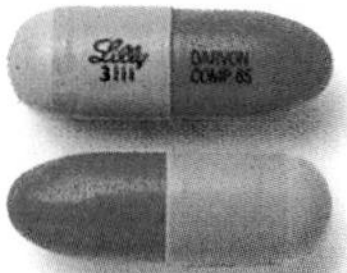

DARVON COMPOUND – 65

Aspirin 389mg
Propoxyphene 65mg
Caffeine 32.4mg

N

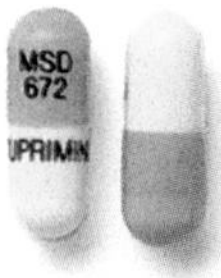

CUPRIMINE

Penicillamine 125mg

O

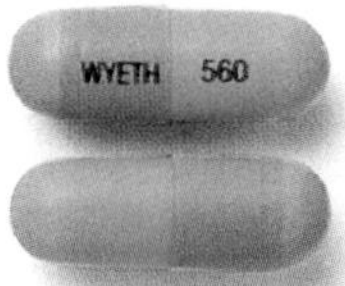

WYMOX

Amoxicillin 500mg

P

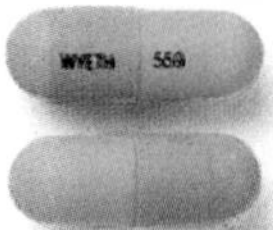

WYMOX

Amoxicillin 250mg

Q

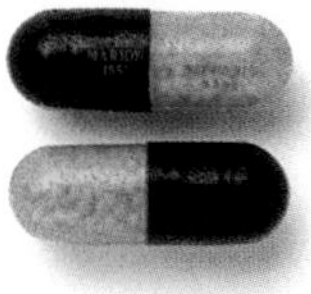

NITRO-BID

Nitroglycerin 6.5mg

R

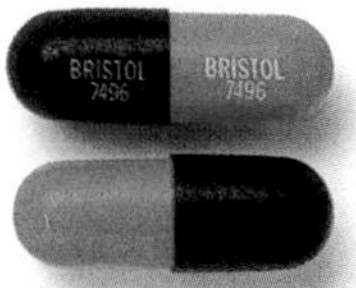

TEGOPEN

Cloxacillin 500mg

S

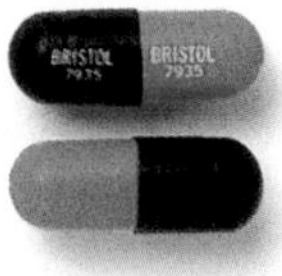

TEGOPEN

Cloxacillin 250mg

T

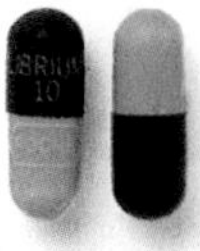

LIBRIUM

Chlordiazepoxide 10mg

MULTICOLOR CAPSULES continued

A

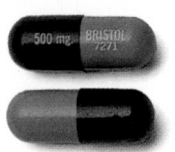

ULTRACEF
Cefadroxil 500mg

E

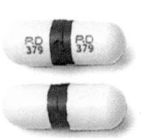

CHLOROMYCETIN
Chloramphenicol 250mg

B

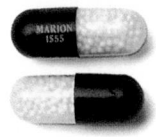

PAVABID
Papaverine 150mg

C

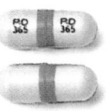

DILANTIN
Phenytoin 30mg

D

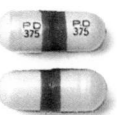

DILANTIN WITH PHENOBARBITAL

Phenytoin 100mg
Phenobarbital 16mg

WHITE CAPSULES

A

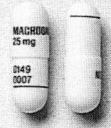

MACRODANTIN

Nitrofurantoin 25mg

B

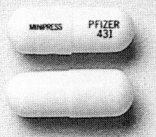

MINIPRESS

Prazosin 1mg

C

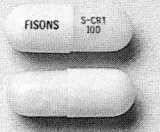

SOMOPHYLLIN CRT

Theophylline 100mg

D

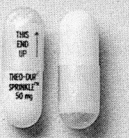

THEO-DUR SPRINKLE

Theophylline 50mg

E

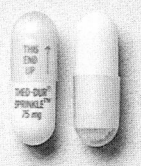

THEO-DUR SPRINKLE

Theophylline 75mg

F

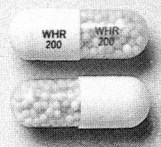

SLO-BID R

Theophylline 200mg

G

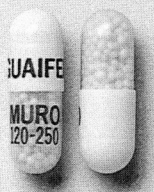

GUAIFED

Guaifenisin 250mg
Pseudoephedrine 120mg

INDEX OF GENERIC AND BRAND-NAME DRUGS

This index contains the names of approximately 2,500 individual drug products and substances. It provides the entry point to the book for readers who are interested in learning about a specific drug or medication. There is no need for you to know before using this index whether the name you want to look up is a brand name or a generic name, or whether it is a prescription or over-the-counter drug; all types of drugs are listed.

What the index contains

The drugs listed include all major generic drugs and many less widely used substances. A broad range of brand names is also included. The index contains, in addition, the names of vitamins and minerals that may be prescribed medically. This comprehensive selection of drugs is designed to reflect the wide diversity of products available for the treatment and prevention of disease. It does not imply AMA endorsement of any of the drugs or products listed, nor does the exclusion of a particular product from the index indicate AMA disapproval.

How the entries are ordered

All entries are listed in alphabetical order, regardless of whether the substance is a generic or brand name. Brand-name products can be distinguished by their initial capital letter.

How the references work

References are either to the pages in Part 4 containing the drug profiles of each principal generic ingredient, or to the section in Part 3 that describes the relevant drug group. Some entries for generic drugs that have not been given a full-page profile contain a brief description. Where an entry for a brand-name product gives the name of a drug but no page number, go to the entry for that drug within this index, which will then direct you to further information as appropriate.

Color Identification Guide

Brand-name tablets and capsules that are pictured in the Color Identification Guide contain a reference in italic type to the page and grid letter where the photograph of that product may be found.

A

Accubron see theophylline 506

Accutane *56H, 57R* (illus.); see isotretinoin 370

acebutolol 214

acecainide an anti-arrhythmic drug 128

aceclidine a *miotic* drug used in the treatment of glaucoma. See Drugs for glaucoma 196

acetaminophen 215

acetazolamide 216

acetic acid the acid found in vinegar. Used medically to inhibit infection in the vagina

acetohexamide 217

acetophenazine a phenothiazine antipsychotic drug 113

acetylcholine a chemical *neurotransmitter* that stimulates the parasympathetic nervous system (107). Used as a *miotic* drug. See Drugs affecting the pupil 198

acetylcysteine 218

Achromycin *60M* (illus.); see tetracycline 504

acid mantle cream a non-greasy oil-in-water preparation used to relieve dry skin conditions

aclarubicin an *investigational* anticancer drug 182

acrisorcin an antifungal drug used in the treatment of tinea versicolor. See Antifungal drugs 166

A

acrivastine a non-sedative antihistamine drug. See Antihistamines 152

Actagen a combined preparation. See pseudoephedrine (472) and triprolidine (527)

ACTH adrenocorticotropic hormone. See corticotropin

Acthar see corticotropin

Acticort see hydrocortisone 358

Actidil see triprolidine 527

Actifed a combined preparation. See pseudoephedrine (472) and triprolidine (527)

Activase see TPA 511

acyclovir 219

Adalat see nifedipine 425

Adapettes an artificial tear preparation 198

Adapin *56 O, 57E* (illus.); see doxepin 322

Adeflor a multivitamin preparation with fluoride. See Vitamins 177

Adipex-P see phentermine

Adrenalin see epinephrine 328

adrenocorticotropic hormone see corticotropin

Adriamycin see doxorubicin 323

Adrucil see fluorouracil 341

Adsorbocarpine see pilocarpine 451

Advil *45L* (illus.); see ibuprofen 360

AeroBid see flunisolide

Aerolate see theophylline 506

Aerolone see isoproterenol 368

A

Aeroseb-Dex see dexamethasone 306

Aerosporin see polymyxin B

Afrin see oxymetazoline 434

Afrinol see pseudoephedrine 472

Agoral a laxative preparation containing mineral oil and phenolphthalein. See Laxatives 139

Akarpine see pilocarpine 451

AK-Cide a combined preparation. See prednisolone (456) and sulfacetamide (491)

AK-Dilate see phenylephrine 447

Akne-Mycin see erythromycin 331

AK-Neo-Cort a combined preparation. See hydrocortisone (358) and neomycin (421)

AK-Pred see prednisolone 456

AK-Sulf see sulfacetamide 491

AK-Sulf Forte see sulfacetamide 491

AK-Tate see prednisolone 456

AK-Tracin see bacitracin 243

AK-Trol see dexamethasone 306

AK-Zol see acetazolamide 216

Alatone see spironolactone 487

Albalon-A a combined preparation. See naphazoline (419) and antazoline

Albalon Liquifilm see naphazoline 419

albuterol 220

alcohol, rubbing ethyl alcohol. Used as a *rubefacient* and as a skin antiseptic. See Anti-infective skin preparations 203

Alconefrin see phenylephrine 447

Aldactazide *46K* (illus.); a combined preparation. See hydrochlorothiazide (357) and spironolactone (487)

Aldactone *40B, 46J* (illus.); see spironolactone 487

Aldoclor a combined preparation. See chlorothiazide (273) and methyldopa (405)

Aldomet *40E, 40F* (illus.); see methyldopa 405

Aldoril *45Q, 45R, 49D* (illus.); a combined preparation. See hydrochlorothiazide (357) and methyldopa (405)

alfacalcidol a vitamin D drug. See Vitamin D 545

Algicon a combined preparation. See aluminum hydroxide 224

Alka-Mints see calcium carbonate

Alka-Seltzer a combined preparation. See aspirin (238), sodium bicarbonate (486), and citric acid (557)

Alkeran *52B* (illus.); see melphalan 394

allantoin a uric acid derivative. Applied *topically,* is said to encourage healing of minor wounds

Allbee C-800 a multivitamin preparation. See Vitamins 177

Allbee with C a multivitamin preparation. See Vitamins 177

Aller-Chlor see chlorpheniramine 274

Allerest a combined preparation. See chlorpheniramine (274), naphazoline (419), and phenylpropanolamine (448)

Allerfrin see triprolidine 527

A

Allergen Ear Drops a combined preparation. See benzocaine (247), antipyrine, glycerin, and oxyquinoline

Allersone a combined preparation. See hydrocortisone (358), diperodon, and zinc oxide

allopurinol 221

Alphaderm see hydrocortisone 358

Alpha Keri a mineral oil and lanolin bath additive for dry, itchy skin. See Antipruritic medications 201

alphaprodine a narcotic analgesic 108

AlphaRedisol see hydroxocobalamin

alpha-tocopherol a form of vitamin E 545

Alphatrex see betamethasone 250

Alphosyl see coal tar

alprazolam 222

alprostadil 223

alseroxylon an antihypertensive drug 130

AlternaGel see aluminum hydroxide 224

altretamine an *investigational* anticancer drug 182

Alu-Cap see aluminum hydroxide 224

aluminum acetate an *astringent* substance applied to soothe inflammation of the skin or outer ear

aluminum carbonate a drug used to reduce phosphate levels in the blood and occasionally used as an antacid. See Antacids 136

aluminum chloride an *antiperspirant*

aluminum hydroxide 224

Alupent *50J, 51M* (illus.); a combined preparation. See metaproterenol 399

Alurate see aprobarbital

Alu-Tab see aluminum hydroxide 224

amantadine 225

ambenonium a drug used to treat myasthenia gravis 149

Ambenyl a combined preparation. See codeine (291) and bromodiphenhydramine

Amcill *60E, 60F* (illus.); see ampicillin 236

amcinonide a corticosteroid used in *topical* preparations. See Topical corticosteroids 202

amdinocillin a penicillin antibiotic. See Antibiotics 156

Amen *47E* (illus.); see medroxyprogesterone 391

Americaine see benzocaine 247

Amicar *48C* (illus.); see aminocaproic acid 227

amikacin an aminoglycoside antibiotic 156

Amikin see amikacin

amiloride a potassium-sparing diuretic 127

aminacrine an *antiseptic* dye used in *topical* preparations. See Anti-infective skin preparations 203

aminoacetic acid a substance occasionally used as an antacid 136

aminocaproic acid 227

aminoglutethimide 228

aminophylline 229

aminosalicylate sodium see aminosalicylic acid

aminosalicylic acid 230

AMINOTHIADIAZOLE – BENDYLATE

A

aminothiadiazole an *investigational* anticancer drug 182

amiodarone 231

Amitril see amitriptyline 232

amitriptyline 232

ammoniated mercury an agent used in treatment of skin conditions such as impetigo and dermatitis

ammonium chloride a drug used to increase the acidity of urine and to speed the excretion of certain poisons in the urine

amobarbital a barbiturate sleeping drug 110

amodiaquine an antimalarial drug not available in the US. See Antimalarial drugs 165

amoxapine 233

amoxicillin 234

Amoxil *60K, 60L* (illus.); see amoxicillin 234

amphetamine 549

Amphojel see aluminum hydroxide 224

amphotericin B 235

ampicillin 236

amrinone a drug used in the treatment of congestive heart failure

amsacrine an *investigational* anticancer drug 182

amyl nitrite a vasodilator drug formerly used in the treatment of angina, now considered a drug of abuse. See Nitrites 553

Amytal see amobarbital

Anacin a combined preparation. See aspirin (238) and caffeine

Anacin 3 see acetaminophen 215

Anadrol-50 see oxymetholone

anagrelide an *investigational* antiplatelet drug. See Drugs that affect blood clotting 132

Anamine a combined preparation. See chlorpheniramine (274) and pseudoephedrine (472)

Anaprox *44 I* (illus.); see naproxen 420

Anaspaz see hyoscyamine

Anatuss a combined preparation. See acetaminophen (215), chlorpheniramine (274), dextromethorphan (307), phenylephrine (447), phenylpropanolamine (448), and guaifenesin

Anavar *54P* (illus.); see oxandrolone 431

Anbesol see benzocaine 247

Ancef see cefazolin 262

Android see methyltestosterone

Anectine see succinylcholine

Anergan see promethazine 468

Anestacon see lidocaine 378

Anexsia-D a combined preparation. See aspirin (238) and hydrocodone

Anhydron see cyclothiazide

anisindione an anticoagulant drug. See Drugs that affect blood clotting 132

anistropine an *anticholinergic, antispasmodic* drug used to relieve irritable bowel syndrome 138

Anorex see phendimetrazine

A

ansamycin an *investigational* antibacterial drug related to rifampin 482

Anspor *56 I, 58P* (illus.); see cephradine

Antabuse see disulfiram 321

antazoline a decongestant 121

Anthra-Derm see anthralin 237

anthralin 237

Antiminth see pyrantel 474

antipyrine an analgesic drug used in ear drops for outer ear inflammation. See Analgesics 108

Antispas dicyclomine 310

Antivert *47D, 47F* (illus.); see meclizine 389

Anturane *50E* (illus.); see sulfinpyrazone 494

Anuject a combined preparation. See procaine (463) and isobutylbenzoate

Anusol cream and suppositories containing benzyl benzoate, zinc oxide, and other ingredients for the relief of anal irritation. See Drugs for rectal and anal disorders 141

Apap see acetaminophen 215

A.P.L. see HCG 355

Apresazide *60H* (illus.); a combined preparation. See hydralazine (356) and hydrochlorothiazide (357)

Apresoline *43K, 44B* (illus.); see hydralazine 356

Apresoline with Esidrix *37S* (illus.); a combined preparation. See hydralazine (356) and hydrochlorothiazide (357)

aprobarbital a barbiturate sleeping drug 110

Aquacare HP moisturizing cream or lotion containing urea for dry skin conditions

Aquamephyton see phytonadione 450

Aquasol A see vitamin A 543

Aquatag see benzthiazide

Aquatar see coal tar

Aquatensen see methyclothiazide

arachis oil refined peanut oil applied *topically* to treat scaly skin conditions

Aralen *35F* (illus.); see chloroquine 272

Aralen Phosphate with Primaquine Phosphate a combined preparation. See chloroquine (272) and primaquine (458)

Aramine see metaraminol

Arfonad see trimethaphan

Aristocort, Aristocort Forte see triamcinolone 519

Aristospan see triamcinolone 519

Arlidin see nylidrin

Armour Thyroid see thyroid 509

arnica a herbal preparation used to treat bruising. Widely employed in homeopathic medicine

Artane *50H, 51K* (illus.); see trihexyphenidyl 523

artemisinine an *investigational* antimalarial drug not available in the US 165

Arthropan see choline salicylate

A.S.A. see aspirin 238

Asbron a combined preparation. See theophylline (506) and guaifenesin

A

ascorbic acid see vitamin C 544. See also A–Z of additives 556

Ascriptin a combined preparation. See aluminum hydroxide (224) and codeine (291)

Asendin *38R, 53F* (illus.); see amoxapine 233

asparaginase a drug used to treat leukemia. See Anticancer drugs 182

Aspercreme lotion or cream containing tolamine salicylate for relief of minor aches and pains

Aspergum preparation containing aspirin 238

aspirin 238

astemizole an antihistamine 152

Atabrine *40N* (illus.); see quinacrine 478

Atarax *37B* (illus.); see hydroxyzine 359

atenolol 239

Ativan *53N, 53 O* (illus.); see lorazepam 384

atracurium a drug used in surgical procedures to induce muscle relaxation. See Muscle-relaxant drugs 148

Atromid-S see clofibrate 284

atropine an *anticholinergic* drug related to belladonna (246). Used in eye drops to dilate the pupil (198) and as *premedication* to dry secretions. It can also be inhaled as a bronchodilator (120)

A/T/S see erythromycin 331

Attenuvax measles vaccine. See Vaccines and immunization 162

Augmentin *54B, 54D* (illus.); a combined preparation. See amoxicillin (234) and potassium clavulanate

Auralgan a combined preparation. See benzocaine (247) and antipyrine

auranofin 240

Aureomycin see chlortetracycline

aurothioglucose a gold-based antirheumatic drug 145

Aventyl see nortriptyline

Axotal a combined preparation. See aspirin (238) and butalbital

Aygestin see norethindrone

azacitidine an anticancer drug 182

azatadine 241

azathioprine 242

azidothymidine see zidovudine 533

azlocillin a penicillin antibiotic 156

Azmacort see triamcinolone 519

Azo Gantanol *45 I* (illus.); a combined preparation. See phenazopyridine (443) and sulfisoxazole (495)

Azo Gantrisin a combined preparation. See phenazopyridine (443) and sulfamethoxazole (492)

Azolid *39M* (illus.); see phenylbutazone 446

Azo-Sulfisoxazole a combined preparation. See phenazopyridine (443) and sulfisoxazole (495)

AZT see zidovudine 533

aztreonam an *investigational* antibiotic 156

Azulfidine, Azulfidine EN-tabs *38N* (illus.); see sulfasalazine 493

B

B&O Supprettes a combined preparation. See belladonna (246) and opium

bacampicillin a penicillin antibiotic 156

Bacarate see phendimetrazine

Baciguent see bacitracin 243

bacitracin 243

baclofen 244

Bactine a combined preparation. See benzalkonium chloride and lidocaine

Bactocill see oxacillin

Bactrim *42J* (illus.); a combined preparation. See sulfamethoxazole (492) and trimethoprim (526)

Bactrim DS *55A* (illus.); a combined preparation. See sulfamethoxazole (492) and trimethoprim (526)

Balmex ointment a combined preparation. See bismuth and zinc oxide

Balneol cleansing lotion for the anogenital area

Balnetar see coal tar

Bancap HC a combined preparation. See acetaminophen (215) and hydrocodone

Banflex see orphenadrine 430

Banthine see methantheline

Baratol see indoramin

Barbidonna a combined preparation. See phenobarbital (445), atropine, hyoscyamine, and scopolamine

Barbita see phenobarbital 445

Basaljel see aluminum hydroxide 224

Bayer 205 see suramin

beclomethasone 245

Beclovent see beclomethasone 245

Beconase see beclomethasone 245

Beepen-VK see penicillin V 440

Belap a combined preparation. See belladonna (246) and phenobarbital (445)

Belganyl see suramin

Belladenal a combined preparation. See belladonna (246) and phenobarbital (445)

belladonna 246

bellafoline see belladonna 246

Bellergal a combined preparation. See belladonna (246), ergotamine (330), and phenobarbital (445)

Bellergal-S *46F, 47 O* (illus.); a combined preparation. See belladonna (246), ergotamine (330), and phenobarbital (445)

Beminal-500 a multivitamin preparation. See Vitamins 177

Benacen see probenecid 460

benactyzine an *anticholinergic* drug used to relieve anxiety. See Anti-anxiety drugs 111

Benadryl see diphenhydramine 317

bendroflumethiazide a thiazide diuretic 127

Bendylate see diphenhydramine 317

BENEMID – CALCIUM CARBONATE

B

Benemid *41 I* (illus.); see probenecid 460

Ben Gay a *topical* preparation containing methyl salicylate and menthol used for the relief of joint and muscle pain

Benisone see betamethasone 250

Benoquin see monobenzone

benoxaprofen a non-steroidal anti-inflammatory drug withdrawn from use in the US in 1982

benoxinate a local anesthetic 108

Benoxyl see benzoyl peroxide 248

Bentyl *57 O* (illus.); see dicyclomine 310

Bentyl with Phenobarbital a combined preparation. See dicyclomine (310) and phenobarbital (445)

Benylin see diphenhydramine 317

Benylin DM see dextromethorphan 307

Benylin DME a combined preparation. See dextromethorphan (307) and guaifenesin

Benzac W see benzoyl peroxide 248

Benzagel see benzoyl peroxide 248

benzalkonium chloride a skin *antiseptic*. See Anti-infective skin preparations 203

Benzamycin a combined preparation. See benzoyl peroxide (248) and erythromycin (331)

benzathine penicillin G see penicillin G 439

Benzedrex see propylhexedrine

benznidazole a drug used in the treatment of trypanosomiasis. See Antiprotozoal drugs 164

benzocaine 247

benzoic acid a *topical* antifungal drug 166

benzoin tincture an aromatic resin added to steam inhalations for the treatment of sinusitis and nasal congestion. See Decongestants 121

benzonatate a cough suppressant. See Drugs to treat coughs 122

benzoyl peroxide 248

benzphetamine a drug related to the amphetamines used as an appetite- suppressant. See Nervous system stimulants 116

benzquinamide an anti-emetic drug 118

benzthiazide a thiazide diuretic 127

benztropine 249

benzyl alcohol a local anesthetic for *topical* application. See Local anesthetics 108

benzyl benzoate an antiparasitic agent used to treat scabies. See Drugs to treat skin parasites 204

benzylpenicillin see penicillin G 439

bephenium an anthelmintic drug 167

Berocca C, Berocca-PN a multivitamin preparation. See Vitamins 177

Berotec see fenoterol

Berubigen see vitamin B$_{12}$ 544

Besta a vitamin preparation. See Vitamins 177

beta carotene see vitamin A 543

Betadine see povidone-iodine

Betagan see levobunolol

B

betahistine a *vasodilator* drug used in the treatment of Ménière's disease. See Vertigo and Ménière's disease 118

Betalin S see thiamine 543

Betalin 12 see vitamin B$_{12}$ 544

betamethasone 250

Betapen-VK see penicillin V 440

Betatrex see betamethasone 250

Beta-Val see betamethasone 250

betaxolol a beta blocker (125) used in the treatment of glaucoma. See Drugs for glaucoma 196

bethanechol a *parasympathomimetic* drug used to treat urinary retention. See Drugs used for urinary disorders 194

Betoptic see betaxolol

bevantolol a beta blocker 125

bezafibrate a lipid-lowering drug 131

bichloracetic acid an antiviral agent used to treat warts

Bicillin, Bicillin L-A see penicillin G 439

Bicillin C-R a combined preparation. See penicillin G (439) and procaine (463)

BiCNU see carmustine

Bi-K see potassium 540

Bilarcil see metrifonate

bile salts substances derived from bile, sometimes included in combination preparations for the treatment of digestive disorders

Biltricide see praziquantel 454

Biopar Forte a combined preparation. See vitamin B$_{12}$ (544) and intrinsic factor

biotin 535

biperiden an *anticholinergic* drug used in Parkinson's disease. See Antiparkinsonism drugs 115

Biphetamine a combined preparation. See amphetamine (549) and dextroamphetamine

bisacodyl 251

bismuth a metal whose salts are used to treat inflammatory diseases of the stomach and bowel. See Antidiarrheal drugs (138) and Drugs for rectal and anal disorders (141)

Bithin see bithionol

bithionol an anthelmintic drug 167

bitolterol a *sympathomimetic* bronchodilator 120

Blenoxane see bleomycin

bleomycin an antibiotic anticancer drug 182

Blephamide, Blephamide S.O.P. a combined preparation. See prednisolone (456), sulfacetamide (491), and benzalkonium chloride

Bleph-10 Liquifilm see sulfacetamide 491

Bleph-10 S.O.P. see sulfacetamide 491

Blocadren *43H, 43 I* (illus.); see timolol 510

Bluboro an *astringent* soaking solution. See aluminum sulfate and calcium acetate

Bonine *37R* (illus.); see meclizine 389

Bontril see phendimetrazine

B

boric acid a skin and eye antiseptic now rarely used because of risk of excessive absorption through the skin

Borofax a combined preparation. See boric acid and lanolin

BranchAmin an amino acid solution used in the treatment of liver disorders

Brasivol see aluminum hydroxide 224

Breonesin see guaifenesin

Brethaire see terbutaline 500

Brethine *51J, 54H* (illus.); see terbutaline 500

bretylium an anti-arrhythmic drug 128

Bretylol see bretylium

Brevibloc see esmolol

Brevicon a combined preparation. See ethinyl estradiol (334) and norethindrone. See also Oral contraceptives 189

Brevital see methohexital

Brexin a combined preparation. See pseudoephedrine (472), carbinoxamine, and guaifenesin

Bricanyl *51N, 53K* (illus.); see terbutaline 500

Bromfed a combined preparation. See brompheniramine (253) and pseudoephedrine (472)

bromides a group of *sedative* drugs now used only rarely as anticonvulsant drugs 114

bromocriptine 252

bromodiphenhydramine an antihistamine 152

bromovinyldeoxyuridine an antiviral agent used to treat herpes simplex. See Antiviral drugs 161

Bromphen see brompheniramine 253

brompheniramine 253

Brondecon *37K* (illus.); a combined preparation. See oxtriphylline (433) and guaifenesin

Bronkaid Mist see epinephrine 328

Bronkodyl S-R see theophylline 506

Bronkolixir a combined preparation. See ephedrine (327), phenobarbital (445), and theophylline (506)

Bronkometer see isoetharine

Bronkosol see isoetharine

Bronkotabs a combined preparation. See ephedrine (327), phenobarbital (445), theophylline (506), and guaifenesin

Bucladin-S see buclizine

buclizine an antihistamine used for motion sickness. See Anti-emetic drugs 118

budesonide an *investigational* corticosteroid drug used principally in asthma. See Corticosteroids 169

Buff-A Comp a combined preparation. See aspirin (238), butalbital, and caffeine

Bufferin see aspirin 238

Buf-Oxal 10 see benzoyl peroxide 248

bumetanide 254

Bumex *41R* (illus.); see bumetanide 254

bupivacaine a long-lasting local anesthetic often used for epidural *anesthesia* during labor. See Local anesthetics 108

B

Buprenex see buprenorphine

buprenorphine a narcotic analgesic 109

Buspar see buspirone

buspirone an *investigational* non-benzodiazepine anti-anxiety drug. See Anti-anxiety drugs 111

busulfan an alkylating agent used in the treatment of certain leukemias. See Anticancer drugs 182

butabarbital a barbiturate sleeping drug 110

butalbital a barbiturate sleeping drug (110) sometimes included in combined analgesic preparations

butamben a local anesthetic (108) applied to the skin to relieve itching. See Antipruritic medications 201

Butazolidin *35B, 58R* (illus.); see phenylbutazone 446

Butesin Picrate see butamben

Butibel *36 O* (illus.); a combined preparation. See belladonna (246) and butabarbital

Butisol see butabarbital

butoconazole a drug applied *topically* to treat vaginal thrush. See Antifungal drugs 166

butorphanol a narcotic analgesic 109

butyl aminobenzoate a local anesthetic 108

C

Cafergot a combined preparation. See ergotamine (330) and caffeine

Cafergot P-B *42P, 46E* (illus.); a combined preparation. See belladonna (246), ergotamine (330), caffeine, and pentobarbital

caffeine a stimulant drug that occurs in coffee, tea, and cola. It is sometimes added to *analgesic* medications

Caladryl a combined preparation. See diphenhydramine (317) and calamine

calamine a lotion containing zinc oxide and ferric oxide used to soothe irritated skin. See Antipruritic medications 201

Calan *39F, 45 O* (illus.); see verapamil 530

Calcet a combined preparation. See calcium (535) and vitamin D (545)

Calcibind see sodium cellulose phosphate

Calcidrine a combined preparation. See codeine (291) and calcium iodide

calcifediol see vitamin D 545

Calcimar see calcitonin 255

Calciparine see heparin 354

calcitonin 255

Calcitrel a combined preparation. See magnesium hydroxide (386) and calcium carbonate

calcitriol see vitamin D 545

calcium 535

calcium carbonate a calcium salt prescribed mainly as an antacid 136

CALCIUM CHLORIDE – CLEMASTINE

C

calcium chloride see calcium 535

calcium citrate see calcium 535

calcium glubionate see calcium 535

calcium gluceptate see calcium 535

calcium gluconate see calcium 535

calcium iodide a calcium compound occasionally used as an *expectorant*

calcium lactate see calcium 535

Calderol see calcifediol

Caldesene anti-infective skin preparation 203

Calel-D a combined preparation. See calcium carbonate and vitamin D (545). See also Vitamins 177

Calmol 4 a drug for anal and rectal disorders 141

Caltrate 600 see calcium carbonate

Cama see aspirin 238

Camalox a combined preparation. See aluminum hydroxide (224), magnesium hydroxide (386), and calcium carbonate

cambendazole a drug used to treat strongyloidiasis. See Anthelmintic drugs 167

camphor a substance applied to the skin to reduce itching. See Antipruritic medications 201

cannabis see marijuana 551

cantharidin an antiviral drug (161) used to treat warts

Cantharone see cantharidin

Cantharone Plus a combined preparation. See cantharidin, podophyllin, and salicylic acid

Cantil see mepenzolate

Capastat sulfate see capreomycin

Capoten *53L, 55L* (illus.); see captopril 256

Capozide a combined preparation. See captopril (256) and hydrochlorothiazide (357)

capreomycin an antituberculous drug 160

captopril 256

Carafate *45A* (illus.); see sucralfate 490

caramiphen a cough suppressant. See Drugs to treat coughs 122

carbachol 257

carbamazepine 258

carbamide peroxide an agent used in drops for softening ear wax

carbaryl a drug used to treat louse infestation. See Drugs to treat skin parasites 204

carbenicillin a penicillin antibiotic 156

carbenoxolone a licorice derivative used in the treatment of ulcers. See Anti-ulcer drugs 137

carbetapentane a cough suppressant. See Drugs to treat coughs 122

carbidopa a drug used to enhance the effect of levodopa (376) in the treatment of Parkinson's disease. See Antiparkinsonism drugs 115

carbimide a drug similar to disulfiram 321

carbinoxamine an antihistamine 152

Carbocaine see mepivacaine

carbocysteine a *mucolytic* decongestant 121

C

carbol-fuchsin an ingredient of Castellani's Paint

carboplatin an *investigational* anticancer drug (182) similar to cisplatin (282)

carboprost 259

carboxymethylcellulose a bulk-forming laxative. See Laxatives 139

Cardec DM a combined preparation. See dextromethorphan (307), pseudoephedrine (472), and carbinoxamine

Cardilate see erythrityl tetranitrate

Cardioquin *46M* (illus.); see quinidine 479

Cardizem *42B, 43B* (illus.); see diltiazem 315

Cardovar see trimazosin

carisoprodol 260

Carmol a lotion (Carmol 10) or cream (Carmol 20). See urea

Carmol HC a cream. See hydrocortisone (358) and urea

carmustine a drug used in the treatment of tumors of the central nervous system and lymphatic system. See Anticancer drugs 182

carphenazine a phenothiazine antipsychotic drug 113

carteolol an *investigational* beta blocker 125

Cartrol see carteolol

casanthranol a stimulant laxative 139

cascara a stimulant laxative 139

Castellani's Paint a mixture of carbol-fuchsin, phenol, resorcinol, acetone, and alcohol applied locally as an antifungal agent. See also Antifungal drugs 166

castor oil a stimulant laxative 139

Catapres *37 I, 46D* (illus.); see clonidine 287

Catapres-TTS see clonidine 287

Ceclor *60P, 60Q* (illus.); see cefaclor 261

cefaclor 261

cefadroxil a cephalosporin antibiotic 156

Cefadyl see cephapirin

cefamandole a cephalosporin antibiotic 156

cefazolin 262

Cefizox see ceftizoxime

Cefobid see cefoperazone 263

Cefol a multivitamin preparation. See Vitamins 177

cefonicid a cephalosporin antibiotic 156

cefoperazone 263

ceforanide a cephalosporin antibiotic 156

cefotaxime a cephalosporin antibiotic 156

cefotetan a cephalosporin antibiotic 156

cefoxitin 264

ceftazidime a cephalosporin antibiotic 156

ceftizoxime a cephalosporin antibiotic 156

ceftriaxone a cephalosporin antibiotic 156

cefuroxime a cephalosporin antibiotic 156

Celestone see betamethasone 250

Celontin see methsuximide

Cenocort see triamcinolone 519

Centrax *57D* (illus.); see prazepam 453

C

Centrum a multivitamin preparation. See Vitamins 177

cephalexin 265

cephalothin 266

cephapirin a cephalosporin antibiotic 156

cephradine a cephalosporin antibiotic 156

Cephulac see lactulose 375

Cerespan see papaverine 437

Cerose-DM Expectorant a combined preparation. See dextromethorphan (307), phenylephrine (447), guaiacolsulfonate, and phenindamine

Cesamet see nabilone

Cetacaine a combined preparation. See benzocaine (247) and tetracaine (503)

Cetacort see hydrocortisone 358

Cetamide see sulfacetamide 491

Cetaphil an oil-in-water ointment

Cetapred a combined preparation. See prednisolone (456) and sulfacetamide (491)

cetrimide a skin antiseptic. See Anti-infective skin preparations 203

Cevalin see vitamin C 544

charcoal activated charcoal is sometimes given to absorb and inactivate poisons or drug overdoses that have been taken by mouth. It has also been used to treat diarrhea

Chardonna-2 a combined preparation. See belladonna (246) and phenobarbital (445)

Chealamide see edetate disodium

Chenix *48N* (illus.); see chenodiol 267

chenodiol 267

Cheracol a combined preparation. See codeine (291) and guaifenesin

CHIP an *investigational* anticancer drug 182

chloral hydrate 268

chlorambucil 269

chloramphenicol 270

Chloraseptic a combined preparation. See phenol and menthol

chlorcyclizine an antihistamine 152

chlordiazepoxide 271

chlorhexidine a skin antiseptic. See Anti-infective skin preparations 203

chlormezanone an anti-anxiety drug 111

chlorobutanol a preservative

Chlorofon-F see chlorzoxazone 278

chloroform a general anesthetic

chloroguanide a drug used in the treatment of malaria. See Antimalarial drugs 165

Chloromycetin *62E* (illus.); see chloramphenicol 270

chlorophenothane an insecticide otherwise known as DDT

chloroprocaine a local anesthetic 108

Chloroptic see chloramphenicol 270

chloroquine 272

chlorothiazide 273

C

chlorotrianisene an estrogen drug used primarily to treat cancer. See Female sex hormones (175) and Anticancer drugs (182)

chloroxylenol a skin antiseptic. See Anti-infective skin preparations 203

chlorphenesin a muscle-relaxant drug 148

chlorpheniramine 274

chlorphentermine an appetite suppressant

chlorpromazine 275

chlorpropamide 276

chlorprothixene a phenothiazine antipsychotic drug 113

chlortetracycline a tetracycline antibiotic 156

chlorthalidone 277

Chlor-Trimetron chlorpheniramine 274

chlorzoxazone 278

Chlorzoxazone with APAP *42C* (illus.); a combined preparation. See acetaminophen (215) and chlorzoxazone (278)

Choledyl *35A, 40R* (illus.); see oxtriphylline 433

cholestyramine 279

choline magnesium trisalicylate a drug similar to aspirin (238) used in arthritic conditions

choline salicylate a drug similar to aspirin (238) used in arthritic conditions

Choloxin see dextrothyroxine

chorionic gonadotropin see HCG (human chorionic gonadotropin) 355

Chromagen capsules a combined preparation. See iron (538), vitamin B_{12} (544), and vitamin C (544)

chromium 536

Chronulac see lactulose 375

chymopapain an *enzyme* used to treat sciatica

Chymoral a combined preparation. See trypsin and chymotrypsin

chymotrypsin an *enzyme* used in the treatment of cataracts

ciclopirox 280

cilastatin-imipenem an antibiotic 156

cimetidine 281

cinnamates a drug used as a sunscreen 207

cinnarizine an antihistamine 152

Cinobac see cinoxacin

cinoxacin a urinary tract antiseptic. See Antibacterial drugs 159

ciprofibrate a lipid-lowering drug 131

cisplatin 282

Citracal see calcium citrate

Citra forte a combined preparation. See vitamin C (544), hydrocodone, and pheniramine

citric acid 557

Citrocarbonate a combined preparation. See sodium bicarbonate (486) and sodium citrate

Claforan see cefotaxime

clavulanic acid see potassium clavulanate

clemastine an antihistamine 152

CLEOCIN – DAPSONE

C

Cleocin *57P, 61C* (illus.); see clindamycin 283

Cleocin T see clindamycin 283

Clerz see hydroxyethylcellulose

clidinium bromide an *antispasmodic* drug used in irritable bowel syndrome 138

clindamycin 283

Clinoril *39P, 39 Q* (illus.); see sulindac 496

clioquinol a *topical* antibacterial and antifungal agent. See Anti-infective skin preparations 203

clobetasol a corticosteroid for *topical* application. See Topical corticosteroids 202

clocortolone a corticosteroid for *topical* application. See Topical corticosteroids 202

Cloderm see clocortolone

clofazimine a drug used in the treatment of leprosy 159

clofibrate 284

Clomid *50L* (illus.); see clomiphene 285

clomiphene 285

clomipramine a tricyclic antidepressant 112

clonazepam 286

clonidine 287

clorazepate 288

clotrimazole 289

cloxacillin 290

Cloxapen *59D* (illus.); see cloxacillin 290

clozapine an antipsychotic drug 113

Clusivol a multivitamin preparation. See Vitamins 177

Clysodrast see bisacodyl 251

Coactin see amdinocillin

coal tar a substance included in many *topical* preparations for the treatment of psoriasis and dandruff. See Drugs for psoriasis (206) and Treatment for dandruff and hair loss (207)

cobalt edetate an *antidote* used in cyanide poisoning

cocaine 550

codeine 291

Codiclear a combined preparation. See hydrocodone and guaiacosulfonate

Codimal LA a combined preparation. See chlorpheniramine (274) and pseudoephedrine (472)

cod liver oil oil obtained from the liver of cod that is rich in vitamin A (543) and vitamin D (545)

Cogentin *52P, 54M* (illus.); see benztropine 249

Co-Gesic a combined preparation. See acetaminophen (215) and hydrocodone

Colace see docusate

ColBenemid *55C* (illus.); a combined preparation. See probenecid (460) and colchicine (292)

colchicine 292

Colestid see colestipol 293

colestipol 293

colistin 294

C

collodion a substance that dries to form a sticky film. It is used to protect broken skin. See Bases for skin preparations 203

Collyrium 2 a combined preparation. See tetrahydrozoline (505), glycerin, and sodium borate

Cologel see methylcellulose 404

Colrex a combined preparation. See acetaminophen (215), chlorpheniramine (274), codeine (291), and phenylephrine (447)

Coly-Mycin S colistin 294

Coly-Mycin S Otic a combined preparation. See colistin (294) and hydrocortisone (358)

Colyte a drug used for clearing the bowel. See Laxatives 139

Combid a combined preparation. See prochlorperazine (465) and isopropamide

Combipres *35 O* (illus.); a combined preparation. See clonidine (287) and chlorthalidone (277)

Comhist LA a cold relief preparation. See chlorpheniramine (274), phenylephrine (447), atropine, and phenyltoloxamine

compactin an *investigational* lipid-lowering drug 131

Compal a combined preparation. See acetaminophen (215), caffeine, and dihydrocodeine

Compazine *42G, 42H* (illus.); see prochlorperazine 465

Compete a multivitamin preparation with iron (538) and zinc (546). See Vitamins 177

Compound W a combined preparation. See salicylic acid, menthol, acetic acid, and camphor

Comtrex a cold relief preparation. See acetaminophen (215), chlorpheniramine (274), dextromethorphan (307), and phenyl-propanolamine

Conar A a cough medication. See acetaminophen (215), phenylephrine (447), guaifenesin, and noscapine

Conex DA a combined preparation. See phenylpropanolamine (448) and phenyltoloxamine

Congespirin see dextromethorphan 307

Congess a cough medication. See pseudoephedrine (472) and guaifenesin

conjugated estrogens 295

Constant-T *36H, 43P* (illus.); see theophylline 506

Contac a cold relief preparation. See chlorpheniramine (274) and phenylpropanolamine (448)

Cophene PL a combined preparation. See chlorpheniramine (274), phenylephrine (447), and phenylpropanolamine (448)

copper 536

Co-Pyronil a combined preparation. See cyclopentamine and pyrrobutamine

Cordran see flurandrenolide

Corgard *44E, 44L* (illus.); see nadolol 415

Coricidin a combined preparation. See aspirin (238) and chlorpheniramine (274)

C

Corilin a combined preparation. See chlorpheniramine (274), sodium salicylate, and aminoacetic acid

Cortaid see hydrocortisone 358

Cort-Dome see hydrocortisone 358

Cortef *50M* (illus.); see hydrocortisone 358

Cortenema see hydrocortisone 358

Corticaine a combined preparation. See hydrocortisone (358) and dibucaine

corticotropin a *hormone* released from the pituitary gland. See Drugs for pituitary disorders 173

Cortifoam see hydrocortisone 358

Cortinal see hydrocortisone 358

cortisol see hydrocortisone 358

cortisone 296

Cortisporin Cream a combined preparation. See bacitracin (243), hydrocortisone (358), neomycin (421), and polymyxin B

Cortisporin Otic a combined preparation. See hydrocortisone (358) and neomycin (421)

Cortone see cortisone 296

Cortrophin Zinc see corticotropin

Cortrosyn see cosyntropin 297

Coryban-D a combined preparation. See chlorpheniramine (274), phenylpropanolamine (448), and caffeine

corynebacterium parvum a drug derived from bacteria that stimulates the immune response used in the treatment of certain cancers. See Anticancer drugs 182

Corzide *47K, 47L* (illus.); a combined preparation. See nadolol (415) and bendroflumethiazide

cosyntropin 297

Cotazym see pancrelipase

Cotrim a combined preparation. See sulfamethoxazole (492) and trimethoprim (526)

CoTylenol a combined preparation. See acetaminophen (215), chlorpheniramine (274), and pseudoephedrine (472)

Coumadin *37M, 37Q* (illus.); see warfarin 531

cresol an *antiseptic* preservative

cromolyn sodium 298

crotamiton an agent applied *topically* used to treat scabies. See Drugs to treat skin parasites 204

Crysticillin a combined preparation. See penicillin G (439) and procaine (463)

Crystodigin *36G* (illus.); see digitoxin 313

Cuprimine *56T, 61N* (illus.); see penicillamine 438

Curretab see medroxyprogesterone 391

cyanocobalamin see vitamin B$_{12}$ 544

Cyanoject see vitamin B$_{12}$ 544

cyclacillin an antibiotic 156

cyclandelate a drug used in the treatment of cerebrovascular and peripheral vascular disorders. See Vasodilators 126

Cyclapen-W *41L* (illus.); see cyclacillin

C

cyclizine an antihistamine used mainly as an anti-emetic. See Antihistamines (152) and Anti-emetic drugs (118)

cyclobenzaprine 299

Cyclocort see amcinonide

Cyclogyl see cyclopentolate

cyclomethycaine a local anesthetic 108

Cyclomydril a combined preparation. See phenylephrine (447) and cyclopentolate

Cyclopar see tetracycline 504

cyclopentamine a decongestant 121

cyclopentolate a *mydriatic* and *cycloplegic* drug. See Drugs affecting the pupil 198

cyclophosphamide 300

cycloserine an antibiotic used to treat tuberculosis. See Antituberculous drugs 160

Cyclospasmol *38M, 57L* (illus.); see cyclandelate

cyclosporine 301

cyclothiazide a thiazide diuretic 127

Cylert see pemoline

cyproheptadine an antihistamine (152) that is also used to stimulate appetite

Cyronine see liothyronine 381

Cystospaz see hyoscyamine

Cytadren *49N* (illus.); see aminoglutethimide 228

cytarabine a drug used in the treatment of leukemia. See Anticancer drugs 182

Cytomel *51P, 52G* (illus.); see liothyronine 381

Cytosar-U see cytarabine

Cytosin Arabinoside see cytarabine

Cytoxan *47M, 47N* (illus.); see cyclophosphamide 300

D

dacarbazine a *cytotoxic* drug used in the treatment of Hodgkin's disease. See Anticancer drugs 182

dactinomycin a *cytotoxic* antibiotic. See Anticancer drugs 182

Dalalone see dexamethasone 306

Dalalone DP see dexamethasone 306

Dalicote see dexamethasone 306

Dalidyne see dexamethasone 306

Dallergy a combined preparation. See chlorpheniramine (274), phenylephrine (447), and methscopolamine

Dalmane *58F, 58M* (illus.); see flurazepam 343

Damason-P see hydrocodone

danazol 302

Danocrine *56Q, 59B* (illus.); see danazol 302

danthron a stimulant laxative 139

Dantrium *58L, 58N* (illus.); dantrolene 303

dantrolene 303

dapsone 304

DARANIDE – DISODIUM AZODISALICYCLIC ACID

D

Daranide see dichlorphenamide

Daraprim see pyrimethamine 477

Darbid see isopropamide

Daricon see oxyphencyclimine

Darvocet-N 50 a combined preparation. See acetaminophen (215) and propoxyphene (469)

Darvocet-N 100 a combined preparation. See acetaminophen (215) and propoxyphene (469)

Darvon *56E* (illus.); see propoxyphene 469

Darvon Compound 65 *61M* (illus.); a combined preparation. See aspirin (238), propoxyphene (469), and caffeine

Darvon-N see propoxyphene 469

daunorubicin a *cytotoxic* antibiotic. See Anticancer drugs 182

Dazamide see acetazolamide 216

DDAVP see desmopressin

Debrox see carbamide peroxide

Decaderm see dexamethasone 306

Decadron *39B, 43 O* (illus.); see dexamethasone 306

Decadron LA see dexamethasone 306

Deca-durabolin see nandrolone 418

Decaject see dexamethasone 306

Decapryn see doxylamine

Decaspray see dexamethasone 306

Decholin see dehydrocholic acid

Declomycin see demeclocycline

Deconade a combined preparation. See chlorpheniramine (274) and phenylpropanolamine (448)

Deconamine SR *60N* (illus.); a combined preparation. See chlorpheniramine (274) and pseudoephedrine (472)

Deconsal see phenylephrine 447

deferoxamine a *chelating* agent used in iron poisoning

dehydrocholic acid a laxative 139

dehydroemetine an antiprotozoal drug 164

Deladumone a combined preparation. See estradiol (332) and testosterone (502)

Delatestryl see testosterone 502

Delatulin see hydroxyprogesterone

Delestrogen see estradiol 332

Delfen a spermicidal foam. See nonoxynol 9

Delsym see dextromethorphan 307

Delta-cortef see prednisolone 456

Deltasone *36B, 52 O* (illus.); see prednisone 457

Demazin a combined preparation. See chlorpheniramine (274) and phenylpropanolamine (448)

demecarium a *miotic* drug used in the treatment of glaucoma. See Drugs for glaucoma 196

demeclocycline a tetracycline antibiotic. See Antibiotics 156

Demerol see meperidine 396

D

Demi-Regroton *52K* (illus.); a combined preparation. See chlorthalidone (277) and reserpine

Demulen a combined preparation. See ethinyl estradiol (334) and ethynodiol

Depakene see valproic acid 528

Depakote see valproic acid 528

Depen see penicillamine 438

Depo-Estradiol see estradiol 332

Depo-Estrone see estrone

Depo-Medrol see methylprednisolone 406

Depo-Provera see medroxyprogesterone 391

Depo-Testadiol a combined preparation. See estradiol (332) and testosterone (502)

deprenyl see selegiline

Deprol a combined preparation. See meprobamate (397) and benactyzine

Dermacort see hydrocortisone 358

Dermolate see hydrocortisone 358

Dermoplast see benzocaine 247

DES see diethylstilbestrol 311

Desenex see undecylenic acid

deserpidine an antihypertensive drug 130

desipramine 305

Desitin a combined preparation. See zinc oxide, cod liver oil, and talc

deslanoside a cardiac glycoside. See Digitalis drugs 124

desmopressin a drug used for the long-term treatment of diabetes insipidus. See Drugs for pituitary disorders 173

desonide a corticosteroid used to treat skin conditions. See Topical corticosteroids 202

DesOwen see desonide

desoximetasone a corticosteroid used in eye and skin preparations. See Topical corticosteroids 202

desoxycorticosterone a corticosteroid 169

Desoxyn see methamphetamine

Desquam-X see benzoyl peroxide 248

Desyrel see trazodone 517

Dexacidin a combined preparation. See dexamethasone (306), neomycin (421), and polymyxin B

dexamethasone 306

Dexatrim see phenylpropanolamine 448

dexbrompheniramine an antihistamine 152

dexchlorpheniramine an antihistamine 152

Dexedrine see dextroamphetamine

Dexone see dexamethasone 306

dexpanthenol a drug related to pantothenic acid (540). Used to relieve flatulence, and applied topically for various skin conditions such as burns and eczema

dextroamphetamine an amphetamine. See Nervous system stimulants (116) and Amphetamines (549)

dextromethorphan 307

D

dextrothyroxine a lipid-lowering drug 131

Dey-Dose Atropine Sulfate see atropine

DHE-45 see dihydroergotamine

DHS Zinc see zinc pyrithione

DHT see dihydrotachysterol

DiaBeta *36K, 55J* (illus.); see glyburide 348

Diabinese *43S, 44C* (illus.); see chlorpropamide 276

diacetylmorphine see heroin

Dia-Gesic see hydrocodone

Dialose see docusate

Dialume see aluminum hydroxide 224

diamidine an antiprotozoal drug 164

Diamox *48P, 50S* (illus.); see acetazolamide 216

Diapid see lypressin 385

diazepam 308

diazoxide an antihypertensive drug that is used to treat hypoglycemia. See Drugs used in diabetes 170

Dibenzyline see phenoxybenzamine

dibucaine a local anesthetic 108

Dical-D a combined preparation. See calcium (535) and vitamin D (545)

dichloralphenazone a sedative drug similar to chloral hydrate 268

dichlorphenamide a carbonic anhydrase inhibitor used in the treatment of glaucoma 196

dicloxacillin a penicillin antibiotic 156

dicumarol 309

dicyclomine 310

Didronel see etidronate

dienestrol an estrogen drug. See Female sex hormones 175

diethylcarbamazine an anthelmintic drug 167

diethylpropion an appetite suppressant

diethylstilbestrol 311

diflorasone a corticosteroid used to treat skin disorders. See Topical corticosteroids 202

diflunisal 312

difluoromethylornithine a drug used to treat protozoal infections and certain cancers. See Antiprotozoal drugs (164) and Anticancer drugs (182)

Di-Gel see simethicone

digitalis a drug derived from foxglove leaves. See Digitalis drugs 124

digitoxin 313

digoxin 314

dihydrocodeine a narcotic analgesic. See Analgesics 108

dihydroergotamine a drug used to treat migraine and cluster headaches. See Drugs used for migraine 117

dihydrotachysterol see vitamin D 545

dihydroxyaluminum an aluminum antacid. See Antacids 136

diiodohydroxyquin see iodoquinol

D

Dilantin *41K, 62C* (illus.); see phenytoin 449

Dilantin with phenobarbital *62D* (illus.); a combined preparation. See phenobarbital (445) and phenytoin (449)

Dilatrate-SR see isosorbide dinitrate 369

Dilaudid see hydromorphone

Dilor see dyphylline

diloxanide an antiprotozoal drug used in the treatment of amebiasis. See Antiprotozoal drugs 164

diltiazem 315

Dimacol see dextromethorphan 307

dimenhydrinate 316

dimercaprol a *chelating* agent used to treat metal poisoning

dimercaptosuccinic acid an agent used in the treatment of lead poisoning

Dimetane-DC Cough see brompheniramine 253

Dimetane Decongestant see brompheniramine 253

Dimetane Elixir see brompheniramine 253

Dimetane Extentab see brompheniramine 253

Dimetane Tabs see brompheniramine 253

Dimetapp a combined preparation. See brompheniramine (253) and phenylpropanolamine (448)

dimethicone a water-repellent substance used in barrier creams

dimethindene an antihistamine 152

dimethisoquin a local anesthetic 108

dimethyl sulfoxide a drug administered into the bladder to treat interstitial cystitis

dimethyl turbocurarine see metocurine

dinoprost a prostaglandin drug used to stimulate contractions of the uterus. See Drugs used in labor 193

dinoprostone a prostaglandin drug used to stimulate contractions of the uterus. See Drugs used in labor 193

diperodon a local anesthetic 108

Diphenatol a combined preparation. See diphenoxylate (318) and atropine

diphenhydramine 317

diphenidol an anti-emetic drug 118

diphenoxylate 318

diphenylpyraline an antihistamine 152

dipivalyl epinephrine see dipivefrin

dipivefrin a drug related to epinephrine used to reduce pressure inside the eye in the treatment of glaucoma 196

Diprolene see betamethasone 250

Diprosone see betamethasone 250

dipyridamole 319

Disalcid see salsalate

Disipal *42S* (illus.); see orphenadrine 430

disodium azodisalicyclic acid an *investigational* drug used for ulcerative colitis. See Drugs for inflammatory bowel disease 140

DISOPHROL – ESTRATEST

E

E

Econopred see prednisolone 456

Ecotrin see aspirin 238

Edecrin see ethacrynic acid

edetate calcium disodium a *chelating* agent used to treat poisoning from lead and other metals

edetate disodium a *chelating* agent used to reduce calcium levels in the blood

edrophonium a drug used to diagnose myasthenia gravis 149

EDTA see edetate disodium

EES *48B* (illus.); see erythromycin 331

Effersyllium see psyllium 473

Efodine see povidone-iodine

Efudex see fluorouracil 341

Elavil *40J, 44H* (illus.); see amitriptyline 232

Eldepryl see selegiline

Eldopaque see hydroquinone

Eldoquin see hydroquinone

Elixicon see theophylline 506

Elixophyllin see theophylline 506

E-lonate PA estradiol 332

Embolex see heparin 354

Emcyt see estramustine

Emete-con see benzquinamide

emetine a drug used to treat amebiasis. See Antiprotozoal drugs 164

Emko a spermicidal vaginal foam containing nonoxynol 9

Empirin see aspirin 238

E-Mycin *37G, 48M* (illus.); see erythromycin 331

E-Mycin 333 erythromycin 331

enalapril 326

Enarax a combined preparation. See hydroxyzine (359) and oxyphencyclimine

encainide an anti-arrhythmic drug 128

Encaprin see aspirin 238

Encare spermicidal vaginal suppositories containing nonoxynol 9

Endep *39J, 39K* (illus.); see amitriptyline 232

Enduron see methyclothiazide

Enduronyl a combined preparation. See methyclothiazide and deserpidine

enflurane a general anesthetic

Enovid E, Enovid 5, Enovid 10 a combined preparation. See mestranol and norethynodrel

Entex LA *44D* (illus.); a combined preparation. See phenylpropanolamine (448) and guaifenesin

Entozyme a combined preparation. See pancreatin, pepsin, and bile salts. See Digestion of fats 142

Entuss a combined preparation. See pseudoephedrine (472), guaifenesin, and hydrocodone

Enuclene an artificial tear preparation (198) containing benzalkonium chloride and tyloxapol

enviroxime an *investigational* antiviral drug 161

ephedrine 327

E

Epifoam a combined preparation. See hydrocortisone (358) and pramoxine

Epifrin see epinephrine 328

E-Pilo a combined preparation. See epinephrine (328) and pilocarpine (451)

Epinal see epinephryl borate

epinephrine 328

epinephryl borate an epinephrine-like drug. See 328

EpiPen see epinephrine 328

Epitrate see epinephrine 328

epoprostenol an *investigational* vasodilator and antiplatelet drug. See Vasodilators (126) and Drugs that affect blood clotting (132)

Eppy N see epinephryl borate

Equagesic *47C* (illus.); a combined preparation. See aspirin (238) and meprobamate (397)

Equanil *49H, 53 I* (illus.); see meprobamate 397

ergocalciferol see vitamin D 545

ergoloid mesylates a drug used occasionally to treat senile dementia

Ergomar *42K* (illus.); see ergotamine 330

ergonovine 329

Ergostat see ergotamine 330

ergotamine 330

Ergotrate maleate *52M* (illus.); see ergonovine 329

ERYC *59A* (illus.); see erythromycin 331

ERYC 125 see erythromycin 331

Erycette see erythromycin 331

EryDerm see erythromycin 331

Erymax see erythromycin 331

Ery-Tab *35R, 54F* (illus.); see erythromycin 331

erythrityl tetranitrate a nitrate anti-angina drug. See Anti-angina drugs 129

Erythrocin *35 I, 36N* (illus.); see erythromycin 331

erythromycin 331

Esgic a combined preparation. See acetaminophen (215), butalbital, and caffeine

Esidrix *36F, 41P* (illus.); see hydrochlorothiazide 357

Esimil see hydrochlorothiazide 357

Eskalith CR *40D, 46P* (illus.); see lithium 382

esmolol an *investigational* beta blocker 125

Estar see coal tar

esterified estrogens an estrogen preparation. See Female sex hormones 175

Estinyl *35K, 46H* (illus.); see ethinyl estradiol 334

Estrace *42L, 44S* (illus.); see estradiol 332

Estraderm an *investigational* transdermal preparation of ethinyl estradiol 334

estradiol 332

Estradurin see polyestradiol

Estra-L see estradiol 332

estramustine an anticancer drug 182

Estratab see esterified estrogens

Estratest a combined preparation. See esterified estrogens and methyltestosterone

ESTRONE – GLUTETHIMIDE

E

estrone an estrogen preparation. See Female sex hormones 175

estropipate an estrogen drug. See Female sex hormones 175

Estrovis see quinestrol

ethacrynate sodium a loop diuretic. See Diuretics 127

ethacrynic acid a loop diuretic. See Diuretics 127

ethambutol 333

ethchlorvynol a sleeping drug 110

ethinamate a sleeping drug 110

ethinyl estradiol 334

ethionamide 335

ethopropazine a phenothiazine antiparkinsonism drug. See Antiparkinsonism drugs 115

ethosuximide 336

ethotoin an anticonvulsant drug 114

Ethrane see enflurane

ethylestrenol an anabolic steroid. See Male sex hormones 174

ethynodiol a progestin drug. See Female sex hormones 175

etidocaine a local anesthetic 108

etidronate a drug used to treat Paget's disease

etofibrate an *investigational* lipid-lowering drug 131

etomidate a general anesthetic

etoposide an anticancer drug 182

Etrafon *36P, 40M* (illus.); a combined preparation. See amitriptyline (232) and perphenazine (442)

etretinate 337

eucatropine an *anticholinergic mydriatic* drug. See Drugs affecting the pupil 198

Eucerin a water-in-oil emulsion used for dry skin conditions. See Bases for skin preparations 203

Eurax see crotamiton

Euthroid a combined preparation known as liotrix. See levothyroxine (377) and liothyronine (381)

Evac Q kit a combined preparation. See magnesium citrate and phenolphthalein

Excedrin a combined preparation. See acetaminophen (215), aspirin (238), and caffeine

Ex-Lax see phenolphthalein

Exsel see selenium 542

Extendryl a combined preparation. See chlorpheniramine (274), phenylephrine (447), and methscopolamine

Extend 12 see dextromethorphan 307

F

famotidine an H$_2$ blocker. See Anti-ulcer drugs 137

Fansidar a combined preparation. See pyrimethamine (477) and sulfadoxine

Fastin see phentermine

F

Fedahist a combined preparation. See chlorpheniramine (274) and pseudoephedrine (472)

Fedrazil a combined preparation. See pseudoephedrine (472) and chlorcyclizine

Feen-a-Mint see phenolphthalein

Feldene *57Q, 61B* (illus.); see piroxicam 452

Feminone see ethinyl estradiol 334

Femiron see ferrous fumarate

Femstat see butoconazole

fenfluramine an appetite suppressant related to the amphetamines. See Nervous system stimulants 116

fenofibrate a lipid-lowering drug 131

fenoprofen 338

fenoterol an *investigational* bronchodilator 120

fentanyl a narcotic analgesic (108) often used to induce general *anesthesia*

Feosol see ferrous sulfate

Feostat see ferrous fumarate

F-E-P Creme a combined preparation. See hydrocortisone (358) and pramoxine

Ferancee a combined preparation. See vitamin C (544) and ferrous fumarate

Fergon see ferrous gluconate

Fer-In-Sol see ferrous sulfate

Fermalox a combined preparation. See aluminum hydroxide (224), magnesium hydroxide (386), and ferrous sulfate

Fero-Folic-500 a combined preparation. See folic acid (537), ferrous sulfate, and sodium ascorbate

Fero-Grad-500 see ferrous sulfate

Fero-Gradumet see ferrous sulfate

Ferralet Plus see ferrous gluconate

Ferro-Sequels a combined preparation. See docusate and ferrous fumarate

ferrous fumarate an iron preparation. See Iron 538

ferrous gluconate an iron preparation. See Iron 538

ferrous sulfate an iron preparation. See Iron 538

Festal II see pancrelipase

Fiberall see psyllium 473

fibrinolysin a preparation containing plasmin, an agent that breaks down blood clots. Used *topically* to treat skin ulcers

Fiogesic a combined preparation. See aspirin (238), phenylpropanolamine (448), pheniramine, and pyrilamine

Fiorinal a combined preparation. See aspirin (238), butalbital, and caffeine

Fiorinal with codeine a combined preparation. See aspirin (238), codeine (291), and butalbital

Flagyl *44N, 44R* (illus.); see metronidazole 411

flavoxate 339

flecainide an anti-arrhythmic drug 128

Fleet Bisacodyl see bisacodyl 251

Fleet relief see pramoxine

Fletcher's Castoria for Children see senna

F

Flexeril *40A* (illus.); see cyclobenzaprine 299

Flexoject see orphenadrine 430

Flintstones a multivitamin preparation. See Vitamins 177

Florinef see fludrocortisone

Florone see diflorasone

Floropryl see isoflurophate

Florvite a vitamin supplement. See Vitamins 177

floxuridine an anticancer drug 182

flubendazole an *investigational* anthelmintic drug 167

flucytosine an antifungal drug 166

fludarabine an anticancer drug 182

fludrocortisone a corticosteroid 169

Fluidil see cyclothiazide

flunarizine an *investigational* calcium channel blocker 129

flunisolide a corticosteroid mainly used to treat bronchial disorders. See Corticosteroids 169

fluocinolone 340

fluocinonide a drug mainly used in *topical* preparations. See Topical corticosteroids 202

fluocortin an *investigational* corticosteroid 169

Fluonid see fluocinolone 340

fluoride 537

Fluoritab see fluoride 537

fluorometholone a drug mainly used *topically* to treat eye disorders. See Corticosteroids 169

Fluoroplex see fluorouracil 341

fluorouracil 341

Fluothane see halothane

fluoxymesterone an anticancer drug 182

fluphenazine 342

Flura see fluoride 537

flurandrenolide a corticosteroid 169

flurazepam 343

flurbiprofen a non-steroidal anti-inflammatory drug 144

Flurosyn see fluocinolone 340

FML see fluorometholone

Foille a combined preparation. See bacitracin (243), benzocaine (247), neomycin (421), and polymyxin B

Foldan see thiabendazole 507

Folex see methotrexate 402

folic acid 537

Folvite see folic acid 537

formaldehyde a disinfectant

Formula 44 a combined preparation. See benzocaine (247) and dextromethorphan (307)

Fortaz see ceftazidime

Fostex a combined preparation. See benzoyl peroxide (248), salicylic acid, and sulfur

Fototar see coal tar

FUDR see floxuridine

Fulvicin U/F *48K, 49K* (illus.); see griseofulvin 350

F

Fungizone see amphotericin B 235

Furacin see nitrofurazone

Furadantin *40S, 41T* (illus.); see nitrofurantoin 426

furazolidone an antiprotozoal drug 164

furosemide 344

G

G-1 Capsules a combined preparation. See acetaminophen (215), butalbital, and caffeine

gallamine a muscle-relaxant drug 148

Gamimune an immune globulin. See Vaccines and immunization 162

gamma benzene hexachloride see lindane 380

Gammacorten see dexamethasone 306

gamma globulin immune globulin. See Vaccines and immunization 162

Gantanol *43A* (illus.); see sulfamethoxazole 492

Gantrisin see sulfisoxazole 495

Garamycin see gentamicin 346

Gaviscon a combined preparation. See aluminum hydroxide (224) and sodium bicarbonate (486)

Gelusil see simethicone

gemfibrozil 345

Gemnisyn a combined preparation. See acetaminophen (215) and aspirin (238)

Genapax vaginal tampons containing gentian violet

Genoptic see gentamicin 346

gentamicin 346

gentian violet a dye used *topically* to treat skin infections. See Anti-infective skin preparations 203

Geocillin see carbenicillin

Geopen see carbenicillin

Geravite a multivitamin preparation. See Vitamins 177

Gerimed a multivitamin and multimineral supplement. See Vitamins 177

Geriplex a multivitamin preparation with iron (538). See Vitamins 177

Geritol Tonic Liquid a multivitamin preparation with iron (538). See Vitamins 177

Ger-O-Foam a combined preparation. See benzocaine (247) and methyl salicyclate

Glaucon see epinephrine 328

gliclazide an oral antidiabetic drug. See Drugs used in diabetes 170

glipizide 347

glucagon a pancreatic *enzyme* used to treat hypoglycemia. See Drugs used in diabetes 170

Glucamide see chlorpropamide 276

Glucotrol *53Q, 53R* (illus.); see glipizide 347

glutaral a skin antiseptic. See Anti-infective skin preparations 203

glutethimide a sleeping drug 110

GLYBURIDE – IMMUNE SERUM GLOBULIN

H

Histosal a combined preparation. See acetaminophen (215), phenylpropanolamine (448), caffeine, and pyrilamine

HMS Liquifilm see medrysone

homatropine a *mydriatic* and *cycloplegic* drug used in certain eye conditions. See Drugs affecting the pupil 198

Homicebrin a multivitamin preparation. See Vitamins 177

human chorionic gonadotropin see HCG 355

human insulin 364

Humorsol see demecarium

Humulin L see insulin 364

Humulin N see insulin 364

Humulin R see insulin 364

Hurricaine see benzocaine 247

hyaluronidase an *enzyme* used in *topical* skin preparations to reduce bruising

hycanthone an anthelmintic drug 167

Hycodan a combined preparation. See hydrocodone and homatropine

Hycodaphen see hydrocodone

Hycomine a combined preparation. See phenylpropanolamine (448) and hydrocodone

Hycotuss a combined preparation. See alcohol, guaifenesin, and hydrocodone

Hydeltrasol see prednisolone 456

Hydeltra TBA see prednisolone 456

Hydergine *54 O* (illus.); see ergoloid mesylates

Hydoril see hydrochlorothiazide 357

hydralazine 356

Hydrea see hydroxyurea

Hydrocet a combined preparation. See acetaminophen (215) and hydrocodone

hydrochlorothiazide 357

Hydrocil see psyllium 473

hydrocodone a narcotic drug mainly used in the treatment of coughs. See Drugs to treat coughs 122

Hydrocort see hydrocortisone 358

hydrocortisone 358

Hydrocortone *54K, 54L* (illus.); see hydrocortisone 358

HydroDIURIL *38B, 38C* (illus.); see hydrochlorothiazide 357

hydroflumethiazide a thiazide diuretic 127

hydrogen peroxide a skin antiseptic. See Anti-infective skin preparations 203

Hydromal see hydrochlorothiazide 357

hydromorphone a narcotic analgesic 108

Hydromox see quinethazone

hydrophilic ointment an oil-in-water emulsion used as a base for skin preparations 203

Hydropres-25 a combined preparation. See hydrochlorothiazide (357) and reserpine

Hydroprin a combined preparation. See hydrochlorothiazide (357) and reserpine

hydroquinone a drug used to bleach the skin

H

Hydroserpine a combined preparation. See hydrochlorothiazide (357) and reserpine

Hydrotensin-50 a combined preparation. See hydrochlorothiazide (357) and reserpine

hydroxocobalamin see vitamin B$_{12}$ 544

hydroxyamphetamine a *mydriatic* drug used to diagnose glaucoma. See Drugs affecting the pupil 198

hydroxychloroquine an antimalarial drug (165) and antirheumatic drug (145)

hydroxydopamine an *investigational* drug used to treat glaucoma 196

hydroxyethylcellulose a substance used in artificial tear preparations 198

hydroxyprogesterone a progestin. See Female sex hormones 175

hydroxypropylcellulose a substance used in artificial tear preparations 198

hydroxypropylmethylcellulose a substance used in artificial tear preparations 198

hydroxyurea an anticancer drug 182

hydroxyzine 359

Hygroton *43R, 52J* (illus.); see chlorthalidone 277

Hylorel see guanadrel

hyoscine see scopolamine

hyoscyamine an *anticholinergic* drug used as an antispasmodic in irritable bowel syndrome (138) and in urinary incontinence (194)

Hyperetic see hydrochlorothiazide 357

Hyperstat see diazoxide

Hytakerol see dihydrotachysterol

Hytinic see iron 538

Hytone see hydrocortisone 358

I

Iberet a multivitamin preparation with iron (538). See Vitamins 177

Iberol a multivitamin preparation with iron (538). See Vitamins 177

ibuprofen 360

idoxuridine 361

ifosfamide an *investigational* alkylating agent. See Anticancer drugs 182

Iletin see insulin 364

Ilopan see dexpanthenol

Ilosone *39E, 58K* (illus.); see erythromycin 331

Ilotycin *38 I* (illus.); see erythromycin 331

Ilozyme see pancrelipase

Imferon see iron 538

imipenem/cilastatin an antibiotic 156

imipramine 362

immune serum globulin an *antibody* preparation injected to prevent certain infectious diseases. See Vaccines and immunization 162

IMODIUM – LEVLEN

J K

K

karaya gum a vegetable gum used as a bulk-forming laxative 139

Kasof see docusate

Kato see potassium chloride 540

Kay Ciel see potassium chloride 540

Keflex *59 I, 59N* (illus.); see cephalexin 265

Keflin see cephalothin 266

Kefzol see cefazolin 262

Kemadrin see procyclidine 466

Kenacort see triamcinolone 519

Kenalog see triamcinolone 519

Keralyt see salicylic acid

Keri Lotion an oil-in-water emulsion. See Bases for skin preparations 203

Kerodex a skin barrier

Ketalar see ketamine

ketamine a non-barbiturate *sedative* drug used to induce general *anesthesia*

ketanserin an *investigational* antihypertensive drug 130

ketoconazole 372

ketoprofen 373

Ketrax see levamisole

Kie Syrup a combined preparation. See ephedrine (327) and potassium iodide

Kinesed a combined preparation. See phenobarbital (445), atropine, hyoscyamine, and scopolamine

Klebcil see kanamycin

Kleer compound a combined preparation. See chlorpheniramine (274), phenylephrine (447), phenylpropanolamine (448), methscopolamine, and salicylamide

Klonopin *44M* (illus.); see clonazepam 286

K-Lor see potassium chloride 540

Klor-con see potassium chloride 540

Klorvess see potassium chloride 540

Klotrix see potassium chloride 540

K-Lyte a combined preparation. See potassium bicarbonate (540) and potassium citrate

Kolantyl a combined preparation. See aluminum hydroxide (224) and magnesium hydroxide (386)

Kolyum a potassium supplement containing potassium gluconate (540) and potassium chloride (540)

Komed a combined preparation. See sodium thiosulfate, salicylic acid, and isopropyl alcohol

Konakion see phytonadione 450

Kondremul Plain a lubricant laxative containing mineral oil. See Laxatives 139

Konsyl see psyllium 473

Koromex Foam, Cream, Jelly a combined preparation. See nonoxynol 9 and octoxynol

K-Phos a combined preparation. See potassium (540), sodium (542), and phosphorus

Kronofed a combined preparation. See chlorpheniramine (274) and pseudoephedrine (472)

K

Kronohist a combined preparation. See chlorpheniramine (274), phenylpropanolamine (448), and pyrilamine

K-Tab see potassium chloride 540

Kudrox a combined preparation. See aluminum hydroxide (224) and magnesium hydroxide (386)

KU Zyme see pancrelipase

Kwell see lindane 380

Kwildane see lindane 380

KY Jelly a vaginal lubricant

L

labetalol 374

LaBID see theophylline 506

Lac-Hydrin see propylene glycol

Lacril see hydroxypropylmethylcellulose

Lacrisert see hydroxypropylcellulose

LactiCare an oil-in-water emulsion. See Bases for skin preparations 203

Lactinex an over-the-counter *medication* containing material from bacteria that are naturally present in milk. It is used in the treatment of diarrhea. See Antidiarrheal drugs 138

Lactocal-F a multivitamin preparation. See Vitamins 177

lactose a constituent of milk sometimes used as a laxative (139) or diuretic (127)

lactulose 375

Lanacort see hydrocortisone 358

Laniazid see isoniazid 367

lanolin a fatty substance obtained from sheep wool and used as a base for *emollient* ointments and cosmetics. See Bases for skin preparations 203

Lanorinal a combined preparation. See aspirin (238), butalbital, and caffeine

Lanoxicaps see digoxin 314

Lanoxin *41G, 52C* (illus.); see digoxin 314

Larobec a multivitamin preparation. See Vitamins 177

Larodopa *35N* (illus.); see levodopa 376

Larotid see amoxicillin 234

Larylgan a spray with an analgesic effect that relieves a dry or irritated throat

Lasan Cream see anthralin 237

Lasan HP see anthralin 237

Lasix *51Q, 54S* (illus.); see furosemide 344

Ledercillin VK *49E, 50F* (illus.); see penicillin V 440

Lente see insulin 364

leucovorin an injectable form of folic acid 537

Leukeran see chlorambucil 269

leuprolide a hormonal anticancer drug 182

levamisole an anthelmintic drug 167

Levlen a combined preparation. See ethinyl estradiol (334) and levonorgestrel

LEVOBUNOLOL – METHARBITAL

METHAZOLAMIDE – NASALCROM

M

methazolamide a carbonic anhydrase inhibitor diuretic (127) used primarily to treat glaucoma (196)

methdilazine an antihistamine 152

methenamine a drug used to treat infections of the urinary tract. See Drugs used for urinary disorders 194

Methergine see methylergonovine

methicillin a penicillin antibiotic 156

methimazole 400

methocarbamol 401

methohexital a barbiturate drug used to induce general *anesthesia*

methotrexate 402

methoxsalen 403

methoxyflurane a volatile substance the fumes of which are inhaled to induce general *anesthesia*

methscopolamine an *anticholinergic, antispasmodic* drug used to treat irritable bowel syndrome 138

methsuximide an anticonvulsant drug 114

methyclothiazide a thiazide diuretic 127

methylbenzethonium a skin antiseptic. See Anti-infective skin preparations 203

methyl-CCNU see semustine

methylcellulose 404

methyldopa 405

methylene blue a dye used in preparations for urinary tract infections 194

methylergonovine a uterine stimulant. See Drugs used in labor 193

methylformamide an *investigational* anticancer drug 182

methyl-glyoxalbis-guanylhydrazone an anticancer drug 182

methylparaben a preservative included in some skin preparations

methylphenidate an amphetamine-like drug used by some physicians in the treatment of hyperactive children. See Nervous system stimulants 116

methylprednisolone 406

methyl salicylate an analgesic in *rubefacient* preparations to relieve muscle and joint pain

methyltestosterone a testosterone drug. See Male sex hormones 174

methyprylon a non-barbiturate, non-benzodiazepine sleeping drug 110

methysergide a drug used to prevent migraine. See Drugs used for migraine 117

Meticorten see prednisone 457

Metimyd a combined preparation. See prednisolone (456) and sulfacetamide (491)

metoclopramide 408

metocurine a muscle-relaxant drug used in surgical procedures. See Muscle-relaxant drugs 148

metolazone 409

Metopirone see metyrapone

metoprolol 410

M

Metreton see prednisolone 456

metrifonate an *investigational* anthelmintic drug 167

Metronid see metronidazole 411

metronidazole 411

Metryl *50 O, 55F* (illus.); see metronidazole 411

metyrapone an *investigational* drug used to block production of adrenal hormones in Cushing's syndrome

metyrosine an antihypertensive drug 130

Mevacor see lovastatin

Mexate, Mexate AQ see methotrexate 402

mexiletine an *investigational* anti-arrhythmic drug. See Anti-arrhythmic drugs 128

mezlocillin a penicillin antibiotic 156

Micatin see miconazole 412

miconazole 412

Micrainin a combined preparation. See aspirin (238) and meprobamate (397)

Micro-K see potassium 540

Micronase *43J* (illus.); see glyburide 348

Micronefrin see epinephrine 328

Micronor see norethindrone

Midamor *41E* (illus.); see amiloride 226

midazolam a benzodiazepine drug used mainly as *premedication*

Midol 200 see ibuprofen 360

Midrin a combined preparation. See acetaminophen (215), dichloralphenazone, and isometheptene

Milkinol a lubricant laxative containing mineral oil. See Laxatives 139

Milk of Magnesia see magnesium hydroxide 386

Milpath a combined preparation. See meprobamate (397) and tridihexethyl chloride

Milprem a combined preparation. See conjugated estrogens (295) and meprobamate (397)

milrinone a drug used to treat heart failure. See Digitalis drugs 124

Miltown *48R* (illus.); see meprobamate 397

mineral oil also known as liquid petrolatum. Used as a lubricant laxative (139) and in skin preparations (203)

Minipress *60G, 63B* (illus.); see prazosin 455

Minocin *39G, 56M* (illus.); see minocycline

minocycline a tetracycline antibiotic 156

minoxidil 413

Mintezol *48A* (illus.); see thiabendazole 507

Miochol see acetylcholine

misoprostol a prostaglandin drug under investigation for the treatment of peptic ulcers

mitolactol an *investigational* anticancer drug 182

mitomycin a cytotoxic antibiotic. See Anticancer drugs 182

mitotane an anticancer drug 182

mitoxantrone an anticancer drug 182

Mitrolan see polycarbophil calcium

M

Mity-Quin a combined preparation. See hydrocortisone (358) and clioquinol

Mixtard see insulin 364

Moban see molindone

Mobidin see magnesium salicylate

Mobigesic a combined preparation. See magnesium salicylate and phenyltoloxamine

Modane see danthron

Modicon a combined preparation. See ethinyl estradiol (334) and norethindrone

Modrastane see trilostane

Moduretic *38P* (illus.); a combined preparation. See amiloride (226) and hydrochlorothiazide (357)

Moisturel an oil-in-water emulsion. See Bases for skin preparations 203

molindone an antipsychotic drug 113

Mol-Iron see ferrous sulfate

Monistat see miconazole 412

monobenzone a *topically* applied drug used to remove skin pigmentation in the treatment of severe vitiligo

Monocid see cefonicid

Mono-Gesic see salsalate

monosulfiram a drug used to treat scabies. See Drugs to treat skin parasites 204

moricizine an *investigational* phenothiazine drug used to treat abnormal heart rhythms. See Antiarrhythmic drugs 128

morphine 414

Motrin *36R, 38T* (illus.); see ibuprofen 360

moxalactam a cephalosporin antibiotic 156

Moxam see moxalactam

MS Contin see morphine 414

Mucomyst see acetylcysteine 218

Murine Plus see tetrahydrozoline 505

Murocel see methylcellulose 404

Murocoll-2 see phenylephrine 447

muromonab CD3 an immunosuppressant drug (184) used to prevent organ rejection following transplant surgery

Muro's Opcon-A a combined preparation. See naphazoline (419) and pheniramine

Muro tears see hydroxypropylmethylcellulose

Mutamycin see mitomycin

Myadec a multivitamin and mineral preparation. See Vitamins 177

Myambutol *48E* (illus.); see ethambutol 333

Mycelex see clotrimazole 289

Mycifradin see neomycin 421

Myciguent see neomycin 421

Mycitracin a combined preparation. See bacitracin (243) and neomycin (421)

Mycolog see triamcinolone 519

Mycolog II Cream a combined preparation. See nystatin (429) and triamcinolone (519)

Mycostatin *45K* (illus.); see nystatin 429

M

Myco-Triacet a combined preparation. See triamcinolone (519) and nystatin (429)

Mydfrin see phenylephrine 447

Mydriacyl see tropicamide

Myidil see triprolidine 527

Myidone see primidone 459

Mykinac see nystatin 429

Mylanta a combined preparation. See aluminum hydroxide (224), magnesium hydroxide (539), and simethicone

Myleran see busulfan

Mylicon see simethicone

Myobid see papaverine 437

Myochrysine see gold sodium thiomalate

Myoflex see trolamine

Mysoline *49P, 52 I* (illus.); see primidone 459

Mysteclin-F *61 I* (illus.); a combined preparation. See amphotericin B (235) and tetracycline (504)

Mysteclin-F Syrup a combined preparation. See amphotericin B (235) and tetracycline (504)

Mytrex see triamcinolone 519

N

nabilone a drug used to treat nausea caused by anticancer drugs. See Anti-emetic drugs 118

nadolol 415

nafcillin a penicillin antibiotic 156

nalbuphine a narcotic analgesic 108

Naldecon *47J* (illus.); a combined preparation. See chlorpheniramine (274), codeine (291), dextromethorphan (307), phenylpropanolamine (448), and guaifenesin

Nalfon *39 O, 61L* (illus.); see fenoprofen 338

nalidixic acid 416

naloxone 417

naltrexone a drug used in the treatment of narcotic dependence. See Drug dependence 23

Nandrolin see nandrolone 418

nandrolone 418

naphazoline 419

Naphcon see naphazoline 419

Naprosyn *38J, 41C, 41D* (illus.); see naproxen 420

naproxen 420

Naqua see trichlormethiazide

Naquival a combined preparation. See reserpine and trichlormethiazide

Narcan see naloxone 417

Nardil *36S* (illus.); see phenelzine (444)

Nasahist a combined preparation. See chlorpheniramine (274), phenylephrine (447), and phenylpropanolamine (448)

Nasahist B see brompheniramine 253

Nasalcrom see cromolyn sodium 298

NASALIDE – OTIC-HC

N

Nasalide see flunisolide

Natabec a multivitamin and mineral preparation. See Vitamins 177

Natafort a multivitamin and mineral preparation. See Vitamins 177

Natalins a multivitamin and mineral preparation. See Vitamins 177

natamycin a drug used to treat fungal infections of the eye. See Antifungal drugs 166

Naturacil see psyllium 473

Nature's Remedy see cascara

Naturetin see bendroflumethiazide

Navane see thiothixene

ND-Stat see brompheniramine 253

Nebcin see tobramycin 512

NegGram *41J, 41M* (illus.); see nalidixic acid 416

Nembutal see pentobarbital

Neo-Calglucon see calcium glubionate

Neo-Cortef a combined preparation. See hydrocortisone (358) and neomycin (421)

NeoDecadron see dexamethasone 306

neomycin 421

Neo-Polycin see neomycin 421

Neoquess see dicyclomine 310

Neosar see cyclophosphamide 300

Neosporin a combined preparation. See bacitracin (243) and neomycin (421)

Neosporin Ophthalmic Solution a combined preparation. See gramicidin (349), neomycin (421), and polymyxin B

neostigmine 422

Neo-Synalar a combined preparation. See fluocinolone (340) and neomycin (421)

Neo-Synephrine 12 Hour see oxymetazoline 434

Neo-Tears see hydroxyethylcellulose with thimerosal and edetate disodium

Neotep a combined preparation. See chlorpheniramine (274) and phenylephrine (447)

Neothylline see dyphylline

Nephrocaps a multivitamin and mineral preparation. See Vitamins 177

Neptazane see methazolamide

Nesacaine see chloroprocaine

Nestabs FA a multivitamin and mineral preparation. See Vitamins 177

netilmicin 423

Netromycin see netilmicin 423

Neutrogena see coal tar

niacin 539

niacinamide see niacin 539

Niclocide see niclosamide 424

niclosamide 424

Nicobid see niacin 539

Nico-400 see niacin 539

nicotine 553

Nico-vert see dimenhydrinate

nifedipine 425

N

Niferex a multivitamin and mineral preparation. See Vitamins 177

nifurtimox an antiprotozoal drug 164

Nilstat see nystatin 429

nimodipine a calcium channel blocker (129). See Drugs used for migraine 117

niridazole an *investigational* anthelmintic drug 167

Nisentil see alphaprodine

Nitoman see tetrabenazine

Nitro-Bid *60T, 61Q* (illus.); see nitroglycerin 427

Nitrodisc see nitroglycerin 427

Nitro-Dur see nitroglycerin 427

nitrofurantoin 426

nitrofurazone a *topical* antibacterial drug (159). See Anti-infective skin preparations 203

nitrogen mustard see mechlorethamine

nitroglycerin 427

Nitrol see nitroglycerin 427

Nitrolingual spray see nitroglycerin 427

Nitropress see sodium nitroprusside

Nitrospan see nitroglycerin 427

Nitrostat *53C* (illus.); see nitroglycerin 427

nitrous oxide a gas used to induce *anesthesia*. See Drugs used in labor 193

Nivea an oil-in-water emulsion. See Bases for skin preparations 203

Nizoral *50A* (illus.); see ketoconazole 372

Noctec *56A* (illus.); see chloral hydrate 268

Nolahist see phenindamine

Nolamine *35G* (illus.); a combined preparation. See chlorpheniramine (274), propanolamine (448), and phenindamine

Noludar see methyprylon

Nolvadex see tamoxifen 498

nonoxynol 9 a spermicide used in contraceptive foams, creams, and gels

Norcet a combined preparation. See acetaminophen (215) and hydrocodone

Nordette 28, Nordette *36A, 38G* (illus.); a combined preparation. See ethinyl estradiol (334) and levonorgestrel

norepinephrine a naturally occurring *neurotransmitter* given to treat shock

norethindrone a progestin drug. See Female sex hormones 175

norethisterone an *investigational* progestin drug. See Female sex hormones 175

norethynodrel a progestin drug. See Female sex hormones 175

Norflex *50P* (illus.); see orphenadrine 430

norfloxacin an *investigational* urinary tract antiseptic. See Antibacterial drugs 159

Norgesic, Norgesic Forte a combined preparation. See aspirin (238), orphenadrine (430), and caffeine

norgestrel 428

Norinyl a combined preparation. See mestranol and norethindrone

N

Norlestrin a combined preparation. See ethinyl estradiol (334) and norethindrone

Norlutate see norethindrone

Norlutin see norethindrone

Normodyne *46C* (illus.); see labetalol 374

Noroxin *38K* (illus.); see norfloxacin

Norpace *58Q, 61H* (illus.); see disopyramide 320

Norpace CR *59H* (illus.); see disopyramide 320

Norpramin *39L, 42Q* (illus.); see desipramine 305

Nor-Q-D see norethindrone

nortriptyline a tricyclic antidepressant 112

noscapine a cough suppressant. See Drugs to treat coughs 122

Nostrilla see oxymetazoline 434

Notezine see diethylcarbamazine

Novafed see pseudoephedrine 472

Novafed A *58E* (illus.); a combined preparation. See chlorpheniramine (274) and pseudoephedrine (472)

Novahistine DMX a combined preparation. See dextromethorphan (307), pseudoephedrine (472), and guaifenesin

Novocain see procaine 463

Novolin L, N, R see insulin 364

NPH Insulin see insulin 364

Nubain see nalbuphine

Nucofed a combined preparation. See codeine (291) and pseudoephedrine (472)

Numorphan see oxymorphone

Nupercainal see dibucaine

Nuprin *40L* (illus.); see ibuprofen 360

Nutracort see hydrocortisone 358

Nutraderm Cream an oil-in-water emulsion. See Bases for skin preparations 203

Nutraplus see urea

Nydrazid see isoniazid 367

nylidrin a drug used to improve blood flow to the limbs in peripheral vascular disease. See Vasodilators 126

nystatin 429

Nystex see nystatin 429

O

Obermine see phentermine

Obetrol an appetite suppressant containing amphetamine and dextroamphetamine. See Nervous system stimulants 116

Occlusal see salicylic acid

octoxynol a spermicide used in vaginal contraceptive creams

Ocusert Pilo see pilocarpine 451

Ogen see estropipate

omeprazole an *investigational* anti-ulcer drug 137

Omnipen *60R, 60S* (illus.); see ampicillin 236

O

Omnipen-N see ampicillin 236

Oncovin see vincristine

Ophthaine see proparacaine

Ophthetic see proparacaine

Ophthochlor see chloramphenicol 270

Ophthocort a combined preparation. See chloramphenicol (270), hydrocortisone (358), and polymyxin B

opium a natural substance containing morphine (414). Opium, derived from the opium poppy, was formerly used in many medications. Highly addictive, opium is now seldom used, but its derivatives and synthetic versions of these (narcotics) are used as analgesics (108), cough suppressants (122), and antidiarrheal drugs (138)

Opti-clean a contact lens cleaning solution

Opticrom see cromolyn sodium 298

Optigene 3 see tetrahydrozoline 505

Optilets-M-500 a multivitamin and mineral preparation. See Vitamins 177

Optimine see azatadine 241

Optimyd a combined preparation. See prednisolone (456) and sulfacetamide (491)

Orabase HCA see hydrocortisone 358

Orajel see benzocaine 247

Oramide see tolbutamide 514

Orap see pimozide

Orasone *43M* (illus.); see prednisone 457

Orazinc see zinc 546

Oretic see hydrochlorothiazide 357

Oreticyl a combined preparation. See hydrochlorothiazide (357) and deserpidine

Oreton Methyl see methyltestosterone

Orgatrax see hydroxyzine 359

Orinase *48 I, 49R* (illus.); see tolbutamide 514

Ornade a combined preparation. See chlorpheniramine (274) and phenylpropanolamine (448)

Ornex a combined preparation. See acetaminophen (215) and phenylpropanolamine (448)

ornidazole an antiprotozoal drug 164

orphenadrine 430

Ortho-Novum 1/35 a combined preparation. See ethinyl estradiol (334) and norethindrone

Ortho-Novum 1/50 *41Q* (illus.); a combined preparation. See ethinyl estradiol (334), norethindrone, and mestranol

Ortho-Novum 7/7/7 *38E* (illus.); a combined preparation. See ethinyl estradiol (334) and norethindrone

Ortho-Novum 10/11 *38F* (illus.); a combined preparation. See ethinyl estradiol (334) and norethindrone

Orudis *59J, 59 O* (illus.); see ketoprofen 373

Os-Cal a combined preparation. See calcium (535) and vitamin D (545)

Osmoglyn see glycerin

Otic-HC a combined preparation. See hydrocortisone (358), chloroxylenol, and pramoxine

OTOBIOTIC – PILOPINE HS GEL

O

Otobiotic a combined preparation. See hydrocortisone (358) and polymyxin B

Otocort a combined preparation. See hydrocortisone (358) and neomycin (421)

Otrivin see xylometazoline 532

ouabain see digitalis drugs 124

Ovcon a combined preparation. See ethinyl estradiol and norethindrone

Ovral *52L* (illus.); a combined preparation. See ethinyl estradiol (334) and norgestrel (428)

Ovrette see norgestrel 428

O-V Statin see nystatin 429

Ovulen a combined preparation. See ethynodiol and mestranol

oxacillin a penicillin antibiotic 156

Oxalid see oxyphenbutazone

oxandrolone 431

oxazepam 432

oxprenolol a beta blocker 125

Oxsoralen *56F* (illus.); see methoxsalen 403

oxtriphylline 433

oxybenzone a sunscreening agent 207

oxybutynin an *anticholinergic* drug used to treat incontinence. See Drugs used for urinary disorders 194

oxychlorosene a *topical* antiseptic. See Drugs used for urinary disorders 194

oxycodone a narcotic analgesic 108

oxymetazoline 434

oxymetholone an anabolic steroid 174

oxymorphone a narcotic analgesic 108

oxyphenbutazone a non-steroidal anti-inflammatory drug 144

oxyphencyclimine an *anticholinergic antispasmodic* used in the treatment of irritable bowel syndrome 138

oxyphenonium an *anticholinergic antispasmodic* used in the treatment of irritable bowel syndrome 138

oxyquinoline a preservative with antimicrobial properties used in *topical* preparations

oxytetracycline 435

oxytocin 436

P

P-200 see papaverine 437

Pamabrom a weak diuretic (127) often combined with an analgesic to relieve premenstrual syndrome. See Drugs used to treat menstrual disorders 188

Pamelor *58S* (illus.); see nortriptyline

Pamine see methscopolamine

Pancrease see pancrelipase

pancreatin a preparation of pancreatic hormones. See Agents used in disorders of the pancreas 142

P

pancrelipase a preparation of pancreatic hormones. See Agents used in disorders of the pancreas 142

pancuronium a muscle-relaxant drug 148

Panmycin see tetracycline 504

Panoxyl, Panoxyl AQ see benzoyl peroxide 248

panthenol see pantothenic acid 540

Pantopon a combined preparation. See morphine (414) and opium

pantothenic acid 540

Panwarfin see warfarin 531

papaverine 437

para-aminobenzoic acid a sunscreening agent 207

Paraflex *37P* (illus.); see chlorzoxazone 278

Parafon Forte *42E* (illus.); a combined preparation. See acetaminophen (215) and chlorzoxazone (278)

paraldehyde an anticonvulsant drug 114

paramethadione an anticonvulsant drug 114

paramethasone a corticosteroid drug 169

paregoric a narcotic analgesic drug, also called camphorated opium tincture. See Antidiarrheal drugs 138

Parlodel *52E, 61K* (illus.); see bromocriptine 252

Parmine see phentermine

Parnate see tranylcypromine

paromomycin an anthelmintic drug 167

Parsidol see ethopropazine

P.A.S. para-aminosalicylic acid. See Aminosalicylic acid 230

Pathibamate see meprobamate 397

Pathocil see dicloxacillin

Pavabid *62B* (illus.); see papaverine 437

Pavacen see papaverine 437

Paveral see codeine 291

Pavulon see pancuronium

Paxipam see halazepam

PBZ see tripelennamine

PCNU an *investigational* anticancer drug 182

pectin a natural gelling agent often included in antidiarrheal medications

PediaCare 1 see dextromethorphan 307

Pediacof a combined preparation. See chlorpheniramine (274), codeine (291), phenylephrine (447), and potassium iodide

Pediaflor see sodium fluoride

Pediamycin see erythromycin 331

Pediazole a combined preparation. See erythromycin (331) and sulfisoxazole (495)

Peganone see ethotoin

pemoline a nervous system stimulant 116

Penapar VK see penicillin V 440

penbutolol a beta blocker 125

Penecort see hydrocortisone 358

penfluridol an antipsychotic drug 113

penicillamine 438

penicillin G 439

P

penicillin V 440

Penntuss see codeine 291

pentaerythritol tetranitrate a nitrate anti-angina drug 129

pentamidine an antiprotozoal drug 164

pentazocine a narcotic analgesic 108

pentetic acid an antidote used in certain types of radioactive isotope poisoning

Pentids *54E* (illus.); see penicillin G 439

pentobarbital a barbiturate sleeping drug 110

pentostatin an anticancer drug 182

Pentothal see thiopental

pentoxyfylline 441

Pentrax see coal tar

Pen-Vee-K *50K* (illus.); see penicillin V 440

Pepcid *46B, 46L* (illus.); see famotidine

peppermint oil used in medicine to treat indigestion and calm spasm of the bowel. See Drugs for irritable bowel syndrome 138

pepsin a digestive enzyme added to some combined preparations for the treatment of digestive disorders

Pepto Bismol see bismuth

Percocet-5 a combined preparation. See acetaminophen (215) and oxycodone

Percodan a combined preparation. See aspirin (238) and oxycodone

Percogesic a combined preparation. See acetaminophen (215) and phenyltoloxamine

Percorten see desoxycorticosterone

Perdiem see psyllium 473

pergolide an *investigational* antiparkinsonism drug 115

Pergonal see menotropins 395

Periactin *52H* (illus.); see cyproheptadine

Peri-Colace a combined preparation. See casanthranol and docusate

Peritrate see pentaerythritol tetranitrate

Permapen see penicillin G 439

permethrim a drug used in preparations for the treatment of head lice. See Drugs to treat skin parasites 204

Permitil see fluphenazine 342

perphenazine 442

Persa-gel see benzoyl peroxide 248

Persantine *35C, 35D, 36T* (illus.); see dipyridamole 319

Pertofrane *61A* (illus.); see desipramine 305

Pertussin see dextromethorphan 307

Peruvian balsam an ingredient of *topical* treatments for hemorrhoids. See Drugs for rectal and anal disorders 141

PETN see pentaerythritol tetranitrate

Petrogalar a lubricant laxative preparation containing mineral oil

petrolatum see mineral oil

Pfizerpen VK see penicillin V 440

P

Phazyme see simethicone

phenacemide an anticonvulsant drug 114

phenacetin a non-narcotic analgesic no longer used because of its adverse effects

Phenaphen see acetaminophen 215

Phenazine see phendimetrazine

phenazopyridine 443

phendimetrazine an appetite suppressant similar to the amphetamines. See Nervous system stimulants 116

phenelzine 444

Phenergan *51E* (illus.); see promethazine 468

Phenergan-D *47B* (illus.); a combined preparation. See promethazine (468) and pseudoephedrine (472)

Phenergan-VC a combined preparation. See phenylephrine (447) and promethazine (468)

phenformin an *investigational* oral antidiabetic drug. See Drugs used in diabetes 170

phenindamine an antihistamine 152

pheniramine an antihistamine 152

phenobarbital 445

phenol a skin antiseptic. See Anti-infective skin preparations 203

phenolphthalein a stimulant laxative 139

phenoxybenzamine a vasodilator used to treat hypertension. See Antihypertensive drugs 130

phenprocoumon a long-acting anticoagulant drug. See Drugs that affect blood clotting 132

phensuximide an anticonvulsant drug 114

phentermine an appetite suppressant similar to the amphetamines. See Nervous system stimulants 116

phentolamine an antihypertensive drug 130

Phenurone see phenacemide

phenylbutazone 446

phenylephrine 447

phenylpropanolamine 448

phenyl salicylate a non-narcotic analgesic similar to aspirin 238

phenyltoloxamine an antihistamine 152

phenytoin 449

pHisoHex see hexachlorophene

Phospholine Iodide see echothiophate

phosphorus a mineral occasionally included in vitamin and mineral supplements. See Vitamins 177

Phrenilin a combined preparation. See acetaminophen (215) and butalbital

Phyllocontin see aminophylline 229

physostigmine a *miotic* drug used to treat glaucoma 196

phytonadione 450

Pilocair see pilocarpine 451

pilocarpine 451

Pilocel see pilocarpine 451

Pilopine HS Gel see pilocarpine 451

PIMOZIDE – QUELIDRINE

P

pimozide an antipsychotic drug (113) used to treat movement disorders

pindolol a beta blocker 125

piperacillin a penicillin antibiotic 156

piperazine an anthelmintic drug 167

piperonyl butoxide a drug used in combination with pyrethrins to treat skin parasites 204

Pipracil see piperacillin

pirenzepine an *anticholinergic* drug sometimes used to treat peptic ulcers. See Anti-ulcer drugs 137

pirmenol an anti-arrhythmic drug 128

piroxicam 452

Pitocin see oxytocin 436

Pitressin see vasopressin 529

Placidyl see ethchlorvynol

Plaquenil see hydroxychloroquine

Platinol see cisplatin 282

Plegine see phendimetrazine

plicamycin an anticancer drug (182) also used to treat hypercalcemia (abnormally high levels of calcium in the blood)

podophyllin a drug used *topically* to treat warts

Polaramine see dexchlorpheniramine

polycarbophil calcium a laxative 139

Polycillin see ampicillin 236

Polycillin-PRB a combined preparation. See ampicillin (236) and probenecid (460)

Polycitra a combined preparation. See potassium (540), sodium citrate, and citric acid

polyestradiol an estrogen drug used to treat cancer of the prostate. See Anticancer drugs 182

polyethylene glycol an emulsifying agent used in skin preparations and in certain preparations for clearing the bowel. See Bases for skin preparations (203) and Laxatives (139)

Poly-Histine CS a combined preparation. See brompheniramine (253), codeine (291), and phenylpropanolamine (448)

Poly-Histine D a combined preparation. See phenylpropanolamine (448), pheniramine, phenyltoloxamine, and pyrilamine

Poly-Histine DM a combined preparation. See brompheniramine (253), dextromethorphan (307), and phenylpropanolamine (448)

Polymox amoxicillin 234

polymyxin B an antibacterial drug (159) mainly used *topically* to treat infections of the skin, eyes, and ears

Poly-Pred see prednisolone 456

polythiazide a thiazide diuretic 127

Poly-Vi-Flor a multivitamin preparation with fluoride and iron. See Vitamins 177

polyvinyl alcohol an ingredient of artificial tear preparations

Poly-Vi-Sol a multivitamin preparation with iron. See Vitamins 177

Pondimin see fenfluramine

P

Ponstel see mefenamic acid 392

Pontocaine see tetracaine 503

Posture a combined preparation. See calcium (535) and vitamin D (545)

potassium 540

potassium chloride a salt. See Potassium 540

potassium citrate an antacid (136) and mineral supplement. See Vitamins (177) and Potassium (540)

potassium clavulanate a drug added to some penicillin antibiotic products to prevent inactivation and increase antibacterial activity of the antibiotic. See Antibiotics 156

potassium gluconate a potassium salt. See Potassium 540

potassium iodide an antifungal drug (166) also used to treat thyrotoxicosis (172)

potassium permanganate a skin antiseptic. See Anti-infective skin preparations 203

Povan see pyrvinium

povidone-iodine a skin antiseptic. See Anti-infective skin preparations 203

Pragmatar a combined preparation. See coal tar, sulfur, and salicylic acid

pralidoxime an antidote used in cases of poisoning by certain pesticides

Pramet a multivitamin and mineral preparation. See Vitamins 177

Pramilet a multivitamin and mineral preparation. See Vitamins 177

Pramosone a combined preparation. See hydrocortisone (358) and pramoxine

pramoxine a local anesthetic 108

Prax see pramoxine

prazepam 453

praziquantel 454

prazosin 455

Precef see ceforanide

Pred Forte, Pred Mild see prednisolone 456

prednisolone 456

prednisone 457

Prefrin see phenylephrine 447

Pregnyl see HCG 355

Prelone see prednisolone 456

Preludin see phendimetrazine

Prelu-2 see phendimetrazine

Premarin *39S, 45D* (illus.); see conjugated estrogens 295

prenalterol a *sympathomimetic* drug used to treat heart failure

Prenate 90 a multivitamin and mineral preparation. See Vitamins 177

Presalin a combined preparation. See acetaminophen (215), aspirin (238), and salicylamide

prilocaine a local anesthetic 108

primaquine 458

Primatene Mist see epinephrine 328

P

Primaxin see cilastatin/imipenem

primidone 459

Principen *57T* (illus.); see ampicillin 236

Pro-Banthine *38H, 52R* (illus.); see propantheline

probenecid 460

probucol 461

procainamide 462

procaine 463

Procan SR *35E, 37D, 42R* (illus.); see procainamide 462

procarbazine 464

Procardia *56K* (illus.); see nifedipine 425

procaterol an *investigational* adrenergic bronchodilator 120

Prochlor-Iso see prochlorperazine 465

prochlorperazine 465

Proctocort see hydrocortisone 358

Proctofoam HC a combined preparation. See hydrocortisone (358) and pramoxine

procyclidine 466

Progens see conjugated estrogens 295

Proglycem see diazoxide

Progynon see estradiol 332

Pro-Iso see prochlorperazine 465

Prolamine see phenylpropanolamine 448

Prolixin *35L, 40K* (illus.); see fluphenazine 342

Proloprim *40T* (illus.); see trimethoprim 526

promazine 467

promethazine 468

Promist a combined preparation. See pseudoephedrine (472) and guaifenesin

Prompt see psyllium 473

Pronestyl SR see procainamide 462

Propacet 100 a combined preparation. See acetaminophen (215) and propoxyphene (469)

propafenone an anti-arrhythmic drug 128

propantheline an *anticholinergic antispasmodic* drug used to treat irritable bowel syndrome (138) and urinary incontinence (194)

proparacaine a local anesthetic 108

Prophene 65 see propoxyphene 469

Propine see dipivefrin

propoxyphene 469

propranolol 470

propylene glycol a moisturizing agent used in skin preparations 203

propylhexedrine a nasal decongestant 121

propylparaben a preservative added to skin preparations

propylthiouracil 471

Prorex see promethazine 468

ProSobee a multivitamin and mineral preparation. See Vitamins 177

Prostaphlin see oxacillin

Prostigmin see neostigmine 422

Prostin/15 see carboprost 259

P

Prostin VR Pediatric see alprostadil 223

protirelin a drug used to test thyroid and pituitary function. See Drugs for thyroid disorders 172

Protostat *55B, 55H* (illus.); see metronidazole 411

protriptyline a tricyclic antidepressant drug 112

Protropin see growth hormone (somatrem) 351

Proventil *50R, 52Q* (illus.); see albuterol 220

Provera *52A, 53G* (illus.); see medroxyprogesterone 391

Pseudo Bid a combined preparation. See pseudoephedrine (472) and guaifenesin

pseudoephedrine 472

Pseudo hist a combined preparation. See chlorpheniramine (274) and pseudoephedrine (472)

Psorigel see coal tar

psyllium 473

Purinethol *50G* (illus.); see mercaptopurine 398

Purodigin see digitoxin 313

PV Carpine see pilocarpine 451

P V Tussin a combined preparation. See chlorpheniramine (274), phenylephrine (447), guaifenesin, hydrocodone, phenindamine, and pyrilamine

Pyocidin-Otic a combined preparation. See hydrocortisone (358) and polymyxin B

pyrantel 474

pyrazinamide 475

pyrethrins a drug used in combination with piperonyl butoxide to treat skin parasites 204

Pyridiate see phenazopyridine 443

Pyridium *45F, 45G* (illus.); see phenazopyridine 443

Pyridium Plus a combined preparation. See phenazopyridine (443), butabarbital, and hyoscyamine

pyridostigmine 476

pyridoxine 541

pyrilamine an antihistamine 152

pyrimethamine 477

pyrrobutamine an antihistamine 152

Pyrroxate a combined preparation. See acetaminophen (215), chlorpheniramine (274), and phenylpropanolamine (448)

pyrvinium an anthelmintic drug 167

Q

Quadrinal a combined preparation. See ephedrine (327), phenobarbital (445), theophylline (506), and potassium iodide

quazepam a benzodiazepine sleeping drug 110

Quelidrine a combined preparation. See chlorpheniramine (274), dextromethorphan (307), ephedrine (327), phenylephrine (447), ammonium chloride, and ipecac

QUESTRAN – SINULIN

Q

Questran see cholestyramine 279

Quibron *56S* (illus.); a combined preparation. See theophylline (506) and guaifenesin

Quibron-T SR *53T* (illus.); see theophylline 506

quinacrine 478

Quinaglute *48F* (illus.); see quinidine 479

Quinamm *48H* (illus.); see quinine 480

Quindan see quinine 480

quinestrol an estrogen drug. See Female sex hormones 175

quinethazone a thiazide-type diuretic 127

quinfamide an *investigational* antiprotozoal drug 164

Quinidex *46 O* (illus.); see quinidine 479

quinidine 479

quinine 480

Quinora see quinidine 479

Quiphile see quinine 480

R

R & C a combined preparation. See pyrethrins and piperonyl butoxide

Racet a combined preparation. See hydrocortisone (358) and clioquinol

ranitidine 481

Raudixin see rauwolfia serpentina

Rauwiloid see alseroxylon

rauwolfia serpentina an antihypertensive drug 130

Rauzide a combined preparation. See rauwolfia serpentina and bendroflumethiazide

razoxane an *investigational* anticancer drug 182

Rectal Medicone see benzocaine 247

Redisol see vitamin B₁₂ 544

Regitine see phentolamine

Reglan *39C* (illus.); see metoclopramide 408

Regonol see pyridostigmine 476

Regroton *36J* (illus.); see chlorthalidone 277

Rela see carisoprodol 260

Remegel a combined preparation. See aluminum hydroxide (224) and magnesium carbonate

Remsed see promethazine 468

Renacidin a solution used to dissolve kidney stones

Renese see polythiazide

rescinnamine an antihypertensive drug 130

reserpine an antihypertensive drug 130

resorcinol an ingredient of skin preparations for the treatment of acne, dermatitis, and fungal infections. See Anti-infective skin preparations 203

Respbid see theophylline 506

Respinol-G a combined preparation. See phenylephrine (447), phenylpropanolamine (448), and guaifenesin

Restoril *58C, 58G* (illus.); see temazepam 499

R

Retet see tetracycline 504

Reticulogen a combined preparation. See thiamine (543) and vitamin B₁₂ (544)

Retin-A see tretinoin 518

retinoic acid a derivative of vitamin A 543

Retrovir see zidovudine 533

Rhindecon see phenylpropanolamine 448

Rhinolar a combined preparation. See chlorpheniramine (274) and phenylpropanolamine (448)

Rhinosyn a combined preparation. See chlorpheniramine (274) and pseudoephedrine (472)

ribavirin a drug used in the prevention and treatment of viral infections. See Antiviral drugs 161

riboflavin 541

Rid a combined preparation. See piperonyl butoxide and pyrethrins

Ridaura see auranofin 240

Rifadin *58D, 61F* (illus.); see rifampin 482

Rifamate a combined preparation. See isoniazid (367) and rifampin (482)

rifampin 482

Rimactane *58H* (illus.); see rifampin 482

Rimactane INH a combined preparation. See isoniazid (367) and rifampin (482)

Rimso-50 see dimethyl sulfoxide

Ritalin see methylphenidate

ritodrine 483

Robaxin *37J, 39H* (illus.); see methocarbamol 401

Robaxisal a combined preparation. See aspirin (238) and methocarbamol (401)

Robicillin see penicillin V 440

Robimycin see erythromycin 331

Robinul see glycopyrrolate

Robitet see tetracycline 504

Robitussin DM a combined preparation. See dextromethorphan (307) and guaifenesin

Rocaltrol see calcitriol

Rocephin see ceftriaxone

Roferon-A see interferon 365

Ronase see tolazamide 513

Rondec-S a combined preparation. See carbinoxamine and pseudoephedrine (472)

Rondomycin see methacycline

Roxanol see morphine 414

RP-Mycin see erythromycin 331

Rubramin see cyanocobalamin

Rufen *35H, 54T* (illus.); see ibuprofen 360

Rubramin see cyanocobalamin

Ru-Tuss a combined preparation. See chlorpheniramine (274) and phenylephrine (447)

Ru-Vert-M see meclizine 389

Rynatan a combined preparation. See chlorpheniramine (274), phenylephrine (447), and pyrilamine

Rynatuss a combined preparation. See chlorpheniramine (274), ephedrine (327), phenylephrine (447), and carbetapentane

S

Safeguard an antimicrobial soap containing triclocarban. See Anti-infective skin preparations 203

SalAc see salicylic acid

salicylamide a non-narcotic analgesic similar to aspirin 238

salicylic acid a keratolytic drug applied *topically* to treat acne (205) and warts

salicylsalicylic acid see salsalate

Saligel see salicylic acid

salsalate a drug similar to aspirin used to treat arthritic disorders. See Non-steroidal anti-inflammatory drugs 144

Saluron see hydroflumethiazide

Salutensin a combined preparation. See hydroflumethiazide and reserpine

Sandimmune see cyclosporine 301

Sanorex see mazindol

Sansert *40 I* (illus.); see methysergide 407

Sarna Lotion menthol and camphor. See Antipruritic medications 201

SAS 500 see sulfasalazine 493

SAStid a combined preparation. See salicylic acid and sulfur

Satric 500 see metronidazole 411

Savacort-50 see prednisolone 456

Scabene see lindane 380

Schamberg's Lotion menthol and camphor. See Antipruritic medications 201

scopolamine an *anticholinergic, antispasmodic* drug used to treat motion sickness and irritable bowel syndrome. See Anti-emetic drugs (118) and Drugs for irritable bowel syndrome (138)

Scot-Tussin a cough relief preparation containing chlorpheniramine (274), dextromethorphan (307), and guaifenesin

Sebulex a combined preparation. See salicylic acid and sulfur

Sebulon an antidandruff shampoo containing zinc pyrithione

Sebutone a shampoo containing coal tar, salicylic acid, and sulfur

secnidazole an antiprotozoal drug 164

secobarbital 484

Seconal see secobarbital 484

Sectral *60 O, 61 G* (illus.); see acebutolol 214

Sedapap-10 a combined preparation. See acetaminophen (215) and butalbital

Seffin see cephalothin 266

Seldane *49J* (illus.); see terfenadine 501

selegiline an *investigational* dopamine-boosting drug related to the monoamine oxidase inhibitors. See Antiparkinsonism drugs 115

selenium 542

S

selenium sulfide an agent included in antidandruff shampoos and applied to the skin for the treatment of tinea versicolor. See Treatment for dandruff and hair loss 207

Selsun see selenium sulfide

Semets see benzocaine 247

Semicid spermicidal suppositories. See nonoxynol 9

semustine an alkylating agent. See Anticancer drugs 182

senna a stimulant laxative. See Laxatives 139

Senokot see senna

Septisol see triclosan

Septra *35P* (illus.); a combined preparation. See sulfamethoxazole (492) and trimethoprim (526)

Septra DS *35Q* (illus.); a combined preparation. See sulfamethoxazole (492) and trimethoprim (526)

Ser-Ap-Es *36L* (illus.); a combined preparation. See hydralazine (356), hydrochlorothiazide (357), and reserpine

Serax *58B, 58J* (illus.); see oxazepam 432

Serentil see mesoridazine

Serophene *51B* (illus.); see clomiphene 285

Serpasil see reserpine

Serpasil-Apresoline a combined preparation. See hydralazine (356) and reserpine

Serpate see reserpine

sevin see carbaryl

Shepard's Skin Cream an oil-in-water emulsion. See Bases for skin preparations 203

Silain-Gel a combined preparation. See aluminum hydroxide (224), magnesium hydroxide (386), and simethicone

Silvadene see silver sulfadiazine 485

silver nitrate a *topical* antibacterial drug. See Anti-infective skin preparations 203

silver sulfadiazine 485

Simeco see simethicone

simethicone a silicone-based substance included as an antifoaming agent in many medications for the relief of excess gas and indigestion. See Types of antacids 136

Simron see ferrous gluconate

Sine-Aid a combined preparation. See acetaminophen (215) and pseudoephedrine (472)

Sinemet *41B, 44G, 44K* (illus.); a combined preparation. See levodopa (376) and carbidopa

Sinequan *58A, 60J* (illus.); see doxepin 322

Singlet a combined preparation. See acetaminophen (215), chlorpheniramine (274), and phenylephrine (447)

Sinubid a combined preparation. See acetaminophen (215), phenylpropanolamine (448), and phenyltoloxamine

Sinufed see pseudoephedrine 472

Sinulin a combined preparation. See acetaminophen (215), chlorpheniramine (274), and phenylpropanolamine (448)

SINUTAB – TESTRED

S | **Sinutab** a combined preparation. See acetaminophen (215), chlorpheniramine (274), and pseudoephedrine (472)

Skelaxin see metaxolone

Slo-Bid *63F* (illus.); see theophylline 506

Slo-Phyllin *51G, 51 I* (illus.); see theophylline 506

Slo-Phyllin GG *57B* (illus.); a combined preparation. See theophylline (506) and guaifenesin

Slow FE see ferrous sulfate

Slow-K see potassium 540

sodium common (table) salt. See Sodium 542

sodium ascorbate a form of vitamin C 544

sodium bicarbonate 486

sodium biphosphate a drug used to reduce high calcium levels in the blood, as a laxative, and to increase acidity of the urine. See Laxatives (139) and Drugs used for urinary disorders (194)

sodium borate a substance with weak *astringent* and antibacterial properties often included in mouthwashes and gargles

sodium cellulose phosphate an agent used for reducing calcium in the urine

sodium citrate an antacid. See Antacids 136

sodium fluoride see fluoride 537

sodium iodide a form of iodine used to treat thyrotoxicosis (172) and thyroid cancers

sodium nitrate an injectable antidote to cyanide poisoning

sodium nitroprusside a vasodilator 126

sodium salicylate a drug similar to aspirin used to treat arthritic disorders. See Non-steroidal anti-inflammatory drugs 144

sodium thiosulfate a drug used *topically* to treat tinea infection of the skin, and given intravenously to treat cyanide poisoning

Solatene see beta carotene

Solfoton see phenobarbital 445

Solganal see aurothioglucose

Solu-Cortef see hydrocortisone 358

Solu-Medrol see methylprednisolone 406

Soma *48L* (illus.); see carisprodol 260

Soma Compound *47A* (illus.); a combined preparation. See aspirin (238) and carisoprodol (260)

Somophyllin, Somophyllin-DF see aminophylline 229

Somophyllin-CRT see theophylline 506

Somophyllin-T *57C* (illus.); see theophylline 506

Soothe see tetrahydrozoline 505

Soprodol see carisprodol 260

Sorbitrate see isosorbide dinitrate 369

sotalol a beta blocker 125

Sparine see promazine 467

Spectazole see econazole 325

spectinomycin an antibiotic used to treat gonorrhea. See Antibiotics 156

Spectrobid *55D* (illus.); see bacampicillin

S | **Spectrocin** a combined preparation. See gramicidin (349) and neomycin (421)

spironolactone 487

Spirozide see spironolactone 487

S-P-T see thyroid 509

SSKI see potassium iodide

Stadol see butorphanol

stanozolol an anabolic steroid 174

Staphcillin see methicillin

Staticin see erythromycin 331

Statobex see phendimetrazine

Statrol a combined preparation. See neomycin (421), benzalkonium chloride, methylparaben, and propylparaben

Stelazine *44 O, 44P, 44Q* (illus.); see trifluoperazine

Sterane see prednisolone 456

stibocaptate a drug used to eradicate blood fluke infections. See Anthelmintic drugs 167

stibogluconate a drug used to treat leishmaniasis. See Antiprotozoal drugs 164

Stilphostrol see diethylstilbestrol 311

Stoxil see idoxuridine 361

Streptase see streptokinase 488

streptokinase 488

streptomycin 489

streptozocin an anticancer antibiotic 182

Stuart Natal, Stuart Prenatal multivitamin and mineral preparations. See Vitamins 177

Sublimaze see fentanyl

succinylcholine a muscle-relaxant drug 148

sucralfate 490

Sucrets Cold Decongestant Formula see phenylpropanolamine 448

Sucrets Cough Control Formula see dextromethorphan 307

Sudafed see pseudoephedrine 472

sufentanil a narcotic analgesic 108

Sulamyd see sulfacetamide 491

Sulf-10 see sulfacetamide 491

sulfabenzamide an antibacterial drug 159

sulfacetamide 491

Sulfacet-R a combined preparation. See sulfacetamide (491) and sulfur

sulfacytine an antifungal drug 166

sulfadiazine an antifungal drug 166

sulfadoxine a drug used in combination with pyrimethamine in the prevention and treatment of malaria. See Antimalarial drugs 165

sulfamerazine a sulfonamide antibacterial drug 159

sulfamethazine a sulfonamide antibacterial drug 159

sulsulfamethizole a sulfonamide antibacterial drug 159

sulfamethoxazole 492

sulfamethoxazole-trimethoprim a combined preparation. See sulfamethoxazole (492) and trimethoprim (526)

S

sulfapyridine a sulfonamide antibacterial drug 159

sulfasalazine 493

sulfathiazole an antibacterial drug 159

sulfinpyrazone 494

sulfisoxazole 495

Sulfoxyl a combined preparation. See benzoyl peroxide (248) and sulfur

sulfur a mild *topical* antibacterial and antifungal agent used in preparations for acne (205) and dandruff (207)

sulindac 496

Sulphrin a combined preparation. See prednisolone (456) and sulfacetamide (491)

Sulqui see niclosamide 424

Sultrin a combined preparation. See sulfacetamide (491), sulfabenzamide, sulfathiazole, and urea

Sumox see amoxicillin 234

Sumycin *56D* (illus.); see tetracycline 504

Supen see ampicillin 236

Supprettes see belladonna 246

suprofen 497 (withdrawn in the US in 1987)

Suprol *59R* (illus.); see suprofen 497 (withdrawn in the US in 1987)

suramin an antiprotozoal (164) and anthelmintic drug (167)

Surbex a multivitamin preparation. See Vitamins 177

Surfak see docusate

Surital see thiamylal

Surmontil see trimipramine

Sus-Phrine see epinephrine 328

Sustaire see theophylline 506

Sutilains an agent applied *topically* to treat infected burns and skin ulcers. See Anti-infective skin preparations 203

Syllact see psyllium 473

Symmetrel *56B* (illus.); see amantadine 225

Synacort see hydrocortisone 358

Synalar see fluocinolone 340

Synalgos-DC a combined preparation. See aspirin (238), caffeine, and dihydrocodeine

Synemol see fluocinolone 340

Synkayvite see menadiol

Synophylate see theophylline 506

Synthroid see levothyroxine 377

Syntocinon see oxytocin 436

T

Tabloid see thioguanine

Tabron a multivitamin and mineral preparation. See Vitamins 177

Tacaryl see methdilazine

TACE see chlorotrianisene

Tagamet *43C, 43D* (illus.); see cimetidine 281

T

Talacen a combined preparation. See acetaminophen (215) and pentazocine

talbutal a barbiturate drug. See Sleeping drugs 110

Talwin see pentazocine

Talwin NX *37T* (illus.); a combined preparation. See naloxone (417) and pentazocine

Tambocor see flecainide

tamoxifen 498

Tandearil see oxyphenbutazone

TAO see troleandomycin

Tapar see acetaminophen 215

Tapazole *51A, 53B* (illus.); see methimazole 400

Taractan see chlorprothixene

Tavist-1 *55K* (illus.); see clemastine

Tazicef see ceftazidime

Tazidime see ceftazidime

Tear-Efrin see phenylephrine 447

Tearisol see hydroxypropylmethylcellulose

Tears Naturale see hydroxypropylmethylcellulose

Tedral *51 O* (illus.); a combined preparation. See ephedrine (327) and theophylline (506)

Teebacin aminosalicylate sodium. See aminosalicylic acid 230

Teebaconin see isoniazid 367

tegafur an antimetabolite anticancer drug 182

Tegison see etretinate 337

Tegopen *61R, 61S* (illus.); see cloxacillin 290

Tegretol *35T, 47 I* (illus.); see carbamazepine 258

Tegrin see coal tar

Teldrin see chlorpheniramine 274

Temaril *46R* (illus.); see trimeprazine 524

temazepam 499

Tempra see acetaminophen 215

teniposide an anticancer drug 182

Tenoretic *49Q, 51C* (illus.); a combined preparation. See atenolol (239) and chlorthalidone (277)

Tenormin *50Q, 52F* (illus.); see atenolol 239

Tensilon see edrophonium

Tenuate see diethylpropion

Tepanil see diethylpropion

Teramine see phentermine

terazosin a *sympatholytic* antihypertensive 130

terbutaline 500

terfenadine 501

Terfonyl see trisulfapyrimidines

terpin hydrate an expectorant. See Drugs to treat coughs 122

Terra-Cortril a combined preparation. See hydrocortisone (358) and oxytetracycline (435)

Terramycin see oxytetracycline 435

Tessalon see benzonatate

testolactone a hormonal anticancer drug 182

testosterone 502

Testred see methyltestosterone

TETRABENAZENE – TROFAN

T

tetrabenazene an *investigational* drug for the treatment of movement disorders such as chorea

tetracaine 503

tetrachloroethylene a drug used in hookworm infections. See Anthelmintic drugs 167

tetracycline 504

Tetracyn see tetracycline 504

tetrahydrozoline 505

Tetrex see tetracycline 504

Texacort see hydrocortisone 358

T/Gel see coal tar

Thalitone see chlorthalidone 277

Theo-24 *58 O, 58T* (illus.); see theophylline 506

Theobid see theophylline 506

Theoclear see theophylline 506

Theo-Dur *50B, 54J, 63D, 63E* (illus.); see theophylline 506

Theolair *49A* (illus.); a combined preparation. See theophylline (506) and guaifenesin

Theo-Organidin see theophylline 506

Theophyl see theophylline 506

theophylline 506

Theospan see theophylline 506

Theostat see theophylline 506

Theovent see theophylline 506

Theozine see hydroxyzine 359

Theragesic a combined preparation. See methyl salicylate and menthol

Theragran a multivitamin preparation with iron (538). See Vitamins 177

thiabendazole 507

thiamine 543

thiamylal a barbiturate used in general *anesthesia*

thiethylperazine an anti-emetic drug (118) often used with anticancer drugs (182)

thimerosal a mercury compound with antimicrobial and antiseptic properties. See Anti-infective skin preparations 203

thioguanine an anticancer drug 182

thiopental a fast-acting barbiturate used to induce general *anesthesia*

thioridazine 508

Thiosulfil see phenazopyridine 443

thiotepa an alkylating agent. See Anticancer drugs 182

thiothixene an antipsychotic drug 113

Thiuretic see hydrochlorothiazide 357

Thorazine *45T, 46A* (illus.); see chlorpromazine 275

thymoxamine a *miotic* drug used in the treatment of glaucoma. See Drugs for glaucoma 196

Thyrar see thyroid 509

thyroid 509

Thyroid Strong see thyroid 509

Thyrolar see liotrix

T

ticarcillin a penicillin antibiotic used for septicemia and skin, genitourinary, and respiratory infections. See Antibiotics 156

ticlopidine an antiplatelet drug. See Drugs that affect blood clotting 132

Tigan *57N, 60 I* (illus.); see trimethobenzamide 525

Timentin a combined preparation. See potassium clavulanate and ticarcillin

Timolide a combined preparation. See hydrochlorothiazide (357) and timolol (510)

timolol 510

Timoptic see timolol 510

Tinactin see tolnaftate 516

Tinactin Cream see tolnaftate 516

Tindal see acetophenazine

tinidazole an antiprotozoal drug 164

Tinver a combined preparation. See salicylic acid and sodium thiosulfate

tioconazole an *investigational* antifungal drug used in the treatment of tinea infections. See Antifungal drugs 166

tiopronin an *investigational* drug for the treatment of stones in the urinary tract

tissue-type plasminogen activator see TPA 511

Titralac see calcium carbonate.

tixocortol an *investigational* drug used in the treatment of inflammatory bowel disease 140

T-Ionate P.A. see testosterone 502

tobramycin 512

Tobrex see tobramycin 512

tocainide an anti-arrhythmic drug 128

tocopherol see vitamin E 545

tocopheryl acetate a vitamin E drug. See vitamin E 545

Tofranil *45M, 45N, 57S, 61J* (illus.); see imipramine 362

tolazamide 513

tolazoline a drug given to treat pulmonary hypertension in newborn infants

tolbutamide 514

Tolectin *48J, 56L* (illus.); see tolmetin 515

Tolinase *49M* (illus.); see tolazamide 513

tolmetin 515

tolnaftate 516

Tonocard *39T* (illus.); see tocainide

Topicort see desoximetasone

Topicycline see tetracycline 504

Topsyn see fluocinonide

Torecan see thiethylperazine

Tornalate see bitolterol

Totacillin see ampicillin 236

TPA 511

Trancopal see chlormezanone

Trandate *38L* (illus.); see labetalol 374

Transderm-Nitro see nitroglycerin 427

T

Transderm-Scop see scopolamine

Tranxene see clorazepate 288

tranylcypromine a monoamine oxidase inhibitor (MAOI). See Antidepressant drugs 112

Trasicor see oxprenolol

Travase see sutilains

trazodone 517

Trecator-SC see ethionamide 335

Tremin see trihexyphenidyl 523

Trental *35M* (illus.); see pentoxyfilline 441

tretinoin 518

Trexan see naltrexone

triacetin an antifungal agent used to treat tinea pedis. See Antifungal drugs 166

Triad a combined preparation. See acetaminophen (215), butalbital, and caffeine

Triafed-C see triprolidine 527

triamcinolone 519

Triaminic see phenylpropanolamine 448

triamterene 520

Triaprin a combined preparation. See acetaminophen (215) and butalbital

Triavil a combined preparation. See amitriptyline (232) and perphenazine (442)

triazolam 521

trichlormethiazide a thiazide diuretic 127

trichloroacetic acid a *topical* preparation containing salicylic acid used to treat warts

triclocarban an antimicrobial agent with antibacterial and antifungal actions used in bar soap. See Anti-infective skin preparations 203

triclosan an antimicrobial agent used in bar soap and wound-cleansing products

Tricodene a combined preparation. See chlorpheniramine (274), dextromethorphan (307), and phenylpropanolamine (448)

Tridesilon a combined preparation. See acetic acid and desonide

tridihexethyl chloride an *anticholinergic, antispasmodic* drug used in the treatment of irritable bowel syndrome 138

Tridil see nitroglycerin 427

Tridione see trimethadione

trientine a *chelating* agent used to remove excess copper in Wilson's disease

triethylenetetramine a *chelating* agent used to remove excess copper in Wilson's disease

trifluoperazine an antipsychotic drug 113

triflupromazine a phenothiazine antipsychotic (113) and anti-emetic drug (118)

trifluridine 522

Trigesic a combined preparation. See acetaminophen (215), aspirin (238), and caffeine

Trihexane see trihexyphenidyl 523

trihexyphenidyl 523

T

Tri-Hydroserpine a combined preparation. See hydralazine (356), hydrochlorothiazide (357), and reserpine

Trilafon *46Q* (illus.); see perphenazine 442

Tri-Levlen a combined preparation. See ethinyl estradiol (334) and levonorgestrel

Trilisate see sodium salicylate

trilostane a synthetic corticosteroid drug given to treat Cushing's syndrome. See Corticosteroids 169

trimazosin an antihypertensive drug 130

trimeprazine 524

trimethadione a drug used to treat absence seizures. See Anticonvulsant drugs 114

trimethaphan a drug given to reduce blood pressure in an emergency. See Antihypertensive drugs 130

trimethobenzamide 525

trimethoprim 526

trimipramine a tricyclic antidepressant drug 112

Trimox *57H, 59M* (illus.); see amoxicillin 234

Trimpex *54 I* (illus.); see trimethoprim 526

Trinalin *36Q* (illus.); a combined preparation. See azatadine (241) and pseudoephedrine (472)

Trind a combined preparation. See chlorpheniramine (274), dextromethorphan (307), and phenylpropanolamine (448)

Tri-Norinyl a combined preparation. See ethinyl estradiol (334) and norethindrone

Trinsicon a multivitamin and mineral preparation. See Vitamins 177

trioxsalen a psoralen drug used in PUVA treatment of psoriasis 206

tripelennamine an antihistamine 152

Triphasil *45P, 46G, 53A* (illus.); a combined preparation. See ethinyl estradiol (334) and levonorgestrel

Triphed see triprolidine 527

Tri-Phen-Chlor a combined preparation. See chlorpheniramine (274), phenylephrine (447), phenylpropanolamine (448), and phenyltoloxamine

triple antibiotic a combined preparation. See bacitracin (243), neomycin (421), and polymyxin B

Triple Sulfas a combined preparation. See sulfacetamide (491), sulfabenzamide, and sulfathiazole

triprolidine 527

Trisoralen see trioxsalen

trisulfapyrimidines a combined preparation. See sulfadiazine, sulfamerazine, and sulfamethazine

Tri-Vi-Flor a multivitamin preparation with fluoride (537). See Vitamins 177

Tri-Vi-Sol a multivitamin preparation. See Vitamins 177

Trobicin see spectinomycin

Trofan see tryptophan

TROLAMINE – VYTONE

T

trolamine an ingredient in ear drops for the removal of ear wax. See Drugs for ear disorders 199

troleandomycin a macrolide antibiotic 156

tromethamine a drug used to dissolve certain types of stones in the urinary tract

Tronolane see pramoxine

Tronothane see pramoxine

Tropicacyl see tropicamide

tropicamide a *mydriatic* drug. See Drugs affecting the pupil 198

Trymex see triamcinolone 519

trypsin an *enzyme* formed in the intestine that is administered as a drug in the treatment of indigestion

Tryptacin see tryptophan

tryptophan a non-benzodiazepine, non-barbiturate drug with effects and risks similar to those of the barbiturates. See Sleeping drugs 110

Trysul a combined preparation. See sulfacetamide (491), sulfabenzamide, and sulfathiazole

T-Stat see erythromycin 331

tubocurarine a muscle-relaxant drug 148

Tuinal a combined preparation. See secobarbital (484) and amobarbital

Tums see calcium carbonate

Tussagesic a combined preparation. See acetaminophen (215), dextromethorphan (307), phenylpropanolamine (448), pheniramine, and pyrilamine

Tussanil a combined preparation. See chlorpheniramine (274), phenylephrine (447), phenylpropanolamine (448), and pyrilamine

Tussar a combined preparation. See chlorpheniramine (274), codeine (291), dextromethorphan (307), and guaifenesin

Tussend a combined preparation. See pseudoephedrine (472) and hydrocodone

Tussionex a combined preparation. See hydrocodone and phenyltoloxamine

Tussi-Organidin a combined preparation. See chlorpheniramine (274) and codeine (291)

Tussi-Organidin DM see dextromethorphan 307

Tussirex a combined preparation. See codeine (291), phenylephrine (447), caffeine, pheniramine, sodium citrate, and sodium salicylate

Tuss-Ornade *60B* (illus.); a combined preparation. See phenylpropanolamine (448) and caramiphen

Twin-K see guaifenesin

Tylenol see acetaminophen 215

Tylenol with codeine *49 I* (illus.); a combined preparation. See acetaminophen (215) and codeine (291)

T

Tylox a combined preparation. See acetaminophen (215), and oxycodone

tyloxapol a mucolytic

Tympagesic Otic Solution a combined preparation. See benzocaine (247), phenylephrine (447), and antipyrine

Tyzine see tetrahydrozoline 505

U

Ultracef *62A* (illus.); see cefadroxil

undecylenic acid an antifungal agent effective in tinea pedis (athlete's foot). See Antifungal drugs 166

Unibase a combined preparation. See lanolin and petrolatum

Unilax a combined preparation. See danthron and docusate

Unipen see nafcillin

Uniphyl see theophylline 506

Unipres a combined preparation. See hydralazine (356), hydrochlorothiazide (357), and reserpine

Unisom see doxylamine

Unproco a combined preparation. See dextromethorphan (307) and guaifenesin

urea a natural breakdown product of proteins excreted in the urine. It is included in skin preparations for the treatment of dry, scaling skin conditions

Urecholine see bethanechol

Urex see methenamine

Urised *45E* (illus.); a combined preparation. See atropine, benzoic acid, hyoscyamine, methenamine, methylene blue, and phenyl salicylate

Urispas *49G* (illus.); see flavoxate 339

Uritabs a combined preparation. See atropine, benzoic acid, hyoscyamine, methenamine, methylene blue, and phenyl salicylate

Urobiotic-250 *59E* (illus.); a combined preparation. See oxytetracycline (435) and phenazopyridine (443)

Urodine see phenazopyridine 443

Urogesic a combined preparation. See phenazopyridine (443), atropine, hyoscyamine, and scopolamine

urokinase a thrombolytic drug. See Drugs that affect blood clotting 132

Uro-Phosphate a combined preparation. See methenamine and sodium biphosphate

ursodeoxycholic acid a drug used in the treatment of gallstones 142

Uticillin VK a combined preparation. See penicillin V (440) and potassium (540)

Uticort see betamethasone 250

Utimox see amoxicillin 234

V

Vacon see phenylephrine 447

Vagilia a combined preparation. See sulfisoxazole (495), allantoin, and aminacrine

Vaginex a cream for the relief of genital itching; contains tripelennamine. See Antipruritic medications 201

Vagitrol a vaginal cream containing sulfanilamide

Valdrene see diphenhydramine 317

Valergen see estradiol 332

Valertest, Valertest 1 a combined preparation. See estradiol (332) and testosterone (502)

Valisone see betamethasone 250

Valium *41F, 50T* (illus.); see diazepam 308

Valmid see ethinamate

valproic acid 528

Valrelease see diazepam 308

Vancenase see beclomethasone 245

Vanceril see beclomethasone 245

vancomycin an antibiotic used for certain penicillin and methicillin-resistant infections. See Antibiotics 156

Vanoxide-HC a combined preparation. See benzoyl peroxide (248) and hydrocortisone (358)

Vanseb a combined preparation. See salicylic acid and sulfur

Vaponefrin see epinephrine 328

Vaseline Petroleum Jelly a water-in-oil emulsion used to protect and lubricate dry skin

Vasocidin a combined preparation. See prednisolone (456) and sulfacetamide (491)

VasoClear see naphazoline 419

Vasocon see naphazoline 419

Vasocon-A a combined preparation. See naphazoline (419) and antazoline

Vasodilan *49L, 50N* (illus.); see isoxsuprine 371

vasopressin 529

Vasosulf see sulfacetamide (491)

Vasotec *45S, 53P* (illus.); see enalapril 326

Vatronol see ephedrine 327

V-Cillin-K *54G* (illus.); see penicillin V 440

vecuronium a muscle-relaxant drug 148

Veetids *38S, 55E* (illus.); see penicillin V 440

Velban see vinblastine

Velosef *60C* (illus.); see cephradine

Velosulin see (pork) insulin 364

Velvachol a combined preparation. See lanolin and petrolatum

Ventolin *52N* (illus.); see albuterol 220

Vepesid see etoposide

verapamil 530

Vermox *38D* (illus.); see mebendazole 388

V

Verrex a combined preparation. See podophyllin and salicylic acid

Verrusol a combined preparation. See cantharidin, salicylic acid, and podophyllin

Vesprin see promazine 467

Vibramycin *57 I, 59Q* (illus.); see doxycycline 324

Vibramycin IV see doxycycline 324

Vibra-Tabs *37N* (illus.); see doxycycline 324

Vicks a combined preparation. See dextromethorphan (307) and pseudoephedrine (472)

Vicodin a combined preparation. See acetaminophen (215) and hydrocodone

Vicon-C a multivitamin preparation. See Vitamins 177

vidarabine a drug applied *topically* and administered *systemically* to treat viral infections. See Antiviral drugs 161

Vi-Daylin a multivitamin preparation. See Vitamins 177

viloxazine a nervous system stimulant 116

vinblastine an anticancer drug 182

vincristine an anticancer drug 182

vindesine an anticancer drug 182

vioform see clioquinol

Viokase see pancrelipase

Vira-A see vidarabine

Viranol see salicylic acid

Virazole see ribavirin

viroptic see trifluridine 522

Visine a combined preparation. See tetrahydrozoline (505) and zinc sulfate

Visken see pindolol

Vistaril *59K, 59P* (illus.); see hydroxyzine 359

vitamin A 543

vitamin B$_1$ see thiamine 543

vitamin B$_2$ see riboflavin 541

vitamin B$_6$ see pyridoxine 541

vitamin B$_{12}$ 544

vitamin C 544

vitamin D 545

vitamin E 545

vitamin K$_1$ phytonadione. See Vitamin K 546

vitamin K$_3$ menadione. See Vitamin K 546

Vitron-C a combined preparation. See iron (538) and vitamin C (544)

Vivactil see protryptyline

Vivalin see viloxazine

Vi-Zac a multivitamin preparation with zinc (546). See Vitamins 177

Vontrol see diphenidol

Vosal Otic see acetic acid

Vosol HC a combined preparation. See hydrocortisone (358) and acetic acid

Voxsuprine see isoxsuprine 371

Vytone a combined preparation. See hydrocortisone (358) and iodoquinol

WANS – ZYMENOL

W

Wans a combined preparation. See pentobarbital and pyrilamine

warfarin 531

Wart-Off see salicylic acid

Wehless see phendimetrazine

Wellcovorin see leucovorin

Westcort see hydrocortisone 358

Whitfield's ointment a combined preparation. See benzoic acid and salicylic acid

Wigraine *48T* (illus.); see ergotamine 330

Wigrettes see ergotamine 330

Wilpowr see phentermine

Winstrol see stanozolol

witch hazel a soothing, mildly astringent agent used to alleviate irritation in genital and rectal areas

Wyamycin S *35J* (illus.); see erythromycin 331

Wyanoids a combined preparation. See belladonna (246), ephedrine (327), bismuth, boric acid, and Peruvian balsam

Wycillin see penicillin G 439

Wydase see hyaluronidase

Wygesic *42N* (illus.); a combined preparation. See acetaminophen (215) and propoxyphene (469)

Wymox *61 O, 61P* (illus.); see amoxicillin 234

Wytensin *53M* (illus.); see guanabenz

X

Xanax *54Q* (illus.); see alprazolam 222

Xerac see aluminum chloride

Xerac BP see benzoyl peroxide 248

X-Otag see orphenadrine 430

X-Prep see senna

X Seb see salicylic acid

Xylocaine, Xylocaine IM, Xylocaine IV, Xylocaine Oral Spray, Xylocaine Viscous Solution see lidocaine 378

Xylocaine with Epinephrine a combined preparation. See epinephrine (328) and lidocaine (378)

xylometazoline a decongestant 121

Y

Y-Itch see tetracaine 503

Yocon see yohimbine

Yodoxin see iodoquinol

yohimbine an antihypertensive drug 130

Yohimex see yohimbine

Yomesan see niclosamide 424

Yutopar *40C* (illus.); see ritodrine 483

Z

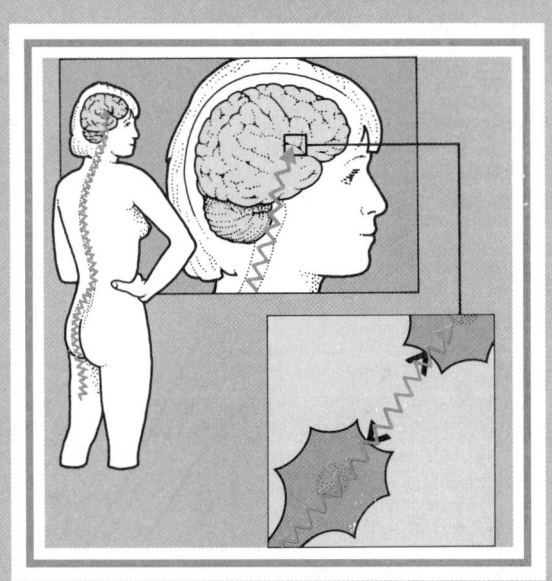

MAJOR DRUG GROUPS

BRAIN AND NERVOUS SYSTEM
RESPIRATORY SYSTEM
HEART AND CIRCULATION
GASTROINTESTINAL TRACT
MUSCLES, BONES AND JOINTS
ALLERGY
INFECTIONS AND INFESTATIONS
HORMONES AND ENDOCRINE SYSTEM
NUTRITION
MALIGNANT AND IMMUNE DISEASE
REPRODUCTIVE AND URINARY TRACTS
EYES AND EARS
SKIN

BRAIN AND NERVOUS SYSTEM

Relying on billions of nerve cells (neurons), the brain is the supervisory center of the nervous system. Receiving electro-chemical impulses from everywhere in the body, interpreting them and sending responsive signals back to various glands and muscles, the brain functions continuously as a switchboard for the human communications system. At the same time, it serves as the seat of emotions and mood, of memory, personality and thought. Extending from the brain is an additional cluster of nerve cells that forms the spinal cord. Together, these two elements compose the central nervous system.

Radiating from the central nervous system is the peripheral nervous system, which has three parts. One branches off the spinal cord and extends to muscles throughout the body. Another, in the head, links the brain to the eyes, ears, nose and taste buds. The third is a semi-independent network called the autonomic, or involuntary, nervous system. This is the part of the nervous system that controls unconscious body functions such as breathing, digestion, and glandular activity (see facing page).

Signals traverse the nervous system by electrical and chemical means. Electrical impulses carry signals from one end of a nerve cell to the other. To cross the gap between cells, chemical *neurotransmitters* are released from one cell to bind on to the *receptor* sites of nearby cells. *Excitatory* transmitters stimulate action; *inhibitory* transmitters reduce it.

What can go wrong

Disorders of the brain and nervous system range from conditions that are generally understood and frequently respond well to drug treatment – for example, epilepsy – to others, including psychoses such as schizophrenia, whose origins remain mysterious. These disorders yield to medical intervention only marginally.

Many authorities believe that an imbalance between the excitatory and inhibitory neurotransmitters usually explains such conditions as depression, anxiety, and prolonged insomnia. The same may be said about Parkinson's disease, caused by a deficiency of dopamine, an excitatory neurotransmitter. Electrical disturbances in certain brain neurons produce the seizures of epilepsy. Poor circulation of blood to the brain hastens the death of neurons and leads to everything from absent-mindedness to certain forms of dementia and senility. Temporary changes in blood circulation

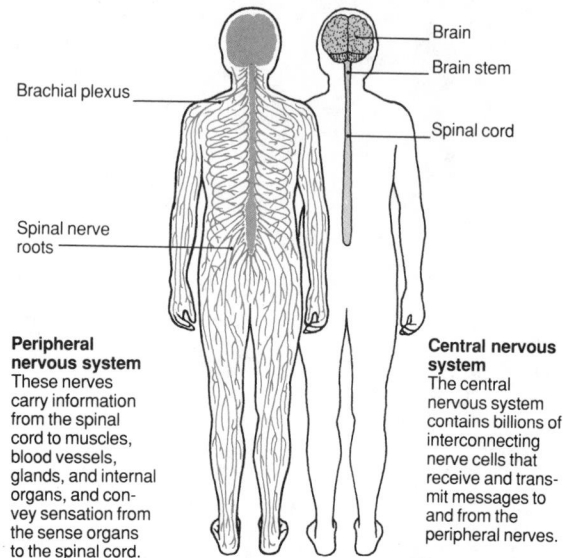

Peripheral nervous system
These nerves carry information from the spinal cord to muscles, blood vessels, glands, and internal organs, and convey sensation from the sense organs to the spinal cord.

Central nervous system
The central nervous system contains billions of interconnecting nerve cells that receive and transmit messages to and from the peripheral nerves.

How nerve signals are transmitted
A nerve signal is an electrical impulse produced by chemical reactions on the surface of the cell body of a neuron (nerve cell). The signal is transmitted by a neurotransmitter, released from the ends of a nerve fiber, that binds to a receptor on the neighboring cell body. This, in turn, transmits the signal to another neuron or triggers a response in a muscle or organ.

within and around the brain are thought to be the principal cause of migraine headaches.

Why drugs are used

By and large, the drugs described in this section do not eliminate nervous system disorders. What they do is correct or modify the communication of the signals that traverse the nervous system. By doing so they can relieve symptoms or restore normal functioning and behavior.

In some cases, such as anxiety and insomnia,

AUTONOMIC NERVOUS SYSTEM

The autonomic, or involuntary, nervous system governs the actions of the muscles of the organs and glands. Such vital functions as heartbeat, salivation, and digestion continue without conscious direction, whether we are awake or asleep.

The autonomic system is divided into two parts, the effects of one generally balancing those of the other. The *sympathetic* nervous system has an *excitatory* effect. It widens the airways to the lungs, for example, and increases the flow of blood to the arms and legs. The *parasympathetic* system, by contrast, has an opposing effect. It slows the heart rate and stimulates the flow of the digestive juices.

Although the functional pace of most organs results from the interplay between the two systems, the muscles surrounding the blood vessels respond only to the signals of the sympathetic system. What decides between the constriction or dilation of the vessels is the relative stimulation of two sets of receptor sites: alpha sites and beta sites.

Neurotransmitters

The parasympathetic nervous system depends on the neurotransmitter acetyl-choline to transmit signals from one cell to another. The sympathetic nervous system relies on epinephrine and norepinephrine, products of the adrenal glands that act as both hormones and neurotransmitters.

Drugs that act on the sympathetic nervous system

Drugs that stimulate the sympathetic nervous system are called adrenergics (or sympathomimetics, see chart). They either promote the release of epinephrine and norepinephrine or mimic their effects. Drugs which interfere with the action of the sympathetic nervous system are called sympatholytics. Alpha blockers act on alpha receptors; beta blockers act on beta receptors (see also Beta blockers, p.125).

Drugs that act on the parasympathetic nervous system

Drugs that stimulate the parasympathetic nervous system are called cholinergics (or parasympathomimetics), and drugs which oppose its action are called anticholinergics. Many drugs prescribed medically have anticholinergic properties (see chart, right).

Effects of stimulation of the autonomic nervous system

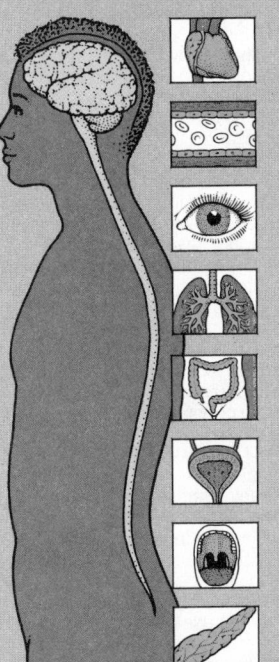

	Sympathetic	Parasympathetic
Heart	The rate and strength of the heartbeat are increased.	The rate and strength of the heartbeat are reduced.
Blood vessels in skin	These are constricted by stimulation of alpha receptors.	No effect.
Pupils	The pupils are dilated.	The pupils are constricted.
Airways	The bronchial muscles relax and widen the airways.	The bronchial muscles contract and narrow the airways.
Intestines	Activity of the muscles of the intestinal wall is reduced.	Activity of the muscles of the intestinal wall is increased.
Bladder	The bladder wall relaxes and the sphincter muscle contracts.	The bladder wall contracts and the sphincter muscle relaxes.
Salivary glands	Secretion of thick saliva increases.	Secretion of watery saliva increases.
Pancreas	Insulin secretion is increased (beta receptors) or reduced (alpha receptors).	Insulin secretion is increased.

Drugs that act on the autonomic nervous system

		Sympathetic	Parasympathetic
Stimulated by			
	Natural neurotransmitters	Epinephrine Norepinephrine	Acetylcholine
	Drugs	Adrenergic drugs (including alpha agonists, beta agonists) Sympathomimetics	Cholinergic drugs Parasympathomimetics
Blocked by			
	Drugs	Alpha blockers (antagonists) Beta blockers (antagonists)	Anticholinergic drugs

drugs encourage the action of inhibitory neuro-transmitters, lowering the level of activity. In other disorders – depression is an example – the excitatory neurotransmitters are stimulated.

Drugs that act on the nervous system are also used for conditions that outwardly have nothing to do with nervous system disorders. Migraine headaches, for example, are often treated with drugs which cause the autonomic nervous system to send out signals constricting the dilated blood vessels that cause the migraine.

MAJOR DRUG GROUPS

Analgesics
Sleeping drugs
Anti-anxiety drugs
Antidepressant drugs
Antipsychotic drugs

Anticonvulsant drugs
Antiparkinsonism drugs
Nervous system stimulants
Drugs used for migraine
Anti-emetic drugs

ANALGESICS

Analgesics are drugs that relieve pain. For many disorders, the relief of pain is one of the most important aspects of treatment. Since pain is not a disease but a symptom, long-term relief depends on treatment of the underlying cause. For example, the pain of toothache can be relieved by drugs but can only be cured by appropriate dental treatment.

Damage to body tissue as a result of disease or injury is detected by nerve endings that transmit signals to the brain, where they are interpreted. The interpretation of these sensations can be affected by the psychological state of the individual, so that pain is worsened by anxiety and fear, for example. Often a reassuring explanation of the cause of discomfort can make pain easier to bear and may even relieve it altogether. Because of these psychological factors, sleeping drugs, anti-anxiety drugs, or antidepressants are often prescribed in addition to, or instead of, analgesics.

Types of analgesics

Narcotics and non-narcotics are the two principal types of analgesics. Another group of drugs that are commonly used to relieve pain are the local anesthetics (see below). Narcotics are related to morphine and they are the most powerful analgesic drugs. Non-narcotic drugs are less powerful, and they include aspirin, acetaminophen, and non-steroidal anti-inflammatory drugs (NSAIDs).

SITES OF ACTION

Narcotic drugs (and acetaminophen) act on the brain and spinal cord to reduce the perception of a painful stimulus. Non-narcotic drugs act at the site of pain to prevent the stimulation of nerve endings.

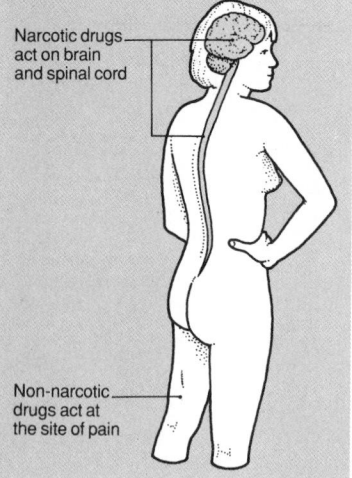

Narcotic drugs act on brain and spinal cord

Non-narcotic drugs act at the site of pain

Narcotics and acetaminophen act directly on the brain and spinal cord to alter the perception of pain. They thus act like the endorphins, local tissue hormones naturally produced in the brain that stop the cell-to-cell transmission of pain sensation. Non-narcotics (except for acetaminophen) prevent stimulation of the nerve endings at the site of the pain.

When pain is treated under medical supervision, it is common to start with a non-narcotic, and if this provides inadequate relief, to change to a combination drug (a mixture of a mild narcotic and a non-narcotic). A strong narcotic may be used if the less powerful drugs are ineffective. More severe (e.g., postoperative) or long-lasting continuous pain may be treated by injections of narcotics.

When treating pain with an over-the-counter preparation, for example, taking aspirin for a headache, you should seek medical advice if pain persists for longer than 48 hours, recurs, or is worse or different from previous pain.

Non-narcotic analgesics
Aspirin

Used for many years to relieve pain and reduce fever, aspirin also reduces inflammation by blocking the production of chemicals called prostaglandins, which contribute to swelling and pain in inflamed tissue (see Action of analgesics, facing page). Aspirin is useful for headaches, toothaches, mild rheumatic pain, sore throat, and discomfort caused by feverish illnesses. Given regularly, it can also relieve the pain and inflammation of chronic rheumatoid arthritis (see Antirheumatic drugs, p.145).

Aspirin is often found in combination with other substances in a variety of medicines (see Cold cures, p.122). Another use is in the treatment of some blood disorders, since an important effect of aspirin is that it helps to prevent abnormal clotting of blood (see Drugs that affect blood clotting, p.132). For this reason, it is not suitable for people whose blood does not clot normally.

LOCAL ANESTHETICS

These are used to prevent pain, usually in minor surgical procedures (for example, dental treatment and suturing lacerations). They can also be injected into the space around the spinal cord to numb the lower half of the body. This is called spinal or epidural anesthesia. Local anesthetics block the passage of nerve impulses at the site of administration, deadening all feeling at that site. They do not interfere with consciousness. Local anesthetics are usually given by injection, but they can also be applied to the skin to relieve pain caused by burns.

Local anesthetics occasionally cause the skin at the site of application to become red

ASPIRIN AND STOMACH IRRITATION

Regular aspirin can irritate the stomach, but buffered or coated aspirin preparations may offer some protection against this. Buffered aspirin is released in the stomach like regular aspirin, but contains drugs that reduce acidity and irritation. Coated preparations do not release aspirin until in the small intestine.

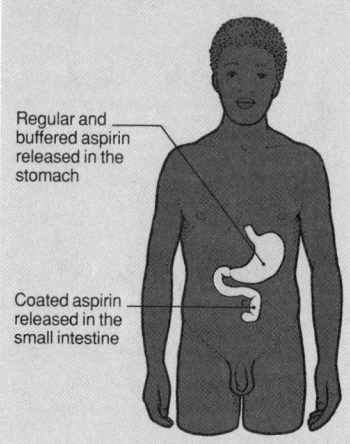

Regular and buffered aspirin released in the stomach

Coated aspirin released in the small intestine

Aspirin's major drawback is that it can cause irritation and even ulceration of the stomach and duodenum, possibly leading to bleeding. For this reason it is best taken after a meal. Specially formulated aspirin preparations designed to avoid irritating the stomach are available. These include buffered aspirin and coated aspirin. Buffered aspirin contains substances which reduce the acidity of the stomach contents and so may lessen irritation. The same or a similar effect may be obtained by taking regular aspirin with a regular dose of an antacid or a glass of milk. Coated aspirin and certain special aspirin capsules do not release the aspirin until they have passed through the stomach

and itchy, and if high doses of the anesthetic enter the bloodstream it may cause a number of adverse effects – restlessness, nausea, and tremors. Because such drugs may also lower blood pressure and disturb heart rhythm, they are given carefully to people with heart problems.

In order to restrict the anesthetic to the site of injection it is often given together with a *vasoconstrictor* drug such as epinephrine, which cuts down the blood supply at the site of injection and prevents the drug being carried away. This prolongs the action and minimizes the likelihood of side effects.

and have entered the small intestine (see Aspirin and stomach irritation, facing page). Aspirin in the form of soluble tablets, dissolved in water before being taken, is absorbed into the bloodstream quickly, relieving pain faster than tablets. Soluble aspirin is not, however, less irritating to the stomach.

Aspirin is available in many formulations, all of which have a similar effect. But because the amount of aspirin in a tablet of each type varies, it is important to read the packet for the correct dosage. Aspirin is not recommended for children suffering acute viral illnesses because its use has been linked to Reye's syndrome, a potentially fatal liver and brain disorder.

Acetaminophen

This is thought to act by reducing the production of prostaglandins in the brain. But, unlike aspirin, it does not affect prostaglandin production in the rest of the body and so does not reduce inflammation. Acetaminophen can be used for everyday aches and pains, such as headaches, toothache, and joint pains. It is given as a liquid for treating pain and reducing fever in children.

It is one of the safest of all analgesics when taken correctly. It does not usually irritate the stomach, and allergic reactions are rare. However, an overdose can cause severe and possibly irreversible liver and kidney damage that may be fatal. For this reason it is used with caution for people with kidney or liver disease. Drinking large quantities of alcohol may increase its toxic potential.

Non-steroidal anti-inflammatory drugs (NSAIDs)

These can relieve both pain and inflammation. NSAIDs are related to aspirin and also work by blocking the production of prostaglandins. They are most commonly used to treat muscle and joint pain and may also be prescribed for menstrual period pain. Like aspirin, NSAIDs can irritate the stomach lining and they are not usually given to people with stomach ulcers. For further information on these drugs, see p.144.

Narcotic analgesics

These are also called opioids and are related to opium, an extract of poppy seeds. They act directly on several sites in the central nervous system involved in pain perception, and block the transmission of pain signals (see Action of analgesics, above). Because they act directly on the parts of the brain where pain is perceived, narcotics are the most effective analgesics and are used to treat the pain arising from surgery, serious injury, and disease.

Morphine is the best known narcotic analgesic. Others include meperidine and

ACTION OF ANALGESICS

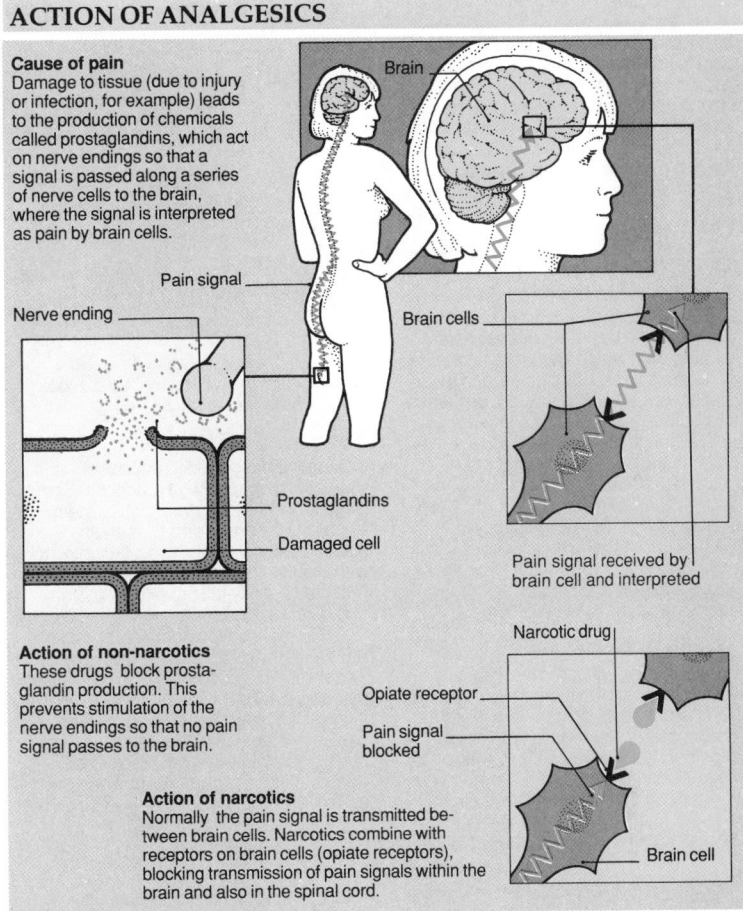

Cause of pain
Damage to tissue (due to injury or infection, for example) leads to the production of chemicals called prostaglandins, which act on nerve endings so that a signal is passed along a series of nerve cells to the brain, where the signal is interpreted as pain by brain cells.

Brain

Pain signal

Nerve ending

Brain cells

Prostaglandins

Damaged cell

Pain signal received by brain cell and interpreted

Action of non-narcotics
These drugs block prostaglandin production. This prevents stimulation of the nerve endings so that no pain signal passes to the brain.

Narcotic drug

Opiate receptor

Pain signal blocked

Action of narcotics
Normally the pain signal is transmitted between brain cells. Narcotics combine with receptors on brain cells (opiate receptors), blocking transmission of pain signals within the brain and also in the spinal cord.

Brain cell

methadone. These powerful narcotics are classified as controlled drugs because they may produce euphoria, which can lead to abuse and addiction. When they are given under medical supervision to treat severe pain for a few days the risk of addiction is negligible.

Narcotic analgesics may cloud consciousness and prevent clear thought. Other drawbacks are that they can produce drowsiness, nausea, vomiting, constipation, and depressed breathing. When taken in overdose, narcotics may induce a deep coma and produce fatal breathing difficulties.

In addition to the powerful narcotics, there are less powerful drugs in this group that are used to relieve mild to moderate pain. They include codeine and propoxyphene.

Combined analgesics

Mild narcotics, such as codeine, are often found combined with non-narcotics, such

as aspirin or acetaminophen. These mixtures may combine the advantages of analgesics that act on the brain with those acting at the site of pain. However, there is little evidence that two analgesics combined in one preparation are more effective than a single drug. A combined preparation may also combine the side effects of both classes of drug. For these reasons it is usually advisable to use a single ingredient preparation which you find effective.

COMMON DRUGS

Non-narcotics	Narcotics
Acetaminophen	Codeine
Aspirin	Meperidine
NSAIDs	Morphine
	Propoxyphene

SLEEPING DRUGS

Difficulty in getting to sleep or staying asleep (insomnia) has many causes. Most people suffer from sleepless nights from time to time, usually as a result of a temporary worry or discomfort from a minor illness. Persistent sleeplessness can be caused by psychological problems including anxiety or depression, or by pain and discomfort arising from a physical disorder.

Why they are used

For occasional bouts of sleeplessness, simple, common remedies to promote relaxation – for example, taking a warm bath or a hot milk drink before bedtime – are usually the best form of treatment. Sleeping drugs (also known as hypnotics) are normally prescribed only when these self-help remedies have failed, and when lack of sleep is beginning to affect your general health. Drugs are used to re-establish the habit of sleeping, but because their effectiveness diminishes rapidly after the first few nights, they are best used for limited periods only (see also Risks and special precautions, below). Long-term treatment of sleep-lessness depends on resolving the underlying cause of the problem.

How they work

Most sleeping drugs promote sleep by depressing brain function. They interfere with chemical activity in the brain and nervous system by reducing communi-cation between nerve cells. This leads to a reduction in brain activity, allowing you to fall asleep more easily. The action of

the main class of sleeping drugs, the benzodiazepines, is described in more detail on the facing page.

How they affect you

A sleeping drug rapidly produces drowsiness and slowed reactions. Some people find that the drug makes them appear to be drunk and slurs their speech, especially if they delay going to bed after taking their dose. Most people find they usually fall asleep within one hour of taking the drug.

Because the sleep induced by drugs is not the same as normal sleep, many people find they do not feel as well rested by it as by a night of natural sleep. This is the result of suppressed brain activity. Sleeping drugs also suppress the sleep during which dreams occur, and both dream sleep and non-dream sleep are essential components for a good night's

sleep (see The effect of drugs on sleep patterns, below).

Some people experience a variety of "hangover" effects the following day. The benzodiazepines may produce minor side effects, such as daytime drowsiness, dizziness, and unsteadiness, that can impair the ability to drive or operate dangerous machinery. Elderly people are especially likely to become confused; for them, selection of an appropriate drug is particularly important.

Risks and special precautions

Most sleeping drugs, other than the antihistamines, can produce psycho-logical and physical dependence (see p.23) when taken regularly for more than a few weeks, especially if taken in larger than normal doses. If they are withdrawn abruptly, sleeplessness, anxiety, seizures, and hallucinations can arise. Nightmares and vivid dreams may occur because the amount of time spent in dream sleep increases. Anyone who has been using sleeping drugs regularly for a long time and wishes to stop taking them should seek his or her physician's advice on how to reduce dosage gradually so as to avoid withdrawal symptoms.

One of the risks of taking sleeping drugs for a prolonged period is that there may be a temptation to exceed the prescribed dose, especially if the person has been taking them for some weeks and their effect has diminished. While it is inadvis-able to take more than the prescribed dose of any drug, overdose can be a particular risk with the barbiturates.

THE EFFECT OF DRUGS ON SLEEP PATTERNS

Normal sleep can be divided into three types: light sleep, deep sleep, and dream sleep. The proportion of time spent in each type of sleep changes with age and is altered by sleeping drugs. Dramatic changes in sleep patterns also occur in the first few days following abrupt withdrawal of sleeping drugs after regular, prolonged use.

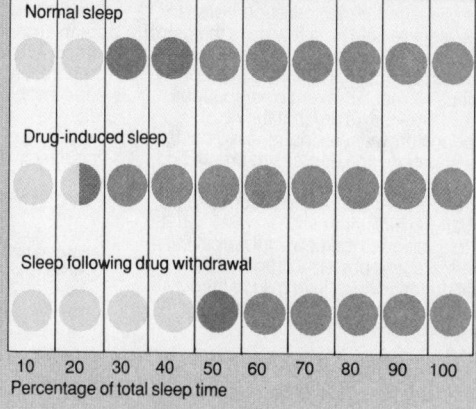

Normal sleep Young adults spend most sleep time in light sleep with roughly equal proportions of dream and deep sleep.

Drug-induced sleep has less dream sleep and less deep sleep with relatively more light sleep.

Sleep following drug withdrawal There is a marked increase in dream sleep, causing nightmares, following withdrawal of drugs used regularly for a long time.

○ Dream sleep

● Deep sleep

● Light sleep

Normal sleep

Drug-induced sleep

Sleep following drug withdrawal

10 20 30 40 50 60 70 80 90 100
Percentage of total sleep time

COMMON DRUGS

Benzodiazepines
Flurazepam
Temazepam
Triazolam

Non-benzodiazepine/non-barbiturate
Chloral hydrate

Barbiturate
Secobarbital

ANTI-ANXIETY DRUGS

A certain amount of stress can be beneficial, providing a stimulus to action. But too much will often result in anxiety, which might be described as fear or apprehension not caused by real danger.

Clinically, anxiety arises when the balance between certain chemicals in the brain is disturbed. The fearful feelings increase brain activity, stimulating the sympathetic nervous system (see p.107), often inducing physical symptoms: shaking, palpitations, breathlessness, digestive distress, and headaches.

Why they are used

Anti-anxiety drugs (also called anxiolytics or minor tranquilizers) are used to alleviate persistent feelings of nervousness and tension caused by stress or other psychological problems. But they cannot resolve the causes. Tackling the underlying problem through counseling and perhaps psychotherapy offers the best hope of a long-term solution. Anti-anxiety drugs are also used in hospitals to calm and relax people who are undergoing uncomfortable medical procedures.

There are two main classes of drugs for relieving anxiety: benzodiazepines and beta blockers. Benzodiazepines are the most widely used, given as a regular treatment for short periods to promote relaxation. Most benzodiazepines have a strong sedative effect, helping to relieve the insomnia that accompanies anxiety (see also Sleeping drugs, facing page).

Beta blockers are mainly used to reduce physical symptoms of anxiety, such as shaking and palpitations. They are commonly prescribed for people who feel excessively anxious in certain situations, for example, at interviews or public appearances. Other drugs used to relieve anxiety include certain antidepressants – prescribed for anxiety arising out of a depressive illness (see p.112) – and meprobamate, a drug with effects similar to those of barbiturates, often causing dependency and withdrawal reactions.

How they work
Benzodiazepines

These drugs depress activity in the part of the brain that controls emotion, by promoting the action of a chemical called gamma-aminobutyric acid (GABA). GABA attaches itself to brain cells, blocking transmission of electrical impulses. This reduces communication between brain cells. Benzodiazepines are thought to increase the inhibitory effect of GABA on brain cells (see Action of benzodiazepines, above), thus preventing excessive brain activity, which causes anxiety.

Beta blockers

The physical symptoms of anxiety are produced by an increase in the activity of the sympathetic nervous system. Sym-

ACTION OF BENZODIAZEPINES

Action on the brain

The reticular activating system (RAS) in the brain stem controls the level of mental activity by stimulating the higher centers of the brain responsible for consciousness. Benzodiazepines depress the RAS, so relieving anxiety. In larger doses they depress the RAS sufficiently to cause drowsiness and sleep.

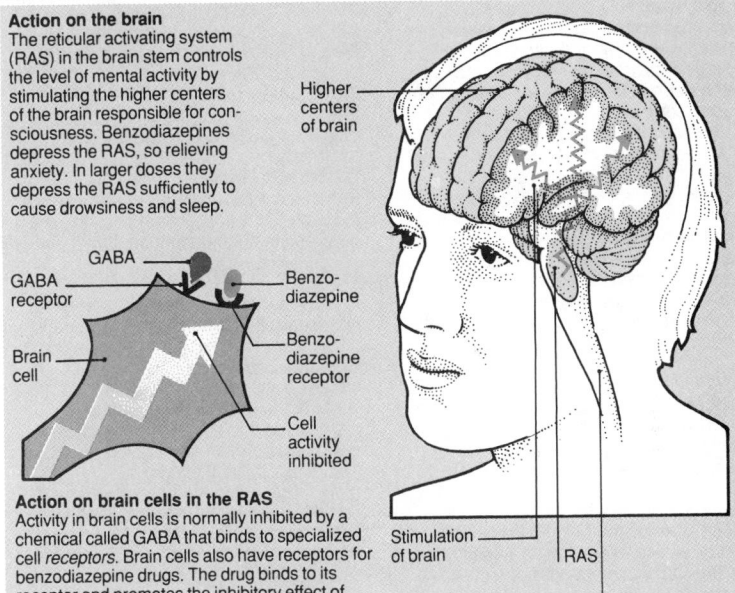

GABA

GABA receptor

Benzo- diazepine

Benzo- diazepine receptor

Brain cell

Cell activity inhibited

Higher centers of brain

Stimulation of brain

RAS

Brain stem

Action on brain cells in the RAS

Activity in brain cells is normally inhibited by a chemical called GABA that binds to specialized cell *receptors*. Brain cells also have receptors for benzodiazepine drugs. The drug binds to its receptor and promotes the inhibitory effect of GABA. This depresses activity in the RAS.

pathetic nerve endings release a chemical transmitter called norepinephrine that stimulates the heart, digestive system, and other organs. Beta blockers block the action of norepinephrine in the body, reducing the physical symptoms of anxiety. For more information on beta blockers, see p.125.

How they affect you

Benzodiazepines reduce feelings of agitation and restlessness, slow mental activity, and often produce drowsiness. They are said to reduce motivation and, if taken in large doses, may lead to apathy. They also have a relaxing effect on the muscles, and some benzodiazepines are used specifically for that purpose (see Muscle relaxants, p.148). Minor adverse effects of these drugs include dizziness and forgetfulness. People who need to drive or operate dangerous machinery should be aware that their reactions may be slowed. Because the brain soon becomes tolerant to their effects, benzodiazepines are usually effective only for a few weeks.

Risks and special precautions

The benzodiazepines are considered safe for most people. They are not known to be fatal or poisonous in overdose. The main risk is that people who take them regularly may become psychologically and physically dependent, particularly when larger

doses have been used. For this reason they are usually given for courses of two weeks or less. If a person has been taking them for a longer period, they are normally withdrawn gradually under medical supervision. If they are stopped suddenly, withdrawal symptoms, including excessive anxiety, nightmares, and restlessness, may occur. Benzodiazepines have been abused for their sedative effect, and they are therefore prescribed with particular caution for people with a history of drug or alcohol abuse.

COMMON DRUGS

Benzodiazepines
Alprazolam
Chlordiazepoxide
Clonazepam
Clorazepate
Diazepam
Lorazepam
Oxazepam

Beta blockers
Oxprenolol
Propranolol

Other drugs
Meprobamate
Phenobarbital

ANTIDEPRESSANT DRUGS

Occasional moods of sadness or discouragement are normal and usually pass quickly. But more severe depression, accompanied by despair, lethargy, loss of sex drive, apathy, and often poor appetite, may call for medical attention. Such depression can arise from the death of someone close, an illness, or sometimes from no apparent cause.

There are two main types of drug used to treat depression: tricyclics and monoamine oxidase inhibitors (see Types of antidepressant, below). Lithium, which is used to treat manic depression, is discussed under Antimanic drugs (facing page). Other antidepressants include the tetracyclic drug maprotiline – which has actions and effects similar to those of the tricyclics – and trazodone.

Why they are used

Minor depression does not usually require drug treatment, and physicians usually avoid prescribing antidepressants when it is likely that the depression will soon pass. In such cases support and help in coming to terms with the cause is often more effective than drugs. Severe depression, however, may be helped by antidepressant drugs. Antidepressants may have to be taken for many months or years. However, they can sometimes be withdrawn gradually after prolonged treatment without relapse.

How they work

Depression is thought to be caused by a reduction in the level of certain chemicals in the brain, called *neurotransmitters*, that affect mood by stimulating brain cells. Antidepressants increase the level of these *excitatory* neurotransmitters.

Tricyclics

When excitatory neurotransmitters are released by brain cells they are normally rapidly taken up again into the cells.

TYPES OF ANTIDEPRESSANT

Monoamine oxidase inhibitors (MAOIs)

These are usually given to people who do not respond to the tricyclics, or for whom tricyclics are not suitable. MAOIs are especially effective in people who are anxious as well as depressed, or who suffer from phobias.

Tricyclics

Tricyclics are the most widely used group of antidepressants and usually the first to be tried. Some of them, such as amitriptyline, are mainly sedative and are commonly given to people with sleeping difficulties as a single dose at night. This results in improved sleep at once, even before the depression is relieved. Other tricyclics, such as imipramine, have a stimulant effect and are given to people who feel lethargic.

Tricyclics block this re-uptake of neurotransmitters, and the level outside the brain cell therefore increases, so prolonging their stimulatory effect on the brain (see Action of antidepressants, right).

Monoamine oxidase inhibitors

These drugs block the action of a brain enzyme that normally breaks down the excitatory neurotransmitters. By blocking this breakdown, MAOIs allow the neurotransmitters to build up to a high level and produce a greater stimulation of the brain (see Action of antidepressants, right).

How they affect you

The beneficial effect of antidepressants is not usually noticeable for 10 to 14 days after the initial dose, and it may be 6 to 8 weeks before you feel the full effect. However, within the first day of treatment some of the tricyclics can produce drowsiness and a variety of *anticholinergic* effects, including dry mouth, blurred vision, and difficulty urinating.

Risks and special precautions

Tricyclics and MAOIs are dangerous in overdose: tricyclics can produce coma, cause seizures, and disturb heart rhythm, which may be fatal; MAOIs can also cause seizures and even death. Both types are prescribed with caution for people with heart problems or epilepsy.

Monoamine oxidase inhibitors have numerous side effects because they deactivate enzymes in the body that normally break down certain chemicals (particularly tyramine) found in some foods. MAOIs taken with certain drugs or foods rich in tyramine (for example, cheese, meat, yeast extracts, and red wine) can produce a dramatic rise in blood pressure, even two weeks after stopping the drug. Symptoms of rising blood pressure include headache, palpitations, and vomiting. People taking these drugs are given a treatment card listing prohibited drugs and foods.

Symptoms, including anxiety and difficulty in sleeping, may arise when MAOI or tricyclic treatment is stopped, even when the drug is withdrawn under medical supervision. These symptoms are short-lived.

COMMON DRUGS

Tricyclics	Other drugs
Amitriptyline	Maprotiline
Amoxapine	Trazodone
Desipramine	
Doxepin	
Imipramine	

Monoamine oxidase inhibitors
Isocarboxazid
Phenelzine

ACTION OF ANTIDEPRESSANTS

Normally brain cells release sufficient quantities of excitatory chemicals (neurotransmitters) to stimulate neighboring cells. The neurotransmitters are constantly reabsorbed into the brain cells, where they are broken down by an enzyme called monoamine oxidase. In depression fewer neurotransmitters are released. Antidepressant drugs act to raise the levels of neurotransmitters in the brain.

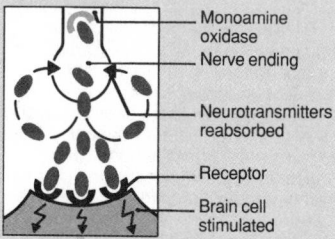

- Monoamine oxidase
- Nerve ending
- Neurotransmitters reabsorbed
- Receptor
- Brain cell stimulated

Normal brain activity
In a normal brain neurotransmitters are constantly being released, reabsorbed, and broken down.

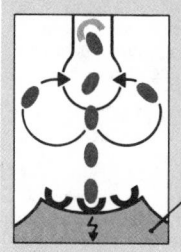

Brain activity in depression
Fewer neurotransmitters than normal are released, leading to reduced stimulation.

- Brain cell poorly stimulated

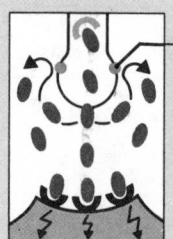

- Drug blocks reabsorption of neurotransmitters

Action of tricyclics
Tricyclic drugs increase the levels of neurotransmitters by blocking their reabsorption.

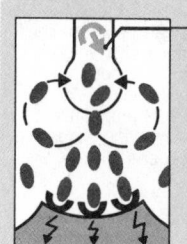

- Drug blocks enzyme

Action of MAOIs
MAOIs increase the levels of neurotransmitters by blocking the action of the enzyme (monoamine oxidase) that breaks them down.

ANTIPSYCHOTIC DRUGS

"Psychosis" is a term used to describe mental disorders that prevent the sufferer from thinking clearly, recognizing reality, and acting rationally. These disorders include schizophrenia, manic depression, and paranoia. The precise causes of these disorders are unknown, although a number of factors, including stress, heredity, and brain injury, may be involved. Temporary psychosis can also arise as a result of alcohol withdrawal or the abuse of mind-altering drugs (see Drugs of abuse, p.547). A variety of drugs are used to treat psychotic disorders (see Common drugs, below), most of which have similar actions and effects. One exception is lithium, which is particularly useful for manic depression (see Antimanic drugs, right).

Why they are used
Because a person with a psychotic illness may recover spontaneously, a drug will not always be prescribed immediately. Long-term treatment is started only when normal life is seriously interfered with. Antipsychotic drugs (also called major tranquilizers or neuroleptics) do not cure the underlying disorder, but they can restore normal behavior.

The drug given to a particular individual depends on the nature of his or her illness and the side effects experienced. Drugs differ in the amount of sedation that they produce; the need for sedation also influences the choice.

Antipsychotics may also be given to calm or sedate a highly agitated or aggressive person, whatever the cause. Some antipsychotic drugs also have a powerful action against nausea and vomiting (see p.118), and are sometimes used as *premedication* before surgery.

How they work
It is thought that some forms of mental illness are caused by an increase in communication between brain cells due to overactivity of a chemical called dopamine. This may disturb normal thought processes and produce abnormal behavior. Dopamine combines with *receptors* on the brain cells. Antipsychotics reduce the transmission of nerve signals by binding to these receptors, thus making the brain cells less sensitive to dopamine (see Action of antipsychotics, below).

How they affect you
By modifying abnormal behavior, the antipsychotics enable the sufferer to live outside of a mental institution, where psychotics were usually confined up until the 1950s.

Because antipsychotics depress the action of dopamine, they can disturb its balance with another chemical in the brain, acetylcholine. If that occurs, signs like those of parkinsonism can appear – the expressionless face and shaky hands (see Antiparkinsonism drugs, p.115).

In those circumstances, a change in medication becomes necessary. Rather than prescribe a drug specifically to counteract the adverse effects of the antipsychotic, a physician will usually try treatment with drugs of a different class.

Antipsychotics may also block the action of another neurotransmitter, norepinephrine. This lowers the blood pressure, especially when you stand up, causing dizziness. It may also prevent ejaculation.

Risks and special precautions
It is important to continue taking these drugs even if all symptoms have gone, because symptoms are controlled only by taking the prescribed dose.

Because these drugs can have permanent as well as temporary side effects, the minimum necessary dosage is used.

This is found by starting with a low dose and increasing it until symptoms are controlled. Sudden withdrawal of antipsychotics after more than a few weeks can cause nausea, vomiting, sweating, headache, and restlessness. For this reason the dose is reduced gradually when drug treatment needs to be stopped.

The most serious long-term risk of antipsychotic treatment is a disorder known as *tardive dyskinesia*, which may develop after one to five years. This consists of repeated jerking movements of the mouth, tongue, and face, and sometimes the hands and feet.

Some physicians have suggested that periodic withdrawal of the drug for several months may reduce the severity of this condition, but the value of such "drug holidays" has not been proved.

How they are administered
Antipsychotics may be injected, or given as tablets, capsules, or syrup. They can also be given in the form of a *depot injection* that releases the drug slowly over several weeks. This is helpful for people who might forget to take their drugs or who might take an overdose.

COMMON DRUGS

Phenothiazine antipsychotics
Chlorpromazine
Fluphenazine
Perphenazine
Prochlorperazine
Thioridazine

Butyrophenone antipsychotic
Haloperidol

Antimanic drug
Lithium

ACTION OF ANTIPSYCHOTICS

Brain activity is partly governed by the action of a chemical called dopamine, which transmits signals between brain cells. In psychotic illness the brain cells release too much dopamine, causing excessive stimulation. Antipsychotic drugs help to reduce the adverse effects of excess dopamine.

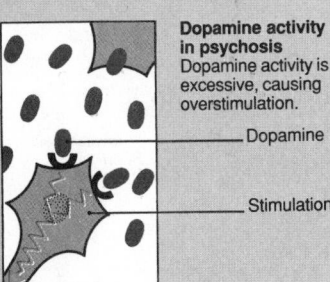

Dopamine activity in psychosis
Dopamine activity is excessive, causing overstimulation.

Dopamine

Stimulation

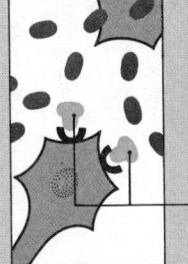

Dopamine activity blocked by drugs
Antipsychotic drugs occupy dopamine receptors and prevent the effects of excess dopamine from being felt.

Drug

ANTICONVULSANT DRUGS

Electrical signals from nerve cells in the brain are normally finely coordinated to produce smooth movements of arms and legs. But these signals can become paroxysmal and chaotic, and trigger the disorderly muscular activity and mental changes which are characteristic of a seizure (also called a fit or convulsion). The most common cause of seizures is the disorder known as epilepsy. However, seizures may also be brought on by outside stimuli – such as flashing lights – or caused by brain disease or injury, by the toxic effects of certain drugs, or, in young children, by a high temperature.

Anticonvulsant drugs are used to reduce the risk of a seizure and to stop one that is in progress.

Why they are used

Isolated seizures seldom require drug treatment, but anticonvulsant drugs are the usual treatment for controlling epileptic seizures. They permit epileptics to lead a normal life, reducing the possibility of brain damage, which can result from recurrent seizures.

ACTION OF ANTICONVULSANTS

Normally there is a relatively low level of electrical activity in the brain. In a seizure, excessive electrical activity builds up, causing uncontrolled stimulation of the brain. Anticonvulsant drugs have an inhibitory effect which neutralizes excessive electrical activity in the brain.

Normal brain activity

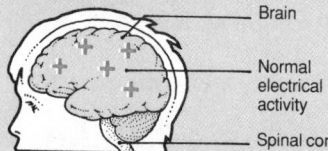

- Brain
- Normal electrical activity
- Spinal cord

Brain activity in a seizure

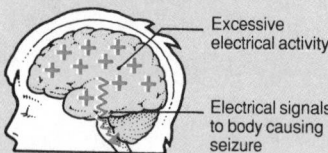

- Excessive electrical activity
- Electrical signals to body causing seizure

Drug action on brain activity

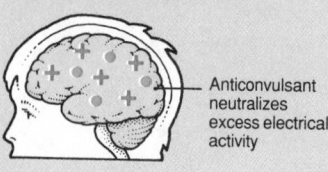

- Anticonvulsant neutralizes excess electrical activity

Most people with epilepsy need to take anticonvulsants on a regular basis to prevent seizures. Usually a single drug is used, and treatment continues until there have been no attacks for at least two years. The particular drug prescribed depends on the kind of epilepsy (see Types of epilepsy, right). If one drug alone is not effective, a combination of drugs may be given. Even when under treatment a person can suffer seizures. A prolonged seizure can be halted by injection of diazepam or a similar drug.

How they work

Brain cells bring about body movement by a form of electrical activity which passes through the nerves to the muscles. In a seizure, excessive electrical activity starts in one part of the brain and spreads to other parts, causing uncontrolled stimulation of brain cells. Most anticonvulsant drugs have an *inhibitory* effect on brain cells and damp down electrical activity, preventing the excessive build-up which causes a seizure (see Action of anticonvulsants, left).

How they affect you

Ideally, the only effect an anticonvulsant should have is to reduce or prevent seizures. Unfortunately, no drug prevents seizures without potentially affecting normal brain function, leading to poor memory, inability to concentrate, lack of coordination, and lethargy. It is important, therefore, to find a dosage that is sufficient to prevent seizures without causing unacceptable side effects. The dose has to be carefully tailored to the individual – there is no standard dose for anticonvulsants. It is usual to start with a low dose of a selected drug and to increase it gradually until a balance is achieved between the effective control of seizures and the occurrence of side effects, many of which wear off after the first few weeks of treatment. Blood tests to monitor levels of the drug in the body are usually carried out periodically. Finding the correct dose may take several months.

Risks and special precautions

Each anticonvulsant drug has its own specific adverse effects and risks. In addition, most of them affect the liver's ability to break down other drugs (see Drug interactions, p.16) and so may influence the action of other drugs you are taking. Physicians try to use the minimum number of anticonvulsants in any one person in order to reduce the risk of such interactions occurring.

People taking anticonvulsants need to be particularly careful to take their medication regularly as prescribed. If the levels of the anticonvulsant in the body are allowed to fall suddenly, seizures are very likely to occur. The reason for this is

TYPES OF EPILEPSY

The selection of anticonvulsant drug depends on the type of epilepsy, although the age and particular response to drug treatment of the individual is also important.

Tonic/clonic (grand mal) seizures This type of seizure is characterized by a warning sensation such as flashing lights or a noise, which is followed by a sudden loss of consciousness during which convulsions occur, and the sufferer may urinate uncontrolledly or foam at the mouth. The seizure usually lasts for a few minutes only, but it can occasionally last for up to an hour. Prolonged attacks are called status epilepticus.

The principal drugs used to prevent tonic/clonic seizures are phenytoin, phenobarbital, primidone, and carbamazepine. Physicians try to avoid prescribing phenytoin for young children because of its unpleasant side effects, such as overgrowth of the gums, acne, and increased body hair. These effects are less prominent in adults. Status epilepticus is usually treated by injection of a benzodiazepine drug such as diazepam.

Absence (petit mal) seizures This form of epilepsy most commonly affects children. The seizures consist of a momentary loss of consciousness, during which the child may seem to go blank. Convulsions do not occur. The following drugs are used for the prevention of this type of seizure: ethosuximide, valproic acid, and, less commonly, clonazepam.

Partial seizures There are a number of different variations of this form of epilepsy. Most partial seizures cause a sudden severe disturbance of the senses and/or muscle spasm without loss of consciousness. Phenytoin, phenobarbital, and carbamazepine are the drugs most commonly used to prevent partial seizures.

that without the inhibitory drug, there is little to stop the building of electrical activity that brings on seizures. Accordingly, the dose should not be reduced or the treatment stopped except on the advice of a physician. If, for any reason, treatment with anticonvulsants needs to be stopped, the dose should be reduced gradually over a period of one to two years. People on anticonvulsant therapy are advised to carry an identification tag that gives full details of their condition and treatment.

COMMON DRUGS

Carbamazepine	Phenobarbital
Clonazepam	Phenytoin
Clorazepate	Primidone
Diazepam	Valproic acid
Ethosuximide	

ANTIPARKINSONISM DRUGS

Antiparkinsonism drugs are used in the treatment of parkinsonism. This is the general term used to describe shaking of the head and limbs, muscular stiffness, an expressionless face, and inability to control or initiate movement. It is caused by an imbalance between the chemicals dopamine and acetylcholine in the brain. These chemicals transmit nerve signals in the part of the brain that coordinates movement. They have opposing actions and are normally finely balanced. In parkinsonism there is a reduction in the action of dopamine, so that the effect of acetylcholine is increased.

Parkinsonism has a variety of causes, but the most common is degeneration of the dopamine-producing cells in the brain, known as Parkinson's disease. Other causes include the side effects of certain drugs, notably antipsychotics (see p.113), brain damage, and narrowing of the blood vessels to the brain.

Why they are used
Antiparkinsonism drugs can help to relieve the symptoms of parkinsonism, but they cannot cure the underlying cause of the chemical imbalance. The degeneration of brain cells in Parkinson's disease cannot be halted, although drugs can minimize symptoms of the disease for many years.

How they work
Antiparkinsonism drugs restore the balance between dopamine and acetylcholine. They fall into two main groups: those drugs that act by reducing the effect of acetylcholine (*anticholinergic* drugs) and those that act by boosting the effect of dopamine.

Anticholinergic drugs
Acetylcholine acts by combining with *receptors* on brain cells and stimulating them. Anticholinergic drugs combine with these receptors and prevent acetylcholine from binding to them. This reduces acetylcholine's relative overactivity and restores the balance with dopamine.

Drugs that boost the effect of dopamine
Dopamine levels in the brain cannot be boosted by giving dopamine directly because it is poorly absorbed through the digestive tract, and cannot pass from the bloodstream into the brain. Levodopa – the chemical from which dopamine is naturally produced in the brain – can be absorbed well through the digestive tract. It increases the level of dopamine and so restores the balance with acetylcholine.

Because a high proportion of each dose of levodopa is broken down in the body before it reaches the brain, it is usually combined with a drug called carbidopa, which prevents this breakdown. Dopamine

ACTION OF ANTIPARKINSONISM DRUGS

Normal movement depends on a balance in the brain between dopamine and acetyl-choline, which combine with receptors on brain cells. In parkinsonism there is less dopamine, so that acetylcholine is relatively overactive. The balance between acetylcholine and dopamine may be restored by anticholinergic drugs, which combine with the receptors for acetylcholine and block acetylcholine's action on the brain cell, or by dopamine-boosting drugs, which increase the level of dopamine activity in the brain.

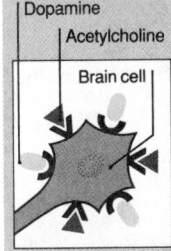
| Dopamine
| Acetylcholine
| Brain cell

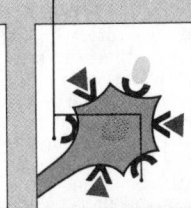
| Reduced dopamine

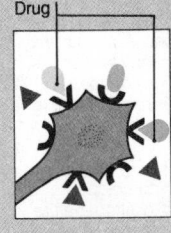
Drug

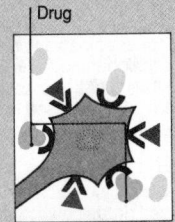
Drug

Normal chemical balance
Normally dopamine and acetylcholine are balanced.

Chemical imbalance in parkinsonism
When dopamine activity is reduced, acetylcholine is overactive.

Action of anticho-linergic drugs
Anticholinergic drugs displace acetylcholine and restore balance.

Action of dopamine-boosting drugs
These drugs increase dopamine activity and restore balance.

is broken down in the brain. To reduce this breakdown levodopa may be given with an investigational drug (deprenyl) to prolong the action of dopamine.

Amantadine (also used as an antiviral agent, see p.161) boosts the levels of dopamine in the brain by stimulating its release. Dopamine action can also be boosted by bromocriptine, which mimics the action of dopamine.

How they affect you
Each type of drug relieves some symptoms of parkinsonism better than others, although it is difficult to control symptoms in the more advanced stage of the disease. Anticholinergics improve stiffness more than shaking or the inability to initiate movement, and benefit is felt within a few days. They also reduce excessive salivation: dribbling is often a problem in Parkinson's disease.

Levodopa often produces a dramatic improvement in all symptoms. Side effects of levodopa include nausea, vomiting, and flushing. When given in excess it can also cause involuntary movements in the face and the body. Although these problems may be alleviated by reducing the dose, as the disease progresses it becomes increasingly difficult to give sufficient levodopa to improve symptoms without causing side effects. Also, in the later stage of the disease, the effect of each dose wears off before the next one is taken, and it may be necessary to take the drug more frequently.

Amantadine relieves all symptoms of parkinsonism in people with mild to moderate cases. It has few side effects but the beneficial effect may wear off over a few months. The most common side effects of bromocriptine are the same as those produced by levodopa.

Choice of drug
The particular drug prescribed depends on both the severity of the disease and the potential adverse effects of the drug.

Anticholinergic drugs are often effective in the early stages of Parkinson's disease, when they may control symptoms adequately without any other antiparkinsonism drugs. They are often used to treat parkinsonism caused by antipsychotic drugs. If a person cannot take anticholinergic drugs because of their side effects, amantadine may be given. Levodopa is usually prescribed when the disease impairs walking. The effectiveness of levodopa usually wanes after two to five years; if this happens, bromocriptine or amantadine may be prescribed as well. People who do not benefit from levodopa or who cannot be given it because of side effects, may be given bromocriptine or amantadine.

COMMON DRUGS

Anticholinergic drugs	Dopamine-boosting drugs
Benztropine	Amantadine
Orphenadrine	Bromocriptine
Procyclidine	Levodopa
Trihexyphenidyl	

NERVOUS SYSTEM STIMULANTS

A person's state of mental alertness varies throughout the day and is under the control of chemicals in the brain, some of which are depressant (causing drowsiness) and others that are stimulant (heightening awareness).

It is thought that an increase in the activity of the depressant chemicals may be responsible for a condition called narcolepsy, a tendency to fall asleep during the day for no obvious reason. Nervous system stimulants are administered to increase wakefulness. They include the amphetamines and related drugs, notably methylphenidate. Respiratory stimulants, including caffeine (found in coffee, tea, and cola), are used to improve breathing (see Respiratory stimulants, right).

Why they are used

In adults who suffer from narcolepsy these drugs can be used to stimulate the brain and prevent excessive drowsiness during the day. Stimulants do not cure narcolepsy, and since the disorder usually lasts throughout the sufferer's lifetime, they may have to be taken indefinitely. Nervous system stimulants are also occasionally given to hyperactive children who have a short attention span.

Because reduced appetite is a side effect of amphetamines, they have also been used as part of the treatment for obesity. However, because of the risk of addiction, sometimes accompanied by paranoid delusions, this use is generally condemned (see Risks and special precautions, below).

Caffeine is sometimes added to analgesic preparations. Various reasons have been offered to justify this combination.

Unfortunately, apart from their use in narcolepsy, stimulants are not useful in the long term because the brain soon becomes tolerant to them. Unless the dose is increased, no stimulation is felt.

How they work

The level of wakefulness is controlled by a part of the brain stem called the reticular activating system (RAS). Activity here depends on the balance between chemicals, some of which are *excitatory* (including norepinephrine) and some *inhibitory* (such as gamma amino butyric acid). Stimulants promote the release of norepinephrine by brain cells, increasing activity in the RAS and other parts of the brain, so raising the level of alertness.

How they affect you

In adults, central nervous system stimulants taken in the prescribed dose for narcolepsy increase wakefulness, allowing normal concentration and thought processes to occur. They may also reduce appetite and cause tremors. In hyperactive children they reduce the general level of activity to a more normal level and increase the attention span.

RESPIRATORY STIMULANTS

Some stimulants (for example, aminophylline, theophylline and caffeine) act on the part of the brain – the respiratory center – that controls respiration. They are sometimes used in hospitals to help people who have difficulty breathing, mainly very young babies and adults with severe bronchitis.

Risks and special precautions

Some people, especially the elderly or those with previous psychiatric problems, are particularly sensitive to stimulants and may experience adverse effects, even when the drugs are given in comparatively low doses. They are used with caution in children because they can retard growth if taken for prolonged periods. In a child, an excess of these drugs depresses the nervous system, producing drowsiness or possibly loss of consciousness. Palpitations may also occur.

These drugs reduce the level of natural stimulants in the brain, so that after regular use for a few weeks a person may become physically dependent on them for normal function. If they are abruptly withdrawn after regular use, the excess of natural inhibitory chemicals in the brain depresses activity in the central nervous system, producing withdrawal symptoms. These may include lethargy, depression, and increased appetite.

If used by adults in excess or inappropriately, stimulants can produce overactivity in the brain, resulting in extreme restlessness, sleeplessness, and feelings of nervousness or anxiety. They also stimulate the sympathetic branch of the autonomic nervous system (see p.107), causing shaking, sweating, and palpitations. More serious risks of exceeding the prescribed dose are seizures and a disturbance in mental functioning that may result in delusions and hallucinations. Since amphetamines have been abused, they are classified as controlled substances (see p.549).

COMMON DRUGS

Amphetamines
Dextroamphetamine

Respiratory stimulants
Aminophylline
Theophylline
Caffeine

Other drugs
Methylphenidate

ACTION OF NERVOUS SYSTEM STIMULANTS

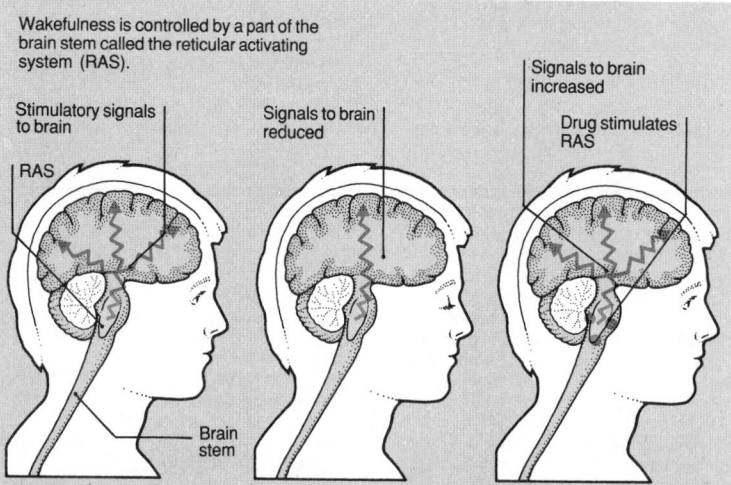

Wakefulness is controlled by a part of the brain stem called the reticular activating system (RAS).

Stimulatory signals to brain

RAS

Signals to brain reduced

Signals to brain increased

Drug stimulates RAS

Brain stem

Normal brain activity
When the brain is functioning normally, signals from the RAS stimulate the upper parts of the brain, which control thought processes and alertness.

Brain activity in narcolepsy
In narcolepsy the level of signals from the RAS is greatly reduced.

Normal brain activity restored
Central nervous system stimulants act on the RAS to increase the level of stimulatory signals to the brain.

DRUGS USED FOR MIGRAINE

"Migraine" is a term applied to recurrent severe headaches affecting only one side of the head and caused by changes in the blood vessels. They may be accompanied by nausea and vomiting and preceded by warning signs, usually flashing lights or numbness and tingling in the arms. Occasionally speech may be impaired, and the attack may be disabling. The exact cause of migraine is unknown, but an attack may be triggered by emotional factors including excitement, tension, shock, physical exertion, a blow to the head, some foods, and some drugs. A family history of migraine also increases the likelihood that an individual will suffer from migraine.

Why they are used

Drugs are used either to relieve symptoms or to prevent attacks. Different drugs are used in each approach, but none cures the underlying disorder. However, the migraine can clear up spontaneously, and if you are taking drugs regularly to prevent attacks, your physician may recommend that you stop them after a few months to see whether this has happened.

In most people migraine headaches can be relieved by a mild analgesic such as aspirin or acetaminophen, or a stronger one like codeine (see Analgesics, p.108). But because the migraine may be accompanied by nausea and vomiting, these drugs may not be absorbed sufficiently to provide relief. Thus suppository forms of these drugs may be used. Preparations containing caffeine have been used for decades to suppress the headache when the early warning symptoms are present but before the pain is manifest. Ergotamine, a more powerful drug, is prescribed in this combination or alone by injection once the headache begins.

When attacks occur more often than once a month, daily drug therapy for a period of weeks or months with methysergide (a drug similar to ergotamine) or propranolol (a beta blocker) may be advised to prevent them.

One of the antidepressant drugs, amitriptyline, is sometimes prescribed regularly for a while to prevent migraine attacks, even for people who are not suffering from depression (see p.112).

Anxiety or depression which can accompany migraine may be treated with other drugs (see Anti-anxiety drugs, p.111, and Antidepressant drugs, p.112). Nausea and vomiting may be controlled with an anti-emetic drug (see p.118).

How they work

A migraine attack begins when blood vessels surrounding the brain constrict, producing the typical migraine warning signs. This is thought to be caused by certain chemicals in food or produced in the body. Methysergide and propranolol

ACTION OF DRUGS USED FOR MIGRAINE

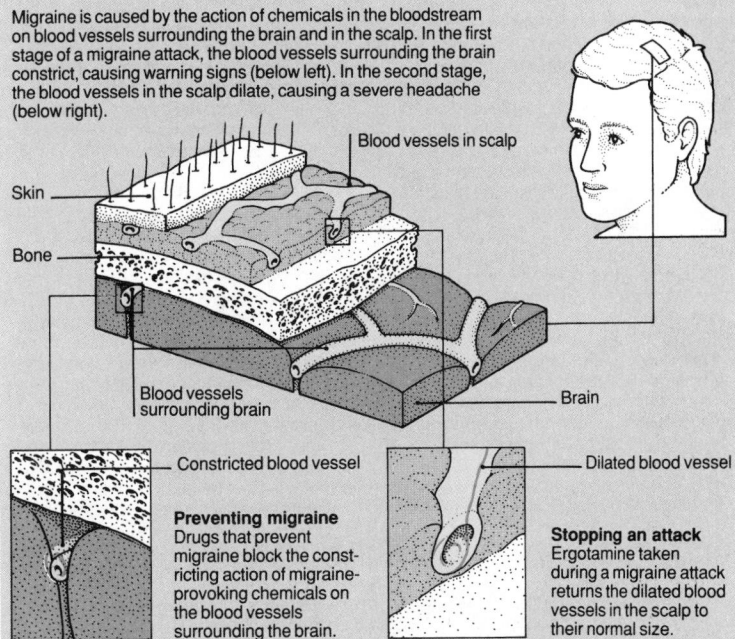

Migraine is caused by the action of chemicals in the bloodstream on blood vessels surrounding the brain and in the scalp. In the first stage of a migraine attack, the blood vessels surrounding the brain constrict, causing warning signs (below left). In the second stage, the blood vessels in the scalp dilate, causing a severe headache (below right).

Blood vessels in scalp

Skin

Bone

Blood vessels surrounding brain

Brain

Constricted blood vessel

Dilated blood vessel

Preventing migraine
Drugs that prevent migraine block the constricting action of migraine-provoking chemicals on the blood vessels surrounding the brain.

Stopping an attack
Ergotamine taken during a migraine attack returns the dilated blood vessels in the scalp to their normal size.

block the effect of the chemicals on blood vessels and so prevent attacks (see Action of drugs used for migraine, above).

The next stage occurs when blood vessels in the scalp and around the eyes dilate. This causes the release of chemicals called prostaglandins which produce pain. Aspirin and acetaminophen relieve pain by blocking the production of prostaglandins, while codeine acts directly on the brain to alter the perception of pain (see Action of analgesics, p.109). Ergotamine relieves pain by narrowing the dilated blood vessels.

How they affect you

All these drugs have their own side effects. Ergotamine may cause drowsiness, and by constricting blood vessels throughout the body, often produces a variety of side effects including burning and tingling sensations in the skin (paresthesia), cramps, weakness in the legs, and pain in the abdomen, arms, and legs.

For more information about the effects of propranolol, see Beta blockers, p.125, and for more information on the effects of analgesics, see p.108.

Risks and special precautions

Ergotamine is used with caution if you have poor circulation because it can damage blood vessels through prolonged overconstriction. Frequent use can lead

to dependence and numerous adverse effects, including headache. For these reasons it is used only for the short-term treatment of severe migraine, and you should not take more than your physician advises in any one week. Ergotamine should not be used if you have an infection because it can restrict blood flow to the site of infection and delay recovery.

Methysergide can produce pain in the abdomen or lower back, and also shortness of breath due to an unusual type of damage to tissues.

How they are administered

They are usually taken by mouth as tablets or capsules. When an attack is advanced or vomiting is present, dihydroergotamine, a drug similar to ergotamine, may be given by injection. Ergotamine may also be taken by aerosol inhalation, or as tablets to be dissolved under the tongue.

COMMON DRUGS

Drugs to relieve migraine	Drugs to prevent migraine
Acetaminophen	Amitriptyline
Aspirin	Methysergide
Codeine	Propranolol
Ergotamine	

ANTI-EMETIC DRUGS

Anti-emetic drugs are used to suppress vomiting and nausea. Vomiting (emesis) is a reflex action that protects the body by expelling harmful substances. Common causes of vomiting and nausea are digestive tract infection, pregnancy, motion sickness, and vertigo. It can also occur as a side effect of a medication, or drug or radiation therapy for cancer.

The main anti-emetic drugs are metoclopramide, the antihistamines, and phenothiazine drugs, which are also used to treat mental illness (see Antipsychotic drugs, p.113). Dronabinol, containing the active ingredient of marijuana, is now approved as an anti-emetic drug for cancer patients.

Why they are used
Physicians usually diagnose the cause of vomiting before prescribing an anti-emetic because vomiting may be the reaction to infection, or to an abdominal condition that might require surgery. Suppressing vomiting and nausea may delay diagnosis, consequently delaying a needed operation. Anti-emetics are often taken to

prevent motion sickness (antihistamines) and nausea resulting from other drug treatment (metoclopramide and phenothiazines), to suppress nausea in vertigo (see right), and occasionally to relieve severe vomiting in pregnancy (antihistamines and phenothiazines).

You should not take an anti-emetic drug for longer than a couple of days without consulting your physician.

How they work
Nausea and vomiting occur when a specialized part of the brain called the vomiting center is stimulated by signals which may arise from various points in the brain and body: from the digestive system, from the part of the brain that is responsible for consciousness, or from the inner ear. Signals may also arise from an area of the brain called the chemoreceptor trigger, which stimulates the vomiting (emetic) center if it detects any harmful substances present in the blood. Anti-emetic drugs may act at one or more of these places in the body. In addition, these drugs may also promote the normal

emptying of the stomach contents into the intestine (see Action of anti-emetics, left).

How they affect you
In addition to reducing or preventing vomiting and nausea, most anti-emetics may make you feel drowsy. Certain nonsedating antihistamines (see p.153) may therefore be preferred for the prevention of motion sickness.

Because the antihistamines block the parasympathetic system (see p.107) they can produce many *anticholinergic* side effects, including dry mouth, blurred vision, and difficulty passing urine. Phenothiazine drugs – which also may produce anticholinergic side effects – can lower blood pressure, leading to dizziness.

Risks and special precautions
Because antihistamines can make you drowsy, it may not be advisable to drive while taking them.

Phenothiazines and metoclopramide can produce uncontrolled movements of the face and tongue, and for this reason they are used with caution in people who suffer from movement disorders such as *parkinsonism*.

ACTION OF ANTI-EMETICS

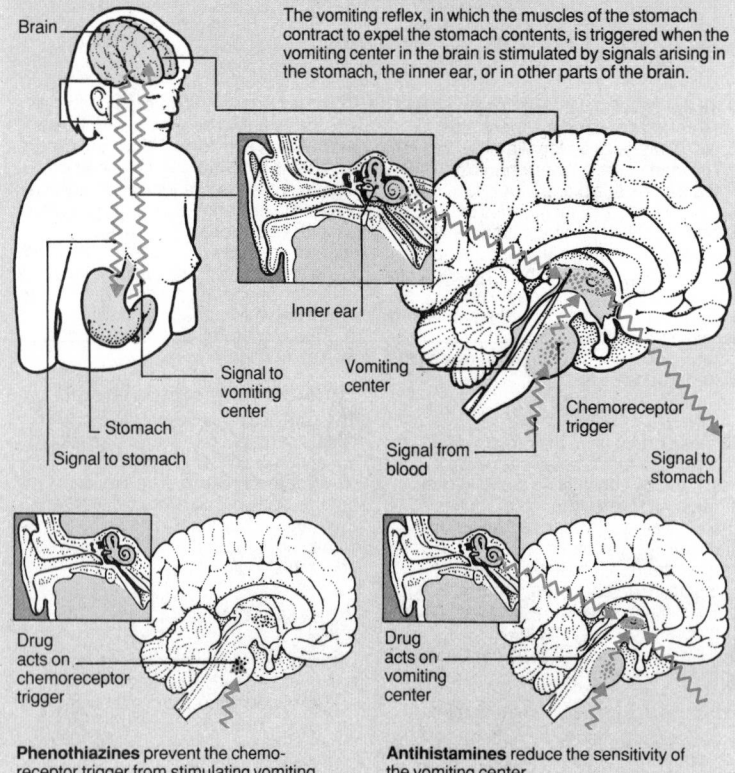

The vomiting reflex, in which the muscles of the stomach contract to expel the stomach contents, is triggered when the vomiting center in the brain is stimulated by signals arising in the stomach, the inner ear, or in other parts of the brain.

Brain

Inner ear

Signal to vomiting center

Stomach

Signal to stomach

Vomiting center

Signal from blood

Chemoreceptor trigger

Signal to stomach

Drug acts on chemoreceptor trigger

Phenothiazines prevent the chemoreceptor trigger from stimulating vomiting.

Drug acts on vomiting center

Antihistamines reduce the sensitivity of the vomiting center.

COMMON DRUGS

Antihistamines
Dimenhydrinate
Meclizine
Promethazine
Trimethobenzamide

Phenothiazines
Fluphenazine
Perphenazine
Prochlorperazine
Promazine

Other drugs
Dronabinol
Metoclopramide
Scopolamine

RESPIRATORY SYSTEM

Comprising the lungs and the passageways by which air reaches them, the respiratory system performs a vital function. Through the process of inhaling and exhaling air – breathing – the body is able to obtain necessary oxygen and expel carbon dioxide, the waste product of man's basic biological process.

What can go wrong

Difficulty in breathing can arise in many ways, including partial blockage of an airway by a physical object, damage to the alveoli (emphysema), and the destruction of lung tissue by tuberculosis or other diseases. The most common problems, however, occur because of allergic reactions (usually in the nasal passages), spasmodic contractions of the bronchi (asthma), or an infection. Most infections, usually viral or bacterial in nature, lead to inflammation of various parts of the airways, with consequent fever, irritation, coughing, and phlegm, a gooey combination of mucus and pus. Such inflammations carry the names of their location: rhinitis (nose), pharyngitis (throat), tonsillitis (tonsils), laryngitis (larynx), and bronchitis (bronchial tubes).

The respiratory system is also damaged by long-term exposure to tobacco smoke and other airborne impurities.

Why drugs are used

Drugs with a variety of actions are used to clear the air passages, soothe inflammation, and reduce the production of mucus. Many of these can be bought without a prescription as single-ingredient or combined-ingredient preparations, often with an analgesic.

Decongestants (p.121) reduce the swelling inside the nose, so making it possible to breathe more freely. If the cause of congestion is an allergic response, an antihistamine (p.152) is often recommended to relieve symptoms or to prevent attacks.

Drugs that widen the bronchi – bronchodilators (p.120) – are used to relieve or prevent asthma attacks. The bronchodilators include drugs that relax the muscles surrounding the airways and those, such as corticosteroids (p.169), that widen the air passages by reducing inflammation of the mucous lining. These may also be of limited benefit in chronic respiratory problems.

A variety of drugs may be used to relieve coughs. Some of them make it easier to eliminate phlegm; others suppress coughing by inhibiting the cough reflex itself.

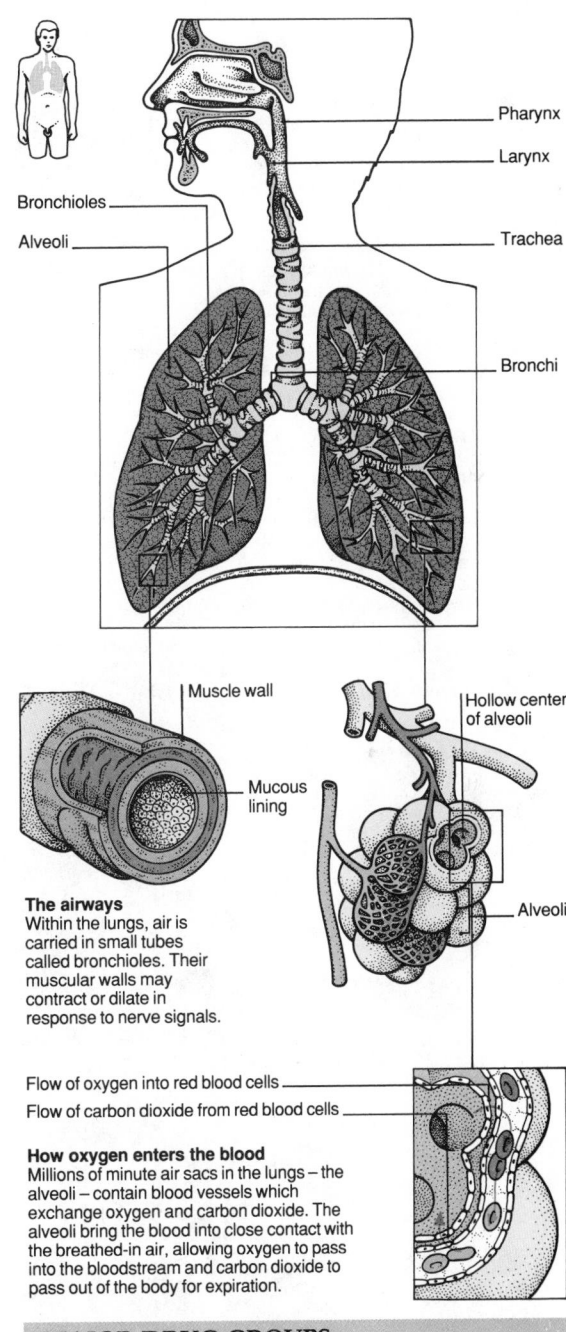

Pharynx

Larynx

Bronchioles

Alveoli

Trachea

Bronchi

Muscle wall

Hollow center of alveoli

Mucous lining

Alveoli

The airways
Within the lungs, air is carried in small tubes called bronchioles. Their muscular walls may contract or dilate in response to nerve signals.

Flow of oxygen into red blood cells

Flow of carbon dioxide from red blood cells

How oxygen enters the blood
Millions of minute air sacs in the lungs – the alveoli – contain blood vessels which exchange oxygen and carbon dioxide. The alveoli bring the blood into close contact with the breathed-in air, allowing oxygen to pass into the bloodstream and carbon dioxide to pass out of the body for expiration.

MAJOR DRUG GROUPS

Bronchodilators
Decongestants
Drugs to treat coughs

BRONCHODILATORS

When air enters the lungs it passes through narrow tubes called bronchioles. In certain conditions the bronchioles become narrower, either as a result of contraction of the muscles in their walls or as a result of mucous congestion. This tightening of the bronchioles obstructs the flow of air into and out of the lungs and causes breathlessness.

Bronchodilators are prescribed to widen the bronchioles and improve breathing. There are three main groups of bronchodilators: *sympathomimetic* drugs, *anticholinergics*, and xanthine drugs, which are related to caffeine.

Why they are used

Bronchodilators are commonly used to relieve asthma and to compensate for narrowing of the bronchioles as a result of accumulation of mucus in chronic bronchitis. However, they are of little benefit when damage to the bronchioles is severe.

Bronchodilators can either be taken as needed to relieve an attack of breathlessness that is in progress, or on a regular basis to prevent such attacks from occurring. Some people find it helpful to take an extra dose of their bronchodilator immediately before any activity

INHALERS

Inhalation of a bronchodilator drug directly into the lungs is usually the most effective method of ensuring maximum beneficial effect without excessive side effects. The main devices for delivering the drug into the airways are described below.

Inhalers or **puffers** release a small dose when they are pressed, but require some skill to use effectively.

Insufflation cartridges deliver larger amounts of drug than inhalers and are easier to use because the drug is taken in as you breathe normally.

Nebulizers pump compressed air through a solution of drug to produce a fine mist which is inhaled through a face mask. They deliver large doses of the drug to the lungs, rapidly relieving breathing difficulty.

likely to provoke an attack of breathlessness. Sympathomimetic drugs are mainly used for the rapid relief of breathlessness; anticholinergic and xanthine drugs are more often used for the long-term prevention of attacks.

How they work

Bronchodilator drugs act by relaxing the muscles surrounding the bronchioles. Sympathomimetic and anticholinergic drugs achieve this by interfering with nerve signals passed to the muscles through the autonomic nervous system (see p.107). Xanthine drugs are thought to relax the muscles in the bronchioles by a direct effect on the muscle fibers, but their precise action is not known.

How they affect you

When taken for the immediate relief of breathlessness, bronchodilators usually improve breathing within a few minutes. Taken to prevent attacks, bronchodilators usually start to increase one's capacity for exercise within a few days, and most people find that the frequency of breathless attacks is reduced.

Bronchodilators can produce minor side effects, especially if taken too frequently or in too large a dose. Because sympathomimetic drugs stimulate a branch of the autonomic nervous system that controls heart rate, they may sometimes cause palpitations and trembling. Typical side effects of anticholinergic drugs include dry mouth, blurred vision, and difficulty in passing urine. Xanthine drugs may cause headaches and palpitations.

Risks and special precautions

Since bronchodilators are not often taken by mouth but inhaled (see Inhalers, above), they do not commonly cause serious side effects. However, because of their possible effect on heart rate, sympathomimetic and xanthine drugs are prescribed with caution for those with heart problems, high blood pressure, or an overactive thyroid gland. Anticholinergic drugs may not be suitable for people with urinary retention or who have a tendency to glaucoma.

ACTION OF BRONCHODILATORS

When bronchioles become narrow following contraction of the muscle layer and swelling of the mucous lining, the passage of air is impeded. Bronchodilators act on the nerve signals that govern muscle activity. Sympathomimetics enhance the action of neurotransmitters that encourage muscle relaxation. Anticholinergics block the neurotransmitters that trigger muscle contraction. Xanthines promote muscle relaxation by a direct effect on the muscles.

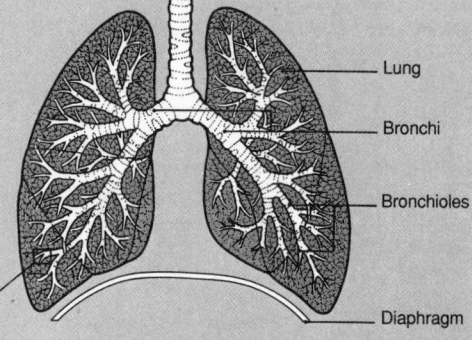

Trachea

Lung

Bronchi

Bronchioles

Diaphragm

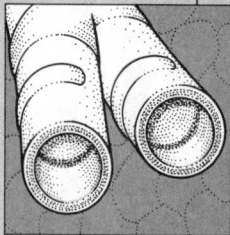

Normal bronchioles
The muscles surrounding the bronchioles are relaxed, leaving the airway open.

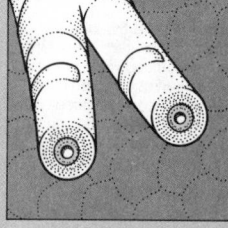

Asthmatic spasm
The muscles contract and the lining swells, narrowing the airway.

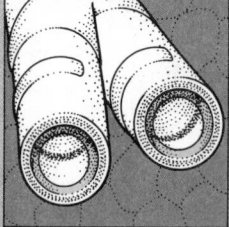

After drug treatment
The muscles relax, opening the airway, but the mucous lining remains swollen.

COMMON DRUGS

Sympathomimetics
Albuterol
Ephedrine
Epinephrine
Isoproterenol
Metaproterenol
Terbutaline

Anticholinergics
Atropine
Ipratropium

Xanthines
Aminophylline
Oxtriphylline
Theophylline

DECONGESTANTS

The usual cause of a blocked nose is swelling of the delicate mucous membrane that lines the nasal passages and excessive production of mucus as a result of inflammation. This may be caused by an infection (usually a common cold) or it may be caused by an allergy – for example, to pollen – a condition known as allergic rhinitis or hay fever. Congestion can also occur in the sinuses (the air spaces in the skull), resulting in sinusitis. Decongestants are drugs that reduce swelling of the mucous membrane and suppress the production of mucus, therefore helping to clear blocked nasal passages and sinuses. Antihistamines, which counter the allergic response in allergy-related conditions, are discussed on p.152.

Why they are used

Most common colds do not need to be treated with decongestants. Simple home remedies such as steam inhalation, possibly with the addition of an aromatic oil – such as menthol or eucalyptus – are often effective. Decongestants are used when such measures are ineffective, or when there is a risk from untreated congestion – for example, in people who suffer from recurrent middle ear or sinus infections.

Decongestants can be taken by mouth. They also are available in the form of drops that are applied directly into the nose (*topical* decongestants). Small quantities of decongestant drugs are often added to over-the-counter cold remedies (see Cold cures, p.122).

How they work

When the mucous membrane lining the nose is irritated by infection or allergy, the blood vessels supplying the membrane become enlarged. This leads to fluid accumulation in the surrounding tissue and encourages the production of larger than normal amounts of mucus.

Most decongestants belong to the *sympathomimetic* group of drugs which stimulate the sympathetic branch of the autonomic nervous system (see p.107). One effect of this action is to constrict the blood vessels, so reducing swelling

ACTION OF DECONGESTANTS

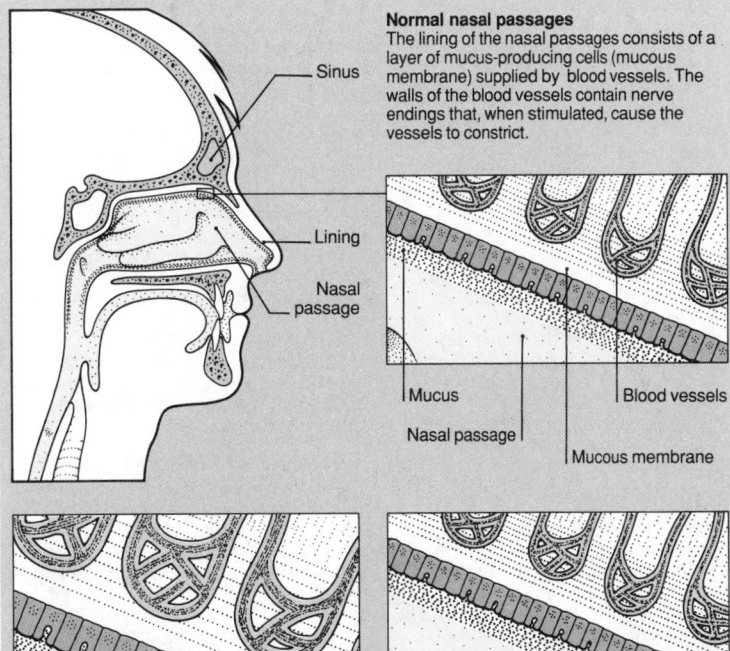

Normal nasal passages
The lining of the nasal passages consists of a layer of mucus-producing cells (mucous membrane) supplied by blood vessels. The walls of the blood vessels contain nerve endings that, when stimulated, cause the vessels to constrict.

Sinus

Lining

Nasal passage

Mucus

Nasal passage

Blood vessels

Mucous membrane

Congested nasal lining
When the blood vessels enlarge in response to infection or irritation, increased amounts of fluid pass into the mucous membrane, which swells and produces more mucus.

Effect of decongestants
Decongestants enhance the action of chemicals that stimulate constriction of the blood vessels. Narrowing of the blood vessels reduces swelling and mucus production.

of the lining of the nose and sinuses.

How they affect you

When applied topically in drops these drugs start to relieve congestion within a few minutes. Decongestants by mouth take a little longer to act, but their effect may last longer.

Topical decongestants used in moderation have few adverse effects because they are not absorbed by the

body in large amounts. Decongestants taken by mouth are more likely to cause symptoms related to their action on the sympathetic nervous system, including increased heart rate and trembling. For these reasons they should be used with caution by those with heart problems, high blood pressure, or an overactive thyroid gland.

Used for too long or in excess, decongestants can, after giving initial relief, do more harm than good, causing a "rebound congestion" (see left). This can be avoided by taking the minimum effective dose and by using decongestant preparations only when absolutely necessary.

REBOUND CONGESTION

This can happen when decongestants are suddenly withdrawn after an extended period of treatment, or when decongestant nose drops are overused. The result is a sudden increase in congestion due to widening of the blood vessels in the nasal lining because blood vessels are no longer constricted by the decongestant.

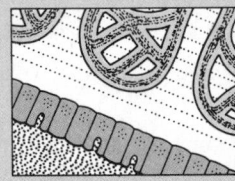

Congestion before drug treatment

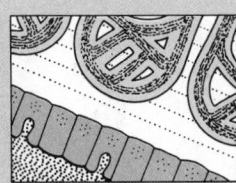

Congestion after stopping drug treatment

COMMON DRUGS

Ephedrine	Pseudoephedrine
Oxymetazoline	Xylometazoline
Phenylephrine	
Phenylpropanolamine	

DRUGS TO TREAT COUGHS

Coughing is a natural response to irritation of the lungs and air passages, designed to expel harmful substances from the respiratory tract. Common causes of coughing include infection of the respiratory tract (for example, bronchitis or pneumonia), inflammation of the airways caused by asthma, or exposure to certain irritant substances such as smoke or chemical fumes. Depending on their cause, coughs may be productive – that is, phlegm-producing – or they may be dry.

In most cases coughing is a helpful reaction that assists the body to get rid of excess phlegm or irritant substances; suppressing the cough may actually delay recovery. However, repeated bouts of coughing can be distressing, sometimes increasing irritation of the air passages. In such cases, medication to ease the cough may be recommended.

There are two main groups of cough remedies, according to whether the cough is productive or dry.

Productive coughs

Mucolytics and expectorants are the groups of drugs most commonly recommended for productive coughs when simple home remedies such as steam inhalation have failed to "loosen" the cough and make it easier to cough up phlegm. Mucolytics alter the consistency of the phlegm, making it less sticky and easier to cough up. These are often given by inhalation.

Expectorants are drugs that are frequently included in over-the-counter cough and cold remedies. These are said to encourage the production of phlegm, but the overall benefits of such drugs are doubtful.

Dry coughs

In dry coughs there is no advantage to be gained from promoting the expulsion of phlegm. Drugs used for dry coughs are given to suppress the coughing mechanism by calming the part of the brain that governs the coughing reflex. Antihistamines are often given for mild coughs, particularly in children. For persistent coughs, mild narcotic drugs such as codeine are prescribed (see also Analgesics, p.108). All cough suppressants have a generally sedating effect on the brain and nervous system and commonly cause drowsiness and other side effects.

Selecting a cough medication

There is a bewildering variety of over-the-counter medications available for treating coughs. Most consist of a syrupy base to which active ingredients and flavorings are added. Many contain a number of different active ingredients, sometimes with contradictory effects: it is not uncommon to find an expectorant (for a productive cough) and a cough suppressant (for a dry cough) included in the same preparation.

It is important to select the correct

COLD CURES

Many preparations are available over the counter to treat different symptoms of the common cold. The main ingredient is usually a mild analgesic such as acetaminophen or aspirin, and is often accompanied by a decongestant (p.121), an antihistamine (p.152), and sometimes caffeine. Often the dose of each added ingredient is too low to provide any benefit. Vitamin C (see p.544) is often included in cold relief products, but there is no evidence that it speeds recovery.

While some people find these preparations help to relieve symptoms, over-the-counter "cold cures" do not alter the course of the illness. Most physicians recommend preparations containing a single analgesic, as the best (and cheapest) way of alleviating the symptoms of the common cold. Additional decongestants or antihistamines may be taken as necessary if this does not provide adequate relief.

type of medication for your cough to avoid the risk that you may make your condition worse. For example, using a cough suppressant for a productive cough may prevent you from getting rid of excess phlegm and may thereby delay your recovery. It is best to choose a preparation with a single active ingredient that is appropriate for your type of cough. Diabetics may need to select a sugar-free product. If you are in any doubt ask your physician or pharmacist for advice. Because there is a danger that use of over-the-counter cough remedies to alleviate symptoms may delay the diagnosis of a more serious underlying disorder, it is important to seek medical advice for any cough that persists for longer than two days or if a cough is accompanied by additional symptoms such as fever or blood in the phlegm.

COMMON DRUGS

Expectorant
Ammonium chloride

Mucolytic
Acetylcysteine

Narcotic cough suppressant
Codeine

Non-narcotic cough suppressants
Antihistamines (see p.152)
Dextromethorphan
Isoproterenol

ACTION OF COUGH REMEDIES

Cough remedies are divided into two main groups: those that alter the consistency or production of phlegm (mucolytics and expectorants); and those that suppress the coughing reflex (narcotic and non-narcotic cough suppressants). Mucolytics are usually given by inhalation and act directly on the lungs and airways. Expectorants are taken by mouth, and are supposed to help bring up phlegm. Cough suppressants are taken by mouth and they act on the coughing center in the brain.

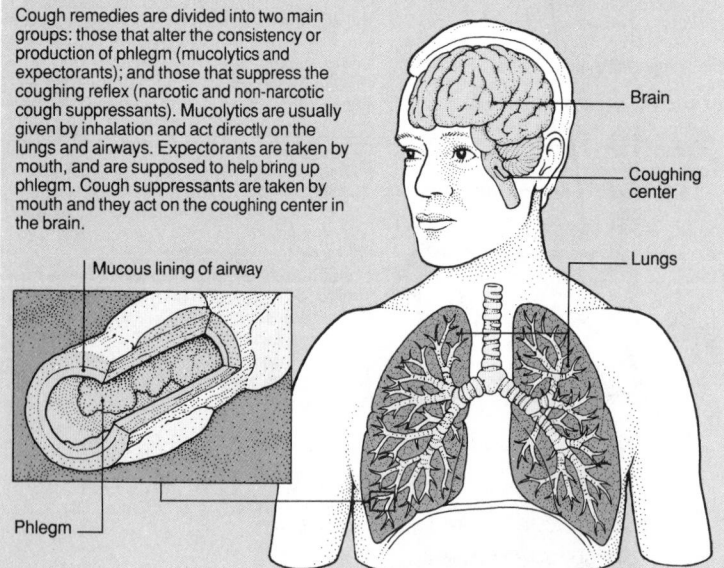

Brain

Coughing center

Lungs

Mucous lining of airway

Phlegm

HEART AND CIRCULATION

The blood transports oxygen, nutrients, and heat, contains chemical messages in the form of drugs and hormones, and carries away waste products for excretion by the liver and kidneys. Pumped by the heart and carried in blood vessels (veins, arteries, and capillaries), blood circulates continuously around the body.

What can go wrong

Efficiency of the circulation may be impaired by a weakening of the heart's pumping action (heart failure) or irregularity of heartbeat (arrhythmias). In addition, the blood vessels may be narrowed and clogged by fatty deposits (atherosclerosis). This may reduce blood supply to the brain, the extremities (peripheral vascular disease), or to the heart muscle (coronary heart disease), causing angina. These last disorders can be complicated by the formation of clots which may block a blood vessel. In the arteries supplying the heart muscle, this is known as coronary thrombosis, and inside the brain it is the most frequent cause of stroke.

One common circulatory disorder is abnormally high blood pressure (hypertension), in which the pressure of the circulating blood on the vessel walls is increased for reasons not yet fully understood. One factor may be loss of elasticity of the blood vessel walls (arteriosclerosis).

A number of other conditions are caused by temporary alterations to blood vessel size. These include migraine and Raynaud's disease.

Why drugs are used

Because those suffering from heart disease often have more than one problem, several drugs may be prescribed at once. Many act directly on the heart to alter the rate and rhythm of the heartbeat. These are known as anti-arrhythmics and include beta blockers and digitalis drugs.

Other drugs affect the blood vessel diameter, either dilating them (vasodilators) to improve blood flow and reduce blood pressure and strain, or constricting them (vasoconstrictors).

Drugs may also reduce blood volume and fat levels, and alter clotting ability. Diuretics (used in the treatment of hypertension and heart failure) increase the body's excretion of water. Lipid-lowering drugs reduce blood fat levels, thereby minimizing the risk of atherosclerosis. Drugs to reduce blood clotting are administered when there is a risk of abnormal blood clots forming in the veins or arteries. Drugs that increase clotting are given when the body's natural clotting mechanism is defective.

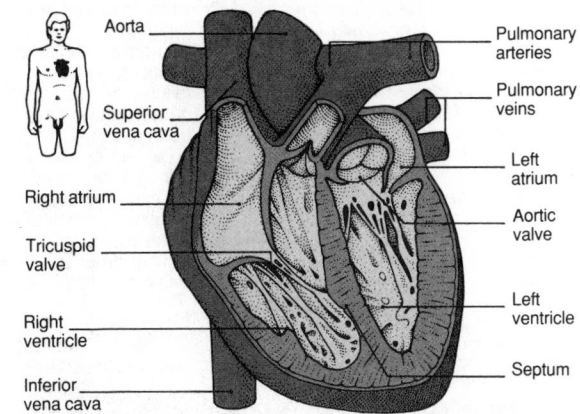

The heart
The heart is a pump containing four chambers. The atrium and ventricle on the left side pump oxygenated blood, while the corresponding chambers on the right pump de-oxygenated blood. Backflow of blood is prevented by valves at the chamber exits.

How blood circulates
De-oxygenated blood is carried to the heart from all parts of the body. It is then pumped to the lungs where it becomes oxygenated. The oxygenated blood returns to the heart and from there is pumped throughout the body.

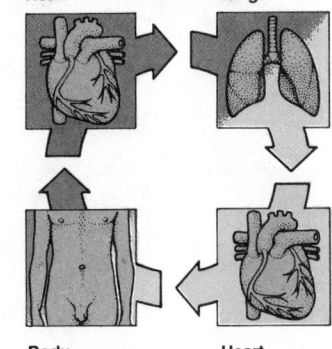

De-oxygenated blood

Oxygenated blood

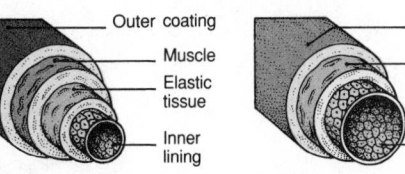

Arteries
Arteries carry blood away from the heart. Muscle walls contract and dilate in response to nerve signals.

Veins
Veins carry de-oxygenated blood back to the heart. The walls are less elastic than artery walls.

MAJOR DRUG GROUPS

Digitalis drugs
Beta blockers
Vasodilators
Diuretics
Anti-arrhythmic drugs

Anti-angina drugs
Antihypertensive drugs
Lipid-lowering drugs
Drugs that affect blood clotting

DIGITALIS DRUGS

"Digitalis" is the collective term for a number of naturally occurring substances (also called cardiac glycosides) found in the leaves of plants of the foxglove family and used for certain heart disorders. The principal drugs in this group are digoxin and digitoxin. Digoxin is more commonly used because it is shorter-acting and dosage is easier to adjust (see also Risks and special precautions, below).

Why they are used

Digitalis drugs do not cure heart disease but improve the heart's pumping action and so relieve many of the symptoms that result from poor heart function. They are useful for treating conditions in which the heart beats irregularly or too rapidly (notably in atrial fibrillation, see Anti-arrhythmic drugs, p.128), when it pumps too weakly (in congestive heart failure), or when the heart muscle is damaged and weakened following a heart attack.

Digitalis drugs can be used for a short period when the heart is working poorly, but in many cases they have to be taken indefinitely. Their effect may begin to wane after a time. In heart failure, digitalis drugs are often given together with a diuretic (see p.127).

How they work

The normal heartbeat results from electrical impulses generated in nerve tissue within the heart. These cause the heart muscle to contract and pump blood. By reducing the passage of electrical impulses in the heart, digitalis makes the heart beat more slowly.

The force with which the heart muscle contracts depends on chemical changes in the muscle. By promoting these chemical changes, digitalis increases the force of muscle contraction each time the heart is stimulated. This compensates for the loss of power that occurs when some of the muscle is damaged following a heart attack. The stronger heartbeat increases the flow of blood to the kidneys. This increases urine production and helps to remove the excess fluid that often accumulates as a result of heart failure.

How they affect you

Digitalis relieves symptoms of heart failure – fatigue, breathlessness, and swelling of the legs – and increases your capacity for exercise. The frequency with which you need to pass urine is also increased initially.

Risks and special precautions

Digitalis drugs can be toxic and, if blood levels rise too high, may produce symptoms of digitalis poisoning. These include excessive tiredness, confusion, loss of appetite, nausea, vomiting, and diarrhea. If such symptoms occur, it is important to report them to your physician promptly.

Digoxin is normally removed from the body by the kidneys; if kidney function is impaired, the drug is more likely to accumulate in the body and cause toxic effects. Digitoxin, which is broken down in the liver, is sometimes preferred in such cases. Digitoxin can accumulate after repeated doses, especially if liver function is reduced.

Both digoxin and digitoxin are more toxic when blood potassium levels are low. Potassium deficiency is commonly caused by diuretic drugs, so that people taking these along with digitalis drugs need to have the effects of both drugs and blood potassium levels carefully monitored. Potassium supplements may be required.

ACTION OF DIGITALIS DRUGS

The heartbeat is triggered by electrical impulses that are generated by a small mass of nerve tissue in the right atrium called the pacemaker. Electrical signals pass from the pacemaker to the atrio-ventricular node. From here a wave of impulses spreads through the heart muscle, causing it to contract and pump blood to the body. The pumping action of the heart can become weak if the heart muscle is damaged or if the ventricles beat too fast, as in atrial fibrillation. In this condition (shown right), rapid signals from the pacemaker trigger fast and inefficient contractions of the ventricles.

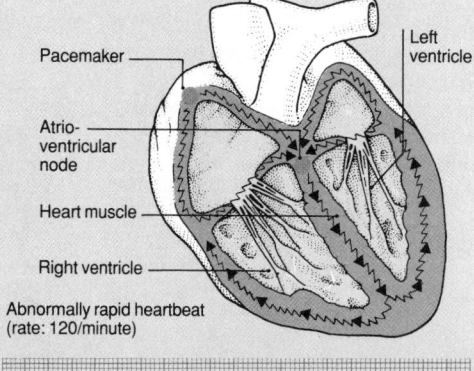

Pacemaker

Atrio-ventricular node

Heart muscle

Right ventricle

Left ventricle

Abnormally rapid heartbeat (rate: 120/minute)

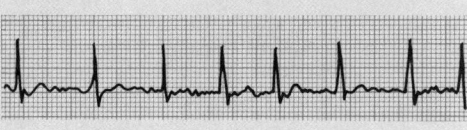

The effect of digitalis
Digitalis drugs reduce the flow of electrical impulses from the atrioventricular node so that the ventricles contract less often. In addition, by promoting the chemical changes in muscle cells necessary for muscular contraction, these drugs increase the force with which the heart muscle contracts and so improve the efficiency of each heartbeat.

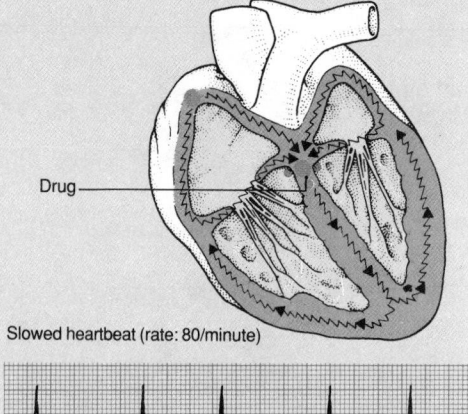

Drug

Slowed heartbeat (rate: 80/minute)

COMMON DRUGS

Digoxin
Digitoxin

BETA BLOCKERS

Beta blockers are drugs that interrupt the transmission of stimuli through the beta *receptors* of the body. Since what they block originates in the adrenal glands (and elsewhere) they are also sometimes called beta adrenergic blocking agents. Used mainly in heart disorders, they are occasionally prescribed for other conditions.

Why they are used

Beta blockers are used in the treatment of angina (see p.129), hypertension (see p.130), and irregular heart rhythms (see p.128). They are sometimes given after a heart attack to reduce the likelihood of fatal arrhythmia or further damage to the heart muscle. These drugs are also prescribed to improve heart function in obstructive cardiomyopathy.

Beta blockers may also be given to prevent migraine headaches (see p.117) or reduce anxiety (see p.111) including stage fright and "butterflies" in the stomach. They may be given to control symptoms of an overactive thyroid gland. A beta blocker is sometimes given in the form of eye drops in glaucoma to lower fluid pressure inside the eye (see p.196).

How they work

By occupying the beta receptors, beta blockers nullify the stimulating action of norepinephrine. Thus they reduce the force and speed of the heartbeat,

BETA RECEPTORS

Signals from the sympathetic nervous system are carried by norepinephrine, a *neurotransmitter* produced in the adrenal glands and at the ends of sympathetic nerve fibers. Beta blockers stop the signals from the neurotransmitter.

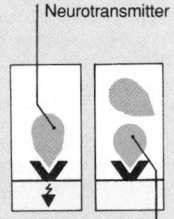

Neurotransmitter

Beta blocker

Types of beta receptor
There are two types of beta receptor: beta 1 and beta 2. Beta 1 receptors are located mainly in the heart muscle; beta 2 receptors are found in the airways and blood vessels. Cardioselective drugs act mainly on beta 1 receptors; non-cardioselective drugs act on both types.

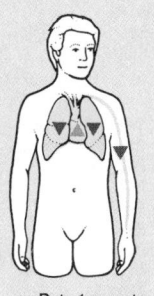

▲ Beta 1 receptors
▼ Beta 2 receptors

THE USES AND EFFECTS OF BETA BLOCKERS

The blockade of the transmission of signals through beta receptors in different parts of the body produces a wide variety of benefits and side effects according to the disease being treated. The illustration (right) shows the main areas and body systems affected by the action of beta blockers.

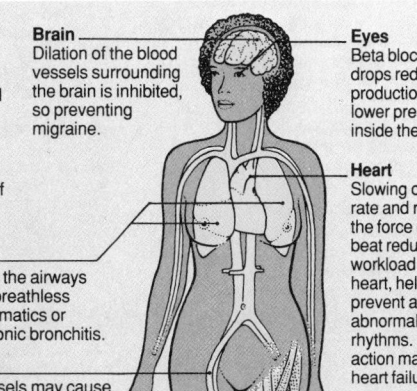

Brain
Dilation of the blood vessels surrounding the brain is inhibited, so preventing migraine.

Eyes
Beta blocker eye drops reduce fluid production and so lower pressure inside the eye.

Heart
Slowing of the heart rate and reduction of the force of the heartbeat reduce the workload of the heart, helping to prevent angina and abnormal heart rhythms. But this action may worsen heart failure.

Lungs
Constriction of the airways may provoke breathless attacks in asthmatics or those with chronic bronchitis.

Muscles
Muscle tremor in anxiety and overactivity of the thyroid gland is reduced.

Blood vessels
Constriction of the blood vessels may cause coldness of the hands and feet.

Blood pressure
This is lowered because the rate and force at which the heart pumps blood into the circulatory system is reduced.

prevent the dilation of the airways to the lungs, and prevent the dilation of the blood vessels surrounding the brain and leading to the extremities. The effect of this "beta blockade" in a variety of disorders is shown in the box above.

How they affect you

Taken to treat angina, beta blockers reduce the frequency and severity of attacks. As part of the treatment for hypertension, they help to lower blood pressure and thus reduce the risks that are associated with this condition. Beta blockers help to prevent severe attacks of arrhythmia or wild, uncontrolled heartbeats.

Because beta blockers affect many parts of the body, they commonly produce minor side effects. By reducing heart rate and air flow to the lungs, they may reduce capacity for strenuous exercise, although this is unlikely to be noticed by somebody whose physical activity was previously limited by heart problems. Many people experience cold hands and feet while taking these drugs, due to the reduction in blood supply to the limbs. Reduced circulation can also lead to temporary impotence during beta blocker treatment.

Risks and special precautions

The main risk of beta blockers is that of provoking breathing difficulties as a result of their blocking effect on beta receptors in the lungs. Cardioselective beta blockers, which act principally on the heart, are thought to be less likely than non-cardioselective ones to cause

such problems. But all beta blockers are prescribed with caution for people with asthma, bronchitis, or other forms of respiratory disease.

Beta blockers are not usually prescribed for people who have poor circulation in the limbs because they reduce the flow of blood and may aggravate such conditions. They are not normally given to people who are subject to heart failure because they may further reduce the force of the heartbeat. Diabetics who need to take beta blockers should be aware that they may notice a change in the warning signs of low blood sugar – in particular, symptoms such as palpitations and tremor may be suppressed.

Beta blockers should not be stopped suddenly after prolonged use; this may provoke a sudden and severe recurrence of symptoms of the original disorder, even a heart attack. Blood pressure may also rise markedly. When the treatment needs to be stopped, it should be withdrawn gradually under medical supervision.

COMMON DRUGS

Non-cardioselective	Cardioselective
Acebutolol	Atenolol
Labetalol	Esmolol
Nadolol	Metoprolol
Oxprenolol	
Propranolol	
Timolol	

VASODILATORS

Vasodilators – drugs that dilate blood vessels – are commonly prescribed for disorders in which narrowing of the blood vessels leads to reduced blood flow and a consequent lower oxygen supply to parts of the body. Disorders of this type include angina, when a narrowing of the coronary arteries reduces the supply of blood, thereby causing painful spasm. They also include peripheral vascular disease, a group of disorders in which blood vessels in the arms and legs cannot supply sufficient blood to the extremities. Vasodilators are also widely used in the treatment of high blood pressure (hypertension).

Several classes of vasodilator drugs are prescribed, including nitrates, *sympatholytics*, calcium channel blockers, and ACE (angiotensin-converting enzyme) inhibitors.

Why they are used

Vasodilators improve blood flow and oxygen supply to areas of the body where they are most needed. In angina, dilation of the blood vessels throughout the body reduces the force with which the heart needs to pump and therefore eases its workload (see also Anti-angina drugs, p.129). This effect is sometimes helpful in the treatment of congestive heart failure when other treatments are not effective. In peripheral vascular disease, vasodilators are usually taken on a continuing basis in order to improve blood circulation.

Because blood pressure depends partly on the diameter of the blood vessels, vasodilators are often helpful in treating hypertension (see p.130).

Vasodilator drugs have also been used for senile dementia, theoretically increasing the supply of oxygen needed by healthy brain cells. The benefits of this treatment have not been proven.

ACTION OF VASODILATORS

The diameter of blood vessels is governed by the contraction of the surrounding muscle. The muscle contracts in response to signals from the sympathetic nervous system (p.107). Vasodilators encourage the muscles to relax, thus increasing the size of blood vessels.

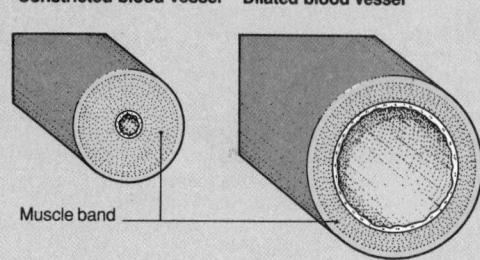

Constricted blood vessel   Dilated blood vessel

Muscle band

Where they act
Each type of vasodilator acts on a different part of the mechanism controlling blood vessel size to prevent contraction of the surrounding layer of muscles.

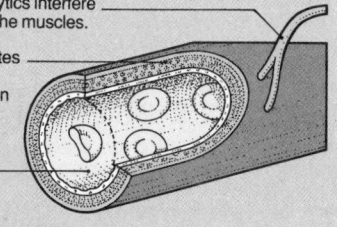

Nerves – Sympatholytics interfere with nerve signals to the muscles.

Muscle layer – Nitrates and calcium channel blockers act directly on the muscle to inhibit contraction.

Blood – ACE inhibitors block enzyme activity in the blood (see box below).

How they work

Vasodilators widen the blood vessels by relaxing the muscles that surround them. They achieve this either by affecting the action of the muscles directly (nitrates and calcium channel blockers) or by interfering with the nerve signals that govern contraction of the blood vessels (sympatholytics). ACE inhibitors act by blocking enzyme activity in the blood (see the box below).

How they affect you

In addition to relieving the symptoms of the disorders for which they are taken, vasodilators can have a number of minor adverse effects related to their action on the blood circulation. Flushing and headaches are common at the start of treatment. Attacks of dizziness and fainting may also occur as a result of lowered blood pressure. Dilation of the blood vessels can also cause a fluid buildup, leading to swelling, particularly of the ankles.

Risks and special precautions

The major risk is that blood pressure may sometimes fall too low. For this reason these drugs are prescribed with caution for those with unstable blood pressure. It may also be advisable to take the first dose of vasodilator drugs at a time when you are able to sit or lie down afterwards.

ACE INHIBITORS

ACE (angiotensin-converting enzyme) inhibitors are powerful vasodilators. They act by blocking the action of an enzyme in the bloodstream that is responsible for converting a chemical called angiotensin I into angiotensin II. Angiotensin II encourages constriction of the blood vessels and its absence permits them to dilate (see right).

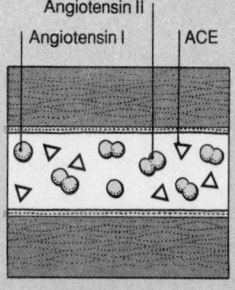

Angiotensin II
Angiotensin I   ACE

Before drug
Angiotensin I is converted by the enzyme into angiotensin II. The blood vessel constricts.

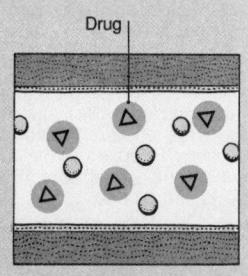

Drug

Drug action
ACE inhibitors block enzyme activity, thereby preventing the formation of angiotensin II. The blood vessel dilates.

COMMON DRUGS

Nitrates
Isosorbide dinitrate
Nitroglycerin

Calcium channel blockers
Nifedipine
Verapamil

ACE inhibitors
Captopril
Enalapril
Lisinopril

Sympatholytics
Guanethidine
Hydralazine
Minoxidil
Prazosin

DIURETICS

Diuretic drugs help to turn excess body water into urine. As the urine is expelled, two disorders are relieved: tissues become less water-swollen (edema) and heart action improves because a smaller volume of blood is circulating. There are several classes of diuretics, each of which has different uses, modes of action, and effects (see Types of diuretic, below). But all act on the kidneys, the organs that govern the water content of the body.

Why they are used

One of the most common uses of diuretics is in the treatment of high blood pressure (hypertension). By removing larger than usual amounts of water from the bloodstream, the kidneys reduce the total volume of blood circulating. This in turn reduces the pressure within the blood vessels (see Antihypertensive drugs, p.130).

Diuretics are also widely used to treat heart failure in which the heart's pumping mechanism has become weak. In this disorder they remove fluid that has accumulated in the tissues and lungs. The resulting drop in blood volume reduces the work of the heart.

Other conditions for which diuretics are often prescribed include nephrotic syndrome (a kidney disorder that causes edema), cirrhosis of the liver (in which fluid may accumulate in the abdominal cavity), and premenstrual syndrome (when hormonal activity can lead to fluid retention and bloating).

Less common uses for diuretics include treating glaucoma (see p.196) and Ménière's disease (see p.118).

How they work

The normal filtration process of the kidneys takes water, salts (mainly potassium and sodium), and waste products out of the bloodstream. Most of the salts and water are returned to the bloodstream, but certain amounts are expelled from the body together with the waste products in the urine. Diuretics interfere with this normal kidney action

ACTION OF DIURETICS

As blood passes through the kidney, water, sodium and potassium salts, and waste products are filtered out of the bloodstream. Most of the water and filtered salts are then reabsorbed by the bloodstream from the tubule, and the remainder is excreted as urine.

By blocking the movement of sodium back into the bloodstream, diuretics prevent the reabsorption of water, so that more is expelled from the body as urine. Different diuretic drugs act on different parts of the tubule (see right).

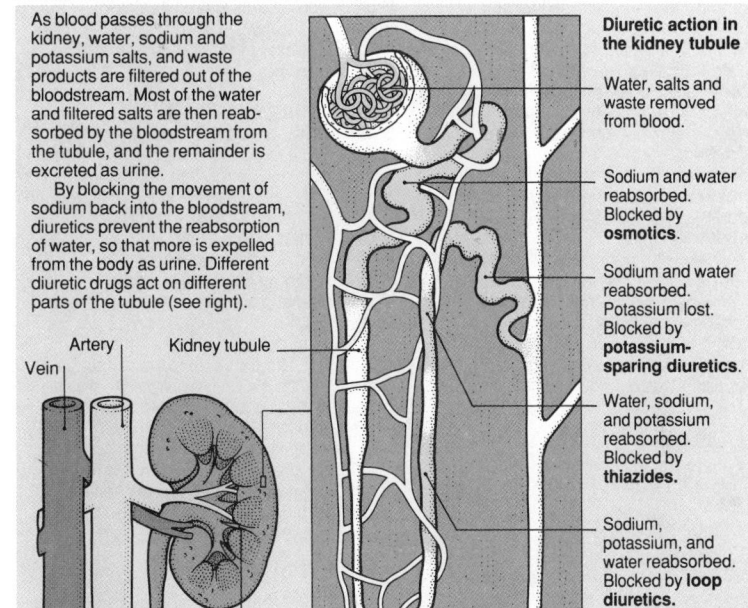

Diuretic action in the kidney tubule

Water, salts and waste removed from blood.

Sodium and water reabsorbed. Blocked by **osmotics**.

Sodium and water reabsorbed. Potassium lost. Blocked by **potassium-sparing diuretics**.

Water, sodium, and potassium reabsorbed. Blocked by **thiazides**.

Sodium, potassium, and water reabsorbed. Blocked by **loop diuretics**.

Artery Kidney tubule
Vein
Kidney

by reducing the amounts of sodium and water taken back into the bloodstream, thus increasing the volume of urine produced. In this way the water content of the blood is reduced and excess water is drawn out of the tissues for elimination as urine.

How they affect you

All diuretics increase the frequency with which you need to pass urine. This is most noticeable at the start of treatment. People who have suffered from edema may notice that swelling – particularly of the ankles – is reduced, and those with heart failure may find that breathlessness is relieved.

Risks and special precautions

Diuretics can cause chemical imbalances in the blood. Most common of these is a fall in potassium levels in the blood (hypokalemia), which can cause weakness and confusion, particularly in the elderly. Low potassium can also trigger abnormal heart rhythms, especially in those taking digitalis drugs. The imbalance can usually be corrected by potassium supplements (see p.540) or by a potassium-sparing diuretic. A diet that is rich in potassium (containing plenty of fresh fruits and vegetables) may be helpful.

Some diuretics may increase levels of uric acid in the blood and thus the risk of gout in susceptible people. They may also raise blood sugar level, which can cause problems for diabetics.

TYPES OF DIURETIC

Thiazides The type most commonly prescribed, thiazides may lead to potassium deficiency and they are, therefore, often given together with a potassium supplement or in conjunction with a potassium-sparing diuretic (see right).

Loop diuretics These fast-acting, powerful drugs increase the output of urine for a few hours; they are sometimes used in emergencies. They may cause excessive loss of potassium, which may need to be countered as is done with thiazides. Large doses may disturb hearing.

Potassium-sparing diuretics These mild diuretics are usually used in conjunction with a thiazide or a loop diuretic to prevent excessive potassium loss.

Osmotic diuretics Prescribed only rarely, these are used to maintain the flow of urine through the kidneys after surgery or injury, and to rapidly reduce pressure within fluid-filled cavities.

Acetazolamide This mild diuretic drug is used principally in the treatment of glaucoma (see p.196).

COMMON DRUGS

Thiazides
Chlorothiazide
Chlorthalidone
Hydrochlorothiazide
Metolazone

Loop diuretics
Bumetanide
Furosemide

Potassium-sparing diuretics
Amiloride
Spironolactone
Triamterene

ANTI-ARRHYTHMIC DRUGS

The heart contains two upper and two lower chambers (see p.123). The pumping actions of these two sets of chambers are normally coordinated by electrical impulses so that the heart beats with a regular rhythm. If this coordination breaks down, the heart may beat abnormally, either irregularly or faster or slower than usual. The general term for abnormal heart rhythm is arrhythmia. There are several types of arrhythmia, depending on the part of the heart that is affected (see Types of arrhythmia, right).

The heart's rhythm can be disrupted in any disorder that affects the heart's mechanism for controlling its beat. Other conditions, including overactivity of the thyroid gland, and certain drugs – for example, *anticholinergic* drugs and caffeine – can also disturb heart rhythm.

SITES OF DRUG ACTION

Anti-arrhythmic drugs either impede the flow of electrical impulses to the heart muscle, or inhibit the ability of the muscle to contract. Beta blockers reduce the ability of the pacemaker to pass electrical signals to the atria. Digitalis drugs reduce the passage of signals from the atrio-ventricular node. Calcium channel blockers interfere with the ability of the heart muscle to contract by impeding the flow of calcium into muscle cells. Other drugs such as quinidine and disopyramide reduce the sensitivity of muscle cells to electrical impulses.

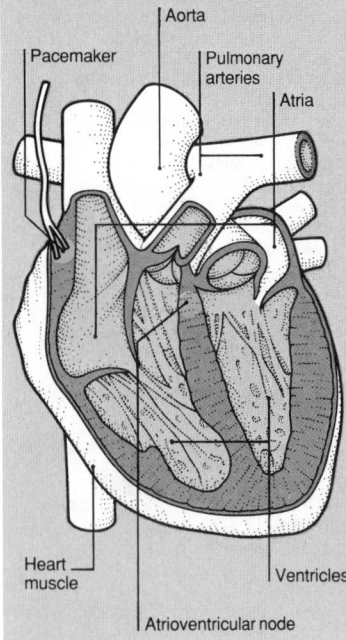

A broad range of drugs is used to regulate heart rhythm, including digitalis drugs, beta blockers, and calcium channel blockers. Other drugs used are lidocaine, disopyramide, procainamide, and quinidine.

Why they are used

Minor disturbances of heart rhythm are common and do not usually require drug treatment. However, if the pumping action of the heart is seriously affected, the circulation of blood throughout the body may become inefficient, and drug treatment may be necessary.

Drugs may be taken to treat individual attacks of arrhythmia, or they may be taken on a regular basis to prevent or control abnormal heart rhythms. The particular drug prescribed depends on the type of arrhythmia to be treated, but because people differ in their response, it may be necessary to try several in order to find the most effective one. When the arrhythmia is sudden and severe, it may be necessary to inject a drug immediately to restore normal heart function.

How they work

The heart's pumping action is governed by electrical impulses under the control of the sympathetic nervous system (see Autonomic nervous system, p.107). These signals pass through the heart muscle and cause each of the two pairs of heart chambers – the atria and the ventricles – to contract in turn (see Sites of drug action, left).

All anti-arrhythmic drugs alter the conduction of electrical signals in the heart, but each drug or drug group affects this sequence of events in a different way. Some block the trans-mission of signals to the heart (beta blockers); some affect the way signals are conducted within the heart (digitalis drugs); others affect the response of the heart muscle to the signals received (calcium channel blockers, disopyramide, procainamide, and quinidine).

How they affect you

These drugs usually prevent symptoms of arrhythmia and may restore a regular heart rhythm. Although they do not prevent all arrhythmias, they usually reduce the frequency and severity of any symptoms.

Unfortunately, as well as suppressing arrhythmias, many of these drugs tend to depress normal heart function, and may produce dizziness on standing up, or increased breathlessness on exertion. Mild nausea and visual disturbances are also fairly frequent. Verapamil can cause constipation, especially in high doses. Disopyramide

TYPES OF ARRHYTHMIA

Atrial fibrillation In this common arrhythmia, the atria contract irregularly at such a high rate that the ventricles cannot keep pace. It is treated with digoxin, sometimes in combination with quinidine.

Ventricular tachycardia This arises from abnormal electrical activity in the ventricles that causes the ventricles to contract rapidly. Regular treatment with disopyramide, procainamide or quinidine is usually given.

Supraventricular tachycardia This occurs when extra electrical impulses arise in the atria or in the atrioventricular node. These extra impulses stimulate the ventricles to contract rapidly. Attacks may disappear on their own without treatment, but drugs such as digoxin, verapamil, or propranolol may be given.

Heart block When signals are not conducted from the atria to the ventricles, the ventricles start to beat at a slower rate. Some cases of heart block do not require treatment. For more severe heart block accompanied by dizziness and fainting, physicians sometimes give atropine to provide temporary relief, but in the long term it is usually necessary to fit an artificial pacemaker.

may interfere with the parasympathetic nervous system (see p.107), resulting in a number of *anticholinergic* effects.

Risks and special precautions

These drugs may further disrupt heart rhythm under certain circumstances and therefore they are used only when the likely benefit outweighs the risks.

Quinidine can be toxic in overdose, resulting in a syndrome called cinchonism, which includes disturbed hearing, giddiness, and impaired vision (even blindness). Because some people are particularly sensitive to this drug, a test dose is usually given before regular treatment is started.

COMMON DRUGS

Beta blockers
(See p.125)

Calcium channel blockers
Diltiazem
Nifedipine
Verapamil

Digitalis drugs
Digitoxin
Digoxin

Other drugs
Disopyramide
Lidocaine
Procainamide
Quinidine
Tocainide

ANTI-ANGINA DRUGS

Angina is chest pain produced when insufficient oxygen reaches the heart muscle. This is usually caused by a narrowing of the blood vessels (coronary arteries) that carry blood and oxygen to the heart muscle. In the most common type of angina (classic angina), pain typically occurs during exertion or emotional stress. In variant angina, pain may also occur at rest. In classic angina, narrowing of the coronary arteries results from deposits of fat – called atheroma – on the walls of the arteries, whereas in variant angina it is caused by contraction (spasm) of muscle fibers in the artery wall.

Atheroma deposits build up in the arteries, especially in smokers and in people who eat high-fat meals. This is why, as a basic part of angina treatment, physicians recommend that you stop smoking and change your diet. Overweight people are also advised to lose weight in order to reduce the demands placed on their hearts. While such changes in lifestyle often produce an improvement in symptoms, drug treatment to relieve angina is also frequently necessary.

Three types of drugs are used to treat angina: beta blockers, nitrates, and calcium channel blockers.

Why they are used

Frequent episodes of angina can be disabling, and if left untreated can lead to an increased risk of a heart attack. Drugs can be used both to relieve angina attacks and to reduce their frequency. People who suffer from only occasional episodes are usually prescribed a rapid-acting drug to take at the first signs of an attack, or prior to an activity that is

known to bring one on. A rapid-acting nitrate – nitroglycerin – is usually prescribed for this purpose.

If attacks become more frequent or more severe, regular treatment to prevent them may be advised. Beta blockers, slow-acting nitrates, and calcium channel blockers are used as regular medication to prevent attacks. The introduction of adhesive patches for administering nitrates through the skin has extended the duration of action of nitroglycerin, making treatment easier on the individual.

Drug treatment can often control angina for many years, but it cannot cure the disorder. When severe angina cannot be controlled by drugs, heart surgery may be necessary.

How they work

Nitrates and calcium channel blockers dilate blood vessels by relaxing the muscle layer in the blood vessel wall (see also Vasodilators, p.126). This reduces strain on the heart by making it easier to pump blood.

Beta blockers interrupt the transmission of signals in the heart and so reduce stimulation of the heart muscle during exercise or stress. This also reduces the oxygen requirement of the heart muscle and makes angina attacks less likely to occur. For further information on beta blockers, see p.125.

How they affect you

Treatment with one or more of these drugs is usually effective in controlling angina. Drugs to prevent attacks allow sufferers to undertake more strenuous activities without provoking pain, and if an attack does occur, nitrates usually

ACTION OF ANTI-ANGINA DRUGS

The pain of angina arises when the heart muscle cannot pump sufficient blood through the circulatory system. By dilating blood vessels, nitrates and calcium channel blockers make this easier. Beta blockers impede the stimulation of heart muscle, reducing its oxygen requirement, thus relieving or preventing angina pain.

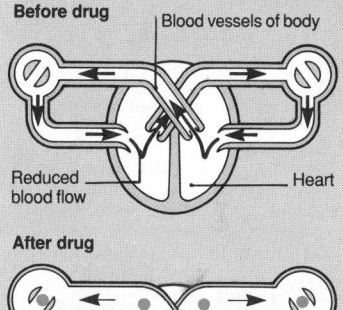

Before drug | Blood vessels of body

Reduced blood flow | Heart

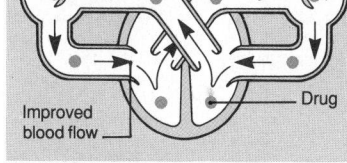

After drug

Improved blood flow | Drug

provide effective relief.

These drugs do not usually cause serious adverse effects, but they can produce a variety of minor symptoms. By dilating blood vessels throughout the body, nitrates and calcium channel blockers can cause dizziness and sometimes fainting (especially when standing). Other possible side effects are headaches at the start of treatment, flushing of the skin – especially of the face – and swelling of the ankles. Beta blockers often cause cold hands and feet, and can produce tiredness and a feeling of heaviness in the legs.

COMMON DRUGS

Beta blockers
(see p.125)

Calcium channel blockers
Diltiazem
Nifedipine
Verapamil

Nitrates
Isosorbide dinitrate
Nitroglycerin

CALCIUM CHANNEL BLOCKERS

The passage of calcium through special channels into muscle cells is an essential part of the mechanism of muscle contraction (see right). This relatively new class of drugs prevents movement of calcium in the muscles of the blood vessels and so encourages them to dilate (see far right). The action helps to reduce blood pressure and relieves the strain on the heart muscle in angina by making it easier for the heart to pump blood throughout the body (see the box above right). Calcium channel blockers also slow the passage of nerve signals through the heart muscle. This can be helpful for correcting certain types of abnormal heart rhythm.

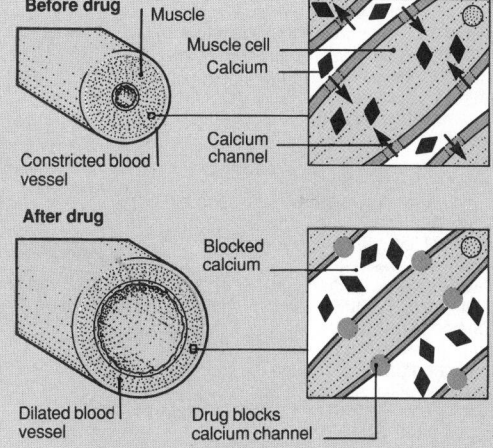

Before drug | Muscle

Muscle cell
Calcium

Calcium channel

Constricted blood vessel

After drug

Blocked calcium

Dilated blood vessel

Drug blocks calcium channel

ANTIHYPERTENSIVE DRUGS

Blood pressure is a measurement of the force exerted by the blood circulating in the arteries. Two readings are taken: one indicates force while the heart's ventricles are contracting (systolic pressure). It is a higher figure than the other reading, which measures the blood-flow push during ventricle relaxation (diastolic pressure). Blood pressure varies among individuals and normally increases with age. If a person's blood pressure is higher than normal on at least three separate occasions, a physician may diagnose hypertension.

Blood pressure may be raised as a result of an underlying disorder, which a physician will try to identify. Usually, however, it is not possible to find a cause. This condition is essential hypertension.

Although hypertension is usually without symptoms, severely raised pressure may produce headaches, palpitations, and general feelings of ill health. It is important to reduce high blood pressure, because it can have serious consequences, including stroke, heart attack, heart failure, and kidney damage. Certain groups are particularly at risk from high blood pressure. These include diabetics, smokers, people with pre-existing heart damage, and those whose blood contains a high level of fat. High blood pressure is more common among black people than among whites.

A small reduction in blood pressure may be brought about by reducing weight, exercising regularly, and keeping to a low-salt diet. But for more severely raised blood pressure, one or more antihypertensive drugs may be prescribed. Several different classes of drugs have antihypertensive properties, including centrally acting antihypertensives, diuretics (p.127), beta blockers (p.125), calcium channel blockers, ACE (angiotensin-converting enzyme) inhibitors, and sympatholytics. See also Vasodilators, p.126.

Why they are used

These drugs are prescribed when diet, exercise, and other simple remedies have not brought about an adequate reduction in blood pressure, and your physician sees a risk of serious consequences if the condition is not treated. Antihypertensive drugs do not cure hypertension and may have to be taken indefinitely. However, it is sometimes possible to taper off drug treatment when blood pressure has been reduced to a normal level for a year or more.

How they work

Blood pressure depends not only on the force with which the heart pumps blood, but also on the diameter of blood vessels and the volume of blood in circulation: blood pressure is increased if the vessels are narrow or the volume of blood is high. Antihypertensive drugs lower blood pressure either by dilating the blood vessels or by reducing blood volume. Antihypertensive drugs work in different ways and some have more than one action (see Action of antihypertensive drugs, left).

Choice of drug

Drug treatment depends on the severity of hypertension. At the beginning of treatment for mild or moderately high blood pressure a single drug is used. A thiazide diuretic is often chosen for initial treatment, but it is also becoming common to use a beta blocker, a calcium channel blocker, or an ACE inhibitor. If a single drug does not reduce the blood pressure sufficiently, a diuretic in combination with one of the other drugs may be used. Some people with moderate hypertension require a third

drug, in which case a sympatholytic or centrally acting antihypertensive may also be given.

Severe hypertension is usually controlled with a combination of a diuretic, a beta blocker, and a centrally acting antihypertensive. If these do not reduce blood pressure sufficiently, a sympatholytic drug may also be added to the treatment.

How they affect you

Treatment with antihypertensive drugs relieves symptoms such as headache and palpitations. However, since most people with hypertension have few, if any, symptoms, side effects may be more noticeable than any immediate beneficial effect. Some antihypertensive drugs may cause dizziness and fainting at the start of treatment because they can sometimes produce an excessive fall in blood pressure. It may take a while for the physician to determine a dosage that avoids such effects. For detailed information on the adverse effects of drugs used to treat hypertension, consult the individual drug profiles in Part 4.

Risks and special precautions

Since your physician needs to know exactly how treatment with a particular drug affects your hypertension – the benefits as well as side effects – it is important to keep using antihypertensive medication as prescribed, even though you may feel the problem is under control. Sudden withdrawal of some of these drugs may cause a dangerous rebound in blood pressure; when treatment is stopped the dose needs to be reduced gradually under medical supervision.

ACTION OF ANTI-HYPERTENSIVE DRUGS

Each type of antihypertensive drug acts on a different part of the body to lower blood pressure.

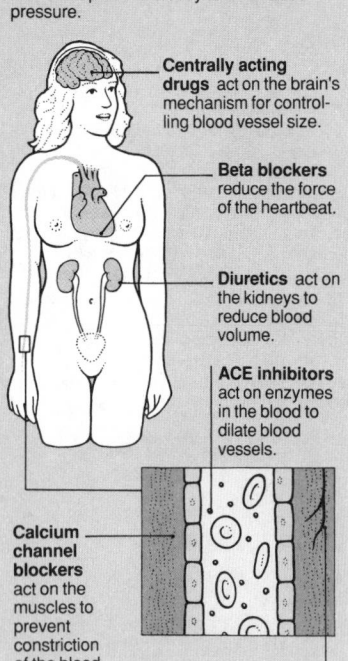

Centrally acting drugs act on the brain's mechanism for controlling blood vessel size.

Beta blockers reduce the force of the heartbeat.

Diuretics act on the kidneys to reduce blood volume.

ACE inhibitors act on enzymes in the blood to dilate blood vessels.

Calcium channel blockers act on the muscles to prevent constriction of the blood vessels.

Sympatholytics block nerve signals that trigger constriction of blood vessels.

COMMON DRUGS

Diuretics
(see p.127)

Beta blockers
(see p.125)

Calcium channel blockers
(See p.129)

ACE inhibitors
(see p.126)

Centrally acting antihypertensives
Clonidine
Methyldopa

Sympatholytics
Guanethidine
Hydralazine
Minoxidil
Prazosin

LIPID-LOWERING DRUGS

The blood contains several types of fats (also known as lipids). Some of these are beneficial but others – particularly saturated fats such as cholesterol, found in meat and dairy products – can be damaging if present in excess. The main risk is atherosclerosis, in which fatty deposits, called atheroma, build up in the arteries, restricting and disrupting the flow of blood. This in turn can lead to a greater likelihood of the formation of abnormal blood clots, leading to potentially fatal disorders such as stroke and heart attack.

For most people, cutting down the amount of fat in the diet is sufficient to reduce the risk of atherosclerosis. However, for others, often those with an inherited tendency to high levels of fat in the blood (hyperlipidemia), treatment with lipid-lowering drugs may also be recommended.

Why they are used
Lipid-lowering drugs are generally prescribed only when dietary measures have failed to control hyperlipidemia. They may also be given when an individual is considered to be at particular risk from atherosclerosis – for example, diabetics and people already suffering from circulatory disorders. Drugs do not remove existing atheroma in the blood vessels, but may prevent the accumulation of new deposits.

For maximum benefit, these drugs need to be used in conjunction with a low-fat diet and a reduction in other risk factors such as obesity and smoking. Because the choice of drug depends to some extent on the particular type of lipid that is causing problems, a full medical history and laboratory analysis of blood samples are needed before drug treatment is prescribed.

How they work
Bile salts, which contain large amounts of cholesterol, are normally released into the bowel to aid digestion and are then reabsorbed into the bloodstream. By blocking the reabsorption of cholesterol-carrying bile salts, some drugs, notably cholestyramine, colestipol, and neomycin, increase the loss of cholesterol from the body and thus help to lower the level of fat in the bloodstream. Other drugs – clofibrate, gemfibrozil, niacin and probucol – prevent conversion of fatty acids to lipids in the liver (see Action of lipid-lowering drugs, above right).

Lipid-lowering drugs do not correct the underlying cause of raised levels of fat in the blood; therefore it is usually necessary to continue drug treatment indefinitely. Withdrawal of treatment almost always leads to a return of high blood lipid levels.

ACTION OF LIPID-LOWERING DRUGS

Lipid-lowering drugs reduce the levels of fats in the blood by interfering with the absorption of bile salts in the bowel, or by altering the way in which the liver converts fatty acids in the blood into different types of lipids.

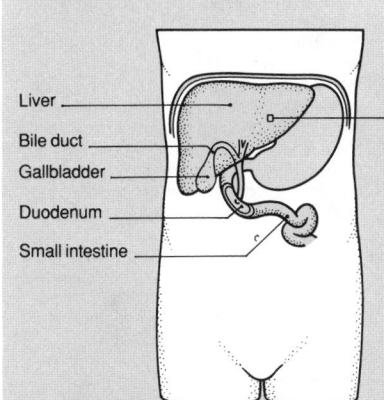

Liver
Bile duct
Gallbladder
Duodenum
Small intestine

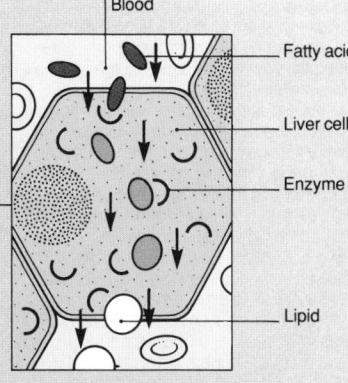

Blood
Fatty acid
Liver cell
Enzyme
Lipid

Drugs that act on the liver
Fatty acids in the blood are normally converted into a variety of lipids by enzyme activity in the liver (above). Several drugs alter enzyme activity in the liver to prevent the manufacture of one or more lipids.

Drugs that act on bile salts
Bile is produced by the liver and released into the small intestine via the bile duct to aid digestion. Salts in the bile carry large amounts of cholesterol and are normally reabsorbed into the bloodstream from the intestine during digestion (right). Some drugs combine with bile salts in the intestine and prevent their reabsorption (far right). This action reduces the levels of bile salts in the blood, and triggers the liver to convert more cholesterol into bile salts, thus reducing cholesterol levels in the blood.

Before drug

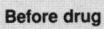

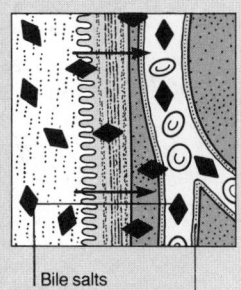

Bile salts
Blood vessel

After drug

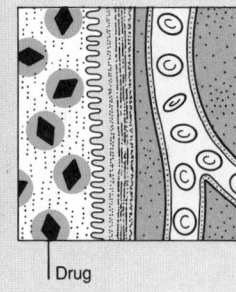

Drug

How they affect you
Because hyperlipidemia and atherosclerosis are without symptoms, you are unlikely to notice any short-term benefits from these drugs. By increasing the amount of bile in the digestive tract, some of these drugs can cause nausea and constipation (colestipol and cholestyramine) or diarrhea (clofibrate, niacin, and probucol), especially at the beginning of treatment.

Risks and special precautions
Cholestyramine, colestipol, and neomycin are not absorbed from the bowel into the bloodstream and therefore have few adverse effects. They may, however, limit absorption of certain fat-soluble vitamins; supplements may be recommended (see Vitamins, p.177).

Other lipid-lowering drugs that act in the liver, in particular clofibrate, can increase susceptibility to gallstones. They can occasionally upset the balance of different types of lipids in the bloodstream. Regular monitoring of blood samples is often advised. They are used with caution in those with reduced liver function.

COMMON DRUGS

Drugs that act on the liver	Drugs that act on bile salts
Clofibrate	Cholestyramine
Gemfibrozil	Colestipol
Lovastatin	Neomycin
Niacin	
Probucol	

DRUGS THAT AFFECT BLOOD CLOTTING

When bleeding occurs from injury or surgery, the body normally acts swiftly to stem the flow by sealing the breaks in the blood vessels. This occurs in two stages – first when cells called platelets accumulate as a plug at the opening in the blood vessel wall, and then when these platelets produce chemicals that activate clotting factors in the blood to form a protein called fibrin. Vitamin K plays an important role in this process (see The clotting mechanism, below). An enzyme in the blood called plasmin ensures that clots are broken down when the injury has been repaired.

Some disorders interfere with this process, either preventing clot formation or creating clots uncontrolledly. There is a danger that a lack of blood clotting will result in excessive blood loss; inappropriate development of clots can lead to blockage of the blood to a vital organ.

Drugs used to promote blood clotting

Fibrin formation depends on the presence in the blood of several clotting-factor proteins. When Factor VIII or Factor IX is absent or at low levels, an inherited disease called hemophilia exists, the symptoms almost always appearing only in males. Factor IX deficiency causes another bleeding condition called Christmas disease, named after the person in whom it was first identified. Lack of these clotting factors can lead to uncontrolled bleeding or excessive bruising following injury.

Regular drug treatment for hemophilia is not normally required. But if severe bleeding or bruising occurs, a concentrated form of the missing factor, extracted from normal blood, may be injected in order to promote clotting and so halt bleeding. Injections may need to be repeated for several days after injury.

It is sometimes useful to promote blood clotting in non-hemophiliacs when bleeding is difficult to stop (for example, after surgery). In such cases, blood clots are sometimes stabilized by reducing the action of plasmin with an antifibrinolytic (or hemostatic) drug such as aminocaproic acid; this is also occasionally given to hemophiliacs prior to minor surgery such as tooth extraction.

A tendency to bleed may also occur as a consequence of vitamin K deficiency (see the box below).

Drugs used to prevent abnormal blood clotting

Blood clots normally form only in response to injury. In some people, however, there is a tendency for clots to form in the blood vessels without apparent cause. Disturbed blood flow as a result of the presence of fatty deposits – atheroma – inside the blood vessels increases the risk of the formation of this type of abnormal clot (or thrombus). In addition, a portion of a blood clot (known as an embolus) formed in response to injury or surgery may sometimes break off and be carried away in the bloodstream. The likelihood of this occurring is increased by long periods of little or no activity. When an abnormal clot forms, there is a risk that it may become lodged in a blood vessel,

THE CLOTTING MECHANISM

When a blood vessel wall is damaged, platelets accumulate at the site of damage and form a plug (1). Platelets clumped together release chemicals that activate blood clotting factors (2). These factors together with vitamin K act on a substance called fibrinogen and convert it to fibrin (3). Strands of fibrin become enmeshed in the platelet plug to form a blood clot (4).

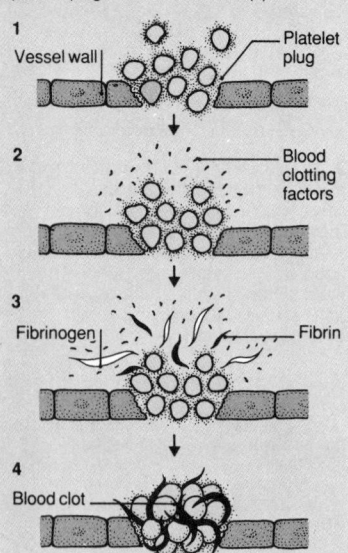

1
Vessel wall — Platelet plug

2
— Blood clotting factors

3
Fibrinogen — Fibrin

4
Blood clot

VITAMIN K

Vitamin K is required for the production of several blood clotting factors. It is absorbed from the intestine in fats, but in some diseases of the small intestine or pancreas in which fat is poorly absorbed, the level of vitamin K in the circulation is low, resulting in impaired blood clotting. A similar problem sometimes occurs in newborn babies due to an absence of the vitamin. Injections of a vitamin K preparation called phytonadione are used to restore normal levels.

ACTION OF ANTIPLATELET DRUGS

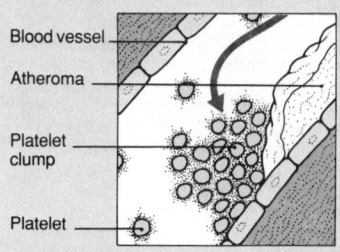

Blood vessel
Atheroma
Platelet clump
Platelet

Before drug
When blood flow is disrupted by atheroma in the blood vessels, platelets tend to clump together.

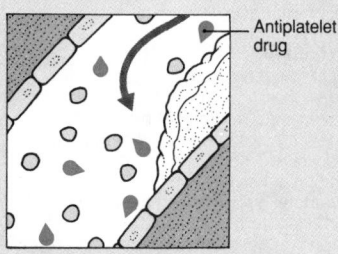

Antiplatelet drug

After drug
Antiplatelet drugs reduce the ability of platelets to stick together and so prevent clot formation.

thus blocking the blood supply to a vital organ such as the brain or heart.

Three main types of drugs are used to prevent and disperse clots: antiplatelet drugs, anticoagulant drugs, and thrombolytic drugs.

Antiplatelet drugs

Taken regularly by people with a tendency to form clots in the fast-flowing blood of the heart and arteries, these are also given to prevent clots from forming after heart surgery. They reduce the tendency of platelets to stick together when blood flow is disrupted (see Action of antiplatelet drugs, above).

The most widely used antiplatelet drug is aspirin (see also Analgesics, p.108). Aspirin has an antiplatelet action only when given in much lower doses than would be necessary to reduce pain. In these low doses adverse effects that may occur when the drug is given in pain-relieving doses are unlikely. Other less common antiplatelet drugs include dipyridamole and sulfinpyrazone.

Anticoagulants

Anticoagulant drugs help to maintain normal blood flow in people who are at risk from clot formation. They can either prevent the formation of blood clots in the veins, or stabilize an existing clot so that it does not break away and become a circulation-stopping embolism. All anticoagulant drugs reduce the activity of certain blood-clotting factors, although the precise mode of action of each drug differs (see Action of anticoagulant drugs, right). They do not, however, dissolve clots that have already formed; these are treated with thrombolytics (below).

Anticoagulants fall into two groups: those that are given by intravenous injection and act immediately, and those that are given by mouth and take effect after a few days.

Intravenous anticoagulants
Heparin is the most widely used drug of this type and it is used mainly in the hospital during or after surgery. In addition, it is also given during kidney dialysis to prevent clots from forming in the dialysis equipment. Because heparin cannot be given by mouth, it is an unsuitable drug for long-term treatment in the home.

Heparin is sometimes given prior to starting regular treatment with an oral anticoagulant.

Oral anticoagulants
These drugs are mainly used to prevent the formation of clots in veins – they are less likely to prevent the formation of blood clots in arteries. Oral anticoagulants may be given following injury or surgery (in particular, heart valve replacement) when there is a high risk of embolism. They are also given as a preventive treatment to people who are at risk from strokes.

ACTION OF ANTICOAGULANT DRUGS

Anticoagulants block the action of certain blood-clotting factors which convert fibrinogen into fibrin, the protein that binds platelets into blood clots.

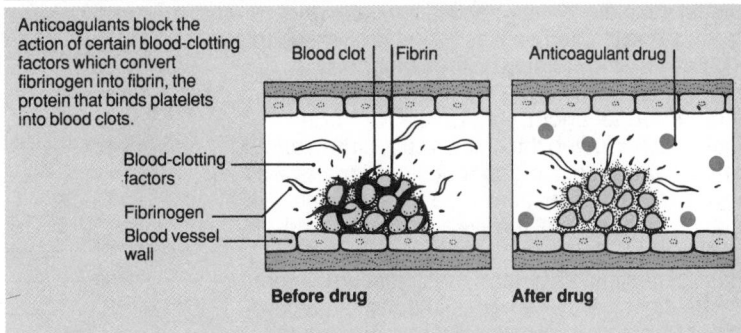

Before drug

After drug

A common problem with these drugs is that overdosage may lead to bleeding from the nose, gums, or in the urinary tract. For this reason the dosage needs to be carefully calculated; regular blood tests are performed to ensure that the clotting mechanism is correctly adjusted. Warfarin is the most widely used drug of this type.

The action of oral anticoagulant drugs may be affected by many other drugs, and it may therefore be necessary to alter the dosage of anticoagulant when other drugs also are needed. People who have been prescribed anticoagulants should carry a warning list of drugs which should not be administered. Aspirin in particular should not be taken together with anticoagulants except on the direction of a physician.

Thrombolytics
Also known as fibrinolytics, these drugs are used to dissolve clots that have already formed. They are usually administered in the hospital by intravenous injection to clear a blocked blood vessel – for example, in coronary thrombosis. As well as being given intravenously, thrombolytic drugs may also be administered directly into a blocked blood vessel.

The main thrombolytic drugs are streptokinase and the recently introduced tissue-type plasminogen activator (TPA), both of which act by increasing the blood level of plasmin, the naturally occurring enzyme that normally breaks down fibrin (see Action of thrombolytic drugs, below). TPA appears to be tolerated better and is quite effective when administered promptly.

The most common problems with the use of these drugs are increased susceptibility to bleeding and bruising, and allergic reactions which often take the form of rashes, breathing difficulty, or general weakness or discomfort.

ACTION OF THROMBOLYTIC DRUGS

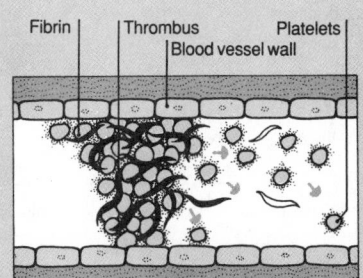

Before drug
When platelets accumulate in a blood vessel and are reinforced by strands of fibrin, the resultant blood clot, called a thrombus, cannot be dissolved either by antiplatelet drugs or anticoagulant drugs.

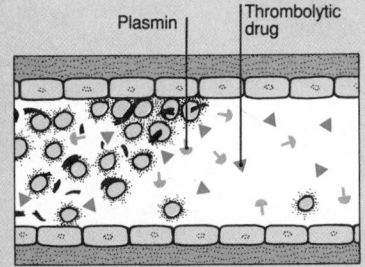

After drug
Thrombolytic drugs boost the action of plasmin, an enzyme in the blood that breaks up the strands of fibrin that bind the clot together. This allows the accumulated platelets to disperse, and restores normal blood flow.

COMMON DRUGS

Normal blood extracts
Antihemophilic factor
Factor IX complex

Antifibrinolytic drug
Aminocaproic acid

Vitamin K
Phytonadione

Antiplatelet drugs
Aspirin
Dipyridamole
Sulfinpyrazone

Anticoagulant drugs
Dicumarol
Heparin
Warfarin

Thrombolytic drugs
Streptokinase
Tissue plasminogen activator (TPA)

GASTROINTESTINAL TRACT

The gastrointestinal tract (also known as the digestive or alimentary tract) is the pathway through which food passes as it is processed to enable the body to absorb the nutrients it contains. It consists of the mouth, esophagus, stomach, duodenum, small intestine, large intestine (including the colon and rectum), and anus. In addition, a number of other organs are involved in the digestion of food: the salivary glands in the mouth, the liver, pancreas, and gallbladder. These organs, together with the gastrointestinal tract, form the digestive system.

The digestive system breaks down large complex chemicals (proteins, fats, carbohydrates) present in the food we eat into simpler molecules that can be used by the body (see also Nutrition, p.176). Undigested or indigestible material, together with some of the body's waste products, pass to the large intestine. When a sufficient mass has reached the rectum, the contents are expelled from the body as feces.

What can go wrong

A common disorder is the inflammation of the lining of the stomach or intestine (gastroenteritis), usually the result of an infection or parasitic infestation. Damage can also be done by the inappropriate production of digestive juices, leading to minor complaints like acidity and major disorders like peptic ulcer. The lining of the intestines can be damaged by abnormal functioning of the immune system (inflammatory bowel disease).The rectum and anus can become painful and irritated by damage to the lining, tears in the skin at the opening of the anus (anal fissure), or enlarged veins (hemorrhoids).

The most frequent gastrointestinal disorders, constipation and diarrhea, occur when something disrupts the normal muscle contractions that propel food residue through the bowel.

Why drugs are used

Many drugs for gastrointestinal disorders are taken by mouth and act directly on the digestive tract without entering the bloodstream. Such drugs include certain antibiotics and other drugs to treat infestation. Some antacids for peptic ulcers and excess stomach acidity, and bulk-forming agents for constipation and diarrhea, also pass through the system unabsorbed.

However, for many disorders drugs with a systemic effect are required, including anti-ulcer drugs, narcotic antidiarrheal drugs, and some of the drugs for inflammatory bowel disease.

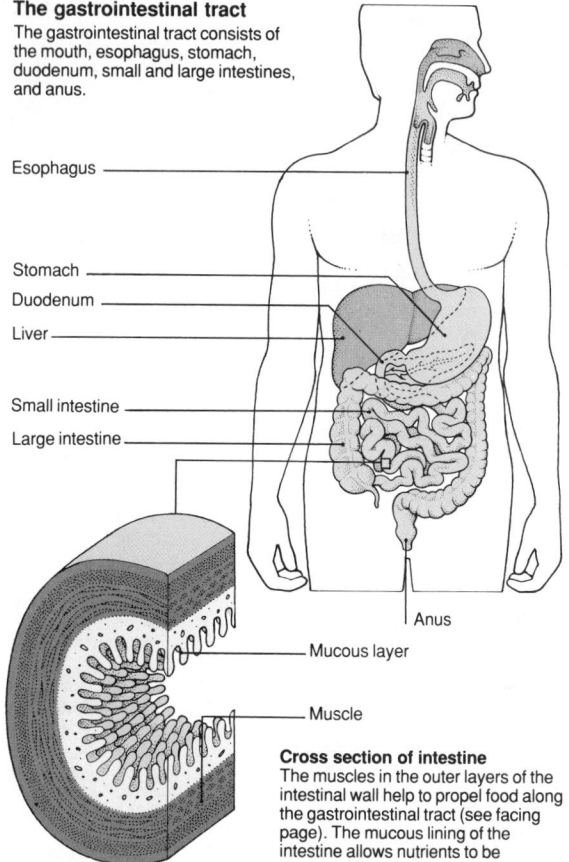

The gastrointestinal tract
The gastrointestinal tract consists of the mouth, esophagus, stomach, duodenum, small and large intestines, and anus.

Esophagus

Stomach
Duodenum
Liver

Small intestine
Large intestine

Anus
Mucous layer
Muscle

Cross section of intestine
The muscles in the outer layers of the intestinal wall help to propel food along the gastrointestinal tract (see facing page). The mucous lining of the intestine allows nutrients to be absorbed into the bloodstream.

Pancreas
The pancreas produces *enzymes* that digest fats, proteins and carbohydrates into simpler substances. Pancreatic juices neutralize acidity of the stomach contents.

Gallbladder
Bile produced by the liver is stored in the gallbladder and released into the small intestine. Bile improves the digestion of fats by reducing them to smaller units that are more easily acted upon by digestive enzymes.

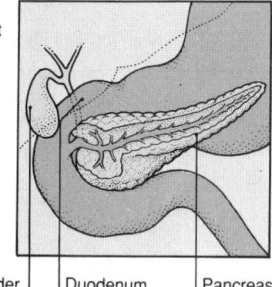

Gallbladder | Duodenum | Pancreas

MAJOR DRUG GROUPS

Antacids	Drugs for rectal and
Anti-ulcer drugs	anal disorders
Antidiarrheal drugs	Drug treatment
Laxatives	for gallstones
Drugs for inflammatory	
bowel disease	

The lining of the gastrointestinal tract

The internal lining of the different sections of the gastro-intestinal tract varies according to the function of that part, depending, for example, on whether its principal role is to secrete digestive juices or to absorb nutrients.

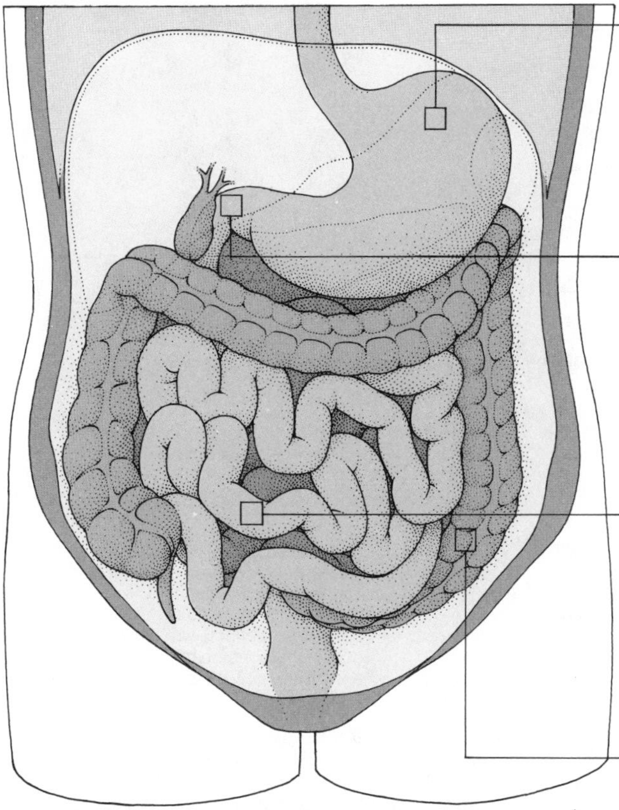

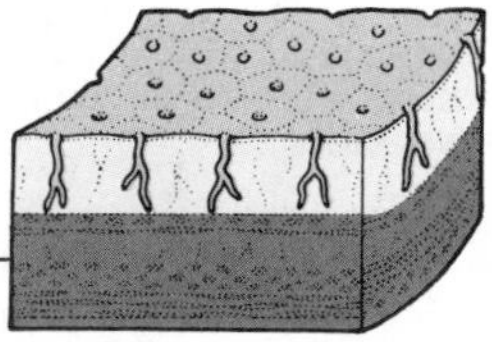

Stomach
Its main job is to store meals and pass food to the intestine. The lining of the stomach releases gastric juice that partly digests food. The stomach wall continuously produces thick mucus that forms a protective coating.

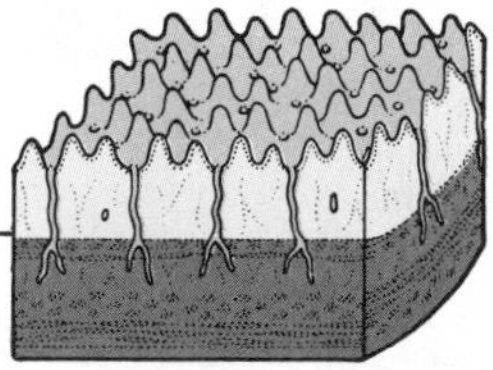

Duodenum
This is the tube that connects the stomach to the intestine. Its lining may be damaged by excess acid produced by the stomach.

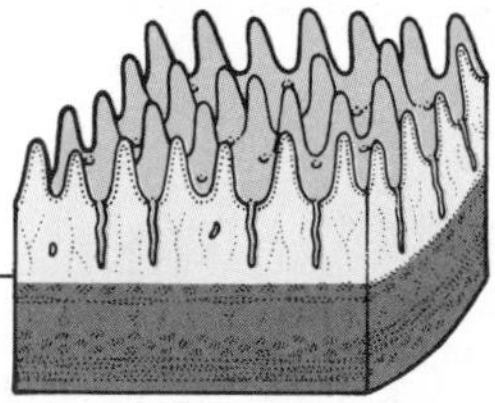

Small intestine
The small intestine is a long tube in which food is broken down by digestive juices. The mucous lining is covered with tiny projections called villi that provide a large surface area through which the products of digestion are absorbed into the bloodstream.

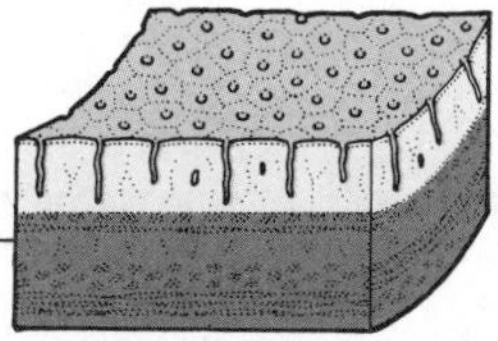

Large intestine
The large intestine receives undigested food and indigestible material from the small intestine. Water and mineral salts pass through the lining into the bloodstream.

MOVEMENT OF FOOD THROUGH THE GASTROINTESTINAL TRACT

Food is propelled through the gastrointestinal tract by rhythmic waves of muscular contraction known as peristalsis. The illustration (right) shows how peristaltic contractions of the bowel wall push food through the intestine.

Muscle contraction in the tract is controlled by the autonomic nervous system (p.107), and is therefore easily disrupted by drugs that either stimulate or inhibit the activity of the autonomic nervous system. Excessive peristaltic action may cause diarrhea; slowed peristalsis may cause constipation.

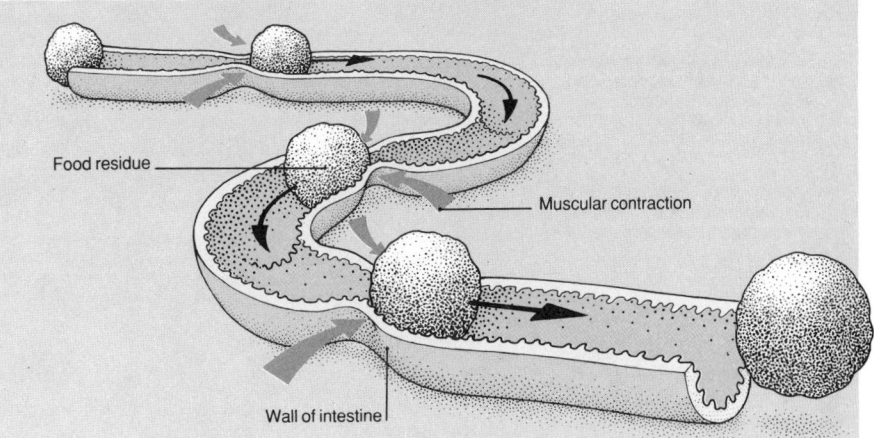

Food residue

Muscular contraction

Wall of intestine

ANTACIDS

Digestive juices in the stomach contain acid and enzymes that break down food before it passes into the intestine. The wall of the stomach is normally protected from the action of digestive acid by a layer of mucus that is constantly secreted by the stomach lining. Problems arise when the stomach lining is damaged or when too much acid is produced and eats away at the mucous layer. Excess acid leading to discomfort, commonly referred to as indigestion, may result from overeating, drinking coffee or alcohol, smoking, anxiety, or, in some people, from eating certain foods. Some drugs, notably aspirin and non-steroidal anti-inflammatory drugs, can also irritate the stomach lining and cause ulcers.

Antacids are used to neutralize acid and thus relieve pain. The types most regularly used are those that contain sodium, those that contain magnesium, and those that contain aluminum. Some antacids contain calcium, but they are not commonly prescribed today.

Why they are used

Antacids may be needed when simple remedies such as a change in diet or a glass of milk fail to relieve indigestion. They are especially useful one to three hours after meals to neutralize after-meal acid surge.

Physicians prescribe these drugs to relieve dyspepsia (pain in the chest or upper abdomen caused or aggravated by acid) in a number of disorders. Such disorders include inflammation of the esophagus, stomach lining, and duodenum. Pain from peptic ulcers in the esophagus, stomach, or duodenum may also be relieved by antacids, which reduce the attack made by acid on the ulcer. The action of the drugs may occasionally lead to the complete healing of an ulcer.

ACTION OF ANTACIDS

Excess acid in the stomach may eat away at the protective layer of mucus that lines the stomach. When this occurs, or when the mucous lining is damaged, for example, by an ulcer, stomach acid comes into contact with the underlying tissues, causing pain and inflammation (right). Antacids react with stomach acid to reduce the acidity of the digestive juices. This helps to prevent pain and inflammation, and allows the mucous layer to repair itself (far right).

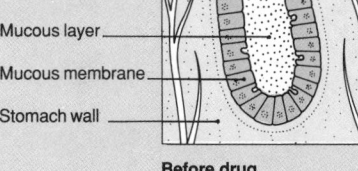

Acid   Drug

Mucous layer

Mucous membrane

Stomach wall

Before drug
Acid damages mucous layer and mucous membrane.

After drug
Acid is neutralized by antacid action.

How they work

By neutralizing stomach acid, antacids prevent inflammation, relieve pain, and allow the mucous layer and lining to mend. When used in the treatment of ulcers, they prevent acid from attacking damaged stomach lining and so allow the ulcer to heal.

How they affect you

If antacids are taken according to instructions, they are usually effective in relieving abdominal discomfort caused by acid. The speed of action varies, depending on the ability to neutralize acid. Their duration of action also varies; short-acting drugs may have to be taken quite frequently.

Although most antacids have few serious side effects when used only occasionally, some may cause diarrhea, and others may cause constipation (see Types of antacids, below).

Risks and special precautions

Antacids should not be taken to prevent abdominal pain on a regular basis except under medical supervision, as they may suppress the symptoms of a serious disorder. Prolonged use of any antacid can cause an increase in the production of stomach acid when treatment is stopped suddenly.

All antacids can interfere with the absorption of other drugs. For this reason, if you are taking a prescription medicine, you should check with your physician before taking an antacid.

COMMON DRUGS

Aluminum hydroxide
Calcium carbonate
Magnesium hydroxide
Sodium bicarbonate

TYPES OF ANTACIDS

Aluminum compounds These have a prolonged action and are widely used, especially for the treatment of peptic ulcers. They may cause constipation, but this is often countered by combining this type of antacid with one that contains magnesium. Aluminum compounds can interfere with the absorption of phosphate from the diet, causing weakness and bone damage if taken in high doses over a long period.

Magnesium compounds Like the aluminum compounds, these have a prolonged action. In large doses they can cause diarrhea, and in people who have impaired kidney function, a high blood magnesium level may build up, causing weakness, lethargy, and drowsiness.

Sodium bicarbonate Sodium bicarbonate, the only sodium compound used as an antacid, acts quickly, but its effect soon passes. It reacts with stomach acids to produce gas, which may cause bloating and belching. This antacid is not advised for people with heart or kidney disease, as it can lead to the accumulation of water (edema) in the legs and lungs, or serious changes in the acid-base balance of the blood.

Combined preparations Antacids may be combined with other substances called alginates and antifoaming agents. Alginates are intended to float on the contents of the stomach and produce a neutralizing layer to subdue acid that can rise into the esophagus, causing heartburn.

Antifoaming agents, usually simethicone, are intended to relieve flatulence. In some preparations a local anesthetic is combined with the antacid to relieve discomfort in esophagitis. None of these additives is of primary benefit.

ANTI-ULCER DRUGS

Normally, the linings of the esophagus, stomach, and duodenum are protected from the irritant action of stomach acids by a layer of mucus. If this layer becomes damaged, stomach acid may erode the underlying tissue, causing a peptic ulcer. A peptic ulcer usually leads to episodes of abdominal pain, vomiting, and loss of appetite. Duodenal ulcers are the most common type of peptic ulcer and are usually less of a problem than other types. The exact diagnostic cause of peptic ulcers is not understood, but a number of predisposing risk factors have been identified; these include heavy smoking, the regular use of aspirin or similar drugs, the overuse of alcohol and coffee, and a stressful lifestyle combined with irregular and rushed meals.

Ulcers may respond to simple measures, particularly rest, giving up smoking, and stopping alcohol intake. Antacids may also relieve symptoms (see facing page). If these measures do not produce satisfactory results, a physician may prescribe treatment with

SITES OF PEPTIC ULCERS

Peptic ulcers most commonly occur in the walls of the stomach or duodenum when damage to the mucous lining allows stomach acid to erode the underlying tissue. Ulcers may also form in the esophagus if acid backs up into the esophagus. Peptic ulcers also occur at the margin where the stomach has been sewn to the intestine after ulcer surgery. Similar drugs are prescribed for all three types of peptic ulcer.

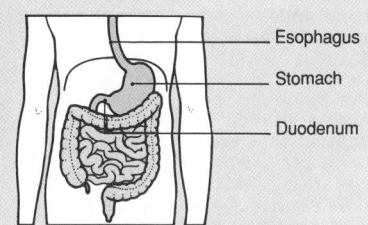

— Esophagus
— Stomach
— Duodenum

an anti-ulcer drug, either an H_2 receptor blocker or sucralfate.

Why they are used
Anti-ulcer drugs are prescribed both to relieve symptoms and to heal the ulcer. Left untreated, ulcers may erode the walls of blood vessels or even perforate the wall of the stomach or duodenum.

Because none of the available drugs can cure a tendency to ulcers, repeated courses of drug treatment may be

required, especially for duodenal ulcers.

Surgical treatment is reserved for complications such as obstruction, perforation, and hemorrhage, and the possibility of malignancy in the case of stomach ulcers.

How they work
Drugs protect ulcers from the action of stomach acid, thereby allowing the underlying tissue to heal. H_2 blockers reduce the amount of acid released into the stomach, whereas sucralfate forms a protective coating over the ulcer (see Action of anti-ulcer drugs, left).

How they affect you
These drugs begin to reduce pain within a few hours, and in most cases allow the ulcer to heal in four to eight weeks. They produce few side effects, although one of the H_2 blockers, cimetidine, can cause confusion in the elderly, particularly if the stated dose is exceeded. Sucralfate may cause constipation. Because these drugs may mask the symptoms of cancer when the ulcer is in the stomach, they are normally prescribed only when tests have ruled out this disorder.

Risks and special precautions
The H_2 receptor blockers are not usually prescribed for courses of more than six months because their safety over prolonged periods is not established. Sucralfate is prescribed for up to eight weeks at a time; it may interfere with absorption of fats and so reduce the absorption of vitamins A, D, E, and K, which are dissolved in fat. Prolonged use may require vitamin supplements.

ACTION OF ANTI-ULCER DRUGS

H_2 blockers
Histamine is a chemical released by mast cells (see Allergy, p.151). It can produce a number of effects, including dilation of the blood vessels in the nose and eyes, constriction of the airways, skin rashes (hives), and increased secretion of stomach acid. Antihistamines (p.152), used medically for many years to block the effects of histamine

in allergic disorders, act only on *receptors* known as H_1 receptors. They do not block the effect of histamine on stomach acid production, which is triggered by the action of histamine on H_2 receptors. A new type of drug was therefore developed to block this action. Since their introduction in the 1970s, the H_2 blockers have been among the most widely prescribed drugs in the United States.

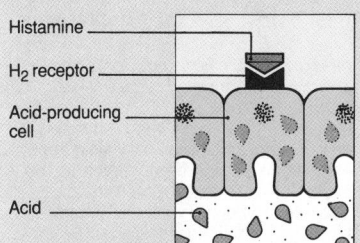

Histamine
H_2 receptor
Acid-producing cell
Acid

The action of histamine on the stomach
Histamine binds to specialized H_2 receptors and stimulates acid-producing cells in the stomach wall to release acid.

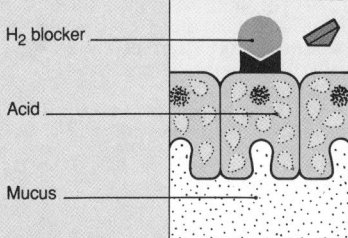

H_2 blocker
Acid
Mucus

The action of H_2 blockers
H_2 blockers occupy H_2 receptors, preventing histamine from triggering the production of acid. This allows the mucous lining to heal.

Sucralfate
This drug forms a coating over the ulcer, protecting it from the action of stomach acid and thus allowing it to heal.

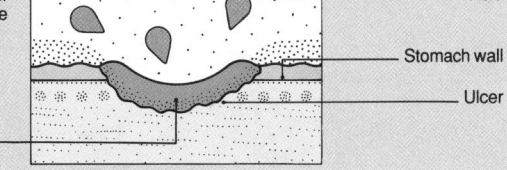

— Acid
— Stomach wall
— Ulcer
Sucralfate

COMMON DRUGS

H_2 blockers
Cimetidine
Famotidine
Ranitidine

Other drugs
Antacids (see facing page)
Sucralfate

ANTIDIARRHEAL DRUGS

Diarrhea is an increase in the fluidity and frequency of bowel movements. In some cases diarrhea protects the body from harmful substances in the intestine by hastening their removal. The most common causes of diarrhea are viral infection, food poisoning, and parasites. But diarrhea also occurs in other illnesses. It can be a side effect of some drugs and may follow radiation therapy for cancer. Diarrhea may also be caused by anxiety.

An attack of diarrhea usually clears up quickly without medical attention. The best treatment is to abstain from food and to drink plenty of clear fluids. Rehydration solutions containing sugar and potassium and sodium salts are widely recommended for preventing dehydration and chemical imbalances, particularly in children. You should consult your physician if: the condition does not improve within 48 hours; the diarrhea contains blood; there is severe abdominal pain and vomiting; you have just returned from a foreign country; or the diarrhea occurs in a small child or an elderly person.

Severe diarrhea can impair absorption of drugs, and anyone taking a prescription medicine should call a physician. A woman taking oral contraceptives may need to take additional contraceptive measures (see p.191).

The main types of drugs used to relieve non-specific diarrhea are narcotics, and bulk-forming and adsorbent agents. Antispasmodic drugs may also be used to relieve pain (see Drugs for irritable bowel syndrome, below).

Why they are used

An antidiarrheal drug may be prescribed when simple remedies do not provide relief. They are generally prescribed to provide relief once it is certain that the diarrhea is neither infectious nor toxic.

ACTION OF ANTIDIARRHEAL DRUGS

Narcotic antidiarrheals
Narcotics reduce the transmission of nerve signals to the intestinal muscles, thus reducing muscle contraction. This allows more time for water to be absorbed from the food residue and therefore reduces the fluidity as well as the frequency of bowel movements.

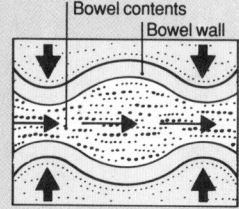
Bowel contents
Bowel wall

Before drug
Rapid bowel contraction prevents water from being absorbed.

After drug
Slowed bowel action allows more water to be absorbed.

Bulk-forming agents
These preparations contain particles that swell up as they absorb water from the large intestine. This makes bowel movements firmer and less fluid. It is thought that these agents may absorb irritants and harmful chemicals along with excess water.

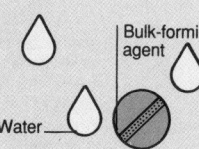
Bulk-forming agent
Water

Water is attracted by bulk-forming agent.

Bulk-forming agent swells as water is absorbed.

Narcotics are the most effective antidiarrheals. They are used when diarrhea is severe and debilitating. Bulking and adsorbent agents have a milder effect and are often used when it is necessary to regulate bowel action over a prolonged period – for example, in those with colostomies or ileostomies.

How they work

Each type of antidiarrheal drug works differently. Narcotic drugs decrease the propulsive activity of the muscles so that fecal matter passes more slowly through the bowel.

Bulk-forming agents and adsorbents take on water and irritants present in the bowel, thus producing larger and firmer bowel movements less frequently.

How they affect you

Drugs used to treat diarrhea reduce the urge to move the bowels. Narcotic drugs and antispasmodics may relieve abdominal pain. All antidiarrheals may cause constipation if used in excess.

Risks and special precautions

Used in relatively low doses for a limited period of time, the narcotic drugs are unlikely to produce adverse effects. However, these drugs should be used with caution when diarrhea is caused by an infection, since they may slow the elimination of microorganisms from the intestine. All antidiarrheals should be taken with plenty of water. It is important not to take a bulk-forming agent together with a narcotic or antispasmodic drug, because a bulky mass could form and obstruct the bowel.

COMMON DRUGS

Antispasmodics
Belladonna
Dicyclomine

Bulk-forming and adsorbent agents
Kaolin
Methylcellulose
Psyllium

Narcotics
Codeine
Diphenoxylate (with atropine)
Loperamide

DRUGS FOR IRRITABLE BOWEL SYNDROME

Irritable bowel syndrome is a common stress-related condition in which the coordinated waves of muscular contraction responsible for moving the bowel contents smoothly through the intestines become strong and irregular, often causing pain. There may also be diarrhea or constipation.

Symptoms are often relieved by adjusting the amount of fiber in the diet, but medication may also be required. Bulk-forming agents may be given to regulate the consistency of the bowel contents. If pain is severe, an antispasmodic drug may be prescribed. These *anticholinergic* drugs reduce the transmission of nerve signals to the bowel wall, thus preventing spasm. Because irritable bowel is often made worse by anxiety, an anti-anxiety drug (p.111) may also be prescribed.

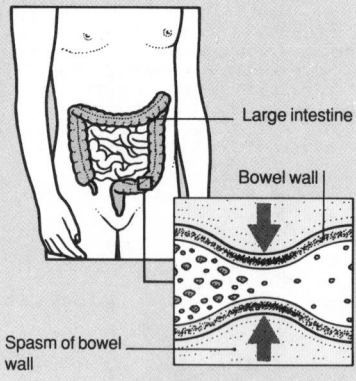
Large intestine
Bowel wall
Spasm of bowel wall

LAXATIVES

When your bowels do not move as frequently as usual and the movements are hard and difficult to pass, you are suffering from constipation. The most common cause is the lack of sufficient fiber in your diet; fiber supplies the bulk that makes the feces soft and easy to pass. The simple remedy is more fluid and a diet higher in fiber, i.e., more fruits, vegetables, and whole grain breads. Constipation is commonly relieved by laxatives, although some physicians advise occasional enemas.

Ignoring the urge to defecate can also cause constipation, the feces becoming dry (and hard to pass) and too small to stimulate the muscles that propel them through the intestine. Certain drugs may be constipating: narcotic analgesics, tricyclic antidepressants, and antacids containing aluminum. Some diseases, such as hypothyroidism and scleroderma (a rare disorder of the connective tissues characterized by hardening of the skin), can lead to constipation.

Because constipation may be a symptom of something serious, consult your physician about any change in bowel habits that lasts more than a week.

Why they are used
Since prolonged use is harmful, laxatives should be used for very short periods only. They may prevent pain and straining in people with aneurysms or hemorrhoids (p.141). Physicians may prescribe laxatives for the same reason after childbirth or abdominal surgery. Laxatives are also used to clear the bowel before such investigative procedures as colonoscopy. They may also be administered to the elderly and bedridden, because lack of exercise can lead to constipation.

How they work
Laxatives act on the large intestine – by increasing the speed with which fecal matter passes through the bowel, or

ACTION OF LAXATIVES

Bulk-forming agents
Taken after a meal, these agents are not absorbed as they pass through the digestive tract. They contain particles that absorb many times their own volume of water. By doing so they increase the bulk of the bowel movements and thus encourage bowel action.

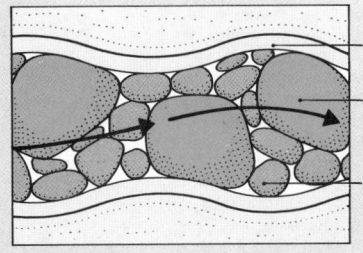

Bowel wall

Bulk-forming agent swollen with water

Fecal matter

Stimulant laxatives
These laxatives are thought to encourage bowel movement by acting on nerve endings in the wall of the intestines that trigger contraction of the intestinal muscles. This speeds the passage of fecal matter through the large intestine, allowing less time for water to be absorbed. Thus bowel movements become more frequent and more liquid.

Before drug

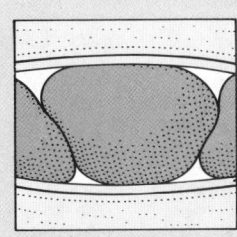

Increased contractions speed passage of fecal matter

After drug

increasing its bulk and/or water content.

Stimulants cause the bowel muscle to contract, increasing the speed with which fecal matter passes through the intestine. Bulk-forming laxatives absorb water in the bowel, thereby increasing the volume of fecal matter and making bowel movements softer and easier to pass. Lactulose also causes fluid to accumulate in the intestine. Saline laxatives prevent water from passing out of the large intestine by osmotic action without increasing the bulk of bowel movements. Lubricant mineral oil preparations make the bowel movements

softer and easier to pass without increasing their bulk. But prolonged use leaves a coating that can interfere with absorption of some essential vitamins.

Risks and special precautions
Laxatives can cause diarrhea if taken in overdose, and constipation if overused. The most serious risk of prolonged use of most laxatives is developing dependence on the laxative for normal bowel action. Use of a laxative should therefore be discontinued as soon as normal bowel movements have been re-established. Children should not be given laxatives except in special circumstances on the advice of a physician.

TYPES OF LAXATIVES

Bulk-forming agents These are relatively slow acting, but are less likely to interfere with normal bowel action. Only after consultation with your doctor should they be taken for constipation accompanied by abdominal pain, because of the risk of intestinal obstruction.

Stimulant (contact) laxatives These are suitable for occasional use when other treatments have failed or when a rapid onset of action is required. Stimulant laxatives should not normally be used for longer than a week, as they can cause abdominal cramps and diarrhea.

Lubricants Mineral oil (also called liquid petrolatum) is used as a fecal softener when

hard bowel movements cause pain on defecation – for example, if hemorrhoids are present. It is often recommended for elderly or debilitated people and for the relief of fecal impaction (blockage of the bowel by fecal material).

Saline laxatives A variety of mineral salts are used to evacuate the bowel prior to surgery or investigative procedures. They are not used for the long-term relief of constipation because they can cause chemical imbalances in the blood.

Lactulose This is an alternative to bulk-forming laxatives for the long-term treatment of chronic constipation. It may cause stomach cramps and flatulence.

COMMON DRUGS

Stimulant laxatives
Bisacodyl
Senna

Bulk-forming agents
Methylcellulose
Psyllium

Others
Lactulose
Magnesium hydroxide
Mineral oil

DRUGS FOR INFLAMMATORY BOWEL DISEASE

"Inflammatory bowel disease" is the term used to describe certain disorders in which the wall of the intestine and other parts of the gastrointestinal tract become inflamed, causing symptoms that include periodic attacks of pain, general feelings of ill-health, and often diarrhea that is sometimes bloody. Loss of appetite and poor absorption of food often result in weight loss.

Although the exact cause of these disorders is unknown, the risks and severity of attacks are increased by some infections, antibiotics, and excessive stress.

Physicians identify two main types of inflammatory bowel disease: Crohn's disease and ulcerative colitis. In Crohn's disease (also called regional enteritis), any part of the digestive tract may be inflamed, although the small intestine is the most commonly affected site. In ulcerative colitis the large intestine becomes inflamed and ulcerated, often producing blood-stained diarrhea (see the box, below).

Establishing a proper diet and a less stressful lifestyle may help to alleviate these conditions. Bed rest during attacks is also advisable. However, these simple measures do not usually suffice to relieve or prevent attacks, and drugs are often necessary.

Three types of drug are used to treat inflammatory bowel disease: corticosteroids (p.169), immunosuppressants (p.184), and sulfasalazine. Safer derivatives of sulfasalazine are currently under investigation. Other drugs that may be given to treat inflammatory bowel

SITES OF BOWEL INFLAMMATION

The two main types of bowel inflammation are called ulcerative colitis and Crohn's disease. The former occurs in the large intestine. Crohn's disease can occur anywhere along the gastrointestinal tract. It is typically found in the small intestine.

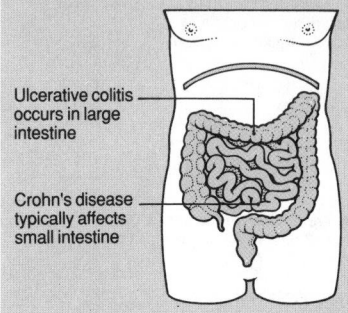

Ulcerative colitis occurs in large intestine

Crohn's disease typically affects small intestine

disease include nutritional supplements (used especially for Crohn's disease) and antidiarrheal drugs (p.138). In very severe cases surgery may be necessary in order to remove damaged areas of the intestine.

Why they are used
Drugs cannot cure inflammatory bowel disease. However, drug treatment can control symptoms and prevent complications, especially severe anemia and perforation of the intestinal wall.

Sulfasalazine is used both to treat attacks and to prevent ulcerative colitis. People who suffer from severe bowel inflammation are usually prescribed a course of corticosteroids, particularly during a sudden flare-up. Once the disease is under control an immunosuppressant drug may be given to prevent a relapse.

How they work
Corticosteroids and sulfasalazine depress the inflammatory process, thus allowing the damaged tissue to recover. They act in different ways to prevent migration of white blood cells into the bowel wall, which may be responsible in part for the inflammation of the bowel.

How they affect you
Taken to treat attacks, these drugs relieve symptoms within a few days, and general health improves gradually over a few weeks. Sulfasalazine is usually effective in providing longer-term relief from symptoms of ulcerative colitis.

The first course of treatment with an immunosuppressant drug may take several months before improving the condition. However, they act more quickly in treating subsequent attacks.

Risks and special precautions
Immunosuppressant and corticosteroid drugs can cause serious adverse effects, and they are thus only prescribed when potential benefits outweigh the risks involved.

It is important to continue taking these drugs as instructed because stopping them abruptly may cause a sudden flare-up of the disorder. Physicians usually supervise a gradual reduction in dosage when stopping the drug, even when given as a short course to treat an attack. Antidiarrheal drugs should not be taken on a routine basis because they may mask signs of deterioration or even aid sudden bowel dilation or rupture.

How they are administered
These drugs are usually taken in tablet form, although mild ulcerative colitis in the last part of the large intestine may be treated with suppositories or an enema containing a corticosteroid.

ACTION OF DRUGS IN ULCERATIVE COLITIS

Ulcerative colitis is the most common form of inflammatory bowel disease. It affects the large intestine, causing ulceration of the lining and producing pain and violent blood-stained diarrhea. It is often treated with corticosteroids and sulfasalazine.

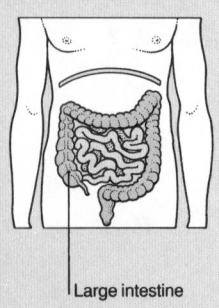

Large intestine

Bowel wall
Ulcerated area
Prostaglandins

White blood cells
Blood vessel

Corticosteroid drug
Sulfasalazine

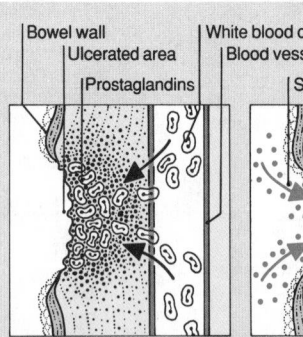

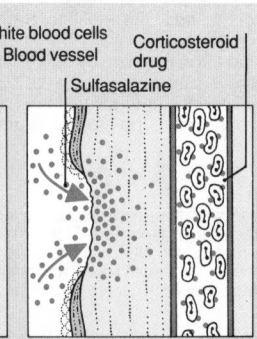

Before drug
Damage to the intestinal lining provokes the formation of chemicals known as prostaglandins which trigger the migration of white blood cells into the ulcerated area. The accumulation of white blood cells in the bowel wall causes inflammation.

Drug action
Sulfasalazine passes into the ulcerated area from inside the bowel. It prevents the formation of prostaglandins around the damaged tissue. Corticosteroids act in the bloodstream to reduce the ability of white blood cells to pass into the bowel wall.

COMMON DRUGS

Corticosteroids
Hydrocortisone
Prednisone

Immunosuppressants
Azathioprine
Mercaptopurine

Other drugs
Sulfasalazine

DRUGS FOR RECTAL AND ANAL DISORDERS

The most common disorder affecting the rectum (the last part of the large intestine) and anus (the opening from the rectum) is hemorrhoids, commonly called piles. They occur when hemorrhoidal veins become swollen, irritated, or clotted, often the result of prolonged local back pressure such as that caused by a pregnancy or a job requiring long hours of sitting. Hemorrhoids may cause irritation and pain, especially on defecation. The condition is aggravated by constipation and straining while passing a bowel movement. Sometimes hemorrhoids may bleed and occasionally clots may form in the swollen veins, leading to severe pain, a condition called thrombosed hemorrhoids.

Other common disorders affecting the anus include anal fissure (painful cracks in the anus), and pruritus ani (itching around the anus).

A number of over-the-counter and prescription-only preparations are available for the relief of such disorders. Warm sitz baths also help.

Why they are used

Preparations for relief of hemorrhoids and anal discomfort fall into two main groups: creams or suppositories that act locally to relieve inflammation and irritation; and measures that relieve constipation, which contributes to the formation of, and discomfort from, hemorrhoids and anal fissure.

Preparations from the first group often contain a soothing agent with *antiseptic*, *astringent*, or *vasoconstrictor* properties. Ingredients of this type include zinc oxide, bismuth, hamamelis (witch hazel), Peruvian balsam, and

DISORDERS OF THE RECTUM AND ANUS

The rectum and anus form the last part of the digestive tract. Common conditions affecting the area include swelling of the veins around the anus (hemorrhoids), cracks in the anus (anal fissure), and inflammation and irritation of the anus and surrounding area (pruritus ani).

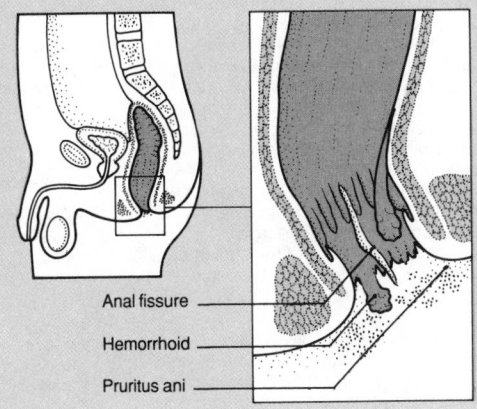

Anal fissure
Hemorrhoid
Pruritus ani

ephedrine. Some products also include a mild local anesthetic such as tetracaine (see p.108). In some cases a physician may prescribe an ointment containing a corticosteroid to relieve inflammation around the anus (see Topical corticosteroids, p.202).

People who suffer from hemorrhoids or anal fissure are generally advised to include in their diets plenty of fluids and fiber-rich foods (such as fresh fruits, vegetables, and whole grain products) to prevent constipation and to ease defecation. A mild bulk-forming or lubricant laxative may also be prescribed (see p.139).

Neither type of treatment can shrink large hemorrhoids, although they may provide relief while healing occurs natu-

rally in anal fissure. Severe, persistently painful hemorrhoids that continue to be troublesome in spite of these measures may need to be removed surgically or, more commonly, by banding with specially applied small rubber bands (see below left).

How they affect you

The treatments described above usually relieve discomfort, especially during defecation. Most people experience no adverse effects, although preparations containing local anesthetics may cause irritation or even a rash in the anal area. It is rare for ingredients in locally acting preparations to be absorbed into the body in sufficient quantities to cause generalized side effects.

The main risk is that self-treatment of hemorrhoids may delay diagnosis of a more serious bowel disorder. It is therefore always wise to consult your physician if you have symptoms of hemorrhoids, especially if you have noticed rectal bleeding.

SITES OF DRUG ACTION

The illustration below shows how and where drugs for the treatment of rectal disorders act to relieve symptoms.

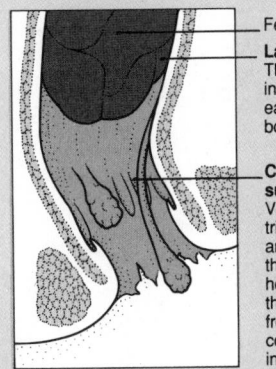

Fecal matter

Laxatives
These act in the large intestine to soften and ease the passage of bowel movements.

Creams and suppositories
Vasoconstrictors and astringents reduce swelling and restrict blood supply, thus helping to relieve hemorrhoids. Local anesthetics numb pain signals from the anus. Topical corticosteroids relieve inflammation.

Banding treatment
A small rubber band is applied to a hemorrhoid, thereby blocking off its blood supply. The hemorrhoid will eventually wither away.

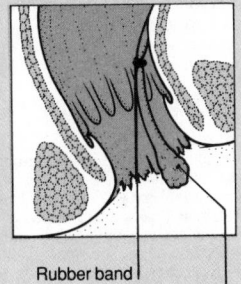

Rubber band
Hemorrhoid

COMMON DRUGS

Soothing and astringent agents
Bismuth
Hamamelis
Peruvian balsam
Zinc oxide

Vasoconstrictors
Ephedrine

Topical corticosteroids
Fluocinolone
Hydrocortisone

Local anesthetics
See p.108

Laxatives
See p.139

DRUG TREATMENT FOR GALLSTONES

The formation of gallstones is the most common disorder of the gallbladder, which is the storage and concentrating unit for bile, a digestive juice produced by the liver. During digestion, bile passes from the gallbladder via the bile duct into the small intestine, where it aids the digestion of fats. Bile is made up of several ingredients, including bile acids, bile salts, and bile pigments. It also contains significant amounts of cholesterol dissolved in bile acid. If the amount of cholesterol in the bile increases or if that of bile acid is reduced, a proportion of the cholesterol cannot remain dissolved. This excess may accumulate in the gallbladder as gallstones.

Another cause of gallstones is infection in the gallbladder. Gallstones may be present in the gallbladder for years without causing symptoms. However, if they become lodged in the bile duct they cause pain and block the flow of bile, which could result in infection and inflammation.

Drugs can be used to dissolve stones that are made principally of cholesterol. However, when they contain significant amounts of other material, or if a stone becomes lodged in the bile duct, surgical removal may be required. The most commonly used gallstone-dissolving drug is chenodiol, but ursodeoxycholic acid is under investigation.

Why they are used

Even if you do not have any symptoms, once gallstones have been diagnosed your physician may advise treatment because of the risk of blockage of the bile duct. Drug treatment is usually preferred to surgery for small cholesterol stones and when it is considered that surgery may be risky.

How they work

Chenodiol is a substance that is naturally present in bile. It acts on chemical processes in the liver to regulate the amount of cholesterol in the blood, by controlling the amount that passes into the bile. Once the level of cholesterol in the bile is reduced, the bile acids are able to start dissolving the stones in the gallbladder. For maximum

DIGESTION OF FATS

The digestion of fats (or lipids) in the small intestine is assisted by the action of bile, a digestive juice produced by the liver and stored in the gallbladder. A complex sequence of chemical processes enables fats to be absorbed through the intestinal wall, broken down in the liver and converted for use in the body. Cholesterol, a lipid present in bile, plays an important part in this chain.

2 Bile salts act on fats to enable them to pass from the small intestine into the bloodstream, either directly or via the lymphatic system.

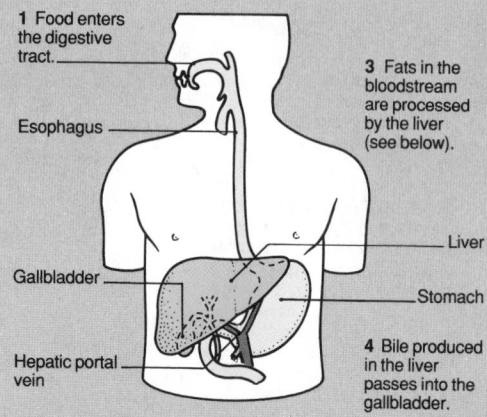

1 Food enters the digestive tract.

Esophagus

Gallbladder

Hepatic portal vein

3 Fats in the bloodstream are processed by the liver (see below).

Liver

Stomach

4 Bile produced in the liver passes into the gallbladder.

How fats are processed in the liver

Fat molecules are broken down in the liver into fatty acids and glycerol. Glycerol and some of the fatty acids pass back into the bloodstream. Other fatty acids are used to form cholesterol, some of which in turn is used to make bile salts. Unchanged cholesterol is dissolved in the bile, which then passes into the gallbladder.

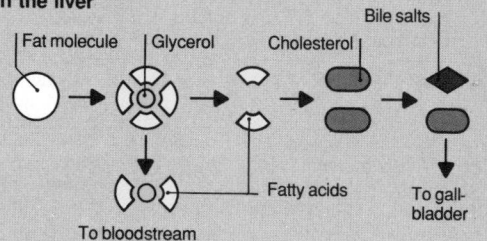

Fat molecule · Glycerol · Cholesterol · Bile salts

To bloodstream · Fatty acids · To gallbladder

effect, chenodiol treatment usually needs to be accompanied by adherence to a low-cholesterol, high-fiber diet.

How they affect you

Drug treatment often takes years to dissolve gallstones completely. You will not, therefore, feel any immediate benefit from the drugs, but you may have some minor side effects, the most usual of which is diarrhea. If this occurs, your physician may adjust the dosage. The effect of drug treatment on the gallstones is usually monitored at regular intervals by means of ultrasound or X-ray examinations.

Even after successful treatment with drugs this condition can recur when

chenodiol is stopped. In some cases drug treatment and dietary restrictions may be continued after the gallstones have dissolved, in order to prevent a recurrence of the problem.

Although these drugs reduce the amount of cholesterol in the gallbladder, they increase the level of cholesterol in the blood. Physicians therefore prescribe them with caution to people with atherosclerosis (fatty deposits in the blood vessels). They are not usually given to people with liver disorders because they can interfere with the normal liver function.

COMMON DRUGS

For gallstones
Chenodiol
Ursodeoxycholic acid (under investigation)

Pancreatic enzymes
Pancreatin
Pancrelipase

AGENTS USED IN DISORDERS OF THE PANCREAS

The pancreas releases certain *enzymes* into the small intestine, which are necessary for digestion of a range of foods. If the release of pancreatic enzymes is impaired, for example by chronic pancreatitis or cystic fibrosis, enzyme replacement therapy may be necessary. Replacement of enzymes does not cure the underlying disorder, but restores normal digestion. Pancreatic enzymes should

be taken just before or with meals, and usually take effect immediately. Your physician will probably advise you to eat a diet that is high in protein and carbohydrates and low in fat.

The most frequently used replacements are pancreatin and pancrelipase, both of which are extracted from pig pancreas. Both must be taken indefinitely as long as the pancreatic disorder persists.

MUSCLES, BONES, AND JOINTS

The basic architecture of the human body relies on bones (206 of them), a variety of muscles, and a complex assortment of other tissues – ligaments, tendons and cartilage – that enable them to function with remarkable efficiency.

What can go wrong

Though tough, these structures often suffer damage. Muscles, tendons, and ligaments can be strained or torn by violent movement. Such injury may cause inflammation, making the affected tissue swollen and painful. Joints, especially those that bear the body's weight – hips, knees, ankles, and vertebrae – are prone to wear and tear. The cartilage covering the bone ends may tear, causing pain and inflammation. Joint damage also occurs in rheumatoid arthritis, thought to be a form of autoimmune disorder. Gout, in which uric acid crystals form in some joints, may also cause inflammation, a condition known as gouty arthritis.

Other problems affecting the muscles, bones, and joints include those in which nerve control over muscle contraction is altered due to injury or a neurological disorder, or by poor nerve signals as in myasthenia gravis. The mineral composition of bone may be weakened by vitamin, mineral, or hormone deficiencies.

Why drugs are used

A simple analgesic drug or one that has an anti-inflammatory effect will provide pain relief in most of the above conditions. For more severe inflammation a physician may inject a drug with a more powerful anti-inflammatory effect – such as a corticosteroid – into the affected site. In cases of severe progressive rheumatoid arthritis, anti-rheumatic drugs may halt the disease process as well as relieving symptoms.

Drugs that help to eliminate excess uric acid from the body are often prescribed to treat gout. Muscle relaxants that inhibit transmission of nerve signals to the muscles are used to treat muscle spasm. Drugs that increase nervous stimulation of the muscle are prescribed for myasthenia gravis. Bone disorders in which the mineral content of the bone is reduced are treated with supplements of minerals, vitamins, and hormones.

MAJOR DRUG GROUPS

Non-steroidal anti-inflammatory drugs
Antirheumatic drugs
Locally acting corticosteroids
Drugs for gout

Muscle-relaxant drugs
Drugs used for myasthenia gravis
Drugs for bone disorders

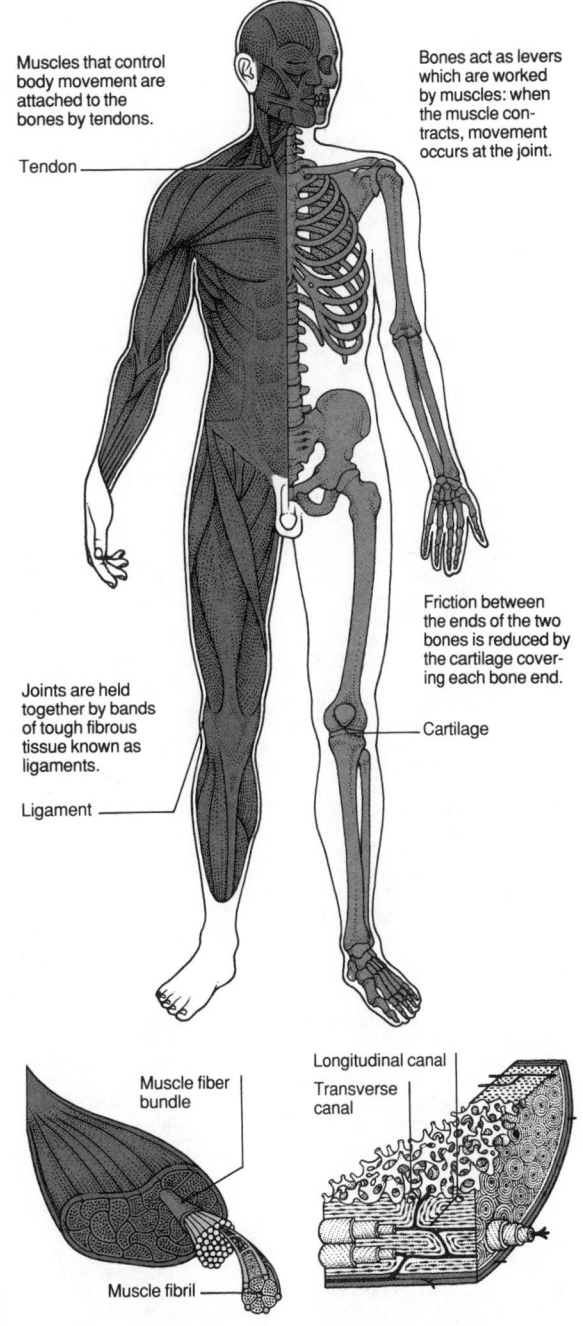

Muscles that control body movement are attached to the bones by tendons.

Tendon

Bones act as levers which are worked by muscles: when the muscle contracts, movement occurs at the joint.

Friction between the ends of the two bones is reduced by the cartilage covering each bone end.

Cartilage

Joints are held together by bands of tough fibrous tissue known as ligaments.

Ligament

Muscle fiber bundle

Muscle fibril

Longitudinal canal

Transverse canal

Muscle
Each muscle is made of thick bundles of fibers; each bundle in turn is made of fibrils. Tiny nerves and blood vessels enable the muscle to function.

Bone
Long bones (e.g., the femur) contain a network of longitudinal and transverse canals to carry blood, nerves, and lymph vessels through the bone.

NON-STEROIDAL ANTI-INFLAMMATORY DRUGS

Drugs in this group are used to relieve pain, stiffness, and inflammation associated with a wide variety of conditions, particularly those affecting the muscles, bones, and joints. NSAIDs are called non-steroidal to distinguish them from corticosteroid drugs (see p.169), which also have an anti-inflammatory effect. Many drugs of this class are already available; others are in various stages of investigation.

Why they are used

NSAIDs are widely prescribed in the treatment of rheumatoid arthritis, osteoarthritis, and other rheumatic conditions. They do not alter the progress of those diseases, but reduce inflammation and thus relieve pain and swelling of joints.

An NSAID may be used as the first line of treatment, or may be given when a simple analgesic such as aspirin does not provide adequate relief or is unsuitable for other reasons. The response to the various drugs in this group varies between individuals, and the first drug chosen may not be effective. It is therefore sometimes necessary for the physician to prescribe a number of different NSAIDs before finding the one which best suits a particular individual.

Because NSAIDs do not alter the progress of the disease, additional treatment may be required, particularly in the case of rheumatoid arthritis (see facing page).

NSAIDs are also commonly prescribed to relieve back pain, gout (p.147), menstrual pain (p.188), headaches, mild pain following surgery, and pain from soft tissue injuries such as sprains and strains (see also Analgesics, p.108).

How they work

Prostaglandins are chemicals released at the site of an injury. They are believed to be the substances responsible for producing pain and inflammation following tissue damage and in immune reactions. All the NSAIDs block the production of prostaglandins and thus reduce pain and inflammation (see p.109).

How they affect you

NSAIDs are usually effective in reducing joint pain and swelling. They are rapidly absorbed from the digestive system and most start to relieve symptoms within an hour. When used regularly for long-term treatment, they reduce stiffness and may improve the function of a joint if this has been impaired. Common side effects include nausea, indigestion, and altered bowel action. However, the potential of most NSAIDs to irritate the stomach is less than that of aspirin.

ACTION OF NSAIDs IN OSTEOARTHRITIS

Non-steroidal anti-inflammatory drugs are commonly prescribed to diminish the pain and stiffness associated with osteoarthritis, a disorder in which, typically, a weight-bearing joint such as the hip is damaged by wear and tear or other factors.

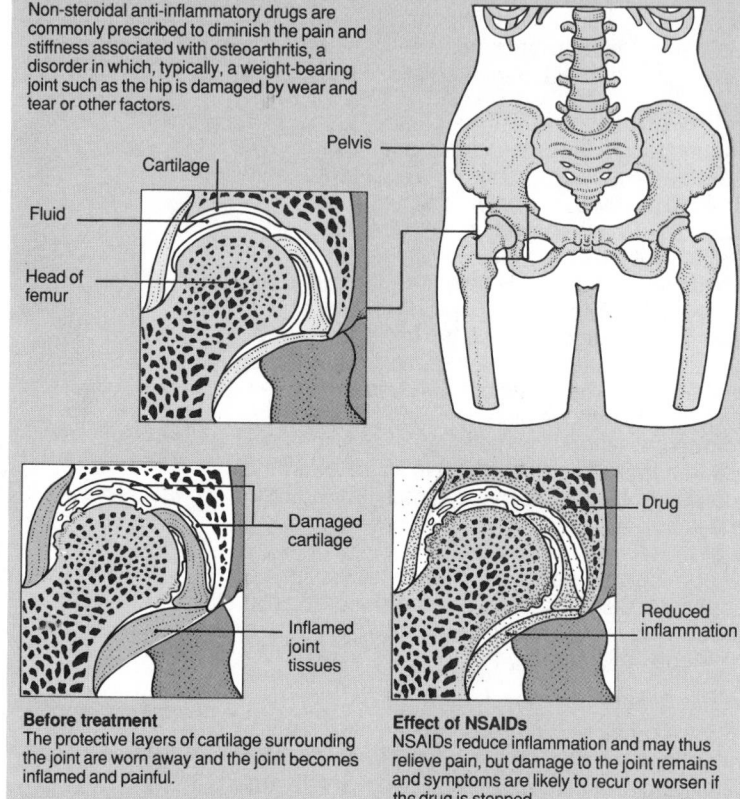

Before treatment
The protective layers of cartilage surrounding the joint are worn away and the joint becomes inflamed and painful.

Effect of NSAIDs
NSAIDs reduce inflammation and may thus relieve pain, but damage to the joint remains and symptoms are likely to recur or worsen if the drug is stopped.

A majority of the NSAIDs are short-acting and need to be taken several times a day in order to provide optimal relief of pain. Some need to be taken only twice daily. Others such as piroxicam are very slowly eliminated from the body and are effective when taken once a day.

Risks and special precautions

With a few exceptions, most NSAIDs are free from serious adverse effects. The main danger is that they can occasionally cause bleeding in the stomach or duodenum. They should normally be avoided by people who have suffered from peptic ulcers.

Most are not recommended during pregnancy or for nursing mothers. Caution is also advised for those with kidney or liver abnormalities or with a history of hypersensitivity to other drugs.

NSAIDs may also impair normal blood clotting and are, therefore, prescribed with caution for people with bleeding disorders or who are taking drugs that reduce blood clotting. At least one NSAID, phenylbutazone, may cause serious adverse effects. It can impair the bone marrow's ability to produce blood cells. Early signs of this include sore throat or fever, and must be reported. Phenylbutazone is usually prescribed for short periods only. Regular blood tests are carried out if it is needed longer.

COMMON DRUGS

Diflunisal
Fenoprofen
Ibuprofen
Indomethacin
Ketoprofen
Meclofenamate
Mefenamic acid
Naproxen
Phenylbutazone
Piroxicam
Sulindac
Tolmetin

ANTIRHEUMATIC DRUGS

These drugs are used in the treatment of various rheumatic disorders, the most crippling and deforming of which is rheumatoid arthritis. It is thought to be a form of auto-immune disease in which the body's mechanism for fighting infection contributes to the damage of its own joint tissue. The disease causes pain, stiffness, and swelling of the joints that over many months can lead to deformity. Flare-ups of rheumatoid arthritis also cause a generalized feeling of being unwell.

Treatments include drugs, rest, changes in diet, immobilization of joints, and physical therapy. Rheumatoid arthritis cannot yet be cured, although in many cases it does not progress far enough to cause permanent disability. The disease may subside spontaneously for prolonged periods.

Why they are used

The aim of drug treatment is to relieve pain and stiffness, maintain mobility, and prevent deformity. There are two main approaches to drug treatment for rheumatoid arthritis: (1) to alleviate symptoms, and (2) to modify, halt, or slow the underlying disease process. Drugs in the first category include aspirin (p.238) and the non-steroidal anti-inflammatory drugs (NSAIDs, facing page). These are often prescribed as a first treatment. However, when rheumatoid arthritis is severe or when the initial drug treatment is inadequate, the second category of drugs may be given. These can be of benefit where the disease is progressive because they may impede further joint damage and disability. They are not prescribed automatically because they have potentially severe adverse effects (see Types of antirheumatic drugs, below) and because the disease may stop spontaneously. Antirheumatic drugs include gold, penicillamine, chloroquine, and the immunosuppressant drugs methotrexate, azathioprine, chlorambucil, and cyclophosphamide. Corticosteroids (p.169) may be used for limited periods.

THE EFFECTS OF ANTIRHEUMATIC DRUGS

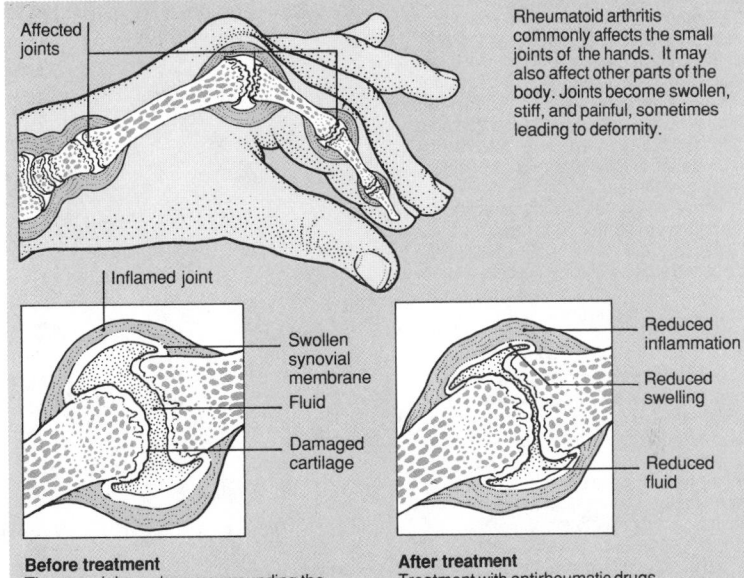

Affected joints

Rheumatoid arthritis commonly affects the small joints of the hands. It may also affect other parts of the body. Joints become swollen, stiff, and painful, sometimes leading to deformity.

Inflamed joint

Swollen synovial membrane

Fluid

Damaged cartilage

Reduced inflammation

Reduced swelling

Reduced fluid

Before treatment
The synovial membrane surrounding the joint is inflamed and thickened, producing increased fluid within the joint. The surrounding tissue is inflamed and joint cartilage damaged.

After treatment
Treatment with antirheumatic drugs relieves pain, swelling, and inflammation. Damage to cartilage and bone may be halted so that further deformity is minimized.

How they work

It is not known precisely how most antirheumatic drugs stop or slow the disease process. Some may reduce the body's immune response, which is thought to be partly responsible for the disease (see also Immunosuppressant drugs, p.184). When effective, such drugs prevent damage to the cartilage and bone, thereby reducing progressive deformity and disability. The effectiveness of each drug varies depending on individual response.

How they affect you

These drugs are generally slow-acting; it may be weeks or even months before benefit is noticed. Treatment with NSAIDs or aspirin is usually continued. After this time, however, antirheumatic drugs can cause a marked improvement in symptoms. Pain is reduced, joint mobility increased, and generalized symptoms of ill health fade. Side effects, which vary between drugs, may be noticed before any beneficial effect, so patience is required. Severe adverse effects may occasionally necessitate abandoning the treatment.

TYPES OF ANTIRHEUMATIC DRUGS

Gold Gold-based drugs are often considered to be the most effective. Given by mouth or injection, these drugs may be prescribed for many years. Possible side effects include skin rash and digestive disturbances. Occasionally gold may cause kidney damage, so regular urine tests are usually carried out. Gold can also suppress production of blood cells in the bone marrow. For this reason, periodic blood tests are also carried out.

Penicillamine This drug (unrelated to penicillin antibiotics) may be used when rheumatoid arthritis is progressing rapidly, or when gold cannot be given. Improvement in symptoms may take 3 to 6 months. It has similar side effects to gold, and periodic blood and urine tests are usually performed.

Chloroquine Originally developed to treat malaria (see p.165), chloroquine and related drugs are less effective than penicillamine or gold. Since prolonged use may cause eye damage, regular eye checks are needed.

Immunosuppressants These may be prescribed if other drugs do not provide relief, and if rheumatoid arthritis is severe and disabling. Regular observation and blood tests must be carried out because immunosuppressants can cause severe undesired complications.

COMMON DRUGS

Immunosuppressants
Azathioprine
Chlorambucil
Cyclophosphamide
Methotrexate

Gold-based drugs
Auranofin
Gold sodium thiomalate

Others
Chloroquine
Penicillamine

LOCALLY ACTING CORTICOSTEROIDS

The adrenal glands, one atop each of the kidneys, produce a number of important hormones. Among them are the corticosteroids, so named because they are made in the outer part (cortex) of the glands. These hormones play an important role, influencing the immune system and regulating the carbohydrate and mineral *metabolism* of the body. A number of drugs that mimic the effects of natural corticosteroid hormones have been developed.

These drugs have many uses and are discussed in more detail under Corticosteroids (p.169). This section concentrates on corticosteroids given by injection into an affected site to treat various joint disorders.

Why they are used

Corticosteroids given by injection are particularly useful for treating joint disorders – notably rheumatoid arthritis and osteoarthritis – when one or only a few joints are involved and pain and inflammation have not been relieved. In such cases it is possible to relieve symptoms by injecting each of the affected joints individually. Cortico-steroids may also be injected to relieve pain and inflammation caused by strained or contracted muscles, ligaments and/or tendons – for example, in frozen shoulder or tennis elbow. They may also be given for bursitis, tendinitis, or swelling that may be compressing a nerve. Corticosteroid injections are sometimes used to relieve pain and stiffness sufficiently to allow physical therapy to be undertaken.

How they work

These drugs have two main actions that are thought to account for their effective-

ness. They depress the activity of the white blood cells, which are responsible for inflammation (below), and also block the production of chemicals called prostaglandins, which are responsible for triggering pain and inflammation. Administration by injection concentrates the effects of the corticosteroids at the site of the problem, producing maximum benefit where it is most needed.

COMMON INJECTION SITES

Corticosteroids are often injected into joints affected by osteo- and rheumatoid arthritis. Joints commonly treated in this way are knee, shoulder and finger joints.

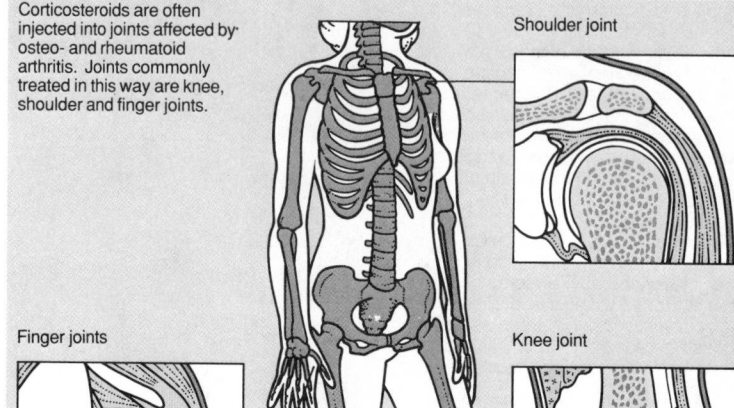

Shoulder joint

Finger joints

Knee joint

How they affect you

Corticosteroids usually produce dramatic relief from symptoms when they are injected into a joint. Often a single injection is sufficient to relieve pain and swelling, and to improve mobility. When used to treat muscle or tendon pain they may not always be effective because it is difficult to position the needle so that the drug reaches the right spot. In some cases repeated injections are necessary.

Because these drugs are concentrated in the affected area, and are not dispersed in significant amounts in the body, the generalized adverse effects that may occur with corticosteroids taken by mouth are unlikely. Minor side effects such as loss of skin pigment at the injection site are uncommon. Occasionally, a temporary increase in pain (steroid flare) may occur. In such cases, local application of ice, rest, and analgesic medication may relieve the condition. Sterile injection technique is critically important.

COMMON DRUGS

Hydrocortisone
Methylprednisolone
Prednisone
Triamcinolone

ACTION OF CORTICOSTEROIDS ON INFLAMED JOINTS

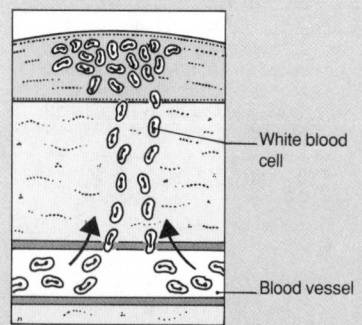

White blood cell

Blood vessel

Inflamed tissue
Inflammation occurs when disease or injury causes large numbers of white blood cells to accumulate in the affected area. In joints this leads to swelling and stiffness.

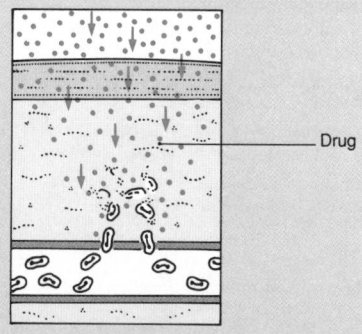

Drug

Action of corticosteroids
Corticosteroids injected into the area per-meate the joint lining (synovial membrane) and prevent accumulation of white blood cells.

DRUGS FOR GOUT

Gout is a disorder that arises when the blood contains increased levels of uric acid, a by-product of *metabolism* which is excreted in urine. When its concentration in the blood is excessive, uric acid crystals may form in various parts of the body, especially in the joints of the foot (most often the big toe), the knee, and the hand, causing intense pain and inflammation known as gouty arthritis. Crystals may form as white masses, known as tophi, in soft tissue, and in the kidneys as stones. Attacks of gouty arthritis can recur, and may lead to damaged joints and deformity. Kidney stones can cause kidney damage.

An excess of uric acid can be caused either by increased production or by an impairment in the kidney function that removes it from the body. The disorder tends to run in families and is far more common in men. The risk of attack is increased by high alcohol intake, obesity, and the consumption of certain foods (including red meat, sardines, anchovies, liver, and brains). An attack may be triggered by drugs such as thiazide diuretics (see p.127), anti-cancer drugs (see p.182), or excessive drinking. Changes in diet and a reduction in alcohol consumption may be an important part of treatment.

Drugs used to treat acute gout include non-steroidal anti-inflammatory drugs (see p.144), colchicine, and, less commonly today, corticosteroids and corticotropin (ACTH), which controls the production and release of adrenal corticosteroid hormones. Others which lower the blood level of uric acid are allopurinol and the uricosuric drugs, probenecid and sulfinpyrazone. Aspirin is not prescribed for pain relief because it slows the excretion of uric acid.

Why they are used

Drugs may be prescribed to treat an attack of gout or to prevent recurrent attacks that could lead to deformity of affected joints and kidney damage. Colchicine can halt an attack of gout; NSAIDs may also ease the symptoms. Either type of drug should be taken as soon as an attack begins. Because colchicine is relatively specific in relieving the pain and inflammation arising from gout, physicians sometimes administer it in order to confirm their diagnosis of the condition before prescribing an NSAID.

If symptoms recur, your physician may advise long-term treatment with allopurinol or uricosuric drugs.

These drugs usually have to be taken indefinitely. Since they can trigger attacks of gout at the beginning of treatment, colchicine is also given with these drugs for a few months.

How they work

Allopurinol reduces the level of uric acid in the blood by interfering with the activity of xanthine oxidase, an *enzyme* that is involved in the production of uric acid in the body. Probenecid and sulfinpyrazone increase the rate at which uric acid is excreted by the kidneys. It is not known how colchicine reduces inflammation and relieves pain. The actions of NSAIDs are described on p.144.

How they affect you

Drugs used in the long-term treatment of gout are usually successful in preventing attacks and joint deformity. However, response may be slow.

Colchicine can disturb the digestive system, causing abdominal pain, which your physician can manage.

Risks and special precautions

Since they increase the output of uric acid through the kidneys, uricosuric drugs can cause uric acid crystals to form in the kidneys. They are not, therefore, usually prescribed for those who already have kidney problems. In such cases allopurinol may be preferred. It is always important to drink plenty of fluids while taking anti-gout drugs to prevent kidney crystals from forming. Regular blood tests to monitor levels of uric acid in the blood may be required.

ACTION OF URICOSURIC DRUGS

Uric acid is removed from the blood by the kidneys and excreted in the urine. Excess uric acid, caused by increased production or impaired kidney function, requires treatment with uricosuric drugs, which increase the rate at which uric acid is expelled.

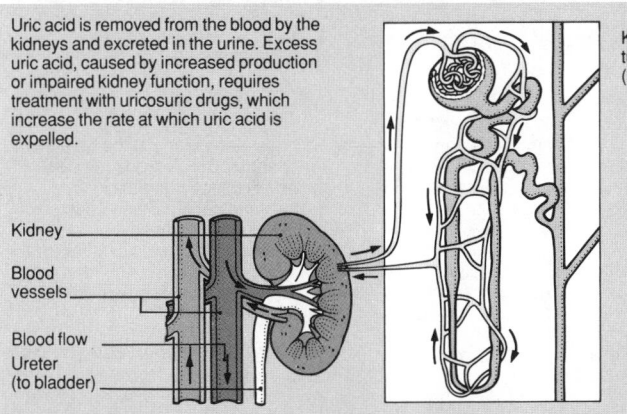

Kidney

Blood vessels

Blood flow

Ureter (to bladder)

Kidney tubule (enlarged)

Uric acid and gouty arthritis

Gouty arthritis occurs when uric acid crystals form in a joint, often in the toe, knee, or hand, causing inflammation and pain. This is the result of excessively high levels of uric acid in the blood. In some cases this is caused by over-production of uric acid, while in others it is the result of reduced excretion of uric acid by the kidneys.

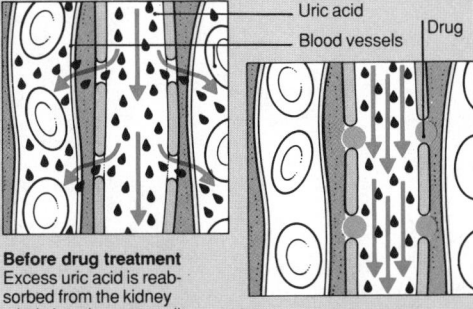

Uric acid

Blood vessels

Drug

Before drug treatment
Excess uric acid is reabsorbed from the kidney tubule into the surrounding blood vessels. This leads to the formation of uric acid crystals, which can cause gouty arthritis.

After drug treatment
When the reabsorption of uric acid into the blood vessels is blocked, the amount of uric acid excreted in the urine is increased.

COMMON DRUGS

Drugs to treat attacks
Colchicine
Corticosteroids (see p.169)
NSAIDs (see p.144)

Drugs to prevent attacks
Allopurinol
Probenecid
Sulfinpyrazone

MUSCLE-RELAXANT DRUGS

Several drugs are available to treat muscle spasm: the involuntary, painful contraction of a muscle or a group of muscles that can stiffen an arm or leg, or make it nearly impossible to straighten your back. There are various causes of muscle spasm. It can follow an injury, arise spontaneously, or be brought on by a disorder like osteoarthritis, the pain in the affected joint triggering abnormal tension in a nearby muscle.

Spasticity is another form of muscle tightness seen in some neurological disorders such as multiple sclerosis, stroke, or cerebral palsy. This can sometimes be helped by physical therapy but in severe cases drugs may be used to relieve symptoms.

Why they are used

Painful muscle spasm resulting from direct injury is usually and most effectively treated with an analgesic (see p.108) or non-steroidal anti-inflammatory drug (see p.144). However, if the spasm is severe, as it may be following a back injury, a muscle relaxant may be tried for a short period to relieve the symptoms. Muscle relaxants are frequently added to analgesic preparations for the relief of spasm caused by conditions of this type.

In spasticity, the sufferer's legs may become so stiff and uncontrollable that it is impossible to walk unaided. In such cases a drug may be prescribed which relieves symptoms without taking all the strength away from the muscles. Relaxation of the muscles often permits physical therapy to be given for longer-term relief in certain spastic conditions.

How they work

Muscle-relaxant drugs work in one of two ways: the centrally acting drugs slow down the passage of the nerve signals from the brain and spinal cord that cause muscles to contract, thus

SITES OF ACTION OF MUSCLE RELAXANTS

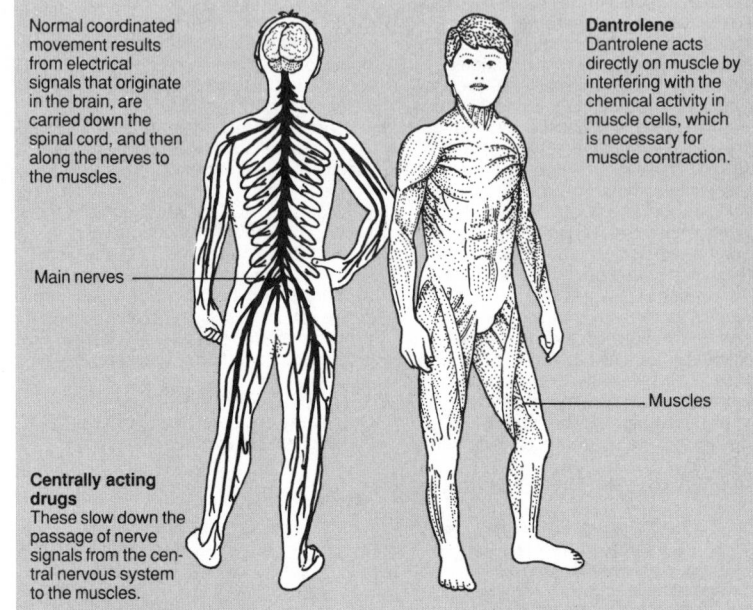

Normal coordinated movement results from electrical signals that originate in the brain, are carried down the spinal cord, and then along the nerves to the muscles.

Main nerves

Centrally acting drugs
These slow down the passage of nerve signals from the central nervous system to the muscles.

Dantrolene
Dantrolene acts directly on muscle by interfering with the chemical activity in muscle cells, which is necessary for muscle contraction.

Muscles

reducing stimulation of muscles and unwanted muscular contraction. Dantrolene reduces the sensitivity of the muscles to nerve signals.

How they affect you

Drugs taken regularly for a spastic disorder of the central nervous system usually reduce stiffness and improve mobility. They may restore the use of the arms and legs when this has been impaired by muscle spasm.

Unfortunately, most centrally acting drugs can have a generally depressant effect on nervous activity and produce

drowsiness, particularly at the beginning of treatment. Too high a dosage can excessively reduce the muscles' ability to contract and can therefore cause weakness. For this reason, the dosage must be carefully adjusted in order to find a level that controls symptoms and at the same time maintains sufficient muscular strength.

Risks and special precautions

The main long-term risk associated with centrally acting muscle relaxants is that the body may become dependent on the drug for depressing the excessive nervous activity responsible for muscle spasm. If the drug is withdrawn suddenly, the stiffness may become worse than it was before drug treatment began.

Dantrolene can, in rare cases, cause serious liver damage, and for this reason those taking this drug should have their blood tested regularly to assess liver function.

ACTION OF CENTRALLY ACTING DRUGS

Centrally acting muscle relaxants restrict the passage of nerve signals to the muscles by occupying a proportion of the *receptors* in the central nervous system that are normally used by chemical *neurotransmitters* to transmit such impulses. Reduced nervous stimulation allows the muscles to relax; however, if the dose of the drug is too high, this action may give rise to excessive muscle weakness.

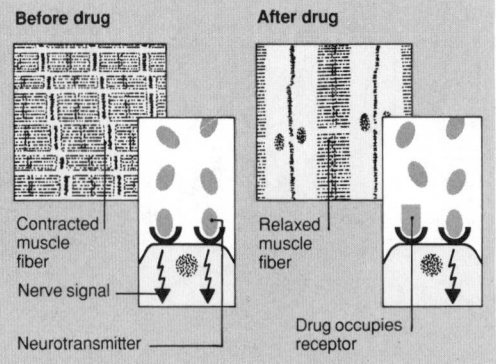

Before drug

Contracted muscle fiber

Nerve signal

Neurotransmitter

After drug

Relaxed muscle fiber

Drug occupies receptor

COMMON DRUGS

Centrally-acting drugs	Others
Baclofen	Dantrolene
Carisoprodol	
Chlorzoxazone	
Cyclobenzaprine	
Diazepam	
Methocarbamol	
Orphenadrine	

DRUGS USED FOR MYASTHENIA GRAVIS

Myasthenia gravis is a disorder that occurs when the immune system (see p.180) becomes defective and produces antibodies that disrupt the signals being transmitted between the nervous system and the muscles under voluntary control. The result is a progressive weakening of muscular response. The muscles first affected are those controlling the eyes, eyelids, face, pharynx, and larynx, with muscles in the arms and legs becoming involved as the disease progresses. The disease is often linked to a disorder of the thymus gland, the source of the destructive antibodies concerned.

Treatment of myasthenia gravis can take several forms. It may involve the removal of the thymus gland (thymectomy). Temporary relief may be obtained by clearing the blood of antibodies, a procedure known as plasmapheresis. Drugs are available that improve muscle function, principally neostigmine and pyridostigmine. They may be used alone or together with other drugs that depress the immune system – usually corticosteroids (see p.169) or azathioprine (see Immunosuppressant drugs, p.184).

Why they are used

Drugs may be given when it is not feasible to remove the thymus gland, or when surgery does not provide adequate relief. Drugs may be taken in the long term to improve muscular strength, but these have no effect on the disease process itself. One of these, edrophonium, acts very rapidly and is used to confirm the diagnosis. When administered, it brings about a dramatic improvement in symptoms, but as the benefits last for only a few minutes, it is not prescribed for regular treatment.

These drugs may also be given following surgery to counteract the effects of a muscle-relaxant drug given prior to certain surgical procedures.

THE EFFECTS OF MYASTHENIA GRAVIS

Myasthenia gravis initially causes weakness of the muscles in the face and throat, affecting the muscles around the eyes and the mouth. In the later stages, arms and legs may be affected.

Late stages

Early stages

The thymus gland
Located in the upper part of the chest, this gland is thought to be partly responsible for the abnormal antibody activity in this disease.

Principal muscles affected

How they work

Normal muscle action occurs when a nerve impulse triggers a nerve ending to release a *neurotransmitter*, which combines with a specialized *receptor* on the muscle cells and causes the muscles to contract. In myasthenia gravis, the body's immune system destroys many of these receptors, so that the muscle is less responsive to nervous stimulation. Drugs used to treat the disorder, like neostigmine, increase the amount of neurotransmitter at the nerve ending by blocking the action of an *enzyme* which normally breaks it down. Increased levels of the neurotransmitter permit the remaining receptors to function more efficiently (see

Action of drugs used for myasthenia gravis, below left).

How they affect you

These drugs usually restore muscle function to a normal or near normal level, particularly when the disease takes a mild form. Unfortunately, they can produce unwanted muscular activity by enhancing the transmission of nerve impulses elsewhere in the body.

Common side effects include vomiting, nausea, diarrhea, and muscle cramps in the arms, legs, and abdomen.

Risks and special precautions

Muscle weakness can suddenly worsen even when it is being treated with drugs. Should this occur, it is important not to take larger doses of the drug in an attempt to relieve the symptoms, because excessive levels can interfere with the transmission of nerve impulses to muscles, causing further weakness. The administration of other drugs, including some antibiotics, can also markedly increase the symptoms of myasthenia gravis. If your symptoms become any worse, your physician should be consulted.

COMMON DRUGS

Neostigmine
Pyridostigmine

ACTION OF DRUGS USED FOR MYASTHENIA GRAVIS

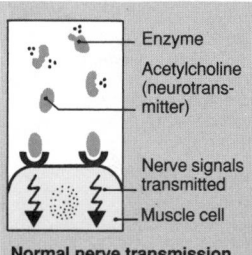

Enzyme
Acetylcholine (neurotransmitter)
Nerve signals transmitted
Muscle cell

Normal nerve transmission
Muscles contract when a neurotransmitter (acetylcholine) binds to receptors on muscle cells. An enzyme breaks down acetylcholine.

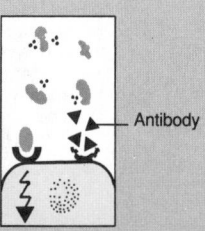

Antibody

In myasthenia gravis
Abnormal antibody activity destroys many receptors, reducing stimulation of muscle cells and weakening muscle action.

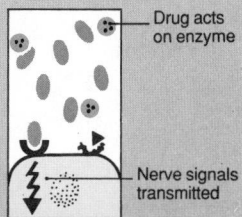

Drug acts on enzyme

Nerve signals transmitted

Drug action
Drugs block enzyme action, increasing acetylcholine and prolonging the muscle cell response to nervous stimulation.

DRUGS FOR BONE DISORDERS

Bone is a biologically active tissue of the body, its hard, mineralized quality created by the action of the bone cells. These continuously deposit and remove converted calcium and phosphorus stored in the pockets of a honeycombed protein framework called the matrix. Because the rates of deposit and removal are about equal in adults, the bone mass remains fairly constant.

That process of removal and renewal, i.e., the bone *metabolism*, is regulated by various hormones and influenced by many factors, notably the level of calcium in the blood. That, in turn, depends on the intake of calcium and vitamin D from the diet, the actions of various hormones, plus the movement and weight-bearing stress involved in everyday activities. When normal bone metabolism is altered, various bone disorders are the result.

Osteoporosis

In osteoporosis the strength and density of bone is reduced. Such wasting occurs when the rate of removal of mineralized bone by the active cells exceeds the rate of renewal. In most people, bone density begins to decrease very gradually from the age of 30 onwards. But bone loss can dramatically increase when a person is immobilized or bed-ridden for a prolonged period, and this is an important cause of osteoporosis in elderly people. Hormone deficiency is another important cause of osteoporosis, commonly occurring in women with lowered estrogen levels following the menopause or removal of the ovaries. Osteoporosis also occurs in disorders in which there is excess production of adrenal or thyroid hormones. It can be a result of long-term treatment with corticosteroid drugs.

People with osteoporosis often have no symptoms. But if the vertebrae become so weakened that they are unable to bear the body's weight, or if the person is injured in a fall, he or she may collapse. Subsequently, the individual suffers from back pain,

reduced height and a round-shouldered appearance. Osteoporosis also increases the likelihood of a fracture of the long bone in the arm or leg as a result of an injury or fall.

Most physicians emphasize the need to prevent the disorder by ensuring adequate intake of protein and calcium in the diet and regular exercise throughout adult life. Estrogen supplements during and after the menopause may help to prevent osteoporosis from occurring in older women. For a full discussion of the benefits and risks of such hormone replacement therapy, see p.175. Calcitonin injections and sodium fluoride tablets are being tried on an *investigational* basis.

The condition of bones damaged by osteoporosis cannot usually be improved, although drug treatment can help prevent further deterioration and help fractures heal. If lack of calcium in the diet is a major cause, supplements are usually prescribed, possibly with vitamin D. Any underlying hormonal imbalance is usually corrected.

Osteomalacia and rickets

In osteomalacia – called rickets when it affects children – lack of vitamin D leads to loss of calcium, resulting in softening of the bones. Sufferers experience pain and tenderness, and there is a risk of fracture and bone deformity. In children, growth is retarded.

The commonest cause of osteomalacia is lack of vitamin D. This can be caused by inadequate diet, inability to absorb the vitamin, or by insufficient exposure of the skin to sunlight (the action of the sun on the skin produces vitamin D inside the body). People at special risk include those confined to bed for long periods who may not be exposed to sufficient sunlight and those whose absorption of vitamin D from the diet is impaired by an intestinal disorder – for example, Crohn's disease or celiac disease. Chronic kidney disease is an important cause of rickets in children and of osteomalacia in adults, since healthy kidneys play an essential role in the body's metabolism of vitamin D.

Long-term relief depends on treating the underlying disorder whenever possible. Treatment may in rare cases need to be lifelong.

BONE WASTING

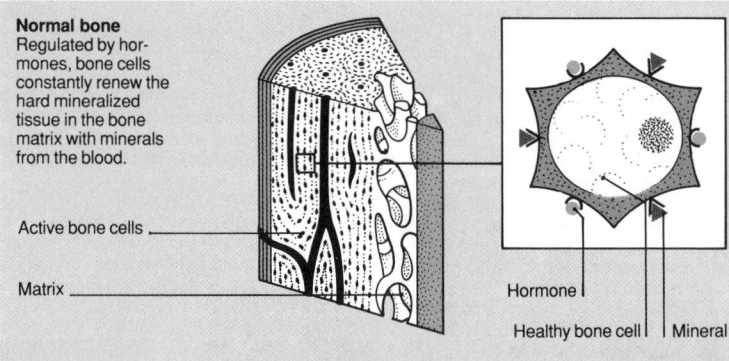

Normal bone
Regulated by hormones, bone cells constantly renew the hard mineralized tissue in the bone matrix with minerals from the blood.

Active bone cells

Matrix

Hormone

Healthy bone cell | Mineral

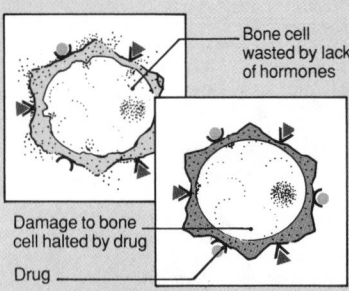

Bone cell wasted by lack of hormones

Damage to bone cell halted by drug

Drug

In osteoporosis
Hormonal disturbance leads to wasting of active bone cells. The bones become less dense and more fragile. Drug treatment with hormone and mineral supplements usually only prevents further bone loss.

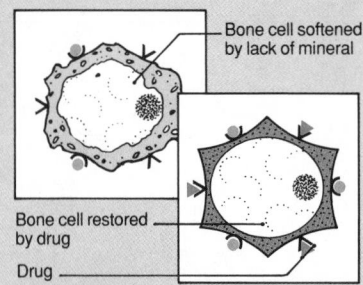

Bone cell softened by lack of mineral

Bone cell restored by drug

Drug

In osteomalacia
Deficiency of calcium or vitamin D causes softening of the bone tissue. The bones become weaker and sometimes deformed. Drug treatment with vitamins and minerals usually restores bone strength.

COMMON DRUGS

Calcitonin
Calcium carbonate
Estrogens (see p.175)
Sodium fluoride
Vitamin D

ALLERGY

Allergy – a hypersensitivity to certain substances – reflects an excessive reaction of the body's immune system. Acting by means of a variety of mechanisms (see Malignant and immune disease, p.180), the immune system protects the body by trying to eliminate foreign substances that it does not recognize, such as invading bacteria or viruses.

One way in which it acts is through the production of *antibodies*. When a particular foreign substance (or allergen) is encountered for the first time, white blood cells known as lymphocytes produce antibodies that attach themselves to other white blood cells known as mast cells. If the same substance is encountered again, the allergen binds to the antibodies on the mast cells, causing the release of chemicals called mediators, the most important of which is histamine. This chemical can produce rash, swelling, narrowing of the airways, and a drop in blood pressure.

What can go wrong

People differ widely in their response to allergens, and while some suffer severe allergic (hypersensitivity) reactions to insect bites or particular foods, others suffer no ill effects from exposure to the same substances.

One of the most common allergic disorders, hay fever, is caused by an allergic reaction to inhaled grass pollen, leading to allergic rhinitis – swelling and irritation of the nasal passages and watering of the nose and eyes. Other substances, such as house-dust mites, animal fur, and feathers, may cause a similar reaction in susceptible people. Asthma, another allergic disorder, may result from the action of mediators other than histamine. Other allergic conditions include urticaria (hives) and other rashes (sometimes in response to a drug), some forms of eczema and dermatitis, and allergic alveolitis (farmer's lung).

Why drugs are used

Antihistamines and drugs that inhibit mast-cell activity are used to prevent and treat allergic reactions. Other drugs are useful for treating allergic symptoms, such as decongestants (p.121) to clear the nose in allergic rhinitis and bronchodilators (p.120) to widen the airways of those with asthma.

MAJOR DRUG GROUPS

Antihistamines

Allergic response

Lymphocytes produce antibodies to allergens, which attach to mast cells. If the allergen enters the body again, it binds to the antibodies, and the mast cells release histamine.

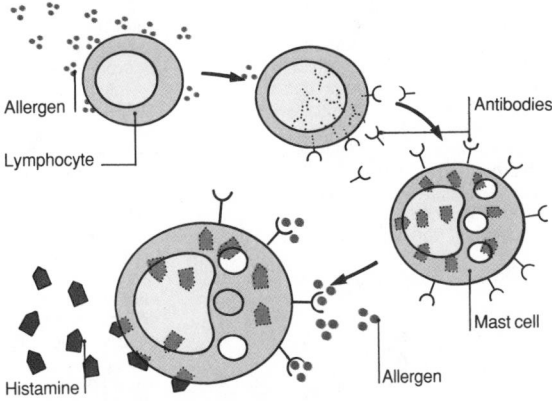

Allergen
Lymphocyte
Antibodies
Mast cell
Allergen
Histamine

Histamine and histamine receptors

Histamine, released in response to injury or the presence of allergens, acts on H_1 *receptors* in the skin, blood vessels, nasal passages, and airways, and on H_2 receptors in the stomach lining, salivary and lacrimal (tear) glands. It provokes dilation of blood vessels, inflammation and swelling of tissues, and narrowing of the airways. Sometimes a reaction termed anaphylactic shock occurs, caused by a dramatic fall in blood pressure and leading to collapse. Antihistamine drugs block H_1 receptors, and H_2 antagonists block H_2 receptors (see also Antihistamines, p.152, and Antiulcer drugs, p.137).

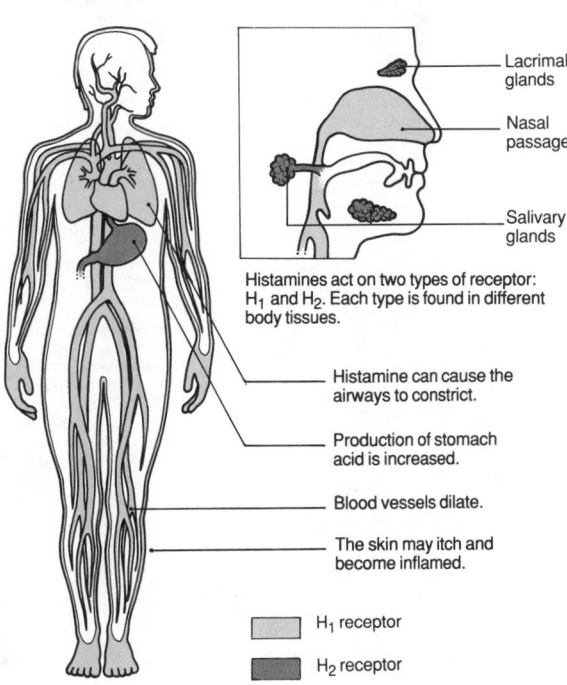

Lacrimal glands
Nasal passage
Salivary glands

Histamines act on two types of receptor: H_1 and H_2. Each type is found in different body tissues.

Histamine can cause the airways to constrict.

Production of stomach acid is increased.

Blood vessels dilate.

The skin may itch and become inflamed.

■ H_1 receptor
■ H_2 receptor

ANTIHISTAMINES

Antihistamines are the most widely used drugs in the treatment of allergic reactions of all kinds. They can be sub-divided according to chemical structure, each subgrouping with slightly different actions and characteristics (see the table on the facing page). Their main action is to counter the effects of histamine, one of the chemicals released in the body when there is an allergic reaction. (For a full explanation of the allergy mechanism, see p.151.)

Histamine is also involved in a number of other body functions, including blood vessel dilation and constriction, the contraction of the muscles of the respiratory and gastrointestinal tracts, and the release of digestive juices in the stomach. The antihistamine drugs described here are also known as H_1 blockers because they only block the action of histamine on certain *receptors*, known as H_1 receptors. Another group of antihistamines, known as H_2 blockers, are used in the treatment of peptic ulcers (see Anti-ulcer drugs, p.137).

Most antihistamines have a significant *anticholinergic* action. This is used to advantage in a variety of conditions, but it also accounts for certain undesired side effects.

Why they are used

Antihistamines relieve allergy-related symptoms when it is not possible or practical to prevent exposure to the substance that has provoked the re-action. Their most common use is in the prevention of allergic rhinitis, inflam-mation of the nose and upper airways resulting from an allergic reaction to a substance such as pollen, house dust, or animal fur. They are more effective when taken before the start of an attack. If they are taken only after an attack has already started, beneficial effects may be delayed.

Antihistamines are not generally effective in asthma caused by similar allergens because the symptoms of this allergic disorder are not solely caused by the action of histamine, but are likely to be the result of more complex mech-anisms. When antihistamines fail to provide adequate relief, alternative treatments may be prescribed (see Other allergy treatments, below).

Antihistamines are also useful for relieving the itching, swelling, and red-ness characteristic of allergic reactions involving the skin – for example, urti-caria (hives), infantile eczema, and other forms of dermatitis. Irritation from chicken pox may be reduced by these drugs. In addition, allergic reactions to insect stings may also be reduced by antihistamines. In such cases the drug may be taken by mouth or applied *topically*. Applied as drops, antihis-tamines also reduce inflammation and irritation of the eyes and eyelids in allergic conjunctivitis.

An antihistamine is often included as an ingredient in cough and cold prep-arations (see p.122), when the anti-cholinergic effect of drying mucus secretions and the sedative effect on the coughing mechanism may be helpful.

Because most antihistamines have a depressant effect on the brain, they are sometimes used to promote sleep, especially when discomfort from itching is disturbing sleep (see also Sleeping drugs, p.110). Because the depressant effect on the brain also extends to the centers that control nausea and vomit-ing, antihistamines are therefore often effective for controlling these symptoms (see Anti-emetic drugs, p.118).

Occasionally, antihistamines are used to treat fever, rash, and breathing difficulties that may occur in adverse reactions to blood transfusions and allergic reactions to drugs. One of the common antihistamines, diphenhydra-mine, is sometimes prescribed in the early stages of Parkinson's disease. Promethazine and hydroxyzine are also used as *premedication*.

How they work

Antihistamines block the action of his-tamine on H_1 receptors. These are found

SITES OF ACTION

Antihistamines act on a variety of sites and systems throughout the body. Their main action is on the muscles surrounding the small blood vessels that supply the skin and mucous membranes. They also act on the airways in the lungs and on the brain.

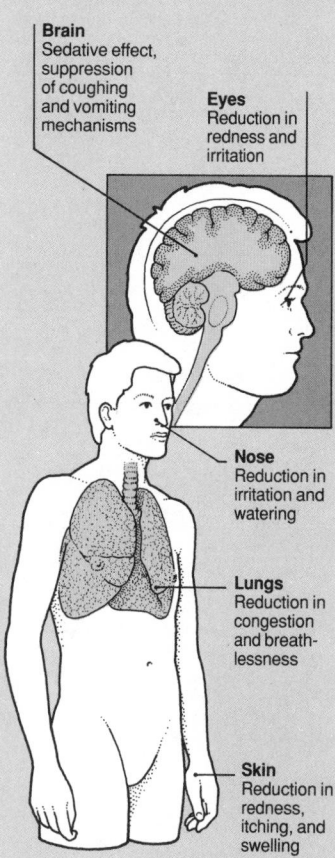

Brain
Sedative effect, suppression of coughing and vomiting mechanisms

Eyes
Reduction in redness and irritation

Nose
Reduction in irritation and watering

Lungs
Reduction in congestion and breath-lessness

Skin
Reduction in redness, itching, and swelling

OTHER ALLERGY TREATMENTS

Antihistamines are usually the first drugs to be tried in the treatment of allergic disorders. When these fail to control symptoms ad-equately, or when they are unsuitable, other drugs may be prescribed.

Cromolyn sodium
This drug is a mast cell inhibitor, one that curbs the release of histamine from mast cells (see p. 151) in response to exposure to an allergen, thus preventing the physical symptoms of allergies. It is most commonly given by inhaler for the prevention of seasonal allergic rhinitis (hay fever) and allergy-induced asthma attacks. For further information on this drug, see p.298.

Desensitization
This may be tried in such allergic conditions as allergic rhinitis and asthma, when anti-histamines have not been effective and tests have shown one or two specific allergens to be responsible.

Desensitization is less likely to be effec-tive when a large number of factors seem to provoke the allergic response. Also, because such treatment often provides only incomplete relief, it is usually attempted only when simpler measures such as avoidance of the allergen have been tried unsuccess-fully. Desensitization to pollen and house dust has been the most effective form.

The treatment involves giving a series of injections containing gradually increasing doses of an extract of the allergen. The precise mechanism by which this prevents allergic reactions is not fully understood. One explanation is that such controlled exposure to the substance triggers the immune system to produce increasing levels of antibodies to the allergen, so that the body no longer responds dramatically when the allergen is encountered naturally.

Desensitization needs to be carried out under careful medical supervision, because it can occasionally provoke a severe allergic response. It is important to remain within close range of emergency medical facilities for at least 20 minutes after each injection.

COMPARISON OF ANTIHISTAMINES

Although antihistamines have broadly similar effects and uses, differences in their strength of anticholinergic action, the amount of drowsiness they produce, and also in their duration of action, affect the uses for which each drug is commonly selected. The table below indicates the main uses of each of the common antihistamines and gives an indication of the relative strengths of their anticholinergic and sedative effects and of their duration of action.

- ■   Strong
- ◣   Medium
- □   Minimal
- ▲   Long (over 12 hours)
- ◮   Medium (6 – 12 hours)
- △   Short (4 – 6 hours)

Drug	Common uses Allergic rhinitis	Skin allergy	Sedation	Parkinson's disease	Nausea/vomiting	Actions and effects Drowsiness	Anticholinergic action	Duration of action
Azatadine	●	●				■	◣	▲
Brompheniramine	●	●				◣	□	△
Chlorpheniramine	●	●				◣	□	◮
Dimenhydrinate					●	◣	◣	△
Diphenhydramine			●	●	●	■	◣	△
Hydroxyzine		●	●			◣	□	△
Meclizine					●	◣	□	△
Promethazine	●	●	●			■	◣	△
Terfenadine	●	●				□	□	▲
Trimeprazine		●	●			■	◣	◮
Triprolidine	●	●				◣	□	◮

on various body tissues, particularly the small blood vessels in the skin, nose, and eyes. This helps prevent the dilation of the vessels, thus reducing the redness and swelling. The anticholinergic action of these drugs also contributes to this effect.

Antihistamines pass from the blood into the brain, where their blocking action on histamine activity produces general sedation and depression of various brain functions, including the vomiting and coughing mechanisms.

How they affect you

Treatment with these drugs relieves symptoms and helps to induce sleep if allergic symptoms have been causing insomnia. Antihistamines frequently cause a degree of daytime drowsiness and may adversely affect coordination, leading to clumsiness. Some of the newer drugs, for example terfenadine, have little or no sedative effect.

Anticholinergic side effects, including dry mouth, blurred vision, and difficulty passing urine, are common. Most side effects diminish with continued use and can often be helped by an adjustment in dosage or a change to a different drug.

Risks and special precautions

Because most antihistamines have a pronounced sedative effect, it may be advisable to avoid driving or operating potentially dangerous machinery while taking them. It is also important to be aware that they can increase the sedative effects of other drugs, such as alcohol and anti-anxiety drugs, that also have a depressant effect on the central nervous system.

People with a history of glaucoma or prostate trouble should seek medical advice before taking antihistamines because the anticholinergic action of these drugs may make such conditions worse. Antihistamines interact dangerously with monoamine oxidase inhibitors (MAOIs), a type of antidepressant drug, and should never be taken within 14 days of MAOI treatment.

ANTIHISTAMINES AND ALLERGIC RHINITIS

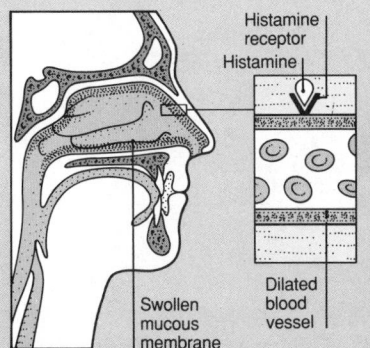

Histamine receptor
Histamine
Swollen mucous membrane
Dilated blood vessel

Before drug treatment
In allergic rhinitis, histamine released in response to an allergen acts on histamine receptors and produces dilation of the blood vessels supplying the lining of the nose, leading to swelling and increased mucus production. There is also irritation that causes sneezing, and often redness and watering of the eyes.

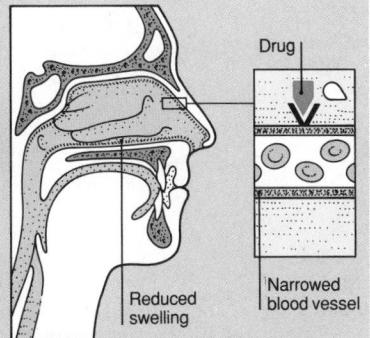

Drug
Reduced swelling
Narrowed blood vessel

After drug treatment
Antihistamine drugs prevent histamine from attaching to histamine receptors, thereby preventing the body from responding to allergens. Over a period of time, the blood vessels in the lining of the nose become narrower, and swelling, irritation, and watery discharge are reduced.

COMMON DRUGS

Azatadine
Brompheniramine
Chlorpheniramine
Dimenhydrinate
Diphenhydramine
Hydroxyzine
Meclizine

Promethazine
Terfenadine
Trimeprazine
Triprolidine

INFECTIONS AND INFESTATIONS

The human body is a suitable environment for many types of microorganism, including bacteria, viruses, fungi, yeasts, and protozoa. It may also become the host for animal parasites such as insects, worms, and flukes.

Microorganisms (microbes) exist all around us and can be transmitted from person to person in many ways: direct contact, inhalation of infected air, and consumption of contaminated food or water (see Transmission of infection, facing page). Not all microorganisms cause disease; many types of bacteria exist on the skin surface or in the bowel without causing ill effects, while others cannot live either in or on the body.

Normally the immune system protects the body from infection. Invading microbes are killed before they can multiply in sufficient numbers to produce the symptoms of disease. (See also Malignant and immune disease, p.180.)

What can go wrong

Infectious diseases occur when the body is invaded by microbes against which its natural defenses are ineffective. This may be because the body has little or no natural immunity to the infection in question, or because the number of invading microbes is too great for the immune system to overcome. Serious infections can occur when the immune system does not function properly or when a disease weakens or destroys the immune system. That is what happens in AIDS (acquired immune deficiency syndrome).

Infections can be generalized (such as flu-like viruses and childhood infectious diseases) or they may affect one part of the body (as in wound infections). Some parts of the body are more susceptible to infection than others: respiratory tract infections are relatively common, whereas infections of the bones and muscles are rare.

Symptoms and consequences depend on the infecting organism and the parts of the body affected. Some are the result of damage to body tissues by the infection, others may be caused by *toxins* released by the microbes. In many cases, symptoms are the result of the activity of the body's immune system.

Most bacterial and viral infections cause fever. Bacterial infections may also cause inflammation and pus formation in the affected area.

Why drugs are used

Antibacterial and antibiotic drugs are frequently used to treat bacterial infections. They either kill the bacteria or prevent them from multiplying.

Types of infecting organisms

Bacteria

A typical bacterium (right) consists of a single cell with a protective wall. Some bacteria are aerobic – that is, they require oxygen – and therefore are more likely to infect surface areas such as the skin or respiratory tract. Others are anaerobic and multiply in oxygen-free surroundings such as the bowel or deep puncture wounds.

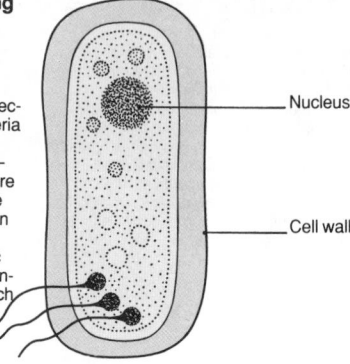

Nucleus

Cell wall

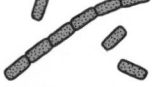

Cocci (spherical)
Streptococcus (above) can cause sore throats and pneumonia.

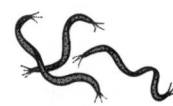

Bacilli (rod-shaped)
Mycobacterium tuberculosis (illustrated above) causes tuberculosis.

Spirochete (spiral-shaped) This group includes those bacteria that cause syphilis and infections of the gums.

Viruses

The smallest known infectious agents, viruses consist simply of a core of genetic material (RNA or DNA) surrounded by a protein coat. A virus can multiply only in a living cell, using the host tissue's replicating enzymes.

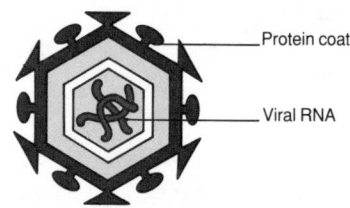

Protein coat

Viral RNA

Protozoa

These single-celled parasites are slightly bigger than bacteria. Many live in the human intestine and are harmless. However, some types cause malaria, sleeping sickness, and dysentery.

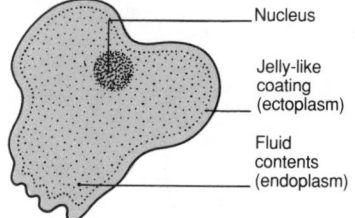

Nucleus

Jelly-like coating (ectoplasm)

Fluid contents (endoplasm)

Treatment is necessary because the appearance of symptoms shows that the immune system has failed to overcome the infection. Many antibiotics can be used for a broad range of applications, while others have a specific effect against particular types of bacteria.

Antiviral drugs are usually less effective than those used for bacterial infection. They are principally used in *topical* preparations for the treatment of viral infections of the skin and eyes.

How bacteria affect the body

Bacteria can cause symptoms of disease in two principal ways: first, by releasing toxins that harm body cells; second, by provoking immune system activity that leads to inflammation.

Effects of toxins

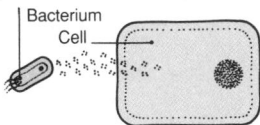
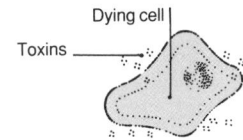

The invading bacterium gives off poisons (toxins) which attack the body cell.

The toxins emanating from the bacterium break through the cell structure and destroy the cell.

Immune system reactions

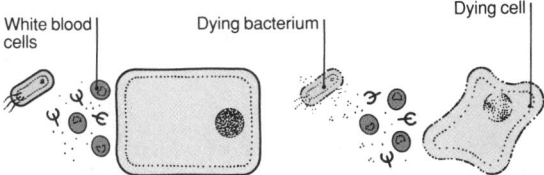

White blood cells of the immune system attack the bacterium directly by releasing inflammatory substances and, later, antibodies.

A side effect of this attack of the immune system on the bacterium is damage and inflammation to the body's own cells.

Transmission of infection

Infecting organisms can enter the human body through a variety of routes, including direct contact between an infected person and another, and eating or breathing in infected material.

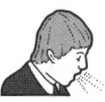
Droplet infection
Coughing and sneezing spread infected secretions.

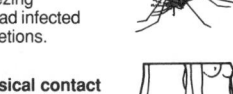
Insects
Insect bites may transmit infection.

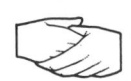
Physical contact
Everyday contact may spread infection.

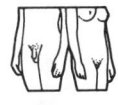
Sexual contact
Certain infections and infestations may be spread by genital contact.

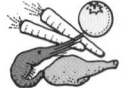
Food
Many infecting organisms can be ingested in food.

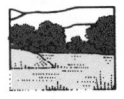
Water
Infections can be spread in polluted water.

Luckily, many viral infections are overcome by the body's natural resistance mechanisms.

Other groups of drugs used in the fight against infection include antiprotozoal drugs (including antimalarials) used for protozoal infections, antifungal drugs used for infection by fungi and yeasts, and anthelmintic drugs that eradicate worm and fluke infestation. Infestation by skin parasites is usually treated with topical application of insecticides (see p.204).

INFESTATIONS

Invasion by parasites that live on the body (such as lice) or in the body (such as tapeworm) is known as infestation. Because the body does not have strong natural defenses against infestation, antiparasitic treatment is necessary. Infestations are associated with tropical climates and poor standards of hygiene.

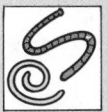
Tapeworms and roundworms live in the intestines and may cause diarrhea and anemia. Roundworm eggs may be passed in feces. Larvae in infected soil penetrate the skin and grow into hookworms. Other worm infestations enter the body via undercooked meat.

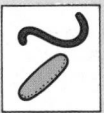
Flukes are of various types. The liver fluke (acquired from infected vegetation) lives in the bile duct in the liver and can lead to jaundice. Another more serious type (which lives in small blood vessels supplying the bladder or intestines) causes schistosomiasis, and is acquired from swimming in infected water.

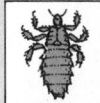
Lice and scabies spread by direct contact. Head, body, and crab lice need human blood to survive, and die away from the body. The dried feces of lice spread typhus by being inhaled or infecting wounds. Scabies (caused by a tiny mite which does not carry disease) makes small, itchy tunnels in the skin.

Life cycle of a worm

Many worms have a complex life cycle. The life cycle of the worm that causes the group of diseases known as filariasis is illustrated below.

A mosquito ingests the filarial larvae and bites a human, thereby transmitting the larvae.

The mature larvae enter the lymph glands and vessels and reproduce there, often causing no ill effects.

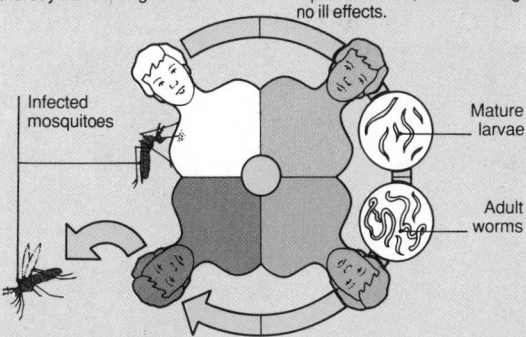

Infected mosquitoes

Mature larvae

Adult worms

The infestation is spread by mosquitoes biting infected people and restarting the cycle.

The larvae grow into adult worms. The severity of the infestation depends on the number of these in the body.

MAJOR DRUG GROUPS

Antibiotics
Antibacterial drugs
Antituberculous drugs
Antiviral drugs
Vaccines and immunization

Antiprotozoal drugs
Antimalarial drugs
Antifungal drugs
Anthelmintic drugs

ANTIBIOTICS

Of the billion or more prescriptions that United States physicians write each year, some 15 percent call for the use of antibiotics. Usually safe and effective in the treatment of bacterial disorders – ranging from minor infections like conjunctivitis to life-threatening diseases like pneumonia, meningitis, and septicemia – the antibiotics have played a major role in broadening the horizons of modern medicine. Similar in function to the antibacterial drugs (see p.159), the antibiotics have a botanical origin in molds and fungi, although they are now largely synthesized.

Many different classes of antibiotics have been developed since 1941, when the first antibiotic – penicillin – was introduced. Each has a different chemical composition and is effective against a particular range of bacteria. None is effective against viral infections (see Antiviral drugs p.161). Some have a broad spectrum of activity against a wide variety of bacteria. Others are used in the treatment of infection by only a few specific organisms. For a description of each class of antibiotic, see the box on page 158.

Why they are used

A human being lives surrounded by bacteria – in the air he or she breathes, in the mucous membranes of the mouth and nose, on the skin, in the intestines. But we are protected, most of the time,

ANTIBIOTIC RESISTANCE

The increasing use of antibiotics in the treatment of infection over the past half century has led to the development of resistance in certain types of bacteria to the effects of particular antibiotics. This resistance to the drug usually occurs when bacteria develop mechanisms of growth and reproduction that are not disrupted by the effects of the antibiotics. In other cases, bacteria produce *enzymes* that neutralize the antibiotics.

Antibiotic resistance may develop in an individual during prolonged treatment when a drug has failed to eliminate the infection

quickly, sometimes because the drug was not taken regularly. The resistant strain of bacteria is able to multiply, thereby prolonging the illness. It may also infect other people, causing the spread of resistant infection within a community.

Physicians try to prevent the development of antibiotic resistance by selecting the drug most likely to eliminate the bacteria present in each individual case as quickly and as thoroughly as possible. Failure to complete a course of antibiotics as prescribed by your physician increases the likelihood that the infection will recur in a resistant form.

by our immunological defenses. When these break down, when bacteria already present migrate to a vulnerable new site, or when harmful bacteria not usually present invade the body, infectious disease sets in.

The bacteria multiply uncontrollably, destroying tissue, releasing toxins, and in some cases threatening to spread via the bloodstream to such vital organs as the heart, brain, lungs, and kidneys. The symptoms of infectious disease, although they almost always include fever, vary widely, depending on the site of the infection and the type of bacteria.

Confronted with a sick person and suspecting a bacterial infection, the physician has an array of infection-destroying drugs that he can prescribe.

Ideally, he should identify the organism causing the disease before prescribing any of them. But tests to analyze the blood, sputum, urine, stool, or pus usually take 24 hours or more. In the meantime, especially if the person is in discomfort or pain, the physician makes a preliminary drug choice, something of an educated guess. In starting this empiric treatment, as it is called, the physician is guided by the site of the infection, the severity of the symptoms, the likely source of infection, and the prevalence of similar illnesses in the community at that time.

In such circumstances, pending laboratory identification of the trouble-making bacteria, the physician may initially prescribe a broad-spectrum antibiotic – one effective against a wide variety of bacteria. As soon as tests provide more exact information, the physician may then switch to an antibiotic that is the recommended treatment for the identified bacteria. Sometimes more than one antibiotic is prescribed to be sure of eliminating all strains of bacteria.

In most cases, antibiotics can be given by mouth. However, in serious infections when high blood levels of the drug are needed rapidly, or when a type of antibiotic is needed that cannot be given by mouth, the drug may be given by injection. Antibiotics are also included in *topical* preparations for localized skin, eye, and ear infections (see also Anti-infective skin preparations, p.203, and Drugs for ear disorders, p.199).

How they work

Depending on the type of drug and the dosage, antibiotics are either bactericidal, killing organisms directly, or bacteriostatic, halting the multiplication of bacteria and enabling the body's natural defenses to overcome the remaining infection.

There are two main mechanisms of action: penicillins and cephalosporins destroy bacteria by preventing them

ACTION OF ANTIBIOTICS

Penicillins and cephalosporins
Drugs from these groups are bactericidal, that is, they kill bacteria. They interfere with the chemicals that bacteria need to form normal cell walls (right). As the cell swells, its outer lining disintegrates and the bacterium dies (far right).

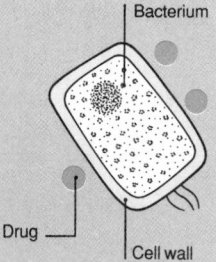
Bacterium

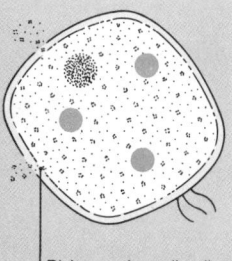

Drug

Cell wall | Disintegrating cell wall

Other antibiotics
These alter chemical activity inside the bacteria, thereby preventing the production of proteins that the bacteria need in order to multiply and survive (right). This may have a lethal effect in itself, or it may prevent reproduction (bacteriostatic action) (far right).

Drug

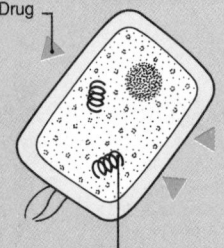

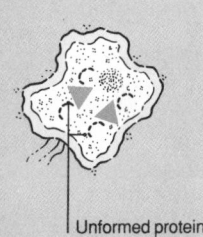

Protein | Unformed protein

THE USES OF ANTIBIOTICS

The table below shows which common drugs in each class of antibiotic are used for the treatment of infections in different parts of the body. For the purposes of comparison, the table also includes at the bottom some of the antibacterial drugs discussed on p.159.

This is not intended to be used as a guide to prescribing, but broadly to indicate the range of applications of each drug.

Some drugs have a wide range of theoretical applications, but this table concentrates on the most common uses of each drug. Selection of

the most suitable antibiotic for any individual is determined by the physician's assessment of the condition, the medical history of the person concerned, and also by the results of laboratory findings (see Why they are used, facing page).

Antibiotic — Site of infection	Ear, nose, throat, and mouth	Respiratory tract	Skin and soft tissue	Gastrointestinal tract	Eye	Kidney and urinary tract	Brain and nervous system	Heart	Bones and joints	Genital tract
Penicillins										
Amoxicillin	●	●		●		●		●	●	●
Ampicillin	●	●		●		●	●	●	●	●
Cloxacillin		●	●						●	
Penicillin G	●	●	●			●	●	●	●	●
Penicillin V	●	●	●							
Cephalosporins										
Cefaclor	●	●				●				
Cefazolin		●	●			●		●	●	
Cefoperazone		●	●	●		●			●	●
Cefoxitin		●	●	●		●				●
Cephalexin		●	●			●				
Cephalothin		●	●			●		●	●	
Aminoglycosides										
Gentamicin		●	●	●	●	●	●	●	●	
Neomycin			●	●						
Netilmicin		●	●	●		●	●		●	
Streptomycin		●						●		
Tobramycin		●	●	●		●	●		●	
Tetracyclines										
Doxycycline	●	●		●		●				●
Oxytetracycline	●	●								
Tetracycline	●	●			●	●				●
Sulfonamides										
Sulfacetamide					●					
Sulfamethoxazole						●				
Sulfisoxazole	●	●				●				
Lincosamides										
Clindamycin		●	●	●					●	
Lincomycin		●	●						●	
Other drugs										
Bacitracin			●							
Chloramphenicol	●			●	●		●			
Colistin		●				●				
Dapsone			●							
Erythromycin	●	●	●		●				●	●
Gramicidin					●					
Metronidazole	●		●	●			●	●	●	●
Nalidixic acid						●				
Nitrofurantoin						●				
Trimethoprim						●				
Trimethoprim/sulfamethoxazole	●	●		●		●				

ANTIBIOTICS continued

from making normal cell walls; most other antibiotics act inside the bacteria, interfering with the chemical activities essential to their life cycle.

How they affect you

Antibiotics stop most common types of infection within days. Because they do not relieve symptoms directly, your physician may advise additional medication such as analgesics (see p.108) to relieve pain and fever until the antibiotics start to take effect. It is important to complete the course of medication as prescribed by your physician even if all symptoms seem to have disappeared. Failure to do this can lead to a resurgence of the infection in an antibiotic-resistant form (see Antibiotic resistance, p.156).

Most antibiotics used in the home do not cause side effects if taken in the recommended dosage. But digestive disturbances such as nausea and diarrhea are among the more common reactions. Some people may be sensitive to particular types of antibiotics, and this can lead to serious adverse reactions.

Risks and special precautions

Most antibiotics prescribed for short periods outside a hospital setting are safe for the majority of people. The most common risk, particularly with penicillins and cephalosporins, is a severe allergic reaction to the drug that can cause rashes and sometimes swelling of the face and throat. If this happens the drug should be stopped and immediate medical advice sought. A previous allergic reaction to an antibiotic means that all other drugs in that class and related classes should be avoided. It is therefore important to inform your physician if you have previously suffered an adverse reaction to an antibiotic treatment.

Another risk of antibiotic treatment, especially if it is prolonged, is that the balance among microorganisms that normally inhabit the body may be disturbed. In particular, antibiotics may destroy the bacteria that normally limit the growth of candida, a yeast that is often present in the body in small amounts. This can lead to overgrowth of candida (also known as thrush) in the mouth, vagina, or bowel. In such cases an antifungal drug (p.166) may need to be prescribed. A rarer, but more serious, consequence of disruption of normal bacterial activity in the body is a disorder called pseudomembranous colitis, in which bacteria that are resistant to the antibiotic multiply in the bowel, causing violent bloody diarrhea. Although this potentially fatal disorder can occur with any antibiotic, it is most common with the lincosamides.

Most antibiotics taken by mouth or injection are eliminated from the body by the kidneys via the urine. Therefore, like many drugs, they should be prescribed with caution for those people who have reduced kidney function (see also Kidney and liver disease, p.22). Less common risks associated with particular types of antibiotics are described under Classes of antibiotics, below.

COMMON DRUGS

Penicillins
Amoxicillin
Ampicillin
Cloxacillin
Penicillin G
Penicillin V

Cephalosporins
Cefaclor
Cefazolin
Cefoperazone
Cefoxitin
Cephalexin
Cephalothin

Aminoglycosides
Gentamicin
Neomycin
Netilmicin
Streptomycin
Tobramycin

Tetracyclines
Doxycycline
Oxytetracycline
Tetracycline

Macrolides
Erythromycin

Lincosamides
Clindamycin
Lincomycin

Other drugs
Bacitracin
Chloramphenicol
Colistin

CLASSES OF ANTIBIOTICS

Penicillins The first antibiotic drugs to be developed, penicillins are still widely used to treat many common infections. Some penicillins are not effective when they are taken by mouth and therefore have to be given by injection in the hospital. Unfortunately, certain strains of bacteria are resistant to penicillin treatment, and other drugs may have to be substituted. Penicillins may often cause allergic reactions.

Cephalosporins These are broad-spectrum antibiotics similar to the penicillins. They are often used when penicillin treatment has proved ineffective. Some cephalosporins can be given by mouth, but others are effective only when they are given by injection. Many people who are allergic to penicillins are also potentially allergic to cephalosporins. The most serious, although rare, adverse effect of a few cephalosporins is their occasional interference with normal blood clotting and consequent bleeding, especially in the elderly.

Macrolides Erythromycin is the only common drug in this group. It is a broad-spectrum antibiotic that is often prescribed as an alternative to penicillins or cephalo-sporin antibiotics. Erythromycin is also effective for some diseases, such as Legionnaires' disease (a rare type of pneumonia), that cannot be treated with other antibiotics. The main risk with erythromycin is that it can occasionally impair liver function.

Tetracyclines These have a broader spectrum of activity than any other class of antibiotic. However, increasing bacterial resistance to their effects (see Antibiotic resistance, p.156) has limited their use, although they remain widely prescribed. In addition to the treatment of infections, tetracyclines are also used in the long-term treatment of acne, although this application is probably not related to their antibacterial action. A major drawback to the use of tetracycline antibiotics in young children and in pregnant women is that they can discolor developing teeth.

With the exception of doxycycline, these drugs are poorly absorbed through the intestines, and when given by mouth they have to be administered in high doses in order to reach effective levels in the blood. Such high doses increase the likelihood of diarrhea as a side effect. The absorption of tetracyclines can be further reduced by interaction with calcium and other minerals. Drugs from this group therefore should not be taken with iron tablets or milk products. Tetracyclines deteriorate and may become poisonous with time. Leftover tablets or capsules should therefore always be discarded.

Aminoglycosides These potent drugs are effective against a broad range of bacteria, but they are not as widely used as some other antibiotics because when given by injection, they have potentially serious side effects. Aminoglycosides are also used in much smaller doses for eye and ear infections. They are often given in conjunction with other antibiotics.

Possible adverse effects include damage to the nerves in the ear, damage to the kidneys, and severe skin rashes.

Lincosamides These drugs are not commonly used because they are more likely to cause serious disruption of bacterial activity in the bowel than other antibiotics. They are mainly reserved for the treatment of bone, joint, and abdominal infections that do not respond well to safer antibiotics.

ANTIBACTERIAL DRUGS

This broad classification of drugs comprises agents that are similar to the antibiotics in function but dissimilar in origin, being chemical rather than botanical in their early development. First used to cure human disease in 1935, the early antibacterials (the so-called sulfa drugs) were derived from a deep red industrial dye called prontosil, metabolized by the body into sulfanilamide, the active antibacterial ingredient. The sulfa drugs quickly proved to be so effective against so many bacterial infections that the U.S. Army included a sulfanilamide in the small first-aid pouches that World War II infantrymen wore into combat.

Why they are used

Sulfonamides, the largest group of drugs within the antibacterial group, are today's successors to the original sulfa drugs. Because of the appearance of strains of bacteria resistant to their actions (see Antibiotic resistance, p.156), sulfonamides have in many cases been superseded by antibiotics that are more effective and safe. Yet there are many circumstances in which physicians believe the sulfonamides to be more effective than antibiotics.

Because they reach high concentrations in the urine, sulfonamides are particularly useful in treating many infections of the urinary tract. They are frequently used for chlamydial pneumonia and for some middle ear infections; sulfacetamide is often included in *topical* preparations for skin, eye, and outer-ear infections. Sulfamethoxazole, in combination with trimethoprim, is used for bladder infections, certain types of bronchitis, and some gastrointestinal infections.

DRUG TREATMENT FOR LEPROSY

Leprosy (also known as Hansen's disease) is a bacterial infection caused by an organism called *Mycobacterium leprae*. It is rare in the United States, but relatively common in parts of Africa, Asia, and Latin America.

The disease progresses slowly, first affecting the peripheral nerves and causing loss of sensation in the hands and feet. This leads to frequent unnoticed injuries and consequent scarring. Later, the nerves of the face may also be affected.

Treatment with dapsone, an antibacterial drug related to the sulfonamides, rapidly halts infectivity and eventually eradicates the disease (courses of treatment usually last about two years). However, because resistance to this drug is increasing, other drugs, such as the antituberculous drugs rifampin and ethionamide, may also be prescribed.

ACTION OF SULFONAMIDES

Before drug treatment
Folic acid, a chemical that is necessary for growth of bacteria, is produced within bacterial cells by the action of an *enzyme* on a chemical called para-aminobenzoic acid.

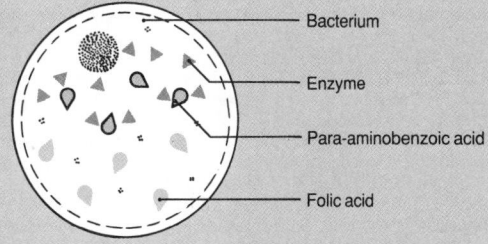

- Bacterium
- Enzyme
- Para-aminobenzoic acid
- Folic acid

After drug treatment
Sulfonamides interfere with the release of the enzyme. This prevents folic acid from being formed. The bacterium is therefore unable to function properly and dies.

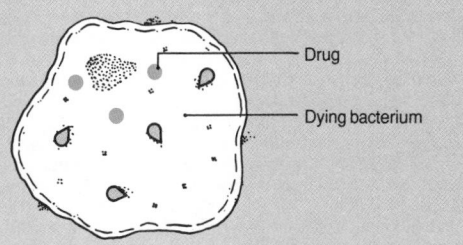

- Drug
- Dying bacterium

Not all antibacterials are sulfonamides, of course. The antibacterials used for tuberculosis are discussed on p.160. Other antibacterials are used against protozoal infections (see Antiprotozoal drugs, p.164). Others, sometimes classified as antimicrobials, include metronidazole, prescribed for a variety of genital infections, some serious infections in the abdomen, pelvic region, the heart, and central nervous system. Nalidixic acid and nitrofurantoin are effective as antiseptics for the urinary tract, and are used to cure or prevent recurrent infections.

How they work

Most antibacterials rid the body of bacteria by preventing the growth and multiplication of the organisms (see also Action of antibiotics, p.156, and Action of sulfonamides, above).

How they affect you

Antibacterials usually take several days to eliminate bacteria. During this time your physician may recommend additional medication to alleviate pain and fever. Sulfonamides can cause loss of appetite, rash, nausea, and drowsiness.

Risks and special precautions

Like antibiotics, most antibacterials can cause allergic reactions in susceptible people. Possible symptoms that should always be brought to your physician's attention include rashes and fever. If such a reaction occurs, a change to another drug is likely to be necessary.

Treatment with sulfonamides carries a number of serious but rare risks. Some drugs in this group can cause crystals to form in the kidneys, a risk that can be reduced by drinking adequate amounts of fluid during prolonged treatment. Because sulfonamides may also occasionally damage the liver, they are not usually prescribed for people with impaired liver function. There is also a slight risk of damage to bone marrow, lowering the production of white blood cells and increasing the chances of infection. Physicians therefore try to avoid prescribing sulfonamides for prolonged periods. Liver function and blood composition are often monitored during unavoidable long-term treatment.

COMMON DRUGS

Sulfonamides
Sulfacetamide
Sulfamethoxazole
Sulfisoxazole

Urinary antiseptics
Nalidixic acid
Nitrofurantoin

Other drugs
Dapsone
Metronidazole
Trimethoprim

ANTITUBERCULOUS DRUGS

Tuberculosis is a contagious bacterial disease acquired, often in childhood, by inhaling the tuberculosis bacilli (long, tube-shaped bacteria) present in the spray caused by a sneeze or cough from someone who is actively infected. Starting in a lung, tuberculosis takes one of two forms: primary infection or reactivation infection.

In 90 to 95 percent of those with primary infection, the body's immune system renders the bacilli quiescent. They remain alive, however, and they may spread via the lymphatic system and the bloodstream throughout the body (see Sites of infection, below).

Aside from some scarring and inflammation of the lungs, almost the only indication of infection is a reaction to an injection of tuberculin, a sterile extraction from the tuberculosis bacilli. When this is injected into or under the skin, only those people who have the latent primary infection show a reaction. Preventive measures are then undertaken (see box, right).

Reactivation tuberculosis (the gradual emergence of the destructive, progressive and sometimes fatal disease in adults) occurs in five to 10 percent of those with a primary infection. The cause is not known. A clinically identical form of the disease, called reinfection tuberculosis, occurs when someone with the dormant primary form of the disease is reinfected.

SITES OF INFECTION

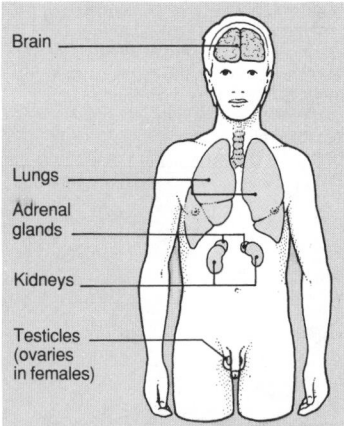

Brain

Lungs

Adrenal glands

Kidneys

Testicles (ovaries in females)

Tuberculosis usually affects only part of the lung at first. However, later outbreaks generally spread to both lungs and may also affect the kidneys, leading to pyelonephritis; the adrenal glands, causing Addison's disease; and the membranes surrounding the brain, which may lead to meningitis. The testicles (in men) and the ovaries (in women) may also be affected.

The symptoms of reactivation (or reinfection) tuberculosis can be deceiving, for the disease may start in any part of the body originally seeded with bacilli. The disease is most often first seen in the upper lobes of the lung, and it is often diagnosed after a chest X-ray. The early symptoms, which appear gradually, commonly include generally poor health, loss of appetite and weight, recurrent fever, and cough.

Why they are used

Left untreated, tuberculosis continues to destroy tissue, spreading and eventually causing death. As recently as 1940, it was the fourth-leading cause of death in the United States.

Like other antibacterial drugs, the antituberculous drugs can successfully eradicate the infection but they cannot, of course, restore destroyed tissue or the scarring that occurs as a result.

A person diagnosed as having tuberculosis is likely to be treated with two or more antituberculous drugs. This helps overcome the danger that the bacteria may develop resistance to one of the drugs (see Antibiotic resistance, p.156).

The drugs that are most likely to be prescribed first are rifampin and isoniazid, but the choice of drug is determined by the areas of the body that are affected, and by the results of sensitivity tests. These tests may take up to two months to confirm whether the infection is sensitive or resistant to the drugs initially used. If the infection is found to be resistant, the initial treatment fails, or serious adverse effects are experienced, the treatment may be changed.

Drug treatment usually continues until the symptoms have subsided and laboratory investigations, such as sputum tests, have shown the person to be clear of infection for one year. Short courses of nine months are sometimes given for otherwise healthy people with uncomplicated disease, but one-year courses of treatment are required for those who have reduced resistance to infection, diabetes, or silicosis.

How they work

Antituberculous drugs act in the same way as antibiotics, either by directly killing the bacteria or by preventing them from multiplying (see Action of antibiotics, p.156).

How they affect you

Although the drugs start to combat the disease within days, benefits of drug treatment are not likely to be noticeable for a few weeks. As the infection is gradually eradicated, the body's healing processes repair the damage caused by the disease. Symptoms such as fever

TUBERCULOSIS PREVENTION

There are two circumstances under which preventive measures are usually undertaken. Uninfected people who are regularly exposed to someone with active pulmonary tuberculosis are at risk, and are given a year-long course of isoniazid and, except in children, pyridoxine. However, if the contact with the infected person ceases within that period, the therapy is stopped, provided that tests are negative.

People with a primary tuberculosis infection are treated with the same drugs for a year or more. The preventive therapy is especially important for those taking certain drugs (especially corticosteroids or immunosuppressants) or those with other serious medical conditions (diabetes, leukemia, Hodgkin's disease, silicosis). A vaccine called BCG (Bacille Calmette-Guerin) is sometimes given to people who are not infected but who are exposed frequently. However, many US physicians are unconvinced of its effectiveness.

and coughing gradually subside, and weight is gained as appetite and general health improve.

Risks and special precautions

Some antituberculous drugs may cause adverse effects (nausea, vomiting, and abdominal pain), and they occasionally lead to serious allergic reactions. These are most likely to occur during the second month of treatment and may parallel the symptoms of the disease itself – fever and general ill health, for instance. When this happens, another drug is substituted.

Some drugs may affect liver function (rifampin and isoniazid); others may adversely affect the nerves (isoniazid). Ethambutol can cause changes in vision, and for this reason is not generally prescribed for young children because they are unable to report the warning symptoms. Other drugs can cause pyridoxine deficiency, and this vitamin is usually given with the drug.

Because the occurrence of adverse effects is usually related to levels of the drug in the bloodstream, dosage is carefully monitored. Special care is needed for children, the elderly, and those with reduced kidney function.

COMMON DRUGS

Aminosalicylic acid
Ethambutol
Isoniazid
Pyrazinamide
Rifampin
Streptomycin

ANTIVIRAL DRUGS

A simpler and smaller organism than the bacterium, the virus is less able to sustain itself. It can survive and multiply only by penetrating body cells (see box, right). Because the virus performs so few functions independently, medicines that disrupt or halt its life cycle without harming human cells have been difficult to develop.

There are many different types of viruses, and viral infections cause illnesses with various symptoms and degrees of severity. Common viral illnesses include the cold, influenza and flu-like illnesses, and the usual child-hood diseases such as mumps and chicken pox. Throat infections, acute bronchitis, pneumonia, gastroenteritis, and meningitis are often, but not always, caused by a virus.

Fortunately, the body's natural defenses are usually strong enough to overcome infections such as these, with drugs given to ease pain and lower fever. However, the more serious viral diseases, such as pneumonia and meningitis, require close medical supervision.

Another difficulty with viral infections is the speed with which the virus multiplies. By the time symptoms appear, the viruses are so numerous that drugs may have little effect. Antiviral agents should be given early in the course of an infection or they may be used prophylactically, i.e., as a preventive. Some viral infections can be prevented by vaccination (see p.162).

In recent years, a few drugs have been introduced that have a partial effect against certain specific viruses.

Why they are used

Antiviral drugs are useful in the treatment of herpes virus infections. Some drugs are applied *topically* to treat herpes eye infections; topical acyclovir may be used to treat the first outbreak of genital herpes. An oral form of this drug is more effective for genital herpes. Acyclovir also can be given by injection, and sometimes by mouth, to treat or prevent severe herpes infections (e.g., cold sores, chicken pox, shingles) in people who have a weakened immune system. Although antiviral drugs can re-duce the severity and duration of herpes virus infections, they do not perma-nently eliminate the virus from the body.

Another antiviral agent is amantadine, which is used to prevent, and in some people to treat, symptoms caused by the influenza A virus. This drug is also used to treat parkinsonism.

AIDS (acquired immune deficiency syndrome) is a viral infection that reduces the body's resistance to infection by other viruses, bacteria, and protozoa, as well as some types of

ACTION OF ANTIVIRAL DRUGS

In order to reproduce, a virus requires a living cell. The invaded cell eventually dies and the new viruses are released, spreading and infecting other cells. Many antiviral drugs act to prevent the virus from replicating its genetic material, DNA. Thus, the virus cannot multiply. Unable to divide, the virus dies and the spread of infection is halted.

Before drug

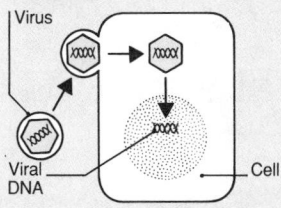
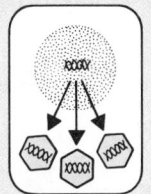
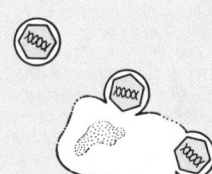

Virus attaches to and penetrates body cell and viral DNA is uncoated.

Viral DNA is replicated in order to produce new viruses.

Cell dies and new viruses are released.

After drug

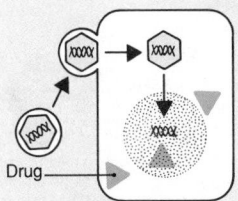
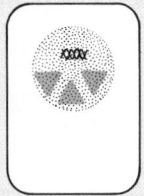

Virus enters cell that has absorbed antiviral drug.

Drug prevents viral DNA replication and new viruses are not produced.

Virus dies and spread of infection is halted.

cancer. Some antiviral drugs may be effective in limiting the progress of this disease. Drug treatment for AIDS is discussed more fully on p.185.

How they work

Many antiviral drugs, such as acyclovir, idoxuridine, trifluridine, and vidarabine act by preventing the formation of viral genetic material (i.e., they inhibit viral DNA replication). Thus, the virus cannot multiply. Halting multiplication of the virus prevents its spread to uninfected cells and improves symptoms rapidly, but in the case of herpes infections, does not completely eradicate the virus from the body. Infection may therefore flare up again on another occasion.

Other antiviral agents have different actions. Amantadine appears to prevent the influenza A virus from entering the host's cells. This drug is most effective when given before the infection has spread widely.

How they affect you

With early treatment, an outbreak of genital herpes can be cut short by taking acyclovir by mouth. Taking oral acyclovir for several months can

prevent or reduce the frequency and/or severity of recurrences. However, active infections will reappear once the drug is stopped. Side effects of oral acyclovir are nausea and headache.

Risks and special precautions

Because some antiviral drugs are removed from the body by the kidneys, they are prescribed with caution for people with reduced kidney function. Some antiviral drugs can adversely affect the activity of normal body cells, particularly those in the bone marrow. Idoxuridine is for this reason available only for topical application.

COMMON DRUGS

Acyclovir
Amantadine
Idoxuridine
Ribavirin
Trifluridine
Vidarabine

VACCINES AND IMMUNIZATION

Many infectious diseases, including most of the common viral infections, occur only once during a person's lifetime. The reason for this is that the antibodies produced in response to the disease remain afterwards, prepared to repel any future invasion as soon as the first infectious germs appear. The duration of such natural immunity varies, but it can last a lifetime.

Protection against many infections can now be provided artificially by the use of vaccines derived from altered forms of the infecting organism. These vaccines stimulate the immune system in the same way as a genuine infection, and provide lasting, active immunity. Because each type of microbe stimulates the production of a specific type of antibody, a different vaccine must be given for each disease.

Another type of immunization, called passive immunization, relies on the introduction of antibodies from someone who has recovered from a particular infectious disease. The transfer is made by means of serum (a part of the blood) containing antibodies (see Immune globulins, below).

Why they are used

Some infectious diseases cannot be treated effectively or are potentially so serious that prevention is the best treatment. The aim of routine immunization is not only to protect the individual, but gradually to eradicate the disease completely, as has been achieved with smallpox. Most children between the ages of 3 months and 15 years are routinely vaccinated against the common childhood infectious diseases. Newborn babies receive antibodies for many diseases from their mothers, but this protection lasts only for about three months. In addition, travelers to many underdeveloped countries are often urged to be vaccinated against the diseases common in those regions.

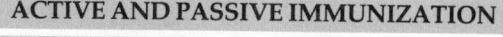

ACTIVE AND PASSIVE IMMUNIZATION

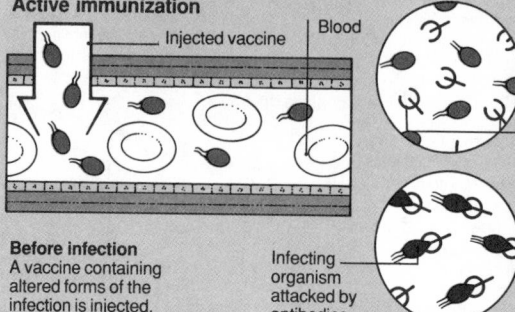

Active immunization

Injected vaccine

Blood

Before infection
A vaccine containing altered forms of the infection is injected.

Infecting organism attacked by antibodies

Antibody formation
The vaccine causes antibodies to form against the infection.

Antibodies

Immunity
Invasion of the body by a similar organism causes antibodies to form as a result of the vaccine and eliminate the infection.

Passive immunization

Injected antibodies

Infecting organisms

Infecting organism attacked by antibodies

After infection
Passive immunization is needed when the infection has entered the blood.

Immune globulin injection
A serum containing antibodies (immune globulin) extracted from donated blood is injected. This helps the body to fight the infection.

Effective lifelong immunization can sometimes be achieved by a single dose of the vaccine. However, in many cases reinforcing doses, commonly called booster shots, are needed later in order to maintain reliable immunity.

Vaccines do not provide immediate protection against infection, and it may be up to four weeks before full immunity develops. When immediate protection from a disease is needed – for example, following exposure to infection – it may be necessary to establish passive immunity with immune globulins.

How they work

Vaccines provoke the immune system into creating antibodies that help the body to resist specific infectious diseases. Many vaccines are made from artificially weakened forms of the disease-causing germ (live vaccine). But these weak germs are nevertheless effective in stimulating sufficient growth of antibodies. Other vaccines rely on inactive (or killed) disease-causing germs, or inactive derivatives. But their effect on the immune system remains the same. Effective antibodies are created; active immunity is established.

How they affect you

The degree of protection varies among different vaccines. Some provide reliable lifelong immunity; others may not give full protection against a disease, and the effects may last for as little as six months. Any vaccine may cause side effects, but when these occur they are usually mild and soon disappear. The most common reactions are a red, slightly raised tender area at the site of injection, and a slight fever or a flu-like illness lasting for one or two days.

Risks and special precautions

Serious reactions with vaccines are rare, and for most children the risk is far

IMMUNE GLOBULINS

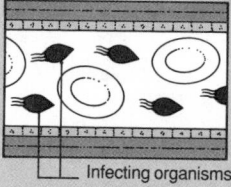

Antibodies, which can result from snake and insect venom as well as infectious disease, permeate the serum of the blood (the part remaining after the red cells and clotting agents are removed). The concentrated serum of people who have survived diseases or poisonous bites is called immune globulin, and given by injection, creates passive immunity. Immune globulin from blood donated by a wide cross section of donors is likely to contain antibodies to most common diseases. Specific immune globulins against rare diseases or toxins are derived from the blood of selected donors likely to have high levels of antibodies to that disease. These are called hyperimmune

globulins. Some immune globulins are extracted from horse blood.

Because immune globulins do not stimulate the body to produce its own antibodies, their effect is not long lasting and diminishes progressively over three or four weeks. Continued protection requires repeated injections.

Adverse effects from immune globulins are uncommon. Some people are sensitive to horse globulins, and about a week after the injection may experience a reaction known as serum sickness, with fever, rash, joint swelling, and pain. This usually ends in a few days, but should be reported to your physician before any further immunization.

outweighed by the value of the protection. Physicians have identified most of the riskiest conditions. Children who have had seizures or who have a family history of epilepsy may not be vaccinated against whooping cough or measles. Children who have an infectious illness will not be given routine vaccination until they have recovered.

Live vaccines should not be given during pregnancy, since they can affect the developing baby, nor should they be given to people whose immune systems are weakened by disease or drug treatment. It is also advisable for those taking corticosteroid drugs (p.169) to delay their vaccination until the end of drug treatment.

Controversy has arisen over the DPT (diphtheria-pertussis-tetanus) vaccination. The vaccine can cause convulsions in about 1 case in 300,000, involving an estimated 40 cases per year of brain damage. However, if no pertussis vaccine were used, it is estimated that 8,000 childhood deaths from pertussis would occur each year.

COMMON VACCINATIONS

Disease	Age	How given	General information
Diphtheria	2 months, 4 months, 6 months, 18 months, 4 – 6 years	Injection	Usually given routinely in infancy as a combined injection with tetanus and whooping cough vaccines. Immunity may diminish in later life.
Tetanus	2 months, 4 months, 6 months, 18 months, 4 – 6 years. Boosters every 5 years	Injection	Given routinely in infancy, this gives protection for 5 to 10 years. Injury likely to result in tetanus infection in a person who has not been vaccinated within the last five years is usually treated immediately with immune globulin (see p.162), and at the same time the physician may start a course of booster injections of the active vaccine. Tetanus boosters in adulthood should not be given within five years of the previous booster; otherwise a hypersensitivity reaction may occur.
Whooping cough (pertussis)	2 months, 4 months, 6 months, 18 months, 4 – 6 years	Injection	The pertussis vaccine may not give complete protection against whooping cough, but reduces the severity of symptoms that may develop following infection. Pertussis vaccine may cause mild fever, irritability, and, rarely, seizures. Children known to be at special risk from seizures – for example, those with a family history of epilepsy – are not usually given this vaccine.
Polio	2 months, 4 months, 18 months, 4 – 6 years. Boosters during adulthood as directed	By mouth	Many physicians recommend a booster every ten years, especially for people likely to be traveling to countries where polio is still prevalent.
Rubella (German measles)	15 months	Injection	Given as a combined injection with measles and mumps vaccine in infancy, immunization against this disease is important because it can damage the developing baby if it affects a woman in early pregnancy. Women of childbearing age who have received the vaccine should be careful to avoid becoming pregnant for at least three months following the injection.
Measles	15 months	Injection	Given together with mumps and rubella vaccine in infancy. It may cause a brief fever or rash, and there is a possibility of seizures. Measles vaccine does not always provide complete protection against the disease, but it does reduce the severity of illness.
Mumps	15 months	Injection	Given in infancy together with measles and rubella vaccines.
Influenza	People of any age who are at risk	Injection	It is impossible to confer long-term immunity against all forms of this disease, but protection against some types may be given to people especially at risk from complications. Protection develops within four weeks and side effects are rare. Annual booster vaccinations may be needed.

ANTIPROTOZOAL DRUGS

Protozoa, single-celled organisms that are often present in soil and may infect animals, can be transmitted to or between humans through contaminated food or water, sexual contact, or bites from insects. There are many types of protozoal infections, each causing a different disease, depending on the organism involved. Trichomoniasis, giardiasis, and pneumocystis pneumonia are probably the most common protozoal infections in the United States. The rarer infections are usually contracted as a result of exposure to infection in another part of the world.

Many types of protozoa infect the bowel, causing diarrhea and generalized symptoms of ill health. Others may infect the genital tract or skin. Some

may penetrate vital organs such as the lungs, brain, and liver. Prompt diagnosis and treatment are important in order to limit the spread of the infection within the body and, in some cases, to others. In many cases, increased attention to hygiene is an important factor in controlling the spread of the disease.

A variety of drugs is used in the treatment of these diseases. Some, such as metronidazole and tetracycline, are also commonly used for their antibacterial action. Others, such as iodoquinol, are rarely used except in specific protozoal infections.

How they affect you
Protozoa are often difficult to eradicate from within the body. Drug treatment

may therefore need to be continued for months in order to eliminate the infecting organisms completely, and thus prevent recurrence of the disease. In addition, unpleasant side effects such as nausea, diarrhea, and abdominal cramps are often unavoidable because of the limited choice of drugs and the need to maintain dosage levels that will effectively cure the disease. For detailed information on the risks and adverse effects of individual anti-protozoal drugs, consult the appropriate drug profile in Part 4.

The table below describes the principal protozoal infections and the drugs used in their treatment. Malaria, probably the most common protozoal disease worldwide, is discussed on the facing page.

SUMMARY OF PROTOZOAL DISEASES

Disease	Protozoa	Description	Drugs
Amebiasis (amebic dysentery)	Entamoeba histolytica	Infection of the bowel by an organism called Entamoeba histolytica. Usually transmitted in contaminated food or water. Major symptom is violent, sometimes bloody diarrhea.	Iodoquinol Metronidazole Chloroquine
Balantidiasis	Balantidium coli	Infection of the bowel by Balantidium coli, usually transmitted through contact with infected pigs. Possible symptoms include diarrhea and abdominal pain.	Tetracycline
Dientamebiasis	Dientamoeba fragilis	A form of amebic dysentery caused by Dientamoeba fragilis, possibly transmitted in the pinworm egg. Causes diarrhea and flu-like symptoms.	Tetracycline Iodoquinol
Giardiasis (lambliasis)	Giardia lamblia	Infection of the bowel by Giardia lamblia, usually transmitted in contaminated food or water, but may also be spread by some types of sexual contact. Major symptoms are general ill health, diarrhea, flatulence, and abdominal pain.	Metronidazole Quinacrine Furazolidone
Leishmaniasis	Leishmania	A mainly tropical and subtropical disease caused by organisms (Leishmania) spread by sand flies. It affects the mucous membranes of the mouth, nose, and throat, and may in its severe form invade organs such as the liver.	Antimony-based agents (stibogluconate) Amphotericin B
Pneumocystis pneumonia	Pneumocystis carinii	Potentially fatal lung infection caused by Pneumocystis carinii. It usually affects only those with reduced resistance to infection, such as AIDS victims. Symptoms include cough, breathlessness, fever, and chest pain.	Trimethoprim/ sulfamethoxazole Pentamidine Difluoromethylornithine (investigational drug)
Toxoplasmosis	Toxoplasma gondii	Infection by Toxoplasma gondii usually spread via contact with cat feces or by eating undercooked meat. It may also be transmitted from mother to baby during pregnancy. May be symptomless, but sometimes causes generalized ill health and low fever, and may affect vision.	Pyrimethamine/ sulfadiazine
Trichomoniasis	Trichomonas vaginalis	Infection by Trichomonas vaginalis most commonly affects the vagina, causing irritation and an offensive discharge. In men infection may occur in the urethra. The disease is usually sexually transmitted.	Metronidazole
Trypanosomiasis	Trypanosoma	African trypanosomiasis (sleeping sickness) is spread by the tsetse fly and causes fever, swollen glands, and drowsiness. South American trypanosomiasis (Chagas' disease) is spread by cone-nosed bugs. It causes inflammation, enlargement of internal organs, and infection of the brain.	Pentamidine, suramin, melarsoprol, nifurtimox, difluoromethylornithine (sleeping sickness), Primaquine (Chagas' disease)

ANTIMALARIAL DRUGS

Of all the infectious diseases that afflict mankind, the one that causes more illness and more deaths worldwide is malaria. Prevalent largely in the tropical zones (see map below), malaria usually strikes only those Americans who travel there or those who happen to receive a transfusion of malaria-infected blood.

Malaria is caused by single-cell protozoa whose life cycle is far from simple. A parasite, the malaria plasmodium, as it is called, lives in and depends on the female anopheles mosquito during one part of its life. It lives in and depends on human beings during other parts of its life cycle.

Transferred to man in the saliva of the mosquito as she penetrates ("bites") the skin, the malaria parasite enters the bloodstream and settles in the liver. Although no symptoms appear yet, the malaria parasite multiplies, asexually.

Following its stay in the liver, the parasite enters another phase of its life cycle, circulating in the bloodstream, penetrating and destroying red blood cells, and reproducing again, the results this time including male and female forms of the parasite. If the plasmodia then transfer back to a female anopheles mosquito via another "bite," they breed once more (bisexually), and are again ready to start a human infection.

It is after the emergence from the liver, when the plasmodia are entering and rupturing the red blood cells, that malaria appears in its classic, symptomatic form: high fever and profuse sweating, alternating with equally agonizing episodes of shivering and chills. One strain of malaria (there are four) produces a single severe attack, which can be fatal. The others cause recurrent attacks, sometimes extending over many years.

A number of drugs are available for malaria, the choice depending on many factors, such as the region in which the disease may have been contracted.

Why they are used

The medical response to malaria takes three forms: prevention, the treatment of symptomatic attacks, and the complete eradication of the plasmodia.

For someone planning a trip to an area where malaria is prevalent, drugs are given that destroy the parasites before they can reach the liver. Treatment begins the week before arrival in the malarial area and will continue for 4 to 8 weeks after return.

The same drugs are effective during the symptomatic period, relieving the episodes of fever and chills. However, these medicines do not destroy the plasmodia remaining in the liver. Future

malarial attacks are probable, sometimes occurring many years later.

To rid someone of the infection completely, a 14-day course of primaquine treatment is administered. Although highly effective in destroying the plasmodia in the liver, the drug is curiously weak against those in the cell-bursting stage. Primaquine treatment is recommended only after a person leaves the malarial area because of the high risk of recurrence. This treatment is advisable whether or not an individual has suffered attacks of malaria, because the infection can be present for several weeks without causing symptoms.

How they work

Most antimalarial drugs act by rapidly killing plasmodia in the bloodstream. Taken as a preventive, the drugs kill the plasmodia before they enter the liver, so stopping them from multiplying. Once the plasmodia have multiplied in the liver, the same drugs given in higher doses kill the parasites that re-enter the bloodstream. Only primaquine destroys the plasmodia in the liver, and it is thus the only drug effective as a radical cure.

How they affect you

The low doses of antimalarial drugs taken to prevent the disease rarely cause noticeable effects. Drugs taken for an attack usually begin to relieve symptoms within a few hours. Most of them can cause nausea, vomiting, and diarrhea. More seriously, quinine can produce giddiness, noises in the ear, and disturbances in vision and hearing.

Risks and special precautions

When drugs are given to prevent or cure malaria the full course of treatment must be taken. No drugs give long-term protection; new treatment is needed for each journey. Because no drug is effective against every type of malaria, a change of antimalarial drug may be necessary when traveling from one malarial area to another where a different form of malaria may be prevalent.

Though most of these drugs do not produce severe adverse effects, primaquine can cause the blood disorder hemolytic anemia, particularly in people with glucose-6-phosphate dehydrogenase (G6PD) deficiency. Blood tests are usually taken during treatment.

CHOICE OF DRUGS

The parts of the world in which malaria is prevalent (illustrated on the map right), and travel to which may make antimalarial drug treatment advisable, can be divided into two groups. Chloroquine is the drug of choice for the prevention of the disease in both groups, but drug treatment of symptomatic attacks may vary between the two groups. Primaquine is the most effective drug for complete cure of the disease. It is advisable to take specific medical advice before traveling to these areas. Pregnant women may need alternative drug treatment.

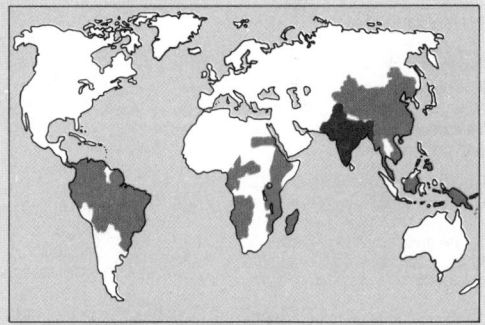

	Group 1 areas	Group 2 areas
	Central and Southern Africa, parts of Central and South America, China, Southeast Asia, and Oceania	Indian subcontinent (Bangladesh, India, Pakistan)

Drug selection	Prevention	Treatment
Group 1 areas	Chloroquine	Chloroquine, pyrimethamine/sulfadoxine, quinine (under medical supervision only)
Group 2 areas	Chloroquine	Pyrimethamine/sulfadoxine, quinine (under medical supervision only)

COMMON DRUGS

Chloroquine
Primaquine
Pyrimethamine
Quinine

ANTIFUNGAL DRUGS

We are continually exposed to fungi – in the air we breathe, the food we eat, and the water we drink. Fortunately, most of them cannot live in the body, and few are harmful. But some can grow in the mouth, skin, hair, or nails, causing irritating or unsightly changes, and a few can cause serious and possibly fatal disease. The most common fungal infections are caused by the tinea group of infections. These include tinea pedis (athlete's foot), tinea cruris (jock itch), and tinea capitis (scalp ringworm). They are caused by a variety of organisms and may be spread by direct or indirect contact with infected humans or animals. Infection is encouraged by warm, moist conditions.

Problems may also result from the proliferation of a fungus normally present in the body; the most common example is excessive growth of candida, a yeast which causes thrush infection of the mouth, vagina, and bowel. It can also infect other organs if it spreads through the body via the bloodstream. Overgrowth of candida may be provoked by antibiotics (p.156), diabetes, immune system disorders such as AIDS, pregnancy, or oral contraceptives (p.189).

Superficial fungal infections – those that attack only the outer layer of the skin and mucous membranes – are common and, although irritating, are not usually a threat to general health. Internal fungal infections – for example, of the lungs, heart, or other organs – are rare, but may be serious and prolonged.

Because antibiotics and other antibacterial drugs have no effect on fungi and yeasts, a different type of drug is needed. Drugs for fungal infections are either applied *topically* to treat minor infections of the skin and mucous membranes, or given by mouth or injection to eliminate serious fungal infections of the internal organs and nails.

Why they are used

Drug treatment is necessary for most fungal infections since they rarely improve alone. Measures such as careful washing and drying of affected areas may help, but are not a substitute for antifungal drugs. The use of over-the-counter preparations to increase the acidity of the vagina is not usually effective except when accompanied by drug treatment.

Fungal infections of the skin and scalp are usually treated with an antifungal cream. Drugs for vaginal thrush are most commonly applied in the form of vaginal suppositories or cream applied with a special applicator. Some preparations may be effective after a single dose; others require repeated applications. Mouth infections are usually eliminated by lozenges dissolved in the mouth or an antifungal solution applied directly to the affected areas. When candida infects the bowel, an antifungal drug that is not absorbed into the bloodstream, such as nystatin, is given in tablet form.

In the rare cases in which fungal infections affect internal organs, or when the nails are severely affected by persistent tinea infection, drugs such as griseofulvin and amphotericin B, which pass into the bloodstream, are given by mouth or injection.

How they work

Most of these drugs alter the permeability of the fungal cell's walls. The chemicals essential for cell life leak out and the cell dies.

ACTION OF ANTIFUNGAL DRUGS

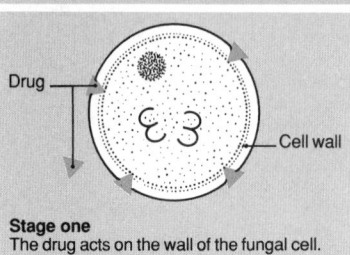

Stage one
The drug acts on the wall of the fungal cell.

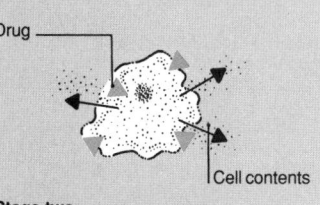

Stage two
The drug damages the cell wall and the cell contents leak out. The cell dies.

How they affect you

The speed with which antifungal drugs provide benefit varies with the type of infection. Thrush and most other fungal or yeast infections of the skin, mouth, and vagina improve within a week. The condition of nails affected by fungal infections improves only when new nail growth occurs, and this takes many months. *Systemic* infections of the internal organs can take weeks to cure.

Antifungal drugs applied topically rarely cause side effects, although they may irritate the skin. However, treatment by mouth or injection for systemic and nail infections may produce more serious side effects. Amphotericin B, injected in cases of life-threatening systemic infections, often causes unpleasant and potentially dangerous effects, notably a severe fever that may require other drugs. Because this drug may also cause kidney damage, sufferers need regular blood tests. Griseofulvin, given for persistent nail infections, carries a risk of liver damage. For this reason it is prescribed only when topical treatments have failed and nail damage is severe.

COMMON DRUGS

Amphotericin B	Ketoconazole
Ciclopirox	Miconazole
Clotrimazole	Nystatin
Econazole	Tolnaftate
Griseofulvin	

CHOICE OF ANTIFUNGAL DRUG

The table below shows the range of uses for each antifungal drug. The particular drug chosen in each case depends on the precise nature and site of the infection. The usual route of administration for each drug is also indicated.

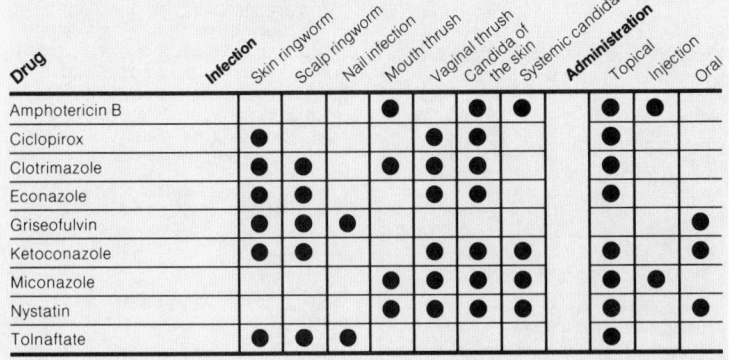

Drug	Infection							Administration		
	Skin ringworm	Scalp ringworm	Nail infection	Mouth thrush	Vaginal thrush	Candida of the skin	Systemic candida	Topical	Injection	Oral
Amphotericin B				●	●		●	●	●	
Ciclopirox	●				●	●		●		
Clotrimazole	●	●		●	●	●		●		
Econazole	●	●			●	●		●		
Griseofulvin	●	●	●							●
Ketoconazole	●	●			●	●		●		●
Miconazole			●	●	●	●		●	●	
Nystatin				●	●	●		●		●
Tolnaftate	●	●	●					●		

ANTHELMINTIC DRUGS

Anthelmintics are drugs that are used to eliminate the many types of worm (helminths) that can enter the body and live there as parasites, producing a general weakness in some cases and serious harm in others. The body may be host to many different worms (see Choice of drug, below). Most species spend part of their life cycle in another animal, and the infestation is often passed on to humans in food contaminated with the eggs or larvae. In some cases, such as hookworm, larvae enter the body through the skin. Larvae or adults may attach themselves to the intestinal wall and feed on the bowel contents; others feed off the intestinal blood supply, causing anemia. Worms can also infest the bloodstream or lodge in the muscles or organs.

Many people have worms at some time during their life, especially during childhood; most can be effectively eliminated with anthelmintic drugs.

Why they are used

Most worms common in the United States cause only mild symptoms and generally do not pose any threat to general health. Anthelmintic drugs are usually necessary, however, because the body's natural defenses against infection are not effective against most worm infestations. Certain types of worm infestation must always be treated since they can cause serious complications. Common roundworm (ascariasis) can block the intestine. In some cases, such as pinworm infestation, physicians may advise anthelmintic treatment for the whole family, to prevent reinfection. If worms that have invaded tissues have formed cysts, they may need to be removed surgically. Laxatives are given with some anthelmintics to hasten expulsion of worms from the bowel. Other drugs may be prescribed to ease symptoms or to compensate for any blood loss or nutritional deficiency.

How they work

The anthelmintic drugs act in several ways. Many of them kill or paralyze the worms, and they pass out of the body in the feces. Others, that act systemically, are used to treat infection in the tissues. Many anthelmintics are specific for particular worms, and the physician must identify the worm before selecting the most appropriate treatment (see Choice of drug). Most common infestations of the intestine are easily treated, often with only one or two doses of the drug. However, tissue infections may require more prolonged treatment.

How they affect you

Once the drug has eliminated the worms, symptoms caused by infestation rapidly disappear. Taken as a single dose, or a short course, anthelmintics do not usually produce side effects. However, treatment can disturb the digestive system, causing abdominal pain, nausea, and vomiting.

COMMON DRUGS

Mebendazole
Niclosamide
Praziquantel
Pyrantel
Thiabendazole

CHOICE OF DRUG

Pinworm (*enterobiasis*)
The most common worm infection in the United States. Commonly affects children. Eggs are usually swallowed in contaminated food or from sucking contaminated fingers or objects. Worms infect the intestines and lay eggs around the skin of the anus, often causing irritation.
Drugs Mebendazole, pyrantel

Common roundworm (*ascariasis*)
The most common worm infection worldwide – transmitted in contaminated raw food or in soil. Infects the intestine. The worms are large and can block the intestine.
Drugs Mebendazole, pyrantel

Threadworm (*strongyloidiasis*)
Mainly occurs in the southern United States and southern Europe. Larvae penetrate skin in contact with contaminated soil, pass into the lungs and later are swallowed into the digestive tract.
Drugs Thiabendazole

Whipworm (*trichuriasis*)
Mainly occurs in tropical areas as a result of eating contaminated raw vegetables. Worms infest the intestines.
Drugs Mebendazole

Hookworm (*uncinariasis*)
Mainly found in tropical areas. Worm larvae penetrate skin and pass via the lymphatic system and bloodstream to the lungs. They then travel up the airways, are swallowed and attach themselves to the intestinal wall.
Drugs Mebendazole, pyrantel

Pork roundworm (*trichinosis*)
Transmitted in infected undercooked pork. Initially worms lodge in the intestines, but larvae may invade muscle to form cysts that are often resistant to drug treatment.
Drugs Mebendazole, thiabendazole

Toxocariasis (*visceral larva migrans*)
Usually occurs as a result of eating soil contaminated by dog or cat feces. Eggs hatch in the intestine and may travel in the bloodstream to the lungs, liver, kidney, brain, and eyes.
Drugs Mebendazole, thiabendazole

Creeping eruption (*cutaneous larva migrans*)
Mainly occurs in tropical areas and coastal areas of southeastern United States as a result of skin contact with larvae from cat and dog feces. Infestation is usually confined to skin.
Drugs Thiabendazole

Filariasis (including onchocerciasis and loiasis)
Tropical areas only. Infection by this group of worms is spread by bites of insects that are carriers of worm larvae or eggs. May affect lymphatic system, blood, eyes, and skin.
Drugs Diethylcarbamazine

Flukes
Sheep liver fluke (fascioliasis) is indigenous to the United States. Infestation usually results from eating watercress grown in contaminated water. Mainly affects the liver and biliary tract. Other flukes found only abroad may infect the lungs, intestines, or blood.
Drugs Praziquantel

Tapeworms (including beef, pork, fish, and dwarf tapeworms)
Depending on type, may be carried by pigs, cattle, or fish and transmitted to humans in undercooked meat. Most types affect the intestines. Larvae of the pork tapeworm may form cysts in muscle and other tissues.
Drugs Niclosamide, praziquantel

Hydatid disease (*echinococciasis*)
Eggs are transmitted in dog feces. Larvae may form cysts over many years, commonly in the liver. Surgery is the usual treatment for cysts.
Drugs Mebendazole

HORMONES AND ENDOCRINE SYSTEM

The endocrine system is a collection of glands located throughout the body that produce *hormones* and release them into the bloodstream. Each endocrine gland produces one or more hormones, each of which governs a particular body function, including growth and repair of tissues, sexual development and reproductive function, and the body's response to stress.

Most hormones are released continuously from birth, but the amount produced fluctuates with the body's needs. Others are produced mainly at certain times: growth hormone is released principally during childhood and adolescence. Sex hormones are produced by the testicles and ovaries from puberty onward (see p.186).

Many endocrine glands release hormones in response to triggering hormones produced by the pituitary gland. The activity of the pituitary gland is partly controlled by the brain through the hypothalamus, which produces "releasing" hormones that stimulate the release of a particular pituitary hormone that in turn stimulates hormone production by the appropriate endocrine gland.

A "feedback" system usually regulates blood hormone levels: if the level rises too high the pituitary releases another hormone that inhibits endocrine gland activity.

What can go wrong

Endocrine disorders, usually resulting in too much or too little of a particular hormone, have a variety of causes. Some are congenital in origin; others may be caused by cancer, autoimmune disease (including some forms of diabetes mellitus), injury, and certain drugs.

Why drugs are used

Natural hormone preparations or their synthetic versions are often prescribed to treat deficiency. Sometimes drugs are given to stimulate increased hormone production in the endocrine gland, such as oral antidiabetic drugs. When too much hormone is produced, drug treatment may reduce the activity of the gland.

Hormones or related drugs are also used to treat other conditions. Corticosteroids are related to adrenal hormones, and are used to relieve inflammation and to suppress immune system activity (see p.184). Several types of cancer are treated with sex hormones (see p.182). Female sex hormones are given as contraceptives (see p.189) and to treat menstrual disorders (p.188).

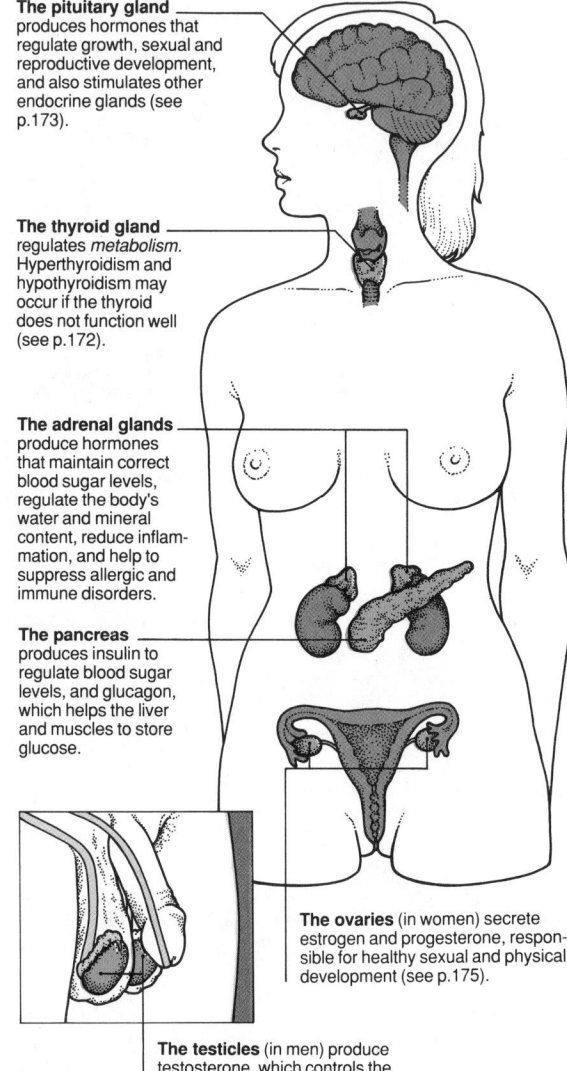

The pituitary gland produces hormones that regulate growth, sexual and reproductive development, and also stimulates other endocrine glands (see p.173).

The thyroid gland regulates *metabolism.* Hyperthyroidism and hypothyroidism may occur if the thyroid does not function well (see p.172).

The adrenal glands produce hormones that maintain correct blood sugar levels, regulate the body's water and mineral content, reduce inflammation, and help to suppress allergic and immune disorders.

The pancreas produces insulin to regulate blood sugar levels, and glucagon, which helps the liver and muscles to store glucose.

The ovaries (in women) secrete estrogen and progesterone, responsible for healthy sexual and physical development (see p.175).

The testicles (in men) produce testosterone, which controls the development of male sexual and physical characteristics (see p.174).

MAJOR DRUG GROUPS

Corticosteroids
Drugs used in diabetes
Drugs for thyroid disorders
Drugs for pituitary disorders
Male sex hormones
Female sex hormones

CORTICOSTEROIDS

The adrenal glands, atop each kidney, produce *hormones* that regulate a variety of body functions. One important group of hormones produced in the outer part of each adrenal gland (cortex) is the corticosteroids. Release of these hormones is governed by the pituitary gland (see p.173). Corticosteroids have two types of effect: glucocorticoid and mineralocorticoid. The glucocorticoid effects include the maintenance of normal levels of sugar in the blood and the promotion of recovery from injury and stress. The main mineralocorticoid effect is the regulation of the balance of mineral salts and the water content of the body. When present in large amounts, corticosteroids reduce inflammation and suppress allergic reactions and immune system activity.

Corticosteroid drugs – often referred to simply as steroids – are derived from or are synthetic variants of the natural corticosteroid hormones. They are distinct from another group of hormones, the anabolic steroids (p.174).

ADVERSE EFFECTS OF CORTICOSTEROIDS

Corticosteroids are effective and useful drugs that often provide benefit when other drugs are ineffective. However, long-term use of high doses can lead to a variety of unwanted effects on the body as shown below.

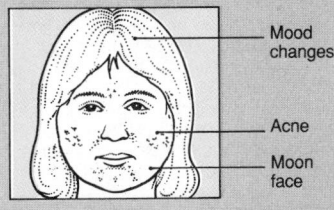
Mood changes
Acne
Moon face

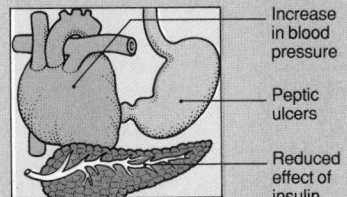
Increase in blood pressure
Peptic ulcers
Reduced effect of insulin

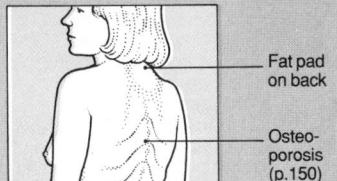
Fat pad on back
Osteoporosis (p.150)

Although corticosteroids have broadly similar actions, they vary in their relative strength and duration of action. The strength of mineralocorticoid effects also varies.

Why they are used

Corticosteroid drugs are used primarily for their anti-inflammatory effect. *Topical* preparations containing corticosteroids are frequently used for the treatment of many inflammatory skin disorders (see p.202). These drugs may also be injected directly into a joint or around a tendon to relieve inflammation caused by injury or disease (see p.146). However, when local administration of the drug is not possible or effective, corticosteroids may be given *systemically*, by mouth or intravenous injection.

An important use of oral corticosteroids is to replace the natural hormones that are deficient when adrenal gland function is reduced, as in Addison's disease. In these cases, drugs that most closely resemble the actions of the natural hormones are selected and a combination of these may be used.

Corticosteroids are an important part of the treatment of many disorders in which inflammation is thought to be caused by excessive or inappropriate activity of the immune system. Such disorders include rheumatoid arthritis (p.145), inflammatory bowel disease (p.140), glomerulonephritis (a kidney disease), and some rare connective tissue disorders such as systemic lupus erythematosus. In these conditions they relieve symptoms and may temporarily halt the disease.

Corticosteroids may be given regularly by mouth or inhaler to treat asthma, although they are not effective for the relief of asthma attacks in progress.

Some cancers of the blood (leukemias) and lymphatic system (lymphomas) may also respond to corticosteroid treatment. These drugs are also widely used to prevent or treat rejection of organ transplants, usually in conjunction with other drugs (see Immunosuppressant drugs, p.184).

How they work

Given in high doses, corticosteroid drugs reduce inflammation by blocking the action of chemicals called prostaglandins that are responsible for triggering the inflammatory response. They also temporarily depress the immune system by reducing the activity of certain types of white blood cells.

How they affect you

Corticosteroid drugs often produce a dramatic improvement in symptoms. Given systemically, corticosteroids

may also act on the brain to produce a heightened sense of well-being and, in some people, a sense of euphoria.

Troublesome day-to-day side effects are rare. However, long-term corticosteroid treatment carries a number of serious risks.

Risks and special precautions

Few risks are associated with these drugs when they are given in low doses by mouth for the treatment of Addison's disease. Expected adverse effects from higher doses depend on the drug used and the duration of treatment.

Drugs with strong mineralocorticoid effects such as hydrocortisone may cause water retention, swelling (particularly of the ankles), and an increase in blood pressure. Because corticosteroids reduce the effect of insulin, they create problems in diabetics. They may even give rise to diabetes in susceptible individuals. They can also cause peptic ulcers.

Since corticosteroids suppress the immune system, they increase susceptibility to infection. They also suppress symptoms of infectious disease. With long-term use, corticosteroids may cause a variety of adverse effects as described in the box on the left. Physicians try to avoid long-term prescription of corticosteroids to children because prolonged use may retard growth.

Long-term use of corticosteroids suppresses the production of the body's own corticosteroid hormones. For this reason, treatment lasting for more than a few weeks should be withdrawn gradually to give the body time to adjust. If the drug is stopped abruptly, the lack of corticosteroid hormones may lead to sudden collapse. People taking corticosteroids by mouth for longer than one month are advised to carry a warning card for two years. In the case of an accident, their defenses against shock may need to be quickly strengthened with extra hydrocortisone.

COMMON DRUGS

Beclomethasone
Betamethasone
Cortisone
Dexamethasone
Fluocinolone
Hydrocortisone
Methylprednisolone
Prednisolone
Prednisone
Triamcinolone

DRUGS USED IN DIABETES

The body obtains most of its energy from glucose, a simple form of sugar broken down in the intestine from starch and other sugars and absorbed into the bloodstream. The hormone insulin, produced by the pancreas, enables body tissues to take up glucose from the blood, either to use it for energy or store it. In diabetes mellitus (also called sugar diabetes) not enough insulin is produced by the pancreas, so that little glucose is taken up by the tissues and glucose in the blood rises to abnormal levels, a condition known as hyperglycemia.

There are two main types of diabetes mellitus. Insulin-dependent or type 1 diabetes, the most severe form, usually first appears in people under 35 and most commonly between the ages of 10 and 16. It develops rapidly when insulin-secreting cells in the pancreas are destroyed, probably as a result of a viral infection. Insulin production ceases almost immediately, leading to symptoms of hyperglycemia: lethargy, general ill health, weight loss, thirst, and increased urination. If treatment is not given, coma and death may result.

The other main form of the disorder, non-insulin-dependent, maturity-onset, or type 2 diabetes, is usually of gradual onset and occurs mainly in people over 40. Insulin is produced, but not in sufficient amounts to meet the body's needs. It is especially common among overweight people who eat large amounts of sugary foods. This form of diabetes may also be caused by chronic pancreatitis and may occasionally be triggered by drugs such as oral contraceptives (p.189) or cortico-steroids (p.169).

In both types of diabetes it is necessary to change the diet to reduce consumption of sugary foods. For many obese type 2 diabetics, control of sugar intake and loss of excess weight reduces the body's insulin requirements to a sufficiently low level without the need for further treatment. However, many type 2 diabetics and all type 1

ADMINISTRATION OF INSULIN

Insulin is given in a way that attempts to mimic the body's production of insulin, which is at a constant overall level with increased production as food is eaten. In practice, the most common and best method of administration is injections twice a day with a mixture of short- and long-acting insulin preparations. The long-acting insulin produces an overall level, while the short-acting one produces the higher level that is needed to cope with the increase in blood sugar following

a meal. Older diabetics may be advised to have injections once a day, which may be necessary if they need someone else to give the injection. Unstable diabetics or those with irregular mealtimes may need to inject short-acting insulin before each meal or snack as well as using a long-acting preparation once or twice a day. In difficult cases a device that continuously delivers insulin into the blood-stream may be needed in order to maintain a finer control over the body's insulin needs.

Duration of action of types of insulin

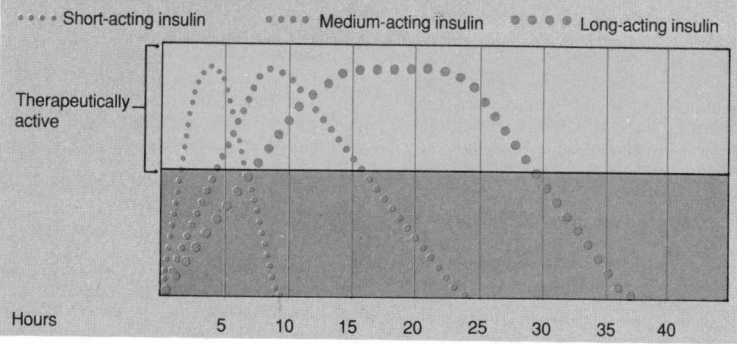

Short-acting insulin   Medium-acting insulin   Long-acting insulin

Therapeutically active

Hours   5   10   15   20   25   30   35   40

diabetics require some form of drug treatment in addition to those simpler measures. Two types of drug can be used – insulin and oral antidiabetic drugs, the sulfonylureas.

Why they are used
Treatment of diabetes is essential to prevent hyperglycemia and to avoid some serious long-term risks. These include an increased likelihood of heart and circulatory problems, and kidney and eye damage.

Oral antidiabetic drugs are prescribed for people with type 2 diabetes who still produce some insulin but whose blood glucose level cannot be adequately

controlled by diet alone. Insulin is prescribed for all sufferers from type 1 diabetes. Treatment must be continued for life. Insulin may also be given to type 2 diabetics to provide control of hyper-glycemia before treatment with oral antidiabetic drugs. Insulin is also used if the oral drugs fail to provide adequate control over the condition. Insulin may also be substituted for other treatments for shorter periods of time when these become temporarily unsuitable or insufficient, for example, during pregnancy, severe illness, or prior to undergoing surgery.

A variety of types of insulin are available. Some have a long duration of action; others are short-acting. Some-times more than one type of insulin is given to provide steady diabetic control (see Administration of insulin, above).

How they work
Sulfonylurea oral antidiabetic drugs encourage the pancreas to produce insulin. They are therefore effective only when some insulin-secreting cells remain active. Insulin treatment directly replaces the natural hormone that is deficient in diabetes mellitus.

By increasing insulin levels in the blood, both types of drug promote the uptake of glucose into body tissues and help to prevent an excessive rise in the level of glucose in the blood.

ACTION OF ORAL ANTIDIABETIC DRUGS

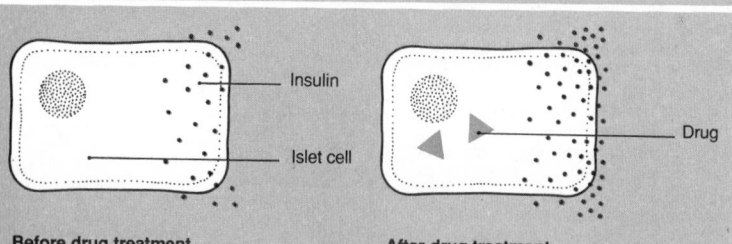

Insulin

Islet cell

Drug

Before drug treatment
In type 2 diabetes the islet cells of the pancreas secrete insufficient insulin to meet the body's needs.

After drug treatment
The drug stimulates the islet cells to release increased amounts of insulin.

Insulin cannot be given by mouth because it is broken down in the digestive tract before it reaches the bloodstream. Regular injections are therefore necessary (see Administration of insulin, facing page).

How they affect you

Antidiabetic drugs rapidly relieve symptoms of diabetes, and in combination with dietary measures, usually permit a diabetic to lead a full and healthy life. Successful control of blood glucose levels helps to reduce the long-term risks of diabetes mellitus.

Because the body's requirement for glucose and therefore for insulin varies according to the level of activity and the rate at which the body burns up energy, the main day-to-day problems arise out of the difficulty in establishing a dosage and schedule to meet individual variations. Symptoms of hyperglycemia may develop if the dose is too low, and those of hypoglycemia (low blood glucose) may arise if the dose is too high.

Insulin dosage is usually established as a part of hospital tests. Physicians sometimes demonstrate the effect of too much insulin by administering a small overdose to cause the warning symptoms of hypoglycemia, including sweating, dizziness, and faintness. Dosage is established for a particular calorie intake and exercise level, making it important to maintain regular eating habits and levels of activity.

Insulin is traditionally extracted from the pancreases of pigs and cattle. Animal insulin may, however, cause allergic reactions in some people. A skin rash at the injection site develops, along with reduced effectiveness of the drug. A human insulin, produced by genetic engineering, is now available and may be prescribed instead. Repeated injection at the same site may disturb the fat layer beneath the skin, producing a swelling or dimpling. This can usually be avoided by regularly changing the injection site.

Risks and special precautions

The most serious risk of treatment with drugs for diabetics is an excessive reduction in the blood glucose level. This is usually caused by insufficient food intake, particularly if a person taking insulin misses a meal or snack, or takes unaccustomed exercise. Unless compensating action is taken, the diabetic may lose consciousness; in rare circumstances prolonged hypoglycemia may result in seizures or brain damage. Diabetics should always carry glucose tablets or candy to take if warning symptoms of hypoglycemia occur. People who take insulin may also be advised to carry glucagon, a drug which rapidly increases the blood glucose level by blocking the effects of insulin, together with instructions for its use in the event of loss of consciousness. As a precaution, family and colleagues should be told about the

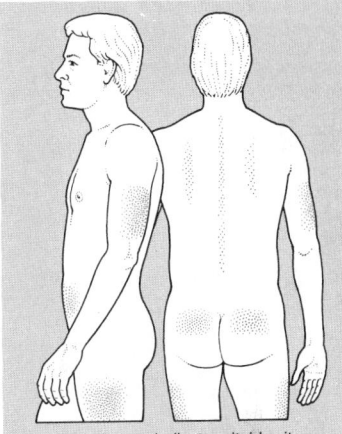

The shaded areas indicate suitable sites for the injection of insulin.

symptoms of hypoglycemia and what treatment to give. If attacks of hypoglycemia occur frequently, a reduction in insulin dosage may be advised.

Because exercise increases the body's glucose requirement, extra insulin and glucose may be needed before undertaking unaccustomed physical activity. Serious illness also increases the need for insulin, and dosage may need to be increased until after recovery. A woman taking sulfonylurea drugs who wishes to become pregnant should discuss her drug treatment with a physician before conceiving because these drugs can cross the placenta and affect the developing baby; a temporary change to insulin treatment until after the baby is born is usually advised.

There are many types of insulin preparations, each available in different strengths. It is important that you receive exactly the same one each time you renew your prescription, since the dosage is tailored for your needs. You will be given an identification card stating type of drug and dosage.

MONITORING BLOOD GLUCOSE

Diabetics need to check either their blood or urine glucose level at home. Blood tests give the most accurate results. The kit illustrated at right consists of a programmable meter that reads the glucose levels of blood samples applied to a special testing strip.

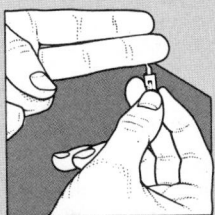

1 Prick your finger to produce a large drop of blood.

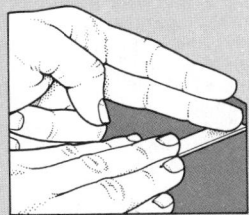

2 Touch the blood onto the test pads of the testing strip.

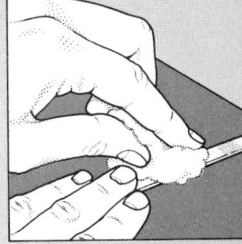

3 Press the time button on the meter. After 60 seconds wipe the blood from the test pads with a clean, dry cotton ball.

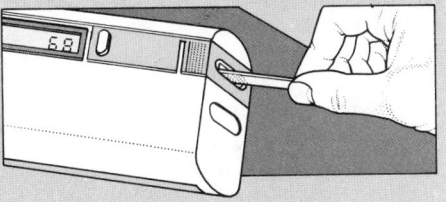

4 Within 120 seconds insert the test strip into the meter as shown. Your reading will appear after 120 seconds.

Sulfonylurea drugs
Acetohexamide
Chlorpropamide
Glipizide
Glyburide
Tolazamide
Tolbutamide

Other drugs
Glucagon
Insulin

DRUGS FOR THYROID DISORDERS

The thyroid gland, located in the lower front part of the neck, produces *hormones* that regulate the body's *metabolism*. During childhood, the hormones from this gland are an essential part of normal mental and physical development. The thyroid also produces calcitonin, a hormone essential to normal calcium balance.

The thyroid gland can become overactive, producing excess amounts of hormones and causing a condition known as hyperthyroidism, also called thyrotoxicosis. The gland can also become underactive, producing insufficient hormones and a condition called hypothyroidism.

Thyrotoxicosis

Overactivity of the thyroid causes thyrotoxicosis. Symptoms include anxiety, trembling, sweating, palpitations, an increased appetite, weight loss, and intolerance to heat. Diarrhea and menstrual disturbances may occur. Thyrotoxicosis can also cause abnormal protrusion of the eyes, exophthalmos.

Drugs for thyrotoxicosis

Antithyroid drugs reduce production of thyroid hormones to near normal levels. These drugs may take about eight weeks to produce any effect, because the thyroid gland contains a store of hormones that is only gradually depleted. Therefore, a beta blocker (p.125) may be prescribed to control symptoms at the beginning of treatment.

A course of antithyroid drug treatment is usually started with a high dose to give a rapid improvement in symptoms; the dosage is gradually reduced, depending on the individual response. Some people recover completely after one course of treatment, but symptoms may return, especially in children, making further treatment necessary. Antithyroid drugs do not improve exophthalmos, although they may prevent it from worsening. To relieve this condition a corticosteroid (p.169) may be given. Surgery may be necessary.

The initial high dose of an antithyroid drug may produce nausea, vomiting, headache, or skin rashes. More serious, these drugs may reduce the white blood cell count, thus increasing susceptibility to infection, and causing recurrent fevers and sore throats. Such symptoms need prompt medical advice.

If drugs do not provide adequate relief, or if the thyroid is dangerously large, radioactive iodine treatment or removal of part of the gland may be advised.

Hypothyroidism

In an adult, a low thyroid hormone level may result in a condition called hypothyroidism. It may be caused by an autoimmune disorder, in which the body's immune system attacks the thyroid gland. Reduced thyroid output may also arise after surgery or radioactive iodine treatment for hyperthyroidism. In newborn babies, hypothyroidism may be the result of an inborn *enzyme* disorder.

Symptoms of adult hypothyroidism usually develop slowly and include tiredness, slowing of mental processes, puffy facial appearance with dry skin and some hair loss, and increased sensitivity to cold. Women may develop heavy or prolonged menstrual periods.

ACTION OF DRUGS FOR THYROID DISORDERS

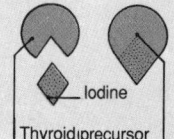

Thyroid hormone production
Iodine combines with other chemicals (precursors) in the thyroid gland to make thyroid hormones.

Iodine

Thyroid precursor

Thyroid hormone

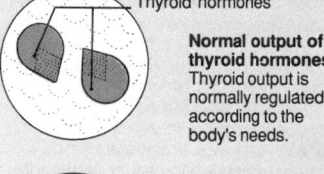

Thyroid hormones

Normal output of thyroid hormones
Thyroid output is normally regulated according to the body's needs.

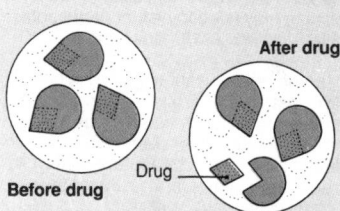

After drug

Drug

Before drug

Action of antithyroid drugs
In thyrotoxicosis, antithyroid drugs reduce the production of thyroid hormones by preventing iodine from combining with thyroid precursors in the thyroid gland.

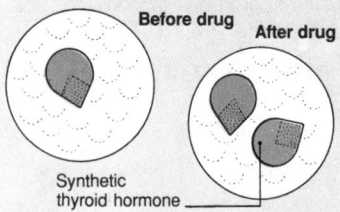

Before drug

After drug

Synthetic thyroid hormone

Action of thyroid hormones
In hypothyroidism, when the thyroid gland is underactive, supplements of synthetic or (rarely) natural thyroid hormones restore hormone levels to normal.

TREATMENT FOR GOITER

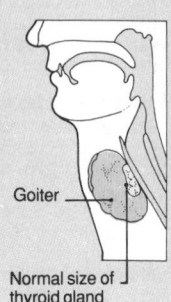

A goiter is a swelling of the thyroid gland. It may occur temporarily during puberty or pregnancy, or may be due to an abnormal growth of thyroid tissue that requires surgical removal. It may rarely be brought about by an iodine deficiency. This last cause is treated with iodine supplements (see also p.538).

Goiter

Normal size of thyroid gland

Drugs for hypothyroidism

Hypothyroidism is usually permanent, necessitating lifelong treatment with synthetic thyroid hormone preparations. These are usually given by mouth, but may be given by injection or by using a nasogastric tube if an individual's level of thyroid hormone falls so low that consciousness is lost.

Babies are routinely checked after birth for thyroid deficiency because low levels may cause cretinism – permanent mental and physical retardation. If the level is low, a thyroid drug is injected immediately and administered at regular intervals thereafter. Prompt treatment should establish normal development.

Thyroid drugs do not usually produce adverse effects, since they are simply supplying a substance that the body would normally produce. However, if the dose is too high, symptoms of thyrotoxicosis may arise. Regular blood tests are usually performed to check that the correct dose is being given. It is common practice to start with a low dose of the drug and to increase it gradually. A sudden rise in hormone levels can put a strain on the heart. For this reason, thyroid drugs are prescribed with caution to the elderly and those with heart disease or high blood pressure. A beta blocker may also be given to reduce adverse effects on the heart.

COMMON DRUGS

Drugs for thyrotoxicosis
Methimazole
Propylthiouracil

Drugs for hypothyroidism
Levothyroxine
Liothyronine
Thyroid

Other drugs
Iodine

DRUGS FOR PITUITARY DISORDERS

The pituitary gland, which lies at the base of the brain, produces a number of *hormones* that regulate physical growth, *metabolism*, sexual development, and reproductive function. Many of these hormones act indirectly by stimulating other glands, such as the thyroid, adrenal glands, ovaries, and testicles, to release their own hormones. A summary of the actions and effects of each pituitary hormone is given below.

An excess or a lack of a pituitary hormone may produce serious effects, the nature of which depends on the hormone involved. Abnormal levels of a particular hormone may be caused by a pituitary tumor, usually treated surgically. In other cases, drugs may be used to correct the hormonal imbalance.

The more common pituitary disorders that can be treated with drugs are those involving growth hormone, antidiuretic hormone, prolactin, adrenal hormones, and the gonadotropins. The first three are discussed below. For information on the use of drugs to treat infertility arising from inadequate levels of gonadotropins, see p.192. Lack of corticotropin, leading to inadequate production of adrenal hormones, is usually treated with corticosteroid drugs (see p.169).

Drugs for growth hormone disorders

Growth hormone (somatropin) is the principal hormone required for normal growth in childhood and adolescence. Lack of growth hormone impairs normal physical growth, a condition known as pituitary dwarfism. Physicians administer growth hormone only after tests have shown that a lack of this hormone is the cause of the disorder. If treatment begins early, regular injections of hormone until the end of adolescence usually allow normal growth and development to take place.

Less often, the pituitary produces an excess of growth hormone. In children this can result in pituitary gigantism; in adults, it can produce a deformity known as acromegaly. Acromegaly is usually the result of a pituitary tumor, and is characterized by thickening of the skull, face, hands, and feet, and the enlargement of some internal organs.

Although these conditions cannot be cured, gigantism may be halted and some of the deformities of acromegaly reversed by reducing the output of growth hormone. This is usually achieved by destroying part of the pituitary gland, either by surgery or radiation treatment. The drug bromocriptine, which reduces growth hormone levels, is also used.

Drugs for diabetes insipidus

Antidiuretic hormone (also known as ADH or vasopressin) acts on the kidneys, controlling the amount of water retained in the body and returned to the blood. A lack of ADH is usually caused by damage to the pituitary, and this in turn causes diabetes insipidus. In this rare condition, the kidneys cannot retain water, and large quantities pass into the urine. The chief symptoms of diabetes insipidus are constant thirst and the production of large volumes of urine.

Diabetes insipidus is treated with vasopressin or lypressin. Vasopressin has to be given by injection. Lypressin, an artificial form of vasopressin, is inhaled from a nasal spray. Mild cases of this disease may be treated either with clofibrate (see also Lipid-lowering drugs, p.131), which increases the amount of ADH released by the pituitary, or chlorpropamide, which also increases ADH release. In addition the drug makes the kidneys more sensitive to the hormone. Alternatively, a thiazide diuretic (such as chlorthalidone) may be prescribed for mild cases (see Diuretics, p.127). The usual effect of such drugs is to increase urine production, but in diabetes insipidus they have the opposite effect, reducing water loss from the body.

Drugs used to reduce prolactin levels

Prolactin, or lactogenic hormone, is produced in both men and women. In women, prolactin controls the secretion of breast milk following childbirth; its function in men is not understood, although it appears to be necessary for normal sperm production. The disorders associated with prolactin are all concerned with overproduction. High levels of prolactin in women can cause lactation unassociated with pregnancy and birth (galactorrhea), lack of menstruation (amenorrhea), and infertility. If excessive amounts are produced in men, the result may be galactorrhea and/or infertility. Some drugs, notably phenothiazine anti-psychotics, estrogen, and methyldopa, can all raise the level of prolactin in the blood. More often, however, increased prolactin results from a pituitary tumor that is usually treated surgically. Bromocriptine inhibits the production of prolactin and is also used in the short term to relieve breast symptoms prior to surgery.

THE EFFECTS OF PITUITARY HORMONES

The pituitary gland produces a large number of hormones, many of which control the activities of other glands. The illustration shows the principal sites of action of the major pituitary hormones.

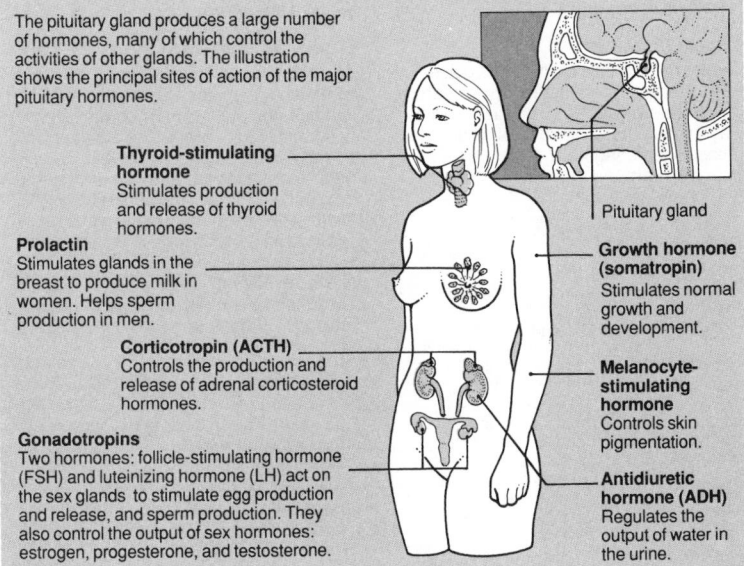

Thyroid-stimulating hormone
Stimulates production and release of thyroid hormones.

Prolactin
Stimulates glands in the breast to produce milk in women. Helps sperm production in men.

Corticotropin (ACTH)
Controls the production and release of adrenal corticosteroid hormones.

Gonadotropins
Two hormones: follicle-stimulating hormone (FSH) and luteinizing hormone (LH) act on the sex glands to stimulate egg production and release, and sperm production. They also control the output of sex hormones: estrogen, progesterone, and testosterone.

Pituitary gland

Growth hormone (somatropin)
Stimulates normal growth and development.

Melanocyte-stimulating hormone
Controls skin pigmentation.

Antidiuretic hormone (ADH)
Regulates the output of water in the urine.

COMMON DRUGS

Drugs for growth hormone disorders
Bromocriptine
Growth hormone

Drugs for diabetes insipidus
Chlorpropamide
Chlorthalidone
Clofibrate
Desmopressin
Lypressin
Vasopressin

Drugs to reduce prolactin levels
Bromocriptine

MALE SEX HORMONES

Male sex hormones – androgens – are responsible for the development of male sexual characteristics. The principal androgen is testosterone, which in men is produced by the testicles from puberty onwards. Women also produce testosterone in small amounts in the adrenal glands, but its exact function in the female body is not known.

Testosterone has two major effects: an androgenic effect and an anabolic effect. Its androgenic effect is to stimulate the appearance of secondary sexual characteristics at puberty, such as the growth of body hair, deepening of the voice, and an increase in the size of the genitals. Its anabolic effect is to increase muscle bulk and accelerate rate of growth.

There are a number of synthetically produced derivatives of testosterone that produce varying degrees of the androgenic and anabolic effects mentioned above. Those having a mainly anabolic effect are known as anabolic steroids (see box below).

Testosterone and its derivatives have been used in both men and women to treat a number of conditions.

Why they are used

Male sex hormones are mainly given to men to promote the development of male sexual characteristics when hormone production is deficient. This may be the result of an abnormality of the testicles or of inadequate production of the pituitary hormones that stimulate the testicles to release testosterone.

A course of treatment with male sex hormones is sometimes prescribed for adolescent boys in whom the onset of puberty is delayed by pituitary problems. This treatment may also help to stimulate the development of secondary male sexual characteristics and to increase sex drive (libido) in adult men who are producing inadequate levels of testosterone. However, such hormone treatment is unlikely to promote the production of sperm. (For information

EFFECTS OF MALE SEX HORMONES

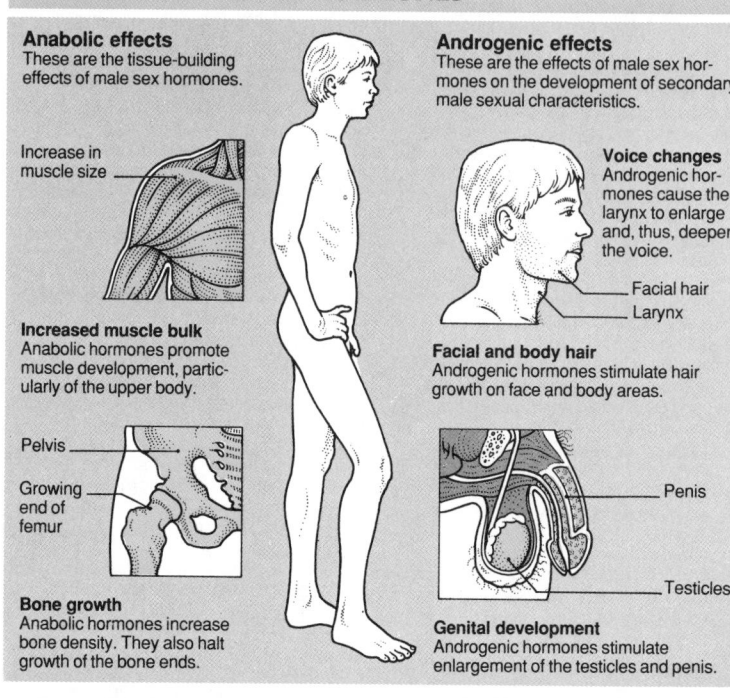

Anabolic effects
These are the tissue-building effects of male sex hormones.

Increase in muscle size

Increased muscle bulk
Anabolic hormones promote muscle development, particularly of the upper body.

Pelvis

Growing end of femur

Bone growth
Anabolic hormones increase bone density. They also halt growth of the bone ends.

Androgenic effects
These are the effects of male sex hormones on the development of secondary male sexual characteristics.

Voice changes
Androgenic hormones cause the larynx to enlarge and, thus, deepen the voice.

Facial hair
Larynx

Facial and body hair
Androgenic hormones stimulate hair growth on face and body areas.

Penis

Testicles

Genital development
Androgenic hormones stimulate enlargement of the testicles and penis.

on the drug treatment of male infertility, see p.192.)

Male sex hormones and mainly some of their synthetic variants may also be prescribed for women to treat certain types of cancer of the breast and uterus (see Anticancer drugs, p.182).

How they work

Taken in low doses as part of replacement therapy when natural production is low, male sex hormones act in the same way as the natural hormones. In adolescents suffering from delayed puberty, hormone treatment produces androgenic and anabolic effects

(above), initiating the development of secondary sexual characteristics over a few months; full sexual development usually takes place over three to four years. In adult men, the effects of hormone treatment may begin to be felt within a few weeks.

Risks and special precautions

The main risks with these drugs occur when they are given to boys with delayed puberty and to women with breast cancer. Given to initiate the onset of puberty, they may stunt growth by prematurely sealing the growing ends of the long bones. Physicians normally try to avoid prescribing hormones in these circumstances until growth is complete. High doses given to women have masculinizing effects – increased facial and body hair, deeper voice. They may also produce enlargement of the clitoris, acne, and changes in libido.

ANABOLIC STEROIDS

Anabolic steroids are synthetically produced variants that mimic the anabolic effects of the natural hormones. They increase muscle bulk and body growth.

Physicians occasionally prescribe anabolic steroids and a high protein diet to promote recovery after serious illness or major surgery. The steroids may also help to increase the production of blood cells in some forms of anemia. They have also been used in the treatment of the bone-wasting disorder osteoporosis in post-menopausal women, but because of the risk of serious side effects alternative forms of treatment are usually given (see p.150).

Anabolic steroids have been widely abused by athletes because they speed up the recovery of muscles after a session of intense exercise. This enables the athlete to go through a more demanding daily exercise program, resulting in a significant improvement in muscle power. The use of anabolic steroids by athletes to improve their performance is condemned by physicians and athletic organizations because of the risks to health, particularly for women. Adverse effects range from acne and baldness to fluid retention, reduced fertility in men and women, hardening of the arteries, a long-term risk of liver disease, and certain forms of cancer.

COMMON DRUGS

Primarily androgenic
Testosterone

Primarily anabolic
Nandrolone
Oxandrolone

FEMALE SEX HORMONES

There are two types of female sex hormones, estrogens and progesterone. In women these are secreted by the ovaries from puberty until after the menopause. Additional estrogens and progesterone are produced by the placenta during pregnancy. Small amounts of estrogens are also produced in the adrenal glands.

Estrogens are responsible for the development of female sexual characteristics including breast development, growth of pubic hair, and widening of the pelvis. Progesterone acts on the lining of the uterus and prepares it for implantation of a fertilized egg. It is also important for the maintenance of pregnancy. On a monthly basis, levels of estrogens and progesterone fluctuate, producing the menstrual cycle (see p.187).

The production of these hormones is regulated by the action of two gonadotropin hormones produced by the pituitary gland (see p.173).

Estrogens and progesterone and synthetic variants of these hormones (synthetic progesterone drugs are known as progestins) are used medically to treat a number of conditions.

Why they are used

The best-known use of these drugs is in oral contraceptive preparations. These are discussed on p.189. Other uses include the treatment of menstrual disorders (p.188) and certain hormone-sensitive cancers (p.182). This page focuses on the use of hormones in conditions in which the levels of natural hormones are deficient.

Hormone deficiency

Deficiency of female sex hormones may occur as a result of deficiency of gonadotropins (caused by a pituitary disorder) or of abnormal development of the ovaries (ovarian failure). This may lead to the absence of menstruation and sexual development. If tests show a deficiency of gonadotropins, preparations of these hormones may be prescribed. These trigger the release of estrogens and progesterone from the ovaries. If pituitary function is normal and ovarian failure is diagnosed as the cause of hormone deficiency, estrogen and progesterone supplements may be given. In this situation, hormone supplements ensure development of normal female sexual characteristics, but cannot stimulate ovulation.

Menopause

A fall in levels of estrogens and progesterone occurs naturally after the menopause, when the menstrual cycle ceases. The sudden reduction in estrogen levels often causes distressing symptoms including sweating, hot flashes, dryness of the vagina, and mood changes. Many physicians advocate the use of hormone supplements following the menopause. Such hormone replacement therapy helps to reduce the symptoms of the menopause and also helps to delay some of the long-term consequences of reduced estrogen levels in old age, including osteoporosis (p.150) and deposition of fat in the arteries (atherosclerosis). When dryness of the vagina is a particular problem, estrogen cream may be prescribed. Hormone replacement therapy is usually maintained for 18 to 24 months, after which the dose is gradually reduced.

Hormone replacement therapy may also be prescribed for women who have undergone a premature menopause as a result of surgical removal of the ovaries or following radiation treatment for ovarian cancer.

How they affect you

Hormones given to treat ovarian failure or delayed puberty may take three to six months to produce a noticeable effect on sexual development. Taken for menopausal symptoms, they can dramatically lessen the number of hot flashes within a week.

Both estrogens and progestins can cause fluid retention, and estrogens may cause nausea, vomiting, breast tenderness, headache, dizziness, and depression. Progestins may cause "breakthrough" bleeding between menstrual periods. In the comparatively low doses used to treat these disorders, however, side effects are unlikely.

Risks and special precautions

Treatment with estrogens and progestins for ovarian failure carries few risks for otherwise healthy young women. However, there are risks linked to long-term estrogen treatment in older women. The hormone increases the risk of abnormal blood clotting (thrombosis) and raised blood pressure (hypertension). For these reasons, estrogen treatment is used with caution in women with heart or circulatory disorders, or who are overweight or smoke. Estrogens may also trigger diabetes mellitus in susceptible people. The risks of estrogen hormones are reduced by prescribing them with progestins, which oppose some of the harmful effects. However, the danger of adverse effects increases with age.

COMPARATIVE HORMONE LEVELS DURING THE MENSTRUAL CYCLE AND PREGNANCY

In an adult woman of child-bearing years the production of female sex hormones fluctuates during a monthly cycle. During pregnancy the levels of both estrogen and progesterone rise dramatically. After the menopause hormone production falls to a level similar to that which occurs during menstruation.

The large graph (right) shows the rise in hormone levels during the 40 weeks of pregnancy. The smaller graph (inset) illustrates hormone levels in a typical 28-day menstrual cycle. Because the hormone levels in pregnancy are so much greater, each unit of measurement on the pregnancy graph represents 100 units in the menstrual cycle graph.

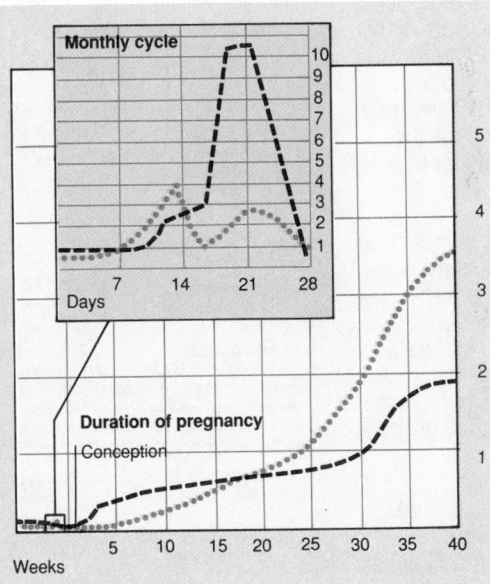

Monthly cycle

Days

Duration of pregnancy

Conception

Weeks

· · · · · · Estrogen

- - - - Progesterone

COMMON DRUGS

Estrogens
Conjugated estrogens
Diethylstilbestrol (DES)
Estradiol
Ethinyl estradiol

Progestins
Medroxyprogesterone
Megestrol
Norgestrel

NUTRITION

Food provides energy (as calories) and materials called nutrients needed for growth and renewal of tissues. Protein, carbohydrate, and fat are the three major nutrient components of food. Vitamins and minerals are found in small amounts in food but are just as important for normal function of the body. Fiber, found only in foods from plants, is needed for a healthy digestive system.

During digestion, large molecules of food are broken down into smaller molecules, releasing nutrients that can be absorbed into the blood-stream. Carbohydrate and fat are then *metabolized* by body cells to produce energy. They may also be incorporated with protein into cell structure. Each metabolic process inside cells is promoted by a specific *enzyme* and often requires the presence of a particular vitamin or mineral.

What can go wrong

Dietary deficiency of essential nutrients can lead to illness. In poorer countries where there is a shortage of food, marasmus (resulting from lack of food energy) and kwashiorkor (from lack of protein) are common. In the developed world, however, excessive food intake leading to obesity is more common. Nutritional deficiencies in developed countries result from poor food choices and usually stem from a lack of a specific vitamin or mineral as in iron-deficiency anemia.

Some nutritional deficiencies may be caused by an inability of the body to absorb a nutrient from food (malabsorption) or to utilize it once it has been absorbed. Malabsorption may be caused by lack of an enzyme or an abnormality of the digestive tract. Errors of metabolism are often inborn and are not yet fully understood. They may be caused by failure of the body to produce the chemicals required to process nutrients for use.

Why supplements are used

Deficiencies of the kwashiorkor or marasmus type are not usually treated by drugs, but by dietary improvement, and perhaps food supplements. Vitamin and mineral deficiencies are usually treated with appropriate supplements. Malabsorption disorders may require continued use of supplements or changes in diet. Metabolic errors are not easily treated with supplements or drugs. Dietary changes may be tried.

Obesity has been treated with appetite suppressants related to amphetamines (p.549), the use of which is now discouraged. The preferred treatment includes reduced food intake, altered eating patterns and increased exercise.

Major food components

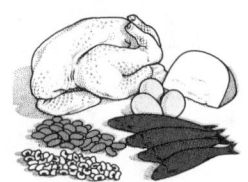

Proteins
Vital for growth and repair of tissue. In meat, fish, dairy products, cereals, and legumes.

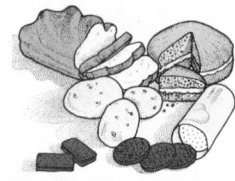

Carbohydrates
A major energy source, stored as fat when taken in excess. In cereals, sugar, and vegetables.

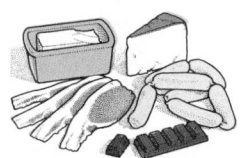

Fats
A concentrated energy form but needed only in small quantities. In animal products and oils.

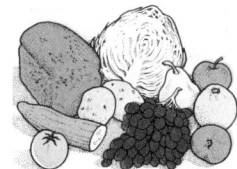

Fiber
The indigestible part of any plant product which, though it contains no nutrients, adds bulk to feces.

Absorption of nutrients
Food passes through the mouth, esophagus, and stomach to the small intestine. The lining of the small intestine secretes many enzymes and is covered by tiny projections (villi) which enable nutrients to pass into the blood.

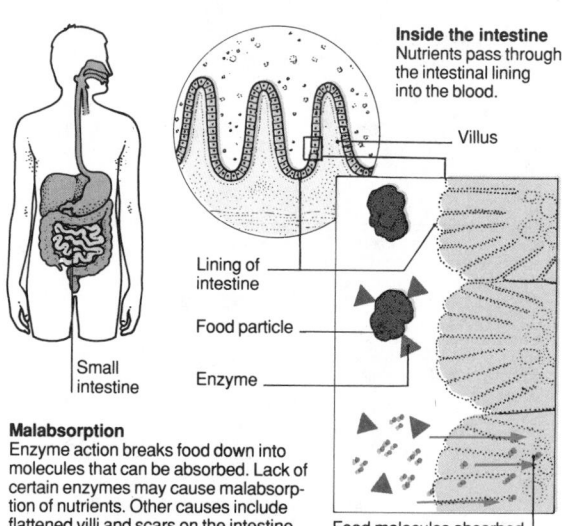

Inside the intestine
Nutrients pass through the intestinal lining into the blood.

Villus

Lining of intestine

Food particle

Enzyme

Small intestine

Malabsorption
Enzyme action breaks food down into molecules that can be absorbed. Lack of certain enzymes may cause malabsorption of nutrients. Other causes include flattened villi and scars on the intestine.

Food molecules absorbed

MAJOR DRUG GROUPS

Vitamins

VITAMINS

Vitamins are complex chemicals that are essential for a variety of body functions. The body is unable to manufacture these substances itself and therefore we need to take them in the diet. There are 13 major vitamins: A, C, D, E, K, and the eight B complex vitamins – thiamine (B_1), riboflavin (B_2), niacin (B_3), folic acid, biotin (vitamin H), pantothenic acid (B_5), pyridoxine (B_6), and cobalamin (B_{12}). Most are required in extremely small amounts, and each vitamin is present in one or more foods (see Main food sources of vitamins and minerals, p.178). Vitamin D is also produced in the body when the skin is exposed to sunlight. Vitamins fall into two groups: those that dissolve in fat and those that dissolve in water (see Fat-soluble and water-soluble vitamins, p.179).

A balanced diet that includes a variety of different types of foods is likely to contain adequate amounts of all the vitamins. Inadequate intake of any vitamin over an extended period can lead to symptoms of deficiency. The nature of these symptoms depends on the vitamin concerned.

A physician may recommend supplements of one or more vitamins in a variety of circumstances: to prevent vitamin deficiency from occurring in people considered at special risk, to treat symptoms of deficiency, and to treat certain medical conditions.

Why they are used
Preventing deficiency
Most people in the United States obtain sufficient quantities of vitamins in their diet, and it is therefore unnecessary in most cases to take additional vitamins in the form of supplements. People who are unsure as to whether their present diet is adequate are advised to look at the table on p.178 to check that foods that are rich in vitamins are eaten regularly. Vitamin intake can often be boosted simply by increasing the quantities of fresh foods and raw fruit and vegetables in the diet.

Certain groups in the population are, however, at increased risk of vitamin deficiency. These include those who have an increased need for certain vitamins that may not be met from dietary sources – in particular, women who are pregnant or nursing, infants, and young children. The elderly who may not be eating a varied diet may also be at risk. Strict vegetarians and others on restricted diets may not receive adequate amounts of all vitamins.

In addition, people being fed intravenously or by stomach tube on artificial nutrients for prolonged periods, those suffering from disorders in which absorption of nutrients from the bowel is impaired, and those who need to take drugs (for example, lipid-lowering drugs) which reduce vitamin absorption, are usually given additional vitamins.

In these cases, a physician is likely to advise supplements of one or more vitamins. Although most vitamin preparations are available without a prescription, it is important to seek specialist advice before starting a course of vitamin supplements, so that a proper assessment can be made of your individual requirements.

Vitamin supplements should not be used as a general tonic to improve well-being – they do not do so – nor should they be used as a substitute for a balanced diet.

Vitamin deficiency
It is rare for a diet to be completely lacking in a particular vitamin. But if

PRIMARY FUNCTIONS OF VITAMINS

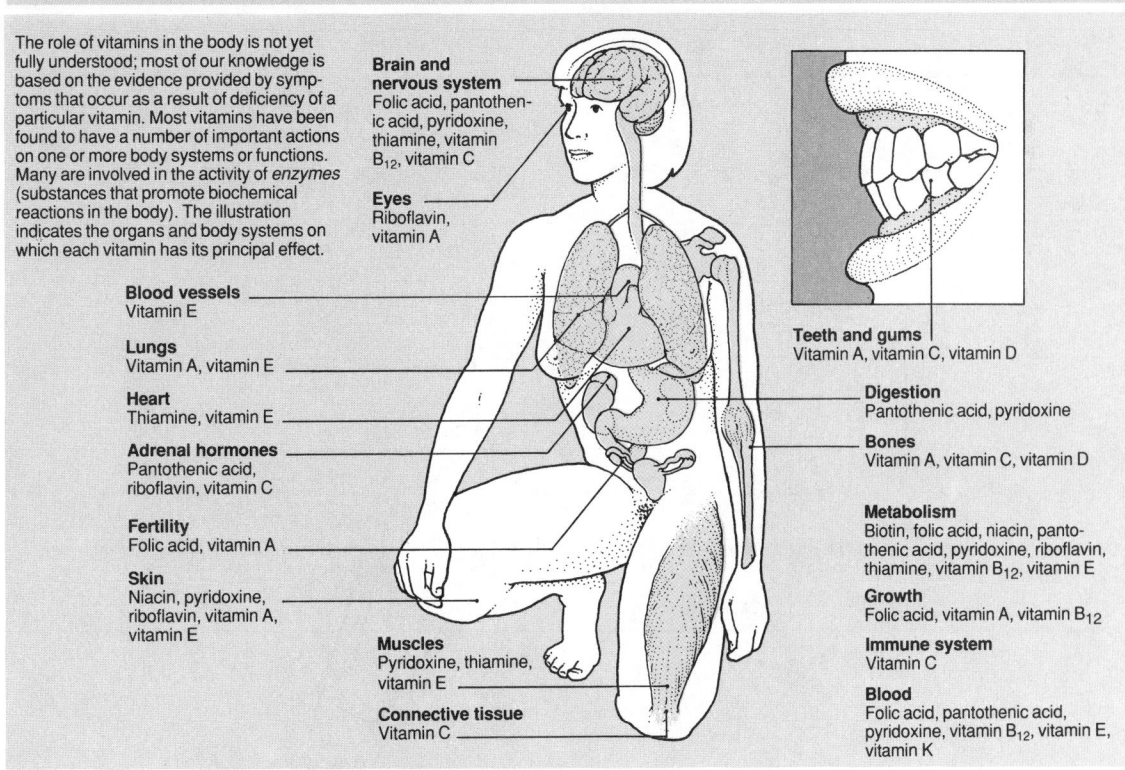

The role of vitamins in the body is not yet fully understood; most of our knowledge is based on the evidence provided by symptoms that occur as a result of deficiency of a particular vitamin. Most vitamins have been found to have a number of important actions on one or more body systems or functions. Many are involved in the activity of *enzymes* (substances that promote biochemical reactions in the body). The illustration indicates the organs and body systems on which each vitamin has its principal effect.

Brain and nervous system
Folic acid, pantothenic acid, pyridoxine, thiamine, vitamin B_{12}, vitamin C

Eyes
Riboflavin, vitamin A

Blood vessels
Vitamin E

Lungs
Vitamin A, vitamin E

Heart
Thiamine, vitamin E

Adrenal hormones
Pantothenic acid, riboflavin, vitamin C

Fertility
Folic acid, vitamin A

Skin
Niacin, pyridoxine, riboflavin, vitamin A, vitamin E

Muscles
Pyridoxine, thiamine, vitamin E

Connective tissue
Vitamin C

Teeth and gums
Vitamin A, vitamin C, vitamin D

Digestion
Pantothenic acid, pyridoxine

Bones
Vitamin A, vitamin C, vitamin D

Metabolism
Biotin, folic acid, niacin, pantothenic acid, pyridoxine, riboflavin, thiamine, vitamin B_{12}, vitamin E

Growth
Folic acid, vitamin A, vitamin B_{12}

Immune system
Vitamin C

Blood
Folic acid, pantothenic acid, pyridoxine, vitamin B_{12}, vitamin E, vitamin K

VITAMINS continued

MAIN FOOD SOURCES OF VITAMINS AND MINERALS

The table below indicates which foods are especially good sources of particular vitamins and minerals. Regularly selecting foods from a variety of categories helps to maintain adequate intake for most people, without a need for supplements. It is important to remember that processed and overcooked foods are likely to contain fewer vitamins than fresh, raw, or lightly cooked foods.

Vitamins	Red meat	Poultry	Liver	Milk	Cheese	Butter/margarine	Eggs	Fish	Cereals and bread	Green vegetables	Root vegetables	Legumes	Nuts	Fruit	Other
Biotin			●				●			●	●				Especially peanut butter. Cauliflower is good vegetable source.
Folic acid			●				●			●				●	Wheat germ and mushrooms are rich sources.
Niacin	●	●	●				●	●		●	●				Protein-rich foods such as milk and eggs contain tryptophan, which can be converted to niacin in the body.
Pantothenic acid			●				●	●							Each food group contributes some pantothenic acid.
Pyridoxine	●	●	●				●	●	●						Especially white meat (chicken, fish) and whole-grain cereals.
Riboflavin			●	●	●		●	●		●	●	●			Found in most foods.
Thiamine	●		●					●		●	●				Brewer's yeast, wheat germ, and bran are also good sources.
Vitamin A			●	●	●	●	●			●				●	Fish liver oil, dark green leafy vegetables such as spinach, and orange or yellow-orange vegetables and fruits such as carrots, apricots, and peaches are especially good sources of vitamin A.
Vitamin B_{12}	●		●	●	●		●	●							Obtained only from animal products.
Vitamin C										●				●	Especially citrus fruits, tomatoes, potatoes, broccoli, strawberries, and cantaloupe.
Vitamin D				●				●							Fortified milk is the only good source. Other dietary sources are unreliable. Also obtained by the body when the skin is exposed to sunlight.
Vitamin E			●			●	●			●	●			●	Vegetable oils, whole-grain cereals, and wheat germ are the best sources.
Vitamin K										●					Found in small amounts in fruits, seeds, tubers, dairy and meat products.
Minerals															
Calcium				●	●					●		●	●		Dark green leafy vegetables, soybean products, and nuts are good non-dairy alternatives. Also present in hard, or alkaline, water supplies.
Chromium	●			●				●	●						Especially unrefined whole-grain cereals.
Copper	●	●	●				●	●	●			●	●		Especially shellfish, whole-grain cereals, and mushrooms.
Fluoride								●							Primarily obtained from fluoridated water supplies. Also in seafood and tea.
Iodine				●	●		●	●							Provided by iodized table salt, but adequate amounts can be obtained from dairy products, saltwater fish, and bread without using table salt.
Iron	●	●	●				●	●	●	●					Especially liver, red meat, and enriched or whole-grains.
Magnesium				●				●	●	●		●	●		Dark green leafy vegetables such as spinach are rich sources. Also present in alkaline water supplies.
Phosphorus	●	●	●	●	●		●	●	●	●	●	●	●	●	Common food additive. Large amounts found in some carbonated beverages.
Potassium								●	●	●				●	Best sources are fruits and vegetables, especially oranges, bananas, and potatoes.
Selenium	●		●	●			●	●							Seafood is the richest source. Amounts in most foods are variable depending on soil where plants were grown and animals grazed.
Sodium	●	●	●	●	●	●	●	●	●	●	●	●	●	●	Sodium is present in all foods, especially table salt, processed foods, potato chips, crackers, and pickled, cured or smoked meats, seafood, and vegetables. Also present in softened water.
Zinc	●						●	●			●				Sufficient amounts only in whole-grain breads and cereals.

intake of a particular vitamin is regularly lower than the body's requirements, over a period of time the body's stores of vitamins may become depleted and symptoms of deficiency may begin to appear. In the United States vitamin deficiency disorders are most common among vagrants and alcoholics and those on low incomes who fail to eat an adequate diet. Deficiencies of water-soluble vitamins are more likely since most of these are not stored in large quantities in the body. For descriptions of individual deficiency disorders, see the appropriate vitamin profile in Part 4.

Dosages of vitamins prescribed to treat vitamin deficiency are likely to be larger than those used to prevent deficiency. Medical supervision is required in these cases.

Other medical uses of vitamins
A number of claims have been made for the value of vitamins in the treatment of a range of medical disorders other than vitamin deficiency. In particular, high doses of vitamin C have been said to be effective in the prevention and treatment of the common cold and in the treatment of cancer. Neither theory has received medical endorsement.

However, certain vitamins have recognized medical uses apart from their nutritional role. At the very high dosages used for these purposes, vitamins have drug-like rather than nutritional effects. Vitamin D has long been used in the treatment of bone-wasting disorders (p.150). Niacin, a B vitamin, is sometimes used as a lipid-lowering drug (p.131). Derivatives of vitamin A (retinoids) are an established part of the treatment of severe acne (p.205). Many sufferers from premenstrual syndrome

MINERALS

Minerals are elements – the simplest form of matter – many of which are essential in trace amounts for normal bodily processes. A balanced diet usually contains all of the minerals that the body requires; mineral deficiency diseases, except iron-deficiency anemia, are uncommon.

Dietary supplements are necessary only as part of the treatment for a medical disorder or when a physician has diagnosed a specific deficiency. Physicians commonly prescribe minerals for people with intestinal diseases that reduce the absorption of minerals from the diet. Iron supplements are advised for women who are pregnant or nursing, and iron-enriched cereals are recommended for infants over 6 months.

Much of the general advice given for vitamins also applies to minerals: taking supplements unless under medical direction is not advisable, exceeding the body's daily requirements is not beneficial, and large doses may be harmful.

CALCULATING DAILY VITAMIN REQUIREMENTS

Two systems of assessing vitamin requirements are in use in the United States. The Food and Nutrition Board of the National Academy of Sciences has established the Recommended Dietary Allowances (RDA) that give the daily intake required to meet the needs of healthy men and women at different ages in the United States. Obtaining at least two-thirds of the RDA is considered adequate to prevent deficiencies in individuals. The United States Recommended Daily Allowances (USRDA) is another system developed by the Food and Drug Administration for use by drug manufacturers and food processors for labeling purposes. The USRDA is the RDA for the group in the population, excluding pregnant or nursing women, with the highest requirement.

Adult daily allowances of vitamins (age 23 – 50)

Vitamin (unit)	RDA Men	Women	USRDA Men and women
Biotin (mg)	Not available		0.3
Folic acid (mcg)	400	400	400
Niacin (mg)	18	15	20
Pantothenic acid (mg)	Not available		10
Pyridoxine (mg)	2.2	2.0	2.0
Riboflavin (mg)	1.6	1.2	1.7
Thiamine (mg)	1.4	1.0	1.5
Vitamin A (mcg)	1,000	800	1,000
(IU)	5,000	4,000	5,000
Vitamin B$_{12}$ (mcg)	3	3	6
Vitamin C (mg)	60	60	60
Vitamin D (mcg)	5	5	10
(IU)	200	200	400
Vitamin E (mg)	10	8	30

take supplements of pyridoxine (vitamin B$_6$) (see also Drugs used to treat menstrual disorders, p.188).

Risks and special precautions
Vitamins are natural substances, and supplements can be taken without risk by most people. It is, however, important to be careful not to exceed the recommended dosage, particularly in the case of fat-soluble vitamins, which may accumulate in the body. Dosage needs to be carefully calculated, taking account of the degree of deficiency, dietary intake, and duration of treatment. Overdosage has at best no therapeutic value and at worst may incur the risk of serious harmful effects. Preparations containing several times the recommended daily intake are best avoided except on medical advice. Multivitamin preparations containing a large number of different vitamins are widely available. Fortunately, the amounts of each vitamin contained in each tablet are not usually large and are not likely to be harmful unless the dose is greatly exceeded. Single vitamin supplements can be harmful because an excess of one vitamin may increase requirements for others. For specific information on each vitamin, see Part 4, pp.534 – 546.

FAT-SOLUBLE AND WATER-SOLUBLE VITAMINS

Fat-soluble vitamins
Vitamins A, D, E, and K are absorbed from the small intestine into the bloodstream together with fat (see also How drugs pass through the body, p.17). Deficiency of these vitamins may occur as a result of any disorder that affects the absorption of fat (for example, sprue). These vitamins are stored in the liver. Reserves of some of them may last for several years. But taking an excess of a fat-soluble vitamin may cause it to build up to a harmful level in the body. Ensuring that foods rich in these vitamins are regularly included in the diet usually provides a sufficient supply without the risk of overdosage.

Water-soluble vitamins
Vitamin C and the B vitamins dissolve in water. Most are stored in the body for only a short period and are rapidly excreted by the kidneys if taken in higher amounts than the body requires. Vitamin B$_{12}$ is the exception; it is stored in the liver, which may hold up to four years' supply. For these reasons foods containing water-soluble vitamins need to be eaten daily. These vitamins are easily lost in cooking, so raw foods containing them should be eaten regularly. An overdose of water-soluble vitamins does not usually cause toxic effects, but adverse reactions to large dosages of vitamin C and pyridoxine (vitamin B$_6$) have been reported.

MALIGNANT AND IMMUNE DISEASE

The creation and growth of new cells are continuously needed by the body – to replace cells that wear out and die naturally, and to repair injured tissue. Under normal circumstances the rate at which cell reproduction takes place is carefully regulated.

But sometimes abnormal cells are formed, and sometimes they multiply uncontrollably. They may form lumps of abnormal tissue (tumors), which are considered benign if they remain in one type of body tissue, malignant if they spread into others. The abnormal cells may also invade tissue and impair function. In any event, the growth and spread of abnormal cells defines cancer.

Opposing such actions, often effectively, are the workings of the immune system. It can recognize unfamiliar cells, not only those of infectious bacteria and viruses but also the cells of transplanted tissues. The immune system relies on different types of white blood cells produced in the lymph glands and the bone marrow. They respond to foreign cells in a variety of ways (facing page).

The activity of the immune system is also responsible for allergic reactions (see page 151).

What can go wrong

There are many different types of cancer, some more deadly than others, and they strike different parts of the body. Although medical science does not identify a single "cause" of cancer, certain outside factors (carcinogens) can often provoke the formation of abnormal cells. Tobacco smoke, for example, is a factor in lung cancer; people with light complexions and long-term exposure to sunlight display a higher-than-average incidence of skin cancer. In one form or another, cancer seems to catch up to nearly everyone who lives to old age, and many physicians now believe that genetic faults increase the risk of certain cancers.

Failure of the immune system can lead to increased susceptibility to infections and to the proliferation of malignant cells. Such failure can result from infection by human immunodeficiency virus (HIV), followed by the various other diseases associated with AIDS. Immune system function can also be reduced by some types of drug, either deliberately or as an unavoidable consequence of necessary drug treatment.

In some cases the immune system triggers an inappropriate attack on the body's own tissue, leading to a wide variety of disorders known collectively as autoimmune diseases. Common conditions that are thought to be caused by auto-

Types of cancer

Uncontrolled multiplication of cells leads to the formation of tumors that may be benign or malignant. Benign tumors do not spread to other tissues; malignant (cancerous) tumors do. Some of the main types of cancer are defined below.

Type of cancer	Tissues affected
Carcinoma	Skin and glandular tissue lining cells of internal organs
Sarcoma	Muscles, bones, and fibrous tissues and lining cells of vessels
Leukemia	White blood cells
Lymphoma	Lymph glands

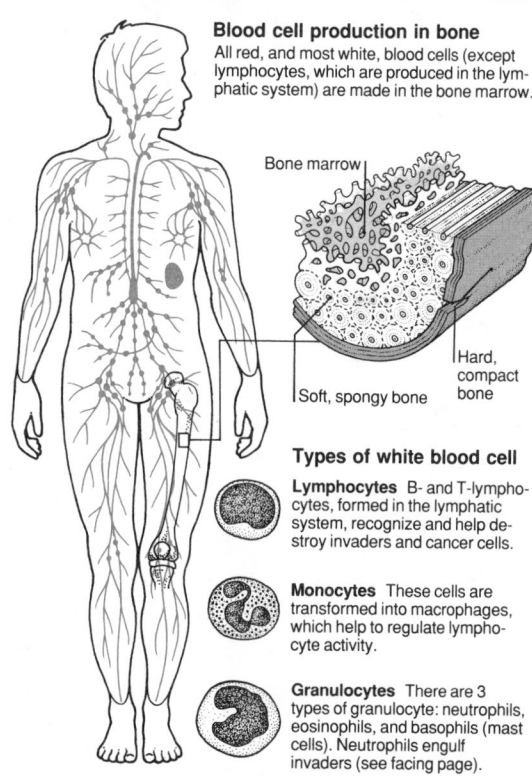

Blood cell production in bone
All red, and most white, blood cells (except lymphocytes, which are produced in the lymphatic system) are made in the bone marrow.

Bone marrow

Hard, compact bone

Soft, spongy bone

Types of white blood cell

Lymphocytes B- and T-lymphocytes, formed in the lymphatic system, recognize and help destroy invaders and cancer cells.

Monocytes These cells are transformed into macrophages, which help to regulate lymphocyte activity.

Granulocytes There are 3 types of granulocyte: neutrophils, eosinophils, and basophils (mast cells). Neutrophils engulf invaders (see facing page).

immune activity include rheumatoid arthritis, inflammatory skin disorders (lupus erythematosus), and some forms of hypothyroidism.

Immune system activity can also be troublesome following an organ or tissue transplant, when it may lead to rejection of the foreign tissue.

Why drugs are used

Drugs act on the mechanisms that lead to malignant and immune disease in a variety of ways. Cytotoxic (cell-killing) drugs are used to

Types of immune response

A specific response occurs when the immune system recognizes an invader. Two types of specific response, humoral and cellular, are described below. Phagocytosis, a non-specific response that does not depend on recognition of the invader, is also described.

Humoral response

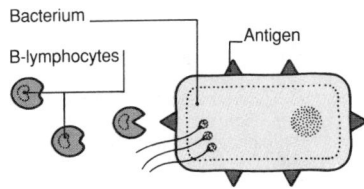

B-lymphocytes are activated by unfamiliar proteins (antigens) on the surface of the invading bacterium.

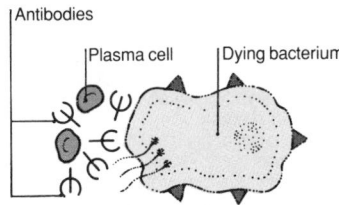

The activated B-lymphocytes form plasma cells, which release antibodies that bind to the invader and kill it.

Cellular response

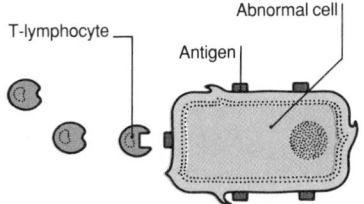

T-lymphocytes recognize the antigens on abnormal or invading cells.

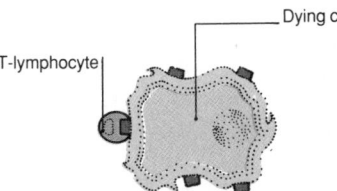

The T-lymphocytes bind to the abnormal cell and destroy it by altering chemical activity within the cell.

Engulfing invaders (phagocytosis)

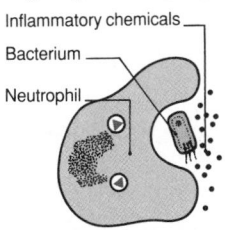

Certain cells such as neutrophils are attracted by inflammatory chemicals to an area of bacterial infection.

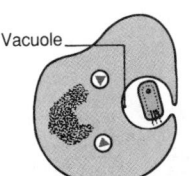

The neutrophil flows around the bacterium, enclosing it within a fluid-filled space called a vacuole.

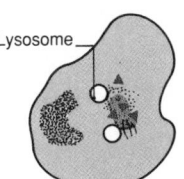

When the vacuole is formed, enzymes from areas called lysosomes within the neutrophil destroy the bacterium.

INTERFERONS

Interferons are natural proteins that limit viral infection by inhibiting viral replication within body cells. These substances also assist in the destruction of cancer cells.

Effect on viral infection

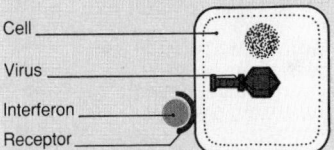

Interferon binds to receptors on a virus-infected cell.

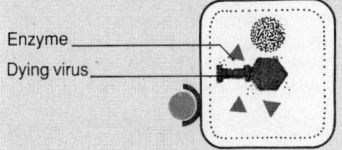

The presence of interferon triggers the release of enzymes that block viral replication. The virus is thus destroyed.

Effect on cancer cells

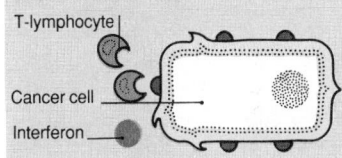

Interferon produced in response to a cancer cell activates T-lymphocytes.

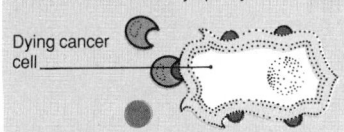

T-lymphocytes attack and destroy the cancer cell.

eliminate abnormally dividing cells in cancer. These drugs act against all rapidly dividing cells. They also reduce the numbers of blood cells being produced by the bone marrow. This can cause serious adverse effects like anemia, but it can also be useful for limiting white blood cell activity in autoimmune disorders. Other drugs also have an immunosuppressant effect, including corticosteroids and cyclosporine, used following transplant surgery.

No drugs are yet available that directly stimulate immune system activity for use in the treatment of immune-deficiency diseases. Drugs are used to treat the consequences of immune deficiency. Examples include antibiotic, antiviral, and anticancer drugs.

MAJOR DRUG GROUPS

Anticancer drugs
Immunosuppressant drugs
Drugs for AIDS and immune deficiency

ANTICANCER DRUGS

The body's cells normally grow and divide in an organized way; cells that are old or damaged are regularly replaced by new, healthy cells. Sometimes, however, a single cell becomes free from the controls that regulate cell division, and it multiplies at an unchecked rate. Such excessive growth usually leads to the production of a tumor, which may be either benign or malignant.

A benign tumor grows slowly and is restricted to a particular area; it produces harmful effects only when it causes pressure on surrounding tissues. A malignant tumor – usually referred to as cancer – tends to spread to other parts of the body; this occurs when the original tumor invades neighboring tissues or when cells break off and are carried to other parts of the body, where they start to grow. The secondary growths that result are known as metastases. Cancerous cells are frequently unable to perform their usual functions, and this leads to progres-

sively impaired function of the organ or area concerned.

There are many different factors that can provoke cancerous changes in cells. A combination of factors may be involved, notably an individual's genetic background, immune system failure, dietary factors, certain viruses, and overexposure to cancer-causing substances (carcinogens) such as strong sunlight, radiation, chemicals, and tobacco smoke.

Treating cancer is a complicated process that depends on the type of cancer, its stage of development, and the patient's condition and wishes. Any of the following treatments may be used on its own or in combination: surgical removal of the cancer, radiation treatment, and chemotherapy (the use of anticancer drugs).

Anticancer drugs that kill cancer cells are sometimes referred to as cytotoxic drugs. They fall into several classes, according to their chemical composition

and principal mode of action: alkylating agents, antimetabolites, and cytotoxic antibiotics are among the most widely used classes. In addition to these drugs, sex hormones and related substances are also used to treat some types of cancer.

Why they are used

Anticancer drugs are the treatment of choice for leukemias, lymphatic cancers, and certain forms of cancer of the testicles. They are particularly useful for rapidly spreading cancers, but are less effective in the treatment of solid tumors. A fuller listing of cancers in which treatment with drugs may be of benefit is included in the box below. Hormone treatment is offered in most cases of hormone-sensitive cancer, including some forms of breast cancer and cancer of the uterus.

Since all anticancer drugs may produce severe adverse effects (see facing page), they are used only when

SUCCESSFUL CHEMOTHERAPY

Not all cancers respond to treatment with anticancer drugs. Some cancers can be cured by drug treatment. In others, drug treatment can slow or temporarily halt the progress of the disease. In a certain number of cases, drug treatment has no beneficial effect, although in some of these cases other treatments, such as surgery, often produce significant benefits. The table at right summarizes the main cancers that fall into each of the three groups described.

Successful drug treatment of cancer normally requires repeated courses of

anticancer drugs, because treatment needs to be halted periodically to allow the blood-producing cells in the bone marrow to recover. The diagram below shows the number of cancer cells and normal blood cells before and after each course of treatment with cytotoxic anticancer drugs during successful chemotherapy. Both cancer cells and blood cells are reduced, but the blood cells recover quickly between courses of drug treatment. When treatment is effective, the number of cancer cells is reduced, so that they no longer cause symptoms.

Response to chemotherapy

Cancers that can be cured by drugs
Some cancers of the lymphatic system (including Hodgkin's disease)
Acute lymphoblastic leukemia (a form of blood cancer)
Choriocarcinoma (cancer of the placenta)
Germ cell tumors (cancers affecting sperm and egg cells)
Wilms' tumor (a rare form of kidney cancer that affects children)
Cancer of the testicles

Cancers in which drugs produce worthwhile benefits
Breast cancer
Ovarian cancer
Some leukemias
Multiple myeloma (a bone marrow cancer)
Small cell cancer of the lung
Cancer of the prostate
Some cancers of the lymphatic system
Cancer of the islet cells of the pancreas
Endometrial cancer (cancer affecting the lining of the uterus)

Cancers in which drugs are unlikely to be of benefit
Bladder cancer
Non-small cell cancer of the lung
Head and neck cancers
Cancer of the stomach
Thyroid cancer
Brain cancer
Malignant melanoma (a form of skin cancer)
Cancer of the soft tissues
Liver cancer
Cancer of the pancreas
Cancer of the cervix
Cancer of the large intestine
Cancer of the esophagus
Kidney cell cancer

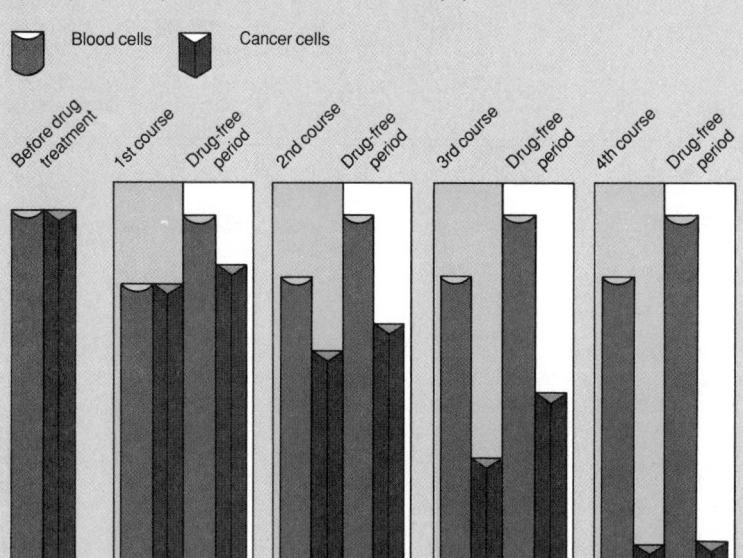

Blood cells   Cancer cells

Before drug treatment | 1st course | Drug-free period | 2nd course | Drug-free period | 3rd course | Drug-free period | 4th course | Drug-free period

there is a reasonable chance of achieving a complete cure, or of significantly prolonging life. Their effectiveness varies a great deal, depending primarily on the type of cancer and the extent of its spread.

Chemotherapy can also be useful after surgical removal of a tumor, or following radiation treatment, to kill any cancer cells that remain.

The choice of anticancer drug depends on the type of cancer and the condition of the person being treated. No class of anticancer drugs is used specifically for a particular cancer; individual drugs have separate properties and uses. Often several drugs are used, either simultaneously or successively.

Certain anticancer drugs are also used for their effect in suppressing immune system activity (see p.184).

How they work

All cytotoxic anticancer drugs kill cancer cells by preventing them from growing or dividing. Cells grow and divide in several stages. Most anticancer drugs act on one specific stage. During treatment, several drugs may be given in sequence in order to eliminate abnormal cells at all stages of development. ·

Hormone treatments work by opposing the effects of the hormone that encourages the growth of the cancer. For example, some breast cancers are stimulated by the female sex hormone estrogen. Spread of the cancer may thus be limited by a drug, such as tamoxifen, that opposes the effects of estrogen. Other hormone-sensitive cancers are damaged by high doses of a particular sex hormone. Diethylstilbestrol, an estrogen, often halts the spread of cancer of the prostate.

How they affect you

At the start of treatment adverse effects of cytotoxic anticancer drugs are likely to be more noticeable than benefits. The most common side effect is nausea and vomiting, for which an anti-emetic drug (see p.118) may be prescribed. Diarrhea is also a common side effect. Many anticancer drugs cause hair loss because of the effect of their activity on the cells of the hair follicles, but the hair usually starts to regrow after chemotherapy has been completed. Individual drugs may produce other side effects, which physicians monitor.

Anticancer drugs are usually administered in the highest doses that can be tolerated in order to kill as many cancer cells as quickly as possible, and therefore to reduce the risk of the cancer spreading to other parts of the body and forming metastases.

Beneficial effects on the underlying

ACTION OF CYTOTOXIC ANTICANCER DRUGS

Each type of cytotoxic drug affects a separate stage of the cancer cell's development, and each type of drug kills the cell by a different mechanism of action. The action of some of the principal classes of cytotoxic drugs is described below.

Alkylating agents and cytotoxic antibiotics
These act within the cell's nucleus to damage the cell's genetic material, DNA. This prevents the cell from growing and dividing.

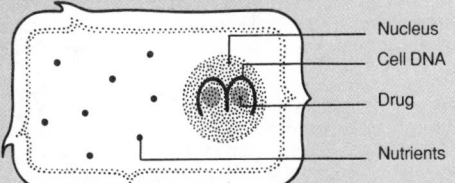

Nucleus
Cell DNA
Drug
Nutrients

Antimetabolites
These drugs prevent the cell from *metabolizing* (processing) nutrients and other substances that are necessary for normal activity in the cell.

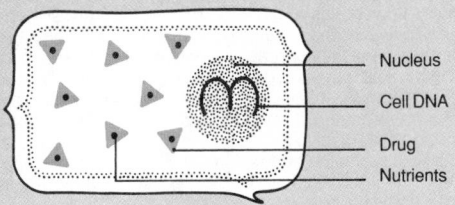

Nucleus
Cell DNA
Drug
Nutrients

disease may not be apparent for several weeks. The unpleasant side effects of intensive cancer chemotherapy, combined with the lack of immediate response to the treatment, often lead to depression among those receiving anticancer drugs. Specialist counseling may be helpful.

Risks and special precautions

All cytotoxic anticancer drugs interfere with the activity of non-cancerous cells, and for this reason they often produce serious adverse effects during long-term treatment. In particular, these drugs often adversely affect the blood-producing cells in the bone marrow. The number of both red and white cells and the number of platelets (particles in the blood which are responsible for clotting) may all be reduced. In some cases, symptoms of anemia (weakness and fatigue) and an increased risk of abnormal or excessive bleeding may develop as a result of treatment. In addition, wounds may take longer to heal, and susceptible people can develop gout as a result of increased release of uric acid (a by-product of cell destruction). Reduction in the number of white blood cells may result in an increased susceptibility to infection.

Because of these problems, anticancer chemotherapy is often given in a hospital, where the effects can be closely monitored. Several short courses of drug treatment are often given, thus allowing the bone marrow time to recover in the intervening period

(see Successful chemotherapy, facing page). Blood tests are performed regularly. Where necessary, blood transfusions, antibiotics, or other forms of treatment are used to overcome the adverse effects. Where relevant, contraceptive advice is given early in treatment, because most anticancer drugs can damage a developing baby.

In addition to these general effects, individual drugs may have adverse effects on particular organs. These are described in the drug profiles in Part 4.

COMMON DRUGS

Alkylating agents
Chlorambucil
Cisplatin
Cyclophosphamide
Melphalan

Antimetabolites
Fluorouracil
Mercaptopurine
Methotrexate

Cytotoxic antibiotic
Doxorubicin

Hormone treatments
Aminoglutethimide
Diethylstilbestrol
Ethinyl estradiol
Medroxyprogesterone
Megestrol
Nandrolone
Tamoxifen

Other drug
Procarbazine

IMMUNOSUPPRESSANT DRUGS

The body is protected against attack from bacteria and viruses by the specialized cells and proteins in the blood and tissues that make up the immune system (see p.180). White blood cells known as lymphocytes either kill these invading organisms directly or produce special proteins (*antibodies*) to destroy them. These mechanisms are also responsible for eliminating abnormal or unhealthy cells that could otherwise multiply and develop into a cancer.

In certain conditions, it is medically necessary to dampen the activity of the immune system. These include a number of autoimmune disorders in which the immune system attacks normal body tissue. Autoimmune disorders may affect a single organ – for example, the kidneys in Goodpasture's syndrome or the thyroid gland in Hashimoto's disease – or may cause widespread damage, as in rheumatoid arthritis or systemic lupus erythematosus.

Immune-system activity may also need to be reduced following an organ transplant, when the body's defenses would otherwise attack and reject the transplanted tissue.

Several types of drugs are used as immunosuppressants: anticancer drugs (p.182), corticosteroids (p.169), and a new drug, cyclosporine.

Why they are used

Immunosuppressant drugs are given in autoimmune disorders such as rheumatoid arthritis when symptoms are severe and other treatments have not provided adequate relief. Cortico-steroids are usually prescribed initially. The pronounced anti-inflammatory effect of these drugs, in addition to their immunosuppressant action, helps to promote healing of tissue damaged by abnormal immune-system activity. Anti-cancer drugs such as azathioprine may be used in addition to corticosteroids if these do not produce sufficient improvement or if their effect wanes (see also Antirheumatic drugs, p.145).

Immunosuppressant drugs are given before and after organ and other tissue transplants. Treatment may have to continue permanently following the transplant to prevent rejection. A number of drugs and drug combinations are used, depending on the organ or tissue being transplanted and the underlying condition of the recipient. Corticosteroids in conjunction with azathioprine were until recently the most widely used therapy. However, cyclo-sporine, a new drug, is now being used increasingly for preventing organ rejection, and is currently being studied to evaluate its possible usefulness in the treatment of autoimmune disorders.

How they work

Immunosuppressant drugs reduce the effectiveness of the immune system, either by depressing the production of lymphocytes or by altering their activity.

How they affect you

When immunosuppressants are given to treat an autoimmune disorder they reduce the severity of the symptoms and in many cases temporarily halt the progress of the disease. However, they cannot restore major tissue damage, such as damage to the joints in rheumatoid arthritis.

Corticosteroids often promote a general feeling of well-being, but given in doses high enough to produce an immunosuppressant effect, they may also produce unwanted effects. These are described in more detail on p.169. Anticancer drugs, when prescribed as immunosuppressants, are given in low doses that produce only mild side effects. They may cause nausea and vomiting, for which an anti-emetic drug (p.118) may be prescribed. Hair loss may occur, but hair growth usually resumes when the drug is discontinued. Cyclosporine may cause increased growth of facial hair, swelling of the gums, and tingling in the hands.

Risks and special precautions

All of these drugs may produce potentially serious adverse effects. By reducing immune system activity, immunosuppressant drugs can affect the body's ability to fight invading micro-organisms, thereby increasing the risk of serious infections, such as those described on the facing page. Because lymphocyte activity is also important for preventing the multiplication of abnormal cells, there is an increased risk of certain types of cancer. A major drawback of anticancer drugs is that, in addition to their effect on the production of lymphocytes, they interfere with the growth and division of other blood cells in the bone marrow. Reduced production of red blood cells can cause *anemia*; when the production of blood platelets is suppressed, blood clotting may be less efficient.

Because cyclosporine is more specific in its action than corticosteroids or anticancer drugs, it produces fewer troublesome side effects. However, it may cause kidney damage, and in too high a dose may affect the brain, causing hallucinations or seizures. Cyclosporine also tends to raise blood pressure, and another drug may be required to counteract this effect (see Antihypertensive drugs, p.130).

ACTION OF IMMUNOSUPPRESSANTS

Before treatment
Many types of blood cell, each with a distinct role, form in the bone marrow. Lymphocytes respond to infection and foreign tissue. B-lymphocytes produce antibodies to attack invading organisms, whereas T-lymphocytes directly attack invading cells. Others help the action of the B- and T-cells.

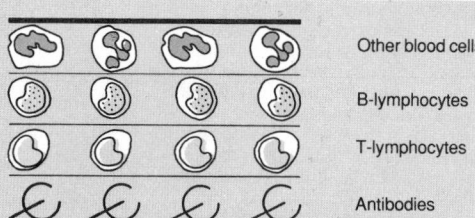

Other blood cells

B-lymphocytes

T-lymphocytes

Antibodies

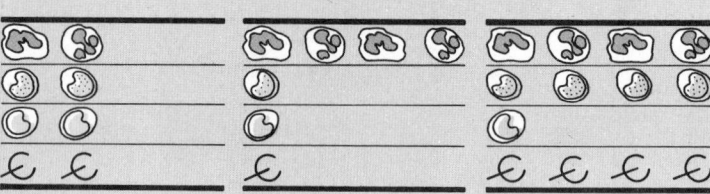

Anticancer drugs
Anticancer drugs slow the production of all cells in the bone marrow.

Corticosteroids
These reduce both B- and T-lymphocyte activity.

Cyclosporine
This inhibits the activity of T-lymphocytes only, and not the activity of B-lymphocytes.

COMMON DRUGS

Anticancer drugs
Azathioprine
Chlorambucil
Cyclophosphamide
Methotrexate

Corticosteroids
See p.169

Other drugs
Antilymphocyte globulin
Cyclosporine

DRUGS FOR AIDS AND IMMUNE DEFICIENCY

Immune deficiency occurs when the body's immune system, which normally protects the body against infecting organisms and the development of cancer, fails. Immune deficiency may be present from birth because the body's immune system has not developed normally, or it may occur during drug treatment (for example, with corticosteroids or anticancer drugs), or as a result of cancer or infection.

AIDS (acquired immune deficiency syndrome) is a disorder caused by infection with HIV (human immunodeficiency virus). The virus invades certain types of cells, particularly the white blood cells known as T-helper lymphocytes. T-helper lymphocytes normally activate other cells in the immune system to produce antibodies to fight infection. Because the AIDS virus kills T-helper lymphocytes, the body is unable to fight the AIDS virus or any subsequent infection.

All immune-deficiency disorders increase susceptibility to certain types of cancer and recurrent or persistent infections. Illnesses that commonly affect people with impaired immunity include gastroenteritis, herpes simplex infections, shingles, Kaposi's sarcoma (a rare form of skin cancer), pneumocystis carinii (a rare form of pneumonia), and dementia.

There is no known cure for any of the immune-deficiency disorders. Drugs can be used to treat the conditions that develop as a result.

Why they are used

Serious infections are the most common consequence of all immune-deficiency disorders. These are treated with a variety of antibiotics (p.156), antibacterial drugs (p.159), antiviral drugs (p.161), and antifungal drugs (p.166). The antiprotozoal drug pentamidine may be used to treat pneumocystis carinii. Kaposi's sarcoma and other cancers are not consistently treated with anticancer drugs, since there is an added risk of depressing the immune system. Radiation therapy may be given instead.

When serious AIDS-related infections have occurred, the new antiviral drug zidovudine, originally known as AZT (azidothymidine), may be prescribed. This does not provide a cure but may prolong life expectancy.

New drugs

Current research into new drug treatment for AIDS is proceeding along two principal lines. Scientists are searching for a vaccine that will provide immunity against the AIDS virus, and they are also trying to develop drugs to eradicate the HIV virus from the body once infection has occurred (see box, right).

AIDS INFECTION AND POSSIBLE TREATMENTS

The illustrations below show how the AIDS virus enters body cells and, once inside, replicates itself to produce new viruses. The stages at which drugs might in the future be used to block the action of AIDS viruses, or destroy them, are also indicated.

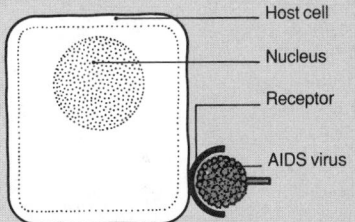

Host cell
Nucleus
Receptor
AIDS virus

Stage 1
The virus binds to a specialized site (receptor) on a body cell.

Possible drug intervention
Binding could be blocked by the production of antibodies to destroy the virus or the cell's receptor.

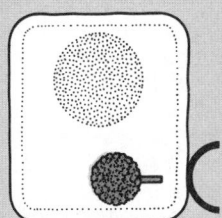

Stage 2
The virus enters the cell.

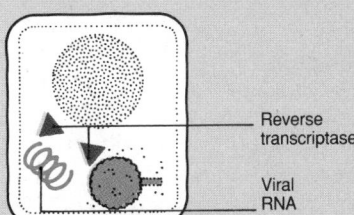

Reverse transcriptase
Viral RNA

Stage 3
The virus loses its protective coat and releases RNA, its genetic material, and an enzyme known as reverse transcriptase.

Possible drug intervention
Drugs may be developed to prevent the virus from losing its protective coat. Amantadine has this effect on the influenza A virus but not on HIV.

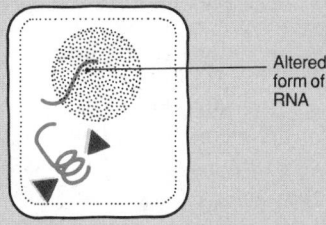

Altered form of RNA

Stage 4
The enzyme reverse transcriptase converts the viral RNA into a form that can then enter the host cell's nucleus and may become integrated with the cell's genetic material.

Possible drug intervention
Zidovudine blocks the action of reverse transcriptase.

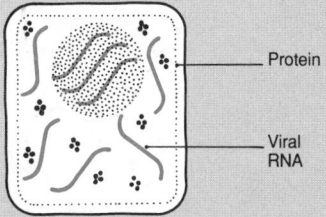

Protein
Viral RNA

Stage 5
The host cell starts to produce new viral RNA and protein from the viral material that has been incorporated into its nucleus.

Possible drug intervention
There is a possibility that in the future drugs may be available to inhibit the production of new viral RNA and proteins by altering genes on the viral material.

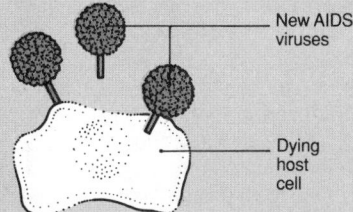

New AIDS viruses
Dying host cell

Stage 6
The new viral RNA and proteins are assembled to produce new viruses. These leave the host cell (which then dies) and are free to attack other cells in the body.

Possible drug intervention
The drug alpha interferon prevents the new viruses from leaving the cell. It is under investigation for limiting the spread of AIDS infection within the body.

REPRODUCTIVE & URINARY TRACTS

The reproductive systems of men and women consist of those organs which produce and release sperm (male), store and release eggs (female), and then nurture a fertilized egg until it becomes a baby (female).

The urinary system filters wastes and water from the blood, producing urine, which is then expelled from the body. The reproductive and urinary systems of men are partially linked, but those of women form two physically close but functionally separate systems.

The female reproductive organs comprise the ovaries, fallopian tubes, and uterus (womb). The uterus opens via the cervix (neck of the uterus) into the vagina. The principal male reproductive organs are the two sperm-producing glands – the testicles (testes) contained in the scrotum – and the penis. Other parts of the male reproductive tract include the prostate gland and several tubular structures: the epididymis, the vas deferens, the seminal vesicles, and the urethra (see right).

The urinary organs in both sexes comprise the kidneys, which filter blood and excrete urine (see also p.127), the ureters down which urine passes, and the bladder, where urine is stored until it is released from the body via the urethra.

What can go wrong

The reproductive and urinary tracts are both subject to infection. Such infections (apart from those transmitted by sexual activity) are relatively uncommon in men because the long male urethra prevents bacteria and other organisms from passing easily to the bladder and upper urinary tract and to the male sex organs. The shorter female urethra allows infection of the urinary tract, especially of the bladder (cystitis) and of the urethra (urethritis), to occur commonly. The female reproductive tract is also vulnerable to infection, sometimes sexually transmitted.

Reproductive function may also be disrupted by hormonal disturbances that lead to reduced fertility. Women may be troubled by symptoms arising from normal activity of the reproductive organs, including menstrual disorders and problems associated with childbirth.

The most common urinary problems apart from infection are those related to bladder function. Urine may be released involuntarily (incontinence) or it may be retained in the bladder. Such disorders are usually the result of abnormal nerve signals to the bladder or sphincter muscle. The filtering action of the kidneys may be disrupted by

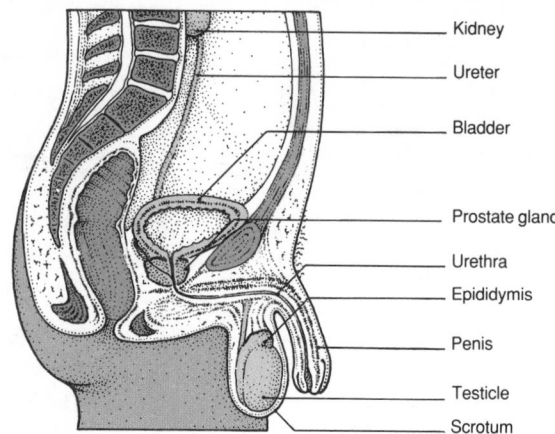

Male reproductive system
Sperm produced in each of the testicles pass into the epididymis, a tightly coiled tube in which the sperm mature before passing along the vas deferens to the seminal vesicles. Sperm are stored in the seminal vesicles until they are ejaculated from the penis via the urethra together with seminal fluid and secretions from the prostate gland.

- Kidney
- Ureter
- Bladder
- Prostate gland
- Urethra
- Epididymis
- Penis
- Testicle
- Scrotum

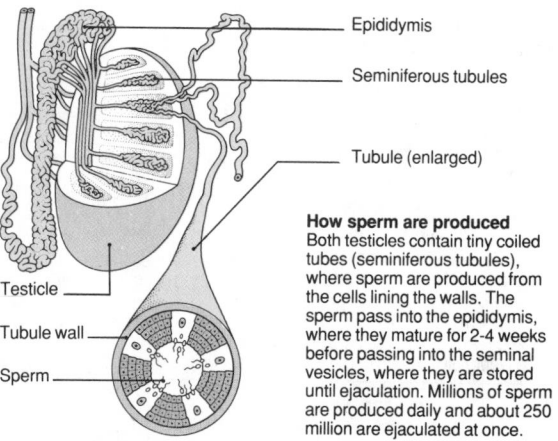

- Epididymis
- Seminiferous tubules
- Tubule (enlarged)
- Testicle
- Tubule wall
- Sperm

How sperm are produced
Both testicles contain tiny coiled tubes (seminiferous tubules), where sperm are produced from the cells lining the walls. The sperm pass into the epididymis, where they mature for 2-4 weeks before passing into the seminal vesicles, where they are stored until ejaculation. Millions of sperm are produced daily and about 250 million are ejaculated at once.

alteration of the composition of the blood or the hormones that regulate urination, or by damage (from infection or inflammation) to the filtering units themselves.

Why drugs are used

Antibiotic drugs (p.156) are used to eliminate both urinary and reproductive tract infections (including sexually transmitted infections). Certain infections of the vagina are caused by fungi or yeasts and require antifungal drugs (p.166).

Hormone drugs are used both to reduce fertility deliberately (oral contraceptives) and to increase fertility in certain conditions that make it impossible

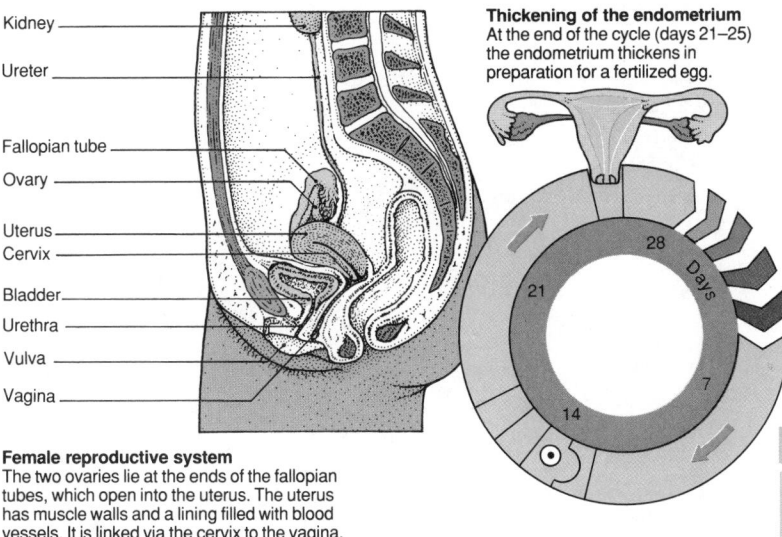

Kidney

Ureter

Fallopian tube

Ovary

Uterus

Cervix

Bladder

Urethra

Vulva

Vagina

Thickening of the endometrium
At the end of the cycle (days 21–25) the endometrium thickens in preparation for a fertilized egg.

Female reproductive system
The two ovaries lie at the ends of the fallopian tubes, which open into the uterus. The uterus has muscle walls and a lining filled with blood vessels. It is linked via the cervix to the vagina.

Menstrual cycle
A monthly cycle of hormone interactions allows an egg to be released and, if it is fertilized, creates the correct environment for it to implant in the uterus. Major body changes occur, most obviously, monthly vaginal bleeding (menstruation). The cycle usually starts between 11 and 14 years, and continues until the menopause, which occurs at around 50. After the menopause, childbearing is no longer possible. The cycle is usually 28 days, but this varies with individuals.

Menstruation
If no egg is fertilized, the endometrium is shed (days 1–5).

Fertile period
Conception may take place in the two days after ovulation (days 14–16).

URINARY SYSTEM

The kidneys extract waste and excess water from the blood. The waste liquid (urine) passes into the bladder, from which it is expelled via the urethra.

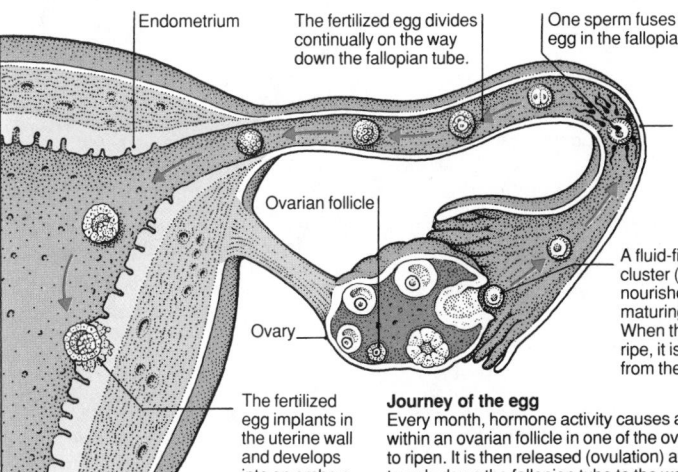

Endometrium

The fertilized egg divides continually on the way down the fallopian tube.

One sperm fuses with the egg in the fallopian tube.

Fallopian tube

Ovarian follicle

A fluid-filled cell cluster (follicle) nourishes the maturing egg. When the egg is ripe, it is released from the follicle.

Ovary

The fertilized egg implants in the uterine wall and develops into an embryo.

Journey of the egg
Every month, hormone activity causes an egg within an ovarian follicle in one of the ovaries to ripen. It is then released (ovulation) and travels down the fallopian tube to the womb.

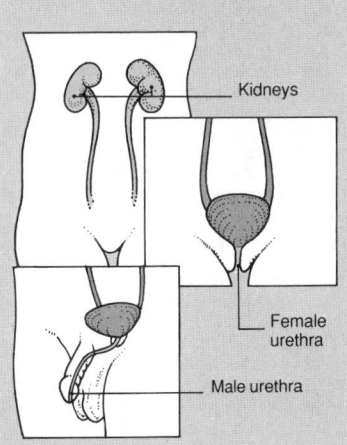

Kidneys

Female urethra

Male urethra

for a couple to conceive. Hormones may also be used to regulate menstruation when this is irregular or excessively painful or heavy. Analgesic drugs (p.108) are used to treat menstrual period pain and are also widely used for pain relief in labor. Other drugs used in labor include those that increase contraction of the muscles of the uterus and those that limit blood loss after the birth. Drugs may also be employed to halt premature labor (see Drugs used in labor, p.193).

Drugs that alter the transmission of nerve signals to the bladder muscles have an important role in the treatment of urinary incontinence and retention. Drugs that increase the filtering action of the kidneys are commonly used to reduce blood pressure and fluid retention (see Diuretics, p.127). Other drugs may alter the composition of the urine, such as the uricosuric drugs used in the treatment of gout (p.147).

MAJOR DRUG GROUPS

Drugs used to treat menstrual disorders
Oral contraceptives
Drugs for infertility
Drugs used in labor
Drugs used for urinary disorders

DRUGS USED TO TREAT MENSTRUAL DISORDERS

The menstrual cycle results from the actions of female sex hormones that each month cause ovulation (release of an egg) and thickening of the endometrium (lining of the uterus) in preparation for pregnancy. Unless the egg is fertilized, the endometrium is shed about two weeks later during menstruation (see also p.187).

The main problems associated with menstruation that may require medical treatment are excessive blood loss (menorrhagia), pain during menstruation (dysmenorrhea), and distressing symptoms prior to menstruation (premenstrual syndrome). Absence of periods (amenorrhea) is discussed under Female sex hormones (p.175).

The drugs most commonly used to treat the menstrual disorders described above include estrogens and progesterone (or synthetic progesterone drugs known as progestins), danazol, and analgesics.

Why they are used

Drug treatment for menstrual disorders is undertaken only when the physician has ruled out the possibility of an underlying gynecological disorder such as pelvic infection or fibroids. In some cases, especially in women over the age of 35, a D and C (dilatation and curettage) may be recommended. When no underlying reason for the problem has been found, drug treatment aimed primarily at the relief of symptoms is usually prescribed.

Dysmenorrhea

Painful menstrual periods are usually treated initially with a simple analgesic (see also p.108). Aspirin and a non-steroidal anti-inflammatory drug (mefenamic acid) are often most effective because they are thought to counter the effects of chemicals called prostaglandins, which are considered to be partly responsible for transmission of pain. Mefenamic acid is also used to reduce blood loss in menorrhagia (below). When these drugs fail to provide sufficient relief of pain, hormonal drug treatment may be advised. If contraception is also required, treatment may take the form of an oral contraceptive pill containing an estrogen and a progestin, or a progestin alone. However, non-contraceptive progestin preparations are also used. These may be taken for only a few days during each month. Treatment of dysmenorrhea caused by endometriosis is described in the box above right.

Menorrhagia

Excessive blood loss during menstruation can sometimes be reduced by mefenamic acid. But in many cases

ENDOMETRIOSIS

Endometriosis is a condition in which fragments of endometrial tissue (uterine lining) occur outside the uterus in the pelvic cavity. This disorder causes severe pain during menstruation and often pain during intercourse; it may sometimes lead to infertility.

Drugs used for this disorder are similar to those prescribed for heavy periods (menorrhagia). However, in this case the intention is to suppress endometrial development for an extended period so that the abnormal tissue eventually withers away. Progesterone supplements that suppress thickening of endometrium may be prescribed throughout the menstrual cycle. Alternatively, danazol, a drug that suppresses endometrial development by reducing estrogen production, may be prescribed. Any drug treatment usually needs to be continued for a minimum of six months.

When drug treatment is unsuccessful, surgical removal of the abnormal tissue is usually necessary.

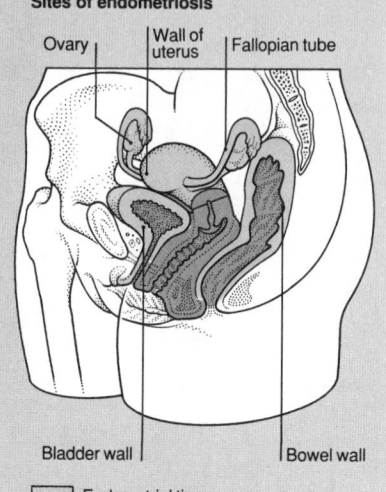

Sites of endometriosis

Ovary | Wall of uterus | Fallopian tube

Bladder wall | Bowel wall

☐ Endometrial tissue

hormone treatment, as described under dysmenorrhea (left), is advised. Alternatively, danazol, a drug that reduces production of the hormone estrogen, may be prescribed.

Premenstrual syndrome

This is a collection of psychological and physical symptoms that affect many women to some degree in the days prior to menstruation. Psychological symptoms include mood changes such as increased irritability, depression, and anxiety. Principal physical symptoms are bloating, headache, and breast tenderness. Because many physicians believe premenstrual syndrome to be the result of a drop in progesterone levels in the last half of the menstrual cycle, non-contraceptive supplements of this hormone may be given in the week or so prior to menstruation. Oral contraceptives may be considered as an alternative. Other drugs sometimes used include pyridoxine (vitamin B_6) for depression, diuretics (p.127) if bloating due to fluid retention is a problem, and bromocriptine when breast tenderness is the major symptom. Anti-anxiety drugs (p.111) may be prescribed in rare cases where severe premenstrual psychological disturbance is experienced.

How they work

Drugs used in menstrual disorders act in a variety of ways. Hormonal treatments are aimed at suppressing the pattern of hormonal changes that is causing troublesome symptoms. Contraceptive

preparations override the normal menstrual cycle. Ovulation does not occur and the endometrium does not thicken normally. Bleeding that occurs at the end of a cycle is less likely to be abnormally heavy, to be preceded by distressing symptoms, or to be accompanied by severe discomfort. For further information on oral contraceptives, see p.189.

Non-contraceptive progesterone preparations taken in the days prior to menstruation do not suppress ovulation. Increased progesterone during this time reduces premenstrual symptoms and prevents excessive thickening of the endometrium.

Danazol, a potent and expensive drug, prevents the thickening of the endometrium, thereby correcting excessively heavy periods. Blood loss is reduced; in some cases menstruation ceases altogether during treatment.

COMMON DRUGS

Estrogens and progestins
(see p.175)

Analgesics
Aspirin
Mefenamic acid

Diuretics
(see p.127)

Others
Bromocriptine
Danazol
Pyridoxine

ORAL CONTRACEPTIVES

There are many different means of ensuring that conception and pregnancy do not follow sexual intercourse, but for most women the oral contraceptive is the most effective method (see Comparison of reliability of different methods of contraception, right); it has the added advantage of being convenient and unobtrusive during lovemaking. About 15 per cent of women seeking contraceptive protection in the United States choose a form of oral contraceptive.

There are three main types of oral contraceptive: the combined pill, the progestin-only pill, and the phased pill. All types contain a progestin (a synthetic form of the female sex hormone progesterone); combined and phased pills also contain a natural or synthetic estrogen (see also Female sex hormones, p.175). All types are taken on a monthly cycle.

Why they are used
The combined pill
The most widely prescribed form of oral contraceptive and that with the lowest failure rate in terms of unwanted pregnancies, the combined pill (usually referred to simply as the "pill") is the type considered most suitable for young women who want to use a hormonal form of contraception. The combined pill is particularly suitable for some women who experience painful, heavy, or prolonged periods (see Drugs used to treat menstrual disorders, p.188).

There are many different products available containing a fixed dose of an estrogen and a progestin drug. They are generally divided into three groupings

COMPARISON OF RELIABILITY OF DIFFERENT METHODS OF CONTRACEPTION

The table (right) indicates the number of pregnancies that occur with each method of contraception among 100 women using that method in a year. The wide variation that occurs with some methods takes into account pregnancies that occur as a result of incorrect use of the method.

Method	Pregnancies*
Combined and phased pills	2 – 3
Progestin-only pill	2.5 – 4
IUCD**	4 – 9
Condom/diaphragm	3 – 20
Rhythm	25 – 30
Contraceptive sponge	9 – 27
Vaginal spermicide alone	2 – 30
No contraception	80 – 85

*Per 100 users per year
**Intra-uterine contraceptive device

according to their estrogen content: low dose, medium dose and high dose (see The hormone content of common oral contraceptives, below). Low dose products are selected whenever possible in order to minimize the risk of adverse effects.

Progestin-only pill
The progestin-only pill is often recommended for women who react adversely to the estrogen in the combined pill or for whom the combined pill is not considered suitable because of their age or medical history (see Risks and special precautions, p.191). It is also prescribed for women who are breast feeding, because it does not reduce milk supply. This form of pill is slightly less reliable

than the combined pill and must be taken at precisely the same time each day for maximum contraceptive effect.

Phased pills
Each pack of phased pills, the newest form of oral contraceptive, contains pills divided into two or three groups, or phases. Each phase contains a different proportion of an estrogen and a progestin. The aim is to provide a hormonal balance that more closely resembles the fluctuations of a normal menstrual cycle. Phased pills, taken in the same way as the combined pill, provide effective contraceptive protection for many women who suffer side effects from the other forms of oral contraceptive available.

How they work
In a normal menstrual cycle the ripening and release of an egg, and the preparation of the uterus for implantation of the fertilized egg, are the result of a complex interplay between the natural female sex hormones, estrogen and progesterone, and the pituitary hormones, follicle-stimulating hormone (FSH) and luteinizing hormone (LH) (see also p.175). Estrogen and progestins contained in oral contraceptives act in a variety of ways to disrupt the normal cycle in such a way as to make conception less likely.

In the combined and phased pills, increased levels of estrogen and progesterone produce effects similar to the hormonal changes of pregnancy. The actions of the hormones inhibit the production of FSH and LH, and thereby prevent the egg from ripening in the ovary and from being released.

The progestin-only pill has a slightly different action. It does not always prevent release of an egg; its main contraceptive effect may be on the

THE HORMONE CONTENT OF COMMON ORAL CONTRACEPTIVES

Oral contraceptive formulations vary according to their hormone content. Estrogen-containing formulations fall into three groups, depending on whether they contain less than

50 micrograms (mcg) of estrogen (low estrogen), 50mcg (medium estrogen), or more than 50mcg (high estrogen). All phased pills are low-estrogen formulations.

Type of pill	Brand names
Combined pills Low estrogen	Brevicon, Modicon, Ovcon-35, Ortho Novum 1/35, Norinyl 1 + 35, Nordette, Lo/Ovral, Loestrin 1.5/30, Loestrin 1/20, Demulen 1/35.
Medium estrogen	Ovcon-50, Ovral, Norlestrin 1/50, Norinyl 1 + 50, Ortho Novum 1/50, Demulen, Norlestrin 2.5/50.
High estrogen	Enovid E, Ovulen, Norinyl 2, Ortho Novum 2, Norinyl 1 + 80, Ortho Novum 1/80.
Phased pills (low estrogen)	Ortho Novum 10/11 + 7/7/7, Tri-Norinyl, Tri-Levlen, Tri-Phasil
Progestin-only pills (no estrogen)	Micronor, Nor QD, Ovrette.

ORAL CONTRACEPTIVES continued

BALANCING THE RISKS AND BENEFITS OF ORAL CONTRACEPTIVES

Oral contraceptives are safe for the vast majority of young women. However, every woman considering using this method of contraception should see her physician to discuss the risks and possible adverse effects of these drugs before deciding that a hormonal method is the most suitable in her case. A variety of factors must be taken into account, including the woman's age, her own medical history, and that of her close relatives, and additional factors such as whether she is a smoker. The importance of these factors varies according to the type of pill. The table below summarizes the main advantages and disadvantages of estrogen-containing and progestin-only pills.

Type of oral contraceptive	Estrogen-containing (combined and phased)	Progestin-only
Advantages	● Very reliable ● Convenient/unobtrusive ● Regularizes menstruation ● Reduced menstrual pain and blood loss ● Reduced risk of: ▼ benign breast disease ▼ endometriosis ▼ ectopic pregnancy ▼ ovarian cysts ▼ pelvic infection ▼ ovarian and endometrial cancer	● Reasonably reliable ● Convenient/unobtrusive ● Suitable during lactation ● Avoids estrogen-related side effects and risks ● Allows rapid return to fertility
Side effects	● Weight gain ● Depression ● Breast swelling ● Reduced sex drive ● Headaches ● Increased vaginal discharge ● Nausea	● Irregular menstruation
Risks	● Thrombosis/embolism ● Heart disease ● High blood pressure ● Jaundice ● Cancer of the liver (rare) ● Gallstones	● Ectopic pregnancy ● Ovarian cysts
Factors that may prohibit use	● Previous thrombosis ● Heart disease ● High levels of fat in blood ● Liver disease ● Blood disorders ● High blood pressure ● Unexplained vaginal bleeding ● Migraine ● Otosclerosis ● Presence of several risk factors (below)	● Previous ectopic pregnancy ● Heart or circulatory disease ● Unexplained vaginal bleeding
Factors that increase risks	● Smoking ● Obesity ● Increasing age ● Diabetes mellitus ● Family history of heart or circulatory disease ● Current treatment with other drugs	● As for estrogen-containing pills, but to a lesser degree

---

How to minimize your health risks while taking the pill

▼ Give up smoking.
▼ Maintain a healthy weight.
▼ Have regular blood pressure and blood fat checks.
▼ Have regular cervical smear tests.

▼ Remind your physician that you are taking oral contraceptives before taking other prescription drugs.
▼ Stop taking estrogen-containing oral contraceptives 4 weeks before planned major surgery (use alternative contraception).

mucus that lines the cervical canal, which thickens and becomes impenetrable to sperm. This effect also occurs to a lesser extent with combined and phased pills.

How they affect you

Each course of combined and phased pills lasts for 21 days, followed by a pill-free seven days during which menstruation occurs. Some brands contain seven additional inactive pills, sometimes containing an iron supplement. This means that the new course directly follows the last, so that the habit of taking the pill daily is not broken. Progestin-only pills are taken for 28 days each month. Menstruation usually occurs during the last few days of the cycle.

Women taking oral contraceptives, especially those containing estrogen, usually find that their menstrual periods are lighter and relatively pain-free. Some women cease to menstruate altogether. This is not a cause for concern in itself, providing no pills have been missed, but it may make it difficult to determine if pregnancy has occurred. An apparently missed period probably indicates a light one, rather than pregnancy. However, if you have missed two consecutive periods and you feel that you are pregnant, it is advisable to have a pregnancy test.

All forms of oral contraceptive may cause spotting of blood in mid-cycle ("breakthrough bleeding") especially at first, but this can be a particular problem

of the progestin-only pill.

The oral contraceptives containing estrogen may produce any of a large number of mild side effects depending on the dose. Symptoms similar to those experienced early in pregnancy may occur, particularly in the first few months of pill use: some women complain of nausea and vomiting, weight gain, depression, altered libido, increased appetite, and cramps in the legs and abdomen. The pill may also affect the circulation, producing minor headaches and dizziness. All these effects usually disappear within a few months, but if they persist, it may be advisable to change to a brand containing a lower dose of estrogen or to another contraceptive method.

Risks and special precautions

All oral contraceptives need to be taken regularly for maximum protection against pregnancy. Contraceptive protection can be reduced by missing a pill (see What to if you miss a pill, below). It may also be reduced by vomiting or diarrhea. If you suffer from either of these symptoms, it is advisable to act as if you had missed your last pill. Many drugs may also affect the action of oral contraceptives, so it is essential to inform your physician that you are taking oral contraceptives before taking additional prescribed medications.

Oral contraceptives, particularly those containing an estrogen, have been found to carry a number of risks. These are summarized in the box on the facing

page. One of the most serious potential adverse effects of estrogen-containing pills is development of a thrombus (blood clot) in a vein or artery, which may travel to the lungs or cause a stroke or heart attack. The risk of thrombus formation increases with age and other factors, notably obesity, high blood pressure, and smoking. Physicians assess these risk factors for each individual when prescribing oral contraceptives. A woman over 35 may be advised against taking a combined pill, especially if she smokes or has an underlying medical condition such as diabetes mellitus.

High blood pressure is a possible complication of oral contraceptives. Measurement of blood pressure before the pill is prescribed and at six-month intervals thereafter is advised for all women taking oral contraceptives.

Despite frequent reports linking the use of oral contraceptives to certain forms of cancer, evidence supporting a direct relationship between the pill and cancer is not conclusive. Some very rare liver cancers have occurred in pill users, but cancers of the ovaries and uterus are less common.

There is no evidence that oral contraceptives reduce a woman's fertility or that they damage babies conceived after they are discontinued, but physicians advise that you wait for at least one normal menstrual period before attempting to become pregnant.

WHAT TO DO IF YOU MISS A PILL

Contraceptive protection may be reduced if blood levels of the hormones in the body fall as a result of missing a pill. It is particularly important to ensure that the progestin-only

pills are taken punctually. If you miss a pill, the action you should take depends on the degree of lateness and the type of pill being used (see below).

	Combined and phased pills	Progestin-only pills
3 – 12 hours late	Take now. No additional precautions necessary.	Take now. Take addition precautions for the next 48 hours.
Over 12 hours late	Omit the missed pill. Take the next on time and take additional precautions for the next 7 days. If the 7 days extend into the pill-free (or inactive pill) period, start the next packet without a break (or without taking the inactive pills).	Omit the missed pill. Take the next on time. Take additional precautions for the next 48 hours.

COMMON DRUGS

Estrogens
Conjugated estrogens
Diethylstilbestrol
Ethinyl estradiol

Progestin
Norgestrel

DRUGS FOR INFERTILITY

Conception and establishment of pregnancy require a healthy reproductive tract in both partners. The man must produce sufficient numbers of healthy sperm; the woman must be able to produce a healthy egg that is able to pass freely down the fallopian tube to the uterus. The lining of the uterus must be in a condition that allows the implantation of the fertilized egg.

Although the cause of infertility sometimes remains undiscovered, in the majority of cases it is found to be due to one of the following factors: intercourse taking place at the wrong time during the menstrual cycle; the man producing too few or unhealthy sperm; the woman failing to ovulate (release an egg), or having blocked fallopian tubes as a result of previous pelvic infection. The production of female hormones necessary for ovulation and implantation of the egg in the uterus may be disturbed by physical illness or psychological stress.

Physicians do not usually begin to investigate the cause of failure to conceive until normal sexual intercourse without contraception has been taking place regularly for over a year. After this time, if no simple explanation can be found, the man's semen will be analyzed to find out if he is producing healthy sperm in sufficient quantity. If these tests show abnormally low numbers of sperm or if a large proportion of the sperm produced are unhealthy, some of the treatments described in the box below may be tried.

If no abnormality of sperm production is found, the woman will be given a thorough medical examination. Ovulation is monitored and blood tests may be performed to assess hormone levels throughout the menstrual cycle. If ovulation does not occur, the woman may be offered treatment with a fertility drug.

Why they are used

Drugs are useful in helping to achieve pregnancy only when a hormone defect

MALE INFERTILITY

When the quality of the sperm is normal but the numbers produced are insufficient, the cause may be excessively low production of FSH and LH by the pituitary gland. In such cases, regular treatment with a pituitary-stimulating drug such as clomiphene, or with menotropins or human chorionic gonadotropin (which mimic the actions of FSH and LH), may be prescribed. Such drug treatment may need to be continued for many months before any increase in sperm production is noticed.

If, however, abnormal sperm production is due to an abnormality of the testicles or another part of the genitourinary tract, drug treatment is unlikely to be helpful.

ACTION OF FERTILITY DRUGS

Menotropins and HCG Menotropins contains FSH and LH. It acts on the ovary to initiate the development of an egg and stimulates the cells surrounding the developing egg (the follicle) to ripen.

HCG mimics the action of the hormone LH, causing the ripened follicle to release the egg into the fallopian tube. It also ensures that after ovulation, progesterone is produced to prepare the uterus for the implantation of a fertilized egg.

Clomiphene Normally, estrogen acts on part of the brain (the hypothalamus) to suppress the output of FSH and LH by the pituitary gland. Clomiphene opposes the action of estrogen, so that FSH and LH continue to be produced.

Comparison of normal hormone fluctuation and timing of drug treatment

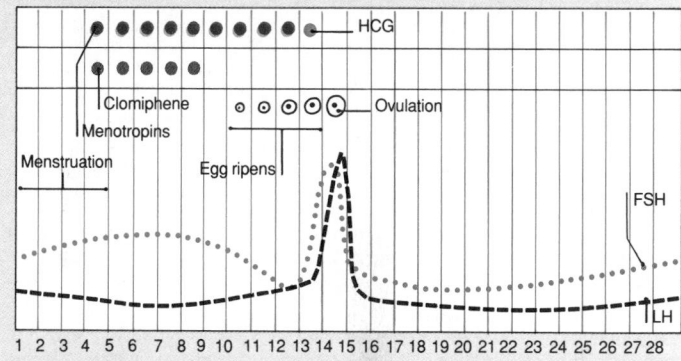

that inhibits ovulation has been diagnosed. Fertility drug treatment may need to be continued for many months and does not always produce a pregnancy.

Women in whom the pituitary gland produces some of the gonadotropin hormones – follicle-stimulating hormone (FSH) and luteinizing hormone (LH) – may be given courses of clomiphene for several days during each month. An effective dose produces ovulation 5 to 10 days after the last tablet is taken. Couples are advised to have intercourse during this phase.

Clomiphene occasionally thickens the cervical mucus, thereby impeding the passage of sperm. If this happens, an estrogen drug that counteracts this effect may be given prior to the course of clomiphene.

If treatment with clomiphene fails to produce ovulation, or if a disorder of the pituitary gland prevents the production of FSH and LH, treatment with menotropins and human chorionic gonadotropin (HCG) may be given.

Menotropins is given during the second week of the menstrual cycle, followed by an injection of HCG. Courses of these drugs may have to be repeated several times before pregnancy occurs.

How they work

Fertility drugs increase the chance of ovulation by boosting the levels of LH and FSH, the pituitary hormones that govern ovulation. Clomiphene stimulates the pituitary gland to increase its output of these hormones. Menotropins acts to stimulate the ripening of the egg in the same way as natural FSH. HCG has an action similar to that of LH; it triggers the release of the egg and promotes the production of progesterone after ovulation has taken place.

How they affect you

Each of these drugs may produce minor adverse effects. Clomiphene may cause hot flashes, nausea, and headache, while HCG can cause tiredness, headache, and mood changes. Menotropins can make the ovaries enlarge, producing abdominal discomfort that may continue for several days.

All these drugs increase the likelihood of multiple births (usually twins). A less common adverse effect is an increased risk of ovarian cysts with clomiphene.

COMMON DRUGS

Clomiphene
HCG (human chorionic gonadotropin)
Menotropins

DRUGS USED IN LABOR

Normal labor has three stages. In the first stage the uterus begins to contract, first irregularly and then gradually more regularly and powerfully, while the cervix dilates until it is fully stretched. During the second stage, powerful contractions of the uterus push the baby down the birth canal and out of the body. The third stage is the delivery of the placenta.

Drugs may be required during one or more stages of labor for any of the following reasons: to induce or augment labor; to delay premature labor (see Uterine muscle relaxants, below right); and to relieve pain. The administration of some drugs may be viewed as part of normal obstetric care; for example, the uterine stimulant ergonovine may be injected routinely before the third stage of labor. Other drugs are administered only when the condition of the mother or baby requires intervention. The possible adverse effects of the drug on both parties are always carefully balanced against the benefits.

Drugs to induce or augment labor

Induction of labor may be advised when a physician considers it risky for the health of the mother or baby for the pregnancy to continue – for example, if natural labor does not occur within two weeks of the due date or when a woman has pre-eclampsia. Other common reasons for inducing labor include premature rupture of the membrane surrounding the baby (breaking of the waters), slow growth of the baby due to poor nourishment by the placenta, or death of the fetus in the uterus.

When labor needs to be induced, oxytocin, a uterine stimulant, is usually administered intravenously. A prostaglandin hormone and laminaria are being investigated for initiation of labor and dilation of the cervix. If these methods are ineffective or cannot be used because of adverse effects (see Risks and special precautions, above right),

DRUGS USED TO TERMINATE PREGNANCY

Drugs may be used in a hospital or clinic to terminate pregnancy up to 20 weeks, or to empty the uterus after the death of the baby. Before the 14th week of pregnancy, a prostaglandin may be given as a vaginal suppository to dilate the cervix before removing the fetus under general anesthetic.

After the 14th week, labor is induced with a prostaglandin drug used as a vaginal suppository or injected into the uterus. These methods may all be supplemented by oxytocin given by intravenous drip (see Drugs to induce or augment labor, above).

a cesarean delivery may have to be performed. Oxytocin may also be used to strengthen the force of contractions in labor that has started spontaneously but is not progressing.

Another uterine stimulant called ergonovine is given to most women as the baby is being born or immediately following birth to prevent excessive bleeding following the delivery of the placenta. Ergonovine encourages the uterus to contract after delivery, which restricts the flow of blood.

Risks and special precautions
When oxytocin is used to induce labor, the dosage is carefully monitored throughout to prevent the possibility of excessively violent contractions. It is administered to women who have had surgery of the uterus only with careful monitoring. The drug is not known to affect the baby adversely. Ergonovine is not given to women who have suffered from high blood pressure during the course of pregnancy.

Drugs used for pain relief
Narcotics
Narcotic drugs such as meperidine may be given once active labor has been established (see Analgesics, p.108). Possible side effects for the mother include drowsiness, nausea, and vomiting. Narcotics may cause respiratory problems for the new baby and are usually not administered within one to two hours of delivery.

Epidural anesthesia
This provides pain relief during labor and birth by numbing the nerves leading to the uterus and pelvic area. It is often used during a planned cesarean delivery, thus enabling the mother to be fully conscious for the birth.

An epidural involves the injection of a local anesthetic drug (see p.108) into the epidural space between the spinal cord and the vertebrae. An epidural may block the mother's urge to push during the second stage, and a forceps delivery may be necessary. Headaches may occasionally occur following epidural anesthesia.

Oxygen and nitrous oxide
These gases are combined to produce a mixture that reduces the pain of contractions. During the first and second stages of labor it is self-administered by inhalation through a mask or mouthpiece. If it is used over too long a period it may produce nausea, confusion, and dehydration in the mother.

Local anesthetics
These drugs are injected inside the vagina or near the vaginal opening and

WHEN DRUGS ARE USED IN LABOR

The drugs used in each stage of labor are described below.

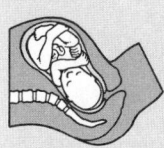

Before labor
Oxytocin
Prostaglandins

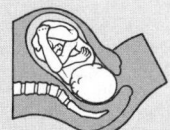

First stage
Epidural anesthetics
Meperidine
Oxytocin

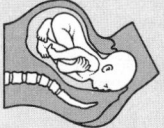

Second stage
Local anesthetics
Nitrous oxide
Oxytocin

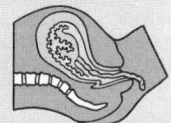

Third stage
Ergonovine
Oxytocin

are used to numb sensation during forceps delivery, before an episiotomy (an incision made to enlarge the vaginal opening), and when stitches are necessary. Side effects are rare.

Uterine muscle relaxants
When contractions of the uterus start before the 34th week of pregnancy, physicians usually advise bed rest and may also administer a drug to relax the muscles of the uterus and thus halt labor. Initially the drug is given by injection in the hospital but may be continued orally at home. These drugs stimulate the sympathetic nervous system (see Autonomic nervous system, p.107) and may cause palpitations and anxiety in the mother. They have not been shown to have adverse effects on the baby.

COMMON DRUGS

Uterine stimulants
Ergonovine
Oxytocin

Prostaglandin
Carboprost

Uterine muscle relaxants
Albuterol
Ritodrine

Narcotic
Meperidine

DRUGS USED FOR URINARY DISORDERS

Urine is produced by the kidneys and stored in the bladder. As urine accumulates, the bladder walls stretch, and pressure within the bladder increases. Eventually, the stretching stimulates nerve endings that produce the urge to urinate. The ring of muscle (sphincter) around the bladder neck normally keeps the bladder closed until it is consciously relaxed, allowing urine to pass via the urethra out of the body.

A number of disorders can affect the urinary tract. The most common are infection in the bladder (cystitis) and urethra (urethritis), and loss of reliable control over urination (urinary incontinence). A less common problem is inability to expel urine (urinary retention). Drugs used to treat these problems include antibiotics and antibacterial drugs, analgesics, drugs to increase the acidity of the urine, and drugs that act on nerve control over the muscles of the bladder and sphincter.

Drugs for urinary infection

Infections of the bladder are almost always caused by bacteria. Symptoms include a continual urge to urinate, although often nothing is passed, pain on urinating, and lower abdominal pain.

Antibiotic and antibacterial drugs are used to eradicate infection. Trimethoprim/sulfamethoxazole, sometimes in a single large dose or in longer courses lasting seven to fourteen days, is one of the most common treatments. A large number of other drugs are also effective, including ampicillin, cephalosporin, and tetracycline antibiotics, and the urinary antiseptics nitrofurantoin and nalidixic

acid (see also Antibiotics, p.156, and Antibacterial drugs, p.159).

Measures are also sometimes taken to increase the acidity of the urine, making it hostile to bacteria. Ascorbic acid (vitamin C) powder in water and acid fruit juices have this effect.

Symptoms may be relieved by a urinary analgesic, phenazopyridine, which concentrates in the urine and has a soothing effect on the lining of the bladder and urethra. It is often combined with an antibacterial drug. For maximum effect, all drug treatments for urinary tract infections need to be accompanied by increased fluid intake.

Drugs for urinary incontinence

Urinary incontinence can occur for a number of reasons. A weak sphincter muscle allows the involuntary passage of urine when abdominal pressure is raised by coughing or physical exertion. This is known as stress incontinence and commonly affects women who have had children. Urgency – the sudden need to urinate – stems from increased sensitivity of the bladder muscle; small quantities of urine stimulate the urge to urinate frequently.

Incontinence can also occur due to loss of nerve control in neurological disorders such as multiple sclerosis. In children, inability to control urination at night (nocturnal enuresis) is also a form of urinary incontinence.

Drug treatment is not necessary or appropriate for all forms of incontinence. In stress incontinence, exercises to strengthen the pelvic floor muscles or surgery to tighten stretched ligaments

may be effective. In urgency, regular emptying of the bladder can often avoid the need for medical intervention. Incontinence caused by loss of nerve control is unlikely to be helped by drug treatment. Stress incontinence may sometimes be helped by *sympathomimetic* drugs, such as ephedrine, that help to constrict the sphincter muscle. Frequency of urination in urgency may be reduced by *anticholinergic* and antispasmodic drugs. These reduce nerve signals from the muscles in the bladder, allowing greater volumes of urine to accumulate without stimulating the urge to pass urine. Tricyclic antidepressants, such as imipramine, have a strong anticholinergic action, and may be prescribed for nocturnal enuresis in children when alternative approaches have failed.

Drugs for urinary retention

Urinary retention is the inability to empty the bladder. This usually results in the failure of the bladder muscle to contract sufficiently to expel accumulated urine. Possible causes include an enlarged prostate gland or tumor, or a long-standing neurological disorder.

Most cases of urinary retention need to be relieved by inserting a tube (catheter) into the urethra, and surgery may be needed to prevent a recurrence of the problem. However, in some cases drug treatment may be prescribed. Phenoxybenzamine, an alpha-adrenergic blocking agent (see Autonomic nervous system, p.107) that relaxes the sphincter, may be used to relieve urinary retention prior to surgery. Bethanechol, a *parasympathomimetic* drug which increases the strength of contraction of the bladder muscle, may relieve urinary retention following surgery. Neither drug is suitable for long-term treatment.

ACTION OF DRUGS ON URINATION

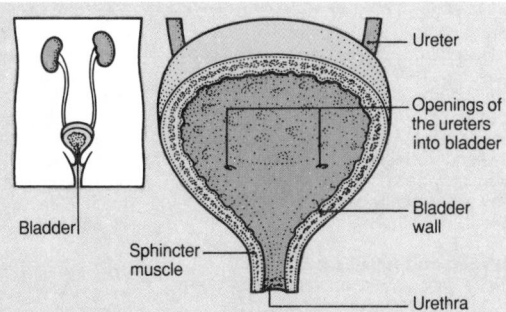

Normal bladder action
Urination occurs when the sphincter that keeps the exit from the bladder into the urethra closed is consciously relaxed in response to signals from the bladder indicating that it is full. As the sphincter opens, the bladder wall contracts and urine is expelled.

Ureter

Openings of the ureters into bladder

Bladder wall

Urethra

Bladder

Sphincter muscle

How drugs act to improve bladder control
Anticholinergics relax the bladder muscle by interfering with the passage of nerve impulses to the muscle.

Sympathomimetics act directly on the sphincter muscle, causing it to contract.

How drugs act to relieve urinary retention
Parasympathomimetics (cholinergics) stimulate contraction of the bladder wall.

Alpha-adrenergic blocking agents relax the muscle of the sphincter.

COMMON DRUGS

Antibiotics and antibacterials
(see pp.156 – 159)

Urinary analgesic
Phenazopyridine

Anticholinergic drug
Flavoxate

Sympathomimetic
Ephedrine

Tricyclic antidepressant
Imipramine

Parasympathomimetic
Bethanechol

Alpha-adrenergic blocker
Phenoxybenzamine

EYES AND EARS

The eyes and ears are the two sense organs that provide us with most information about the world around us. The eye is the organ of vision that converts light images into nerve signals, which are transmitted to the brain for interpretation.

The ear not only provides the means by which sound is detected and communicated to the brain, but it also contains the organ of balance that tells the brain about the position and movement of the body. It is divided into three parts – outer, middle, and inner ear.

What can go wrong

The most common eye and ear disorders are infection and inflammation (sometimes caused by allergy). Many parts of the eye may be affected, notably the conjunctiva (membrane that covers the front of the eye and lines the eyelids) and the iris. The middle and outer ear are more commonly affected by infection than the inner ear.

The eye is subject to a disorder known as glaucoma, in which pressure of fluid within the eye builds up and may eventually threaten vision. Eye problems such as retinopathy (disease of the retina) or cataracts (clouding of the lens) may occur as a result of diabetes and are controlled by treatment of the primary problem. Disorders for which no drug treatment is appropriate are beyond the scope of this book.

Other disorders affecting the ear include build-up of wax (cerumen) in the outer-ear canal and disturbances to the balance mechanism (see Vertigo and Ménière's disease, p.118).

Why drugs are used

Physicians usually prescribe antibiotics (see p.156) to clear ear and eye infections. These may be given by mouth or *topically*. Topical eye and ear preparations may contain a corticosteroid (p.169) to reduce inflammation. When inflammation has been caused by allergy, antihistamines (p.152) may also be taken. Decongestant drugs (p.121) are often prescribed to help clear the eustachian tube in middle-ear infections.

A variety of drugs are used to reduce fluid pressure in glaucoma. These include diuretics (p.127), beta blockers (p.125) and *miotics* to narrow the pupil. In other cases, the pupil may need to be widened by *mydriatic* drugs.

MAJOR DRUG GROUPS

Drugs for glaucoma

Drugs affecting the pupil

Drugs for ear disorders

How the eye works
Light enters the eye through the cornea. The muscles of the iris control pupil size and thus the amount of light passing into the eye. The optic nerve carries signals received by the retina to be interpreted in the brain.

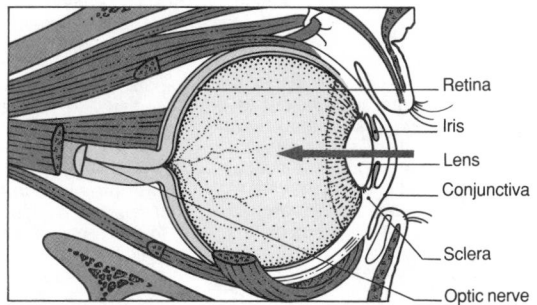

- Retina
- Iris
- Lens
- Conjunctiva
- Sclera
- Optic nerve

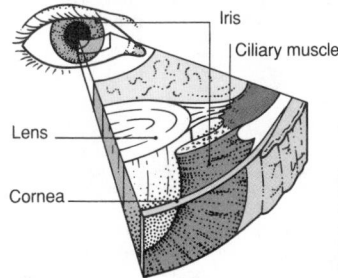

Iris

Ciliary muscle

Lens

Cornea

The eye muscles
Focusing and pupil size are governed by muscles controlled by the autonomic nervous system (p.107), which may be affected by many drugs. Disturbed vision is often a side effect of such drugs.

The ear
The outer-ear canal is separated from the middle ear by the eardrum. Three bones in the middle ear connect it to the inner ear. This contains the cochlea (organ of hearing) and the labyrinth (organ of balance).

Sound is carried to the cochlea and converted to nerve impulses.

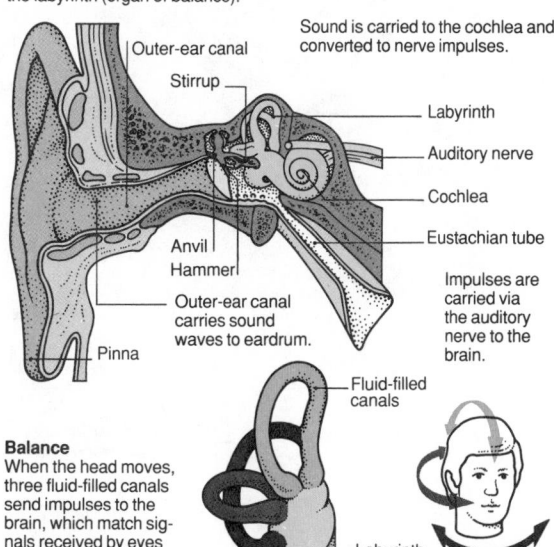

Outer-ear canal

Stirrup

- Labyrinth
- Auditory nerve
- Cochlea
- Eustachian tube

Anvil
Hammer

Outer-ear canal carries sound waves to eardrum.

Pinna

Impulses are carried via the auditory nerve to the brain.

Fluid-filled canals

Balance
When the head moves, three fluid-filled canals send impulses to the brain, which match signals received by eyes and limb muscles.

Labyrinth

DRUGS FOR GLAUCOMA

Glaucoma is the name given to a group of conditions in which the pressure in the eye builds up to an abnormally high level. This compresses the blood vessels supplying the nerve that connects the eye to the brain (optic nerve), and may lead to irreversible nerve damage and permanent loss of vision.

In the most common type of glaucoma, known as chronic (or open-angle) glaucoma, reduced drainage of fluid from the eye causes pressure inside the eye to build up slowly. Progressive reduction in the peripheral field of vision may take months or years to be noticed. Acute (or closed-angle) glaucoma occurs when drainage of fluid is suddenly blocked by the iris. Fluid pressure builds up quite suddenly, blurring vision in the affected eye (see the box below). The eye becomes red and painful, accompanied by a headache and sometimes vomiting. The main attack is often preceded by milder warning attacks such as seeing

halos around lights in the previous weeks or months. Elderly, farsighted people are particularly at risk of developing acute glaucoma. The angle may also narrow suddenly following injury or after taking certain drugs, for example, *anticholinergic* drugs.

Drugs are used in the treatment of both types of glaucoma. These include miotics (see also Drugs affecting the pupil, p.198), beta blockers (p.125), and certain diuretics (carbonic anhydrase inhibitors and osmotics).

Why they are used
Chronic glaucoma
In this form of glaucoma, drugs are used to bring about a reduction in pressure inside the eye and to maintain normal pressure thereafter (lifelong treatment is often necessary). This prevents further deterioration of vision, but cannot restore any damage that has already been sustained.

Initially drops containing a beta blocker (usually timolol) are given to reduce secretion of fluid within the eye. A miotic drug such as pilocarpine may also have to be given, which improves drainage of fluid from the eye. Epinephrine drops may also be helpful. When these measures fail to bring about the necessary reduction of pressure within the eye, acetazolamide, a carbonic anhydrase inhibitor, may be given by mouth to further reduce fluid production. Treatment with acetazolamide is usually continued only until laser treatment or surgery can be arranged.

Acute glaucoma
People who have acute glaucoma need immediate medical treatment in order to prevent total loss of vision. Drugs are used initially to bring down blood pressure within the eye. Laser treatment or eye surgery is then carried out to prevent a recurrence of the problem. It

---

WHAT HAPPENS IN GLAUCOMA

Normal eye
The ciliary body, situated at the root of the iris, continuously produces aqueous humor – a watery fluid that helps maintain the normal shape of the eyeball. Aqueous humor continuously drains via the angle between the cornea and iris through a mesh of fibers (the trabecular meshwork) into a channel in the sclera (white of the eye).

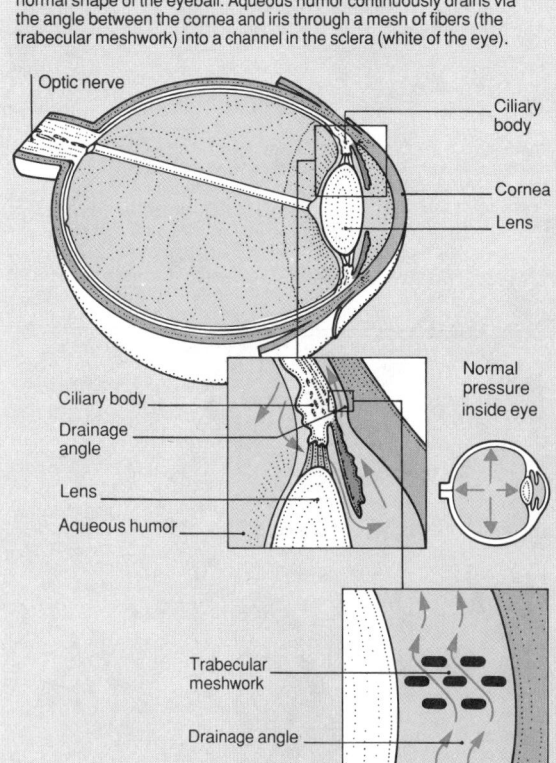

Optic nerve
Ciliary body
Cornea
Lens

Ciliary body
Drainage angle
Lens
Aqueous humor

Trabecular meshwork
Drainage angle

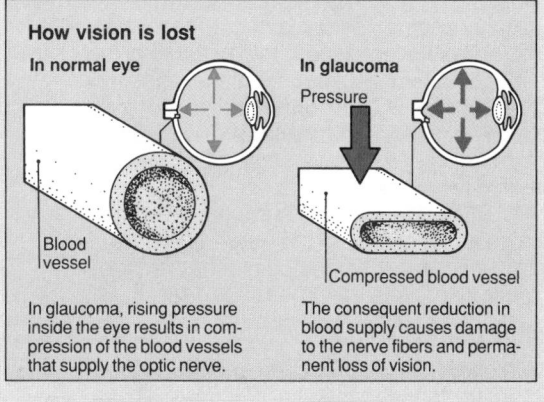

How vision is lost

In normal eye

In glaucoma
Pressure

Blood vessel

Compressed blood vessel

In glaucoma, rising pressure inside the eye results in compression of the blood vessels that supply the optic nerve.

The consequent reduction in blood supply causes damage to the nerve fibers and permanent loss of vision.

Normal pressure inside eye

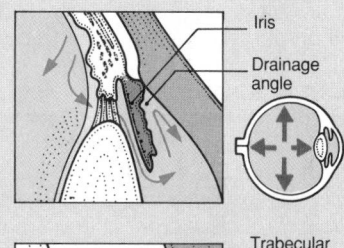

Acute glaucoma
In acute glaucoma, the drainage angle between the cornea and the iris becomes completely closed – so that the pressure inside the eye rises rapidly. This may lead to permanent damage to the nerve fibers.

Iris
Drainage angle

Chronic glaucoma
In chronic glaucoma, the trabecular meshwork through which the aqueous humor normally drains gradually closes off, so that fluid pressure builds up slowly, gradually damaging the optic nerve.

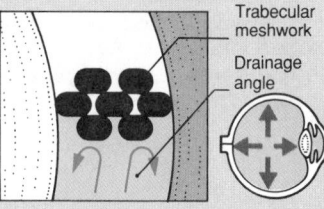

Trabecular meshwork
Drainage angle

is rare for drug treatment to be continued long-term.

Acetazolamide is usually the first drug administered when the condition is diagnosed. This is initially injected for rapid effect and thereafter administered by mouth. Frequent applications are given of eye drops containing pilocarpine or another miotic drug. Occasionally an osmotic diuretic is administered. This draws fluid out of all body tissues, including the eye, and reduces pressure within the eye.

How they work

The drugs used to treat glaucoma act in various ways to reduce the pressure of fluid in the eye. Miotics improve the drainage of the fluid out of the eye. In chronic glaucoma this is achieved by increasing the outflow of aqueous humor through the drainage channel called the trabecular meshwork. In acute glaucoma the pupil-constricting effect of miotics pulls the iris away from the drainage channel, allowing the aqueous humor to flow out normally. Beta blockers and carbonic anhydrase inhibitors act on the fluid-producing cells inside the eye to reduce the output of aqueous humor.

How they affect you

Drugs for acute glaucoma act quickly, relieving pain and other symptoms within a few hours. The benefits of drug treatment in chronic glaucoma may not be immediately apparent since they only halt a further deterioration of vision.

People receiving miotic eye drops are likely to notice darkening of vision and difficulty seeing in the dark. Increased shortsightedness may be noticeable. Some miotics also cause irritation and redness of the eyes.

ACTION OF DRUGS FOR GLAUCOMA

Miotics
These act on the circular muscle in the iris to reduce the size of the pupil. In acute glaucoma this relieves any obstruction to the flow of aqueous humor by pulling the iris away from the cornea (right). In chronic glaucoma, miotic drugs act directly to increase the outflow of aqueous humor.

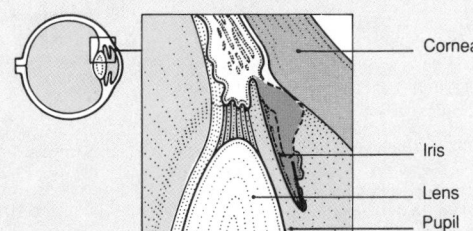

Cornea

Iris

Lens

Pupil

Beta blockers
The fluid-producing cells in the ciliary body are stimulated by signals passed through beta receptors. Beta blocking drugs prevent the transmission of signals through these receptors, thereby reducing the stimulus to produce fluid.

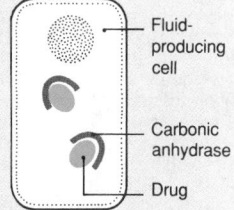

Fluid-producing cell

Carbonic anhydrase

Drug

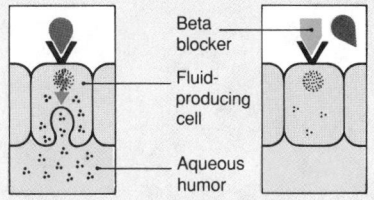

Beta blocker

Fluid-producing cell

Aqueous humor

Before drug

After drug

Carbonic anhydrase inhibitors
These block carbonic anhydrase, an *enzyme* involved in the production of aqueous humor in the ciliary body.

Beta blocker eye drops have few day-to-day side effects but carry risks for a few people (see below). Acetazolamide usually causes an increase in frequency of urination and thirst. Nausea and general malaise are also common.

Risks and special precautions
Miotics are generally risk free. If beta blockers are absorbed into the body they can affect the lungs, heart, and circulation. For this reason, they are prescribed with caution to people with asthma or certain circulatory disorders, and in some cases they are withheld altogether. The amount of the drug absorbed into the body can be reduced by applying the eye drops carefully, as described in the box (left). Acetazolamide is not normally prescribed for prolonged treatment because of its troublesome adverse effects, including painful tingling of the hands and feet. It may encourage the formation of kidney stones and may in rare cases cause kidney damage. People with existing kidney problems are not usually given this drug. For further information on acetazolamide, consult the drug profile in Part 4.

APPLYING EYE DROPS IN GLAUCOMA

To reduce the amount of drug absorbed into the blood via the lacrimal (tear) duct, apply eye drops as described. This also improves the effectiveness of the drug.

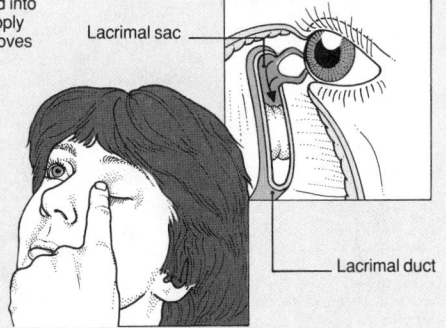

Lacrimal sac

Lacrimal duct

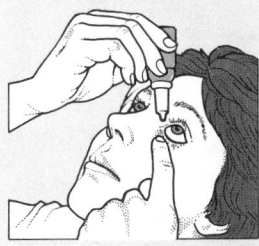

1 Press firmly on the lacrimal sac in the corner of the eye and apply the number of drops prescribed by your physician.

2 Maintain pressure on the lacrimal sac for a few moments after applying the drops.

COMMON DRUGS

Miotic
Pilocarpine

Beta blockers
Betaxolol
Levobunolol
Timolol

Carbonic anhydrase inhibitor
Acetazolamide

DRUGS AFFECTING THE PUPIL

The pupil of the eye is the circular opening in the center of the iris (the colored part of the eye) through which light enters. It continually changes in size to adjust to variations in the intensity of light: in bright light it becomes quite small (constricts), but in dim light it enlarges (dilates).

Eye drops containing drugs that act on the pupil are widely used by eye physicians. They are of two types: those that dilate the pupil, known as *mydriatics*; and those that constrict the pupil, known as *miotics*.

Why they are used

Mydriatics are most often used to allow the physician to view the inside of the eye – particularly the retina, the optic nerve head, and the blood vessels that supply the retina. Many of these drugs cause a temporary paralysis of the eye's focusing mechanism, a state known as cycloplegia. Cycloplegia is sometimes induced to help determine the presence of any focusing errors, especially in babies and young children. By producing cycloplegia, physicians can determine the precise optical prescription required for a small child, especially in the case of a squint.

Dilation of the pupil is part of the treatment for uveitis, an inflammatory disease of the iris and focusing muscle. In uveitis, the inflamed iris may stick to the lens, and thus cause severe damage to the eye. This can be prevented by early dilation of the pupil so that the iris is no longer in contact with the lens.

Constriction of the pupil with miotic drugs is often required in the treatment of glaucoma (see p.196). Miotics can also be used to restore the pupil to a normal size after dilation has been induced artificially.

How they work

The size of the pupil is controlled by two separate sets of muscles in the iris, the circular muscle and the radial muscle. Each set of muscles is governed by a separate branch of the autonomic nervous system (see p.107): the sympathetic nervous system controls the radial muscle, and the parasympathetic nervous system controls the circular muscle.

Individual mydriatic and miotic drugs take effect on different branches of the autonomic nervous system, and will cause the pupil of the eye either to dilate or to contract, depending on the type being used.

ACTION OF DRUGS AFFECTING THE PUPIL

The muscles of the iris
The pupil is made smaller and larger by the coordinated action of the circular and radial muscles in the iris. The circular muscle forms a ring around the pupil; when it contracts, the pupil becomes smaller. The radial muscle is composed of fibers that run from the pupil to the base of the iris like the spokes of a wheel. Contraction of these fibers causes the pupil to become larger.

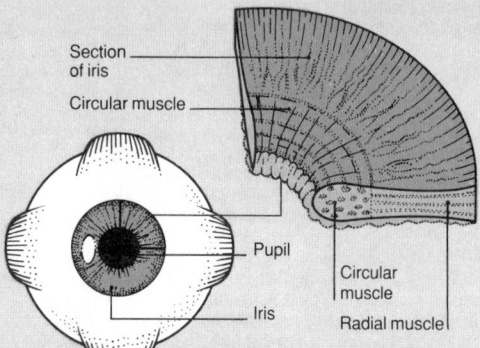

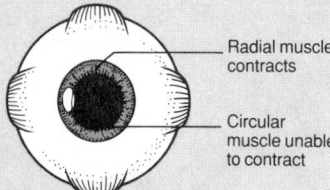

Mydriatics
Mydriatics enlarge the pupil in one of two ways. The *sympathomimetics* stimulate the radial muscle to contract. The *anticholinergics* prevent the circular muscle from contracting.

Miotics
Most miotics reduce size of the pupil by stimulating the activity of the parasympathetic nervous system, which causes the circular muscle to contract.

How they affect you

Mydriatic drugs – especially the long-acting types – impair the ability to focus the eye(s) for several hours after use. This interferes particularly with close activities such as reading. Bright light may cause discomfort. Miotics often interfere with night vision and may cause temporary short sight (myopia).

Normally, these eye drops produce few serious adverse effects. *Sympatho-mimetic* mydriatics may raise blood pressure and are used with caution in people with heart disease or hypertension. Miotics may irritate the eye, but rarely cause generalized effects.

COMMON DRUGS

Sympathomimetic mydriatics
Epinephrine
Phenylephrine

Anticholinergic mydriatics
Atropine
Tropicamide

Miotics
Carbachol
Pilocarpine

ARTIFICIAL TEAR PREPARATIONS

Tears are continually produced to keep the front of the eye covered with a thin moist film. This is essential for clear vision and for keeping the front of the eye free from dirt and other irritants. In some conditions, known collectively as dry eye syndromes (for example, Sjögren's syndrome), inadequate tear production may make the eyes feel dry and sore. Sore eyes can also occur in disorders where the eyelids do not close properly, causing the eye to become dry.

Why they are used
Since prolonged deficiency of natural tears can damage the cornea, regular application of artificial tears in the form of eye drops is recommended in all of the conditions described. Artificial tears may also be used to provide temporary relief from any feeling of discomfort and dryness in the eye caused by irritants, exposure to wind or sun, or the initial wearing of contact lenses.

Although artificial tears are non-irritating, the preparations containing them often include a preservative (for example, thimerosal or benzalkonium chloride) that may cause irritation. This risk is increased for wearers of soft contact lenses, who should ask their physician for advice before using any type of eye drops.

DRUGS FOR EAR DISORDERS

Inflammation and infection of the outer and the middle ear are the most common disorders affecting the ear that are treated with drugs. Drug treatment of Ménière's disease, which affects the inner ear, is described under Vertigo and Ménière's disease, p.118.

The type of drug treatment given for ear inflammation depends on the cause of the trouble and the site affected.

Inflammation of the outer ear

Inflammation of the external ear canal (otitis externa) can be caused by eczema, or by a bacterial or fungal infection. The risk of inflammation is increased by swimming in dirty water, the accumulation of wax in the ear, or by too frequent poking or scratching at the ear.

Symptoms vary, but often there is itching, pain (which may be severe if there is a boil in the ear canal), tenderness, and possibly some loss of hearing. If the ear is infected as well there will probably be a discharge.

Drug treatment

A weak corticosteroid (see p.169), in the form of ear drops, may be used to treat inflammation of the outer ear when there is no infection. Aluminum acetate solution, as drops or applied on a piece of gauze, may also be used. Relief is usually obtained within a day or two. Prolonged use of corticosteroids is not advisable because they may reduce the ear's resistance to infection.

If there is both inflammation and infection, the physician may prescribe ear drops containing an antibiotic (see p.156) combined with a weak corticosteroid to relieve the inflammation. Usually, a combination of antibiotics is prescribed – commonly neomycin with polymyxin B or colistin – to make the treatment effective against a wide range

EAR WAX REMOVAL

Ear wax (or cerumen) is a natural secretion from the outer ear canal that keeps it free from dust and skin debris. Occasionally, wax may build up in the outer ear canal and become hard, leading to irritation and/or hearing loss.

A number of over-the-counter products are available to soften ear wax and hasten its expulsion. Such products may contain irritating substances that can cause inflammation. Physicians advise instead application of mineral oil or glycerin. A cotton plug should be inserted to retain the oil in the outer ear. When ear wax is not dislodged by such home treatment, a physician may syringe the ear with warm water.

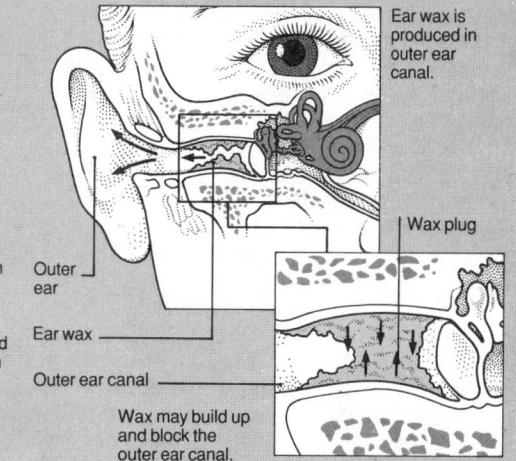

Ear wax is produced in outer ear canal.

Outer ear

Ear wax

Outer ear canal

Wax plug

Wax may build up and block the outer ear canal.

of bacteria. These antibiotics are not usually taken for long periods, since prolonged use can irritate the skin that lines the ear canal.

Sometimes an antibiotic given in the form of drops is not effective, and another type of antibiotic may also have to be taken by mouth.

Infection of the middle ear

Infection of the middle ear (otitis media) often causes severe pain and hearing loss. It is particularly common in young children in whom infecting organisms are able to spread easily into the middle ear from the nose or throat via the eustachian tube.

Viral infections of the middle ear usually cure themselves and are less serious than those caused by bacteria.

Bacterial infections often cause the eustachian tube to swell and become blocked. When a blockage occurs, pus builds up in the middle ear and puts pressure on the eardrum, which may then perforate.

Drug treatment

Physicians usually prescribe a decongestant (see p.121) or antihistamine (see p.152) to reduce swelling in the eustachian tube, thus allowing the pus to drain out of the middle ear. Usually, an antibiotic is then given by mouth to clear the infection.

Antibiotics are not effective against viral infections, but as it is often difficult to distinguish between a viral and a bacterial infection of the middle ear, your physician may prescribe an antibiotic as a precautionary measure. Acetaminophen, an analgesic (see p.108), may be given to relieve pain. When infection is recurrent, antibiotic treatment lasting several weeks may be prescribed.

HOW TO USE EAR DROPS

Ear drops for outer ear disorders are more easily and efficiently administered if you have someone to help you. Lie on your side while the other person drops the medication into the ear cavity, ensuring that the dropper does not touch the ear. If possible, it is advisable to remain lying in that position for a few minutes in order to allow the drops to bathe the ear canal. Ear drops should be discarded when the course of treatment has been completed.

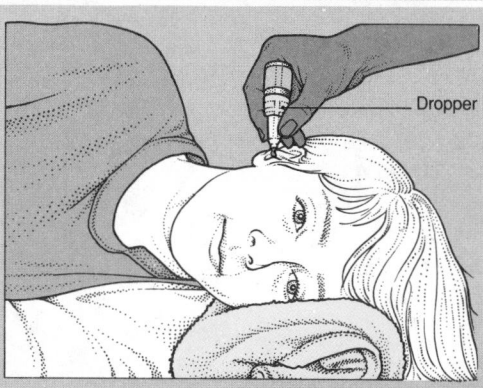

Dropper

COMMON DRUGS

Antibiotic ear drops
Chloramphenicol
Colistin
Gentamicin
Neomycin
Polymyxin B

Oral antibiotics
See p.156

Other drugs
Antihistamines (see p.152)
Corticosteroids (see p.169)
Decongestants (see p.121)

SKIN

The largest organ of the human body, the skin performs a variety of essential tasks. It provides a barrier against innumerable infections and infestations; it helps the body retain its vital fluids; it plays a major role in temperature control; and it houses the sensory nerves of touch.

The skin consists of two main layers: a thin, tough top layer, the epidermis, and below it a thicker layer, the dermis. The epidermis divides into two: the skin surface, or stratum corneum (horny layer) consisting of dead skin cells, and below, a layer of active cells. The active layer cells divide and eventually die, maintaining the horny layer. Living cells produce keratin, which toughens the epidermis and is the basic substance of hair and nails. Some living cells in the epidermis contain melanin, a pigment released following exposure to sunlight, which protects the dermis.

The dermis contains different types of nerve endings for sensing pain, pressure, and temperature; sweat glands to cool the body; sebaceous glands that release an oil (sebum) that lubricates and waterproofs the skin; and white blood cells that help keep the skin clear of infection.

What can go wrong

Most skin complaints are not serious, but they may be distressing if visible. They include infection, inflammation and irritation, infestation by skin parasites, and changes in skin structure and texture (psoriasis and acne).

Why drugs are used

Skin problems often resolve themselves without drug treatment. Over-the-counter preparations containing active ingredients are available, but physicians generally advise against their use without medical supervision because they can aggravate some skin conditions if used inappropriately. Drugs prescribed by physicians are often highly effective: antibiotics (p.156) for bacterial infections; antifungal drugs (p.166) for fungal infections; anti-infestation agents for skin parasites (p.204); and corticosteroids (p.202) for inflammatory conditions. Specialized drugs are available for conditions like psoriasis and acne.

Although many drugs are *topical* medications, you must use them as carefully as drugs taken by mouth, since they too can cause adverse effects.

Structure of the skin
The epidermis contains keratin and melanin, while the dermis contains sweat glands, sebaceous glands, and nerve endings that sense pain, temperature, and pressure.

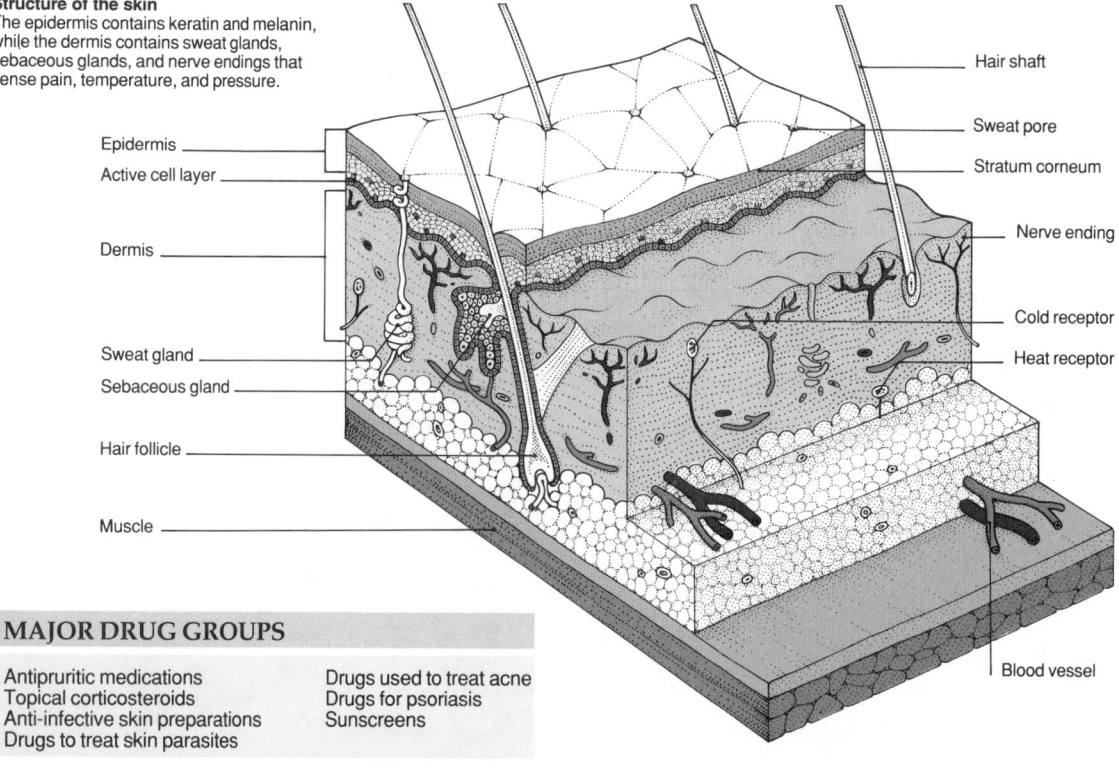

Epidermis

Active cell layer

Dermis

Sweat gland

Sebaceous gland

Hair follicle

Muscle

Hair shaft

Sweat pore

Stratum corneum

Nerve ending

Cold receptor

Heat receptor

Blood vessel

MAJOR DRUG GROUPS

Antipruritic medications
Topical corticosteroids
Anti-infective skin preparations
Drugs to treat skin parasites

Drugs used to treat acne
Drugs for psoriasis
Sunscreens

ANTIPRURITIC MEDICATIONS

Itching (irritation of the skin that creates the urge to scratch), also known as pruritus, probably occurs as a result of chemical changes in the skin caused by disease, allergy, inflammation, or exposure to irritant substances. People differ in their tolerance of itching, and an individual's threshold can be altered by stress and other psychological factors.

Itching is a common symptom of many skin disorders, including eczema and allergic conditions such as urticaria (hives). It may also be caused by local-ized fungal infection or parasitic infestation. Diseases such as chicken pox and psoriasis may also cause itching. Less commonly, itching may also occur in diabetes mellitus, jaundice, and kidney failure.

In many cases, generalized itching is caused by dry skin. Itching in particular parts of the body often has special causes: itching around the anus (pruritus ani) may result from hemor-rhoids or worm infestation; genital itching in women (pruritus vulvae) may be caused by vaginal infection or, in older women, hormone deficiency.

Although scratching provides temporary relief, it often increases skin inflammation and thus may make the condition worse. In some cases, continued scratching of an area of irritated skin can lead to a vicious circle of scratching and itching that continues long after the original cause of the trouble has been removed.

A number of different types of medication are used for the relief of skin irritation. These include soothing preparations that are applied to the affected skin and drugs that are taken by mouth. The principal drugs used in antipruritic medications include corticosteroids (see Topical cortico-steroids, p.202), local anesthetics (p.108), and antihistamines (p.152). Plain *emollient* or cooling creams and ointments containing no active ingredients are often recommended.

Why they are used
For mild itching arising from sunburn, urticaria or insect bites, a cooling lotion such as calamine, perhaps containing menthol, phenol, or camphor, may be the most appropriate treatment. Local anesthetic creams are sometimes helpful for small areas of irritation such as insect bites, but are unsuitable for widespread itching. Itching from dry skin is often soothed by a simple emollient. Avoidance of excessive bathing and use of moisturizing bath oils may also help.

Severe itching from eczema or other inflammatory skin conditions may be treated with a topical corticosteroid preparation. Where the irritation prevents sleep, a physician may prescribe an antihistamine drug to be taken at night to promote sleep as well as relieve itching (see also Sleeping drugs, p.110). Antihistamines are also often included in topical preparations for the relief of skin irritation but their effectiveness when administered in this way is doubtful. For the treatment of pruritus ani, see Drugs for rectal and anal disorders (p.141). Post-meno-pausal pruritus vulvae may be helped by vaginal creams containing estrogen. For further information, see Female sex hormones (p.175). Itching that is caused by an underlying illness cannot be helped by skin creams, and requires treatment for the principal disorder.

Risks and special precautions
The main risk with any of these prepa-rations other than simple emollient and soothing preparations is that prolonged or heavy use may cause skin irritation, thereby aggravating itching. Antihis-tamine and local anesthetic creams are especially likely to cause a reaction, and have to be stopped if they do so. Antihistamines taken by mouth to re-lieve itching are likely to cause drowsi-ness. The special risks of topical corticosteroids are discussed on p.202.

Because itching can be a symptom of many underlying conditions, self-treatment should be continued for no longer than a week before seeking medical advice.

ACTION OF ANTIPRURITICS

Irritation of the skin causes the release of substances from the blood that cause blood vessels to dilate and fluid to accumulate under the skin. This causes itching and inflammation. Antipruritic drugs act either by reducing inflammation and therefore irritation, or by numbing the nerve impulses that transmit sensation to the brain.

Corticosteroids applied to the skin surface reduce itching caused by allergy within a few days, although the soothing effect of the cream may produce an immediate improve-ment. They pass into the underlying tissues and blood vessels and reduce the release of histamine, the chemical that causes itching and inflammation.

Antihistamines act within a few hours to reduce allergy-related skin inflammation. Applied to the skin, they pass into the underlying tissue and block the effects of histamine on the blood vessels beneath the skin. Taken by mouth they also act on the brain to reduce the perception of irritation.

Local anesthetics absorbed through the skin numb the transmission of signals from the nerves in the skin to the brain.

Soothing and emollient creams Calamine lotion and similar preparations applied to the skin surface reduce inflammation and itching by cooling the skin. Emollient creams lubricate the skin surface and prevent dryness.

COMMON DRUGS

Corticosteroids
See p.169

Local anesthetics
Benzocaine
Lidocaine
Procaine
Tetracaine

Antihistamines
See p.152

Emollient and cooling preparations
Hydrophilic ointment USP
Cold cream USP
Calamine lotion USP
Phenolated calamine lotion USP

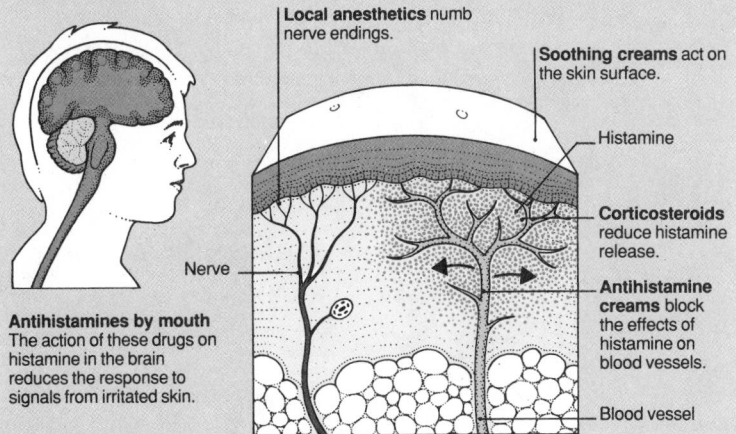

Local anesthetics numb nerve endings.

Soothing creams act on the skin surface.

Histamine

Corticosteroids reduce histamine release.

Antihistamine creams block the effects of histamine on blood vessels.

Blood vessel

Nerve

Antihistamines by mouth
The action of these drugs on histamine in the brain reduces the response to signals from irritated skin.

TOPICAL CORTICOSTEROIDS

Corticosteroid drugs (often simply called steroids) are related to hormones produced by the adrenal glands. For a full description of these drugs, see p.169. *Topical* preparations containing a corticosteroid drug are often used to treat skin conditions in which inflammation is a prominent symptom.

Why they are used

Corticosteroid creams and ointments are most commonly given to relieve itching and inflammation associated with skin diseases such as eczema and dermatitis. These preparations may also be prescribed for psoriasis (see p.206). Corticosteroids do not affect the underlying cause of skin irritation, and the condition is therefore likely to recur unless the substance (allergen or irritant) that has provoked the irritation is itself removed, or the underlying condition treated.

A physician may not prescribe a corticosteroid as the initial treatment, preferring to try a topical medicine that has fewer adverse effects (see Antipruritic medications, p.201).

In most cases treatment is started with a preparation containing a low concentration of a mild corticosteroid drug. A stronger preparation may be prescribed subsequently if the first product is ineffective.

How they affect you

Corticosteroids prevent the release of chemicals that trigger the symptoms of inflammation (see Action of corticosteroids on the skin, above right). Conditions for which topical corticosteroids are prescribed improve within a few days of starting treatment. Applied topically, corticosteroids rarely cause adverse effects, but the stronger drugs used in high concentrations carry certain risks.

ACTION OF CORTICOSTEROIDS ON THE SKIN

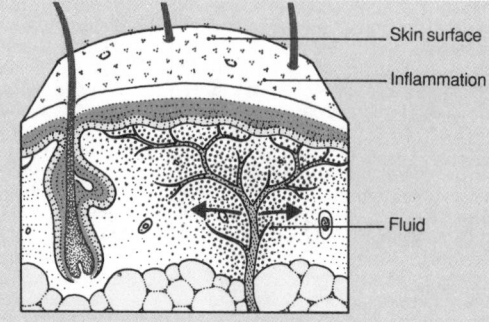

Skin inflammation
Irritation of the skin caused by allergens or irritant substances provokes the release by white blood cells of substances that dilate the blood vessels. This, in turn, causes fluid to accumulate in the skin tissue.

Skin surface

Inflammation

Fluid

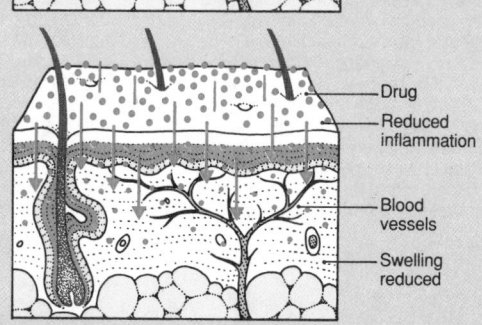

Drug action
Applied to the skin surface, corticosteroids are absorbed into the underlying tissue. There they inhibit the action of the substances that cause inflammation, thereby allowing the blood vessels to return to normal and reducing the swelling.

Drug

Reduced inflammation

Blood vessels

Swelling reduced

Risks and special precautions

Prolonged use of potent corticosteroids in high concentrations can lead to permanent changes in the skin. The most common effect is thinning of the skin, sometimes resulting in stretch marks that may be permanent. Fine blood vessels under the surface of the skin may become prominent (a condition known as telangiectasia). The vessels may become damaged, resulting in a red rash beneath the skin. Because the skin

on the face is especially vulnerable to such damage, topical corticosteroids are not usually prescribed for use on the face. Dark-skinned people sometimes suffer a temporary reduction in pigmentation at the site of application.

When powerful corticosteroid preparations have been used for a prolonged period, abrupt discontinuation of the treatment can result in a general reddening of the skin called "rebound erythroderma." This may be avoided by a gradual reduction in dosage. Corticosteroids suppress the body's immune system (see p.184), thus increasing the risk of infection. For this reason, they are not used alone to treat skin inflammation caused by bacterial or fungal infection. However, they may sometimes be included in a topical preparation that also contains an antibiotic or antifungal agent (see Anti-infective skin preparations, p.203).

LONG-TERM EFFECTS OF TOPICAL CORTICOSTEROIDS

Prolonged use of topical corticosteroids causes drying and thinning of the epidermis, so that tiny blood vessels close to the skin surface become visible. In addition, long-term use of these drugs weakens the underlying connective tissue of the dermis, leading to an increased susceptibility to stretch marks.

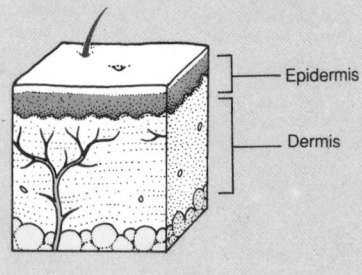

Epidermis

Dermis

Normal skin

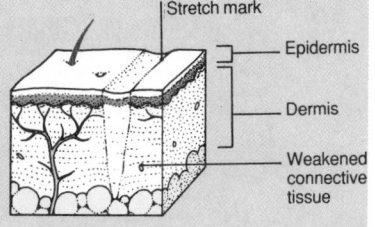

Stretch mark

Epidermis

Dermis

Weakened connective tissue

After prolonged use of topical corticosteroids

COMMON DRUGS

Betamethasone
Fluocinolone
Hydrocortisone
Triamcinolone

ANTI-INFECTIVE SKIN PREPARATIONS

The skin is the body's first line of defense against infection. Yet it can also become infected itself, especially if the outer layer (epidermis) is damaged by a burn, cut, scrape, insect bite, or an inflammatory skin condition such as eczema or dermatitis.

Several different types of organism may infect the skin, including bacteria, viruses, fungi, and yeasts. This page concentrates on drugs applied *topically* to treat bacterial skin infections. These include antiseptics, antibiotics, and other antibacterial agents. Infection by other organisms is covered elsewhere (see Antiviral drugs, p.161, Antifungal drugs, p.166, and Drugs to treat skin parasites, p.204).

Why they are used

Bacterial infections of the skin can usually be prevented by thorough cleansing of an area of skin damage and the application of antiseptic creams and lotions as described in the box (right). Once infection has occurred (causing redness, swelling, and sometimes formation of pus), treatment with an antibiotic preparation may be necessary. An antibiotic or antibacterial skin cream may be used to prevent infection when a physician considers this to be a particular risk – for example, in the case of severe burns.

Other skin disorders in which topical antibiotic treatment may be prescribed include impetigo and infected eczema, skin ulcers, bedsores, and diaper rash.

Usually, a preparation containing two or more antibiotics is used in order to ensure that all bacteria are eradicated. The antibiotics selected for inclusion in topical preparations are usually drugs that are poorly absorbed through the skin (for example, the aminoglycosides). Thus the drug remains concentrated on

ANTISEPTICS

Antiseptics (sometimes called germicides or skin disinfectants) are chemicals that kill or prevent the growth of microorganisms. They are weaker than household disinfectants, which are irritating to the skin.

Antiseptic lotions, creams, and solutions may be effective for preventing infection following surface wounds to the skin. Solutions can be added to water while bathing wounds

(used undiluted they may cause inflammation and increase the risk of infection). Creams may be applied to wounds after cleansing.

Antiseptics are also included in some soaps and shampoos for the prevention of acne and dandruff, but their benefits in these disorders are doubtful. They are also included as ingredients of some throat lozenges but their effectiveness in curing infections is unproven.

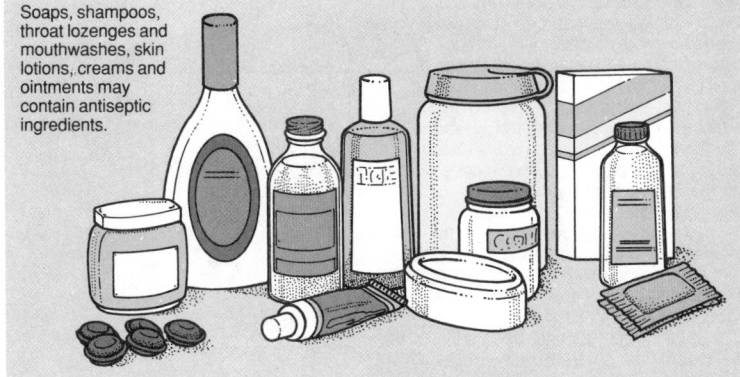

Soaps, shampoos, throat lozenges and mouthwashes, skin lotions, creams and ointments may contain antiseptic ingredients.

the surface and in the skin's upper layers where it is intended that it should have its effect. However, if the infection is deep under the skin, or is causing fever and malaise, antibiotics may need to be administered by mouth or injection.

Risks and special precautions

Some ointments containing antibiotics are available without prescription, but physicians do not encourage the use of these preparations for self-medication because of the risk of encouraging the formation of drug-resistant strains of

bacteria if an inappropriate medication is used (see Antibiotic resistance, p.156). It is always wise to seek medical advice if you suspect that a wound or other skin condition has become infected, and to follow your physician's instructions concerning the duration of treatment even though the infection may appear to have cleared.

Any topical antibiotic product can irritate the skin or cause an allergic reaction. Irritation is often caused by the cream that contains the active drug. Allergic reactions causing swelling and reddening of the skin are more likely to be caused by the antibiotic itself. Any adverse reaction of this kind should be reported to your physician, who may substitute another drug.

BASES FOR SKIN PREPARATIONS

Drugs that are applied to the skin are usually in a preparation known as a base (or vehicle), such as cream, lotion, ointment, or paste. Many bases are beneficial on their own.

Creams These have an *emollient* effect. They are usually composed of an oil-in-water base and are used in the treatment of dry skin disorders, such as psoriasis and certain types of eczema. They may contain other ingredients such as lanolin, camphor, or menthol. Barrier creams protect the skin against water and irritating substances. They may be used in the treatment of diaper rash and to protect the skin around an open sore. They may contain talc and water-repellent substances, such as silicones.

Lotions Thin, semi-liquid preparations often used to cool and soothe inflamed skin. They are most suitable for use on large, hairy areas. Shake lotions contain fine powder which

remains on the surface of the skin when the liquid has evaporated. They are used to encourage scabs to form.

Ointments These are usually greasy and are suitable for treating certain types of eczema. Most ointments contain mineral oil or wax and are insoluble in water.

Pastes Containing large amounts of finely powdered solids such as starch or zinc oxide, pastes protect the skin as well as absorb unwanted moisture and are used for skin conditions that affect clearly defined areas, such as psoriasis.

Collodions These are preparations that, when applied to damaged areas of the skin such as ulcers and minor wounds, dry to form a protective film. They are sometimes used to keep a dissolved drug in contact with the skin.

COMMON DRUGS

Antibiotics
Bacitracin
Clindamycin
Colistin
Gramicidin
Neomycin
Silver sulfadiazine
Tetracycline

Antiseptics
Cetrimide
Chlorhexidine
Potassium permanganate

DRUGS TO TREAT SKIN PARASITES

Mites and lice are the most common parasites that live on the skin. Mites cause the skin disease known as scabies; they burrow into the skin and lay eggs, causing an intense itching. Scratching the affected area results in bleeding and the formation of scabs and increases the risk of infection.

There are three types of lice, each of which infests a different part of the body: the head louse, the body (or clothes) louse, and the crab louse, which often infests the pubic areas but is also sometimes found on other hairy areas such as the eyebrows. All lice cause itching and lay eggs (nits) that look like white grains attached to hairs.

Both mites and lice are passed on by direct contact with an infected person (during sexual intercourse in the case of pubic lice) or, particularly in the case of body lice, by contact with infected bedding or clothing.

The drugs most commonly used to eliminate skin parasites are insecticides that kill both the adult insects and their eggs. The principal drugs are lindane (both scabies and louse infestations), crotamiton (scabies only), and pyrethrins and piperonyl butoxide (louse infestations only).

Why they are used

Skin parasites do not represent a serious threat to health, but require prompt treatment because they can cause severe irritation and spread rapidly if untreated. Drugs are used to eradicate the parasites from the body, but it may also be necessary to disinfect bedding and clothing to avoid the possibility of reinfection.

How they are used

Lotions for the treatment of scabies containing lindane or crotamiton are applied to the whole body – with the exception of the head and neck –

SITES AFFECTED BY SKIN PARASITES

Scabies
The female scabies mite burrows into the skin and lays its eggs under the skin surface. After hatching, the larvae travel to the skin surface, where they mature for 10 – 17 days before starting the cycle again.

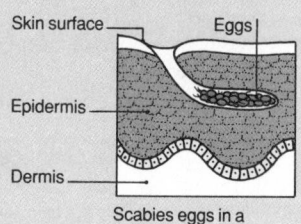

Skin surface — Eggs
Epidermis
Dermis
Scabies eggs in a burrow under the skin.

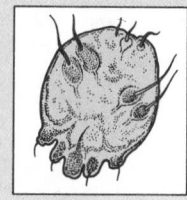

Scabies mite

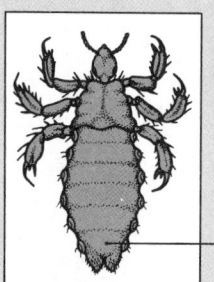

Head louse

Head lice
These tiny brown insects are transmitted from person to person (commonly among children). Their bites often cause itching.

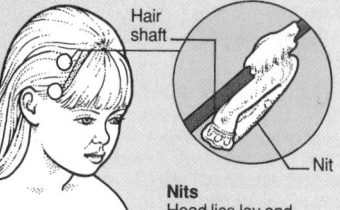

Hair shaft
Nit

Nits
Head lice lay and attach their eggs near the base of the hair shaft, especially around the ears.

following a bath or shower. Many people find these lotions messy to use, but they should not be washed off for 8 to 12 hours (lindane) or 48 hours (crotamiton); otherwise they will not be effective. It is probably most convenient to apply lindane before going to bed. It may then be washed off the following morning.

One or two treatments are normally sufficient to remove the scabies mites. However, the itch associated with scabies may persist after the mite has been removed, so it may be necessary to use a soothing cream or medication containing an antipruritic drug (see p. 201) to ease this. People who have skin-to-skin contact with a sufferer from

scabies – family members and sexual partners – should also undergo treatment at the same time.

Head and pubic lice infestations are usually treated with a shampoo containing lindane or pyrethrins. For full effect these shampoos must be left on the skin for several minutes – four minutes for lindane and ten minutes for pyrethrins. Treatment may need to be repeated after one week. If the skin has become infected as a result of scratching, a *topical* antibiotic (see Anti-infective skin preparations p.203) may also be prescribed.

Risks and special precautions

Lotions prescribed to control parasites can cause irritation and stinging that may be intense if the medication is allowed to come into contact with the eyes, mouth, or other moist membranes. Care is therefore needed when applying lotions and shampoos. Because they are applied *topically*, antiparasitic drugs seldom have generalized effects. Nevertheless, it is important not to apply these preparations more often than directed.

ELIMINATING PARASITES FROM BEDDING AND CLOTHING

Most skin parasites may also infest bedding and clothing that has been next to the skin of an infected person. Therefore, to avoid reinfestation following removal of the parasites from the body, it is essential to eradicate insects and eggs that may be lodged in them.

Washing
Since all skin parasites are killed by heat, washing affected items of clothing and bedding in hot water and drying them in a hot dryer is an effective and convenient method of dealing with the problem.

Non-washable items
Items that cannot be washed should be isolated in plastic bags. The insects and their eggs cannot survive long without their human

hosts and die within days. The length of time they can survive, and therefore the period of isolation, varies depending on the type of parasite (see the table below).

Parasite	Maximum survival time away from host		Isolation period
	Insects	Eggs	
Scabies	2 days	0 days	2 days
Head lice	2 days	10 days	10 days
Crab lice	1 day	10 days	10 days
Body lice	10 days	30 days	30 days

COMMON DRUGS

Crotamiton
Lindane
Pyrethrins

DRUGS USED TO TREAT ACNE

Acne, known medically as acne vulgaris, is a common condition caused by an excess production of the skin's natural oil (sebum), which leads to blockage of hair follicles (see What happens in acne, right). Though it chiefly affects adolescents, acne may occur at any age as a result of taking certain drugs, exposure to industrial chemicals, oily cosmetics, or hot and humid conditions.

Acne primarily affects the skin on the face, neck, back, and chest. The principal skin symptoms are blackheads, papules (inflamed spots), and pustules (raised pus-filled spots with a white center). Mild acne may produce only blackheads and an occasional papule or pustule. Moderate cases are characterized by larger numbers of pustules and papules. In severe cases of acne, painful, inflamed cysts also develop. These can cause permanent pitting and scarring.

Medication for acne can be divided into two groups: *topical* preparations applied directly to the skin and *systemic* treatments taken by mouth.

Why they are used

Mild acne does not normally require medical intervention. It can be controlled by regular washing and moderate exposure to sunlight or ultraviolet light. Over-the-counter antibacterial soaps and lotions have only a limited usefulness and may cause irritation.

CLEARING BLOCKED HAIR FOLLICLES

The most common treatment for acne is the application of keratolytic skin ointments. These encourage the layer of dead and hardened skin cells that form the skin surface to peel off. This action simultaneously clears blocked hair follicles that give rise to the formation of acne spots.

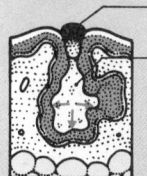

Blackhead

Trapped sebum

Blocked hair follicle
A hair follicle blocked by a plug of skin debris and sebum is ideal for acne spot formation.

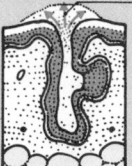

Freed sebum

Cleared hair follicle
Once the follicle is unblocked, sebum can escape and air can enter, thereby limiting bacterial activity.

WHAT HAPPENS IN ACNE

In normal skin, sebum produced by a sebaceous gland attached to a hair follicle is able to flow out of the follicle along the hair. An acne spot forms when the flow of the sebum from the sebaceous gland is blocked by a plug of skin debris and hardened sebum, leading to an accumulation of sebum.

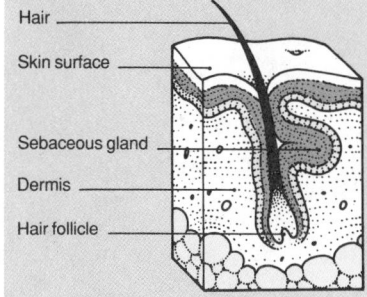

Hair

Skin surface

Sebaceous gland

Dermis

Hair follicle

Acne papules and pustules
Bacterial activity leads to the formation of pustules and papules. Irritant substances may leak into the surrounding skin, causing inflammation.

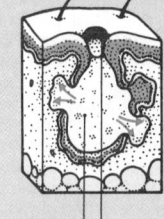

Sebum

Blackhead

Cyst

Cystic acne
When acne is severe, cysts may form in the inflamed dermis. These are pockets of pus enclosed within scar tissue.

When a physician considers acne is severe enough to warrant medical treatment, he or she is likely initially to recommend a topical preparation containing benzoyl peroxide, sulfur, or salicylic acid. If this treatment does not produce an adequate improvement, an ointment containing tretinoin, a drug related to vitamin A, or tetracycline, an antibiotic, may be prescribed.

If acne is severe or does not respond to topical treatments, a physician may prescribe a long course of antibiotics (a tetracycline or erythromycin) by mouth. If all these measures are unsuccessful, the more powerful vitamin A drug isotretinoin may be prescribed by mouth.

Estrogen drugs may have a beneficial effect on acne. A woman who suffers from troublesome acne and who also requires contraceptive protection may therefore be advised to try an estrogen-containing oral contraceptive (p.189).

How they work

Drugs used to treat acne act in different ways. Some have a keratolytic effect – that is they loosen the dead cells on the skin surface (see Clearing blocked hair follicles, left). Other drugs counter bacterial activity in the skin or reduce sebum production.

Topical preparations such as benzoyl peroxide, salicylic acid, tretinoin, and sulfur have a keratolytic effect. Benzoyl peroxide and sulfur also have an antibacterial effect. Tetracyclines applied topically or taken systemically reduce bacterial activity, but may also have a direct anti-inflammatory effect on the skin. Isotretinoin reduces sebum production, soothes inflammation, and also helps to unblock hair follicles.

How they affect you

Keratolytic preparations often cause soreness of the skin, especially at the start of treatment. If this persists, a change to a milder preparation may be recommended. Day-to-day side effects are rare with antibiotics.

Isotretinoin treatment often causes dryness and scaling of the skin, particularly on the lips. The skin may become itchy and some hair loss may occur.

Risks and special precautions

Antibiotic ointments may, in rare cases, provoke an allergic reaction requiring discontinuation of treatment. The tetracyclines, some of the most commonly used antibiotics for acne, are not suitable for use by mouth in pregnancy since they can damage the teeth of the developing baby. Isotretinoin can increase levels of fat in the blood. More seriously, the drug is known to damage the developing baby if taken during pregnancy. Women taking this drug must be certain to use effective contraception during treatment.

COMMON DRUGS

Antibiotics
Erythromycin
Oxytetracycline
Tetracycline

Vitamin A drugs
Isotretinoin
Tretinoin

Topical treatments
Benzoyl peroxide
Clindamycin
Salicylic acid
Sulfur

DRUGS FOR PSORIASIS

The skin is constantly being renewed; as fast as dead cells in the outermost layer (epidermis) are shed, they are replaced by cells from the base of the epidermis. Psoriasis occurs when the production of new cells increases while the shedding of old cells remains normal. As a result, the live skin cells accumulate and produce patches of inflamed, thickened skin covered by silvery scales. In some cases, the area of skin affected is extensive and causes severe embarrassment and physical discomfort. Psoriasis may occasionally be accompanied by arthritis in which the joints become swollen and painful.

The underlying cause of psoriasis is unknown. It usually first occurs between the ages of 10 and 30, and recurs throughout life. Outbreaks may be triggered by emotional stress, skin damage, and physical illnesses. Psoriasis can also be a consequence of the withdrawal of corticosteroid drugs.

There is no complete cure for psoriasis. Simple measures such as careful sunbathing or using an ultraviolet lamp may help to clear mild psoriasis. An *emollient* cream (see p.201) often soothes the irritation. When such measures fail to provide adequate relief, additional drug therapy is needed.

Why they are used

Drugs are used to reduce the size of areas of affected skin and to reduce inflammation and scaling. Mild or moderate psoriasis is usually treated with a *topical* preparation. Coal tar preparations in the form of creams, pastes, and bath additives are often helpful, although some people dislike the smell. Anthralin is also widely used. Applied to the affected areas, it is then left for a few minutes or overnight (depending on the preparation), after which it is washed off. Both anthralin and coal tar can stain clothes and bed linen.

If these agents alone do not produce adequate benefit, ultraviolet light therapy in the form of regulated exposure to natural sunlight or to ultraviolet lamps may be advised. Salicylic acid may be applied to help remove thick scale and crusts, especially from the scalp.

Topical corticosteroids (see p.202) may be used in difficult cases that do not respond to those treatments. They are particularly useful for the skinfold areas and may be given to counter irritation caused by anthralin.

For more severe psoriasis not improved by any of these treatments, your physician may recommend special treatment with more powerful drugs. These include etretinate, a vitamin A derivative that is taken by mouth in courses lasting about 6 months, and methotrexate, an anticancer drug.

PUVA

PUVA is the combined use of a psoralen drug and ultraviolet A light (UVA). The drug is applied *topically* or taken by mouth some hours before exposure to UVA, which enhances the effect of the drug on skin cells.

This therapy is given two to three times a week, producing an improvement in skin condition within about four to six weeks.

Possible adverse effects include nausea, itching, and painful reddening of the normal areas of skin. More seriously, there is a risk of the skin aging prematurely and a long-term risk of skin cancer, particularly in fair-skinned people. For these reasons, PUVA therapy is generally recommended only for severe psoriasis after other treatments have failed.

In psoriasis
Skin cells form at the base of the epidermis faster than they can be shed from the skin surface. This causes the formation of patches of thickened, inflamed skin covered by a layer of flaking dead skin.

Normal skin   **Skin in psoriasis**

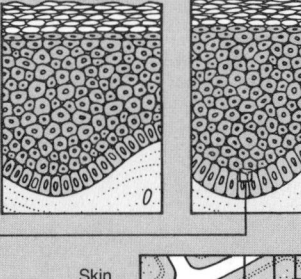
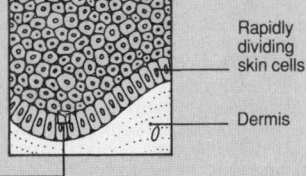

- Epidermis
- Rapidly dividing skin cells
- Dermis

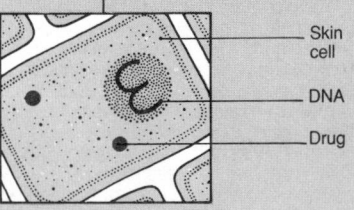
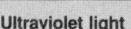

- Skin cell
- DNA
- Drug

- UVA rays
- Drug
- DNA restricted

Psoralen drugs
In PUVA, psoralen drugs administered by mouth or as ointment penetrate the skin cells.

Ultraviolet light
The drug is activated by exposure of the skin to ultraviolet light. It acts on the cell's genetic material (DNA) to regulate its rate of division.

Another form of treatment, using the psoralen drug methoxsalen in conjunction with ultraviolet light therapy (PUVA), is described above.

How they work

Some drug treatments for psoriasis slow down the rapid rate of cell division that is responsible for skin thickening. Drugs that act in this way include anthralin, etretinate, and methotrexate. Etretinate also reduces production of keratin, the hard protein that forms in the outer layer of skin. Other drugs remove the layers of dead skin cells – for example, salicylic acid and coal tar. Corticosteroids reduce inflammation of the underlying skin.

How they affect you

Appropriate treatment of psoriasis usually improves the appearance of the skin. However, because drugs cannot cure the underlying cause of the disorder, psoriasis tends to recur even after successful treatment.

Individual drugs may cause side effects. Topical preparations can cause stinging and inflammation, especially if applied to normal skin. Coal tar and methoxsalen increase the skin's sensitivity to sunlight; excessive sunbathing or over-exposure to artificial ultraviolet light may damage skin and worsen the condition.

Etretinate and methotrexate have a number of possible adverse effects, including liver damage (etretinate), and gastrointestinal upsets and bone marrow damage (methotrexate). For detailed information on specific drugs, consult the relevant drug profile in Part 4.

COMMON DRUGS

Anthralin
Etretinate
Methotrexate
Methoxsalen
Salicylic acid
Topical corticosteroids (see p.202)

SUNSCREENS

Sunscreens are creams or oils containing chemicals that protect the skin from the damaging effects of ultraviolet radiation from the sun.

People vary widely in their sensitivity to sunlight. Fair-skinned people generally have the least tolerance to direct sunlight and tend to burn easily, while people with darker skin can usually withstand exposure to the sun for much longer periods without noticeable harm.

In a few cases the skin is made more sensitive to sunlight by a disease such as pellagra (a form of malnutrition primarily due to a deficiency of niacin; see p.539) or herpes simplex infection. Certain drugs – such as the thiazide diuretics, phenothiazine antipsychotics, sulfonamide antibacterials, tetracycline antibiotics, psoralens, and nalidixic acid – can also increase the skin's sensitivity to sunlight.

Why they are used

Sunscreens are usually applied before sunbathing to prevent burning while allowing the skin to tan. Prolonged exposure of unprotected skin to strong sunlight increases the risk of skin cancer, especially among fair-skinned people, and can cause premature aging of the skin. A sunscreen is therefore particularly advisable for people traveling to tropical and semi-tropical countries who are unaccustomed to strong sunlight.

Sunscreens are graded according to the degree of protection they offer – the

ACTION OF SUNSCREENS

Fair skin unprotected by a sunscreen suffers damage as ultraviolet rays pass through to the layers beneath, causing pain and inflammation. Sunscreens block out some of these ultraviolet rays, while allowing a proportion of them to pass through the skin surface to the epidermis to stimulate the activity of melanin, the pigment that gives the skin a tan and helps to protect it during further exposure to the sun.

Skin unprotected

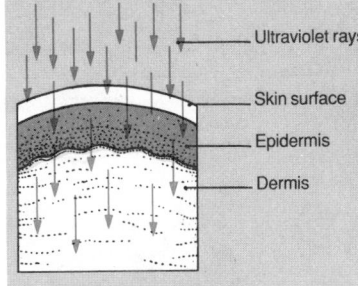

Ultraviolet rays

Skin surface

Epidermis

Dermis

Skin protected by sunscreen

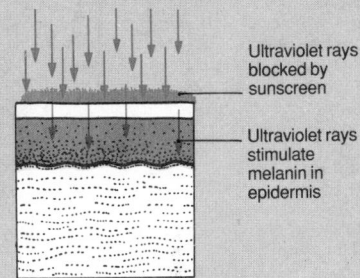

Ultraviolet rays blocked by sunscreen

Ultraviolet rays stimulate melanin in epidermis

sun protection factor (SPF). This is a measure of the amount of ultraviolet radiation that the sunscreen absorbs; the higher the number, the greater the protection afforded. Thus people of various skin types can choose the most suitable sunscreen. Those with fair skin should start with a sunscreen with an SPF of 10 to 15, while those with darker skin may use a screen with an SPF of 6 to 8. As the skin tans, a lower SPF may be adequate.

How they work

Sunlight is composed of different wavelengths of electromagnetic radiation. Of these, ultraviolet radiation can be particularly harmful to the skin. The chemicals in sunscreens absorb ultraviolet radiation, ensuring that a smaller proportion of it reaches the skin.

Risks and special precautions

Sunscreens only form a physical barrier to the passage of ultraviolet radiation. They do not alter the skin to make it more resistant to sunlight. Therefore a sunscreen lotion must be applied frequently to maintain protection.

Even sunscreens with the highest blocking effect do not completely exclude radiation from the sun. Accordingly, people who are fair-skinned or very sensitive to sunlight should never expose themselves to direct sun, even if they are using a sunscreen.

Sunscreens can irritate the skin and some may cause an allergic rash. People who are sensitive to drugs such as procaine and benzocaine, certain hair dyes, and sulfanilamide may develop a rash following application of a preparation containing para-aminobenzoic acid or benzophenones like oxybenzone or sulisobenzone.

COMMON DRUGS

Oxybenzone
Para-aminobenzoic acid
Sulisobenzone

TREATMENT FOR DANDRUFF AND HAIR LOSS

Dandruff treatments

The condition in which dead cells accumulate on the scalp and form white flaky scales is commonly referred to as dandruff. It is not a sign of ill health, but most people find it unsightly and want to get rid of it. In some cases frequent washing (four to six times a week) with a mild shampoo keeps the scalp free of dandruff. Many people, however, find that a medicated shampoo is more effective.

Medicated shampoos usually contain active ingredients such as tar, sulfur, or salicylic acid that soften the dead scales and make them easier to remove.

Shampoos that contain zinc pyrithione, chloroxin, or selenium sulfide are often effective for more severe cases. These reduce the formation of dandruff by slowing down the growth of skin cells. They also have a mild antifungal action. (Some physicians believe that yeast infection is a cause of dandruff.)

If the dandruff is severe and does not respond to any of those treatments, a physician may prescribe a weak corticosteroid lotion or gel (see also Topical corticosteroids, p.202).

Drugs used for hair loss

One of the most common causes of hair loss is male pattern baldness, in which hair lost from the temples and crown is initially replaced by fine downy hair, and finally lost permanently. It is probably caused by hormonal changes and most commonly affects men, although women can also suffer this type of hair loss.

Traditionally, response to male pattern baldness has included the use of wigs and toupees, and hair transplants. Recently, however, minoxidil, a vasodilator and antihypertensive drug, has been found to stimulate hair growth in some people. A topical preparation of the drug is at present being investigated as a possible treatment for hair loss. It acts by increasing blood flow in the skin, and elongating the hair follicles as well as reducing the number of white cells around hair follicles. Unlicensed preparations of minoxidil are available at some clinics, but these should be avoided because of poor control over the concentrations of the drug being used. The drug may be absorbed through the scalp and in excessive concentrations can produce harmful effects.

Temporary thinning of the hair may be caused by fungal infection, stress, serious illness, childbirth, or treatment with anticancer drugs (see p.182). In these cases drug treatment is not effective and hair growth returns to normal once the cause has been removed.

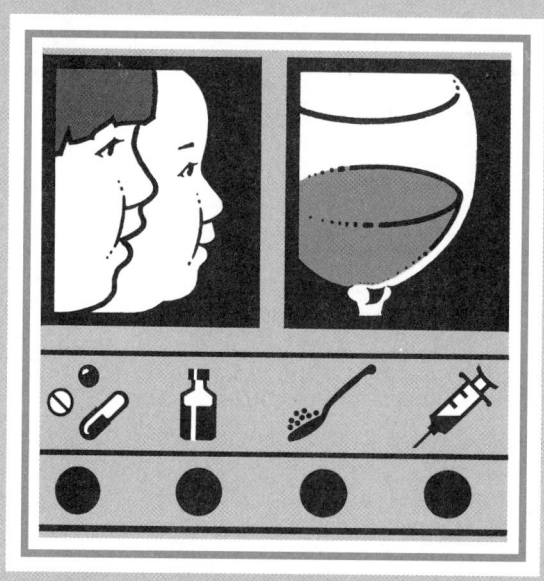

PART
4

A – Z
OF DRUGS

A – Z OF MEDICAL DRUGS
A – Z OF VITAMINS AND MINERALS
DRUGS OF ABUSE
FOOD ADDITIVES

A – Z OF MEDICAL DRUGS

The drug profiles in this section provide information and practical advice on 320 individual drugs. It is intended that these profiles should provide reference and guidance for non-medical readers taking drug treatment. However, it is impossible for a book of this kind to take into account every variation in individual circumstances, and readers should always follow their physician's instructions where these differ from the advice in this section.

The drugs have been selected to provide representative coverage of the principal classes of drugs in medical use today. For disorders where a number of different drugs are available for treatment, the ones which are used most commonly have been selected. Emphasis has also been placed on those drugs which are likely to be used in the home, although in a few cases those that are administered only in the hospital have been included when it has been judged a drug is of sufficient interest. At the end of this section supplementary profiles are provided on vitamins and minerals (pp.534 – 546), drugs of abuse (pp.547 – 554) and food additives (pp.555 –559).

Each drug profile is organized in the same way, using standard headings (see sample page, below). To help you make the most of the information provided, the terms used and the instructions given under each heading are discussed and explained on the following pages.

HOW TO UNDERSTAND THE PROFILES

For ease of reference, the information on each drug is arranged in a consistent format under standard headings.

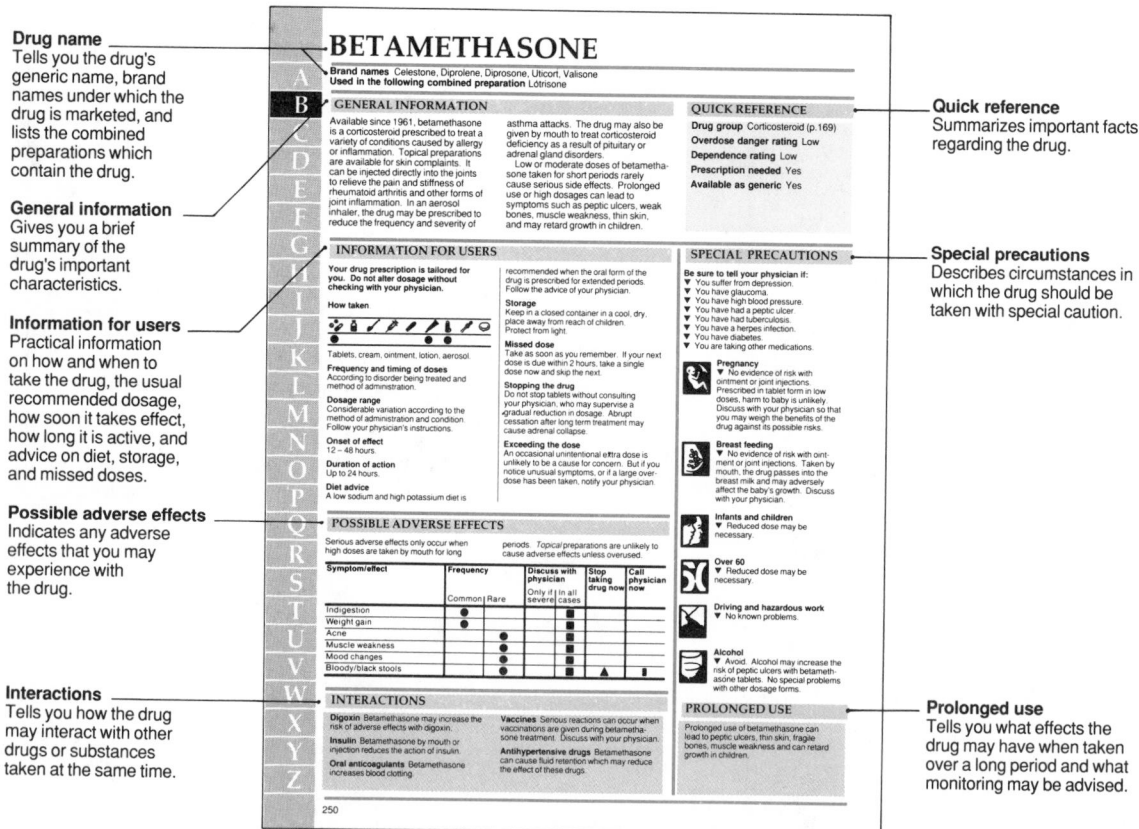

Drug name
Tells you the drug's generic name, brand names under which the drug is marketed, and lists the combined preparations which contain the drug.

General information
Gives you a brief summary of the drug's important characteristics.

Information for users
Practical information on how and when to take the drug, the usual recommended dosage, how soon it takes effect, how long it is active, and advice on diet, storage, and missed doses.

Possible adverse effects
Indicates any adverse effects that you may experience with the drug.

Interactions
Tells you how the drug may interact with other drugs or substances taken at the same time.

Quick reference
Summarizes important facts regarding the drug.

Special precautions
Describes circumstances in which the drug should be taken with special caution.

Prolonged use
Tells you what effects the drug may have when taken over a long period and what monitoring may be advised.

DRUG NAME

Generic name
The main heading on the page is the shortest form of the drug's *generic* name, unless the short form causes confusion with another drug, in which case the full generic name is given. For example, dantrolene sodium, a muscle relaxant, is listed as dantrolene, as there is no other generic drug of this name. However, magnesium hydroxide, an antacid, is listed under its full name to avoid confusing it with the mineral magnesium, or other compounds of the mineral, such as magnesium sulfate.

Brand names
Under the generic name are the brand names of products in which the drug is the major single active ingredient; if there are a number of different brand-name forms of the drug, only the most commonly used ones are given. A maximum of five brand names has been allowed. The names of preparations, if any, in which the drug is combined with other drugs are also listed. For more information about brand names and generic names, see p.13.

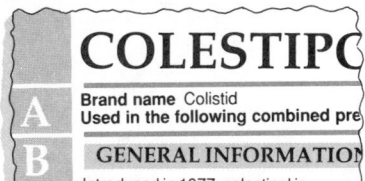

GENERAL INFORMATION

The information here helps you build up an overall picture of the drug. It includes notes on the drug's history (for example, when it was first introduced), and the principal disorders for which it is prescribed. This section also discusses the drug's major possible adverse effects.

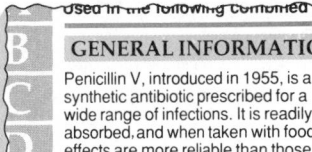

GENERAL INFORMATION

Penicillin V, introduced in 1955, is a synthetic antibiotic prescribed for a wide range of infections. It is readily absorbed, and when taken with food its effects are more reliable than those of other oral penicillins.

QUICK REFERENCE

The text in this box summarizes the important facts regarding your drug, and is organized under five headings, which are explained in detail below.

Drug group
This tells you which of the major groups the drug belongs to, and the page on which you can find out more about the drugs in the group and the various disorders or conditions they are used to treat. Where a drug belongs to more than one group, each group included in the book is listed. For example, interferon is listed as an antiviral drug (p.161) and an anticancer drug (p.182).

Overdose danger rating
Gives a general indication of the seriousness of the drug's effects if the dosage prescribed by your physician, or that recommended on the label of an over-the-counter drug, is exceeded. The ratings – low, medium and high – are explained

> **QUICK REFERENCE**
> **Drug group** Antimalarial drug (p.165) and antirheumatic drug (p.145)
> **Overdose danger rating** High
> **Dependence rating** Low
> **Prescription needed** Yes

below. The rating also determines the advice given under Exceeding the dose.

- **Low** Symptoms unlikely. Death unknown.
- **Medium** Medical advice needed. Death rare.
- **High** Medical attention needed urgently. Potentially fatal.

If you do exceed the dose, advice is given under Exceeding the dose.

Dependence rating
Drugs are classified on the basis of the risk of dependence, and are given a rating of low, medium or high.

- **Low** Dependence unknown.
- **Medium** Rare possibility of dependence.
- **High** Dependence is likely in long-term use.

Prescription needed
This tells you whether a prescription is needed to purchase the drug. Prescription drugs that are controlled substances (see p.13) have been designated by the letter C, with a Roman numeral to denote their category, or schedule. Controlled drugs and their schedules are explained in more detail on p.13.

Available as generic
Tells you if a drug is available as a generic product.

INFORMATION FOR USERS

This section contains information on the following: methods of administration, frequency and amount of dosage, effects and actions, diet advice, practical advice on storage, missed doses, overdose, and stopping drug treatment. All information is generalized and is in no way a recommendation for an individual dosing schedule. Always follow your physician's instructions in the case of prescription drugs, and those of the manufacturer for over-the-counter medication.

How taken
The symbols in the box represent the various ways in which drugs can be administered. The dot that appears below the symbol indicates the form in which the drug is available. This acts as a visual backup to the written information which follows immediately below the box.

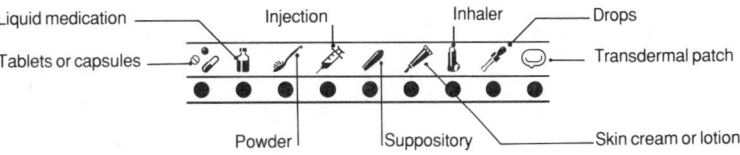

A – Z OF MEDICAL DRUGS continued

INFORMATION FOR USERS continued

Frequency and timing of doses

This refers to the standard number of times each day that the drug should be taken and, where relevant, whether it should be taken with liquid, with meals, or on an empty stomach.

> **Frequency and timing of doses**
> *By mouth* Once daily (prevention of malaria): 1 – 2 x daily (treatment of malaria): once daily (amebic infection and arthritis). *Injections* Every 6 hours (treatment of malaria).

> **Frequency and timing of doses**
> 2 x daily with meals

Dosage range

This is generally given as the normal oral dosage range for an adult; dosages for injection are not usually given. In cases where the dosages for specific age groups vary significantly from the normal adult dosage, these will also be given. Where dosage varies according to use, the dosage for each use is included.

The vast majority of drug dosages are expressed in metric units, usually milligrams (mg) or micrograms (mcg). A few dosages are given in units (u) or international units (IU). See also Weights and measures, facing page.

> **Adult dosage range**
> *Prevention of gout attacks* 0.6 – 1.8mg daily *Relief of gout attacks* 0.5 or 0.6mg per dose up to a maximum of 6mg daily until joint is better or gastrointestinal problems arise.

> **Dosage range**
> *Adults* 500mg – 1g per dose up to a maximum of 4g daily. *Children* Up to 1 year, 60 – 120mg per dose: 1 – 5 years, 120 – 250mg per dose: 6 – 12 years, 320 – 480mg per dose.

Onset of effect

The onset of effect is the time it takes for the drug to become active in the body. This sometimes coincides with the onset of beneficial effects, but there may sometimes be an interval between the time when a drug is pharmacologically active and when you start to notice improvement in your symptoms or your underlying condition.

> **Onset of effect**
> Fat levels in the blood are lowered in 24 – 48 hours, but full benefits may not be apparent for up to 1 – 3 months. When this drug is used for itching or diarrhea, full beneficial effects may not be felt for several days.

> **Onset of effect**
> 2 – 3 days. In rheumatoid arthritis, full effect may not be felt for up to 6 months.

Duration of action

The information given here refers to the length of time that one dose of the drug remains active in the body.

> **Duration of action**
> Up to 6 hours

> **Duration of action**
> 8 hours (tablets, liquid, suppositories): 12 – 24 hours (slow-release tablets).

Diet advice

With some drugs, it is important to avoid certain foods, either because they reduce the effect of the drug or because they interact adversely. This section of the profile tells you what, if any, dietary changes are necessary.

> **Diet advice**
> A low-fat diet may be recommended. Use of this drug may deplete levels of certain vitamins. Supplements may be advised.

Storage

Drugs will deteriorate and may become inactive if they are not stored under suitable conditions. The advice given in the profiles is usually to store in a cool, dry place out of the reach of children. Some drugs must also be protected from light. Some drugs, especially liquid medications, need to be kept in a refrigerator, but should not be frozen. For further advice on storing drugs, see p.29.

> **Storage**
> Keep in a closed container in a cool, dry place away from reach of children. Protect from light.

Missed dose

This section gives advice on what to do if you forget a dose of your drug, so that the effectiveness and safety of your treatment is maintained as far as possible. If you forget to take several doses in succession, consult your physician. You can read more about missed doses on p.28.

> **Missed dose**
> No cause for concern, but take when you remember. If your next dose is due within 2 hours, take a single dose now and skip the next.

> **Missed dose**
> Take as soon as you remember. If your next dose is due within 24 hours (once weekly schedule) or 6 hours (once or twice daily schedule), take a single dose now and skip the next.

Stopping the drug

If you are taking a drug regularly you should know how and when you can safely stop taking it. Some drugs can be safely stopped as soon as you feel better, or as soon as your symptoms have disappeared. Others must not be stopped until the full course of treatment has been completed, or they must be gradually withdrawn under the supervision of a physician. Failure to comply with instructions for stopping a drug may lead to adverse effects, or may cause your condition to worsen or your symptoms to reappear. See also Ending drug treatment, p.28.

> **Stopping the drug**
> Can be safely stopped as soon as you no longer need it.

> **Stopping the drug**
> Do not stop the drug without consulting your physician: stopping the drug may lead to worsening of the underlying condition.

Exceeding the dose

The information in this section expands on that in the quick reference box on the drug's overdose danger rating. It explains the possible consequences of exceeding the dose and what to do if an overdose is taken. Examples of wordings used for low, medium, and high overdose ratings are as follows:

Low
An occasional extra dose is unlikely to be a cause for concern but if you notice unusual symptoms, or if a large overdose has been taken, notify your physician.

Medium
An occasional extra dose is unlikely to cause problems, but if a large overdose has been taken, notify your physician.

High
Seek immediate medical advice in all cases. Take emergency action if [relevant symptoms] occur.

> **Exceeding the dose**
> An occasional unintentional extra dose is unlikely to be a cause for concern. But if you notice unusual symptoms, or if a large overdose has been taken, notify your physician.
>
> **OVERDOSE ACTION**
> Seek immediate medical advice in all cases. Take emergency action if vomiting, confusion, or loss of consciousness occur.
>
> **See Drug poisoning emergency guide (p.590).**

SPECIAL PRECAUTIONS

Many drugs need to be taken with care by people with a history of particular conditions. The profile lists conditions you should tell your physician about when a drug is prescribed for you, and conditions you should discuss with your physician before taking an over-the-counter drug. Certain groups of people (pregnant women, nursing mothers, children, and those over 60) may also be at special risk from drug treatment. Advice for these groups is given in every profile. Information is also included about drinking alcohol, driving, and undertaking hazardous work.

SPECIAL PRECAUTIONS

Be sure to tell your physician if:
▼ You have impaired liver or kidney function.
▼ You have heart problems.
▼ You have a blood disorder.
▼ You have stomach ulcers.
▼ You have chronic inflammation of the bowel.
▼ You are taking other medications.

Pregnancy
▼ No evidence of risk with low doses. High doses may have adverse effects on hearing, balance, and vision in the baby. Discuss with your physician.

Breast feeding
▼ Discuss with your physician. The drug passes into the breast milk and may make the baby irritable.

Infants and children
▼ Not recommended under 6 years. Reduced dose necessary in older children.

Over 60
▼ Reduced dose may be necessary. Increased likelihood of adverse effects.

Driving and hazardous work
▼ Avoid such activities until you have learned how the drug affects you because the drug may cause dizziness in high doses.

Alcohol
▼ Although this drug does not interact with alcohol, your underlying condition may make it inadvisable to take alcohol.

WEIGHTS AND MEASURES

Metric equivalents of measurements used in this book:

1000 mcg (microgram) = 1 mg (milligram)
1000 mg = 1 g (gram)
1000 ml (milliliter) = 1 l (liter)

Units or international units
Units (u) and international units (IU) are also used to express drug dosages. They represent the biological activity of a drug (its effect on the body). This ability cannot be measured in terms of weight or volume, but must be calculated in a laboratory.

POSSIBLE ADVERSE EFFECTS

The adverse effects discussed in the drug profile are symptoms or reactions that may arise when you take the drug. The emphasis is on symptoms that you, the patient, are likely to notice, rather than on the findings of laboratory tests that your physician may order. The bulk of the section is in the form of a table that lists the adverse effects and indicates how commonly they occur, when to tell your physician about them, and when to stop the drug. The headings in the table are explained below.

Frequency
Tells you whether the adverse effect is common or rare. Common effects are listed first.

Discuss with physician
The marker in this section indicates under what circumstances you need to inform your physician about an adverse effect you are experiencing.

Only if severe A marker in this column means that the symptom is unlikely to be serious, but that you should seek your physician's advice if it troubles you.
In all cases Adverse effects marked in this column require prompt, but not necessarily emergency, medical attention. (See also Call physician now, below.)

Stop taking drug now
In cases where certain unpleasant or dangerous adverse effects of a drug may override its beneficial effects, you are advised to stop taking the drug immediately, if necessary before seeing your physician.

Call physician now
Effects marked in this column require immediate medical help. They indicate a potentially dangerous response to the drug treatment, for which you should seek emergency medical attention.

| Symptom/effect | Frequency | | Discuss with physician | | Stop taking drug now | Call physician now |
	Common	Rare	Only if severe	In all cases		
Nausea	●			■		
Diarrhea/abdominal pain	●			■		
Headache/dizziness		●		■		
Rash		●			■	▲	▌
Blurred vision		●			■	▲	▌

INTERACTIONS

The interactions discussed here are those that may occur between the drug under discussion and other drugs. Information includes the name of the interacting drug or drug groups and the effect of the interaction.

INTERACTIONS

Diuretics can lower levels of potassium in the body, and this increases the risk of adverse effects with digitoxin.

Quinidine and verapamil may increase

Sy
epi
incr
the

PROLONGED USE

The information given here concerns the adverse, and sometimes beneficial, effects of the drug which may occur during long-term use. These may differ from those listed under Possible adverse effects. This section of the profile also includes information on monitoring the effects of the drug during long-term treatment, explaining the tests you may be given if your physician thinks they are necessary.

PROLONGED USE

Prolonged use of this drug may lead to hair loss, rashes, tingling in the hands and feet, muscle pain and weakness, and blood disorders.

Monitoring Periodic blood checks are usually required.

ACEBUTOLOL

Brand name Sectral
Used in the following combined preparations None

GENERAL INFORMATION

Acebutolol, introduced in 1985, is a beta blocker that is most commonly prescribed to treat hypertension, angina, and certain types of abnormal heart rhythms. It can also be used to relieve palpitations and tremor caused by overactivity of the thyroid gland or the sort of anxiety that goes with stage fright. Acebutolol may be given following a heart attack to protect the heart from further damage.

Unlike some similar drugs that act on both the heart and lungs, acebutolol is cardioselective – that is, it acts mainly on the heart. This makes it especially suitable for people with asthma, bronchitis, or other lung problems, although special caution is still required. In common with other beta blockers, acebutolol affects the body's response to low blood sugar, which can cause problems for diabetics. It can also reduce circulation to the hands and feet.

INFORMATION FOR USERS

Your drug prescription is tailored for you. Do not alter dosage without checking with your physician.

How taken

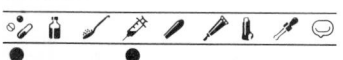

Tablets, capsules, injection.

Frequency and timing of doses
1 – 2 x daily.

Dosage range
400 – 900mg daily.

Onset of effect
1 – 4 hours. Full beneficial effect on blood pressure may take some weeks.

Duration of action
Up to 24 hours.

Diet advice
None.

Storage
Keep in a closed container in a cool, dry place away from reach of children.

Missed dose
Take as soon as you remember. If your next dose is due within 2 hours, take a single dose now and skip the next.

Stopping the drug
Do not stop the drug without consulting your physician; stopping the drug may lead to worsening of the underlying condition.

OVERDOSE ACTION

Seek immediate medical advice in all cases. Take emergency action if collapse or loss of consciousness occurs.

See Drug poisoning emergency guide (p.590).

POSSIBLE ADVERSE EFFECTS

Acebutolol has adverse effects that are common to most beta blockers. Symptoms such as fatigue and nausea are usually temporary and diminish with long-term use.

Acebutolol can occasionally provoke or worsen asthma and heart problems. Fainting may be a sign that the drug has slowed the heartbeat excessively.

Symptom/effect	Frequency		Discuss with physician		Stop taking drug now	Call physician now
	Common	Rare	Only if severe	In all cases		
Lethargy	●			■		
Cold hands and feet	●			■		
Nausea		●		■		
Nightmares/vivid dreams		●		■		
Rash		●			■	▲
Breathlessness/fainting		●		■	▲	∎

INTERACTIONS

Nifedipine can lower the blood pressure excessively if taken with acebutolol.

Anti-arrhythmic drugs Taken with acebutolol, some of these drugs may cause a further reduction in heart rate.

Indomethacin reduces the antihypertensive effect of acebutolol.

Cimetidine can increase the levels of acebutolol in the blood.

SPECIAL PRECAUTIONS

Be sure to tell your physician if:
▼ You have a lung disorder such as asthma or bronchitis.
▼ You have diabetes.
▼ You have circulatory disease.
▼ You are taking other medications.

Pregnancy
▼ No evidence of risk to baby when taken in early pregnancy. Taken in late pregnancy, the drug may affect the baby's heart rate or blood sugar levels adversely.

Breast feeding
▼ Discuss with your physician. The drug passes into the breast milk, but at normal doses adverse effects on the baby are uncommon.

Infants and children
▼ Not usually prescribed.

Over 60
▼ Increased likelihood of adverse effects.

Driving and hazardous work
▼ No known problems.

Alcohol
▼ No known problems.

Surgery and general anesthetics
▼ Acebutolol may need to be stopped before you have a general anesthetic. Discuss this with your physician or dentist before any surgery.

PROLONGED USE

No known problems.

ACETAMINOPHEN

Brand names Anacin-3, Panadol, Tempra, Tylenol, Tylenol Extra Strength
Used in the following combined preparations Parafon Forte, Tylenol w/codeine

GENERAL INFORMATION

Although acetaminophen has been known since the early 1900s, it has been widely used as an analgesic only since 1955. One of a group of drugs known as the non-narcotic analgesics, it is kept in the home to relieve occasional bouts of mild pain and to reduce fever. It is suitable for children as well as adults, and children's syrups are available.

One of the advantages of taking acetaminophen is that it does not cause stomach upset or bleeding problems. That makes it a particularly useful alternative for people who suffer from peptic ulcers or who cannot tolerate aspirin. It can also be safely taken if you are receiving treatment with anticoagulants.

An overdose of acetaminophen is dangerous, capable of causing serious damage to the liver and kidneys. Large dosages of acetaminophen may be toxic in people who are regular consumers of more than 3-4 ounces of alcohol per day.

QUICK REFERENCE

Drug group Non-narcotic analgesic (p.108)

Overdose danger rating High

Dependence rating Low

Prescription needed No

Available as generic Yes

INFORMATION FOR USERS

Follow instructions on the label. Call your physician if symptoms worsen.

How taken

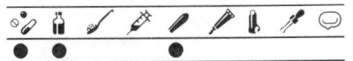

Tablets, capsules, syrup, rectal suppositories.

Frequency and timing of doses
Every 4 – 6 hours as necessary.

Dosage range
Adults 500mg – 1g per dose up to a maximum of 4g daily.
Children Up to 1 year, 60 – 120mg per dose; 1 – 5 years, 120 – 250mg per dose; 6 – 12 years, 320 – 480mg per dose.

Onset of effect
Within 10 – 60 minutes.

Duration of action
Up to 6 hours.

Diet advice
None.

Storage
Keep in a closed container in a cool, dry place, away from reach of children.

Missed dose
Take as soon as you remember if required to relieve pain. Otherwise do not take the missed dose, and take a further dose only when you are in pain.

Stopping the drug
Can be safely stopped as soon as you no longer need it.

OVERDOSE ACTION

 Seek immediate medical advice in all cases. Take emergency action if nausea, vomiting, or stomach pain occurs.

See Drug poisoning emergency guide (p.590).

POSSIBLE ADVERSE EFFECTS

Acetaminophen has rarely been found to produce any side effects if you take the drug as recommended.

Symptom/effect	Frequency		Discuss with physician		Stop taking drug now	Call physician now
	Common	Rare	Only if severe	In all cases		
Nausea		●	■			
Rash		●		■	▲	

INTERACTIONS

General note Interactions with drugs other than alcohol are unreported.

SPECIAL PRECAUTIONS

Be sure to consult your physician before using this drug if:
▼ You have impaired kidney or liver function.
▼ You are taking other medications.

 Pregnancy
▼ Not usually prescribed. Safety in pregnancy not established.

 Breast feeding
▼ In normal doses the drug does not significantly affect the breast milk or baby.

 Infants and children
▼ Reduced dose necessary.

 Over 60
▼ No special problems.

 Driving and hazardous work
▼ No special problems.

 Alcohol
▼ Prolonged heavy intake of alcohol in combination with acetaminophen may substantially increase the risk of injury to the liver.

PROLONGED USE

You should not normally take this drug for a period longer than 48 hours except on the advice of your physician.

ACETAZOLAMIDE

Brand names AK-Zol, Dazamide, Diamox, Diamox Parenteral
Used in the following combined preparations None

GENERAL INFORMATION

Acetazolamide, introduced in 1953, is a carbonic anhydrase inhibitor, a type of diuretic. Because it works differently from most other diuretics, reducing the reabsorption of sodium bicarbonate following the initial filtering action of the kidneys, it produces a more acidic condition in the fluids of the body. Together with other actions of the anhydrase inhibitor, this results in less fluid in the anterior chamber of the eye, making acetazolamide a valuable drug in the treatment of glaucoma (see Drugs for glaucoma, p.196). It is occasionally used to prevent or treat acute mountain (altitude) sickness.

Acetazolamide is sometimes prescribed to prevent a rare hereditary disease (familial periodic paralysis) associated with an elevated potassium level and muscle weakness. It is rarely used as a diuretic to treat the substantial fluid retention of congestive heart failure or liver disease.

QUICK REFERENCE

Drug group Carbonic anhydrase inhibitor diuretic (p.196)

Overdose danger rating Medium

Dependence rating Low

Prescription needed Yes

Available as generic Yes

INFORMATION FOR USERS

Your drug prescription is tailored for you. Do not alter dosage without checking with your physician.

How taken

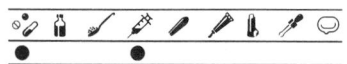

Tablets, injection.

Frequency and timing of doses
4 x daily with food (the drug is not necessarily taken every day) or 2 x daily (sustained release tablets).

Adult dosage range
500 – 1000mg daily.

Onset of effect
Within 30 minutes.

Duration of action
6 – 24 hours.

Diet advice
Use of this drug may reduce potassium in the body. Eat plenty of fresh fruit and vegetables. Also, drink plenty of fluids to help eliminate acetazolamide from the kidneys.

Storage
Keep in a closed container in a cool, dry place away from reach of children.

Missed dose
No cause for concern, but take as soon as you remember.

Stopping the drug
Do not stop the drug without consulting your physician; symptoms may recur.

Exceeding the dose
An occasional unintentional extra dose is unlikely to cause problems. Large overdoses may cause nausea and confusion. Notify your physician.

SPECIAL PRECAUTIONS

Be sure to tell your physician if:
▼ You have impaired kidney function.
▼ You have Addison's disease.
▼ You are taking other medications.

Pregnancy
▼ Not prescribed. May cause abnormalities in the developing baby. Discuss with your physician so that you may weigh the benefits of the drug against its risks.

Breast feeding
▼ The drug passes into the breast milk and may reduce your milk supply. Discuss with your physician.

Infants and children
▼ Not usually prescribed. Reduced dose necessary.

Over 60
▼ Increased likelihood of adverse effects.

Driving and hazardous work
▼ No known problems.

Alcohol
▼ Avoid. Dehydration after consumption of alcohol could lead to kidney damage with this drug.

POSSIBLE ADVERSE EFFECTS

There are a number of troublesome side effects associated with acetazolamide. Nausea can be alleviated by taking the drug at mealtimes, but other side effects can in some cases become severe enough to make stopping the drug necessary.

Symptom/effect	Frequency		Discuss with physician		Stop taking drug now	Call physician now
	Common	Rare	Only if severe	In all cases		
Lethargy	●		■			
Nausea/vomiting/diarrhea	●		■			
Tingling hands and feet	●		■			
Weight loss	●		■			
Confusion	●			■		
Temporary impotence	●			■		
Fever		●		■		
Rash		●		■		▲

INTERACTIONS

Thiazide diuretics Excessive loss of potassium may occur when thiazide diuretics are taken with acetazolamide. The combination is usually avoided.

PROLONGED USE

Serious problems are unlikely, but levels of certain salts in the body may occasionally become disrupted during prolonged use.

Monitoring Periodic tests may be performed to check on kidney function and levels of body salts.

ACETOHEXAMIDE

Brand name Dymelor
Used in the following combined preparations None

GENERAL INFORMATION

Acetohexamide, introduced in 1963, is an oral antidiabetic drug. Like other drugs of this class, it lowers blood sugar by stimulating secretion of insulin from the pancreas and promoting the uptake of sugar into body cells. It is used in the treatment of adult (maturity-onset) diabetes mellitus, together with a special diabetic diet. For overweight people, a reducing diet should also be prescribed.

This is the only oral antidiabetic drug that lowers blood uric acid levels, making it suitable for the treatment of diabetes in people with gout.

Serious side effects occur only rarely, but high doses taken for prolonged periods may lead to excessively low blood sugar levels, causing anxiety, sweating, weakness, tremor, and confusion. Acetohexamide may lose its effect during serious illnesses, injury, or surgery, requiring that insulin be substituted.

QUICK REFERENCE

Drug group Oral antidiabetic drug (p.170)

Overdose danger rating High

Dependence rating Low

Prescription needed Yes

Available as generic No

INFORMATION FOR USERS

Your drug prescription is tailored for you. Do not alter dosage without checking with your physician.

How taken

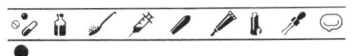

Tablets.

Frequency and timing of doses
Once daily (in the morning), or 2 x daily (in the morning and evening before meals).

Dosage range
250mg – 2g daily.

Onset of effect
Within 1 hour.

Duration of action
12 – 24 hours.

Diet advice
A low-sugar, low-fat diet must be maintained in order for the drug to be fully effective. Follow your physician's advice.

Storage
Keep in a closed container in a cool, dry place away from reach of children.

Missed dose
Take before your next meal.

Stopping the drug
Do not stop the drug without consulting your physician; stopping the drug may lead to worsening of your diabetes.

OVERDOSE ACTION

Seek immediate medical advice in all cases. You may notice symptoms of low blood sugar such as faintness, confusion, sweating, trembling, or headache. If these occur, eat or drink something sugary. Take emergency action if seizures or loss of consciousness occurs.

See Drug poisoning emergency guide (p.590).

SPECIAL PRECAUTIONS

Be sure to tell your physician if:
▼ You have impaired liver or kidney function.
▼ You are allergic to sulfonamide drugs.
▼ You are taking other medications.

Pregnancy
▼ Not usually prescribed. May cause low blood sugar in the newborn baby. Insulin is generally substituted in pregnancy.

Breast feeding
▼ Discuss with your physician. The drug passes into the breast milk and may cause low blood sugar in the baby.

Infants and children
▼ Not prescribed.

Over 60
▼ Signs of low blood sugar may be more difficult to recognize.

Driving and hazardous work
▼ Usually no problem. Avoid these activities if you have warning signs of low blood sugar.

Alcohol
▼ Avoid. Alcoholic drinks upset diabetic control.

Surgery and general anesthetics
▼ Surgery may reduce the beneficial effect of acetohexamide on diabetes. Notify your physician that you are diabetic before any surgery; insulin treatment may need to be substituted.

POSSIBLE ADVERSE EFFECTS

Serious adverse effects are rare. Faintness, sweating, tremor, weakness, and confusion may be signs of low blood sugar due to lack of food or too high a dose of the drug.

Symptom/effect	Frequency		Discuss with physician		Stop taking drug now	Call physician now
	Common	Rare	Only if severe	In all cases		
Faintness/confusion	●			■		
Weakness/tremor	●			■		
Sweating	●			■		
Nausea/vomiting		●	■			
Thirst		●		■		
Rash/itching		●		■		

PROLONGED USE

No problems expected.

Monitoring Regular monitoring of urine and/or blood sugar is required.

INTERACTIONS

General note A variety of drugs may reduce effect of acetohexamide and so may raise blood sugar levels. Such drugs include corticosteroids, estrogens, diuretics, rifampin, phenobarbital, antipsychotic drugs, and phenytoin. Other drugs increase the risk of low blood sugar. These include dicumarol, sulfonamides, anabolic steroids, aspirin, and ketoconazole.

Beta blockers These mask the signs of low blood sugar.

ACETYLCYSTEINE

Brand name Mucomyst
Used in the following combined preparation Mucomyst with Isoproterenol

GENERAL INFORMATION

Acetylcysteine is a mucolytic agent given to relieve mucous congestion of the nose, sinuses, and airways. It is widely used in the treatment of chronic bronchitis and emphysema.

The drug is usually administered as a nebulized (fine) spray, inhaled to liquefy and loosen accumulated mucus so that it can be more easily expelled by coughing. For certain acute illnesses, this is considered a hospital procedure, requiring special suction equipment. For more chronic pulmonary conditions, acetylcysteine inhalations can be carried out effectively when administered by a simple pump with a nebulizer.

Acetylcysteine rarely causes serious adverse effects, but it has an unpleasant odor that sometimes provokes nausea and vomiting.

Because it alters the action of mucus in the stomach, acetylcysteine may also cause indigestion; it is used with caution for people who have had peptic ulcers. The drug can irritate the air passages, occasionally worsening the breathing difficulties of people with asthma.

Acetylcysteine is also used as an antidote to acetaminophen overdose; it is given orally in repeated doses.

QUICK REFERENCE

Drug group Mucolytic decongestant (p.122)

Overdose danger rating Low

Dependence rating Low

Prescription needed Yes

Available as generic No

INFORMATION FOR USERS

Your drug prescription is tailored for you. Do not alter dosage without checking with your physician.

How taken

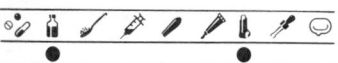

Liquid, inhaler.

Frequency and timing of doses
Every 4 – 6 hours as required.

Dosage range
Adults 2 – 20ml of 10 percent solution or 1 – 10ml of a 20 percent solution.
Children Reduced dose necessary according to age and weight.

Onset of effect
Within 1 hour.

Duration of action
Up to 8 hours.

Diet advice
None.

Storage
Keep in a closed container in a cool, dry place away from reach of children. Once opened, keep for no longer than 96 hours in a refrigerator. Do not freeze. Avoid contact with metal or rubber.

Missed dose
Take as soon as you remember.

Stopping the drug
Can be safely stopped as soon as you no longer need it.

Exceeding the dose
An occasional unintentional extra dose is unlikely to be a cause for concern. But if you notice unusual symptoms, or if a large overdose has been taken, notify your physician.

SPECIAL PRECAUTIONS

Be sure to tell your physician if:
▼ You have had peptic ulcers.
▼ You are taking other medications.

Pregnancy
▼ No evidence of risk to baby.

Breast feeding
▼ Discuss with your physician. Effect on breast feeding uncertain.

Infants and children
▼ Reduced dose necessary according to age and weight.

Over 60
▼ Reduced dose may be necessary.

Driving and hazardous work
▼ No known problems.

Alcohol
▼ No known problems.

POSSIBLE ADVERSE EFFECTS

There are few adverse effects that commonly occur with acetylcysteine. In acute cases, excessive mucus may be produced, requiring removal by suction. In these cases, the drug should not be used unless suction equipment is available.

Symptom/effect	Frequency		Discuss with physician		Stop taking drug now	Call physician now
	Common	Rare	Only if severe	In all cases		
Nausea/vomiting		●		■		
Rash		●		■		
Breathing difficulties		●		■		
Excessive/bloody mucus	●			■		

INTERACTIONS

None.

PROLONGED USE

No special problems.

ACYCLOVIR

Brand name Zovirax
Used in the following combined preparations None

GENERAL INFORMATION

Introduced in 1982, acyclovir is an anti-viral drug used in the treatment of herpes infections of all types. Most commonly given in the form of an ointment, it reduces the severity of out-breaks of cold sores and shingles. It also effectively relieves the pain and itching of genital herpes. However, acyclovir does not prevent the infec-tion from recurring. It also has some effect against the cytomegalovirus (CMV) and Epstein-Barr virus (EBV).

Acyclovir may be given by injection or by mouth for severe or recurrent cases of genital herpes. It is prescribed on a regular basis for people with reduced immunity. The drug is also admin-istered as an ointment for herpes infections of the cornea.
 The injected form is prescribed with caution to those with impaired kidney function because with high doses there is a slight risk of crystals forming in the kidneys.

QUICK REFERENCE

Drug group Antiviral drug (p.161)
Overdose danger rating Low
Dependence rating Low
Prescription needed Yes
Available as generic No

INFORMATION FOR USERS

Your drug prescription is tailored for you. Do not alter dosage without checking with your physician.

How taken

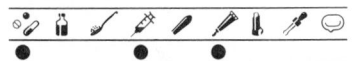

Capsules, injection, ointment.

Frequency and timing of doses
5 x daily (capsules); 6 x daily (ointment).

Dosage range
Capsules 1g daily for 10 days (herpes infec-tion); 600mg – 1g (prevention of infection).
Ointment One-half inch per 4 square inches of affected skin at each application.
Eye drops As directed.

Onset of effect
Within 24 hours.

Duration of action
Up to 8 hours.

Diet advice
None.

Storage
Keep in a closed container in a cool, dry place away from reach of children. Protect from light.

Missed dose
Ointment Do not apply the missed dose. Apply your next dose as usual.
Capsules Take as soon as you remember.

Stopping the drug
Complete the full course as directed.

Exceeding the dose
An occasional unintentional extra dose is unlikely to be a cause for concern. But if you notice unusual symptoms, or if a large over-dose has been taken, notify your physician.

POSSIBLE ADVERSE EFFECTS

Serious adverse effects are rare. Ointment commonly causes discomfort at the site of application. Confusion, hallucinations, and blood in urine occur rarely with injections.

Symptom/effect	Frequency		Discuss with physician		Stop taking drug now	Call physician now
	Common	Rare	Only if severe	In all cases		
Ointment						
Burning/stinging/itching	●		■			
Rash	●			■	▲	
Capsules						
Nausea/vomiting	●		■			
Headache/dizziness	●		■			
Injection						
Blood in urine		●		■	▲	
Confusion/hallucinations		●		■	▲	

INTERACTIONS (capsules and injection only)

General note Any drug that affects the kidneys increases the risk of such effects with acyclovir.

Probenecid This drug increases the level of acyclovir in the blood.

Interferon and methotrexate Taken with acyclovir, these may increase the risk of adverse effects on the nervous system.

SPECIAL PRECAUTIONS

Be sure to tell your physician if:
▼ You have impaired kidney function.
▼ You are taking other medications.

 Pregnancy
▼ The ointment carries no known risk, but oral and injectable forms are not usually prescribed, as the effects on the developing baby are unknown.

 Breast feeding
▼ No evidence of risk with ointment. It is unknown whether the drug passes into the milk if it is taken orally or by injection. Discuss with your physician.

 Infants and children
▼ Reduced dose necessary.

 Over 60
▼ Reduced dose may be necessary.

 Driving and hazardous work
▼ No known problems.

 Alcohol
▼ No known problems.

PROLONGED USE

There is a rare risk of resistance to acyclovir with prolonged use.

A B C D E F G H I J K L M N O P Q R S T U V W X Y Z

ALBUTEROL

Brand names Proventil, Ventolin
Used in the following combined preparations None

GENERAL INFORMATION

Albuterol is a *sympathomimetic* bronchodilator that relaxes the muscle surrounding the bronchioles (airways in the lung).

It is used mainly in the treatment of asthma, chronic bronchitis, and emphysema. Although albuterol can be taken by mouth, inhalation is considered more effective because the drug is delivered directly to the bronchioles, giving rapid relief, allowing smaller doses, and creating fewer side effects.

Compared with some similar drugs, it has little stimulant effect on the heart rate and blood pressure, making it safer for those with heart problems or high blood pressure. Because albuterol relaxes the muscles of the uterus, it is under investigation for use in prevention of premature labor. It is also being investigated for possible use as an adjunct in the treatment of congestive heart failure.

The most common side effect of albuterol is fine tremor of the hands, which may interfere with precise manual work. Anxiety, tension, and restlessness may also occur.

QUICK REFERENCE

Drug group Bronchodilator (p.120) and drug used in labor (p.193)

Overdose danger rating Low

Dependence rating Low

Prescription needed Yes

Available as generic No

INFORMATION FOR USERS

Your drug prescription is tailored for you. Do not alter dosage without checking with your physician.

How taken

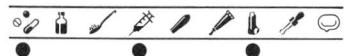

Tablets, injection, inhaler.

Frequency and timing of doses
Two inhalations every 4 – 6 hours (inhaler); 3 – 4 x daily (tablets).

Dosage range
400 – 800 micrograms daily (inhaler); 6 – 16mg daily (tablets).

Onset of effect
Within 5 – 15 minutes (inhaler); within 30 – 60 minutes (tablets).

Duration of action
Up to 6 hours (inhaler); up to 8 hours (tablets).

Diet advice
None.

Storage
Keep in a closed container in a cool, dry place away from reach of children. Protect from light. Do not puncture or burn inhalers.

Missed dose
Do not take the missed dose. Take your next dose as usual.

Stopping the drug
Do not stop the drug without consulting your physician; symptoms may recur.

Exceeding the dose
An occasional unintentional extra dose is unlikely to be a cause for concern. But if you notice any unusual symptoms, or if a large overdose has been taken, notify your physician.

POSSIBLE ADVERSE EFFECTS

Muscle tremor, especially of the hands, anxiety, and restlessness are the most common adverse effects. Palpitations and headache are rare.

Symptom/effect	Frequency		Discuss with physician		Stop taking drug now	Call physician now
	Common	Rare	Only if severe	In all cases		
Anxiety	●		■			
Nausea	●		■			
Tremor	●		■			
Restlessness	●		■			
Headache		●	■			
Palpitations		●		■		

INTERACTIONS

Other sympathomimetic drugs These may increase the effects of albuterol, increasing the risk of adverse effects.

Beta blockers may inhibit the effects of albuterol and vice versa.

Monoamine oxidase inhibitors (MAOIs) These drugs can interact with albuterol to produce a dangerous rise in blood pressure. Do not use albuterol while taking an MAOI or for 14 days thereafter.

SPECIAL PRECAUTIONS

Be sure to tell your physician if:
▼ You have heart problems.
▼ You have high blood pressure.
▼ You have an overactive thyroid gland.
▼ You have diabetes.
▼ You have difficulty in urination.
▼ You are taking other medications.

Pregnancy
▼ Not usually prescribed. Safety in pregnancy not established. Discuss with your physician so that you can weigh the benefits of the drug against its possible risks.

Breast feeding
▼ The drug passes into the breast milk, but at normal doses adverse effects on the baby are unknown. Discuss with your physician.

Infants and children
▼ Reduced dose necessary.

Over 60
▼ Reduced dose may be necessary. Increased likelihood of adverse effects.

Driving and hazardous work
▼ Avoid such activities until you have learned how the drug affects you, because the drug can cause tremors.

Alcohol
▼ No known problems.

PROLONGED USE

Prolonged use may result in tolerance to the effects of albuterol. However, failure to respond to the drug may be a result of worsening asthma that requires urgent medical attention.

ALLOPURINOL

Brand names Lopurin, Zyloprim
Used in the following combined preparations None

GENERAL INFORMATION

Widely used since 1963, allopurinol is prescribed as a long-term preventive for recurrent attacks of gout. It acts by halting the formation in the joints of uric acid crystals, which cause the inflammation characteristic of gout. Because of its inhibitive effect on uric acid formation, allopurinol is also employed to lower high uric acid levels (hyperuricemia) caused by other drugs, especially anticancer drugs.

Its effects tend to be long-term, so

allopurinol is not effective in relieving the pain of an acute flare-up. Actually, gout attacks may increase during the first months of allopurinol treatment, so colchicine is often given initially.

Unlike the gout drugs that reduce uric acid levels by increasing the quantity excreted in the urine, allopurinol does not raise the risk of kidney stones, making it particularly suitable for those with poor kidney function or a tendency to form kidney stones.

QUICK REFERENCE

Drug group Drug for gout (p.147)
Overdose danger rating Medium
Dependence rating Low
Prescription needed Yes
Available as generic Yes

INFORMATION FOR USERS

Your drug prescription is tailored for you. Do not alter dosage without checking with your physician.

How taken

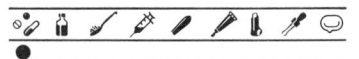

Tablets.

Frequency and timing of doses
1 – 3 x daily with meals.

Adult dosage range
Gout 200 – 600mg daily, usually 300mg.
With anticancer drugs 600 – 800mg daily.

Onset of effect
Within 24 – 48 hours. Full effect may not be felt for several weeks.

Duration of action
Up to 30 hours. Some effect may last for 1 – 2 weeks after the drug has been stopped.

Diet advice
A high fluid intake (3 quarts of fluid daily) is recommended.

Storage
Keep in a closed container in a cool, dry place away from reach of children.

Missed dose
Take as soon as you remember. If your next dose is due within 12 hours, take a dose now and take the next one on time.

Stopping the drug
Do not stop the drug without consulting your physician; symptoms may recur.

Exceeding the dose
An occasional unintentional extra dose is unlikely to cause problems. Large overdoses may cause nausea, vomiting, abdominal pain, and diarrhea. Notify your physician.

SPECIAL PRECAUTIONS

Be sure to tell your physician if:
▼ You have impaired liver or kidney function.
▼ You have hemochromatosis.
▼ You are taking other medications.

Pregnancy
▼ Not usually prescribed. Safety in pregnancy not established. Discuss with your physician so that you can weigh the benefits of the drug against its possible risks.

Breast feeding
▼ Discuss with your physician. The drug passes into the breast milk and may affect the baby adversely.

Infants and children
▼ Reduced dose necessary.

Over 60
▼ Reduced dose may be necessary.

Driving and hazardous work
▼ Avoid such activities until you have learned how the drug affects you, because the drug can cause drowsiness.

Alcohol
▼ Avoid. Alcohol increases the adverse effects of this drug.

POSSIBLE ADVERSE EFFECTS

Adverse effects of allopurinol are not very common. The most serious is an allergic rash that may require the drug to be stopped and an alternative treatment substituted.

Symptom/effect	Frequency		Discuss with physician		Stop taking drug now	Call physician now
	Common	Rare	Only if severe	In all cases		
Nausea	●		■			
Rash/itching	●			■	▲	▮
Drowsiness		●	■			
Headache		●		■		
Tingling hands/feet		●		■		
Metallic taste		●		■		
Fever and chills		●		■		

INTERACTIONS

Iron Iron supplements should not be taken with allopurinol because iron salts may be deposited in the liver.

Mercaptopurine and azathioprine Allopurinol blocks the breakdown of these drugs, so they have to be given in reduced doses.

Anticoagulant drugs Allopurinol may increase the effects of these drugs.

Thiazide diuretics These drugs reduce the effect of allopurinol.

Ampicillin and amoxicillin increase the risk of adverse effects with allopurinol.

PROLONGED USE

Apart from an increased risk of gout in the first weeks or months, no problems are expected.

Monitoring Periodic checks on uric acid levels in the blood are usually performed.

ALPRAZOLAM

Brand name Xanax
Used in the following combined preparations None

GENERAL INFORMATION

Alprazolam, introduced in 1982, belongs to a group of drugs known as benzodiazepines, which are effective in the short-term relief of nervousness and tension, relaxing muscles, and encouraging sleep. See p. 111 for a fuller description of the actions and adverse effects of this category of drugs.

Alprazolam has a particular usefulness in the treatment of panic disorders and anxiety accompanied by agitated depression. Physicians also prescribe it for agoraphobia (fear of open spaces), other phobias, and anxieties of a general nature.

In common with other benzodiazepines, alprazolam can be addictive if taken regularly over a long period. Its effects may also become weaker over time. For those reasons, treatment with alprazolam is reviewed at regular intervals.

QUICK REFERENCE

Drug group Benzodiazepine anti-anxiety drug (p.111)

Overdose danger rating Medium

Dependence rating High

Prescription needed Yes CIV

Available as generic No

INFORMATION FOR USERS

Your drug prescription is tailored for you. Do not alter dosage without checking with your physician.

How taken

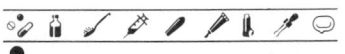

Tablets.

Frequency and timing of doses
2 – 3 x daily.

Adult dosage range
0.75 – 1.5mg daily.

Onset of effect
1 – 2 hours.

Duration of action
Up to 24 hours.

Diet advice
None.

Storage
Keep in a tightly closed container in a cool, dry place away from reach of children. Protect from light.

Missed dose
No cause for concern, but take when you remember. If your next dose is due within 2 hours, take a single dose now and skip the next.

Stopping the drug
If you have been taking the drug continuously for less than 2 weeks, it can be safely stopped as soon as you feel you no longer need it. However, if you have been taking it for longer, consult your physician, who may advise a gradual reduction in dosage. Stopping abruptly may lead to withdrawal symptoms (see p.111).

Exceeding the dose
An occasional unintentional extra dose is unlikely to cause problems. Larger overdoses may cause unusual drowsiness. Notify your physician.

SPECIAL PRECAUTIONS

Be sure to tell your physician if:
▼ You have impaired kidney or liver function.
▼ You have had problems with alcohol or drug abuse.
▼ You are taking other medications.

 Pregnancy
▼ Not usually prescribed. Safety in pregnancy not established. Discuss with your physician so that you can weigh the benefits of the drug against its possible risks.

 Breast feeding
▼ Discuss with your physician. The drug passes into the breast milk. Its effects on the baby are not clearly known.

 Infants and children
▼ Not recommended.

 Over 60
▼ Reduced dose may be necessary. Increased likelihood of adverse effects.

 Driving and hazardous work
▼ Avoid such activities until you have learned how the drug affects you, because the drug can cause reduced alertness and slowed reactions.

 Alcohol
▼ Avoid. Alcohol may increase the sedative effects of this drug.

POSSIBLE ADVERSE EFFECTS

The principal adverse effects of this drug are related to its sedative and tranquilizing properties. These effects normally diminish after the first few days of treatment. If adverse effects persist, they can often be reduced by adjustment of dosage.

Symptom/effect	Frequency		Discuss with physician		Stop taking drug now	Call physician now
	Common	Rare	Only if severe	In all cases		
Daytime drowsiness	●			■		
Dizziness/unsteadiness	●			■		
Blurred vision		●		■		
Forgetfulness/confusion		●		■		
Headache		●		■		
Rash		●			■	▲

INTERACTIONS

Sedatives All drugs that have a sedative effect on the central nervous system are likely to increase the sedative properties of alprazolam. Such drugs include sleeping drugs, antihistamines, antidepressants, narcotic analgesics, and antipsychotics.

PROLONGED USE

Regular use of this drug over several weeks can lead to a reduction in its effect as the body adapts. It may also be habit-forming when taken for extended periods, especially if larger than average doses are taken.

ALPROSTADIL

Brand name Prostin VR Pediatric
Used in the following combined preparations None

GENERAL INFORMATION

Introduced in 1981, alprostadil is used to treat newborn infants with rare congenital heart disorders that impair the flow of blood between heart and lungs. The consequent poor supply of oxygen in the blood causes cyanosis (blueness of the skin) and, in rare cases, death.

Alprostadil is a synthetic prostaglandin – a locally acting body "messenger" between one type of cell and other nearby cells. By duplicating the actions of certain prostaglandins, alprostadil keeps open a blood vessel called the ductus arteriosus that links a newborn's heart and lungs.

Given by injection and closely monitored, alprostadil ensures an adequate level of oxygen in the blood until corrective surgery can be performed.

When the drug is withdrawn, the ductus arteriosus closes normally, and if surgery is successful there are no long-term risks to the baby's health.

Alprostadil is also currently under investigation for use in Raynaud's disease – a circulatory disorder characterized by cold hands and feet.

INFORMATION FOR USERS

This drug is given only in the hospital under medical supervision and is not for self-administration.

How taken

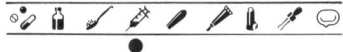

Injection.

Frequency and timing of doses
Alprostadil is given by continuous infusion until heart surgery to repair the defect has been completed, usually within 48 hours.

Dosage range
Dosage is determined according to body weight and response.

Onset of effect
15 – 30 minutes.

Duration of action
As long as infusion is continued. The ductus arteriosus starts to close 1 – 2 hours after infusion is stopped.

Diet advice
Not applicable.

Storage
Not applicable. The drug is not kept in the home.

Missed dose
Not applicable. The drug is given only in a hospital under medical supervision.

Stopping the drug
Not applicable. The drug is usually stopped after corrective heart surgery.

Exceeding the dose
The drug is given only in a hospital under medical supervision, and overdose is extremely unlikely.

SPECIAL PRECAUTIONS

Alprostadil is prescribed only under close medical supervision, taking account of the baby's condition.

Pregnancy
▼ Not applicable.

Breast feeding
▼ Not applicable.

Infants and children
▼ Alprostadil is given only to newborn infants with congenital heart disorders.

Over 60
▼ Not applicable.

Driving and hazardous work
▼ Not applicable.

Alcohol
▼ Not applicable.

POSSIBLE ADVERSE EFFECTS

Alprostadil treatment and its adverse effects are continually monitored under intensive care. Fever, flushing of the face or arms, and stopped or slow breathing occur most frequently at the start of treatment and generally disappear with dose reduction.

Symptom/effect	Frequency		Discuss with physician		Stop taking drug now	Call physician now
	Common	Rare	Only if severe	In all cases		
Fever	●			■		
Flushing	●			■		
Seizures		●		■		
Diarrhea		●		■		

INTERACTIONS

None.

PROLONGED USE

Not usually given for longer than 48 hours.

ALUMINUM HYDROXIDE

Brand names AlternaGel, Alu-Cap, Alu-Tab, Amphojel, Dialume
Used in the following combined preparations Ascriptin, Gaviscon, Maalox, Mylanta, Mylanta II

GENERAL INFORMATION

Commonly used for more than 50 years to neutralize stomach acid, aluminum hydroxide is the ingredient basic to most of the over-the-counter remedies for indigestion and heartburn.
Because it is constipating (it is sometimes used for diarrhea), aluminum hydroxide is usually combined with a magnesium-containing antacid with a balancing laxative effect.

The action of aluminum hydroxide is prolonged, making it particularly useful in preventing the pain caused by stomach and duodenal ulcers or reflux esophagitis. Aluminum hydroxide can

also promote the healing of ulcers.
In the intestine, aluminum hydroxide inactivates phosphate. This makes it helpful in the treatment of high blood phosphate (hyperphosphatemia), a condition of some people suffering impaired kidney function. But prolonged use of aluminum hydroxide can lead to phosphate deficiency and a consequent weakening of the bones.

Some preparations include large amounts of sodium and should be used with caution by those on low-sodium diets. Liquid preparations of the drug may be more effective than tablets.

QUICK REFERENCE

Drug group Antacid (p.136)

Overdose danger rating Low

Dependence rating Low

Prescription needed No

Available as generic Yes

INFORMATION FOR USERS

Follow instructions on the label. Call your physician if symptoms worsen.

How taken

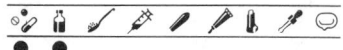

Tablets, liquid (gel suspension). Tablets should be well chewed before swallowing.

Frequency and timing of doses
As antacid 4 – 6 x daily as needed, or 1 hour before and after meals.
Peptic ulcer Every 1 – 2 hours while awake.
Hyperphosphatemia 3 – 4 x daily.
Diarrhea 3 – 6 x daily.

Dosage range
Adults 60 – 180ml daily (liquid),1.5 – 9.5g daily (tablets).
Children over 6 years Reduced dose according to age and weight.

Onset of effect
Within 15 minutes.

Duration of action
2 - 4 hours.

Diet advice
For hyperphosphatemia and kidney stones, aluminum hydroxide may be given with a low-phosphate diet.

Storage
Keep in a closed container in a cool, dry place away from reach of children.

Missed dose
Do not take the missed dose. Take your next dose as usual.

Stopping the drug
Can be safely stopped as soon as you no longer need it (indigestion). When given as ulcer treatment or for kidney failure, do not stop without consulting your physician.

Exceeding the dose
An occasional unintentional extra dose is unlikely to be a cause for concern. But if you notice unusual symptoms, or if a large overdose has been taken, notify your physician.

POSSIBLE ADVERSE EFFECTS

Constipation is common with aluminum hydroxide; nausea and vomiting may occur due to the granular, powdery nature of the

drug. Bone pain and muscle weakness occur only when large doses have been taken regularly for months or years.

Symptom/effect	Frequency		Discuss with physician		Stop taking drug now	Call physician now
	Common	Rare	Only if severe	In all cases		
Constipation	●		■			
Nausea	●		■			
Vomiting		●		■		
Bone pain		●		■		
Muscle weakness		●		■		

INTERACTIONS

General note Aluminum hydroxide interferes with the absorption or excretion of oral anticoagulants, digitalis drugs, antipsychotics, tetracyclines, penicillamine, phenytoin, and corticosteroids.

Enteric-coated tablets This drug may break up the enteric coating of tablets such as bisacodyl, causing stomach irritation.

SPECIAL PRECAUTIONS

Be sure to consult your physician before taking this drug if:
▼ You have impaired kidney function.
▼ You have heart problems.
▼ You have high blood pressure.
▼ You suffer from constipation.
▼ You have a bone disease.
▼ You are taking other medications.

Pregnancy
▼ Not usually prescribed. Safety in pregnancy not established. Discuss with your physician so that you can weigh the benefits of the drug against its possible risks.

Breast feeding
▼ No evidence of risk.

Infants and children
▼ Not recommended in children under 6 years except on the advice of a physician.

Over 60
▼ Reduced dose may be necessary. Increased likelihood of constipation.

Driving and hazardous work
▼ No known problems.

Alcohol
▼ No known problems.

PROLONGED USE

Aluminum hydroxide should not be used for longer than 4 weeks without consulting your physician. Prolonged use in high doses may deplete blood phosphate and calcium levels, leading to weakening of the bones and fractures.

AMANTADINE

Brand name Symmetrel
Used in the following combined preparations None

GENERAL INFORMATION

Amantadine was introduced in the 1960s as an antiviral drug, originally used in the prevention and treatment of influenza A. As a preventive against influenza A it proved very effective, protecting some 70 percent of those not receiving vaccination. As therapy, it is effective when given within 48 hours of the onset of flu.

In 1969 it was found to be moderately useful in parkinsonism, and this is now its most common use. Though amantadine usually produces symptomatic improvement during the first few weeks, its effectiveness wears off in a period of months, requiring replacement by another drug. It is sometimes given with levodopa, another antiparkinsonism drug. Marked adverse effects with amantadine are unusual.

INFORMATION FOR USERS

Your drug prescription is tailored for you. Do not alter dosage without checking with your physician.

How taken

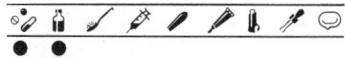

Capsules, liquid.

Frequency and timing of doses
1 – 2 x daily.

Adult dosage range
100 – 200mg daily (Parkinson's disease and viral infections).

Onset of effect
In Parkinson's disease some benefits may be noticed within 1 hour, but full effect may not be felt for up to 2 weeks. In viral infections the severity and duration of symptoms is likely to be reduced during a 2-week course of treatment if the drug is begun within 48 hours of onset of symptoms.

Duration of action
Up to 24 hours.

Diet advice
None.

Storage
Keep in a closed container in a cool, dry place away from reach of children.

Missed dose
Take as soon as you remember. If your next dose is due within 2 hours, take a single dose now and skip the next.

Stopping the drug
Do not stop taking the drug without consulting your physician; symptoms may recur.

Exceeding the dose
An occasional unintentional extra dose is unlikely to cause problems. But if you notice unusual symptoms, or if a large overdose has been taken, notify your physician.

POSSIBLE ADVERSE EFFECTS

Adverse effects are uncommon and often wear off during continued treatment. They are rarely serious enough to require treatment to be stopped.

Symptom/effect	Frequency		Discuss with physician		Stop taking drug now	Call physician now
	Common	Rare	Only if severe	In all cases		
Nervousness/agitation	●		■			
Insomnia	●		■			
Dry mouth	●		■			
Dizziness	●			■		
Blurred vision	●			■		
Digestive disturbances	●			■		
Ankle swelling	●			■		
Rash	●			■	▲	

INTERACTIONS

Anticholinergic drugs Amantadine may add to the effects of *anticholinergic* drugs. In that event your physician will probably reduce the dose of the anticholinergic drugs.

SPECIAL PRECAUTIONS

Be sure to tell your physician if:
▼ You have impaired kidney or liver function.
▼ You have had epileptic seizures.
▼ You are taking other medications.

Pregnancy
▼ Not usually prescribed. Safety in pregnancy not established. Discuss with your physician so that you can weigh the benefits of the drug against its possible risks.

Breast feeding
▼ Discuss with your physician. The drug passes into the breast milk. Its effects on the baby are not clearly known.

Infants and children
▼ Not usually prescribed. Reduced dose necessary.

Over 60
▼ Reduced dose may be necessary. Increased likelihood of adverse effects.

Driving and hazardous work
▼ Avoid such activities until you have learned how the drug affects you because of the possibility of blurred vision and agitation.

Alcohol
▼ Avoid in the first few days of treatment; thereafter keep consumption low.

PROLONGED USE

The beneficial effects of amantadine usually diminish during continuous treatment for parkinsonism. When this happens, another drug may be substituted or given together with amantadine. Sometimes the effectiveness of amantadine can be restored if it is withdrawn for a few weeks and later reintroduced.

AMILORIDE

Brand name Midamor
Used in the following combined preparation Moduretic

GENERAL INFORMATION

Amiloride belongs to the class of drugs known as potassium-sparing diuretics. Combined with thiazide or loop diuretics, amiloride is used in the treatment of hypertension, and for edema (fluid retention) resulting from heart failure or liver disease.

Amiloride's effect on urine flow is apparent within two to four hours. For this reason, avoid taking it after about 4 p.m.; otherwise you may need to pass urine during the night. As with other potassium-sparing diuretics, amiloride can be risky when there are unusually high levels of potassium in the blood. Both the drug and diseased kidneys may contribute to dangerously elevated levels. The drug is prescribed with caution for people with kidney disorders.

QUICK REFERENCE

Drug group Potassium-sparing diuretic (p.127)

Overdose danger rating Low

Dependence rating Low

Prescription needed Yes

Available as generic Yes

INFORMATION FOR USERS

Your drug prescription is tailored for you. Do not alter dosage without checking with your physician.

How taken

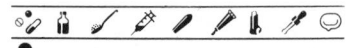

Tablets.

Frequency and timing of doses
Once daily, usually in the morning.

Dosage range
5 – 10mg daily.

Onset of effect
Within 2 – 4 hours.

Duration of action
12 – 24 hours.

Diet advice
Avoid foods that are high in potassium – for example, dried fruit, low-sodium milk, salt substitutes, and bananas.

Storage
Keep in a closed container in a cool, dry place away from reach of children.

Missed dose
Take as soon as you remember. However, if it is late in the day, do not take the missed dose, or you may need to get up at night to pass urine. Take the next scheduled dose as usual.

Stopping the drug
Do not stop the drug without consulting your physician; symptoms may recur.

Exceeding the dose
An occasional unintentional extra dose is unlikely to be a cause for concern. But if you notice unusual symptoms, or if a large overdose has been taken, notify your physician.

POSSIBLE ADVERSE EFFECTS

Amiloride has few adverse effects; the main problem is the possibility that potassium may be retained by the body, causing muscle weakness and numbness.

Symptom/effect	Frequency		Discuss with physician		Stop taking drug now	Call physician now
	Common	Rare	Only if severe	In all cases		
Digestive disturbance		●	■			
Lethargy		●	■			
Muscle weakness		●		■		
Rash		●		■	▲	

INTERACTIONS

Lithium Amiloride may increase the blood levels of lithium, leading to an increased risk of lithium poisoning.

SPECIAL PRECAUTIONS

Be sure to tell your physician if:
▼ You have impaired kidney function.
▼ You have gout.
▼ You are taking other medications.

Pregnancy
▼ Not usually prescribed. May cause a reduction in the blood supply to the developing baby.

Breast feeding
▼ Discuss with your physician. The drug passes into the breast milk and could also reduce your milk supply.

Infants and children
▼ Not usually prescribed. Reduced dose necessary.

Over 60
▼ Reduced dose may be necessary. Increased likelihood of adverse effects.

Driving and hazardous work
▼ No known problems.

Alcohol
▼ No special problems.

PROLONGED USE

Serious problems are unlikely.

Monitoring Blood tests may be performed to check on kidney function and levels of body salts.

AMINOCAPROIC ACID

Brand name Amicar
Used in the following combined preparations None

GENERAL INFORMATION

Introduced in 1964, aminocaproic acid is given to control bleeding. By limiting the action of plasmin, a component of the blood that dissolves clots once they have served their purpose, aminocaproic acid encourages and extends clotting.

The drug is used in a number of situations: after heart surgery, where the bleeding of the stitched tissues is highly undesirable; and in bleeding disorders caused by cirrhosis, aplastic anemia (in which the bone marrow fails to produce blood cells), and certain cancers. Excreted by the kidneys, the drug is particularly effective in urinary tract bleeding. It is sometimes used to halt the further bleeding of a brain hemorrhage or to prevent internal bleeding caused by drugs given for a thrombosis (a clot blocking a blood vessel). In such cases, aminocaproic acid is given in the hospital by injection. However, it may be taken by mouth to control bleeding in hemophiliacs after minor surgery. Nausea and diarrhea occur frequently, but serious adverse effects are rare.

QUICK REFERENCE

Drug group Drug to promote blood clotting (p.132)

Overdose danger rating Medium

Dependence rating Low

Prescription needed Yes

Available as generic Yes

INFORMATION FOR USERS

Your drug prescription is tailored for you. Do not alter dosage without checking with your physician.

How taken

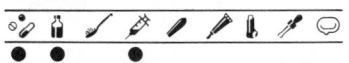

Tablets, syrup, injection.

Frequency and timing of doses
Every 6 hours (by mouth) or by continuous intravenous infusion for about 8 hours or until bleeding has stopped.

Dosage range
By mouth 4 – 5g per dose.
By injection 4 – 5g initially, then 1g per hour for approximately 8 hours, or until bleeding has stopped.

Onset of effect
Within 20 minutes.

Duration of action
4 – 6 hours.

Diet advice
None.

Storage
Keep in a closed container in a cool, dry place away from reach of children.

Missed dose
Take as soon as you remember. If your next dose is due at this time, skip the missed dose and take your next dose as usual.

Stopping the drug
Do not stop taking the drug without consulting your physician; stopping the drug may lead to excessive bleeding.

Exceeding the dose
An occasional unintentional extra dose is unlikely to cause problems. Large over-doses may cause vomiting, diarrhea, and abdominal cramps. Notify your physician.

SPECIAL PRECAUTIONS

Be sure to tell your physician if:
▼ You have impaired kidney function.
▼ You have heart problems.
▼ You have had a previous heart attack, blood clots or a stroke.
▼ You are taking other medications.

 Pregnancy
▼ Not usually prescribed. Safety in pregnancy not established. Discuss with your physician so that you can weigh the benefits of the drug against its possible risks.

 Breast feeding
▼ The drug passes into the breast milk, but at normal doses adverse effects on the baby are unlikely. Discuss with your physician.

 Infants and children
▼ Reduced dose necessary.

 Over 60
▼ Reduced dose may be necessary.

 Driving and hazardous work
▼ No special problems.

 Alcohol
▼ No known problems.

POSSIBLE ADVERSE EFFECTS

The most common adverse effects with this drug are nausea, vomiting, and diarrhea. Unusual tiredness or weakness may occur if aminocaproic acid is injected too rapidly, but persistence of these effects may indicate a muscle disorder.

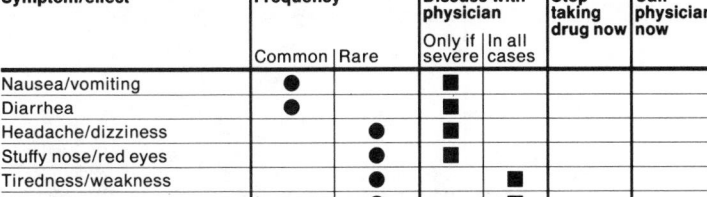

Symptom/effect	Frequency		Discuss with physician		Stop taking drug now	Call physician now
	Common	Rare	Only if severe	In all cases		
Nausea/vomiting	●		■			
Diarrhea	●		■			
Headache/dizziness		●	■			
Stuffy nose/red eyes		●	■			
Tiredness/weakness		●		■		
Itching/rash		●		■		

INTERACTIONS

Oral contraceptives and other estrogen drugs These increase the risk of abnormal blood clots with aminocaproic acid.

PROLONGED USE

Aminocaproic acid is usually given only for short periods. Prolonged use increases the risk of abnormal blood clots occurring.

Monitoring Blood clotting is monitored periodically.

AMINOGLUTETHIMIDE

Brand name Cytadren
Used in the following combined preparations None

GENERAL INFORMATION

Aminoglutethimide has been prescribed since 1960 to treat Cushing's syndrome. The syndrome, characterized by a swelling of the torso and face, is caused by the overproduction of corticosteroids in the adrenal glands. By inhibiting the function of the adrenal glands, aminoglutethimide successfully corrects the symptoms. To prevent relapse, the drug has to be continued.

Research is being done into use of the drug for types of cancerous breast tumors that depend upon estrogen stimulation to grow. It is also under investigation for the treatment of prostate cancer. Adverse effects such as lethargy, drowsiness, nausea, and loss of appetite are reduced by small initial doses, gradually increased as the body adjusts.

QUICK REFERENCE

Drug group Hormone antagonist and anticancer drug (p.182)

Overdose danger rating Medium

Dependence rating Medium

Prescription needed Yes

Available as generic No

INFORMATION FOR USERS

Your drug prescription is tailored for you. Do not alter dosage without checking with your physician.

How taken

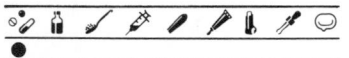

Tablets.

Frequency and timing of doses
2 – 4 x daily (starting dose); 4 x daily (maintenance dose).

Dosage range
500 – 750mg daily (starting dose); 1g daily (maintenance dose).

Onset of effect
Adverse effects may appear within a few days, but full beneficial effects may not be noticed for 2 – 3 months.

Duration of action
12 – 24 hours.

Diet advice
None.

Storage
Keep in a closed container in a cool, dry place away from reach of children.

Missed dose
Take as soon as you remember. If your next dose is due within 2 hours, take a single dose now and skip the next.

Stopping the drug
Do not stop the drug without consulting your physician; stopping the drug may lead to worsening of your underlying condition.

Exceeding the dose
An occasional extra dose is unlikely to cause problems. Large overdoses may cause drowsiness and unsteadiness. Notify your physician.

SPECIAL PRECAUTIONS

Aminoglutethimide is prescribed only under close medical supervision, taking account of your present condition and medical history.

Pregnancy
▼ Not usually prescribed. May cause abnormalities in the unborn baby. Discuss with your physician so that you may weigh the benefits of the drug against its risks.

Breast feeding
▼ Discontinue breast feeding. The drug passes into the breast milk and is likely to affect the baby adversely.

Infants and children
▼ Not usually prescribed.

Over 60
▼ No special problems.

Driving and hazardous work
▼ Avoid such activities until you have learned how the drug affects you, because the drug can cause drowsiness.

Alcohol
▼ Avoid. Alcohol may increase the adverse effects of this drug.

POSSIBLE ADVERSE EFFECTS

Many of the common adverse effects are less severe when the drug is given in gradually increased doses. Deepening of the voice and increased body hair in women tend to occur only if aminoglutethimide is taken for long periods.

Symptom/effect	Frequency		Discuss with physician		Stop taking drug now	Call physician now
	Common	Rare	Only if severe	In all cases		
Drowsiness/lethargy	●		■			
Unsteadiness	●		■			
Rash	●		■			
Increased body hair		●		■		
Deepening of voice		●		■		
Headache		●		■		
Numbness of feet/hands		●		■		

INTERACTIONS

Allopurinol This drug may increase blood levels of aminoglutethimide, leading to an increased risk of adverse effects.

PROLONGED USE

Prolonged use of this drug may lead to deepening of the voice and increased body hair in women. It may also reduce production of blood cells in the bone marrow and may impair thyroid function.

Monitoring Periodic checks on blood composition and thyroid function may be required.

AMINOPHYLLINE

Brand names Phyllocontin, Somophyllin, Somophyllin DF
Used in the following combined preparations Asmacol, Dainite KI

GENERAL INFORMATION

Aminophylline belongs to the xanthine group of bronchodilating drugs that widen the airways and stimulate the respiratory center in the brain.

It is used mainly to ease breathing in bronchial disease, especially asthma. Since there is a relatively narrow margin between the dose required for a beneficial effect and that producing a toxic effect, careful monitoring of aminophylline is usually required.

In addition to bronchodilation, aminophylline produces dilation of the blood vessels and increases the output of the heart, thus making the drug useful in congestive heart failure. Its stimulating effect on the central nervous system helps to treat apnea (transient cessation of breathing) in the newborn.

QUICK REFERENCE

Drug group Bronchodilator (p.120)
Overdose danger rating High
Dependence rating Low
Prescription needed Yes
Available as generic Yes

INFORMATION FOR USERS

Your drug prescription is tailored for you. Do not alter dosage without checking with your physician.

How taken

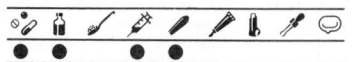

Tablets, liquid, injection, rectal suppositories.

Frequency and timing of doses
Every 6 – 8 hours (tablets, liquid); every 12 – 24 hours (slow-release tablets); 1 – 3 x daily (suppositories or rectal solution).

Dosage range
Considerable variation between different formulations and methods of administration. Follow your physician's instructions.

Onset of effect
Within a few minutes (injection); within 30 minutes (tablets, liquid, suppositories); within 90 minutes (slow-release tablets).

Duration of action
8 hours (tablets, liquid, suppositories); 12 – 24 hours (slow-release tablets).

Diet advice
Avoid charcoal-broiled foods and high-protein, low-carbohydrate meals as these may reduce the effect of the drug.

Storage
Keep in a closed container in a cool, dry place away from reach of children. Protect from light.

Missed dose
Take as soon as you remember. If your next dose is due within 2 hours, for short-acting preparations, take half a dose now and half at the next scheduled time; for long-acting preparations take a single dose now and skip the next dose.

Stopping the drug
Do not stop the drug without consulting your physician; stopping the drug may lead to worsening of the underlying condition.

OVERDOSE ACTION

Seek immediate medical advice in all cases. Take emergency action if vomiting, confusion, or loss of consciousness occurs.

See Drug poisoning emergency guide (p.590).

SPECIAL PRECAUTIONS

Be sure to tell your physician if:
▼ You have impaired liver or kidney function.
▼ You have heart problems.
▼ You have had epileptic seizures.
▼ You have had a peptic ulcer.
▼ You smoke.
▼ You are taking other medications.

 Pregnancy
▼ Not usually prescribed. Safety in pregnancy not established. Discuss with your physician so that you can weigh the benefits of the drug against its possible risks.

 Breast feeding
▼ Discuss with your physician. The drug passes into the breast milk and may make the baby irritable.

 Infants and children
▼ Reduced dose according to age and weight.

 Over 60
▼ Reduced dose may be necessary.

 Driving and hazardous work
▼ No known problems.

 Alcohol
▼ No known problems.

PROLONGED USE

No problems expected.

Monitoring Periodic checks on blood levels of the drug are usually required.

POSSIBLE ADVERSE EFFECTS

Toxic effects such as dizziness, nausea, vomiting and, more rarely, palpitations may be controlled by reducing the dosage of aminophylline.

Symptom/effect	Frequency		Discuss with physician		Stop taking drug now	Call physician now
	Common	Rare	Only if severe	In all cases		
Headache	●		■			
Irritability/insomnia	●		■			
Nausea/vomiting	●			■		▮
Dizziness/palpitations		●		■	▲	
Seizures		●		■	▲	▮

INTERACTIONS

General note Some drugs increase the effect of aminophylline (for example, erythromycin, cimetidine, and beta blockers); others reduce its effect (for example, anticonvulsants, rifampin, and sulfinpyrazone).

Oral anticoagulant drugs Aminophylline may increase their anticoagulant effect.

Tobacco smoking reduces the effect of aminophylline.

AMINOSALICYLIC ACID

Brand name Teebacin
Used in the following combined preparations None

GENERAL INFORMATION

There are three chemically distinct forms of aminosalicylic acid used in medicine: para-aminosalicylic acid (PAS), 4-aminosalicylic acid, and 5-aminosalicylic acid. PAS, introduced in 1948, is an established antituberculous drug often prescribed for the treatment of tuberculosis in young children when other drug treatments have failed and when alternative drugs are unsuitable. It may also be used to treat recurrences of the disease in adults, but is not usually a drug of first choice because it frequently causes side effects such as nausea, vomiting, and diarrhea. PAS is always given with other drugs.

4-aminosalicylic acid and 5-aminosalicylic acid, derivatives of sulfasalazine, are currently under investigation for the treatment of inflammatory bowel diseases.

INFORMATION FOR USERS

Your drug prescription is tailored for you. Do not alter dosage without checking with your physician.

How taken

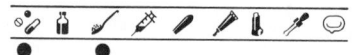

Tablets, powder.

Frequency and timing of doses
2 – 3 x daily after meals.

Dosage range
Adults 10 – 12g daily.
Children Reduced dose according to age and weight.

Onset of effect
Several days.

Duration of action
12 – 24 hours.

Diet advice
None.

Storage
Keep in a closed container in a cool, dry place away from reach of children. Protect from light. Tablets that have turned brown or purple should be discarded.

Missed dose
Take as soon as you remember. If your next dose is due within 2 hours, take a single dose now and skip the next.

Stopping the drug
Take the full course. Even if you feel better the infection may still be present and may recur if treatment is stopped too soon.

Exceeding the dose
An occasional unintentional extra dose is unlikely to be a cause for concern. But if you notice unusual symptoms, or if a large overdose has been taken, notify your physician.

SPECIAL PRECAUTIONS

Be sure to tell your physician if:
▼ You have impaired liver or kidney function.
▼ You have heart problems.
▼ You have a peptic ulcer.
▼ You have glucose-6-phosphate dehydrogenase (G6PD) deficiency.
▼ You are sensitive to streptomycin or isoniazid.
▼ You are taking other medications.

Pregnancy
▼ Not usually prescribed. Safety in pregnancy not established. Discuss with your physician so that you can weigh the benefits of the drug against its possible risks.

Breast feeding
▼ The drug passes into the breast milk, but at normal doses adverse effects on the baby are unlikely. Discuss with your physician.

Infants and children
▼ Reduced dose necessary.

Over 60
▼ No special problems.

Driving and hazardous work
▼ No known problems.

Alcohol
▼ Avoid. Alcohol increases the likelihood of stomach irritation with this drug.

POSSIBLE ADVERSE EFFECTS

Adverse effects occur less frequently in children than in adults. Gastrointestinal disturbances including nausea, vomiting, and diarrhea are common. Hypersensitivity reactions such as rashes, fever, and unusual tiredness or weakness are fairly common, and are occasionally serious. Notify your physician promptly.

Symptom/effect	Frequency		Discuss with physician		Stop taking drug now	Call physician now
	Common	Rare	Only if severe	In all cases		
Nausea/vomiting	●		■			
Diarrhea	●		■			
Rash/itching	●			■	▲	❘
Fever/sore throat		●		■	▲	❘
Weakness/fatigue		●		■	▲	❘
Jaundice		●		■	▲	❘

INTERACTIONS

Rifampin Aminosalicylic acid may impair absorption of rifampin taken by mouth. Spacing of doses may be recommended.

Oral anticoagulant drugs Aminosalicylic acid may increase the effects of these drugs. Dosage may need to be adjusted accordingly.

Probenecid and sulfinpyrazone These drugs increase the blood levels of aminosalicylic acid.

Ethionamide may increase the risk of adverse effects with aminosalicylic acid.

PROLONGED USE

No problems expected.

AMIODARONE

Brand name Cordarone
Used in the following combined preparations None

GENERAL INFORMATION

Amiodarone was introduced in the United States in 1986 to treat various kinds of abnormal heartbeat (arrhythmia). Similar in chemical structure to the thyroid hormone thyroxine, it works by slowing down the transmission of nerve impulses through the heart muscle. Amiodarone is given to prevent the recurrence of atrial fibrillation and ventricular fibrillation, and to treat ventricular and supraventricular tachycardia.

Amiodarone is generally used only when other drugs have proved ineffective, since it can cause a number of serious adverse effects if used for prolonged periods. These effects include liver damage, hypothyroidism, and eye and lung damage.

Treatment with amiodarone is usually started in the hospital, and the dose is then reduced and carefully adjusted so that abnormal heart rhythm is controlled.

INFORMATION FOR USERS

Your drug prescription is tailored for you. Do not alter dosage without checking with your physician.

How taken

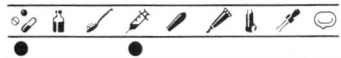

Tablets, injection.

Frequency and timing of doses
3 x daily or by injection initially, then once daily or every other day (maintenance dose).

Adult dosage range
400mg – 1.8g daily.

Onset of effect
Some effects may be noticed within 2 hours, but full benefits may not be felt for up to 3 months.

Duration of action
1 week – 2 months.

Diet advice
None.

Storage
Keep in a closed container in a cool, dry place away from reach of children. Protect from light.

Missed dose
Take as soon as you remember. If your next dose is due within 12 hours, do not take the missed dose. Take your next scheduled dose as usual.

Stopping the drug
Do not stop the drug without consulting your physician; symptoms may recur.

Exceeding the dose
An occasional unintentional extra dose is unlikely to cause problems. Large overdoses may cause nausea, vomiting, dizziness, and abnormal heartbeat. Notify your physician.

SPECIAL PRECAUTIONS

Be sure to tell your physician if:
▼ You have impaired liver function.
▼ You have heart disease.
▼ You have eye disease.
▼ You have a lung disorder such as asthma or bronchitis.
▼ You are taking other medications.

 Pregnancy
▼ Not usually prescribed. May cause thyroid disease and slow heartbeat in newborn infant. Discuss with your physician so that you may weigh the benefits of the drug against its risks.

 Breast feeding
▼ Discuss with your physician. The drug passes into the breast milk and may affect the baby adversely.

 Infants and children
▼ Not recommended.

 Over 60
▼ Reduced dose may be necessary. Increased likelihood of adverse effects.

 Driving and hazardous work
▼ No known problems.

 Alcohol
▼ No known problems.

POSSIBLE ADVERSE EFFECTS

The most common adverse effects of amiodarone such as nausea and vomiting, loss of appetite, and constipation may be relieved by reducing the dose.

Symptom/effect	Frequency		Discuss with physician		Stop taking drug now	Call physician now
	Common	Rare	Only if severe	In all cases		
Nausea/vomiting	●		■			
Constipation	●		■			
Abdominal pain	●			■		
Headache		●		■		
Blurred vision		●		■		
Light-sensitive rash		●		■		
Weakness		●		■		
Depression/hallucinations		●		■		

PROLONGED USE

Prolonged use of this drug may cause a number of adverse effects on the eyes, lungs, thyroid gland, and liver.

INTERACTIONS

Warfarin Amiodarone may increase the anticoagulant effect of warfarin. This interaction may occur for several months after treatment with amiodarone is stopped.

Phenytoin Amiodarone may increase the effects of phenytoin.

Other anti-arrhythmic drugs Amiodarone is likely to increase the effects of drugs such as digoxin, procainamide, and quinidine, causing abnormal heart rhythms.

AMITRIPTYLINE

Brand names Amitril, Elavil, Endep
Used in the following combined preparations Etrafon, Limbitrol, Triavil

GENERAL INFORMATION

Amitriptyline, introduced in 1961, belongs to a class of antidepressant drugs known as the tricyclics. It is used mainly in the long-term treatment of depression. It elevates mood, increases physical activity, improves appetite, and restores interest in everyday activities.

More sedating than some of the other tricyclic antidepressants, amitriptyline is useful when depression is accompanied by anxiety and insomnia. Taken at night, it encourages sleep and helps to eliminate the need for additional sleeping drugs.

In overdose amitriptyline may cause coma and dangerously abnormal heart rhythms.

QUICK REFERENCE

Drug group Tricyclic antidepressant drug (p.112)

Overdose danger rating High

Dependence rating Low

Prescription needed Yes

Available as generic Yes

INFORMATION FOR USERS

Your drug prescription is tailored for you. Do not alter dosage without checking with your physician.

How taken

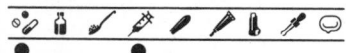

Tablets, capsules, injection.

Frequency and timing of doses
1 – 4 x daily.

Adult dosage range
25 – 300mg daily.

Onset of effect
Can appear within hours, though full antidepressant effect may not be felt for 2 – 6 weeks.

Duration of action
Antidepressant effect may last for 6 weeks; adverse effects, only a few days.

Diet advice
None.

Storage
Keep in a closed container in a cool, dry place away from reach of children.

Missed dose
Take as soon as you remember. If your next dose is due within 3 hours, take a single dose now and skip the next.

Stopping the drug
An abrupt stop can cause withdrawal symptoms and a recurrence of the original trouble. Consult your physician, who may supervise a gradual reduction in dosage.

OVERDOSE ACTION

 Seek immediate medical advice in all cases. Take emergency action if palpitations are noted or consciousness is lost.

See Drug poisoning emergency guide (p.590).

SPECIAL PRECAUTIONS

Be sure to tell your physician if:
▼ You have heart problems.
▼ You have had epileptic seizures.
▼ You have impaired kidney or liver function.
▼ You have had glaucoma.
▼ You have had prostate trouble.
▼ You are taking other medications.

 Pregnancy
▼ Not usually prescribed. Safety in pregnancy not established. Discuss with your physician so that you may weigh the benefits of the drug against its possible risks.

 Breast feeding
▼ The drug passes into the breast milk. Discuss with your physician.

 Infants and children
▼ Not recommended under 6 years. Reduced dose necessary in older children.

 Over 60
▼ Reduced dose may be necessary initially. Increased likelihood of adverse effects.

 Driving and hazardous work
▼ Avoid such activities until you have learned how the drug affects you because of the possibility of blurred vision and reduced alertness.

 Alcohol
▼ Avoid. Alcohol may increase the sedative effects of this drug.

Surgery and general anesthetics
▼ Amitriptyline treatment may need to be stopped before you have a general anesthetic. Discuss this with your physician or dentist before any operation.

POSSIBLE ADVERSE EFFECTS

The possible adverse effects of this drug are mainly the result of its *anticholinergic* action and its blocking action on the transmission of signals through the heart.

Symptom/effect	Frequency		Discuss with physician		Stop taking drug now	Call physician now
	Common	Rare	Only if severe	In all cases		
Drowsiness	●		■			
Sweating/flushing	●		■			
Blurred vision	●			■		
Dizziness/fainting	●			■		
Rash		●		■	▲	
Difficulty passing urine		●		■	▲	
Palpitations		●		■	▲	■

INTERACTIONS

Sedatives All drugs that have sedative effects intensify those of amitriptyline.

Barbiturates These reduce the antidepressant effect of amitriptyline, but may increase its toxic effects in overdose.

Heavy smoking This may reduce the antidepressant effect of amitriptyline.

Antihypertensive drugs Amitriptyline may reduce the effect of some of these drugs.

Monoamine oxidase inhibitors (MAOIs) In the rare cases where these drugs are given with amitriptyline, serious interactions may occur: fever, seizures, and delirium.

PROLONGED USE

No problems expected.

AMOXAPINE

Brand name Asendin
Used in the following combined preparations None

GENERAL INFORMATION

Amoxapine was introduced in 1970. It belongs to a class of antidepressant drugs known as the tricyclics (see Antidepressants p.112).

Often prescribed to treat the depression that accompanies anxiety, amoxapine is also more effective than some other tricyclic antidepressants in treating anxiety and agitation. It elevates mood, increases physical activity, improves appetite, and restores interest in everyday activities. A weaker sedative than some other tricyclic antidepressants, amoxapine causes less interference with normal activities.

Amoxapine can cause a variety of side effects (see below). However, in overdose it is less likely to cause abnormal heart rhythms than other drugs in this group, though it carries a greater risk of causing seizures.

QUICK REFERENCE

Drug group Tricyclic antidepressant drug (p.112)

Overdose danger rating High

Dependence rating Low

Prescription needed Yes

Available as generic No

INFORMATION FOR USERS

Your drug prescription is tailored for you. Do not alter dosage without checking with your physician.

How taken

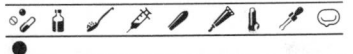

Tablets.

Frequency and timing of doses
1 – 3 x daily.

Dosage range
200 – 300mg daily.

Onset of effect
Some benefits and effects may appear within hours of starting treatment, but full antidepressant effect may not be felt for 2 weeks or more.

Duration of action
24 hours, sometimes longer.

Diet advice
None.

Storage
Keep in a closed container in a cool, dry place away from reach of children. Protect from light.

Missed dose
Take as soon as you remember. If your next dose is due within 4 hours, take a single dose now and skip the next.

Stopping the drug
Do not stop taking the drug without consulting your physician; symptoms may recur.

OVERDOSE ACTION

 Seek immediate medical advice in all cases. Take emergency action if consciousness is lost.

See Drug poisoning emergency guide (p.590).

SPECIAL PRECAUTIONS

Be sure to tell your physician if:
▼ You have heart problems.
▼ You have had epileptic seizures.
▼ You have glaucoma.
▼ You have had prostate trouble.
▼ You are taking other medications.

 Pregnancy
▼ Not usually prescribed. Safety in pregnancy not established. Discuss with your physician so that you can weigh the benefits of the drug against its possible risks.

 Breast feeding
▼ Discuss with your physician. The drug passes into the breast milk. Its effects on the baby are not clearly known.

 Infants and children
▼ Not recommended under 13 years. Reduced dose necessary in adolescents.

 Over 60
▼ Reduced dose may be necessary. Increased likelihood of adverse effects.

Driving and hazardous work
▼ Avoid such activities until you have learned how the drug affects you, because the drug can cause blurred vision and drowsiness.

Alcohol
▼ Avoid. Alcohol may increase the sedative effects of this drug.

Surgery and general anesthetics
▼ Amoxapine treatment may need to be stopped before you have a general anesthetic. Discuss this with your physician or dentist before any operation.

POSSIBLE ADVERSE EFFECTS

The possible adverse effects of this drug are mainly the result of its *anticholinergic* action and its blocking action on the transmission of signals through the heart. Some problems can be overcome by medically supervised adjustment of dosage.

Symptom/effect	Frequency		Discuss with physician		Stop taking drug now	Call physician now
	Common	Rare	Only if severe	In all cases		
Drowsiness	●		■			
Dry mouth	●		■			
Constipation	●		■			
Involuntary movements		●		■		
Nipple discharge		●		■		
Rash		●		■	▲	
Palpitations/seizures		●		■	▲	■

INTERACTIONS

Monoamine oxidase inhibitors (MAOIs) There is a possibility of a serious interaction between these drugs and amoxapine, producing seizures and delirium. Such drugs are prescribed together only under strict supervision.

Heavy smoking This may reduce the antidepressant effect of amoxapine.

Sedatives Amoxapine is likely to increase the effect of drugs that have a sedative effect on the central nervous system.

PROLONGED USE

May produce tremors and abnormal movements (*parkinsonism* or *tardive dyskinesia*) when used for periods of several months or longer.

AMOXICILLIN

Brand names Amoxil, Larotid, Polymox, Trimox, Wymox
Used in the following combined preparation Augmentin

GENERAL INFORMATION

Amoxicillin, a penicillin antibiotic, has been in use since 1969. It is pre-scribed to treat a variety of infections, but is particularly useful for treating ear, nose, and throat infections, respiratory tract infections, cystitis, uncomplicated gonorrhea, and certain skin and soft tissue infections.

When taken by mouth, amoxicillin is absorbed well by the body and it works quickly and effectively.

As with other penicillin antibiotics, the most common side effect of amoxi-cillin is a blotchy skin rash. It can also provoke a more severe allergic reaction, causing symptoms of fever, swelling of the mouth and tongue, itching, and breathing difficulties.

INFORMATION FOR USERS

Your drug prescription is tailored for you. Do not alter dosage without checking with your physician.

How taken

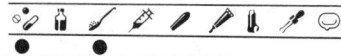

Capsules, powder.

Frequency and timing of doses
3 x daily.

Dosage range
Adults 750mg – 1.5g daily.
Children Reduced dose according to age and weight.

Onset of effect
1 – 2 hours.

Duration of action
Up to 8 hours.

Diet advice
None.

Storage
Keep in a closed container in a cool, dry place away from reach of children.

Missed dose
Take as soon as you remember. If your next dose is due at this time, double the usual dose to make up the missed dose.

Stopping the drug
Take the full course. Even if you feel better, the original infection may still be present and symptoms may recur if treatment is stopped too soon.

Exceeding the dose
An occasional unintentional extra dose is unlikely to be a cause for concern. But if you notice any unusual symptoms, or if a large overdose has been taken, notify your physician.

SPECIAL PRECAUTIONS

Be sure to tell your physician if:
▼ You have impaired kidney function.
▼ You have an allergy (for example, asthma, hay fever, or eczema).
▼ You have had a rash after being given a penicillin or cephalosporin antibiotic.
▼ You have ulcerative colitis.
▼ You have infectious mononucleosis.
▼ You are taking other medications.

Pregnancy
▼ No evidence of risk to baby.

Breast feeding
▼ Discuss with your physician. The drug passes into the milk and may make the baby allergic to the drug in later life.

Infants and children
▼ Reduced dose necessary.

Over 60
▼ No known problems.

Driving and hazardous work
▼ No known problems.

Alcohol
▼ No known problems.

POSSIBLE ADVERSE EFFECTS

If you develop a rash, wheezing, itching, fever, or joint swelling, this may indicate an allergy. Call your physician, who may prescribe a different antibiotic.

Symptom/effect	Frequency		Discuss with physician		Stop taking drug now	Call physician now
	Common	Rare	Only if severe	In all cases		
Rash	●			■		
Diarrhea	●			■		
Nausea/vomiting		●	■			
Unusual thirst		●	■			
Tiredness/weakness		●	■			
Wheezing		●		■	▲	▎
Itching		●		■	▲	▎
Swollen mouth/tongue		●		■	▲	▎

PROLONGED USE

Amoxicillin is usually given only for short courses of treatment.

INTERACTIONS

Oral contraceptives Amoxicillin may reduce the effectiveness of the contra-ceptive pill and also increase the risk of breakthrough bleeding. Discuss with your physician.

AMPHOTERICIN B

Brand name Fungizone
Used in the following combined preparation Mysteclin F

GENERAL INFORMATION

Since its introduction in 1958, amphotericin B has come to be regarded as a highly effective and powerful antifungal drug. Administered by intravenous injection, it is used in cases of potentially fatal systemic fungal infections. Amphotericin B is also used topically for eye and ear infections. It is applied to the skin to combat candida (thrush) infections of the skin or nails. It is not, however, used in vaginal candidiasis.

Treatment by injection is carefully supervised, usually in the hospital, because of adverse effects. Adverse reactions to the ointment are rare.

QUICK REFERENCE

Drug group Antifungal drug (p.166)
Overdose danger rating Low
Dependence rating Low
Prescription needed Yes
Available as generic No

INFORMATION FOR USERS

Your drug prescription is tailored for you. Do not alter dosage without checking with your physician.

How taken

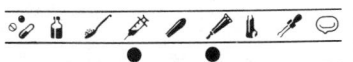

Injection, ointment.

Frequency and timing of doses
Daily, usually over 2 – 4 hours (injection); 2 – 4 x daily (ointment).

Dosage range
The dosage for injection is determined individually. Ointment should be applied as directed.

Onset of effect
In skin infections an improvement may be noticed after 2 – 4 days. Internal (systemic) infections may take several weeks to clear.

Duration of action
Up to 3 days (ointment). Some effect may persist for several weeks after treatment has been stopped (injection).

Diet advice
When given by injection, amphotericin B may reduce the levels of potassium and magnesium in the blood. Mineral supplements may be recommended.

Storage
Keep ointment in a closed container in a cool, dry place away from reach of children.

Missed dose
Apply a missed application of ointment as soon as you remember.

Stopping the drug
Use the full course of ointment. Even if symptoms improve, the original infection may still be present and symptoms may recur if treatment is stopped too soon.

Exceeding the dose
An occasional unintentional extra dose of ointment is unlikely to be a cause for concern. But if you notice unusual symptoms, notify your physician.

SPECIAL PRECAUTIONS

Be sure to tell your physician if:
▼ You have impaired kidney function.
▼ You have previously had an allergic reaction to amphotericin.
▼ You are taking other medications.

Pregnancy
▼ There is no evidence of risk from the ointment. Injections are given only when the infection is life-threatening.

Breast feeding
▼ No evidence of risk from the ointment. Given by injection, the drug passes into the breast milk. Discuss with your physician.

Infants and children
▼ Ointment is safe for children, but the drug is given by injection only in life-threatening conditions.

Over 60
▼ No special problems.

Driving and hazardous work
▼ No known problems.

Alcohol
▼ No known problems.

POSSIBLE ADVERSE EFFECTS

Amphotericin B is given by injection only under close medical supervision. Adverse effects are thus carefully monitored and promptly treated. Given as an ointment, the drug may cause local reactions at the site of application.

Symptom/effect	Frequency		Discuss with physician		Stop taking drug now	Call physician now
	Common	Rare	Only if severe	In all cases		
Injection						
Nausea/vomiting	●			■		
Headache/fever	●			■		
Unusual bleeding		●		■		
Seizures		●		■		
Ointment						
Skin discoloration/irritation	●		■			
Rash		●		■	▲	

INTERACTIONS   (injection only)

Digitalis drugs Amphotericin B increases the toxicity of digitalis.

Diuretics Amphotericin B increases the risk of low potassium levels with diuretics.

Aminoglycoside antibiotics Taken with amphotericin B, these drugs increase the likelihood of kidney damage.

PROLONGED USE

Given by injection the drug may cause a reduction in blood levels of potassium and magnesium. It may also damage the kidneys and cause blood disorders.

Monitoring Regular blood tests to monitor kidney function are advised during treatment by injection.

AMPICILLIN

Brand names Amcill, Omnipen, Omnipen-N, Polycillin, Principen
Used in the following combined preparations Polycillin - PRB, Principen with Probenecid

GENERAL INFORMATION

Ampicillin, a penicillin antibiotic available since 1966, is prescribed to treat a variety of infections.

In common with other penicillin antibiotics, it is particularly useful for treating ear, nose, and throat infections, infections in the respiratory tract, cystitis, uncomplicated gonorrhea, and certain skin and soft tissue infections.

When given in large doses by injection, ampicillin is an effective treatment for more serious infections,

such as meningitis. It may also be prescribed to treat biliary tract infections and typhoid fever.

Gastrointestinal infections caused by salmonella and shigella bacteria may sometimes be treated with ampicillin, but these bacteria are becoming resistant to the drug.

As with other penicillin antibiotics, there is the possibility of a severe allergic reaction, causing fever, swelling of the mouth and tongue, itching, and breathing difficulties.

QUICK REFERENCE

Drug group Penicillin antibiotic (p.156)

Overdose danger rating Low

Dependence rating Low

Prescription needed Yes

Available as generic Yes

INFORMATION FOR USERS

Your drug prescription is tailored for you. Do not alter dosage without checking with your physician.

How taken

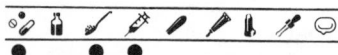

Capsules, powder, injection.

Frequency and timing of doses
4 x daily on an empty stomach.

Dosage range
Adults 1 – 2g daily (by mouth).
Children Reduced dose according to age and weight.

Onset of effect
Within 2 hours.

Duration of action
6 – 8 hours.

Diet advice
None.

Storage
Keep in a closed container in a cool, dry place away from reach of children.

Missed dose
Take as soon as you remember. If your next dose is due at this time, double the usual dose to make up the missed dose.

Stopping the drug
Take the full course. Even if you feel better, the original infection may still be present and symptoms may recur if treatment is stopped too soon.

Exceeding the dose
An occasional unintentional extra dose is unlikely to be a cause for concern. But if you notice unusual symptoms, or if a large overdose has been taken, notify your physician.

SPECIAL PRECAUTIONS

Be sure to tell your physician if:
▼ You have impaired kidney function.
▼ You have an allergy (for example, asthma, hay fever, eczema, or hives).
▼ You have had a rash after taking a penicillin or cephalosporin antibiotic.
▼ You have had ulcerative colitis.
▼ You have recently had infectious mononucleosis.
▼ You are taking other medications.

Pregnancy
▼ No evidence of risk to developing baby.

Breast feeding
▼ Discuss with your physician. The drug passes into the breast milk and may affect the baby adversely.

Infants and children
▼ Reduced dose necessary.

Over 60
▼ No known problems.

Driving and hazardous work
▼ No known problems.

Alcohol
▼ No known problems.

POSSIBLE ADVERSE EFFECTS

If you develop a rash, wheezing, itching, fever, or joint swelling, this may indicate an allergy. Call your physician, who may prescribe a different antibiotic.

Symptom/effect	Frequency		Discuss with physician		Stop taking drug now	Call physician now
	Common	Rare	Only if severe	In all cases		
Diarrhea	●			■		
Rash	●			■		
Nausea/vomiting		●	■			
Unusual thirst		●	■			
Tiredness/weakness		●	■			
Wheezing		●		■	▲	▮
Itching		●		■	▲	▮
Swollen mouth/tongue		●		■	▲	▮

INTERACTIONS

Oral contraceptives Ampicillin may reduce the effectiveness of the contraceptive pill and also increase the risk of breakthrough bleeding. Discuss with your physician.

PROLONGED USE

No known problems. Ampicillin is usually only given for short courses of treatment.

ANTHRALIN

Brand names Anthra-Derm, Drithocreme, Drithocreme HP, Lasan Cream, Lasan HP
Used in the following combined preparation Dritho-Scalp

GENERAL INFORMATION

Anthralin, introduced in 1936, is the most effective *topical* non-steroidal agent for moderately severe psoriasis. Applied as a cream or ointment, it restores excessive skin growth to normal. It is sometimes accompanied by periodic ultraviolet (UVA) treatments to boost its effect.

If psoriasis is particularly severe, treatment at a specialized outpatient center may be recommended. However, most people can use the drug at home, leaving it on either overnight or for up to thirty minutes each day.

Since the drug may stain clothes and bed linen, these should be protected.

Anthralin frequently causes irritation or redness of normal skin around the treated areas, especially at high concentrations. A protective coat of petrolatum applied to normal skin before using the drug helps to minimize such effects; plastic gloves should be worn during application. Raw, blistered, or oozing areas should never be treated, and the drug should not be used on the face, genital area, or skin folds such as those of the neck or groin.

QUICK REFERENCE

Drug group Psoriasis drug (p.206)
Overdose danger rating Low
Dependence rating Low
Prescription needed Yes
Available as generic Yes

INFORMATION FOR USERS

Your drug prescription is tailored for you. Do not alter dosage without checking with your physician.

How taken

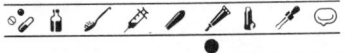

Ointment, cream.

Frequency and timing of doses
Once daily, either low concentration (0.1 – 0.5 percent) at bedtime for 8 – 12 hours (overnight treatment) or high concentration (1 percent) during the day for 10 – 30 minutes as directed (short-contact treatment). Remove the medicine by washing as directed after each application.

Adult dosage range
Apply thinly to the affected area as directed. The strength of the ointment or cream is increased, if required, as treatment continues.

Onset of effect
2 – 3 days. Full beneficial effect of the drug may not be felt for several weeks.

Duration of action
Up to 72 hours.

Diet advice
None.

Storage
Keep in a closed container in a cool, dry place away from reach of children. Protect from light.

Missed dose
Apply as soon as you remember. If not remembered until the next morning (overnight treatment), skip the missed application and apply your next dose as usual. If your next dose is due within 4 hours (short-contact treatment), apply a single dose now and skip the next dose.

Stopping the drug
For best results, apply the full course of treatment.

Exceeding the dose
An occasional unintentional extra application is unlikely to cause problems. If the cream is left on the skin longer than recommended, irritation and redness may result. If this occurs, notify your physician.

SPECIAL PRECAUTIONS

Be sure to tell your physician if:
▼ You have impaired kidney function.
▼ You are taking other medications.

Pregnancy
▼ Not usually prescribed. Safety in pregnancy not established. Discuss with your physician so that you can weigh the benefits of the drug against its possible risks.

Breast feeding
▼ Discuss with your physician. The drug passes into the breast milk, and may affect the baby adversely.

Infants and children
▼ Not recommended under 12 years.

Over 60
▼ No special problems.

Driving and hazardous work
▼ No known problems.

Alcohol
▼ No known problems.

PROLONGED USE

No special problems.

POSSIBLE ADVERSE EFFECTS

Irritation or redness of the skin around the treated areas is fairly common and is usually helped by reducing the amount or frequency of application. Allergic skin rashes are rare.

Symptom/effect	Frequency		Discuss with physician		Stop taking drug now	Call physician now
	Common	Rare	Only if severe	In all cases		
Irritation	●			■		
Redness	●			■		
Rash		●		■	▲	▮

INTERACTIONS

General note Any drug that increases the sensitivity of the skin to light may increase the risk of redness or irritation with anthralin. Such drugs include coal tar or coal tar derivatives, thiazide diuretics, griseofulvin, nalidixic acid, phenothiazine antipsychotic drugs, sulfonamides, and tetracycline antibiotics.

ASPIRIN

Brand names Ascriptin, Bufferin, Easprin, Ecotrin, Zorprin
Used in the following combined preparations Fiorinal, Fiorinal w/codeine, Empirin w/codeine, Percodan

GENERAL INFORMATION

Commonly used since 1899, aspirin is a non-narcotic analgesic that relieves pain, reduces fever, and alleviates the symptoms of arthritis. In small doses, it helps prevent blood clots.

It is present in numerous combination medicines for colds, menstrual period pains, headaches, and joint or muscular aches.

One disadvantage of aspirin is its tendency to irritate the stomach and even cause bleeding. Another is the possibility that it can cause Reye's syndrome, a rare brain and liver disorder usually occurring in children. Only under close medical supervision should it be given to children with fever caused by viral illness.

QUICK REFERENCE

Drug group Non-narcotic analgesic (p.108) and antiplatelet drug (p.132)

Overdose danger rating High

Dependence rating Low

Prescription needed No

Available as generic Yes

INFORMATION FOR USERS

Follow instructions on the label. Call your physician if symptoms worsen.

How taken

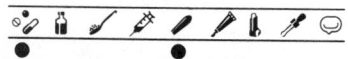

Tablets, capsules, rectal suppositories.

Frequency and timing of doses
Relief of pain and fever Every 4 hours as necessary, with food or milk. (Slow-release capsules every 8 – 12 hours.)
Prevention of blood clots Once daily.

Adult dosage range
Relief of pain and fever 650mg per dose.
Prevention of blood clots Dose uncertain: 25 –150mg daily. Larger doses may be given in arthritis.

Onset of effect
30 – 60 minutes (regular aspirin); 1 1/2 – 8 hours (enteric-coated tablets or slow-release capsules).

Duration of action
Up to 12 hours. Some effect may persist for several days when used to prevent blood clotting.

Diet advice
None.

Storage
Keep in a closed container in a cool, dry place away from reach of children.

Missed dose
Do not make up the dose you missed. Take your next dose on your original schedule. If you are taking the medicine long term, take the missed dose as soon as you remember.

Stopping the drug
If you have been prescribed aspirin by your physician for a long-term condition, you should seek medical advice before stopping the drug. Otherwise it can be safely stopped as soon as you no longer need it.

OVERDOSE ACTION

Seek immediate medical advice in all cases. Take emergency action if there is restlessness, stomach pain, ringing noises in the ears, blurred vision, or vomiting.

See Drug poisoning emergency guide (p.590).

SPECIAL PRECAUTIONS

Be sure to consult your physician before taking this drug if:
▼ You have impaired kidney or liver function.
▼ You have asthma.
▼ You have nasal polyps.
▼ You have a blood clotting disorder.
▼ You have a peptic ulcer.
▼ You are taking other medications.

Pregnancy
▼ Not usually recommended. An alternative drug may be safer. Discuss with your physician.

Breast feeding
▼ Not usually recommended. The drug passes into the breast milk. An alternative drug may be safer. Discuss with your physician.

Infants and children
▼ Not recommended.

Over 60
▼ No special problems.

Driving and hazardous work
▼ No special problems.

Alcohol
▼ Avoid. Alcohol increases the likelihood of stomach irritation with this drug.

Surgery and general anesthetics
▼ Treatment with aspirin may need to be stopped about one week before surgery. Discuss with your physician or dentist before any operation.

POSSIBLE ADVERSE EFFECTS

Adverse effects are more likely to occur with high dosage of aspirin, but may be reduced by taking the drug with food or in buffered or enteric coated forms.

Symptom/effect	Frequency		Discuss with physician		Stop taking drug now	Call physician now
	Common	Rare	Only if severe	In all cases		
Indigestion	●			■		
Nausea/vomiting	●			■		▮
Rash		●		■	▲	
Breathlessness/wheezing		●		■	▲	▮

INTERACTIONS

Anticoagulants Aspirin may add to the anticoagulant effect of such drugs, leading to an increased risk of abnormal bleeding.

Non-steroidal anti-inflammatory drugs These drugs increase the likelihood of stomach irritation when taken with aspirin.

Corticosteroids These drugs increase the likelihood of stomach irritation.

Drugs for gout Aspirin may reduce the effect of these drugs, especially allopurinol.

Oral antidiabetic drugs Aspirin may increase the effect of these drugs.

PROLONGED USE

Aspirin should not be taken for longer than 2 days except on your physician's advice. Prolonged use of aspirin may lead to bleeding in the stomach and to stomach ulcers.

ATENOLOL

Brand name Tenormin
Used in the following combined preparation Tenoretic

GENERAL INFORMATION

Atenolol, in use since 1981, belongs to the class of drugs known as beta blockers (see p.125). Decreasing the heart's oxygen requirements and permitting it to beat more slowly, these drugs are used in the treatment of both angina and hypertension.

Atenolol is particularly useful for people with diabetes, lung problems, and poor circulation, because unlike other beta blockers, it acts mainly on the heart rather than on other parts of the body. It may also be given just after a heart attack to protect the heart from further damage.

Because atenolol does not cure heart disease, but only controls the symptoms, it may have to be taken continuously over a long period, even for the rest of a person's life. It stays in the body for a long time, so it only needs to be taken once a day, an advantage to people who have difficulty remembering to take their medicines.

QUICK REFERENCE

Drug group Beta blocker (p.125)
Overdose danger rating Low
Dependence rating Low
Prescription needed Yes
Available as generic No

INFORMATION FOR USERS

Your drug prescription is tailored for you. Do not alter dosage without checking with your physician.

How taken

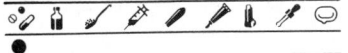

Tablets.

Frequency and timing of doses
Once daily.

Adult dosage range
50 – 200 mg daily.

Onset of action
2 – 4 hours.

Duration of action
20 – 30 hours. Some effects may last for 2 – 3 days in people with impaired kidney function.

Diet advice
None.

Storage
Keep in a tightly closed container in a cool, dry place away from reach of children.

Missed dose
Take as soon as you remember. If your next dose is due within 6 hours, do not take the missed dose but take the next scheduled dose as usual.

Stopping the drug
Do not stop taking the drug without consulting your physician; withdrawal of the drug may lead to severe worsening of the underlying condition.

Exceeding the dose
An occasional unintentional extra dose is unlikely to be a cause for concern. But if you notice unusual symptoms, or if a large overdose has been taken, notify your physician.

SPECIAL PRECAUTIONS

Be sure to tell your physician if:
▼ You have impaired kidney function.
▼ You have poor circulation.
▼ You have diabetes.
▼ You have a lung disorder such as asthma or bronchitis.
▼ You are taking other medications.

Pregnancy
▼ Discuss with your physician. The drug has been used to treat high blood pressure right through late pregnancy with no adverse effects on the baby.

Breast feeding
▼ The drug passes into the breast milk, but at normal doses adverse effects on the baby are uncommon. Discuss with your physician.

Infants and children
▼ Reduced dose necessary.

Over 60
▼ No special problems. Reduced dose may be necessary if there is impaired kidney function. Increased likelihood of adverse effects.

Driving and hazardous work
▼ No special problems.

Alcohol
▼ No special problems.

Surgery and general anesthetics
▼ Atenolol may need to be stopped before you have a general anesthetic. Discuss this with your physician or dentist before any surgery.

POSSIBLE ADVERSE EFFECTS

Atenolol has adverse effects that are common to most beta blockers. Symptoms are usually temporary and diminish with long-term use.

Symptom/effect	Frequency		Discuss with physician		Stop taking drug now	Call physician now
	Common	Rare	Only if severe	In all cases		
Muscle ache	●		■			
Dizziness/lightheadedness		●	■			
Cold hands and feet		●	■			
Nightmares/sleeplessness		●	■			
Rash		●		■		
Digestive disturbance		●		■		
Breathing difficulties		●		■		
Depression/confusion		●		■		

INTERACTIONS

Antacids Antacids reduce the atenolol effect, so the two drugs should be taken at least half an hour apart.

PROLONGED USE

No special problems.

AURANOFIN

Brand name Ridaura
Used in the following combined preparations None

GENERAL INFORMATION

Introduced in 1985, auranofin is the only gold-compound drug for rheumatoid arthritis that can be taken by mouth. The other gold drugs have to be injected, usually in a physician's office or a hospital. Most of the drugs for rheumatoid arthritis ease the pain and soothe the inflammation (aspirin and non-steroidal anti-inflammatory drugs). They do not change the course of the disease.

Auranofin and the other gold compounds, however, are able to do so, arresting or slowing the progression of the disease. The gold drugs are toxic, however, and so long as an arthritic condition remains stable, most physicians prefer to keep a person on the conventional treatment. But when early signs of deformity appear, signaling an increase in the pace of the disease, treatment by auranofin is appropriate. Since it can take 3 – 6 months to work, the use of analgesics and anti-inflammatory drugs is continued for that period.

Such side effects as diarrhea, nausea, and abdominal pain occur early and do not last long. More serious effects – blood disorders, rashes, and impaired kidney function – require that the drug be stopped.

INFORMATION FOR USERS

Your drug prescription is tailored for you. Do not alter dosage without checking with your physician.

How taken

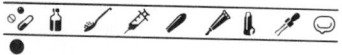

Capsules.

Frequency and timing of doses
1 – 2 x daily.

Dosage range
6mg daily. This may be increased up to a maximum of 9mg daily in some people.

Onset of effect
Adverse effects may be felt within 2 weeks. Beneficial effects may not be felt for 3 – 6 months.

Duration of action
Effects may last for several months after stopping the drug.

Diet advice
None.

Storage
Keep in a closed container in a cool, dry place away from reach of children.

Missed dose
Take as soon as you remember. If your next dose is due within 2 hours, take a single dose now and skip the next.

Stopping the drug
Do not stop the drug without consulting your physician; stopping suddenly could lead to a flare-up of rheumatoid arthritis.

Exceeding the dose
An occasional unintentional extra dose is unlikely to cause problems. Large overdoses may cause vomiting. Notify your physician.

SPECIAL PRECAUTIONS

Be sure to tell your physician if:
▼ You have impaired liver or kidney function.
▼ You have previously had an allergic reaction to gold treatment.
▼ You have inflammatory bowel disease.
▼ You have severe eczema.
▼ You have had a blood disorder.
▼ You have high blood pressure.
▼ You are taking other medications.

Pregnancy
▼ Not usually prescribed. Safety in pregnancy not established. Discuss with your physician so that you can weigh the benefits of the drug against its possible risks.

Breast feeding
▼ Discuss with your physician. The drug may pass into the breast milk and may affect the baby adversely.

Infants and children
▼ Not recommended.

Over 60
▼ No special problems.

Driving and hazardous work
▼ No known problems.

Alcohol
▼ No known problems.

POSSIBLE ADVERSE EFFECTS

The most common adverse effects of this drug include rashes that may sometimes be serious, nausea, and diarrhea. Cloudy urine may be a sign of kidney problems.

Symptom/effect	Frequency		Discuss with physician		Stop taking drug now	Call physician now
	Common	Rare	Only if severe	In all cases		
Diarrhea/nausea	●		■			
Indigestion/abdominal pain	●			■		
Conjunctivitis	●			■		
Mouth ulcers/soreness	●			■		
Cloudy urine		●		■		
Rash/itching	●			■	▲	∎

INTERACTIONS

Non-steroidal anti-inflammatory drugs (NSAIDs) and penicillamine may increase the risk of impaired kidney function with auranofin. Penicillamine may also increase the risk of blood disorders.

PROLONGED USE

Prolonged use may rarely lead to kidney damage and blood disorders.

Monitoring Periodic blood counts, urine examination and tests of kidney function are usually required.

AZATADINE

Brand name Optimine
Used in the following combined preparation Trinalin

GENERAL INFORMATION

Azatadine is an antihistamine used for treating allergic conditions. Introduced in 1977, it relieves the itching, swelling, and redness of the skin caused by allergy, insect bites, or contact with irritant chemicals. Because of its relatively strong sedative effect, it is especially useful for the relief of itching at night. Azatadine is also effective for treating allergic rhinitis, its *anticholinergic* action helping to dry up runny eyes and nose. This drug is occasionally prescribed for the prevention and treatment of allergic reactions to blood transfusions.

Longer acting than many similar drugs, azatadine retains its effect for about 12 hours. Its main disadvantage is that it frequently causes drowsiness.

QUICK REFERENCE

Drug group Antihistamine (p.152)
Overdose danger rating Medium
Dependence rating Low
Prescription needed Yes
Available as generic No

INFORMATION FOR USERS

Your drug prescription is tailored for you. Do not alter dosage without checking with your physician.

How taken

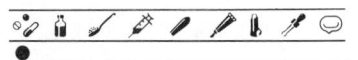

Tablets.

Frequency and timing of doses
2 x daily.

Adult dosage range
2 – 4mg daily.

Onset of effect
15 – 60 minutes.

Duration of action
Up to 12 hours.

Diet advice
None.

Storage
Keep in a closed container in a cool, dry place away from reach of children.

Missed dose
Take as soon as you remember. If your next dose is due within 2 hours, take a single dose now and skip the next.

Stopping the drug
Can be safely stopped as soon as you no longer need it.

Exceeding the dose
An occasional unintentional extra dose is unlikely to cause problems. Large overdoses may cause unusual drowsiness. Notify your physician.

SPECIAL PRECAUTIONS

Be sure to tell your physician if:
▼ You have impaired liver function.
▼ You have glaucoma.
▼ You have difficulty passing urine.
▼ You are taking other medications.

Pregnancy
▼ Not usually prescribed. Safety in pregnancy not established. Discuss with your physician so that you can weigh the benefits of the drug against its possible risks.

Breast feeding
▼ Discuss with your physician. The drug passes into the breast milk and may affect the baby adversely.

Infants and children
▼ Not recommended for children under 12 years.

Over 60
▼ Reduced dose may be necessary.

Driving and hazardous work
▼ Avoid such activities until you have learned how the drug affects you, because the drug may cause drowsiness.

Alcohol
▼ Avoid. Alcohol may increase the sedative effects of this drug.

POSSIBLE ADVERSE EFFECTS

Drowsiness is the most significant adverse effect of this drug. Certain other side effects such as dry mouth and blurred vision are due to its *anticholinergic* action. Nausea and other digestive disturbances can be avoided by taking the drug with food or milk.

Symptom/effect	Frequency		Discuss with physician		Stop taking drug now	Call physician now
	Common	Rare	Only if severe	In all cases		
Drowsiness	●		■			
Dry mouth	●		■			
Blurred vision	●		■			
Nausea/loss of appetite		●	■			
Dizziness/clumsiness		●	■			
Difficulty passing urine		●			■	
Rash		●			■	▲

INTERACTIONS

Sedatives All drugs that have a sedative effect on the central nervous system are likely to enhance the sedative effect of azatadine.

Anticholinergic drugs The anticholinergic effects of azatadine are likely to be increased by all drugs that have anticholinergic effects, including some antiparkinsonism drugs, antipsychotic and tricyclic antidepressant drugs.

Monoamine oxidase inhibitors (MAOIs) There is a risk of a dangerous rise in blood pressure if azatadine is taken within 14 days of MAOIs.

PROLONGED USE

The effect of the drug may become weaker over a period of weeks or months as the body adapts. Transfer to a different antihistamine may be recommended.

AZATHIOPRINE

Brand name Imuran
Used in the following combined preparations None

GENERAL INFORMATION

Azathioprine, approved in 1968, is an immunosuppressant drug which depresses the immune system, whose actions tend to reject transplanted organs. The drug is also given for severe rheumatoid arthritis that has failed to respond to conventional drug therapy.

Autoimmune and collagen diseases (including systemic lupus erythematosus, polymyositis, dermatomyositis, myasthenia gravis, and chronic inflammatory bowel disease) may also

be treated with azathioprine. Often prescribed when corticosteroids have proved insufficient, azathioprine boosts the effects of these drugs, thus allowing a reduction in the dose of corticosteroids in some cases.

Azathioprine is given only under close supervision because of the risk of serious adverse effects. These include suppression of the production of white blood cells, thereby increasing the risk of infection, and the risk of excessive or prolonged bleeding.

QUICK REFERENCE

Drug group Antirheumatic drug (p.145) and immunosuppressant drug (p.184)

Overdose danger rating Medium

Dependence rating Low

Prescription needed Yes

Available as generic No

INFORMATION FOR USERS

Your drug prescription is tailored for you. Do not alter dosage without checking with your physician.

How taken

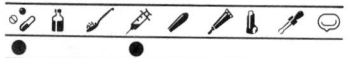

Tablets, injection.

Frequency and timing of doses
Usually once daily.

Dosage range
Initially according to body weight and then adjusted according to the response of the individual.

Onset of effect
2 – 4 weeks. Antirheumatic effect may not be felt for 8 weeks or more.

Duration of action
Immunosuppressant effects may last for several weeks after the drug is stopped.

Diet advice
None.

Storage
Keep in a closed container in a cool, dry place away from reach of children. Protect from light.

Missed dose
Take as soon as you remember, then return to your normal schedule. If more than 2 doses are missed, consult your physician.

Stopping the drug
Do not stop the drug without consulting your physician. If taken to prevent graft transplant rejection, stopping treatment could provoke rejection of the transplant.

Exceeding the dose
An occasional unintentional extra dose is unlikely to cause problems. Large overdoses may cause nausea, vomiting, abdominal pains, and diarrhea. Notify your physician.

SPECIAL PRECAUTIONS

Be sure to tell your physician if:
▼ You have impaired liver or kidney function.
▼ You have recently had shingles or chicken pox.
▼ You have an infection.
▼ You have pancreatitis.
▼ You are taking other medications.

Pregnancy
▼ Not usually prescribed. Safety in pregnancy not established. Discuss with your physician so that you can weigh the benefits of the drug against its possible risks.

Breast feeding
▼ Discuss with your physician. The drug passes into the breast milk and may affect the baby adversely.

Infants and children
▼ No special problems.

Over 60
▼ Increased likelihood of adverse effects.

Driving and hazardous work
▼ No known problems.

Alcohol
▼ No known problems.

POSSIBLE ADVERSE EFFECTS

Digestive disturbances and adverse effects on the blood which could lead to sore throat, fever, and weakness are common with azathioprine. Unusual bleeding or bruising while taking this drug may be a sign of reduced levels of platelets in the blood.

Symptom/effect	Frequency		Discuss with physician		Stop taking drug now	Call physician now
	Common	Rare	Only if severe	In all cases		
Nausea/vomiting	●		■			
Weakness/fatigue	●			■		
Sore throat	●			■		
Fever/chills	●			■		▮
Unusual bleeding/bruising		●		■		▮
Jaundice		●		■		
Rash		●		■	▲	

INTERACTIONS

General note Any drug that affects the breakdown of other drugs in the liver or kidneys may alter the blood levels of azathioprine. These include phenytoin, phenobarbital, rifampin, allopurinol, and certain antibiotics. Dosage adjustment may be necessary.

PROLONGED USE

There may be a slightly increased risk of some cancers with long-term use of azathioprine. Blood changes may also occur, but may be corrected by adjusting the dose.

Monitoring Regular checks on blood composition are usually carried out.

BACITRACIN

Brand names Ak-Tracin, Baciguent
Used in the following combined preparations Cortisporin, Mycitracin, Neo-polycin, Neosporin, Polysporin (ointments)

GENERAL INFORMATION

Introduced in 1948, bacitracin is a *topical* antibiotic used mainly for staphylococcic and streptococcic infections of the skin, outer ear, and eyelids. It is combined with other drugs into ointments that have a wide spectrum of bacteria-killing action. Some bacitracin preparations contain a corticosteroid to help in the relief of skin inflammation.

When applied to the skin, bacitracin rarely causes adverse effects. What harmful reactions do occur usually result from the other drugs in a combined preparation.

Not readily absorbed in the digestive tract, bacitracin has been used on an investigational basis to treat certain inflammatory infections of the large intestine. Other drugs are just as effective, however, and less risky. Bacitracin can cause kidney damage, especially in the rare cases when it is given by injection.

QUICK REFERENCE

Drug group Antibiotic (p.156)
Overdose danger rating Low
Dependence rating Low
Prescription needed No
Available as generic Yes

INFORMATION FOR USERS

Follow instructions on the label. Call your physician if symptoms worsen.

How taken

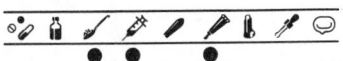

Powder, injection, ointment.

Frequency and timing of doses
1 – 4 x daily.

Dosage range
Enough to cover the affected area at each application (skin preparations).

Onset of effect
1 – 2 hours (skin preparations).

Duration of action
Up to 24 hours.

Diet advice
None.

Storage
Keep topical preparations in a closed container in a cool, dry place away from reach of children.

Missed dose
Apply topical preparations as soon as you remember.

Stopping the drug
Take the full course. Even if you feel better, the original infection may still be present and may recur if treatment is stopped too soon.

Exceeding the dose
An occasional unintentional extra dose is unlikely to be a cause for concern. But if you notice unusual symptoms, or if a large overdose has been taken, notify your physician.

POSSIBLE ADVERSE EFFECTS

Used topically, bacitracin rarely causes adverse effects. Injection treatment is only undertaken in the hospital, where any side effects can be closely monitored.

Symptom/effect	Frequency		Discuss with physician		Stop taking drug now	Call physician now
	Common	Rare	Only if severe	In all cases		
Topical preparations						
Skin irritation/rash		●		■		▲
Injection						
Rash		●		■		❚
Dark/cloudy urine		●		■		❚

INTERACTIONS

None.

SPECIAL PRECAUTIONS

Be sure to consult your physician before using this drug if:
▼ You have impaired kidney function.
▼ You are allergic to bacitracin.
▼ You are taking other medications.

Pregnancy
▼ No evidence of risk with oral or topical preparations. Doses by injection may adversely affect the developing baby. Discuss with your physician so that you may weigh the benefits of the drug against its risks.

Breast feeding
▼ No evidence of risk with oral or topical preparations. Injected, this drug passes into the breast milk and may affect the baby adversely. Discuss with your physician.

Infants and children
▼ No special problems.

Over 60
▼ Prolonged use by injection is avoided because there is an increased likelihood of kidney damage.

Driving and hazardous work
▼ No known problems.

Alcohol
▼ No known problems.

PROLONGED USE

Prolonged use of this drug by injection may lead to kidney damage.

Monitoring Periodic kidney function tests are recommended when the drug is taken by injection.

BACLOFEN

Brand names Lioresal, Lioresal DS
Used in the following combined preparations None

GENERAL INFORMATION

Baclofen is a muscle relaxant drug, introduced in 1978, that acts on the central nervous system, including the spinal cord. It relieves the spasms, cramping, and rigidity of muscles caused by such disorders as multiple sclerosis and spinal cord injury. It is also used to treat spasticity due to brain injury, cerebral palsy, or stroke.

Although this drug does not cure these disorders, it increases mobility, allowing other treatment, such as physical therapy, to be carried out.

Baclofen is also prescribed for attacks of nerve pain in the face (trigeminal neuralgia).

Baclofen is less likely to cause muscle weakness than similar drugs, and its side effects, such as dizziness and drowsiness, are usually temporary. Elderly people who take baclofen may experience unusual excitement; they also are more likely to suffer from confusion or hallucinations.

QUICK REFERENCE

Drug group Muscle-relaxant drug(p.148)

Overdose danger rating Medium

Dependence rating Low

Prescription needed Yes

Available as generic Yes

INFORMATION FOR USERS

Your drug prescription is tailored for you. Do not alter dosage without checking with your physician.

How taken

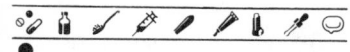

Tablets.

Frequency and timing of doses
3 x daily with food or milk.

Adult dosage range
5 – 10mg daily (starting dose) for 3 days, increased by 5mg every 3 days as required.

Onset of effect
Some benefits may appear after 2 – 3 hours, but full beneficial effects may not be felt for several weeks after maximum effective dose has been reached.

Duration of action
Up to 8 hours.

Diet advice
None.

Storage
Keep in a closed container in a cool, dry place away from reach of children.

Missed dose
Take as soon as you remember. If your next dose is due within 2 hours, take a single dose now and skip the next.

Stopping the drug
Do not stop taking the drug without consulting your physician, who will supervise a gradual reduction in dosage. Abrupt cessation may cause hallucinations and seizures.

Exceeding the dose
An occasional unintentional extra dose is unlikely to cause problems. Large over-doses may cause weakness, vomiting, and severe drowsiness. Notify your physician.

SPECIAL PRECAUTIONS

Be sure to tell your physician if:
▼ You have impaired kidney function.
▼ You have had a peptic ulcer.
▼ You have had epileptic seizures.
▼ You have diabetes.
▼ You are taking other medications.

Pregnancy
▼ Not usually prescribed. Safety in pregnancy not established. Discuss with your physician so that you can weigh the benefits of the drug against its possible risks.

Breast feeding
▼ Discuss with your physician. The drug passes into the breast milk and may affect the baby adversely.

Infants and children
▼ Not recommended under 12 years.

Over 60
▼ Reduced dose necessary. Increased likelihood of adverse effects.

Driving and hazardous work
▼ Avoid such activities until you have learned how the drug affects you, because the drug can cause dizziness and drowsiness.

Alcohol
▼ Avoid. Alcohol may increase the sedative effects of this drug.

Surgery and general anesthetics
▼ Be sure to inform your physician or dentist that you are taking baclofen before you have a general anesthetic.

POSSIBLE ADVERSE EFFECTS

The common adverse effects are related to the sedative effects of the drug. Such effects can be minimized by starting with a low dose that is gradually increased.

Symptom/effect	Frequency		Discuss with physician		Stop taking drug now	Call physician now
	Common	Rare	Only if severe	In all cases		
Dizziness	●		■			
Drowsiness	●		■			
Nausea	●		■			
Constipation		●	■			
Headache		●	■			
Confusion		●		■		
Muscle fatigue/weakness		●		■		

INTERACTIONS

Antidiabetic drugs Baclofen may increase blood sugar levels, so the dosage may need to be adjusted accordingly.

Antihypertensive drugs Baclofen may increase the blood pressure-lowering effect of such drugs.

Sedatives All drugs that have a sedative effect on the central nervous system are likely to increase the sedative properties of baclofen.

PROLONGED USE

This drug may alter liver function.

Monitoring Blood tests to check liver function are usually taken before starting treatment and periodically during prolonged treatment.

BECLOMETHASONE

Brand names Beclovent, Beconase, Vancenase, Vanceril
Used in the following combined preparations None

GENERAL INFORMATION

Beclomethasone is a corticosteroid drug prescribed to relieve the symptoms of allergic rhinitis (as a nasal spray) and to control asthma (as an inhalant). It controls nasal symptoms by reducing inflammation and mucus production in the nose. It also helps to reduce chest symptoms, such as wheezing and coughing, by reducing inflammation in the bronchi. People who suffer from asthma may take beclomethasone to reduce the severity and frequency of attacks. However, once an attack has started, this drug does not relieve symptoms.

Beclomethasone is given primarily to people whose asthma does not respond to bronchodilators alone (p.120). Fungal infection causing

irritation of the mouth and throat is a possible side effect of beclomethasone treatment that can, to a certain degree, be avoided by thoroughly rinsing the mouth and gargling with water after each inhalation.

There are few serious adverse effects associated with beclomethasone because it is given *topically* by nasal spray or inhaler. This means that beclomethasone is not absorbed by the body to any great extent, thus preventing a buildup of the drug and the possibility of a suppression of the adrenocortical gland function, which may lead to shock in a person under severe stress. Instructions must be followed carefully for the drug to be fully effective.

INFORMATION FOR USERS

Your drug prescription is tailored for you. Do not alter dosage without checking with your physician.

How taken

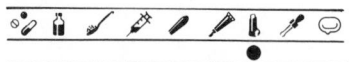

Nasal spray, inhaler.

Frequency and timing of doses
2 – 4 x daily.

Dosage range
Adults 2 sprays 3 – 4 x daily (asthma);
1 spray in each nostril 2 – 4 x daily
(allergic rhinitis).
Children Reduced dose according to age and weight.

Onset of effect
Within 1 week (asthma); 1 – 3 days (allergic rhinitis). Full benefit may not be felt for up to 4 weeks.

Duration of action
Several days after stopping the drug.

Diet advice
None.

Storage
Keep in a closed container in a cool, dry place away from reach of children. Protect from light.

Missed dose
Take as soon as you remember. If your next dose is due within 2 hours, take a single dose now and skip the next.

Stopping the drug
Do not stop the drug without consulting your physician; symptoms may recur. Rare instances of adrenal insufficiency can occur.

Exceeding the dose
An occasional unintentional extra dose is unlikely to be a cause for concern. But if you notice unusual symptoms, or if a large overdose has been taken, notify your physician. Adverse effects may occur if the recommended dose is regularly exceeded over a prolonged period.

SPECIAL PRECAUTIONS

Be sure to tell your physician if:
▼ You have had any nasal ulcers or surgery.
▼ You have had tuberculosis or another respiratory infection.
▼ You are taking other medications.

Pregnancy
▼ Not usually prescribed. Safety in pregnancy not established. Discuss with your physician so that you can weigh the benefits of the drug against its possible risks.

Breast feeding
▼ The drug passes into the breast milk, but at normal doses adverse effects on the baby are uncommon. Discuss with your physician.

Infants and children
▼ Not recommended for children under 6 years. Reduced dose necessary in older children.

Over 60
▼ No known problems.

Driving and hazardous work
▼ No known problems.

Alcohol
▼ No known problems.

POSSIBLE ADVERSE EFFECTS

Adverse effects are unlikely as the dose used is low. The main side effects are irritation of the nasal passages and fungal infection of the throat and mouth.

Symptom/effect	Frequency		Discuss with physician		Stop taking drug now	Call physician now
	Common	Rare	Only if severe	In all cases		
Nasal discomfort/irritation	●		■			
Cough	●		■			
Sore/dry throat	●			■		
Nosebleed		●		■		

PROLONGED USE

No problems expected.

Monitoring Periodic checks to make sure that the adrenal glands are functioning healthily may be required if large doses are being used.

INTERACTIONS

None.

BELLADONNA

Brand names None
Used in the following preparations B&O Supprettes, Bellergal, Bellergal S, Butibel, Wyanoids

GENERAL INFORMATION

Ever since its extraction from deadly nightshade in 1831, belladonna has demonstrated a capability of producing a variety of physical effects. Among the first to be noticed was its ability to dilate the pupil of the eye, thought to enhance female attractiveness, creating the "bella donna" or beautiful lady.

The drug has *antispasmodic* properties, making it useful in easing the abdominal cramps of people with irritable bowel syndrome. It is pre-

scribed to help relieve the tremors and stiffness of Parkinson's disease.

Belladonna also has *anticholinergic* actions. Affecting a part of the involuntary nervous system, these increase the heartbeat, narrow arteries, and constrict certain muscles, making belladonna useful for migraine, motion sickness, and incontinence.

It has a number of the classic anticholinergic adverse side effects, such as heart palpitations and dryness of the mouth (see below).

INFORMATION FOR USERS

Your drug prescription is tailored for you. Do not alter dosage without checking with your physician.

How taken

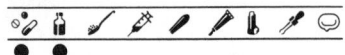

Tablets, liquid.

Frequency and timing of doses
3 – 4 x daily, 30 – 60 minutes before meals and at bedtime.

Adult dosage range
Dosage is determined individually according to condition, response, and preparation used.

Onset of effect
1 – 2 hours.

Duration of action
4 – 6 hours.

Diet advice
None.

Storage
Keep in a closed container in a cool, dry place away from reach of children.

Missed dose
Take as soon as you remember. If your next dose is due within 2 hours, take a single dose now and skip the next.

Stopping the drug
Do not stop the drug without consulting your physician, who may supervise a gradual reduction in dosage.

OVERDOSE ACTION

Seek immediate medical advice in all cases. Take emergency action if palpitations, tremors, delirium, loss of consciousness, or seizures occurs.

See Drug poisoning emergency guide (p.590).

POSSIBLE ADVERSE EFFECTS

The principal adverse effects of belladonna are related to its anticholinergic properties.

These are helped by reducing the dosage, and they diminish after a few days.

Symptom/effect	Frequency		Discuss with physician		Stop taking drug now	Call physician now
	Common	Rare	Only if severe	In all cases		
Blurred vision	●			■		
Dry mouth		●	■			
Constipation		●		■		
Difficulty passing urine		●		■		
Headache/eye pain		●		■		
Palpitations		●		■		

INTERACTIONS

Antacids These drugs may reduce absorption of belladonna. Doses should be spaced 1 hour apart.

Sedatives All drugs that have a sedative effect on the nervous system are likely to increase the sedative properties of belladonna.

SPECIAL PRECAUTIONS

Be sure to tell your physician if:
▼ You have impaired liver or kidney function.
▼ You have heart problems.
▼ You have high blood pressure.
▼ You have glaucoma.
▼ You have urinary difficulties.
▼ You have reflux esophagitis.
▼ You have myasthenia gravis.
▼ You are taking other medications.

Pregnancy
▼ Not usually prescribed.

Breast feeding
▼ The drug passes into the breast milk, but at normal doses adverse effects on the baby are uncommon. Discuss with your physician.

Infants and children
▼ Not usually prescribed for children under 5 years. Reduced dose necessary for older children.

Over 60
▼ Reduced dose necessary.

Driving and hazardous work
▼ Avoid such activities until you have learned how the drug affects you, because the drug can cause blurred vision and may impair your concentration.

Alcohol
▼ No known problems.

PROLONGED USE

No problems expected, but since the body adapts to this drug, a gradual reduction in dose is usually recommended when stopping after prolonged use.

BENZOCAINE

Brand names Americaine, Dermoplast, Foille, Hurricane, Orajel
Used in the following combined preparations Allergen Ear Drops, Auralgan, Cetacaine, Semets, Tympagesic

GENERAL INFORMATION

Benzocaine, introduced in 1905, is one of the earliest local anesthetics. Many preparations can be obtained without a prescription, and they are widely used to relieve sunburn, itching, and the pain of minor burns. A gel formulation is available for short-term relief of toothache in adults and teething pains in infants. Hemorrhoids and other painful anal disorders may be treated with ointment.

Benzocaine is also frequently given to relieve pain and prevent gagging prior to dental treatment, oral surgery, and medical examination of the mouth,

throat, trachea, or esophagus. Occasionally, it may be prescribed as ear drops to relieve pain caused by ear inflammation. It can also be taken as a lozenge for suppressing appetite, although there is no proof of its effectiveness as a diet aid.

Poorly absorbed through the skin and mucous membranes, the drug rarely causes adverse effects, though allergic reactions may occur occasionally. It should not be used for more than a few days except under medical supervision, since it could mask the symptoms of a more serious disease.

QUICK REFERENCE

Drug group Local anesthetic (p.108)

Overdose danger rating Low

Dependence rating Low

Prescription needed No

Available as generic Yes

INFORMATION FOR USERS

Follow instructions on the label. Call your physician if symptoms worsen.

How taken

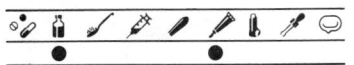

Liquid, ointment, cream, spray, paste, gel, lozenges.

Frequency and timing of doses
As needed. For hemorrhoids, ointment is applied to the rectal area morning and evening and after each bowel movement.

Dosage range
Apply ointment, cream, gel, or paste thinly to the affected area. Apply spray for 1 second, and repeat the application if necessary. For rectal ointment, use one applicatorful per application.

Onset of effect
About 1 minute.

Duration of action
20 – 30 minutes.

Diet advice
Benzocaine by mouth causes numbness of the mouth and throat and may interfere with swallowing. To avoid choking and injury to the inside of your mouth from hot food or drink, do not eat or drink anything for one hour afterwards.

Storage
Keep in a closed container in a cool, dry place away from reach of children.

Missed dose
Take as soon as you remember if still required.

Stopping the drug
Can be safely stopped as soon as you no longer need it.

Exceeding the dose
An occasional unintentional extra application is unlikely to be a cause for concern. But if you notice unusual symptoms, or if a large overdose has been taken, notify your physician.

SPECIAL PRECAUTIONS

Be sure to consult your physician before using this drug if:
▼ You have ever had an allergic reaction to a local anesthetic.
▼ You are taking other medications.

Pregnancy
▼ No evidence of risk to developing baby.

Breast feeding
▼ No evidence of risk. Avoid use on or around nipples.

Infants and children
▼ Not recommended under 6 years except on the advice of a physician.

Over 60
▼ No special problems.

Driving and hazardous work
▼ No known problems.

Alcohol
▼ No known problems.

POSSIBLE ADVERSE EFFECTS

Adverse effects are rare with short-term use of benzocaine. Allergic reactions such as burning, stinging, redness, itching, and sometimes swelling may occasionally occur.

Symptom/effect	Frequency		Discuss with physician		Stop taking drug now	Call physician now
	Common	Rare	Only if severe	In all cases		
Burning/stinging		●		■	▲	
Itching/redness		●		■	▲	
Swelling		●		■	▲	
Rash		●		■	▲	

PROLONGED USE

This drug should not be used for prolonged periods. If your symptoms do not improve within a few days, consult your physician.

INTERACTIONS

None.

BENZOYL PEROXIDE

Brand names Benzac W, Desquam-X, Desquam-X Wash, Panoxyl, Panoxyl AQ
Used in the following combined preparations Sulfoxyl, Vanoxide-HC

GENERAL INFORMATION

Benzoyl peroxide, introduced for medical use in 1931, is used in *topical* preparations for the treatment of acne. Available over the counter and by prescription, it comes in concentrations of varying strengths for moderate acne. It is often added to tinted preparations that camouflage as well as treat the condition.

Benzoyl peroxide works by removing the top layer of skin and unblocking the sebaceous glands. It also reduces inflammation of blocked hair follicles by killing bacteria that infect them.

It may cause irritation due to its drying effect on the skin, but this generally diminishes with time. The drug should be left on the skin for about 15 minutes initially and then washed off. The length of exposure can then be increased as the body adapts. Side effects are less likely if treatment is started with a preparation containing a low concentration of benzoyl peroxide and changed to a stronger preparation only if necessary. Marked dryness and peeling of the skin, which may occur with overuse, can usually be controlled by reducing the frequency of application.

QUICK REFERENCE

Drug group Drug for acne (p.205)

Overdose danger rating Medium

Dependence rating Low

Prescription needed No (most forms)

Available as generic Yes

INFORMATION FOR USERS

Follow instructions on the label. Call your physician if symptoms worsen.

How taken

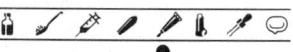

Cream, lotion, gel, cleansing bar.

Frequency and timing of doses
1 – 2 x daily (cream, gel, lotion); 2 – 3 x daily (cleansing bar).

Dosage range
Apply to affected skin sparingly.

Onset of effect
Reduces oiliness of skin immediately. Acne usually improves within 4 – 6 weeks.

Duration of action
24 – 48 hours.

Diet advice
None.

Storage
Keep in a closed container in a cool, dry place away from reach of children.

Missed dose
Apply as soon as you remember.

Stopping the drug
Can be safely stopped as soon as you no longer need it.

Exceeding the dose
A single extra application is unlikely to cause problems. Regular overuse may cause irritation, peeling, redness, and swelling.

POSSIBLE ADVERSE EFFECTS

Application of benzoyl peroxide may cause temporary burning or stinging of the skin. Redness, peeling, and swelling may result from excessive drying of the skin with overuse, and usually clears up if the treatment is stopped or used less frequently. If severe burning, blistering, or crusting occur, stop using the product and consult a physician.

Symptom/effect	Frequency		Discuss with physician		Stop taking drug now	Call physician now
	Common	Rare	Only if severe	In all cases		
Irritation	●		■			
Dryness/peeling		●	■			
Stinging/redness		●	■			
Blistering/crusting/swelling		●		■	▲	∎
Rash		●		■	▲	∎

INTERACTIONS

Skin-drying preparations Medicated cosmetics, soaps, toiletries, and anti-acne preparations increase the likelihood of dryness and irritation of the skin with benzoyl peroxide.

SPECIAL PRECAUTIONS

Be sure to consult your physician before using this drug if:
▼ You have eczema.
▼ You have sunburn.
▼ Your skin is highly sensitive to sunlight.
▼ You are taking other medications.

Pregnancy
▼ Not usually prescribed. Safety in pregnancy not established. Discuss with your physician so that you can weigh the benefits of the drug against its possible risks.

Breast feeding
▼ No evidence of risk.

Infants and children
▼ Not recommended under 12 years.

Over 60
▼ Not usually required.

Driving and hazardous work
▼ No known problems.

Alcohol
▼ No known problems.

PROLONGED USE

Benzoyl peroxide should not be used for longer than 6 weeks except on the advice of your physician.

BENZTROPINE

Brand name Cogentin
Used in the following combined preparations None

GENERAL INFORMATION

Benztropine was introduced for the treatment of Parkinson's disease in the 1940s. It is still used for relieving early symptoms of the disease, and is also used in conjunction with the stronger, levodopa-based drugs for treatment of more advanced cases of Parkinson's disease. It is particularly helpful in treating the rigidity and tremor of Parkinson's disease and in the reduction of excess salivation. However, it does little to improve the slow physical movements that also characterize the disease.

Dosage has to be determined individually in order to find the best balance between relief of symptoms and the occurrence of adverse effects.

QUICK REFERENCE

Drug group Anticholinergic antiparkinsonism drug (p.115)

Overdose danger rating Medium

Dependence rating Low

Prescription needed Yes

Available as generic No

INFORMATION FOR USERS

Your drug prescription is tailored for you. Do not alter dosage without checking with your physician.

How taken

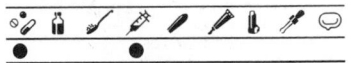

Tablets, injection.

Frequency and timing of doses
1 – 3 x daily.

Adult dosage range
0.5 – 6mg daily.

Onset of effect
Within 30 minutes.

Duration of action
6 – 24 hours.

Diet advice
None.

Storage
Keep in a closed container in a cool, dry place away from reach of children.

Missed dose
Take as soon as you remember. If your next dose is due within 2 hours, take a single dose now and skip the next.

Stopping the drug
Do not stop the drug without consulting your physician; symptoms may recur.

Exceeding the dose
An occasional unintentional extra dose is unlikely to cause problems. Larger overdoses may cause agitation and/or an increase in heart rate. Notify your physician.

SPECIAL PRECAUTIONS

Be sure to tell your physician if:
▼ You have impaired kidney or liver function.
▼ You have had glaucoma.
▼ You have urinary difficulties.
▼ You have high blood pressure.
▼ You suffer from depression.
▼ You have peptic ulcers.
▼ You are taking other medications.

Pregnancy
▼ Unlikely to be required.

Breast feeding
▼ Unlikely to be required.

Infants and children
▼ Not usually prescribed.

Over 60
▼ Reduced dose may be necessary. Increased likelihood of adverse effects.

Driving and hazardous work
▼ Avoid such activities until you have learned how the drug affects you, because the drug can cause blurred vision and drowsiness.

Alcohol
▼ Avoid. Alcohol may increase the sedative effects of this drug.

POSSIBLE ADVERSE EFFECTS

The possible adverse effects of benztropine are mainly the result of its *anticholinergic* action. Some of the more common symptoms, such as dry eyes and mouth, drowsiness, and blurred vision, can be overcome by an adjustment in dosage.

Symptom/effect	Frequency		Discuss with physician		Stop taking drug now	Call physician now
	Common	Rare	Only if severe	In all cases		
Dry mouth/eyes	●		■			
Difficulty in passing urine	●		■			
Constipation	●		■			
Nervousness	●		■			
Blurred vision	●			■		
Confusion		●		■		
Nausea/vomiting		●		■		
Rash		●		■	▲	
Palpitations		●		■	▲	■

INTERACTIONS

Anticholinergic drugs and antihistamines Benztropine adds to the actions of such drugs, so increasing the likelihood of adverse effects.

PROLONGED USE

Prolonged use of this drug may contribute to the onset of glaucoma.

Monitoring Periodic eye examinations are usually required.

BETAMETHASONE

Brand names Celestone, Diprolene, Diprosone, Uticort, Valisone
Used in the following combined preparation Lotrisone

GENERAL INFORMATION

Available since 1961, betamethasone is a corticosteroid prescribed to treat a variety of conditions caused by allergy or inflammation. Topical preparations are available for skin complaints. It can be injected directly into the joints to relieve the pain and stiffness of rheumatoid arthritis and other forms of joint inflammation. In an aerosol inhaler, the drug may be prescribed to reduce the frequency and severity of asthma attacks. The drug may also be given by mouth to treat corticosteroid deficiency as a result of pituitary or adrenal gland disorders.

Low or moderate doses of betamethasone taken for short periods rarely cause serious side effects. Prolonged use or high dosages can lead to peptic ulcers, weak bones, muscle weakness, and thin skin, and may retard growth in children.

QUICK REFERENCE

Drug group Corticosteroid (p.169)
Overdose danger rating Low
Dependence rating Low
Prescription needed Yes
Available as generic Yes

INFORMATION FOR USERS

Your drug prescription is tailored for you. Do not alter dosage without checking with your physician.

How taken

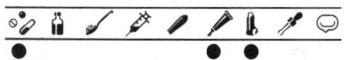

Tablets, cream, ointment, lotion, aerosol.

Frequency and timing of doses
According to disorder being treated and method of administration.

Dosage range
Considerable variation according to the method of administration and condition. Follow your physician's instructions.

Onset of effect
12 – 48 hours.

Duration of action
Up to 24 hours.

Diet advice
A low-sodium, high-potassium diet is recommended when the oral form of the drug is prescribed for extended periods. Follow the advice of your physician.

Storage
Keep in a closed container in a cool, dry place away from reach of children. Protect from light.

Missed dose
Take as soon as you remember. If your next dose is due within 2 hours, take a single dose now and skip the next.

Stopping the drug
Do not stop tablets without consulting your physician, who may supervise a gradual reduction in dosage. Abrupt cessation after long-term treatment may cause adrenal collapse.

Exceeding the dose
An occasional unintentional extra dose is unlikely to be a cause for concern. But if you notice unusual symptoms, or if a large overdose has been taken, notify your physician.

SPECIAL PRECAUTIONS

Be sure to tell your physician if:
▼ You suffer from depression.
▼ You have glaucoma.
▼ You have high blood pressure.
▼ You have had a peptic ulcer.
▼ You have had tuberculosis.
▼ You have a herpes infection.
▼ You have diabetes.
▼ You are taking other medications.

 Pregnancy
▼ No evidence of risk with ointment or joint injections. Prescribed in tablet form in low doses, harm to baby is unlikely. Discuss with your physician so that you may weigh the benefits of the drug against its possible risks.

 Breast feeding
▼ No evidence of risk with ointment or joint injections. Taken by mouth, the drug passes into the breast milk and may adversely affect the baby's growth. Discuss with your physician.

 Infants and children
▼ Reduced dose may be necessary.

 Over 60
▼ Reduced dose may be necessary.

 Driving and hazardous work
▼ No known problems.

 Alcohol
▼ Avoid. Alcohol may increase the risk of peptic ulcers with betamethasone tablets. No special problems with other dosage forms.

POSSIBLE ADVERSE EFFECTS

Serious adverse effects only occur when high doses are taken by mouth for long periods. *Topical* preparations are unlikely to cause adverse effects unless overused.

Symptom/effect	Frequency		Discuss with physician		Stop taking drug now	Call physician now
	Common	Rare	Only if severe	In all cases		
Indigestion	●			■		
Weight gain	●			■		
Acne		●		■		
Muscle weakness		●		■		
Mood changes		●		■		
Bloody/black stools		●		■	▲	■

INTERACTIONS

Digoxin Betamethasone may increase the risk of adverse effects with digoxin.

Insulin Betamethasone by mouth or injection reduces the action of insulin.

Oral anticoagulant drugs Betamethasone increases blood clotting.

Vaccines Serious reactions can occur when vaccinations are given during betamethasone treatment. Discuss with your physician.

Antihypertensive drugs Betamethasone can cause fluid retention, which may reduce the effect of these drugs.

PROLONGED USE

Prolonged use of betamethasone can lead to peptic ulcers, thin skin, fragile bones, and muscle weakness, and can retard growth in children.

BISACODYL

Brand names Ducolax, Fleet Bisacodyl
Used in the following combined preparation Clysodrast

GENERAL INFORMATION

Bisacodyl is a powerful stimulant laxative. It encourages bowel activity by keeping the stool moist and soft and by stimulating the muscle contractions that propel feces through the bowel.

Available without a prescription, it is widely used for relief of constipation. It is also sometimes given after abdominal surgery or a heart attack so that strained efforts for bowel movement are unnecessary. It may also be used to evacuate the bowel prior to surgery or labor or before medical or X-ray examinations of the colon or rectum.

Since bisacodyl can irritate the stomach, tablets are covered with a protective coating to prevent their breakdown before they reach the intestine; they should be swallowed whole to avoid indigestion or nausea. Taken at bedtime with a snack, they stimulate a bowel action in the morning. Rectal suppositories are faster-acting, but sometimes cause stinging and inflammation.

Regular long-term use of this drug may seriously upset normal bowel action, leading to severe, prolonged diarrhea. This may disrupt the balance of potassium in the body and affect nerve and muscle activity, causing weakness and debility.

QUICK REFERENCE

Drug group Laxative (p.139)
Overdose danger rating Medium
Dependence rating Medium
Prescription needed No
Available as generic Yes

INFORMATION FOR USERS

Follow instructions on the label. Call your physician if symptoms worsen.

How taken

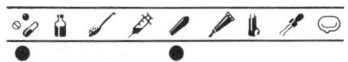

Tablets, rectal suppositories, enema.

Frequency and timing of doses
Tablets Once daily at bedtime with food and water. Do not chew.
Suppositories Once daily, usually in the morning.

Adult dosage range
5 – 15mg daily (tablets); 10mg daily (suppositories); 30ml (enema).

Onset of effect
6 – 8 hours (tablets); 15 – 60 minutes (suppositories, enema).

Duration of action
Several days.

Diet advice
None.

Storage
Keep in a closed container in a cool, dry place away from reach of children.

Missed dose
Do not take the missed dose. Take your next dose only if relief of severe constipation is required.

Stopping the drug
Can be safely stopped as soon as you no longer need it.

Exceeding the dose
An occasional unintentional extra dose is unlikely to cause problems. Large overdoses may cause colicky lower abdominal pain. Notify your physician.

POSSIBLE ADVERSE EFFECTS

Side effects are rarely serious. Tablets may cause irritation of the stomach or bowel, leading to abdominal cramps. Soreness and itching around the anus and rectum are the most common adverse effects of bisacodyl suppositories.

Symptom/effect	Frequency		Discuss with physician		Stop taking drug now	Call physician now
	Common	Rare	Only if severe	In all cases		
Abdominal pain	●		■			
Rectal irritation	●		■			
Belching		●	■			
Nausea		●	■			
Diarrhea		●		■	▲	

INTERACTIONS

Antacids and milk If taken within one hour of bisacodyl tablets, these may cause premature disintegration of the enteric coating, leading to stomach irritation.

SPECIAL PRECAUTIONS

Be sure to consult your physician before taking this drug if:
▼ You have severe abdominal pain.
▼ You have severe constipation and/or hard stools.
▼ You have unexplained rectal bleeding.
▼ You are taking other medications.

Pregnancy
▼ Not usually prescribed. Other laxatives are more widely used and regarded as safer in pregnancy.

Breast feeding
▼ No evidence of risk.

Infants and children
▼ Not recommended except on the advice of a physician.

Over 60
▼ Increased likelihood of adverse effects.

Driving and hazardous work
▼ No known problems.

Alcohol
▼ No known problems.

PROLONGED USE

Not recommended. Bisacodyl should not be taken regularly for longer than one week except on the advice of your physician. Overuse of laxatives – the laxative habit – reduces spontaneous, normal bowel activity and leads to dependence on the drug for bowel movement.

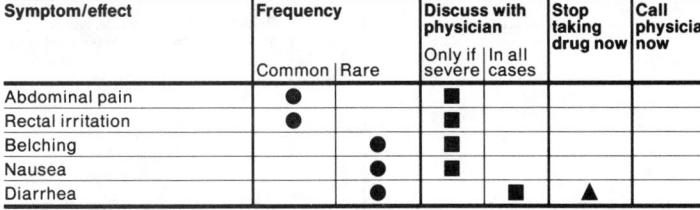

BROMOCRIPTINE

Brand name Parlodel
Used in the following combined preparations None

GENERAL INFORMATION

By inhibiting the secretion of the hormone prolactin from the pituitary gland, bromocriptine is helpful in treating conditions associated with excessive prolactin production. Such conditions include some types of female infertility, premenstrual breast discomfort, occasionally male infertility and impotence, and benign pituitary tumors that cause acromegaly (abnormal bone growth). Bromocriptine is also sometimes used to suppress lactation in women who do not wish to breast feed.

A few years after its development in the 1960s, bromocriptine was found to be effective for relieving the symptoms of parkinsonism, since it has almost the same characteristics as dopamine, the chemical lacking in the brain of someone with Parkinson's disease. Bromocriptine is now widely used to treat those in the advanced stages of parkinsonism when other drugs have failed or are unsuitable .

Serious adverse effects are uncommon when the drug is given in low doses. Nausea and vomiting, the most common problems, can be minimized by taking bromocriptine with meals. Bromocriptine may in rare cases cause ulceration of the stomach, which, if unrecognized, may result in perforation or hemorrhage.

QUICK REFERENCE

Drug group Antiparkinsonism drug (p.115) and pituitary agent (p.173)

Overdose danger rating Low

Dependence rating Low

Prescription needed Yes

Available as generic No

INFORMATION FOR USERS

Your drug prescription is tailored for you. Do not alter dosage without checking with your physician.

How taken

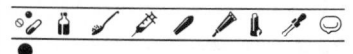

Tablets, capsules.

Frequency and timing of doses
1 – 3 x daily with food or milk.

Adult dosage range
The dose given depends on the condition being treated and your response. In most cases treatment starts with a daily dose of 2.5mg. This is gradually increased until a satisfactory response is achieved.

Onset of effect
Within 1 hour.

Duration of action
About 8 hours.

Diet advice
None.

Storage
Keep in a closed container in a cool, dry place away from reach of children.

Missed dose
Take as soon as you remember. If your next dose is due within 2 hours, take a single dose now and skip the next.

Stopping the drug
Do not stop the drug without consulting your physician; symptoms may recur.

Exceeding the dose
An occasional unintentional extra dose is unlikely to be a cause for concern. But if you notice unusual symptoms, or if a large overdose has been taken, notify your physician.

SPECIAL PRECAUTIONS

Be sure to tell your physician if:
▼ You have an inner ear disorder.
▼ You have poor circulation in hands or feet.
▼ You have a stomach ulcer.
▼ You are taking other medications.

Pregnancy
▼ Not usually prescribed. Safety in pregnancy not established. Discuss with your physician.

Breast feeding
▼ The drug suppresses milk production, and prevents it completely if given within 12 hours of delivery. If you wish to breast-feed, consult your physician.

Infants and children
▼ Not usually prescribed. Reduced dose necessary.

Over 60
▼ Reduced dose may be necessary. Increased likelihood of adverse effects.

Driving and hazardous work
▼ Avoid such activities until you have learned how the drug affects you, because of the possibility of reduced alertness.

Alcohol
▼ Avoid. Alcohol increases the likelihood of confusion while taking this drug.

POSSIBLE ADVERSE EFFECTS

Adverse effects are usually related to dosage level: problems are uncommon with low doses, but the risk of adverse effects increases with higher doses. When taken for Parkinson's disease, bromocriptine may cause abnormal movements of the face and limbs, and hallucinations. Ulceration of the stomach is rare.

Symptom/effect	Frequency		Discuss with physician		Stop taking drug now	Call physician now
	Common	Rare	Only if severe	In all cases		
Nausea/vomiting	●		■			
Confusion/dizziness	●			■		
Headache/constipation		●	■			
Abnormal movements		●		■		
Hallucinations		●		■		
Collapse		●		■	▲	▮

PROLONGED USE

No special problems.

Monitoring Periodic blood tests may be performed to check hormone levels.

INTERACTIONS

Antipsychotic drugs These drugs oppose the action of bromocriptine. When they are taken with bromocriptine, there is an increased risk of the abnormal movements of *parkinsonism*.

BROMPHENIRAMINE

Brand names Bromphen, Dimetane Elixir, Dimetane Extentab, Dimetane Tabs
Used in the following combined preparations Dimetane-DC Cough, Dimetane Decongestant, Dimetapp, Drixoral

GENERAL INFORMATION

Brompheniramine, an antihistamine introduced in 1957, is used for treating allergies such as hay fever, allergic conjunctivitis, urticaria (hives), and angioedema (allergic swellings). It is also a common ingredient of over-the-counter cold remedies (see p.122).

Like other antihistamines, it relieves allergic skin symptoms such as itching, swelling, and redness. It also reduces sneezing and runny nose and the itching eyes in hay fever. It has a mild *anticholinergic* action, which enhances its drying effect on the nose.

Brompheniramine may also be used to prevent or treat allergic reactions to blood transfusions or X-ray contrast material, and to supplement epinephrine injections for people with acute allergic shock (anaphylaxis).

QUICK REFERENCE

Drug group Antihistamine (p.152)
Overdose danger rating Medium
Dependence rating Low
Prescription needed No
Available as generic Yes

INFORMATION FOR USERS

Follow instructions on the label. Call your physician if symptoms worsen.

How taken

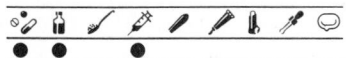

Tablets, slow-release tablets, liquid, injection.

Frequency and timing of doses
4 – 6 x daily (tablets, liquid); 2 – 3 x daily (slow-release tablets); single dose as needed (injection).

Dosage range
Adults 16 – 24mg daily (tablets, liquid); up to 40mg per dose (injection).
Children 4 – 6mg daily (2 – 6 years, liquid); 8 – 12mg daily (6 – 12 years: tablets, liquid).

Onset of effect
Within 60 minutes (orally); within 20 minutes (injection).

Duration of action
4 – 6 hours (tablets, liquid, injection), 10 – 14 hours (slow-release tablets).

Diet advice
None.

Storage
Keep in a closed container in a cool, dry place away from reach of children. Protect from light.

Missed dose
Take as soon as you remember. If your next dose is due within 2 hours, take a single dose now and skip the next.

Stopping the drug
Can be safely stopped as soon as you no longer need it.

Exceeding the dose
An occasional unintentional extra dose is unlikely to cause problems. Large overdoses may cause unusual drowsiness or agitation. Notify your physician.

POSSIBLE ADVERSE EFFECTS

Brompheniramine has few adverse effects. The most common is drowsiness. Other symptoms, such as dryness of the mouth, blurred vision, and difficulty passing urine, are due to the *anticholinergic* effects of brompheniramine. Gastrointestinal irritation may be reduced by taking tablets or liquid with food or drink.

Symptom/effect	Frequency		Discuss with physician		Stop taking drug now	Call physician now
	Common	Rare	Only if severe	In all cases		
Drowsiness	●		■			
Blurred vision		●	■			
Dizziness/incoordination		●	■			
Digestive disturbances		●		■		
Urinary difficulties		●		■		
Dry mouth		●		■		
Excitation (in children)		●		■	▲	

INTERACTIONS

Sedatives All drugs that have a sedative effect are likely to enhance the sedative effect of brompheniramine.

Anticholinergic drugs are likely to increase the anticholinergic effects of brompheniramine.

Monoamine oxidase inhibitors (MAOIs) There is a risk of a dangerous rise in blood pressure if brompheniramine is taken with MAOIs.

SPECIAL PRECAUTIONS

Be sure to tell your physician before taking this drug if:
▼ You have impaired liver function.
▼ You have had epileptic seizures.
▼ You have had glaucoma.
▼ You have urinary difficulties.
▼ You are taking other medications.

Pregnancy
▼ Not usually prescribed. Safety in pregnancy not established. Discuss with your physician so that you can weigh the benefits of the drug against its possible risks.

Breast feeding
▼ No evidence of risk.

Infants and children
▼ Not recommended for newborn or premature infants. Reduced dose necessary for older children.

Over 60
▼ Reduced dose may be necessary. Increased likelihood of adverse effects.

Driving and hazardous work
▼ Avoid such activities until you have learned how the drug affects you, because the drug can cause drowsiness.

Alcohol
▼ Avoid. Alcohol may increase the sedative effects of this drug.

PROLONGED USE

The effect of the drug may become weaker with prolonged use over a period of weeks or months as the body adapts. Transfer to a different antihistamine may be recommended.

A
B
C
D
E
F
G
H
I
J
K
L
M
N
O
P
Q
R
S
T
U
V
W
X
Y
Z

BUMETANIDE

Brand name Bumex
Used in the following combined preparations None

GENERAL INFORMATION

Bumetanide is a powerful, short-acting loop diuretic. Like other diuretics, it is used to treat edema (fluid retention) resulting from heart failure, nephrotic syndrome, and cirrhosis of the liver. It is also employed in the long-term treatment of hypertension. Bumetanide is particularly useful in the treatment of people with impaired kidney function who do not respond well to thiazide diuretics. Because it is fast-acting, it is often injected in emergencies to relieve pulmonary edema.

Bumetanide increases the loss of potassium in the urine, which can result in a wide variety of symptoms (see p.127). For this reason, a potassium supplement or a diuretic that conserves potassium is often given with the drug.

(see p.127)

QUICK REFERENCE

Drug group Loop diuretic (p.127)
Overdose danger rating Low
Dependence rating Low
Prescription needed Yes
Available as generic No

Loop diuretic (p.127)

INFORMATION FOR USERS

Your drug prescription is tailored for you. Do not alter dosage without checking with your physician.

How taken

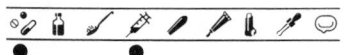

Tablets, injection.

Frequency and timing of doses
Once daily, usually in the morning.

Dosage range
0.5 – 2mg daily. Dose may be increased if kidney function is impaired.

Onset of effect
Within 30 minutes (tablets), immediately (injection).

Duration of action
2 – 4 hours.

Diet advice
Use of this drug may reduce potassium in the body. Eat plenty of fresh fruit and vegetables.

Storage
Keep in a closed container in a cool, dry place away from reach of children.

Missed dose
No cause for concern, but take as soon as you remember. However, if it is late in the day do not take the missed dose, or you may need to get up during the night to pass urine. Take the next scheduled dose as usual.

Stopping the drug
Do not stop the drug without consulting your physician; symptoms may recur.

Exceeding the dose
An occasional unintentional extra dose is unlikely to be a cause for concern. But if you notice unusual symptoms, or if a large overdose has been taken, notify your physician.

SPECIAL PRECAUTIONS

Be sure to tell your physician if:
▼ You have impaired kidney or liver function.
▼ You have diabetes.
▼ You have prostate trouble.
▼ You are taking other medications.

Pregnancy
▼ Not usually prescribed. May cause a reduction in blood supply to the developing baby. Discuss with your physician so that you can weigh the benefits of the drug against its risks.

Breast feeding
▼ Discuss with your physician. This drug may reduce your milk supply.

Infants and children
▼ Not usually prescribed. Reduced dose necessary.

Over 60
▼ Increased likelihood of adverse effects.

Driving and hazardous work
▼ No special problems.

Alcohol
▼ Avoid. Bumetanide increases the likelihood of dehydration and hangovers after consumption of alcohol.

POSSIBLE ADVERSE EFFECTS

Adverse effects are caused mainly by the rapid fluid loss produced by bumetanide. These diminish as the body adjusts to taking the drug.

Symptom/effect	Frequency		Discuss with physician		Stop taking drug now	Call physician now
	Common	Rare	Only if severe	In all cases		
Dizziness	●		■			
Lethargy		●	■			
Cramps		●	■			
Rash		●		■		
Noises in ears (high dose)		●		■		

INTERACTIONS

Non-steroidal anti-inflammatory drugs (NSAIDs) These may reduce the diuretic effect of bumetanide.

Aminoglycoside antibiotics These increase the risk of hearing problems when taken with bumetanide.

Lithium Bumetanide may increase the blood levels of lithium, leading to an increased risk of lithium poisoning.

PROLONGED USE

Serious problems are unlikely, but levels of certain salts in the body may occasionally become disrupted during prolonged use.

Monitoring Periodic tests may be performed to check on kidney function and levels of body salts.

CALCITONIN

Brand name Calcimar
Used in the following combined preparations None

GENERAL INFORMATION

Calcitonin, a hormone produced by the thyroid gland, reduces loss of calcium from the bones and helps maintain normal levels of calcium in the blood. A synthetic form of calcitonin, derived from salmon and available since 1978, is used to treat Paget's disease, a condition involving abnormal, deformed growth of the bones. Paget's disease can cause bone pain and fractures and may lead to compression of the nerves in the spine and skull, sometimes causing deafness or impaired vision.

Calcitonin, given by injection, halts abnormal bone formation and, within a few months, can relieve pain and other symptoms. Although some symptoms of nerve compression may improve, deafness is not usually helped.

Calcitonin is also prescribed for the treatment of osteoporosis. Along with other agents, it reduces high levels of calcium in the blood (hypercalcemia) caused by overactivity of the parathyroid glands or by bone cancer. Because some people are allergic to salmon calcitonin, a skin test may be performed before starting treatment with the drug.

QUICK REFERENCE

Drug group Drug for bone disorders (p.150)

Overdose danger rating Low

Dependence rating Medium

Prescription needed Yes

Available as generic No

INFORMATION FOR USERS

Your drug prescription is tailored for you. Do not alter dosage without checking with your physician.

How taken

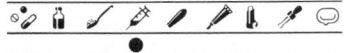

Injection.

Frequency and timing of doses
3 x weekly (Paget's disease); every 12 hours (hypercalcemia); once daily (osteoporosis).

Adult dosage range
Paget's disease 50 – 100 IU (international units) per dose.
Hypercalcemia According to weight.
Osteoporosis 100 IU daily.

Onset of effect
Within a week. Full therapeutic effect may not be felt for several months.

Duration of action
Up to 72 hours.

Diet advice
None.

Storage
Refrigerate, but do not freeze. Keep away from reach of children.

Missed dose
Take as soon as you remember. If your next dose is due within 24 hours (taken on alternate days) or within 6 hours (taken daily or every 12 hours), take a single dose now and skip the next. Resume your normal dosage schedule thereafter.

Stopping the drug
Do not stop taking the drug without consulting your physician; stopping the drug may lead to worsening of the underlying condition.

Exceeding the dose
An occasional unintentional extra dose is unlikely to cause problems. Large overdoses may cause nausea, vomiting, or flushing. Notify your physician.

SPECIAL PRECAUTIONS

Be sure to tell your physician if:
▼ You are prone to allergic reactions.
▼ You are taking other medications.

Pregnancy
▼ Not usually prescribed. Safety in pregnancy not established. Discuss with your physician so that you can weigh the benefits of the drug against its possible risks.

Breast feeding
▼ Discuss with your physician. The drug does not pass into the breast milk, but its safety during breast feeding has not been established.

Infants and children
▼ Not usually prescribed.

Over 60
▼ No special problems.

Driving and hazardous work
▼ No special problems.

Alcohol
▼ No special problems.

POSSIBLE ADVERSE EFFECTS

Adverse effects occur frequently with calcitonin. Nausea, vomiting, and diarrhea usually diminish with continued use. Local reactions at the injection site are common.

Symptom/effect	Frequency		Discuss with physician		Stop taking drug now	Call physician now
	Common	Rare	Only if severe	In all cases		
Nausea/vomiting	●		■			
Flushing	●		■			
Local irritation	●		■			
Unpleasant taste		●	■			
Diarrhea		●	■			
Rash		●			■	▲

INTERACTIONS

Calcium-containing preparations or vitamin D These drugs may counter the beneficial effect of calcitonin.

PROLONGED USE

The effectiveness of the drug may be partially reduced in some people after about a year. Antibodies to the drug can develop.

Monitoring Periodic checks on blood calcium levels and imaging procedures may be required to assess the effectiveness of the drug.

CAPTOPRIL

Brand name Capoten
Used in the following combined preparation Capozide

GENERAL INFORMATION

Captopril, an antihypertensive drug introduced in 1981, is the first of a new class of drugs called ACE inhibitors. Like some other antihypertensive drugs, captopril dilates the blood vessels and eases the flow of blood. But it accomplishes this by blocking the agent that constricts most of the vessels, in contrast to earlier drugs that act on nerve control over the constricting muscles.

Captopril is thus especially useful for people with high blood pressure who have experienced adverse effects from other drugs. It lowers blood pressure rapidly but may require several weeks to achieve maximum effect. People with severe heart failure who have not responded well to diuretics may be given captopril in addition. It can achieve dramatic improvement, relieving vascular muscle spasm and reducing the workload of the heart.

When first used, captopril was given in high doses, requiring careful monitoring under hospital conditions. But now, small initial doses are usually given, allowing treatment on an outpatient basis. Diuretics are often prescribed with it, and in stubborn cases, beta blockers.

A variety of minor adverse effects may occur, such as rashes, nausea, and digestive disturbances, but in lower dosages this drug has little adverse effect on general well-being.

INFORMATION FOR USERS

Your drug prescription is tailored for you. Do not alter dosage without checking with your physician.

How taken

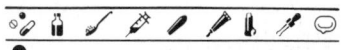

Tablets.

Frequency and timing of doses
2 – 3 x daily one hour before food.

Adult dosage range
12.5 – 37.5mg daily (starting dose), gradually increased to 75 – 150mg daily (maintenance dose).

Onset of effect
30 – 60 minutes.

Duration of action
6 – 8 hours.

Diet advice
None.

Storage
Keep in a closed container in a cool, dry place away from reach of children.

Missed dose
Take as soon as you remember. If your next dose is due within 2 hours, take a single dose now and skip the next.

Stopping the drug
Do not stop the drug without consulting your physician; stopping the drug may lead to worsening of the underlying condition.

Exceeding the dose
An occasional unintentional extra dose is unlikely to cause problems. Large overdoses may cause dizziness or fainting. Notify your physician.

SPECIAL PRECAUTIONS

Be sure to tell your physician if:
▼ You have impaired kidney or liver function.
▼ You have coronary artery disease.
▼ You have an autoimmune disease.
▼ You are taking other medications.

Pregnancy
▼ Not usually prescribed. Safety in pregnancy not established. Discuss with your physician so that you can weigh the benefits of the drug against its possible risks.

Breast feeding
▼ The drug passes into the breast milk, but at normal doses adverse effects on the baby are uncommon. Discuss with your physician.

Infants and children
▼ Not usually prescribed. Reduced dose necessary.

Over 60
▼ Reduced dose may be necessary. Increased likelihood of adverse effects.

Driving and hazardous work
▼ Avoid such activities until you have learned how the drug affects you, because the drug can cause dizziness and fainting.

Alcohol
▼ Avoid. Alcohol may increase the adverse effects of this drug.

POSSIBLE ADVERSE EFFECTS

Captopril may cause a variety of minor adverse effects on the gastrointestinal system. Rashes, which occur frequently, usually disappear when the drug is stopped. Large doses have been associated with altered kidney function.

Symptom/effect	Frequency		Discuss with physician		Stop taking drug now	Call physician now
	Common	Rare	Only if severe	In all cases		
Dizziness/weakness	●		■			
Loss of taste/appetite	●		■			
Rash/itching	●			■		
Mouth ulcers		●		■		
Nausea/vomiting		●		■		

INTERACTIONS

Non-steroidal anti-inflammatory drugs and vasodilators These drugs reduce the blood pressure even further.

Cimetidine increases the risk of adverse effects and reduces the effect of captopril.

PROLONGED USE

No problems expected.

Monitoring Periodic checks on the white blood cell count and the urine are usually performed regularly during the first three months of treatment.

CARBACHOL

Brand name Isopto Carbachol
Used in the following combined preparations None

GENERAL INFORMATION

Carbachol, introduced in 1979, is a pupil-constricting (miotic) drug used in the treatment of glaucoma. Applied in the form of eye drops, it is used mainly to treat chronic glaucoma, particularly in people who have become resistant to other treatments or who can no longer take other drugs because of side effects. It is occasionally given for emergency treatment of acute glaucoma prior to surgery.

Given by injection into the eye, it is also used to induce prolonged constriction of the pupil during cataract removal or other types of eye surgery.

In common with other miotics, carbachol frequently causes visual disturbances such as blurred vision, difficulty with close work, and poor vision in dim light. Spasm of muscles inside the eye may cause eye pain or headache, particularly at the start of treatment.

QUICK REFERENCE

Drug group Miotic drug affecting the pupil (p.198) and drug for glaucoma (p.196)

Overdose danger rating Medium

Dependence rating Low

Prescription needed Yes

Available as generic Yes

INFORMATION FOR USERS

Your drug prescription is tailored for you. Do not alter dosage without checking with your physician.

How taken

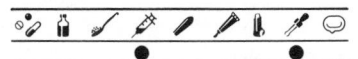

Injection into the eye, eye drops.

Frequency and timing of doses
Every 8 hours (eye drops); as a single dose during surgery (injection).

Dosage range
1 drop per application.

Onset of effect
Within 10 – 20 minutes.

Duration of action
8 – 12 hours (eye drops).

Diet advice
None.

Storage
Keep in a closed container in a cool, dry place away from reach of children.

Missed dose
Take as soon as you remember. If your next dose is due within 2 hours, take a single dose now and skip the next.

Stopping the drug
Do not stop the drug without consulting your physician; symptoms may recur.

Exceeding the dose
An occasional unintentional extra application is unlikely to cause problems. Excessive use may cause facial flushing, an increase in the flow of saliva, and sweating. If accidentally swallowed, seek medical attention immediately.

SPECIAL PRECAUTIONS

Be sure to tell your physician if:
▼ You have asthma.
▼ You have inflamed eyes or an eye injury.
▼ You wear soft contact lenses.
▼ You are taking other medications.

 Pregnancy
▼ No evidence of risk to developing baby.

 Breast feeding
▼ No evidence of risk.

 Infants and children
▼ Not usually prescribed.

 Over 60
▼ No special problems.

 Driving and hazardous work
▼ Avoid such activities until you have learned how the drug affects you, because the drug may cause blurred vision, nearsightedness and poor night vision.

 Alcohol
▼ No known problems.

POSSIBLE ADVERSE EFFECTS

Serious adverse effects are rare with carbachol. Blurred vision, nearsightedness and brow pain may be troublesome, especially at the start of treatment. Headaches and eye irritation are also fairly common symptoms with this drug.

Symptom/effect	Frequency		Discuss with physician		Stop taking drug now	Call physician now
	Common	Rare	Only if severe	In all cases		
Blurred vision	●		■			
Poor night vision	●		■			
Brow pain/headache	●		■			
Stinging/irritation	●		■			
Twitching eye lids		●	■			
Red/watery eyes		●	■			

PROLONGED USE

The effects of carbachol may wear off suddenly or gradually with prolonged use as the body adapts. Other antiglaucoma drugs may need to be substituted.

INTERACTIONS

None.

CARBAMAZEPINE

Brand name Tegretol
Used in the following combined preparations None

GENERAL INFORMATION

Chemically related to the tricyclic antidepressants (see p.112), carbamazepine reduces the likelihood of seizures caused by abnormal nerve signals in the brain. Physicians have used it in the long-term treatment of epilepsy since 1960, and it is considered particularly suitable for treating children because it has only a mild sedative effect. Carbamazepine is also prescribed to relieve the intermittent severe pain caused by damage to the cranial nerves – for example, in trigeminal neuralgia (tic douloureux) or neuralgia of the tongue and throat. Carbamazepine is also occasionally prescribed to treat certain psychological or behavioral disorders.

(see p.112)

QUICK REFERENCE

Drug group Anticonvulsant drug (p.114)

Overdose danger rating Medium

Dependence rating Low

Prescription needed Yes

Available as generic No

INFORMATION FOR USERS

Your drug prescription is tailored for you. Do not alter dosage without checking with your physician.

How taken

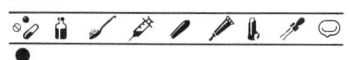

Tablets.

Frequency and timing of doses
2 – 4 x daily with food or milk.

Adult dosage range
Epilepsy 400 – 1200mg daily.
Pain relief 200 – 1200mg daily.

Onset of effect
Within 4 hours.

Duration of action
12 – 24 hours.

Diet advice
None.

Storage
Keep in a closed container in a cool, dry place away from reach of children.

Missed dose
Take as soon as you remember. If your next dose is due within 2 hours, take a single dose now and skip the next.

Stopping the drug
Do not stop the drug without consulting your physician; symptoms may recur.

Exceeding the dose
An occasional unintentional extra dose is unlikely to cause problems. Large overdoses may cause dizziness or drowsiness. Notify your physician.

SPECIAL PRECAUTIONS

Be sure to tell your physician if:
- ▼ You have impaired kidney or liver function.
- ▼ You have heart problems.
- ▼ You have poor circulation.
- ▼ You have prostate trouble.
- ▼ You are hypersensitive to tricyclic antidepressants.
- ▼ You are taking other medications.

 Pregnancy
▼ Not usually prescribed. May cause abnormalities in the unborn baby. Discuss with your physician so that you may weigh the benefits of the drug against its risks.

 Breast feeding
▼ Discuss with your physician. The drug passes into the breast milk, but at normal doses adverse effects on the baby are uncommon.

 Infants and children
▼ Reduced dose necessary.

 Over 60
▼ May cause confused or agitated behavior in the elderly. Reduced dose may be necessary.

 Driving and hazardous work
▼ Discuss with your physician. Your underlying condition, as well as the possibility of reduced alertness while taking this drug, may make such activities inadvisable.

 Alcohol
▼ Avoid. Alcohol may increase the sedative effects of this drug.

POSSIBLE ADVERSE EFFECTS

Most people experience very few adverse effects with this drug, but when blood levels get too high, adverse effects are common and the dose may need to be reduced.

Symptom/effect	Frequency		Discuss with physician		Stop taking drug now	Call physician now
	Common	Rare	Only if severe	In all cases		
Dizziness/unsteadiness	●		■			
Drowsiness	●		■			
Nausea/vomiting	●		■			
Blurred vision	●			■		
Ankle swelling		●		■		
Rash		●		■	▲	

INTERACTIONS

Anticoagulants Carbamazepine may reduce the effect of anticoagulant drugs. The anticoagulant dose may need to be adjusted accordingly.

Oral contraceptives Carbamazepine may reduce the effectiveness of oral contraceptives. An alternative form of contraceptive may need to be used. Discuss with your physician.

Alcohol Alcohol increases the sedative effect of carbamazepine.

Tricyclic antidepressants These may increase the sedative effect of carbamazepine and also reduce its anticonvulsant effect. Dosage adjustments may need to be made to control seizures.

Quinidine The effectiveness of this anti-arrhythmic drug may be reduced when it is taken along with carbamazepine. The dosage of quinidine may need to be adjusted.

PROLONGED USE

There is a slight risk of blood abnormalities occurring during prolonged use.

Monitoring Periodic blood tests may be performed to monitor levels of the drug in the body and the composition of the blood.

CARBOPROST

Brand name Prostin/15M
Used in the following combined preparations None

GENERAL INFORMATION

Introduced in 1979, carboprost is a synthetic form of a naturally occurring prostaglandin (a locally acting chemical "messenger") that stimulates contractions of the uterus. Longer-acting than some similar drugs, it is given by injection for termination of pregnancy between 12 and 20 weeks. Carboprost may also be given to induce labor when the fetus has died in the uterus. It is sometimes used to stop bleeding from the uterus after childbirth or termination of pregnancy, after other treatments have failed.

Vaginal suppositories containing the drug are under investigation for preparing the cervix prior to termination of pregnancy by suction methods.

Adverse effects are rarely serious. Nausea, vomiting, or diarrhea are common. For this reason, anti-emetic and antidiarrheal drugs are often given before or with carboprost as a preventive measure.

QUICK REFERENCE

Drug group Drug used to terminate pregnancy (p.193)

Overdose danger rating Low

Dependence rating Low

Prescription needed Yes

Available as generic No

INFORMATION FOR USERS

This drug is given only in the hospital under medical supervision and is not for self-administration.

How taken

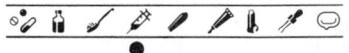

Injection.

Frequency and timing of doses
Every 1.5 – 3.5 hours.

Adult dosage range
Dosage is determined by individual response.

Onset of effect
Contractions start in 1 – 2 hours, and termination is usually completed about 16 hours after the first carboprost injection.

Duration of action
Up to 4 hours.

Diet advice
None.

Storage
Not applicable. The drug is not kept in the home.

Missed dose
Not applicable. The drug is given only in the hospital under medical supervision.

Stopping the drug
Not applicable. The drug is stopped under medical supervision.

Exceeding the dose
The drug is given only in the hospital under medical supervision, and overdose is extremely unlikely to occur.

SPECIAL PRECAUTIONS

Be sure to tell your physician if:
▼ You have impaired liver or kidney function.
▼ You have had heart problems or high blood pressure.
▼ You suffer from asthma or another lung disease.
▼ You have diabetes.
▼ You have had epileptic seizures.
▼ You are anemic.
▼ You have ever had an operation on your uterus or a cesarean section.
▼ You are taking other medications.

 Pregnancy
▼ Not prescribed except for termination of pregnancy.

 Breast feeding
▼ Not prescribed.

 Infants and children
▼ Not prescribed.

 Over 60
▼ Not prescribed.

 Driving and hazardous work
▼ Not applicable.

 Alcohol
▼ Not applicable.

POSSIBLE ADVERSE EFFECTS

Nausea, vomiting, and diarrhea are very common with carboprost; other drugs are routinely given to prevent or control these effects. Fever also occurs fairly frequently. All adverse effects are closely monitored during administration of the drug.

Symptom/effect	Frequency		Discuss with physician		Stop taking drug now	Call physician now
	Common	Rare	Only if severe	In all cases		
Nausea/vomiting	●		■			
Diarrhea	●		■			
Fever/chills	●		■			
Facial flushing	●		■			
Headache		●	■			

INTERACTIONS

None.

PROLONGED USE

Not used for prolonged periods.

CARISOPRODOL

Brand names Rela, Soma, Soprodol
Used in the following combined preparations Soma Compound, Soma Compound with Codeine

GENERAL INFORMATION

Introduced in 1959, carisoprodol is a muscle relaxant related to meprobamate, an anti-anxiety drug. It is prescribed to relieve muscle spasm, rigidity, and pain following injury. It is available on its own or in a combined preparation with an *analgesic*, such as aspirin or codeine. However, this drug does not cure the underlying damage, so drug treatment usually should be accompanied by rest and physical therapy. It is not known exactly how the drug works, but the benefits are probably due to sedation of the central nervous system.

Carisoprodol is not useful for treating muscle spasm due to spasticity. Drowsiness and dizziness, the most common side effects, may be alleviated by dosage reduction.

QUICK REFERENCE

Drug group Muscle-relaxant drug (p.148)

Overdose danger rating Medium

Dependence rating Low

Prescription needed Yes

Available as generic Yes

INFORMATION FOR USERS

Your drug prescription is tailored for you. Do not alter dosage without checking with your physician.

How taken

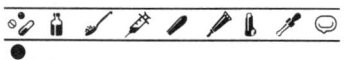

Tablets.

Frequency and timing of doses
4 x daily.

Adult dosage range
1.4g daily.

Onset of effect
Within 30 minutes.

Duration of action
4 – 6 hours.

Diet advice
None.

Storage
Keep in a closed container in a cool, dry place away from reach of children.

Missed dose
Take as soon as you remember. If your next dose is due within 2 hours, take a single dose now and skip the next.

Stopping the drug
Can be safely stopped as soon as you no longer need it.

Exceeding the dose
An occasional unintentional extra dose is unlikely to cause problems. Large overdoses may cause drowsiness, weakness, and breathing problems. Notify your physician.

POSSIBLE ADVERSE EFFECTS

Carisoprodol rarely causes adverse effects. Those that do occur are related to the sedative effects of the drug. They usually diminish with continued treatment and can be minimized by starting with a low dose. Rarely, it can cause attacks of extreme weakness, blurred vision, and confusion in susceptible individuals.

Symptom/effect	Frequency		Discuss with physician		Stop taking drug now	Call physician now
	Common	Rare	Only if severe	In all cases		
Drowsiness/dizziness	●		■			
Headache		●		■		
Insomnia		●		■		
Facial flushing		●		■		
Clumsiness/unsteadiness		●		■		
Blurred vision		●		■	▲	▮
Faintness/weakness		●		■	▲	▮
Confusion		●		■	▲	▮

INTERACTIONS

Sedatives All drugs that have a sedative effect on the nervous system are likely to increase the sedative properties of carisoprodol. Such drugs include anti-anxiety and sleeping drugs, antihistamines, narcotic analgesics, and antidepressant and antipsychotic drugs.

SPECIAL PRECAUTIONS

Be sure to tell your physician if:
▼ You have impaired liver or kidney function.
▼ You suffer from porphyria.
▼ You are taking other medications.

Pregnancy
▼ Not usually prescribed. Safety in pregnancy not established. Discuss with your physician so that you may weigh the benefits of the drug against its risks.

Breast feeding
▼ Discuss with your physician. The drug passes into the breast milk and may affect the baby adversely.

Infants and children
▼ Not recommended.

Over 60
▼ No special problems.

Driving and hazardous work
▼ Avoid such activities until you have learned how the drug affects you, because the drug can cause drowsiness and dizziness.

Alcohol
▼ Avoid. Alcohol may increase the sedative effects of this drug.

PROLONGED USE

No problems expected.

CEFACLOR

Brand name Ceclor
Used in the following combined preparations None

GENERAL INFORMATION

Cefaclor, introduced in 1979, is an antibiotic given by mouth to treat a variety of bacterial infections, mainly those affecting the respiratory tract, sinuses, skin, soft tissue, urinary tract, and middle ear. It has a wider range of effectiveness than many antibiotics against some types of bacteria that are resistant to penicillin.

The main use for cefaclor is in the treatment of childhood ear infections that are resistant to ampicillin. Sometimes it is prescribed as follow-up treatment for more severe infections

after a different cephalosporin has been given by injection.

Unlike many other similar drugs, cefaclor is not affected by the action of digestive juices, so it can be taken on an empty stomach. Food slows down the body's ability to absorb the drug, delaying its onset of action.

Diarrhea is the most common side effect of cefaclor. Some people may suffer from nausea or vomiting, itching, skin rash, and fever especially if they are sensitive to penicillin. In such cases another drug is substituted.

QUICK REFERENCE

Drug group Cephalosporin antibiotic (p.156)

Overdose danger rating Low

Dependence rating Low

Prescription needed Yes

Available as generic No

INFORMATION FOR USERS

Your drug prescription is tailored for you. Do not alter dosage without checking with your physician.

How taken

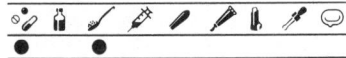

Capsules, powder.

Frequency and timing of doses
3 x daily on an empty stomach.

Dosage range
Adults 750mg – 4g daily.
Children Reduced dose according to age and weight.

Onset of effect
30 – 60 minutes.

Duration of action
8 hours.

Diet advice
None.

Storage
Keep capsules in a closed container in a cool, dry place away from children. Refrigerate liquid, but do not freeze, and keep for no longer than 14 days.

Missed dose
Take as soon as you remember. If your next dose is due at this time, take both doses now.

Stopping the drug
Take the full course. Even if you feel better, the original infection may still be present and may recur if treatment is stopped too soon.

Exceeding the dose
An occasional unintentional extra dose is unlikely to be a cause for concern. But if you notice unusual symptoms, or if a large overdose has been taken, notify your physician.

SPECIAL PRECAUTIONS

Be sure to tell your physician if:
▼ You have impaired kidney function.
▼ You have had a previous allergic reaction to penicillin antibiotics.
▼ You are taking other medications.

 Pregnancy
▼ No evidence of risk to developing baby.

 Breast feeding
▼ Discuss with your physician. May cause the child to become permanently sensitized to this antibiotic and others.

 Infants and children
▼ Reduced dose necessary.

 Over 60
▼ No special problems.

 Driving and hazardous work
▼ No special problems.

 Alcohol
▼ No special problems.

POSSIBLE ADVERSE EFFECTS

Most people do not suffer any adverse effects while taking cefaclor. Diarrhea occurs fairly commonly but it tends not to be severe. Most other adverse effects are due to an allergic reaction that may necessitate stopping the drug.

Symptom/effect	Frequency		Discuss with physician		Stop taking drug now	Call physician now
	Common	Rare	Only if severe	In all cases		
Diarrhea	●		■			
Nausea/vomiting		●	■			
Fever		●		■		
Itching		●		■	▲	▮
Rash		●		■	▲	▮
Joint pain/swelling		●		■	▲	▮

INTERACTIONS

Probenecid This drug increases the level of cefaclor in the blood. The dosage of cefaclor may need to be adjusted accordingly.

PROLONGED USE

Cefaclor is usually given only for short courses of treatment.

CEFAZOLIN

Brand names Ancef, Kefzol
Used in the following combined preparations None

GENERAL INFORMATION

Introduced in 1973, cefazolin is a cephalosporin antibiotic. Available in injection form only, it is mainly given in the hospital to prevent infection in people undergoing major surgery. Also it is given to treat serious infections such as septicemia, and severe gallbladder, respiratory, and urinary tract infections when laboratory tests have shown the bacteria to be sensitive to this drug. Cefazolin is occasionally given in conjunction with an aminoglycoside antibiotic for certain forms of pneumonia.

Cefazolin causes less pain at the site of injection than other similar cephalosporins. Possible side effects include nausea, vomiting, and diarrhea.

INFORMATION FOR USERS

The drug is given only under medical supervision and is not for self-administration.

How taken

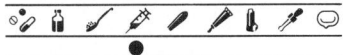

Injection.

Frequency and timing of doses
3 – 4 x daily.

Dosage range
Dosage is determined individually according to condition and response.

Onset of effect
30 – 60 minutes

Duration of action
8 – 24 hours.

Diet advice
None.

Storage
Not applicable. This drug is not normally kept in the home.

Missed dose
A missed dose is unlikely, since treatment is given by a physician or nurse.

Stopping the drug
The course of treatment should be completed as prescribed. Even if you feel better, the original infection may still be present and may recur if treatment is stopped too soon.

Exceeding the dose
Overdosage is unlikely, since treatment is administered by a physician or nurse.

SPECIAL PRECAUTIONS

Be sure to tell your physician if:
▼ You have impaired kidney function.
▼ You have previously suffered an allergic reaction to antibiotics.
▼ You are taking other medications.

Pregnancy
▼ Discuss with your physician so that you can weigh the benefits of the drug against its possible risks.

Breast feeding
▼ The drug passes into the breast milk, but at normal doses adverse effects on the baby are unlikely. Discuss with your physician.

Infants and children
▼ Reduced dose necessary.

Over 60
▼ Reduced dose may be necessary. Increased likelihood of adverse effects.

Driving and hazardous work
▼ No known problems.

Alcohol
▼ No known problems.

POSSIBLE ADVERSE EFFECTS

Cefazolin rarely causes serious adverse effects. Development of a rash or fever is due to an allergic reaction that makes stopping the drug necessary.

Symptom/effect	Frequency		Discuss with physician		Stop taking drug now	Call physician now
	Common	Rare	Only if severe	In all cases		
Nausea/vomiting	●		■			
Diarrhea	●		■			
Fever	●			■		▮
Rash/itching	●			■	▲	▮

INTERACTIONS

Probenecid This drug increases the level of cefazolin in the blood. The dosage of cefazolin may need to be adjusted accordingly.

PROLONGED USE

Cefazolin is usually only given for short courses of treatment.

CEFOPERAZONE

Brand name Cefobid
Used in the following combined preparations None

GENERAL INFORMATION

Introduced in 1982, cefoperazone is one of the newest cephalosporin antibiotics. Given by injection, it is used to treat serious infections of the respiratory tract, urinary tract, skin, and joints that are resistant to other antibiotics. Cefoperazone is also given to treat septicemia and pelvic infections. Unlike many other cephalosporin antibiotics, cefoperazone may be safely given to people with kidney problems. An advantage of this antibiotic is that it need be given only twice a day.

Diarrhea, nausea, and vomiting are the most common adverse effects of cefoperazone. Diarrhea is more common than with the other cephalosporins. Alcohol should not be taken with this drug, since it may react dangerously, like Antabuse (p.321).

INFORMATION FOR USERS

The drug is given only under medical supervision and is not for self-administration.

How taken

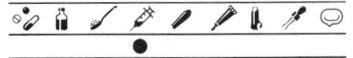

Injection.

Frequency and timing of doses
2 x daily.

Adult dosage range
Dosage is determined individually according to the condition being treated.

Onset of effect
1 – 2 days.

Duration of action
12 – 24 hours.

Diet advice
None.

Storage
Not applicable. This drug is not normally kept in the home.

Missed dose
A missed dose is unlikely, since treatment is given by a physician or nurse.

Stopping the drug
The course of treatment should be completed as prescribed. Even if you feel better, the original infection may still be present and may recur if treatment is stopped too soon.

Exceeding the dose
Overdosage is unlikely, since treatment is administered by a physician or nurse.

POSSIBLE ADVERSE EFFECTS

Gastrointestinal disturbances such as nausea, vomiting, and diarrhea are the most common adverse effects of this drug. Other adverse effects may be caused by an allergic reaction that may make stopping the drug necessary.

Symptom/effect	Frequency		Discuss with physician		Stop taking drug now	Call physician now
	Common	Rare	Only if severe	In all cases		
Nausea/vomiting	●		■			
Diarrhea	●		■			
Abdominal pain		●	■			
Sore mouth/tongue		●		■		
Rash		●		■	▲	▮

INTERACTIONS

Anticoagulant drugs Cefoperazone may increase the effect of these drugs. Anticoagulant dosage may need to be adjusted accordingly.

SPECIAL PRECAUTIONS

Be sure to tell your physician if:
▼ You have previously had an allergic reaction to an antibiotic.
▼ You have a history of bleeding disorders.
▼ You are taking other medications.

Pregnancy
▼ Not usually prescribed. Safety in pregnancy not established. Discuss with your physician so that you can weigh the benefits of the drug against its possible risks.

Breast feeding
▼ The drug may pass into the breast milk, but at normal doses adverse effects on the baby are unlikely. Discuss with your physician.

Infants and children
▼ Not usually prescribed.

Over 60
▼ Reduced dose may be necessary. Increased likelihood of adverse effects.

Driving and hazardous work
▼ No known problems.

Alcohol
▼ Never drink while under treatment with cefoperazone. Alcohol may interact dangerously with this drug, causing flushing, nausea, and possibly collapse.

PROLONGED USE

Prolonged treatment with cefoperazone increases the risk of blood-clotting disorders.

Monitoring Periodic blood tests to check clotting may be performed during prolonged treatment.

CEFOXITIN

Brand name Mefoxin
Used in the following combined preparations None

GENERAL INFORMATION

Introduced in 1978, cefoxitin is a cephalosporin antibiotic. Available in injection form only, it is mainly given in the hospital to prevent infection in people undergoing major surgery. In addition, cefoxitin is used in many cases of serious infection when tests show that the harmful bacteria is sensitive to the drug. Examples include blood poisoning (septicemia), and infections of the abdominal cavity (peritonitis), bone, lung, and urinary tract.

Cefoxitin is also effective against gonorrhea, but drugs that are less expensive or can be taken orally are usually preferred. Possible side effects include nausea, vomiting, and diarrhea.

QUICK REFERENCE

Drug group Cephalosporin antibiotic (p.156)

Overdose danger rating Low

Dependence rating Low

Prescription needed Yes

Available as generic No

INFORMATION FOR USERS

This drug is given only under medical supervision and is not for self-administration.

How taken

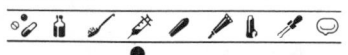

Injection.

Frequency and timing of doses
Every 4 – 8 hours.

Adult dosage range
Up to 12g daily.

Onset of effect
1 – 2 days.

Duration of action
4 – 12 hours.

Diet advice
None.

Storage
Not applicable. This drug is not normally kept in the home.

Missed dose
A missed dose is unlikely, since treatment is given by a physician or nurse.

Stopping the drug
The course of treatment should be completed as prescribed. Even if you feel better, the original infection may still be present and may recur if treatment is stopped too soon.

Exceeding the dose
Overdosage is unlikely, since treatment is administered by a physician or nurse.

SPECIAL PRECAUTIONS

Be sure to tell your physician if:
▼ You have impaired kidney or liver function.
▼ You have previously suffered an allergic reaction to antibiotics.
▼ You are taking other medications.

Pregnancy
▼ Not usually prescribed. Safety in pregnancy not established. Discuss with your physician so that you can weigh the benefits of the drug against its possible risks.

Breast feeding
▼ The drug passes into the breast milk, but at normal doses adverse effects on the baby are uncommon. Discuss with your physician.

Infants and children
▼ Not usually prescribed for babies under 1 month. Reduced dose necessary for older children.

Over 60
▼ Reduced dose may be necessary.

Driving and hazardous work
▼ No known problems.

Alcohol
▼ No known problems.

POSSIBLE ADVERSE EFFECTS

Cefoxitin rarely causes serious adverse effects. Development of a rash or fever may be due to an allergic reaction that makes stopping the drug necessary.

Symptom/effect	Frequency		Discuss with physician		Stop taking drug now	Call physician now
	Common	Rare	Only if severe	In all cases		
Nausea/vomiting		●	■			
Diarrhea		●	■			
Fever		●		■		
Rash/itching		●		■		

INTERACTIONS

Probenecid This drug increases the level of cefoxitin in the blood. The dosage of cefoxitin may need to be reduced.

PROLONGED USE

Cefoxitin is usually only given for short courses of treatment.

CEPHALEXIN

Brand name Keflex
Used in the following combined preparations None

GENERAL INFORMATION

Cephalexin, introduced in 1971, is a cephalosporin antibiotic prescribed for a variety of mild to moderate infections. Cephalexin does not have such a wide range of effectiveness as some other antibiotics, but it is helpful in treating bronchitis, cystitis, and certain skin and soft tissue infections. Sometimes it is prescribed as follow-up treatment for severe infections after a faster-acting cephalosporin has been given by injection.

Some people may not find cephalexin as convenient as some other similar drugs because it has a shorter duration of action and has to be taken four times daily.

Diarrhea is the most common side effect of cephalexin, though it tends to be less severe than with other cephalosporin antibiotics. In addition, some people may find that they are allergic to this drug, especially if they are sensitive to penicillin.

INFORMATION FOR USERS

Your drug prescription is tailored for you. Do not alter dosage without checking with your physician.

How taken

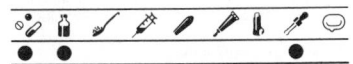

Tablets, capsules, liquid, drops.

Frequency and timing of doses
4 x daily.

Dosage range
Adults 1 – 4g daily.
Children Reduced dose according to age and weight.

Onset of effect
Within 1 hour.

Duration of action
6 hours.

Diet advice
None.

Storage
Keep tablets and capsules in a closed container in a cool, dry place away from reach of children. Refrigerate but do not freeze liquid; discard after 14 days.

Missed dose
Take as soon as you remember. If your next dose is due at this time, take both doses now.

Stopping the drug
Take the full course. Even if you feel better, the original infection may still be present and may recur if treatment is stopped too soon.

Exceeding the dose
An occasional unintentional extra dose is unlikely to be a cause for concern. But if you notice unusual symptoms, or if a large overdose has been taken, notify your physician.

SPECIAL PRECAUTIONS

Be sure to tell your physician if:
▼ You have impaired kidney function.
▼ You have had a previous allergic reaction to penicillin antibiotics.
▼ You are taking other medications.

Pregnancy
▼ No evidence of risk to developing baby.

Breast feeding
▼ Discuss with your physician. May cause the child to become permanently sensitized to this antibiotic and others.

Infants and children
▼ Reduced dose necessary.

Over 60
▼ No special problems.

Driving and hazardous work
▼ No known problems.

Alcohol
▼ No known problems.

POSSIBLE ADVERSE EFFECTS

Most people do not suffer serious adverse effects while taking cephalexin. Diarrhea is common but it tends not to be severe. The rarer adverse effects are usually due to an allergic reaction and may necessitate stopping the drug.

Symptom/effect	Frequency		Discuss with physician		Stop taking drug now	Call physician now
	Common	Rare	Only if severe	In all cases		
Diarrhea	●		■			
Nausea/vomiting		●	■			
Abdominal pain		●		■		
Rash		●		■	▲	▮
Itching/swelling/wheezing		●		■	▲	▮

PROLONGED USE

Cephalexin is usually given only for short courses of treatment.

INTERACTIONS

Probenecid This drug increases the level of cephalexin in the blood. The dosage of cephalexin may need to be adjusted accordingly.

CEPHALOTHIN

Brand names Keflin, Seffin
Used in the following combined preparations

GENERAL INFORMATION

Cephalothin, introduced in 1964, was the first cephalosporin antibiotic. Given by injection, it is used in the hospital for the treatment of a variety of serious infections, particularly in the respiratory tract, urinary tract, skin, and joints. In addition, people undergoing major surgery are often given cephalothin to prevent infection. This drug can also be given as eye drops to treat bacterial conjunctivitis.

The main drawback of cephalothin is that it causes severe pain at the site of injection into a muscle. But this can be avoided by giving it into a vein. Other possible side effects following injection include abdominal pain, nausea, diarrhea, and tiredness.

INFORMATION FOR USERS

Your drug prescription is tailored for you. Do not alter dosage without checking with your physician.

How taken

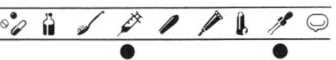

Injection, eye drops.

Frequency and timing of doses
4 – 6 x daily; as directed (eye drops).

Dosage range
Dosage is determined individually according to condition and response.

Onset of effect
30 – 60 minutes.

Duration of action
6 – 24 hours.

Diet advice
None.

Storage
Keep in a closed container in a cool, dry place away from reach of children.

Missed dose
By injection, a missed dose is unlikely, since treatment is given by a physician or nurse. A missed dose of eye drops is no cause for concern. Apply the next dose as soon as possible.

Stopping the drug
The course of treatment should be completed as prescribed. Even if you feel better, the original infection may still be present and may recur if treatment is stopped too soon.

Exceeding the dose
Overdosage by injection is unlikely, since treatment is administered by a physician or nurse. An extra application of eye drops is unlikely to be a cause for concern.

POSSIBLE ADVERSE EFFECTS

Injections of cephalothin into the muscle are usually painful. A rash or fever usually indicates an allergy to the drug, in which case, another antibiotic may need to be substituted. Adverse effects from cephalothin eye drops are rare.

Symptom/effect	Frequency		Discuss with physician		Stop taking drug now	Call physician now
	Common	Rare	Only if severe	In all cases		
Pain at injection site	●			■		
Abdominal pain		●	■			
Diarrhea		●	■			
Tiredness/weakness		●	■			
Joint pain/swelling		●	■		▲	▮
Fever		●		■	▲	▮
Rash		●		■	▲	▮

INTERACTIONS

Aminoglycoside antibiotics
Cephalothin may increase the risk of kidney damage when taken with aminoglycoside antibiotics.

Probenecid This drug increases the level of cephalothin in the blood. The dosage of cephalothin may need to be adjusted accordingly.

SPECIAL PRECAUTIONS

Be sure to tell your physician if:
▼ You have impaired kidney function.
▼ You have previously suffered an allergic reaction to an antibiotic.
▼ You are taking other medications.

Pregnancy
▼ Discuss with your physician so that you can weigh the benefits of the drug against its possible risks.

Breast feeding
▼ The drug passes into the breast milk, but at normal doses adverse effects on the baby are unlikely. Discuss with your physician.

Infants and children
▼ Reduced dose necessary.

Over 60
▼ Reduced dose may be necessary. Increased likelihood of adverse effects.

Driving and hazardous work
▼ No known problems.

Alcohol
▼ No known problems.

PROLONGED USE

Cephalothin is usually given only for short courses of treatment.

CHENODIOL

Brand name Chenix
Used in the following combined preparations None

GENERAL INFORMATION

Chenodiol is a chemical that occurs naturally in bile, where it has an important role in controlling the concentration of cholesterol in the blood. As an orally administered drug, it has been an alternative to surgery in the treatment of gallstones since 1983. It acts by reducing levels of cholesterol in the bile, helping to dissolve gallstones that are made predominantly of cholesterol. Chenodiol is ineffective with stones of a high calcium or bile acid content. Its benefits are increased by weight loss and a diet high in fiber, low in fat. Chenodiol dissolves gallstones in 3 to 18 months. The progress of treatment is assessed regularly by ultrasound or X-ray. Drug treatment may be continued after the stones have disappeared to prevent recurrence of gallstones.

Diarrhea is the most common adverse effect. Regular blood tests are usually carried out to check liver function, which may be temporarily and adversely affected by the drug.

QUICK REFERENCE

Drug group Drug for gallstones (p.142)

Overdose danger rating Low

Dependence rating Low

Prescription needed Yes

Available as generic No

INFORMATION FOR USERS

Your drug prescription is tailored for you. Do not alter dosage without checking with your physician.

How taken

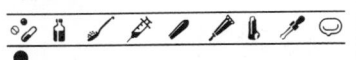

Tablets.

Frequency and timing of doses
2 x daily with food or milk.

Adult dosage range
500mg daily (starting dose), rising to 750 – 1500mg daily (maintenance dose).

Onset of effect
Within 30 minutes. Full beneficial effects may not be felt for up to 18 months.

Duration of action
Up to 12 hours.

Diet advice
A low-cholesterol, high-fiber diet is advisable, as it enhances gallstone dissolution, prevents new stones forming, and reduces circulating cholesterol levels, which are raised by treatment.

Storage
Keep in closed container in a cool, dry place away from reach of children.

Missed dose
No cause for concern. but take as soon as you remember. If your next dose is due within 2 hours, take a single dose now and skip the next.

Stopping the drug
Do not stop the drug without consulting your physician; symptoms may recur.

Exceeding the dose
An occasional unintentional extra dose is unlikely to be a cause for concern. But if you notice unusual symptoms or if a large overdose has been taken, notify your physician.

SPECIAL PRECAUTIONS

Be sure to tell your physician if:
▼ You have impaired liver function
▼ You have pancreatic disease.
▼ You have peptic ulcers.
▼ You are taking other medications.

 Pregnancy
▼ Not usually prescribed. Safety in pregnancy not established. Discuss with your physician so that you can weigh the benefits of the drug against its possible risks.

 Breast feeding
▼ Discuss with your physician. The drug passes into the breast milk and may affect the baby adversely.

 Infants and children
▼ Not recommended.

 Over 60
▼ No special problems.

 Driving and hazardous work
▼ No known problems.

 Alcohol
▼ No known problems.

POSSIBLE ADVERSE EFFECTS

Diarrhea is the most widely experienced adverse effect, particularly at the start of treatment. It can often be minimized by a reduction in dosage.

Symptom/effect	Frequency		Discuss with physician		Stop taking drug now	Call physician now
	Common	Rare	Only if severe	In all cases		
Diarrhea	●		■			
Indigestion		●	■			
Rash		●			■	▲

INTERACTIONS

Cholestyramine, colestipol, and aluminum antacids These reduce the beneficial effect of chenodiol.

Oral contraceptive drugs Estrogen-containing preparations may counter the beneficial effects of chenodiol.

PROLONGED USE

Prolonged use of this drug may in rare cases lead to impairment of liver function. This is reversible on cessation of treatment.

Monitoring Blood tests may be performed to check liver function. Ultrasound or X-ray examinations may be carried out to assess the progress of treatment.

CHLORAL HYDRATE

Brand name Noctec
Used in the following combined preparations None

GENERAL INFORMATION

Chloral hydrate – the chemical ingredient in the classic Mickey Finn, also called knockout drops – is a respected, legitimate and still used sleeping drug (see p.110). It is prescribed by physicians for the short-term treatment of insomnia, for relief of anxiety before a surgical or diagnostic procedure, and for alleviating the unpleasant symptoms associated with alcohol withdrawal. Unlike many sleeping drugs, chloral hydrate is suitable for use with children.

Because it loses effectiveness quickly, however, chloral hydrate is not as commonly used as other sleeping drugs. It also has an unpleasant taste. But its introduction in capsule form recently has provided a solution to that difficulty.

QUICK REFERENCE

Drug group Non-barbiturate, non-benzodiazepine sleeping drug (p.110)

Overdose danger rating High

Dependence rating Medium

Prescription needed Yes CIV

Available as generic Yes

INFORMATION FOR USERS

Your drug prescription is tailored for you. Do not alter dosage without checking with your physician.

How taken

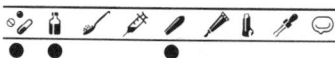

Capsules, liquid, rectal suppositories.

Frequency and timing of doses
Insomnia Once daily 15 – 30 minutes before bedtime.
Anxiety 3 x daily after meals.
Capsules should be taken with a full glass of water. Syrup should be well diluted with milk or water.

Dosage range
Adults 500mg – 1g daily (insomnia); 750 mg daily (anxiety).
Children Reduced dose according to age and weight.

Onset of effect
30 – 60 minutes.

Duration of action
4 – 9 hours.

Diet advice
None.

Storage
Keep in a closed container in a cool, dry place away from reach of children.

Missed dose
If you fall asleep without having taken a dose and wake some hours later, do not take the missed dose. If necessary, return to your normal dose schedule the following night.

Stopping the drug
If you have been taking the drug for less than 4 weeks, it can be safely stopped as soon as you feel that you no longer need it. However, if you have been taking the drug for longer than a few weeks, consult your physician, who may supervise a gradual reduction in dosage. Stopping abruptly may lead to withdrawal symptoms (see p.110).

OVERDOSE ACTION

 Seek immediate medical advice in all cases. Take emergency action if severe confusion, vomiting or loss of consciousness occur.

See Drug poisoning emergency guide (p.590).

SPECIAL PRECAUTIONS

Be sure to tell your physician if:
▼ You have impaired kidney or liver function.
▼ You have heart problems.
▼ You suffer from porphyria.
▼ You have had problems with alcohol or drug abuse.
▼ You are taking other medications.

 Pregnancy
▼ Not usually prescribed. Safety in pregnancy not established. Discuss with your physician so that you can weigh the benefits of the drug against its possible risks.

 Breast feeding
▼ Discuss with your physician. The drug passes into the breast milk. Its effects on the baby are not clearly known.

 Infants and children
▼ Reduced dose necessary.

 Over 60
▼ Reduced dose may be necessary.

 Driving and hazardous work
▼ Avoid such activities until you have learned how the drug affects you. The drug can cause drowsiness.

 Alcohol
▼ Avoid. Alcohol may increase the sedative effects of this drug.

POSSIBLE ADVERSE EFFECTS

The principal adverse effects of this drug are related to its sedative properties. These effects normally diminish after the first few days of treatment.

Symptom/effect	Frequency		Discuss with physician		Stop taking drug now	Call physician now
	Common	Rare	Only if severe	In all cases		
Nausea/vomiting	●		■			
Clumsiness/unsteadiness		●	■			
Daytime drowsiness		●	■			
Unusual excitement		●		■		
Headache		●		■		
Rash		●		■	▲	

PROLONGED USE

Regular use of this drug over several weeks can lead to a reduction in its effect as the body adapts. It may also be habit-forming when taken for extended periods, especially if larger than average doses are taken.

INTERACTIONS

Sedatives All drugs that have a sedative effect on the central nervous system are likely to increase the sedative properties of chloral hydrate.

Anticoagulants Coumarin anticoagulants, such as dicumarol, may be less effective when taken with chloral hydrate.

CHLORAMBUCIL

Brand name Leukeran
Used in the following combined preparations None

GENERAL INFORMATION

Introduced in 1957, this anticancer drug interferes with the growth of cancer cells, thereby helping the immune system overcome the disease. Taken in tablet form, chlorambucil is mainly used to treat certain types of leukemia (cancer of the blood cells) and lymphoma (cancer of the lymph glands), and also cancers of the ovaries and testicles.

Because chlorambucil also has an immunosuppressant action, it is sometimes given to people with such disorders of the immune system as certain types of kidney disease and severe rheumatoid arthritis.

As with other anticancer drugs, chlorambucil may reduce blood cell production by the bone marrow, thereby increasing the risk of abnormal bleeding, anemia, and infection. Long-term use of the drug can also lead to sterility in men and to cessation of periods in women; both these problems may improve after the treatment is stopped. Unlike many anticancer drugs, chlorambucil rarely causes nausea and vomiting.

INFORMATION FOR USERS

Your drug prescription is tailored for you. Do not alter dosage without checking with your physician.

How taken

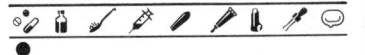

Tablets.

Frequency and timing of doses
Once daily.

Dosage range
Dosage is determined individually according to body height, weight, and response.

Onset of effect
Active in the body within 2 hours. Beneficial effects may not be noticed for 3 – 4 weeks.

Duration of action
24 hours.

Diet advice
None.

Storage
Keep in a closed container in a cool, dry place away from reach of children.

Missed dose
Take as soon as you remember. If your next dose is due within 6 hours, take a single dose now and skip the next. Tell your physician that you missed a dose.

Stopping the drug
Do not stop the drug without consulting your physician; stopping the drug may lead to worsening of the underlying condition.

Exceeding the dose
An occasional unintentional extra dose is unlikely to cause problems. Large overdoses may cause nausea and vomiting. Notify your physician.

POSSIBLE ADVERSE EFFECTS

Noticeable adverse effects are uncommon with chlorambucil, but always require medical attention. Irregular menstruation in women and sterility in men are usually temporary and disappear when treatment is stopped.

Symptom/effect	Frequency		Discuss with physician		Stop taking drug now	Call physician now
	Common	Rare	Only if severe	In all cases		
Nausea/vomiting		●		■		
Seizures		●		■		
Irregular menstruation		●		■		▌
Rash	●			■	▲	▌
Jaundice	●			■	▲	▌

INTERACTIONS

Allopurinol This drug may increase blood levels of chlorambucil, leading to an increased risk of adverse effects.

SPECIAL PRECAUTIONS

Chlorambucil is prescribed only under close medical supervision, taking account of your present condition and medical history.

Pregnancy
▼ Not usually prescribed. May cause abnormalities in the unborn baby. Discuss with your physician so that you may weigh the benefits of the drug against its risks.

Breast feeding
▼ Discontinue breast feeding. The drug passes into the breast milk and may affect the baby adversely.

Infants and children
▼ Reduced dose necessary.

Over 60
▼ No special problems.

Driving and hazardous work
▼ No known problems.

Alcohol
▼ No known problems.

PROLONGED USE

Prolonged use of this drug may reduce production of blood cells, and may cause temporary sterility in men and disrupted periods in women.

Monitoring Periodic checks on blood composition are usually required.

CHLORAMPHENICOL

Brand names Chloromycetin, Chloroptic Ophthalmic, Econochlor Ophthalmic, Ophthochlor Ophthalmic
Used in the following combined preparations Ophthocort, Chloromycetin Hydrocortisone Powder

GENERAL INFORMATION

Chloramphenicol, discovered in 1947, is an antibiotic that is commonly included in *topical* preparations for eye and ear infections. Given by mouth or injection, it is widely distributed in the body and penetrates the brain well, making it useful in the treatment of meningitis and brain abscesses. It is often prescribed for typhoid fever and abdominal infections. It is particularly useful for combating acute infections, such as pneumonia, epiglottitis, or meningitis, caused by a bacterium that is resistant to other antibiotics. Q fever, Rocky Mountain spotted fever, and similar infections may also be treated with the drug.

Although most people experience few adverse effects, chloramphenicol occasionally causes serious or even fatal blood disorders. For this reason, oral or injectable chloramphenicol is reserved for life-threatening infections that do not respond to safer drugs.

QUICK REFERENCE

Drug group Antibiotic (p.156)
Overdose danger rating Low
Dependence rating Low
Prescription needed Yes
Available as generic Yes

INFORMATION FOR USERS

Your drug prescription is tailored for you. Do not alter dosage without checking with your physician.

How taken

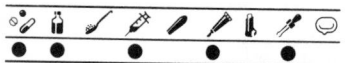

Capsules, liquid, injection, ointment, eye and ear drops.

Frequency and timing of doses
Every 6 – 8 hours (by mouth, injection); every 3 hours (eye preparations); 3 x daily (ear drops).

Adult dosage range
Varies according to preparation and condition. Follow your physician's instructions.

Onset of effect
1 – 3 days, depending on the condition and preparation.

Duration of action
6 – 8 hours.

Diet advice
None.

Storage
Keep in a closed container in a cool, dry place away from reach of children.

Missed dose
Take as soon as you remember (capsules, liquid). If your next dose is due, double the dose to make up the missed dose. For eye and ear preparations, take as soon as you remember.

Stopping the drug
Take the full course. Even if you feel better, the infection may still be present and may recur if treatment is stopped too soon.

Exceeding the dose
An occasional unintentional extra dose is unlikely to be a cause for concern. But if you notice unusual symptoms, or if a large overdose has been taken, notify your physician.

SPECIAL PRECAUTIONS

Be sure to tell your physician if:
▼ You have impaired liver or kidney function.
▼ You have a blood disorder.
▼ You are taking other medications.

 Pregnancy
▼ Taken by mouth or injection in late pregnancy, may cause vomiting, breathing difficulties, and poor circulation in the newborn infant. Discuss with your physician so that you may weigh the benefits of the drug against its risks.

 Breast feeding
▼ No evidence of risk with eye or ear preparations. Taken by mouth the drug passes into the breast milk and may increase the risk of blood disorders in the baby. Discuss with your physician.

 Infants and children
▼ Reduced dose necessary.

 Over 60
▼ Reduced dose may be necessary.

 Driving and hazardous work
▼ No known problems.

 Alcohol
▼ No known problems.

POSSIBLE ADVERSE EFFECTS

Transient irritation may occur with eye or ear drops. Sore throat, fever, and unusual tiredness with any form of chloramphenicol may be signs of blood abnormalities and should be reported to your physician without delay even after treatment has been stopped.

Symptom/effect	Frequency		Discuss with physician		Stop taking drug now	Call physician now
	Common	Rare	Only if severe	In all cases		
Burning/stinging (drops)		●	■			
Numb/tingling hands/feet		●		■		▮
Rash/itching		●		■		▮
Impaired vision		●		■		▮
Sore throat/fever/weakness		●		■	▲	▮
Painful mouth/tongue		●		■	▲	▮

INTERACTIONS

General note Chloramphenicol may increase the effect of certain other drugs, including phenytoin, oral antidiabetics, and oral anticoagulants. Phenobarbital, phenytoin and rifampin may reduce the effect of chloramphenicol.

Anti-anemia drugs Chloramphenicol may delay the body's response to iron, vitamin B₁₂, or folic acid.

Other antibiotics Chloramphenicol may inhibit the antibacterial effects of penicillin and erythromycin antibiotics.

PROLONGED USE

Prolonged use of this drug may increase the risk of serious blood disorders and eye damage.

Monitoring Periodic blood cell counts and eye tests may be performed. Blood levels of the drug are usually monitored in young children given chloramphenicol by mouth or by injection.

CHLORDIAZEPOXIDE

Brand names Libritabs, Librium
Used in the following combined preparations Librax, Limbitrol

GENERAL INFORMATION

Introduced in the mid-1960s, chlordiazepoxide belongs to a group of drugs known as benzodiazepines. These are used to help to relieve nervousness and tension, relax muscles, and encourage sleep. The actions and adverse effects of this group of drugs are described more fully on p.111.

Prescribed primarily to treat anxiety, chlordiazepoxide is also administered to relieve the symptoms of alcohol withdrawal.

As a combined preparation with the tricyclic antidepressant amitriptyline, chlordiazepoxide is sometimes used to treat depression associated with anxiety.

Chlordiazepoxide is also combined with clidinium bromide for the treatment of gastrointestinal disorders such as indigestion and irritable bowel syndrome, which may be made worse by anxiety.

Addictive if taken regularly over a long period, chlordiazepoxide may also lose effectiveness with time. For those reasons, treatment is regularly reviewed.

INFORMATION FOR USERS

Your drug prescription is tailored for you. Do not alter dosage without checking with your physician.

How taken

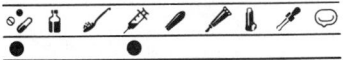

Tablets, injection.

Frequency and timing of doses
1 – 4 x daily with food or milk.

Adult dosage range
10 – 100mg daily. The dosage varies considerably from person to person.

Onset of effect
1 – 3 hours.

Duration of action
12 – 24 hours, but some effect may last up to 4 days.

Diet advice
None.

Storage
Keep in a closed container in a cool, dry place away from reach of children. Protect from light.

Missed dose
No cause for concern, but take when you remember. If your next dose is due within 2 hours, take a single dose now and skip the next.

Stopping the drug
If you have been taking the drug for less than 2 weeks, it can be safely stopped as soon as you feel you no longer need it. However, if you have been taking the drug for longer, consult your physician, who may supervise a gradual reduction in dosage. Stopping abruptly may lead to withdrawal symptoms (see p.111).

Exceeding the dose
An occasional unintentional extra dose is unlikely to cause problems. Large overdoses may cause unusual drowsiness. Notify your physician.

SPECIAL PRECAUTIONS

Be sure to tell your physician if:
▼ You have impaired kidney or liver function.
▼ You have had problems with alcohol or drug abuse.
▼ You are taking other medications.

Pregnancy
▼ Not usually prescribed. Safety in pregnancy not established. Discuss with your physician so that you can weigh the benefits of the drug against its possible risks.

Breast feeding
▼ Discuss with your physician. The drug passes into the breast milk. Its effects on the baby are not clearly known.

Infants and children
▼ Not usually prescribed. Reduced dose necessary.

Over 60
▼ Reduced dose may be necessary. Increased likelihood of adverse effects.

Driving and hazardous work
▼ Avoid such activities until you have learned how the drug affects you, because the drug can cause reduced alertness and slowed reactions.

Alcohol
▼ Avoid. Alcohol may increase the sedative effects of this drug.

POSSIBLE ADVERSE EFFECTS

The principal adverse effects of this drug are related to its sedative and tranquilizing properties. These effects normally diminish after the first few days of treatment.

Symptom/effect	Frequency		Discuss with physician		Stop taking drug now	Call physician now
	Common	Rare	Only if severe	In all cases		
Daytime drowsiness	●		■			
Dizziness/unsteadiness	●		■			
Forgetfulness/confusion		●	■			
Headache		●	■			
Blurred vision		●		■		
Rash		●		■	▲	
Hallucinations		●		■	▲	■

PROLONGED USE

Regular use of this drug over several weeks can lead to a reduction in its effect as the body adapts. It may also be habit-forming when taken for extended periods, especially if larger than average doses are taken.

INTERACTIONS

Cimetidine May cause a buildup of chlordiazepoxide levels in the blood, which increases the likelihood of adverse effects.

Sedatives All drugs that have a sedative effect on the central nervous system are likely to increase the sedative properties of chlordiazepoxide.

A
B
C
D
E
F
G
H
I
J
K
L
M
N
O
P
Q
R
S
T
U
V
W
X
Y
Z

CHLOROQUINE

Brand name Aralen
Used in the following combined preparation Aralen Phosphate with Primaquine Phosphate

GENERAL INFORMATION

Chloroquine was introduced in 1943 for the prevention and treatment of malaria. Taken by mouth, it is rapidly absorbed in high concentrations and usually clears an attack of the disease within three days. Injections may be given when an attack is severe. As a preventive treatment, a low dose of chloroquine is given once weekly starting one week before a trip to a high-risk area and continuing for six weeks after departure. Chloroquine is not suitable for use in all countries because resistance to the drug has developed in some areas.

Chloroquine is occasionally used in the treatment of amebic infections of the liver. It is also used as a treatment for *autoimmune* diseases, including rheumatoid arthritis and lupus erythematosus.

Common side effects include nausea, headache, diarrhea, and abdominal cramps. Occasionally a rash develops. More seriously, chloroquine can damage the retina during prolonged treatment, causing blurred vision sometimes proceeding to blindness. Regular eye examinations are performed to detect early changes.

INFORMATION FOR USERS

Your drug prescription is tailored for you. Do not alter dosage without checking with your physician.

How taken

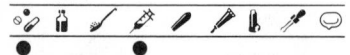

Tablets, injection.

Frequency and timing of doses
By mouth Once weekly (prevention of malaria); 1 – 2 x daily (treatment of malaria); once daily (amebic infection and arthritis). *Injections* Every 6 hours (treatment of malaria).

Adult dosage range
300mg per dose (prevention of malaria); initially 600mg reduced to 300mg per dose (treatment of malaria and amebic infection); according to body weight (arthritis).

Onset of effect
2 – 3 days. In rheumatoid arthritis, full effect may not be felt for up to 6 months.

Duration of action
Up to one week.

Diet advice
None.

Storage
Keep in a closed container in a cool, dry place away from reach of children.

Missed dose
Take as soon as you remember. If your next dose is due within 24 hours (once weekly schedule), or 6 hours (once or twice daily schedule), take a single dose now and skip the next.

Stopping the drug
Do not stop taking the drug without consulting your physician.

OVERDOSE ACTION

 Seek immediate medical advice in all cases. Take emergency action if breathing difficulties, seizures, or loss of consciousness occurs.

See Drug poisoning emergency guide (p.590).

POSSIBLE ADVERSE EFFECTS

Side effects such as nausea, diarrhea, and abdominal pain can be avoided by taking the drug with food. Changes in vision should be reported promptly.

Symptom/effect	Frequency		Discuss with physician		Stop taking drug now	Call physician now
	Common	Rare	Only if severe	In all cases		
Nausea	●		■			
Diarrhea/abdominal pain	●		■			
Headache/dizziness		●	■			
Rash		●		■	▲	▮
Blurred vision		●		■	▲	▮

INTERACTIONS

Rabies vaccine Chloroquine may reduce the effect of this vaccine.

SPECIAL PRECAUTIONS

Be sure to tell your physician if:
▼ You have impaired liver or kidney function.
▼ You have glucose-6-phosphate dehydrogenase (G6PD) deficiency.
▼ You have eye or vision problems.
▼ You have psoriasis.
▼ You suffer from porphyria.
▼ You are taking other medications.

 Pregnancy
▼ No evidence of risk with low doses. High doses may have adverse effects on hearing, balance, and vision in the baby. Discuss with your physician.

 Breast feeding
▼ The drug passes into breast milk, but at normal doses adverse effects on the baby are uncommon. Discuss with your physician.

 Infants and children
▼ Reduced dose necessary.

 Over 60
▼ No special problems.

 Driving and hazardous work
▼ Avoid such activities until you have learned how the drug affects you, because the drug may cause dizziness in high doses.

 Alcohol
▼ Never drink while under treatment with chloroquine. Alcohol may interact with this drug to cause liver problems.

PROLONGED USE

Prolonged use may cause eye damage, cardiac and skeletal muscle damage, and blood disorders.

Monitoring Periodic eye tests and blood counts may be carried out.

CHLOROTHIAZIDE

Brand name Diuril
Used in the following combined preparations Aldoclor, Diupres

GENERAL INFORMATION

Chlorothiazide, introduced in 1958, belongs to the thiazide group of diuretic drugs (p.127). These drugs remove excess water from the body and reduce edema (fluid retention) in people with congestive heart failure, kidney disorders, cirrhosis of the liver, and premenstrual tension. Chlorothiazide is frequently used to treat high blood pressure (see Antihypertensive drugs, p.130), and because it reduces the amount of calcium in the urine, it is sometimes used to prevent the recurrence of some types of kidney stones.

As with all thiazides, chlorothiazide increases the loss of potassium, causing a variety of symptoms (see p.540) and increasing the likelihood of irregular heart rhythms, particularly in those taking drugs such as digoxin for heart failure. Potassium supplements are often prescribed.

INFORMATION FOR USERS

Your drug prescription is tailored for you. Do not alter dosage without checking with your physician.

How taken

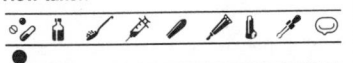

Tablets.

Frequency and timing of doses
Once daily or every 2 days, early in the day.

Adult dosage range
250mg – 1g daily.

Onset of effect
Within 2 hours.

Duration of action
6 – 12 hours.

Diet advice
Use of this drug may reduce potassium in the body. Eat plenty of fresh fruit and vegetables. Discuss the advisability of reducing your salt intake with your physician.

Storage
Keep in a closed container in a cool, dry place away from reach of children.

Missed dose
No cause for concern, but take as soon as you remember. However, if it is late in the day do not take the missed dose, or you may need to get up during the night to pass urine. Take the next scheduled dose as usual.

Stopping the drug
Do not stop taking the drug without consulting your physician; symptoms may recur.

Exceeding the dose
An occasional unintentional extra dose is unlikely to be a cause for concern. But if you notice unusual symptoms, or if a large overdose has been taken, notify your physician.

SPECIAL PRECAUTIONS

Be sure to tell your physician if:
▼ You have impaired kidney or liver function.
▼ You have had gout.
▼ You have diabetes.
▼ You have a high level of fat in your blood (hyperlipidemia).
▼ You are taking other medications.

Pregnancy
▼ Not usually prescribed. No evidence that it harms the baby, but it may cause excessive sodium (salt) loss in the mother.

Breast feeding
▼ Discuss with your physician. The drug passes into the breast milk and may reduce your milk supply.

Infants and children
▼ Not usually prescribed. Reduced dose necessary.

Over 60
▼ Increased likelihood of adverse effects.

Driving and hazardous work
▼ No special problems.

Alcohol
▼ Keep consumption low. Chlorothiazide increases the likelihood of dehydration and hangovers after consumption of alcohol.

POSSIBLE ADVERSE EFFECTS

Most effects are caused by excessive loss of potassium. This can usually be put right by taking a potassium supplement. In rare cases gout may occur in susceptible people, and certain forms of diabetes may become more difficult to control.

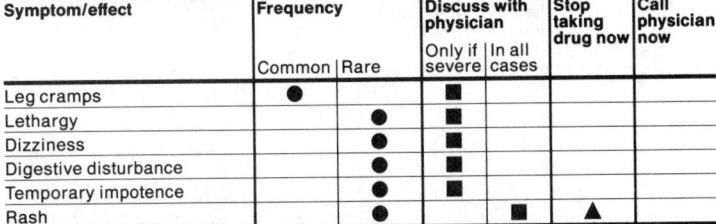

Symptom/effect	Frequency		Discuss with physician		Stop taking drug now	Call physician now
	Common	Rare	Only if severe	In all cases		
Leg cramps	●		■			
Lethargy		●	■			
Dizziness		●	■			
Digestive disturbance		●	■			
Temporary impotence		●	■			
Rash		●		■	▲	

INTERACTIONS

Non-steroidal anti-inflammatory drugs (NSAIDs) may reduce the diuretic effect of chlorothiazide; dosage may need to be adjusted.

Digitalis drugs The adverse effects of such drugs may be increased if excessive amounts of potassium are lost.

Corticosteroids These drugs further increase the loss of potassium from the body when taken with chlorothiazide.

Lithium Chlorothiazide may increase lithium levels in the blood, leading to a risk of serious adverse effects.

PROLONGED USE

Prolonged use of this drug can lead to excessive loss of potassium and imbalances of other salts.

Monitoring Blood tests may be performed periodically to check kidney function and levels of blood sugar, potassium, and other salts.

CHLORPHENIRAMINE

Brand names Alermine, Aller-Chlor, Chlor-Trimeton, Histex, Teldrin
Used in the following combined preparations Deconamine, Naldecon, Ornade, Rynatan, Tussi-Organidin

GENERAL INFORMATION

Chlorpheniramine, an antihistamine used for over 30 years, is given to treat allergies such as hay fever, allergic conjunctivitis, urticaria (hives), and angioedema (allergic swellings). It is a common ingredient of over-the-counter cold remedies (see p.122).

Like other antihistamines, it relieves allergic skin symptoms such as itching, swelling, and redness. It also reduces sneezing and runny nose and itching eyes in hay fever. It has a mild *anticholinergic* action, which suppresses mucus secretion.

Chlorpheniramine may also be used to prevent or treat allergic reactions to blood transfusions or X-ray contrast material, and as a supplement to epinephrine injections for acute allergic shock (anaphylaxis).

QUICK REFERENCE

Drug group Antihistamine (p.152)

Overdose danger rating Medium

Dependence rating Low

Prescription needed No

Available as generic Yes

INFORMATION FOR USERS

Follow instructions on the label. Call your physician if symptoms worsen.

How taken

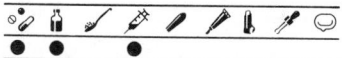

Tablets, slow-release tablets, liquid, injection.

Frequency and timing of doses
3 – 4 x daily (tablets, liquid); 1 – 3 x daily (slow-release tablets); single dose as needed (injection).

Dosage range
Healthy adults 8 – 24mg daily (orally); up to 40mg per dose (injection).
Children over 7 years Reduced dose according to age and weight.

Onset of effect
Within 60 minutes (orally); within 20 minutes (injection).

Duration of action
6 – 8 hours (tablets, liquid, injection), 10 – 14 hours (slow-release tablets).

Diet advice
None.

Storage
Keep in a closed container in a cool, dry place away from reach of children.

Missed dose
Take as soon as you remember. If your next dose is due within 2 hours, take a single dose now and skip the next.

Stopping the drug
Can be safely stopped as soon as you no longer need it.

Exceeding the dose
An occasional unintentional extra dose is unlikely to cause problems. Large overdoses may cause drowsiness or agitation . Notify your physician.

SPECIAL PRECAUTIONS

Be sure to consult your physician before taking this drug if:
▼ You have impaired liver function.
▼ You have had epileptic seizures.
▼ You have had glaucoma.
▼ You have urinary difficulties.
▼ You are taking other medications.

Pregnancy
▼ Not usually prescribed. Safety in pregnancy not established. Discuss with your physician so that you can weigh the benefits of the drug against its possible risks.

Breast feeding
▼ No evidence of risk.

Infants and children
▼ Not recommended in children under 7 years old. Reduced dose necessary in older children.

Over 60
▼ Reduced dose may be necessary. Increased likelihood of adverse effects.

Driving and hazardous work
▼ Avoid such activities until you have learned how the drug affects you, because the drug can cause drowsiness.

Alcohol
▼ Avoid. Alcohol may increase the sedative effects of this drug.

POSSIBLE ADVERSE EFFECTS

Drowsiness is the most common adverse effect of chlorpheniramine. Other side effects are rare. Some of these, such as dryness of the mouth, blurred vision, and difficulty passing urine, are due to its anticholinergic effects. Gastrointestinal irritation may be reduced by taking tablets or liquid with food or drink.

Symptom/effect	Frequency		Discuss with physician		Stop taking drug now	Call physician now
	Common	Rare	Only if severe	In all cases		
Drowsiness	●		■			
Digestive disturbance		●	■			
Urinary difficulties		●	■			
Dry mouth		●	■			
Shaking/tremor		●	■			
Excitation (children)		●		■		▲
Rash		●		■		▲

PROLONGED USE

The effect of the drug may become weaker with prolonged use over a period of weeks or months as the body adapts. Transfer to a different antihistamine may be recommended.

INTERACTIONS

Sedatives All drugs that have a sedative effect are likely to enhance the sedative effect of chlorpheniramine.

Monoamine oxidase inhibitors (MAOIs) There is a risk of a dangerous rise in blood pressure if chlorpheniramine is taken with MAOIs.

Anticholinergic drugs The anticholinergic effects of chlorpheniramine are likely to be increased by all drugs that have anticholinergic effects, including trihexyphenidyl, antipsychotic drugs, and tricyclic antidepressants.

CHLORPROMAZINE

Brand name Thorazine
Used in the following combined preparations None

GENERAL INFORMATION

Chlorpromazine, introduced in the early 1950s, was the first antipsychotic drug to be marketed. It remains one of the most widely used of this group of drugs, effective in suppressing abnormal behavior, reducing aggression, and inducing a generally tranquilizing effect. For further information, see p.113.

Chlorpromazine is used in the treatment of schizophrenia, mania, dementia, and other disorders where confused, aggressive, or abnormal behavior may occur and a degree of sedation is required. It does not cure the underlying disorder, but it does relieve the distressing symptoms. Another use of chlorpromazine is in the treatment of nausea and vomiting, especially when caused by drug or radiation treatment, or anesthetics.

The main drawback to the use of chlorpromazine is that it can produce serious side effects (below).

QUICK REFERENCE

Drug group Phenothiazine antipsychotic (p.113) and anti-emetic drug (p.118)

Overdose danger rating Medium

Dependence rating Low

Prescription needed Yes

Available as generic Yes

INFORMATION FOR USERS

Your drug prescription is tailored for you. Do not alter dosage without checking with your physician.

How taken

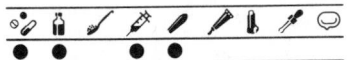

Tablets, liquid, injection, rectal suppository.

Frequency and timing of doses
2 – 4 x daily on an empty stomach.

Adult dosage range
Mental illness 75 – 300mg daily. Dose may be increased in severe illness.
Nausea and vomiting 40 – 150mg daily.

Onset of effect
30 – 60 minutes by mouth; 15 – 20 minutes by injection; up to 30 minutes by suppository.

Duration of action
10 – 12 hours by mouth or injection; 3 – 4 hours by suppository. Some effect may persist for up to 3 weeks when stopping the drug after regular use.

Diet advice
None.

Storage
Keep in a closed container in a cool, dry place away from reach of children. Protect from light.

Missed dose
Take as soon as you remember. If your next dose is due within 2 hours, do not take the missed dose. Take your next scheduled dose as usual.

Stopping the drug
Do not stop the drug without consulting your physician; symptoms may recur.

Exceeding the dose
An occasional unintentional extra dose is unlikely to cause problems. Larger overdoses may cause unusual drowsiness, fainting, muscle rigidity, and agitation. Notify your physician.

SPECIAL PRECAUTIONS

Be sure to tell your physician if:
▼ You have impaired kidney or liver function.
▼ You have had heart problems.
▼ You have had epileptic seizures.
▼ You have an overactive thyroid gland.
▼ You have Parkinson's disease.
▼ You have glaucoma.
▼ You are taking other medications.

Pregnancy
▼ Not usually prescribed. Taken near the time of delivery it can prolong labor and may cause drowsiness in the newborn baby.

Breast feeding
▼ Discuss with your physician. The drug passes into the breast milk and may affect the baby.

Infants and children
▼ Not recommended for children under one year. Reduced dose is necessary for older children.

Over 60
▼ Initial dosage is low; it may be increased if there is no response and no adverse reactions, such as abnormal limb movements or low blood pressure on arising.

Driving and hazardous work
▼ Avoid such activities until you have learned how the drug affects you, because of the possibility of drowsiness and slowed reactions.

Alcohol
▼ Avoid. Alcohol may increase the sedative effects of this drug.

Surgery and general anesthetics
▼ Chlorpromazine treatment may need to be stopped before you have a general anesthetic. Discuss this with your physician or dentist before any operation.

POSSIBLE ADVERSE EFFECTS

Chlorpromazine has a strong *anticholinergic* effect, which can cause symptoms. The most significant adverse effect is abnormal movements of the face and limbs (*parkinsonism*).

Symptom/effect	Frequency		Discuss with physician		Stop taking drug now	Call physician now
	Common	Rare	Only if severe	In all cases		
Drowsiness/lethargy	●		■			
Weight gain	●		■			
Blurred vision	●			■		
Dizziness/fainting	●			■		
Parkinsonism	●			■		
Infrequent periods		●		■		
Rash		●		■		▲

INTERACTIONS

Sedatives All drugs that have a sedative effect on the central nervous system are likely to increase the sedative properties of chlorpromazine.

Antiparkinsonism drugs Chlorpromazine may reduce the effect of these drugs.

Anticholinergic drugs may intensify the *anticholinergic* properties of chlorpromazine.

PROLONGED USE

If used for more than a few months, chlorpromazine may cause *tardive dyskinesia*, a movement disorder. Occasionally, jaundice may occur.

CHLORPROPAMIDE

Brand names Diabinese, Glucamide
Used in the following combined preparations None

GENERAL INFORMATION

Chlorpropamide, introduced in 1958, is an oral antidiabetic drug. Given in conjunction with a diet low in sugar and fats, it is used in the treatment of adult (maturity-onset) diabetes mellitus. It lowers blood sugar by stimulating insulin secretion from the pancreas and by promoting the uptake of sugar into body cells.

The longest acting of the oral antidiabetic drugs, chlorpropamide

need be taken only once daily. It is not given to people with kidney failure and is used with caution in the elderly and children, since it may build up in the body and cause excessive lowering of the blood sugar.

Chlorpropamide is also prescribed for mild forms of diabetes insipidus, in which it reduces the volume of urine produced by increasing water reabsorption in the kidneys.

INFORMATION FOR USERS

Your drug prescription is tailored for you. Do not alter dosage without checking with your physician.

How taken

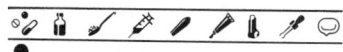

Tablets.

Frequency and timing of doses
Once daily with breakfast.

Dosage range
Adults 100 – 500mg daily.
Children Reduced dose necessary.

Onset of effect
Within 1 hour.

Duration of action
1 – 3 days.

Diet advice
For treatment of diabetes mellitus, a low-sugar, low-fat diet must be maintained. Follow your physician's advice.

Storage
Keep in a closed container in a cool, dry place away from reach of children.

Missed dose
Take before your next meal.

Stopping the drug
Do not stop the drug without consulting your physician; stopping the drug may lead to worsening of your diabetes.

OVERDOSE ACTION

 Seek immediate medical advice in all cases. If symptoms of low blood sugar such as faintness, confusion, sweating, or shaking occur, eat or drink something sugary. Take emergency action if seizures or loss of consciousness occurs.

See Drug poisoning emergency guide (p.590).

SPECIAL PRECAUTIONS

Be sure to tell your physician if:
▼ You have impaired liver or kidney function.
▼ You are allergic to sulfonamide drugs.
▼ You are taking other medications.

 Pregnancy
▼ Not usually prescribed. May cause severe low blood sugar in the newborn baby. Insulin is generally used in pregnancy.

 Breast feeding
▼ Discuss with your physician. The drug passes into the breast milk and may cause low blood sugar in the baby.

 Infants and children
▼ Not prescribed for diabetes mellitus. Reduced dose necessary for diabetes insipidus.

 Over 60
▼ Signs of low blood sugar may be more difficult to recognize.

 Driving and hazardous work
▼ Usually no problem. Avoid these activities if you have warning signs of low blood sugar.

 Alcohol
▼ Avoid. Alcoholic drinks upset diabetic control.

Surgery and general anesthetics
▼ Surgery may reduce the response to this drug. Notify your physician that you are diabetic before any surgery; insulin treatment may need to be substituted.

POSSIBLE ADVERSE EFFECTS

Serious adverse effects are rare. Faintness, sweating, tremor, weakness, and confusion

may be signs of low blood sugar due to lack of food or too high a dose.

Symptom/effect	Frequency		Discuss with physician		Stop taking drug now	Call physician now
	Common	Rare	Only if severe	In all cases		
Faintness/confusion	●			■		
Weakness/tremor	●			■		
Sweating	●			■		
Nausea/vomiting		●		■		
Heartburn/indigestion		●	■			
Thirst		●		■		
Rash/itching		●		■		

INTERACTIONS

General note A variety of drugs may reduce the effect of chlorpropamide and so raise blood sugar levels. Such drugs include corticosteroids, estrogens, diuretics, rifampin, phenobarbital, anti-psychotic drugs, and phenytoin. Other

drugs increase the risk of low blood sugar. These include dicumarol, sulfonamides, anabolic steroids, aspirin, and ketoconazole.

Beta blockers These mask the signs of low blood sugar.

PROLONGED USE

No problems expected.

Monitoring If the drug is taken for diabetes mellitus, regular monitoring of urine or blood sugar is required.

CHLORTHALIDONE

Brand names Hygroton, Thalitone
Used in the following combined preparations Combipres, Cemi-Regroton, Regroton, Tenoretic

GENERAL INFORMATION

Chlorthalidone, introduced in 1960, belongs to the thiazide group of diuretic drugs (p.127). These drugs remove excess water from the body and reduce edema (fluid retention) in people with congestive heart failure, kidney disorders, cirrhosis of the liver, and premenstrual tension.

Chlorthalidone is frequently used to treat high blood pressure (see Antihypertensive drugs, p.130), and because it reduces the amount of calcium in the urine, it is sometimes used to prevent the recurrence of certain types of kidney stones.

It is longer-acting than many other thiazides. But it increases the loss of potassium and other body salts in the urine, which can cause a variety of symptoms (see p.540), increasing the likelihood of irregular heart rhythms, particularly in those taking drugs such as digoxin for heart failure. For this reason potassium supplements are often prescribed along with chlorthalidone.

QUICK REFERENCE

Drug group Thiazide diuretic (p.127)

Overdose danger rating Low

Dependence rating Low

Prescription needed Yes

Available as generic Yes

INFORMATION FOR USERS

Your drug prescription is tailored for you. Do not alter dosage without checking with your physician.

How taken

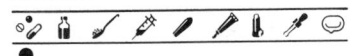

Tablets.

Frequency and timing of doses
Once daily, early in the day, with food.

Adult dosage range
25 – 100mg daily, or three times a week.

Onset of effect
Within 2 hours.

Duration of action
60 hours.

Diet advice
Use of this drug may reduce potassium in the body. Eat plenty of fresh fruit and vegetables. Discuss the advisability of reducing your salt intake with your physician.

Storage
Keep in a closed container in a cool, dry place away from reach of children.

Missed dose
No cause for concern, but take as soon as you remember.

Stopping the drug
Do not stop taking the drug without consulting your physician; symptoms may recur.

Exceeding the dose
An occasional unintentional extra dose is unlikely to be a cause for concern. But if you notice unusual symptoms, or if a large overdose has been taken, notify your physician.

SPECIAL PRECAUTIONS

Be sure to tell your physician if:
▼ You have impaired kidney or liver function.
▼ You have had gout.
▼ You have diabetes.
▼ You have a high level of fat in your blood (hyperlipidemia).
▼ You are taking other medications.

 Pregnancy
▼ Not usually prescribed. No evidence that it harms the baby, but it may cause excessive sodium (salt) loss in the mother.

 Breast feeding
▼ The drug passes into the breast milk, but at normal doses adverse effects on the baby are uncommon. It may reduce your milk supply. Discuss with your physician.

 Infants and children
▼ Not usually prescribed. Reduced dose necessary.

 Over 60
▼ Increased likelihood of adverse effects.

 Driving and hazardous work
▼ No special problems.

 Alcohol
▼ Keep consumption low. Chlorthalidone increases the likelihood of dehydration and hangovers after consumption of alcohol.

POSSIBLE ADVERSE EFFECTS

Most adverse effects are caused by the excessive loss of potassium from the body.

This can usually be put right by taking a potassium supplement.

Symptom/effect	Frequency		Discuss with physician		Stop taking drug now	Call physician now
	Common	Rare	Only if severe	In all cases		
Lethargy		●	■			
Dizziness		●	■			
Rash		●	■			
Digestive disturbance		●	■			
Temporary impotence		●	■			

INTERACTIONS

Non-steroidal anti-inflammatory drugs (NSAIDs) These may reduce the diuretic effect of chlorthalidone. The dosage of chlorthalidone may need to be adjusted accordingly.

Digitalis drugs The effects of such drugs may be increased if excessive amounts of potassium are lost.

Corticosteroids These drugs further increase the loss of potassium from the body when taken with chlorthalidone.

Lithium Chlorthalidone may increase lithium levels in the blood, leading to a risk of serious adverse effects.

PROLONGED USE

Prolonged use of this drug can lead to excessive loss of potassium and imbalances of other salts.

Monitoring Blood tests may be performed periodically to check kidney function and levels of blood sugar, potassium, and other salts.

CHLORZOXAZONE

Brand name Paraflex
Used in the following combined preparations Chlorofon-F, Parafon Forte

GENERAL INFORMATION

Chlorzoxazone acts on nerve cells in the central nervous system to relieve muscle spasm and rigidity; it may also help to relieve pain. Introduced in 1958, it is mainly used to treat symptoms caused by soft tissue injury. Muscle spasm caused by neurological disorders, such as multiple sclerosis, or by injury to the spinal cord is not effectively treated by chlorzoxazone. Treatment usually needs to be accompanied by rest and physical therapy. Chlorzoxazone is also available with acetaminophen in a combination drug when stronger pain relief is needed.

As with other muscle relaxants, there is a risk of liver damage when this drug is taken for long periods.

QUICK REFERENCE

Drug group Muscle-relaxant drug (p.148)

Overdose danger rating Medium

Dependence rating Low

Prescription needed Yes

Available as generic Yes

INFORMATION FOR USERS

Your drug prescription is tailored for you. Do not alter dosage without checking with your physician.

How taken

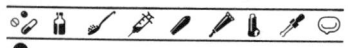

Tablets.

Frequency and timing of doses
3 – 4 x daily.

Adult dosage range
750mg – 3g daily.

Onset of effect
Within 1 hour.

Duration of action
3 – 4 hours.

Diet advice
None.

Storage
Keep in a closed container in a cool, dry place away from reach of children.

Missed dose
Take as soon as you remember. If your next dose is due within 2 hours, take a single dose now and skip the next.

Stopping the drug
If you have been taking the drug for less than 3 weeks, it can be safely stopped as soon as you feel that you no longer need it. However, if you have been taking the drug for longer, consult your physician, who will supervise a gradual reduction in dosage. Stopping abruptly may lead to cramping muscle pains.

Exceeding the dose
An occasional unintentional extra dose is unlikely to cause problems. Large overdoses may cause nausea, vomiting, diarrhea, severe drowsiness, and muscle weakness. Notify your physician.

SPECIAL PRECAUTIONS

Be sure to tell your physician if:
▼ You have impaired liver or kidney function.
▼ You have a history of allergies.
▼ You are taking other medications.

Pregnancy
▼ Not usually prescribed. Safety in pregnancy not established. Discuss with your physician so that you can weigh the benefits of the drug against its possible risks.

Breast feeding
▼ Discuss with your physician. The drug passes into the breast milk, but at normal doses adverse effects on the baby are uncommon.

Infants and children
▼ Not usually prescribed. Reduced dose necessary.

Over 60
▼ Reduced dose may be necessary.

Driving and hazardous work
▼ Avoid such activities until you have learned how the drug affects you, because the drug can cause drowsiness.

Alcohol
▼ Avoid. Alcohol may increase the adverse effects of this drug on the liver.

Surgery and general anesthetics
▼ Be sure to tell your physician or dentist that you are taking chlorzoxazone before you have a general anesthetic.

POSSIBLE ADVERSE EFFECTS

The most common adverse effects of chlorzoxazone are due to the drug's action on the central nervous system. These usually diminish as your body adjusts to the drug, and they disappear when treatment with chlorzoxazone is stopped.

Symptom/effect	Frequency		Discuss with physician		Stop taking drug now	Call physician now
	Common	Rare	Only if severe	In all cases		
Drowsiness	●		■			
Headache	●			■		
Dizziness/lightheadedness		●	■			
Jaundice		●		■		
Discoloration of urine		●		■		
Rash		●		■	▲	

INTERACTIONS

Sedatives All drugs that have a sedative effect on the central nervous system are likely to increase the sedative properties of chlorzoxazone. Such drugs include anti-anxiety and sleeping drugs, antihistamines, antidepressants, narcotic analgesics, and antipsychotic drugs.

PROLONGED USE

There is a risk of damage to the liver when chlorzoxazone is taken over an extended period.

Monitoring Periodic blood tests to check liver function are usually required.

CHOLESTYRAMINE

Brand name Questran
Used in the following combined preparations None

GENERAL INFORMATION

Cholestyramine is a *chelating* agent, attaching itself to bile acids and cholesterol in the intestine before those substances can be absorbed. The action on the bile acids makes bowel movements bulkier, thus creating an antidiarrheal effect. The action on cholesterol helps people with hyperlipidemia (high levels of fat in the blood) who have not responded to a weight-reducing, low-fat diet, or who are at particular risk from heart disease because of diabetes or a family history of death from heart attacks.

If bile salts accumulate in the bloodstream, as sometimes happens in liver disorders such as primary biliary cirrhosis, cholestyramine may be prescribed to deal with the accompanying itching which occurs.

If taken in large doses, cholestyramine often leads to bloating, mild nausea, and constipation. Cholestyramine may also interfere with the body's ability to absorb fat, and certain vitamins dissolved in fat, causing pale, bulky, foul-smelling bowel movements (steatorrhea).

QUICK REFERENCE

Drug group Lipid-lowering drug (p.131)

Overdose danger rating Low

Dependence rating Low

Prescription needed Yes

Available as generic No

INFORMATION FOR USERS

Your drug prescription is tailored for you. Do not alter dosage without checking with your physician.

How taken

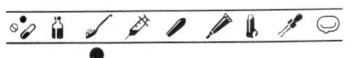

Powder mixed with water, juices, or soft foods.

Frequency and timing of doses
3 – 4 x daily before meals and at bedtime.

Adult dosage range
4g daily (starting dose), increasing to 12 – 32g daily (maintenance dose).

Onset of effect
Some effect is noticed within one week, but full beneficial effects may not be felt for several weeks.

Duration of action
12 – 24 hours.

Diet advice
A low-fat, low-calorie diet may be recommended for those overweight. Use of this drug may deplete levels of certain vitamins. Supplements may be advised.

Storage
Keep in a closed container in a cool, dry place away from reach of children.

Missed dose
Take as soon as you remember.

Stopping the drug
Do not stop taking the drug without consulting your physician.

Exceeding the dose
An occasional unintentional extra dose is unlikely to cause problems. But if you notice unusual symptoms, or if a large overdose has been taken, notify your physician.

SPECIAL PRECAUTIONS

Be sure to tell your physician if:
▼ You suffer from constipation.
▼ You have jaundice.
▼ You have a kidney disorder.
▼ You have a peptic ulcer.
▼ You suffer from hemorrhoids.
▼ You are taking other medications.

 Pregnancy
▼ Not usually prescribed. Safety in pregnancy not established. Discuss with your physician so that you can weigh the benefits of the drug against its possible risks.

 Breast feeding
▼ Discuss with your physician.

 Infants and children
▼ Not recommended for children under 6 years. Reduced dose necessary in older children.

 Over 60
▼ Increased likelihood of adverse effects.

 Driving and hazardous work
▼ No special problems.

 Alcohol
▼ Although this drug does not interact with alcohol, your underlying condition may make it inadvisable to take alcohol.

POSSIBLE ADVERSE EFFECTS

Adverse effects are more likely if large doses are taken by people over 60. Minor side effects such as indigestion and abdominal pain are uncomfortable but rarely a cause for concern. More serious adverse effects are usually the result of vitamin deficiency.

Symptom/effect	Frequency		Discuss with physician		Stop taking drug now	Call physician now
	Common	Rare	Only if severe	In all cases		
Indigestion	●		■			
Abdominal pain	●		■			
Nausea/vomiting	●		■			
Constipation	●				■	
Steatorrhea	●				■	
Loss of weight		●			■	

INTERACTIONS

General note Cholestyramine considerably reduces the body's ability to absorb other drugs. It may be necessary to organize a schedule in consultation with your physician whereby you take other medications at a fixed time before you take cholestyramine. The dosage of other drugs may need to be adjusted.

PROLONGED USE

As this drug reduces vitamin absorption, supplements of vitamins A, D, and K and folic acid may be advised.

Monitoring Periodic blood checks are usually required to monitor the level of cholesterol in the blood.

CICLOPIROX

Brand name Loprox
Used in the following combined preparations None

GENERAL INFORMATION

This antifungal drug, introduced in 1983, is prescribed as a *topical* treatment for fungal and yeast infections of the skin, such as athlete's foot and jock itch. It may also be prescribed to treat the less common skin disease known as tinea versicolor, characterized by fine scales over the skin, usually on the chest. Ciclopirox may also be given to treat Candida (thrush) infections of the vagina or penis.

Ciclopirox has two clear advantages over other topical antifungal preparations. It has a more rapid onset of effect; and its adverse reactions are rare, and tend to be minor.

INFORMATION FOR USERS

Your drug prescription is tailored for you. Do not alter dosage without checking with your physician.

How taken

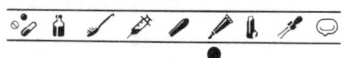

Cream.

Frequency and timing of doses
Skin infections 2 x daily.
Vaginal infection Once daily.

Adult dosage range
Skin infections Sufficient cream to cover the infected and surrounding area at each application.
Vaginal infection One application per dose.

Onset of effect
1 – 2 days.

Duration of action
12 hours.

Diet advice
None.

Storage
Keep in a closed container in a cool, dry place away from reach of children.

Missed dose
No cause for concern, but apply cream as soon as you remember.

Stopping the drug
Take the full course. Even if symptoms disappear, the original infection may still be present and may recur if treatment is stopped too soon.

Exceeding the dose
An occasional unintentional extra application is unlikely to be a cause for concern.

POSSIBLE ADVERSE EFFECTS

Ciclopirox rarely causes adverse effects. It may occasionally cause local irritation, and this may mean that a different antifungal may need to be substituted.

Symptom/effect	Frequency		Discuss with physician		Stop taking drug now	Call physician now
	Common	Rare	Only if severe	In all cases		
Irritation		●		■	▲	
Rash/itching		●		■	▲	■

INTERACTIONS

None.

SPECIAL PRECAUTIONS

Be sure to tell your physician if:
▼ You are taking other medications.

Pregnancy
▼ No evidence of risk to developing baby.

Breast feeding
▼ No evidence of risk.

Infants and children
▼ Safety for children under 10 years not established.

Over 60
▼ No special problems.

Driving and hazardous work
▼ No known problems.

Alcohol
▼ No known problems.

PROLONGED USE

No problems expected.

CIMETIDINE

Brand names Tagamet
Used in the following combined preparations None

GENERAL INFORMATION

Introduced in 1976, cimetidine reduces the secretion of gastric acid and of pepsin, an enzyme which helps the digestion of protein. By reducing levels of acid and pepsin, it promotes healing of ulcers in the stomach and duodenum (see p.137). Cimetidine is also used in reflux esophagitis, a tendency to burp acid stomach contents partway up the esophagus. Treatment is usually given in courses of four to eight weeks, with further short courses if symptoms recur.

Cimetidine also affects the actions of certain enzymes in the liver, where many drugs are broken down. It is therefore prescribed with caution if you are receiving drugs, particularly anti-coagulants and anticonvulsants, whose levels need to be carefully controlled. As cimetidine promotes healing of the stomach lining, it may mask the symptoms of stomach cancer, delaying diagnosis. It is usually prescribed only when this disease has been ruled out.

INFORMATION FOR USERS

Your prescription is tailored for you. Do not alter dosage without checking with your physician.

How taken

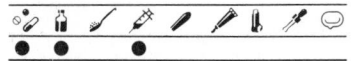

Tablets, liquid, injection.

Frequency and timing of doses
4 x daily (after meals and at bedtime).

Adult dosage range
800 – 1200mg daily.

Onset of effect
Within 90 minutes.

Duration of action
2 – 3 hours.

Diet advice
None.

Storage
Keep in a closed container in a cool, dry place away from reach of children.

Missed dose
Do not take the missed dose. Take your next dose as usual.

Stopping the drug
Do not stop taking the drug without consulting your physician; symptoms may recur.

Exceeding the dose
An occasional unintentional extra dose is unlikely to be a cause for concern. But if you notice unusual symptoms, or if a large overdose has been taken, notify your physician.

SPECIAL PRECAUTIONS

Be sure to tell your physician if:
▼ You have impaired kidney or liver function.
▼ You have arthritis.
▼ You are taking other medications.

Pregnancy
▼ Not usually prescribed. Discuss with your physician so that you can weigh the benefits of the drug against its possible risks.

Breast feeding
▼ Discuss with your physician. The drug passes into the breast milk and may affect the baby adversely.

Infants and children
▼ Not usually prescribed. Reduced dose necessary.

Over 60
▼ Reduced dose may be necessary. Increased risk of confusion.

Driving and hazardous work
▼ Avoid such activities until you have learned how the drug affects you, because the drug may cause dizziness and confusion.

Alcohol
▼ Avoid. Alcohol may aggravate the underlying condition and counter the beneficial effects of cimetidine.

POSSIBLE ADVERSE EFFECTS

Adverse effects of cimetidine are uncommon. They are usually related to dosage level and almost always disappear when the drug is stopped.

Symptom/effect	Frequency		Discuss with physician		Stop taking drug now	Call physician now
	Common	Rare	Only if severe	In all cases		
Diarrhea		●		■		
Dizziness/unsteadiness		●		■		
Muscle pain		●		■		
Breast enlargement (men)		●		■		
Impotence		●		■		
Rash		●		■		

INTERACTIONS

Antacids These may reduce absorption of cimetidine. If you need to take antacids for additional relief of pain, they should be taken at least 1 hour after cimetidine.

Benzodiazepine drugs Cimetidine may cause an increase in blood levels of some of these drugs, leading to an increased risk of adverse effects.

Anticoagulant drugs Cimetidine may increase the effect of these drugs. The dosage of anticoagulants may need to be reduced.

Anticonvulsant drugs Cimetidine may increase the blood levels of such drugs, and the dose may need to be reduced.

PROLONGED USE

Courses of longer than 6 months are not usually necessary. Continuous use of the drug for longer than 1 year is not recommended except in exceptional circumstances, because the safety of this drug for prolonged use has not yet been confirmed.

CISPLATIN

Brand names Platinol
Used in the following combined preparations None

GENERAL INFORMATION

Introduced in 1979, cisplatin is one of the most effective drugs available to treat cancers of the ovaries and testicles. People with cancer of the face, neck, bladder, cervix, and lung have also responded well to cisplatin. And recent research indicates this drug may be an effective treatment against bone cancer in children. Cisplatin is often given along with other anticancer drugs.

The most common and serious adverse effect of cisplatin is impaired kidney function.

To reduce the risk of permanent kidney damage, the drug is usually given only once every four weeks, allowing the kidneys time to recover between courses of treatment. Nausea and vomiting may occur shortly after administration of cisplatin. Because the symptoms may be quite severe, an anti-emetic drug is often given to reduce them.

Damage to hearing is common, and may be more severe in children. Use of this drug may also increase the risk of anemia, disorders of blood clotting, and infection during treatment.

QUICK REFERENCE

Drug group Anticancer drug (p.182)
Overdose danger rating Medium
Dependence rating Low
Prescription needed Yes
Available as generic No

INFORMATION FOR USERS

This drug is given only under medical supervision and is not for self-administration.

How taken

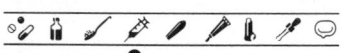

Injection.

Frequency and timing of doses
Once every 4 weeks (on its own); once daily for 5 days every 3 weeks (in combination with other anticancer drugs).

Adult dosage range
Dosage is determined individually according to body height, weight, and response.

Onset of effect
Some adverse effects, such as nausea and vomiting, may appear within hours of starting treatment.

Duration of action
Some adverse effects may last for up to 1 week after treatment has stopped.

Diet advice
It is necessary to drink plenty of water during the 24 hours following treatment to reduce the risk of kidney damage.

Storage
Keep in a closed container in a cool, dry place away from reach of children.

Missed dose
Not applicable. The drug is given only in the hospital under medical supervision.

Stopping the drug
Not applicable. The drug will be stopped under medical supervision.

Exceeding the dose
Overdosage is unlikely, since treatment is carefully monitored.

SPECIAL PRECAUTIONS

Cisplatin is prescribed only under close medical supervision, taking account of your present condition and medical history.

Pregnancy
▼ Not usually prescribed. Cisplatin may cause birth defects or premature birth. Discuss with your physician so that you can weigh the benefits of the drug against its risks.

Breast feeding
▼ Discontinue breast feeding. The drug passes into the breast milk and may affect the baby adversely.

Infants and children
▼ Not usually prescribed. The risk of hearing loss is increased.

Over 60
▼ Reduced dose may be necessary. Increased likelihood of adverse effects.

Driving and hazardous work
▼ No known problems.

Alcohol
▼ No known problems.

POSSIBLE ADVERSE EFFECTS

Most adverse effects appear within a few hours of injection and are carefully monitored in the hospital after each dose.

Some effects wear off within 24 hours. Nausea and loss of appetite may last for up to a week.

Symptom/effect	Frequency		Discuss with physician		Stop taking drug now	Call physician now
	Common	Rare	Only if severe	In all cases		
Nausea/vomiting	●		■			
Loss of appetite/taste	●		■			
Ringing in the ears	●			■		
Breathing difficulties		●		■		▮
Seizures		●		■		▮
Wheezing		●		■		▮
Rash		●		■		▮

INTERACTIONS

General note A number of drugs increase the adverse effects of cisplatin. Because cisplatin is given only under close medical supervision, these interactions are carefully monitored and the dosage is adjusted accordingly.

PROLONGED USE

Prolonged use of this drug increases the risk of damage to the kidneys, nerves, bone marrow, and to hearing.

Monitoring Hearing tests and blood checks to monitor kidney function and bone marrow activity are carried out regularly.

CLINDAMYCIN

Brand names Cleocin Phosphate, Cleocin T
Used in the following combined preparations None

GENERAL INFORMATION

Clindamycin, introduced in 1970, is a powerful antibiotic that can be taken by mouth and is absorbed into the bloodstream in high concentrations. It is used in the treatment of serious infections, particularly those that commonly involve penicillin-resistant bacteria. These include gynecological and pelvic infections in women, peritonitis, serious lung infections, and skin infections, such as abscesses and infected bedsores.

Since clindamycin penetrates bone and joints well, it is also prescribed for bone and joint infections, including osteomyelitis and septic arthritis. Occasionally, it may be given to prevent infection in those undergoing bowel or urinary tract surgery. As a skin preparation, it is used in the treatment of acne.

Although clindamycin can be safely used in most people, it may occasionally cause a potentially fatal disorder called pseudomembranous colitis. This disorder is caused by an overgrowth of clindamycin-resistant bacteria in the bowel, leading to severe bloody diarrhea with cramping abdominal pain and fever.

QUICK REFERENCE

Drug group Lincosamide antibiotic (p.158)

Overdose danger rating Low

Dependence rating Low

Prescription needed Yes

Available as generic No

INFORMATION FOR USERS

Your drug prescription is tailored for you. Do not alter dosage without checking with your physician.

How taken

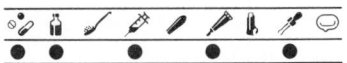

Capsules, liquid, injection, ointment, eye drops.

Frequency and timing of doses
By mouth 3 – 4 x daily with food or water.
Injection 2 – 4 x daily or continuously by infusion.
Topical 2 x daily morning and evening.

Dosage range
Adults 600 – 1800mg daily (by mouth); 15 – 40mg daily (eye drops).
Children Reduced dose according to age and weight.

Onset of effect
2 – 3 days.

Duration of action
8 – 12 hours.

Diet advice
None.

Storage
Keep in a closed container in a cool, dry place away from reach of children.

Missed dose
Take as soon as you remember. If your next dose is due within 2 hours, take a single dose now and skip the next.

Stopping the drug
Take the full course. Even if you feel better the original infection may still be present and may recur if treatment is stopped too soon.

Exceeding the dose
An occasional unintentional extra dose is unlikely to be a cause for concern. But if you notice unusual symptoms, or if a large overdose has been taken, notify your physician.

SPECIAL PRECAUTIONS

Be sure to tell your physician if:
▼ You have impaired liver or kidney function.
▼ You have myasthenia gravis.
▼ You have had a bowel disorder.
▼ You are taking other medications.

Pregnancy
▼ Not usually prescribed. Safety in pregnancy not established. Discuss with your physician so that you can weigh the benefits of the drug against its possible risks.

Breast feeding
▼ The drug passes into the breast milk, but at normal doses adverse effects on the baby are uncommon. Discuss with your physician.

Infants and children
▼ Reduced dose necessary.

Over 60
▼ Reduced dose may be necessary. Increased likelihood of adverse effects.

Driving and hazardous work
▼ No known problems.

Alcohol
▼ No known problems.

POSSIBLE ADVERSE EFFECTS

Adverse effects are rare with clindamycin eye and skin preparations. The most common side effect of clindamycin is mild diarrhea. More severe diarrhea, especially if bloodstained or accompanied by abdominal pain or fever, may be a sign of pseudomembranous colitis and requires immediate medical attention.

Symptom/effect	Frequency		Discuss with physician		Stop taking drug now	Call physician now
	Common	Rare	Only if severe	In all cases		
Diarrhea	●		■			
Nausea/vomiting		●	■			
Rash/itching		●		■	▲	
Fever		●		■		▮
Abdominal cramps		●		■	▲	▮
Blood/mucus in stools		●		■	▲	▮

INTERACTIONS

Drugs for myasthenia gravis Clindamycin may oppose the beneficial effects of these drugs on myasthenia gravis.

PROLONGED USE

No special problems.

CLOFIBRATE

Brand name Atromid-S
Used in the following combined preparations None

GENERAL INFORMATION

Clofibrate, a lipid-lowering drug, reduces the level of triglyceride (a type of fat) in the blood. Hyperlipidemia (raised levels of fat in the blood) is associated with atherosclerosis (fat deposits in arterial walls), which causes coronary heart disease (e.g., angina) and cerebro-vascular disease (e.g., stroke).

Monitored by regular checks of blood fat levels, clofibrate is usually prescribed only when a low-fat diet has failed to reduce levels of fat in the blood. The drug usually succeeds in reducing hyperlipidemia, but there is no evidence yet that clofibrate reduces the risk of death from disorders of the blood fats. Clofibrate can also be used to treat diabetes insipidus, a disorder that causes excessive loss of water from the kidneys.

Common side effects include gastrointestinal upset, such as nausea, vomiting, and indigestion, which usually settles down during continuing treatment. Weight gain and drowsiness are other possible side effects. Clofibrate is also thought to increase susceptibility to gallstones.

QUICK REFERENCE

Drug group Lipid-lowering drug (p.131)

Overdose danger rating Medium

Dependence rating Low

Prescription needed Yes

Available as generic No

INFORMATION FOR USERS

Your drug prescription is tailored for you. Do not alter dosage without checking with your physician.

How taken

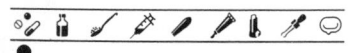

Capsules.

Frequency and timing of doses
3 – 4 x daily after meals.

Adult dosage range
1 – 2g daily.

Onset of effect
1 – 4 hours. Full beneficial effect may not be produced for months or years.

Duration of action
About 6 – 12 hours. This may vary according to the individual.

Diet advice
A low-fat diet is recommended.

Storage
Keep in a closed container in a cool, dry place away from reach of children.

Missed dose
Take as soon as you remember. If your next dose is due within 2 hours, take a single dose now and skip the next.

Stopping the drug
Do not stop the drug without consulting your physician; stopping the drug may lead to a rise in levels of fat in the blood.

Exceeding the dose
An occasional unintentional extra dose is unlikely to cause problems. Large overdoses may cause nausea or indigestion. Notify your physician.

POSSIBLE ADVERSE EFFECTS

Nausea is the most common adverse effect of clofibrate. It is usually temporary and disappears with long-term use. Drowsiness and weight gain may also occur, but are usually no cause for concern unless the symptoms are severe.

Symptom/effect	Frequency		Discuss with physician		Stop taking drug now	Call physician now
	Common	Rare	Only if severe	In all cases		
Nausea/vomiting	●		■			
Rash	●			■	▲	
Drowsiness		●	■			
Weight gain		●	■			
Flu-like illness with pains		●	■			
Bald spots		●		■		
Sore throat		●		■		▮

INTERACTIONS

Oral anticoagulant drugs The effect of these drugs may be increased by clofibrate.

Phenytoin Clofibrate may increase the effects of this drug.

Tolbutamide Clofibrate may interact with this drug to lower blood sugar levels.

Blood tests for coronary thrombosis Clofibrate can cause false positive results.

SPECIAL PRECAUTIONS

Be sure to tell your physician if:
▼ You have impaired kidney or liver function.
▼ You have gallstones.
▼ You have had a heart attack.
▼ You have had peptic ulcers.
▼ You have diabetes insipidus.
▼ You are taking other medications.

Pregnancy
▼ Not usually prescribed. May adversely affect the developing baby. Discuss with your physician so that you may weigh the benefits of the drug against its risks.

Breast feeding
▼ The drug passes into the breast milk, but at normal doses adverse effects on the baby are uncommon. Discuss with your physician.

Infants and children
▼ Not usually prescribed.

Over 60
▼ No special problems.

Driving and hazardous work
▼ No special problems.

Alcohol
▼ Avoid. Alcohol may reduce the effect of this drug.

PROLONGED USE

Gallstones are more common in people on extended clofibrate treatment.

Monitoring Regular tests of blood fat levels and liver and muscle enzymes may be advisable.

CLOMIPHENE

Brand names Clomid, Serophene
Used in the following combined preparations None

GENERAL INFORMATION

Clomiphene, introduced in 1967, increases the output of hormones by the pituitary gland, stimulating ovulation in women (release of egg) and the production of sperm in men. It is also used to test pituitary function in both sexes. If hormone levels in the blood fail to rise after the drug is taken, the gland is not working as it should.

For female infertility, tablets are taken for five consecutive days each month in the middle of the menstrual cycle. This stimulates ovulation. If clomiphene fails to stimulate ovulation after several months, other drugs may be prescribed.

When used in the treatment of infertility in a man, clomiphene is given daily for six to twelve months or until his partner becomes pregnant.

Multiple pregnancies (usually twins) are common in women treated with clomiphene. Adverse effects include an increased risk of ovarian cysts. In rare cases, the ovaries become greatly enlarged, leading to abdominal pain and swelling. Breast enlargement may occur occasionally in men.

QUICK REFERENCE

Drug group Drug for infertility (p.192)

Overdose danger rating Low

Dependence rating Low

Prescription needed Yes

Available as generic No

INFORMATION FOR USERS

Your drug prescription is tailored for you. Do not alter dosage without checking with your physician.

How taken

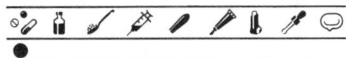

Tablets.

Frequency and timing of doses
Once daily for 5 days during each menstrual cycle (women); once daily on a continuous basis (men).

Dosage range
Women 50mg daily initially; dose may be increased up to 200mg daily.
Men 25mg daily initially; dose may be increased up to 50mg daily.

Onset of effect
In women, ovulation occurs 4 – 10 days after the last dose in any cycle. However, it may be several months before this occurs. In men an improvement in sperm count may occur in 3 – 6 months.

Duration of action
5 days.

Diet advice
None.

Storage
Keep in a closed container in a cool, dry place away from reach of children. Protect from light.

Missed dose
Take as soon as you remember. If your next dose is due at this time, take the missed dose and the next scheduled dose together.

Stopping the drug
Take as directed by your physician. Stopping the drug will reduce the chance of conception.

Exceeding the dose
An occasional unintentional extra dose is unlikely to be a cause for concern. But if you notice unusual symptoms, or if a large overdose has been taken, notify your physician.

SPECIAL PRECAUTIONS

Be sure to tell your physician if:
▼ You have impaired liver function.
▼ You are taking other medications.

Pregnancy
▼ Not prescribed. The drug is stopped as soon as pregnancy occurs.

Breast feeding
▼ Not prescribed.

Infants and children
▼ Not prescribed.

Over 60
▼ Not usually required.

Driving and hazardous work
▼ Avoid such activities until you have learned how the drug affects you, because the drug may cause blurred vision.

Alcohol
▼ Keep consumption low. Alcohol does not interact directly with clomiphene but taken in excess may reduce the chance of conception.

POSSIBLE ADVERSE EFFECTS

In women, abdominal pain and swelling, due to enlargement of the ovaries or the formation of cysts, are fairly common. In rare cases, massive enlargement of the ovaries may occur about a week after ovulation, but usually disappears over several weeks.

Symptom/effect	Frequency		Discuss with physician		Stop taking drug now	Call physician now
	Common	Rare	Only if severe	In all cases		
Hot flashes	●		■			
Abdominal pain/swelling	●			■		
Breast enlargement (men)		●	■			
Breast tenderness		●		■		
Impaired vision		●		■		
Dry skin/hair loss/rash		●		■		
Jaundice		●		■	▲	▮

PROLONGED USE

Prolonged use may cause visual impairment.

Monitoring Eye tests may be recommended if clomiphene is given for more than a year. Monitoring of body temperature and blood or urine hormone levels during each treatment cycle are performed to detect the first signs of pregnancy in women.

INTERACTIONS

None.

CLONAZEPAM

Brand name Klonopin
Used in the following combined preparations None

GENERAL INFORMATION

Clonazepam, introduced in 1975, belongs to a group of drugs known as the benzodiazepines, which are mainly used in the treatment of anxiety and insomnia (see p.111). Clonazepam, however, is almost exclusively used as an anticonvulsant to prevent and treat epileptic seizures. It is particularly useful for the prevention of brief muscle spasms and absence seizures (petit mal) in children, but other forms of epilepsy, such as sudden flaccidity or seizures induced by bright lights, also respond to clonazepam treatment. Being a benzodiazepine, it also has tranquilizing and sedative effects.

Clonazepam is used either on its own or along with other anticonvulsant drugs. Its anticonvulsant effect may begin to wear off after a few months.

INFORMATION FOR USERS

Your drug prescription is tailored for you. Do not alter dosage without checking with your physician.

How taken

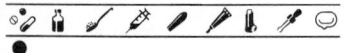

Tablets.

Frequency and timing of doses
1 – 3 x daily with food or milk.

Dosage range
Adults 1.5 – 20mg daily.
Children Reduced dose according to age and weight.

Onset of action
Within 30 minutes.

Duration of action
Approximately 30 hours.

Diet advice
None.

Storage
Keep in a closed container in a cool, dry place away from reach of children.

Missed dose
No cause for concern, but take as soon as you remember. If your next dose is due within 2 hours, take both doses now.

Stopping the drug
Do not stop the drug without consulting your physician; symptoms may recur.

Exceeding the dose
An occasional unintentional extra dose is unlikely to cause problems. Larger overdoses may cause unusual drowsiness. Notify your physician.

POSSIBLE ADVERSE EFFECTS

The principal adverse effects of this drug are related to its sedative and tranquilizing properties. These effects normally diminish after the first few days of treatment and can often be reduced by medically supervised adjustment of dosage.

Symptom/effect	Frequency		Discuss with physician		Stop taking drug now	Call physician now
	Common	Rare	Only if severe	In all cases		
Daytime drowsiness	●		■			
Dizziness/unsteadiness	●		■			
Increased salivation	●		■			
Altered behavior	●			■		
Forgetfulness/confusion		●		■		
Headache		●		■		
Rash		●		■	▲	

INTERACTIONS

Other anticonvulsants Clonazepam may alter the effects of other anticonvulsants you are taking, and adjustment of dosage or change of drug may be necessary. Use of clonazepam and valproic acid may produce absence seizures.

Sedatives All drugs that have a sedative effect on the central nervous system are likely to increase the sedative properties of clonazepam. Such drugs include anti-anxiety and sleeping drugs, antihistamines, antidepressants, narcotic analgesics, and antipsychotics.

SPECIAL PRECAUTIONS

Be sure to tell your physician if:
▼ You have severe respiratory disease.
▼ You have impaired kidney or liver function.
▼ You have had glaucoma.
▼ You have had problems with alcohol or drug abuse.
▼ You are taking other medications.

Pregnancy
▼ Not usually prescribed. Safety in pregnancy not established. Discuss with your physician so that you can weigh the benefits of the drug against its possible risks.

Breast feeding
▼ Discuss with your physician. The drug passes into the breast milk and may affect the baby adversely.

Infants and children
▼ Reduced dose necessary.

Over 60
▼ Reduced dose may be necessary.

Driving and hazardous work
▼ Your underlying condition as well as the possibility of drowsiness while taking this drug may make such activities inadvisable. Discuss with your physician.

Alcohol
▼ Avoid. Alcohol may increase the sedative effects of this drug.

PROLONGED USE

Both beneficial and adverse effects of clonazepam may become less marked during prolonged treatment as the body adapts.

CLONIDINE

Brand names Catapres, Catapres-TTS
Used in the following combined preparation Combipres

GENERAL INFORMATION

Clonidine, a member of a group of drugs known as antihypertensives, is used to treat high blood pressure. By reducing the stimulatory nerve impulses from the brain to the heart and circulatory system, clonidine lowers the blood pressure to a safe level. It is sometimes prescribed together with a diuretic to treat all degrees of high blood pressure.

Clonidine has also been given with variable effectiveness for other conditions such as hot flashes during the menopause and withdrawal symptoms during drug detoxification. Its main drawback is that when used in the doses required to control blood pressure, there may be a severe rise in blood pressure if doses are missed or if the drug is stopped suddenly.

QUICK REFERENCE

Drug group Antihypertensive drug (p.130).

Overdose danger rating Medium

Dependence rating Low

Prescription needed Yes

Available as generic Yes

INFORMATION FOR USERS

Your drug prescription is tailored for you. Do not alter dosage without checking with your physician.

How taken

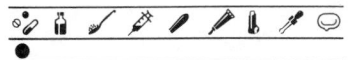

Tablets.

Frequency and timing of doses
2 – 3 x daily.

Adult dosage range
High blood pressure 0.2mg – 0.8mg daily. Doses of up to 2.4mg daily have been used in some resistant cases.

Onset of effect
2 – 5 hours.

Duration of action
6 – 20 hours.

Diet advice
None.

Storage
Keep in a closed container in a cool, dry place away from reach of children.

Missed dose
Take as soon as you remember, then resume your normal schedule. Discuss with your physician if you miss two or more doses.

Stopping the drug
Do not stop the drug without consulting your physician, who will supervise a gradual reduction in dosage. Abrupt withdrawal in people taking over 1.2mg daily may cause a dangerous rise in blood pressure.

Exceeding the dose
An occasional unintentional extra dose is unlikely to cause problems. You may experience vomiting or drowsiness. Notify your physician.

SPECIAL PRECAUTIONS

Be sure to tell your physician if:
▼ You have impaired kidney or liver function.
▼ You have poor circulation.
▼ You have coronary artery disease.
▼ You are taking other medications.

Pregnancy
▼ Not usually prescribed. Safety in pregnancy not established.

Breast feeding
▼ Discuss with your physician. The drug passes into the breast milk.

Infants and children
▼ Not recommended.

Over 60
▼ No special problems.

Driving and hazardous work
▼ Avoid such activities until you have learned how the drug affects you, because the drug can cause drowsiness.

Alcohol
▼ Avoid. Alcohol may increase the sedative effects of this drug.

POSSIBLE ADVERSE EFFECTS

Clonidine may cause drowsiness, dry mouth, and constipation. These effects usually decrease after long-term therapy. An adjustment in dosage may help.

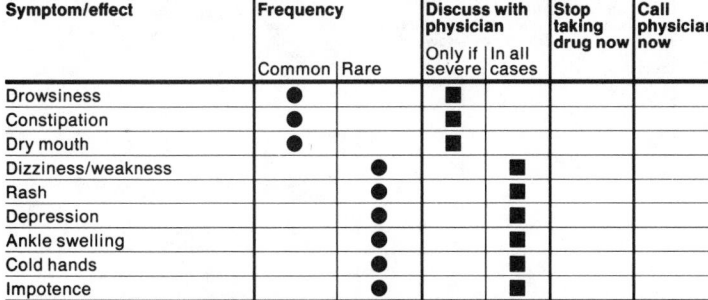

Symptom/effect	Frequency		Discuss with physician		Stop taking drug now	Call physician now
	Common	Rare	Only if severe	In all cases		
Drowsiness	●		■			
Constipation	●		■			
Dry mouth	●		■			
Dizziness/weakness		●		■		
Rash		●		■		
Depression		●		■		
Ankle swelling		●		■		
Cold hands		●		■		
Impotence		●		■		

PROLONGED USE

The more common adverse effects, such as drowsiness, constipation, and dry mouth, may decrease with long-term use.

INTERACTIONS

Tricyclic antidepressant drugs May reduce the effect of clonidine.

Sedatives Clonidine increases the effect of these drugs.

Beta blockers May interact with clonidine to produce a rise in blood pressure.

CLORAZEPATE

Brand name Tranxene
Used in the following combined preparations None

GENERAL INFORMATION

Introduced in 1972, clorazepate is a member of the group of drugs known as the benzodiazepines. These drugs help relieve nervousness and tension, relax muscles, and encourage sleep. The actions and adverse effects of this group of drugs are described more fully on p.111.

Clorazepate is principally used in the treatment of anxiety and anxiety-related insomnia. It is also prescribed in the treatment of alcohol withdrawal and for the relief of epileptic seizures.

Clorazepate can be habit-forming if taken regularly over a long period. Its effects may also diminish with time. Changing medications or tapering off clorazepate for a while may restore desired effects. Treatment with clorazepate is usually reviewed frequently.

INFORMATION FOR USERS

Your drug prescription is tailored for you. Do not alter dosage without checking with your physician.

How taken

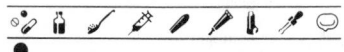

Tablets, capsules.

Frequency and timing of doses
1 – 4 x daily with food or milk.

Adult dosage range
7.5 – 60mg daily.

Onset of action
Within 2 hours.

Duration of action
Up to 24 hours. Some effect may last up to 4 days.

Diet advice
None.

Storage
Keep in a closed container in a cool, dry place away from reach of children.

Missed dose
No cause for concern, but take when you next feel you need the drug. If your next dose is due within 2 hours, take a single dose now and skip the next.

Stopping the drug
If you have been taking the drug continuously for less than 2 weeks, it can be safely stopped as soon as you feel you no longer need it. However, if you have been taking it for longer, consult your physician, who will supervise a gradual reduction in dosage. Stopping abruptly may lead to withdrawal symptoms (see p.111).

Exceeding the dose
An occasional unintentional extra dose is unlikely to cause problems. Larger overdoses may cause unusual drowsiness. Notify your physician.

SPECIAL PRECAUTIONS

Be sure to tell your physician if:
▼ You have severe respiratory disease.
▼ You have impaired kidney or liver function.
▼ You have had problems with alcohol or drug abuse.
▼ You have glaucoma.
▼ You are taking other medications.

Pregnancy
▼ Not usually prescribed. Safety in pregnancy not established. Discuss with your physician so that you can weigh the benefits of the drug against its possible risks.

Breast feeding
▼ Discuss with your physician. The drug passes into the breast milk. Its effects on the baby are not clearly known.

Infants and children
▼ Not usually prescribed. Reduced dose necessary.

Over 60
▼ Reduced dose may be necessary. Increased likelihood of adverse effects.

Driving and hazardous work
▼ Avoid such activities until you have learned how the drug affects you, because the drug can cause reduced alertness and slowed reactions.

Alcohol
▼ Avoid. Alcohol may increase the sedative effects of this drug.

POSSIBLE ADVERSE EFFECTS

The principal adverse effects of this drug are related to its sedative properties. These effects, including drowsiness and dizziness, normally diminish after the first few days and, if troublesome, can often be reduced by adjustment of dosage.

Symptom/effect	Frequency		Discuss with physician		Stop taking drug now	Call physician now
	Common	Rare	Only if severe	In all cases		
Daytime drowsiness	●		■			
Dizziness/unsteadiness	●			■		
Headache		●	■			
Blurred vision		●		■		
Forgetfulness/confusion		●		■		
Rash		●		■		▲

INTERACTIONS

Sedatives All drugs that have a sedative effect on the central nervous system, including alcohol, are likely to increase the sedative properties of clorazepate.

Cimetidine Breakdown of clorazepate in the liver may be inhibited by cimetidine. This can cause a buildup of clorazepate levels in the blood, which increases the likelihood of adverse effects.

PROLONGED USE

Regular use of this drug over several weeks can lead to a reduction in its effect as the body adapts. It may also be habit-forming when taken for extended periods. Severe withdrawal reactions have occurred.

CLOTRIMAZOLE

Brand names Gyne-Lotrimin, Lotrimin, Mycelex, Mycelex-G
Used in the following combined preparations None

GENERAL INFORMATION

Clotrimazole is prescribed for yeast and fungal infections. It is effective for treating tinea (ringworm) infections of the skin, and candida (thrush) infections of the mouth, vagina, or penis. Available since 1976, the drug is given in the form of cream, lozenges, or vaginal suppositories.

Adverse effects from clotrimazole are very rare, although some people may experience burning and irritation on the skin surface where the cream has been applied. Inadvertently swallowing instead of sucking the lozenges may lead to nausea and occasionally to diarrhea.

QUICK REFERENCE

Drug group Antifungal drug (p.166)
Overdose danger rating Low
Dependence rating Low
Prescription needed Yes
Available as generic Yes

INFORMATION FOR USERS

Your drug prescription is tailored for you. Do not alter dosage without checking with your physician.

How taken

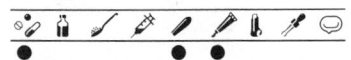

Lozenges, vaginal suppositories, cream.

Frequency and timing of doses
Skin infections 2 x daily (cream).
Vaginal infections Once daily at bedtime (cream or vaginal suppository).
Mouth infections 5 x daily (lozenges).
The drug usually needs to be taken for 2 – 3 weeks in all cases.

Adult dosage range
Skin infections Sufficient cream to cover the infected and surrounding area at each application.
Vaginal thrush 100 – 500mg per dose (vaginal suppository); 1 applicatorful per dose (vaginal cream).
Mouth infections 10mg per dose (lozenges).

Onset of effect
Within 3 – 7 days.

Duration of action
Up to 12 hours.

Diet advice
None.

Storage
Keep in a closed container in a cool, dry place away from reach of children.

Missed dose
No cause for concern, but make up the missed dose or application as soon as you remember.

Stopping the drug
Take the full course. Even if symptoms disappear, the original infection may still be present and symptoms may recur if treatment is stopped too soon.

Exceeding the dose
An occasional unintentional extra dose is unlikely to be a cause for concern. But if you notice unusual symptoms or if a large overdose has been taken, notify your physician.

SPECIAL PRECAUTIONS

Be sure to tell your physician if:
▼ You have impaired liver function.

Pregnancy
▼ No evidence of risk to developing baby.

Breast feeding
▼ No evidence of risk.

Infants and children
▼ Lozenges not recommended for children under 3 years.

Over 60
▼ No special problems.

Driving and hazardous work
▼ No known problems.

Alcohol
▼ No known problems.

POSSIBLE ADVERSE EFFECTS

Clotrimazole rarely causes adverse effects. Skin creams and vaginal applications may occasionally cause localized burning and irritation. Lozenges containing clotrimazole may cause nausea or diarrhea but these symptoms are rarely severe.

Symptom/effect	Frequency		Discuss with physician		Stop taking drug now	Call physician now
	Common	Rare	Only if severe	In all cases		
Nausea/vomiting		●	■			
Diarrhea		●	■			
Local burning or stinging		●	■			
Skin irritation		●	■			

INTERACTIONS

None.

PROLONGED USE

No problems expected.

CLOXACILLIN

Brand names Cloxapen, Tegopen
Used in the following combined preparations None

GENERAL INFORMATION

Cloxacillin, a penicillin antibiotic first available in 1962, is prescribed to treat staphylococcal infections. These are usually resistant to treatment with other forms of penicillin because the bacteria produce an enzyme that breaks down the antibiotic. Cloxacillin, however, is not affected by the enzyme. Common sites where staphylococcal infection may occur include the skin and soft tissues.

For maximum effect, cloxacillin needs to be taken on an empty stomach, because food interferes with absorption of the drug from the digestive tract.

Diarrhea is the most common side effect. As with other penicillin antibiotics, there is a risk of an allergic reaction – rash and possibly fever, itching, swelling of the mouth and tongue, and breathing difficulty.

QUICK REFERENCE

Drug group Penicillin antibiotic (p.156)

Overdose danger rating Low

Dependence rating Low

Prescription needed Yes

Available as generic Yes

INFORMATION FOR USERS

Your drug prescription is tailored for you. Do not alter dosage without checking with your physician.

How taken

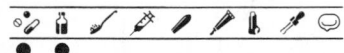

Capsules, liquid.

Frequency and timing of doses
4 x daily at least 1 hour before, or 2 hours after eating.

Dosage range
Adults 1 – 4g daily.
Children Reduced dose according to age and weight.

Onset of effect
1 – 2 hours.

Duration of action
Up to 6 hours.

Diet advice
None.

Storage
Keep in a closed container in a cool, dry place away from reach of children.

Missed dose
Take as soon as you remember. If your next dose is due at this time, take both doses now.

Stopping the drug
Take the full course. Even if you feel better, the original infection may still be present and symptoms may recur if treatment is stopped too soon.

Exceeding the dose
An occasional unintentional extra dose is unlikely to be a cause for concern. But if you notice unusual symptoms, or if a large overdose has been taken, notify your physician.

POSSIBLE ADVERSE EFFECTS

If you develop a rash, wheezing, itching, fever, or joint swelling, this may indicate an allergy to cloxacillin, making it necessary to take a different antibiotic.

Symptom/effect	Frequency		Discuss with physician		Stop taking drug now	Call physician now
	Common	Rare	Only if severe	In all cases		
Rash	●			■	▲	
Nausea/vomiting		●	■			
Unusual thirst		●	■			
Tiredness/weakness		●	■			
Diarrhea		●		■		
Wheezing/breathlessness		●		■	▲	∎
Itching		●		■	▲	∎
Swollen mouth/tongue		●		■	▲	∎

INTERACTIONS

Oral contraceptives Cloxacillin may slightly reduce the effectiveness of the contraceptive pill and also increase the risk of breakthrough bleeding. Discuss with your physician.

SPECIAL PRECAUTIONS

Be sure to tell your physician if:
▼ You have an allergy (for example, asthma, hay fever, eczema, or hives).
▼ You have ulcerative colitis.
▼ You have had a rash after taking a penicillin or cephalosporin antibiotic.
▼ You are taking other medications.

Pregnancy
▼ No evidence of risk to developing baby.

Breast feeding
▼ Discuss with your physician. The drug passes into the breast milk and may affect the baby adversely.

Infants and children
▼ No evidence of risk to baby.

Over 60
▼ Reduced dose necessary.

Driving and hazardous work
▼ No known problems.

Alcohol
▼ No known problems.

PROLONGED USE

Cloxacillin is usually given only for short courses of treatment.

CODEINE

Used in the following combined preparations Empirin with codeine, Phenaphen with codeine, Phenergan with codeine, Tussi-Organdin, Tylenol with codeine

GENERAL INFORMATION

In common medical use since the beginning of the century, codeine is a narcotic analgesic, partly synthesized but still – like all opiates – ultimately derived from the seeds of a particular poppy plant.

It is primarily used to relieve mild to moderate pain, often in combination with a non-narcotic analgesic, but it is an effective cough suppressant too. It is an ingredient in many prescription cold medicines and cough syrups. Like other narcotic drugs, codeine is constipating, a characteristic that makes it sometimes useful in the short-term control of diarrhea.

Codeine is habit-forming, but addiction seldom occurs if the drug is used for a limited period of time and the recommended dosage is followed.

INFORMATION FOR USERS

Your drug prescription is tailored for you. Do not alter dosage without checking with your physician.

How taken

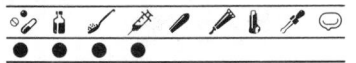

Tablets, liquid, powder, injection.

Frequency and timing of doses
4 – 6 x daily (pain); every 4 – 6 hours when necessary (cough); every 2 – 8 hours when necessary (diarrhea).

Adult dosage range
120 – 360mg daily (pain); 40 – 120mg daily (cough); 30 – 360mg daily (diarrhea).

Onset of effect
30 – 60 minutes.

Duration of action
4 – 6 hours.

Diet advice
None.

Storage
Keep in a closed container in a cool, dry place away from reach of children. Protect from light.

Missed dose
Take as soon as you remember if needed for relief of symptoms. If not needed, do not take the missed dose, and return to your normal dose schedule when necessary.

Stopping the drug
Can be safely stopped as soon as you no longer need it.

OVERDOSE ACTION

Seek immediate medical advice in all cases. Take emergency action if there are symptoms such as slow or irregular breathing, severe drowsiness, or loss of consciousness.

See Drug poisoning emergency guide (p.590).

SPECIAL PRECAUTIONS

Be sure to tell your physician if:
▼ You have impaired liver or kidney function.
▼ You have a lung disorder such as asthma or bronchitis.
▼ You have thyroid disease.
▼ You are taking other medications.

 Pregnancy
▼ No evidence of risk, but may adversely affect the baby's breathing if taken during labor.

 Breast feeding
▼ Discuss with your physician. The drug passes into the breast milk and may affect the baby adversely.

 Infants and children
▼ Reduced dose necessary.

 Over 60
▼ Reduced dose may be necessary.

 Driving and hazardous work
▼ Avoid such activities until you have learned how the drug affects you, because the drug may cause dizziness and drowsiness.

 Alcohol
▼ Avoid. Alcohol may increase the sedative effects of this drug.

POSSIBLE ADVERSE EFFECTS

Serious adverse effects are rare with codeine. Constipation occurs occasionally, but other side effects, such as nausea, vomiting, and drowsiness, are unusual at recommended doses, and usually disappear if the dose is reduced.

Symptom/effect	Frequency		Discuss with physician		Stop taking drug now	Call physician now
	Common	Rare	Only if severe	In all cases		
Constipation	●		■			
Nausea/vomiting		●		■		
Drowsiness		●		■		
Dizziness		●		■		
Agitation/restlessness		●		■	▲	
Rash/hives		●		■	▲	▮
Wheezing/breathlessness		●		■	▲	▮

PROLONGED USE

Codeine is normally used only for short-term relief of symptoms. It can be habit-forming if taken for extended periods, especially if higher than average doses are taken.

INTERACTIONS

Sedatives All drugs that have a sedative effect on the central nervous system are likely to increase sedation with codeine. Such drugs include antidepressant drugs, sleeping drugs, and antihistamines.

Monoamine oxidase inhibitors (MAOIs) Codeine may interact with these drugs to cause a dangerous rise in blood pressure.

COLCHICINE

Brand names None
Used in the following combined preparation ColBenemid

GENERAL INFORMATION

Colchicine, a drug originally extracted from the crocus flower and later synthesized, has been used since the 18th century for gout. Although it has now been to some extent superseded by newer drugs, it is still often used to relieve joint pain and inflammation in flare-ups of gout. It is most effective when taken at the first sign of symptoms, and it almost always produces an improvement. Colchicine is also often given in the first few months of treatment with allopurinol or probenecid (other drugs used for treating gout), because these may at first increase the frequency of gout attacks.

Colchicine is also prescribed for pseudogout (a buildup of calcium deposits), amyloidosis (abnormal protein deposits in the body), and the relief of symptoms of familial Mediterranean fever (a rare congenital condition).

Digestive upset can sometimes be prevented by injecting the drug.

INFORMATION FOR USERS

Your drug prescription is tailored for you. Do not alter dosage without checking with your physician.

How taken

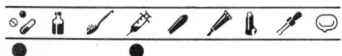

Tablets, injection.

Frequency and timing of doses
Prevention of gout attacks 1 – 2 x daily.
Relief of gout attacks Every 1 – 2 hours.

Adult dosage range
Prevention of gout attacks 0.6 – 1.8mg daily.
Relief of gout attacks 0.5 or 0.6mg per dose up to a maximum of 6mg daily until joint is better or gastrointestinal problems arise.

Onset of effect
Relief of symptoms in an acute attack of gout may be felt in 6 – 24 hours. Full beneficial effect in gout prevention may not be felt for several days.

Duration of action
Up to 2 hours. Some effect may last for several days.

Diet advice
Certain foods are known to make gout worse. Discuss with your physician.

Storage
Keep in a closed container in a cool, dry place away from reach of children. Protect from light.

Missed dose
Take as soon as you remember. If your next dose is due within 30 minutes, take a single dose now and skip the next.

Stopping the drug
When taking colchicine frequently during an acute attack, stop if diarrhea or abdominal pain develop. In other cases do not stop without consulting your physician.

OVERDOSE ACTION

 Seek immediate medical advice in all cases; some reactions can be fatal. Take emergency action if severe nausea, vomiting, bloody diarrhea, severe abdominal pain, or loss of consciousness occurs.

See Drug poisoning emergency guide (p.590).

SPECIAL PRECAUTIONS

Be sure to tell your physician if:
▼ You have impaired liver or kidney function.
▼ You have heart problems.
▼ You have a blood disorder.
▼ You have stomach ulcers.
▼ You have chronic inflammation of the bowel.
▼ You are taking other medications.

 Pregnancy
▼ Not usually prescribed. May cause defects in the unborn baby. Discuss with your physician so that you may weigh the benefits of the drug against its risks.

 Breast feeding
▼ Discuss with your physician. The drug passes into the breast milk and may affect the baby adversely.

 Infants and children
▼ Not recommended.

 Over 60
▼ Increased likelihood of adverse effects.

 Driving and hazardous work
▼ No special problems.

 Alcohol
▼ Avoid. Alcohol may increase stomach irritation caused by colchicine.

POSSIBLE ADVERSE EFFECTS

The appearance of any symptom that may be an adverse effect of the drug is a sign that you should stop the drug until you have received further medical advice. Drugs are sometimes prescribed to relieve adverse effects.

Symptom/effect	Frequency		Discuss with physician		Stop taking drug now	Call physician now
	Common	Rare	Only if severe	In all cases		
Nausea/vomiting	●			■	▲	▮
Diarrhea/abdominal pain	●			■	▲	▮
Numbness and tingling		●		■	▲	
Unusual bleeding/bruising		●		■	▲	
Rash		●		■	▲	▮

PROLONGED USE

Prolonged use of this drug may lead to hair loss, rashes, tingling in the hands and feet, muscle pain and weakness, and blood disorders.

Monitoring Periodic blood checks are usually required.

INTERACTIONS

Sedatives Colchicine may increase the effects of all sedative drugs.

Vitamin B$_{12}$ Colchicine may interfere with vitamin B$_{12}$ absorption.

COLESTIPOL

Brand name Colistid
Used in the following combined preparations None

A
B
C
D
E
F
G
H
I
J
K
L
M
N
O
P
Q
R
S
T
U
V
W
X
Y
Z

GENERAL INFORMATION

Introduced in 1977, colestipol is given to lower fat (lipid) levels in the blood. It is prescribed in conjunction with a low-fat diet for people with high blood lipid levels (hyperlipidemia) who are at risk from coronary heart disease and other disorders associated with fat deposits in the arteries (atherosclerosis).

As with other similar drugs, it is reserved for people who have failed to respond to dietary measures alone. Colestipol may also be given to relieve itching associated with high blood levels of bile acids in people with liver disease.

Since colestipol is not absorbed into the bloodstream, its adverse effects are confined to the gastro-intestinal tract. Bloating, nausea, and constipation are the most frequent problems.

QUICK REFERENCE

Drug group Lipid-lowering drug (p.131)

Overdose danger rating Low

Dependence rating Low

Prescription needed Yes

Available as generic No

INFORMATION FOR USERS

Your drug prescription is tailored for you. Do not alter dosage without checking with your physician.

How taken

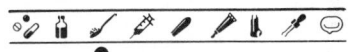

Granules, mixed with liquid such as fruit juice.

Frequency and timing of doses
2 x daily with meals.

Adult dosage range
10g daily (starting dose), gradually increasing to 30g daily (maintenance dose).

Onset of effect
Fat levels in the blood are lowered in 24 – 48 hours, but full benefits may not be apparent for up to 1 – 3 months. Used for itching or diarrhea, full beneficial effects may not be felt for several days.

Duration of action
12 – 24 hours (diarrhea). Effects on fat levels persist for up to a month after stopping treatment.

Diet advice
A low-fat diet may be recommended. Use of this drug may deplete levels of certain vitamins. Supplements may be advised.

Storage
Keep in a closed container in a cool, dry place away from reach of children.

Missed dose
Take as soon as you remember. If your next dose is due within 2 hours, take a single dose now and skip the next.

Stopping the drug
Do not stop the drug without consulting your physician; stopping the drug may lead to worsening of the underlying condition.

Exceeding the dose
An occasional unintentional extra dose is unlikely to be a cause for concern. But if you notice unusual symptoms, or if a large overdose has been taken, notify your physician.

SPECIAL PRECAUTIONS

Be sure to tell your physician if:
▼ You suffer from constipation or hemorrhoids.
▼ You have a peptic ulcer.
▼ You have a blood disorder.
▼ You are taking other medications.

Pregnancy
▼ Not usually prescribed. Safety in pregnancy not established. Discuss with your physician so that you can weigh the benefits of the drug against its possible risks.

Breast feeding
▼ No known evidence of risk.

Infants and children
▼ Not recommended under 6 years. Reduced dose necessary for older children.

Over 60
▼ Increased likelihood of adverse effects.

Driving and hazardous work
▼ No special problems.

Alcohol
▼ Although this drug does not interact with alcohol, your underlying condition may make it inadvisable to take alcohol.

POSSIBLE ADVERSE EFFECTS

Mild constipation is the most common side effect of colestipol. Like bloating and nausea, it usually clears up as treatment continues. Large doses may reduce absorption of fats from the bowel, leading to fatty bowel movements and weight loss.

Symptom/effect	Frequency		Discuss with physician		Stop taking drug now	Call physician now
	Common	Rare	Only if severe	In all cases		
Constipation/bloating	●			■		
Indigestion/excess gas		●	■			
Abdominal pain/heartburn		●	■			
Nausea/vomiting		●	■			
Weight loss		●		■		

PROLONGED USE

As this drug reduces vitamin absorption, supplements of vitamins A, D, and K and folic acid may be advised.

Monitoring Periodic blood tests are usually required to monitor the levels of lipids in the blood.

INTERACTIONS

General note Colestipol considerably reduces the body's ability to absorb other drugs (such as digoxin, warfarin, and thiazide diuretics). It may be necessary to organize a schedule in consultation with your physician, whereby you take other medications at a fixed time before or after you take colestipol.

COLISTIN

Brand name Coly-Mycin S
Used in the following combined preparation Coly-Mycin S Otic

GENERAL INFORMATION

Introduced in 1962, colistin (also known as polymyxin E) is a limited-spectrum antibiotic. It is most commonly used with other antibiotics (neomycin, gramicidin, and bacitracin) and often a corticosteroid for the prevention and treatment of ear, eye, and skin infections. Applied as drops or ointment, the drug acts locally, rarely causing *systemic* side effects.

Not absorbed by the body when taken by mouth, colistin in liquid form is sometimes given to children who have diarrhea caused by a bacterial infection. Since it may cause damage to the nerves and kidneys, colistin is rarely administered by injection to treat *systemic* infections.

QUICK REFERENCE

Drug group Antibiotic (p.156)
Overdose danger rating Low
Dependence rating Low
Prescription needed Yes
Available as generic No

INFORMATION FOR USERS

Your drug prescription is tailored for you. Do not alter dosage without checking with your physician.

How taken

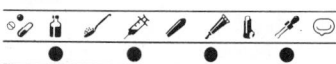

Liquid, injection, ointment, ear/eye drops.

Frequency and timing of doses
Every 3 – 4 hours (eye infections); every 6 – 8 hours (ear infections); 3 x daily (diarrhea).

Dosage range
As directed.

Onset of effect
Symptoms usually improve within 1 – 2 days.

Duration of action
6 – 8 hours (by mouth); up to 8 hours (topically).

Diet advice
None.

Storage
Keep in a closed container in a cool, dry place away from reach of children.

Missed dose
Take as soon as you remember. If your next dose is due within 2 hours, take a single dose now and skip the next.

Stopping the drug
Do not stop the drug without consulting your physician; symptoms may recur.

Exceeding the dose
An occasional unintentional extra dose is unlikely to be a cause for concern. But if you notice unusual symptoms, or if a large overdose has been taken, notify your physician.

SPECIAL PRECAUTIONS

Be sure to tell your physician if:
▼ You suffer from chronic ear infections.
▼ You have impaired hearing.
▼ You are taking other medications.

 Pregnancy
▼ No evidence of risk to developing baby.

 Breast feeding
▼ No evidence of risk.

 Infants and children
▼ Reduced dose necessary.

 Over 60
▼ No special problems.

 Driving and hazardous work
▼ No known problems.

 Alcohol
▼ No known problems.

POSSIBLE ADVERSE EFFECTS

Colistin rarely causes adverse effects. Any symptoms that do occur are usually caused by another ingredient in the preparation.

The adverse effects below indicate an allergy, making it necessary to replace colistin with another antibiotic.

Symptom/effect	Frequency		Discuss with physician		Stop taking drug now	Call physician now
	Common	Rare	Only if severe	In all cases		
Itching		●		■		
Redness/swelling		●		■	▲	
Rash		●		■	▲	

INTERACTIONS

None.

PROLONGED USE

Large doses applied daily to an open wound are not recommended for prolonged periods, since colistin may be absorbed by the body, leading to kidney or nerve damage. There is also a risk that the infection may become resistant to this drug with prolonged use.

CONJUGATED ESTROGENS

Brand names Premarin, Progens
Used in the following combined preparations Esprogyn, Milprem, PMB, Premarin with methyltestosterone

GENERAL INFORMATION

Conjugated estrogen preparations, in use since 1942, consist of naturally occurring estrogens similar to those found in the urine of pregnant mares.

Given by mouth, they are used to relieve menopausal symptoms such as hot flashes and sweating, to treat hypogonadism (underdeveloped ovaries), and to control abnormal bleeding from the womb due to hormone imbalance. They are also used to treat and prevent osteoporosis (brittle bones), which may occur after the menopause, and to treat certain forms of infertility. High doses of conjugated estrogens may be given as post-coital contraception.

As replacement therapy, conjugated estrogens are usually taken on a cyclic dosing schedule, often in conjunction with a progestin, to simulate the hormonal changes of a normal menstrual cycle. They are also prescribed in the form of vaginal cream to relieve pain and dryness of the vagina or vulva after the menopause.

INFORMATION FOR USERS

Your drug prescription is tailored for you. Do not alter dosage without checking with your physician.

How taken

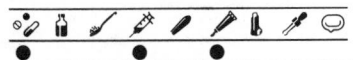

Tablets, injection, cream.

Frequency and timing of doses
Tablets 1 – 3 x daily, with food.
Cream Once daily.

Adult dosage range
Replacement therapy 0.3 – 1.25mg daily (tablets); 2 – 4g daily (cream).
Prostate cancer 3.75 – 7.5mg daily.
Breast cancer 30mg daily.
Post-coital contraception 30mg daily for 5 days.

Onset of effect
Within 5 days (post-coital contraception); 10 – 20 days (other actions).

Duration of action
1 – 2 days.

Diet advice
None.

Storage
Keep in a closed container in a cool, dry place away from reach of children.

Missed dose
Take as soon as you remember.

Stopping the drug
Do not stop the drug without consulting your physician; symptoms may recur. Contraceptive effect may not be reliable if treatment is stopped too soon.

Exceeding the dose
An occasional unintentional extra dose is unlikely to be a cause for concern. But if you notice unusual symptoms, or if a large overdose has been taken, notify your physician.

POSSIBLE ADVERSE EFFECTS

The most common adverse effects of conjugated estrogens are similar to symptoms that occur in the early stages of pregnancy, and generally diminish or disappear after 2 – 3 months of treatment. Sudden, sharp pain in the chest, groin, or legs may indicate an abnormal blood clot and requires urgent medical attention.

Symptom/effect	Frequency		Discuss with physician		Stop taking drug now	Call physician now
	Common	Rare	Only if severe	In all cases		
Nausea	●		■			
Breast swelling/tenderness	●		■			
Reduced sex drive		●	■			
Depression		●		■		
Vaginal bleeding		●		■		
Pain in chest/groin/legs		●		■	▲	∎

INTERACTIONS

Tobacco smoking Smoking increases the risk of serious adverse effects on the heart and circulation with conjugated estrogens.

Oral anticoagulant drugs Conjugated estrogens reduce the anticoagulant effect of these drugs.

SPECIAL PRECAUTIONS

Be sure to tell your physician if:
▼ You have heart failure or high blood pressure.
▼ You have had blood clots or a stroke.
▼ You have impaired liver or kidney function.
▼ You have diabetes.
▼ You are a smoker.
▼ You suffer from migraine or epilepsy.
▼ You are taking other medications.

 Pregnancy
▼ Not prescribed. May adversely affect the development of the baby's sex organs.

 Breast feeding
▼ Not prescribed. The drug passes into the breast milk and may inhibit the flow of milk.

 Infants and children
▼ Not usually prescribed.

 Over 60
▼ No special problems.

 Driving and hazardous work
▼ No known problems.

 Alcohol
▼ No known problems.

Surgery and general anesthetics
▼ Conjugated estrogens may need to be stopped several weeks before you have surgery. Discuss with your physician.

PROLONGED USE

There is a slightly higher risk of cancer of the uterus after the menopause when used without a progestin. The risk of gallstones is also increased.

Monitoring Physical examinations and blood pressure checks may be needed.

CORTISONE

Brand name Cortone
Used in the following combined preparations None

GENERAL INFORMATION

Introduced with much press attention in 1948, cortisone was the first of the synthetic corticosteroids – the great soothers of the human body. Because of its anti-inflammatory actions, cortisone is used for a wide variety of allergic and inflamed conditions – from rashes and hives to ulcerative colitis and rheumatoid arthritis.

When cortisone enters the body it is converted to cortisol, a hormone produced by the adrenal glands that is vital in regulating sugar *metabolism* and balance, blood pressure, and the concentration of mineral salts. Though other drugs are now often preferred, cortisone was and still is used to treat the adrenal insufficiency known as Addison's disease.

When given at a low dose for short periods, cortisone rarely has troublesome side effects. Long-term treatment with high doses can cause unpleasant and serious side effects, such as fluid retention, mood changes, stomach irritation, ulcers, and diabetes.

INFORMATION FOR USERS

Your drug prescription is tailored for you. Do not alter dosage without checking with your physician.

How taken

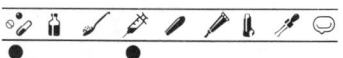

●   ●

Tablets, injection.

Frequency and timing of doses
1 – 2 x daily with food.

Adult dosage range
Adrenal replacement 30 – 70mg daily.
Inflammatory and other disorders 20 – 300mg daily.

Onset of effect
Within 2 – 4 days.

Duration of action
8 – 12 hours.

Diet advice
Salt intake may need to be restricted when the drug is taken by mouth. Potassium levels may be depleted, so you may need to take supplements.

Storage
Keep in a closed container in a cool, dry place away from reach of children.

Missed dose
Take as soon as you remember. If your next dose is due within 2 hours, take a single dose now and skip the next.

Stopping the drug
Do not stop taking the drug without consulting your physician. A gradual reduction in dose is required following prolonged treatment.

Exceeding the dose
An occasional unintentional extra dose is unlikely to be a cause for concern. But if you notice unusual symptoms, or if a large overdose has been taken, notify your physician.

POSSIBLE ADVERSE EFFECTS

The more serious adverse effects usually occur only when cortisone is taken in high doses for long periods. Side effects are carefully monitored during treatment.

Symptom/effect	Frequency		Discuss with physician		Stop taking drug now	Call physician now
	Common	Rare	Only if severe	In all cases		
Indigestion	●		■			
Weight gain	●		■			
Acne	●		■			
Fluid retention		●		■		
Muscle weakness		●		■		
Mood changes		●		■		

INTERACTIONS

Antidiabetic drugs Cortisone increases the actions of these drugs, so dosage may need to be adjusted.

Antihypertensive drugs Cortisone may reduce the effects of these drugs.

Barbiturates These drugs reduce the effectiveness of cortisone by increasing its rate of metabolism.

Vaccines Cortisone may interact dangerously with some vaccines.

SPECIAL PRECAUTIONS

Be sure to tell your physician if:
▼ You have had a peptic ulcer.
▼ You have suffered from depression or mental illness.
▼ You have glaucoma.
▼ You have had tuberculosis.
▼ You have a herpes infection.
▼ You are taking other medications.

Pregnancy
▼ Not usually prescribed. High doses may affect the developing baby. Discuss with your physician so that you may weigh the benefits of the drug against its risks.

Breast feeding
▼ Discuss with your physician. The drug passes into the breast milk and may affect the baby adversely.

Infants and children
▼ Reduced dose necessary.

Over 60
▼ Reduced dose may be necessary.

Driving and hazardous work
▼ No known problems.

Alcohol
▼ Avoid. Alcohol may increase the risk of peptic ulcer.

PROLONGED USE

Prolonged use of this drug is recommended only when essential, because it can lead to adverse effects such as peptic ulcer, diabetes, glaucoma, cataracts, fragile bones, and thin skin, and may retard growth in children.

COSYNTROPIN

Brand name Cortrosyn
Used in the following combined preparations None

GENERAL INFORMATION

Cosyntropin, introduced in 1971, is a synthetic form of corticotropin, a hormone secreted by the pituitary gland. Like the natural hormone, cosyntropin stimulates the release of corticosteroid hormones from the adrenal glands, but is less likely to cause an allergic reaction than natural corticotropin.

The drug is used to diagnose adrenal insufficiency (inadequate production of adrenal hormones). If hormone production does not follow an injection of cosyntropin, a diagnosis of underactive adrenal glands is confirmed. A single injection is usually sufficient to enable a diagnosis to be made, but with some people, injections may be continued for several days. Cosyntropin may sometimes be administered by intravenous infusion to determine whether an insufficiency of corticosteroid hormones stems from a problem in the pituitary or adrenal glands.

QUICK REFERENCE

Drug group Pituitary hormone (p.173)

Overdose danger rating Low

Dependence rating Low

Prescription needed Yes

Available as generic No

INFORMATION FOR USERS

This drug is given only under medical supervision and is not for self-administration.

How taken

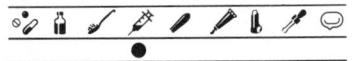

Injection.

Frequency and timing of doses
A single injection given over 2 minutes or an intravenous infusion administered over 4 – 8 hours.

Dosage range
Adults 0.25mg (single injection); 0.25mg – 0.75mg (infusion).
Children Reduced dose necessary according to age and weight.

Onset of effect
Within 2 minutes.

Duration of action
Up to 4 hours.

Diet advice
None.

Storage
Not applicable. The drug is not kept in the home.

Missed dose
Not applicable. The drug is given under strict medical supervision.

Stopping the drug
Not applicable.

Exceeding the dose
The drug is always injected by a trained nurse or physician. Overdose is unlikely.

POSSIBLE ADVERSE EFFECTS

Adverse effects are extremely rare with cosyntropin and can be quickly dealt with under close medical supervision. There is a very small risk of an allergic reaction.

Symptom/effect	Frequency		Discuss with physician		Stop taking drug now	Call physician now
	Common	Rare	Only if severe	In all cases		
Fever		●		■		
Dizziness/lightheadedness		●		■		
Nausea/vomiting		●		■		
Rash/itching		●		■		
Seizures		●		■	▲	
Breathing difficulties		●		■		▲

INTERACTIONS

Corticosteroids may interfere with the measured effects of cosyntropin and reduce the accuracy of results.

Spironolactone may interfere with the accuracy of results from cosyntropin.

SPECIAL PRECAUTIONS

Be sure to tell your physician if:
▼ You are taking other medications.

Pregnancy
▼ Only given when benefit to mother outweighs possible risk to the baby. Discuss with your physician.

Breast feeding
▼ No evidence of risk.

Infants and children
▼ Reduced dose necessary.

Over 60
▼ No special problems.

Driving and hazardous work
▼ No known problems.

Alcohol
▼ No known problems.

PROLONGED USE

This drug is not used for prolonged periods.

CROMOLYN SODIUM

Brand names Intal, Nasalcrom, Opticrom
Used in the following combined preparations None

GENERAL INFORMATION

Cromolyn sodium, introduced in the 1970s, is used primarily as a preventive for asthma and allergic conditions.

Taken by inhaler as a powder (spinhaler) or a spray, it is commonly prescribed to prevent mild to moderate asthma in children. It also reduces the frequency and severity of adult allergic asthma attacks induced by exercise or cold air. Cromolyn sodium has a slow onset of action, taking from a few days to up to six weeks of regular dosage to produce its anti-asthmatic effect. It is not effective for the relief of an asthma attack in progress.

Aside from its use in asthma, cromolyn sodium is also given as eye drops to prevent allergic conjunctivitis. Taken as a nasal spray, it is also helpful in preventing allergic rhinitis (hay fever). It has been given for gastrointestinal food allergy and for diarrhea due to a rare disease called systemic mastocytosis.

Side effects are mild. Coughing and wheezing on inhalation may be prevented by using a *sympathomimetic* bronchodilator (p.120) first. Hoarseness and throat irritation can be avoided by rinsing the mouth with water after inhalation.

INFORMATION FOR USERS

Your drug prescription is tailored for you. Do not alter dosage without checking with your physician.

How taken

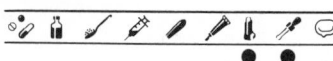

Inhaler (various types), nasal spray, eye drops.

Frequency and timing of doses
4 – 6 x daily (eye drops, nasal spray); 4 x daily at regular intervals (inhaler).

Dosage range
80mg daily (spinhaler, nebulizer); 6.4mg daily (metered-dose inhaler); one spray into each nostril (nasal spray); one drop into each eye per dose.

Onset of effect
Varies with dosage, form and condition treated. Eye conditions and allergic rhinitis may respond after several days' treatment with drops, while asthma and chronic allergic rhinitis may take take 2 – 6 weeks to show improvement.

Duration of action
4 – 6 hours. Some effect persists for several days after treatment is stopped.

Diet advice
None.

Storage
Keep in a closed container in a cool, dry place away from reach of children. Protect from light.

Missed dose
Take as soon as you remember. If your next dose is due within 2 hours, take a single dose now and skip the next.

Stopping the drug
Do not stop the drug without consulting your physician; symptoms may recur.

Exceeding the dose
An occasional unintentional extra dose is unlikely to be a cause for concern. But if you notice unusual symptoms, or if a large overdose has been taken, notify your physician.

POSSIBLE ADVERSE EFFECTS

Coughing and hoarseness are common with inhalation of cromolyn sodium, and local irritation such as burning and stinging may occur with all dosage forms. Nasal spray may cause sneezing. All these symptoms diminish with continued use.

Symptom/effect	Frequency		Discuss with physician		Stop taking drug now	Call physician now
	Common	Rare	Only if severe	In all cases		
Coughing/hoarseness	●		■			
Local irritation	●		■			
Nausea/vomiting		●		■		
Dizziness/headache		●		■		
Wheezing/breathlessness		●		■		
Rash/itching		●		■	▲	

INTERACTIONS

None.

SPECIAL PRECAUTIONS

Be sure to tell your physician if:
▼ You have impaired liver or kidney function.
▼ You are taking other medications.

Pregnancy
▼ No evidence of risk to developing baby.

Breast feeding
▼ No evidence of risk.

Infants and children
▼ Not recommended for children under 5 years, except in the form of eye drops.

Over 60
▼ No special problems.

Driving and hazardous work
▼ No known problems.

Alcohol
▼ No known problems.

PROLONGED USE

No problems expected.

CYCLOBENZAPRINE

Brand name Flexeril
Used in the following combined preparations None

GENERAL INFORMATION

Chemically similar to the tricyclic antidepressant drugs (p.112), cyclobenzaprine acts on nerve cells in the central nervous system to relieve spasm and rigidity of the muscles. It may also help to relieve pain. It is mainly used in the short term to treat painful symptoms caused by injury. Cyclobenzaprine treatment is usually accompan-

ied by rest and physical therapy.
Because cyclobenzaprine is not recommended for prolonged treatment, it is not useful for neurological disorders, such as multiple sclerosis, or after injury to the spinal cord. As with all muscle relaxants, drowsiness is one of the most common side effects of cyclobenzaprine.

INFORMATION FOR USERS

Your drug prescription is tailored for you. Do not alter dosage without checking with your physician.

How taken

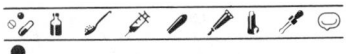

Tablets.

Frequency and timing of doses
3 x daily.

Adult dosage range
20 – 40mg daily. Larger doses may be given in some cases.

Onset of effect
Within 1 hour.

Duration of action
Up to 24 hours.

Diet advice
None.

Storage
Keep in a closed container in a cool, dry place away from reach of children.

Missed dose
Take as soon as you remember. If your next dose is due within 2 hours, take a single dose now and skip the next.

Stopping the drug
Do not stop the drug without consulting your physician; symptoms may recur.

OVERDOSE ACTION

 Seek immediate medical advice in all cases. Take emergency action if abnormal heart rhythm, breathing difficulties, loss of consciousness, or coma occurs.

See Drug poisoning emergency guide (p.590).

POSSIBLE ADVERSE EFFECTS

Most adverse effects of cyclobenzaprine are due to its sedative and *anticholinergic* properties and disappear when a course of treatment with the drug is stopped.

Symptom/effect	Frequency		Discuss with physician		Stop taking drug now	Call physician now
	Common	Rare	Only if severe	In all cases		
Drowsiness	●		■			
Dizziness	●		■			
Dry mouth	●		■			
Blurred vision		●		■		
Nausea/indigestion		●		■		
Weakness		●		■	▲	
Palpitations		●		■	▲	■

INTERACTIONS

Sedatives All drugs that have a sedative effect on the central nervous system are likely to increase the sedative properties of cyclobenzaprine.

Anticholinergic drugs There is an increased risk of side effects if these drugs are taken with cyclobenzaprine.

Monoamine oxidase inhibitors (MAOIs) There is a risk of severe high blood pressure if these drugs are taken within 14 days of cyclobenzaprine.

Guanethidine Cyclobenzaprine interferes with the blood pressure-lowering effect of guanethidine.

SPECIAL PRECAUTIONS

Be sure to tell your physician if:
▼ You have had a recent heart attack or heart problems.
▼ You have had glaucoma.
▼ You have an overactive thyroid gland.
▼ You have urinary difficulties.
▼ You are taking other medications.

 Pregnancy
▼ Not usually prescribed. Safety in pregnancy not established. Discuss with your physician so that you can weigh the benefits of the drug against its possible risks.

 Breast feeding
▼ Discuss with your physician. The drug passes into the breast milk and may make the baby drowsy.

 Infants and children
▼ Not recommended.

 Over 60
▼ Reduced dose may be necessary.

 Driving and hazardous work
▼ Avoid such activities until you have learned how the drug affects you, because the drug can cause drowsiness.

 Alcohol
▼ Avoid. Alcohol may increase the adverse effects of this drug.

Surgery and general anesthetics
▼ Cyclobenzaprine may need to be stopped before you have a general anesthetic. Discuss this with your physician or dentist before any surgery.

PROLONGED USE

Cyclobenzaprine is not prescribed for prolonged periods and should probably not be taken for longer than two or three weeks.

CYCLOPHOSPHAMIDE

Brand names Cytoxan, Neosar
Used in the following combined preparations None

GENERAL INFORMATION

Used since 1959, cyclophosphamide is the most widely used of the anti-cancer drugs known as alkylating agents. It interferes with the growth of cancer cells, which are later destroyed by the immune system.

Alone, or together with other anti-cancer drugs, it is effective against lymphomas (lymph gland cancers), including Hodgkin's disease, and cancers of the ovary, testicles, breast, and lung. Because of its strong immunosuppressive action, it is sometimes given to treat severe rheumatoid arthritis, Wegener's granulomatosis (a kidney disorder), and nephrotic syndrome in children. It is also used after a bone marrow transplant to prevent rejection of donated bone marrow.

Cyclophosphamide causes nausea, vomiting, and loss of hair; it can affect the heart, lungs, liver, and bladder. Because cyclophosphamide often reduces blood cell production, the drug may lead to abnormal bleeding and increased risk of infection, and reduced fertility in men.

INFORMATION FOR USERS

Your drug prescription is tailored for you. Do not alter dosage without checking with your physician.

How taken

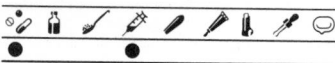

Tablets, injection.

Frequency and timing of doses
Once daily (tablets); once every 2 – 4 weeks (injection).

Dosage range
Dosage is determined individually according to body weight and response.

Onset of effect
Some effects may appear within hours of starting treatment. Full beneficial effects may not be felt for up to 6 weeks.

Duration of action
Several weeks.

Diet advice
None.

Storage
Keep in a closed container in a cool, dry place away from reach of children. Protect from light.

Missed dose
Injections are given only in the hospital. If you are taking tablets, take the missed dose as soon as you remember. If your next dose is due within 6 hours, take a single dose now and skip the next. Tell your physician that you missed a dose.

Stopping the drug
The drug will be stopped under medical supervision (injection). Do not stop taking the drug without consulting your physician (tablets); stopping the drug may lead to worsening of the underlying condition.

Exceeding the dose
An occasional unintentional extra dose is unlikely to cause problems. Large overdoses may cause nausea and vomiting. Notify your physician.

SPECIAL PRECAUTIONS

Cyclophosphamide is prescribed only under close medical supervision, taking account of your present condition and medical history.

Pregnancy
▼ Not usually prescribed. May cause birth defects or premature birth. Discuss with your physician.

Breast feeding
▼ Discontinue breast feeding. The drug passes into the breast milk and may affect the baby adversely.

Infants and children
▼ Reduced dose necessary.

Over 60
▼ No special problems.

Driving and hazardous work
▼ No known problems.

Alcohol
▼ No known problems.

POSSIBLE ADVERSE EFFECTS

Cyclophosphamide often causes nausea and vomiting, which usually diminish as your body adjusts. Also, women often experience irregular periods. Blood in the urine may be a sign of bladder damage and requires prompt medical attention.

Symptom/effect	Frequency		Discuss with physician		Stop taking drug now	Call physician now
	Common	Rare	Only if severe	In all cases		
Nausea/vomiting	●		■			
Hair loss	●		■			
Irregular menstruation	●			■		
Mouth ulcers		●		■		
Bloodstained urine		●		■		▌

PROLONGED USE

Prolonged use of this drug may reduce production of blood cells and may impair liver function.

Monitoring Periodic checks on blood composition and on all effects of the drug are usually required.

INTERACTIONS

Allopurinol This drug may increase blood levels of cyclophosphamide, leading to an increased risk of adverse effects.

CYCLOSPORINE

Brand name Sandimmune
Used in the following combined preparations None

GENERAL INFORMATION

Cyclosporine was introduced in 1984. It belongs to a group of drugs known as immunosuppressants. These drugs suppress the body's natural defenses against infection and foreign cells. This action is of particular use following organ transplants, when the immune system may start to reject the transplanted organ unless the immune system is controlled.

Cyclosporine is now widely used following many different types of transplant surgery including heart, kidney, bone marrow, liver, and pancreas. Its use has considerably reduced the risk of tissue rejection and

the need for large doses of corticosteroids. It may need to be taken for an indefinite period following surgery. Its effect on other illnesses such as rheumatoid arthritis and diabetes is also being studied.

Because cyclosporine reduces the effectiveness of the immune system, people being treated with this drug are more susceptible than usual to infections. Cyclosporine has also been found to cause kidney damage in some people. If signs of kidney damage are noticed, the dose of cyclosporine may need to be reduced or another drug substituted.

QUICK REFERENCE

Drug group Immunosuppressant drug (p.184)

Overdose danger rating Low

Dependence rating Low

Prescription needed Yes

Available as generic No

INFORMATION FOR USERS

Your drug prescription is tailored for you. Do not alter dosage without checking with your physician.

How taken

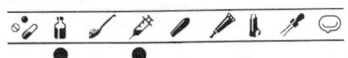

Liquid, injection.

Frequency and timing of doses
1 – 2 x daily.

Dosage range
The dosage of this drug is calculated on an individual basis according to age and weight.

Onset of effect
Within 12 hours.

Duration of action
Up to 3 days.

Diet advice
None.

Storage
Keep in a closed container in a cool, dry place away from reach of children.

Missed dose
Take as soon as you remember. If your dose is more than 36 hours late, consult your physician.

Stopping the drug
Do not stop taking the drug without consulting your physician; stopping the drug may lead to transplant rejection.

Exceeding the dose
An occasional unintentional extra dose is unlikely to be a cause for concern. But if you notice any unusual symptoms or if a large overdose has been taken, notify your physician.

SPECIAL PRECAUTIONS

Cyclosporine is prescribed only under close medical supervision, taking account of your present condition and medical history.

Pregnancy
▼ Not usually prescribed. Safety in pregnancy not established. Discuss with your physician.

Breast feeding
▼ Discuss with your physician. The drug passes into the breast milk and may affect the baby adversely.

Infants and children
▼ Reduced dose necessary.

Over 60
▼ Reduced dose may be necessary.

Driving and hazardous work
▼ No known problems.

Alcohol
▼ No known problems.

POSSIBLE ADVERSE EFFECTS

The main adverse effect of this drug is increased susceptibility to infections of all kinds. Any flu-like illness or localized infection should be brought to your physician's attention. Most other adverse effects of cyclosporine are minor compared

with the risks of the conditions that it is used to treat and prevent. Because of the seriousness of such conditions, anyone receiving cyclosporine will be under regular specialist supervision, and possible adverse effects of the drug will be carefully monitored.

Symptom/effect	Frequency		Discuss with physician		Stop taking drug now	Call physician now
	Common	Rare	Only if severe	In all cases		
Swelling of gums	●			■		
Increased body hair		●	■			
Tremor		●		■		
Nausea/vomiting		●		■		

PROLONGED USE

Long-term use of this drug, especially in high doses, can cause reduced kidney function.

Monitoring Regular checks on blood samples – to measure cyclosporine levels and to monitor kidney function – are normally carried out.

INTERACTIONS

Ketoconazole This drug may increase blood levels of cyclosporine.

Rifampin This drug may reduce blood levels of cyclosporine.

Anticonvulsant drugs Certain anticonvulsants may reduce blood levels of cyclosporine.

DANAZOL

Brand name Danocrine
Used in the following combined preparations None

GENERAL INFORMATION

Introduced in 1976, danazol is a synthetic hormone that opposes the effects of estrogen and strengthens secondary male sexual characteristics. Its main use is in the long-term treatment of endometriosis, a condition where fragments of the endometrial tissue (uterine lining) grow outside the uterus. Danazol is also used to relieve pain, tenderness, and lumpiness in the breast caused by fibrocystic disease.

Danazol is occasionally prescribed to treat excessive bleeding during menstruation (menorrhagia), and to reduce breast swelling in men (gynecomastia). Danazol may also be prescribed for people who are susceptible to hereditary angiodema (a rare disorder that causes facial swelling).

Danazol treatment commonly disrupts normal menstrual periods. Cessation of menstruation is normal during treatment for endometriosis. Other adverse effects include nausea, dizziness, rash, back pain, weight gain, and flushing. Women taking high doses may notice unusual hair growth and deepening of the voice.

INFORMATION FOR USERS

Your drug prescription is tailored for you. Do not alter dosage without checking with your physician.

How taken

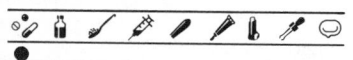

Capsules.

Frequency and timing of doses
2 – 4 x daily with food.

Adult dosage range
Endometriosis 100 – 800mg daily, depending on the severity of the disorder. *Fibrocystic disease* 100 – 400mg daily. *Hereditary angiodema* 400 – 600mg daily.

Onset of effect
Adverse effects and benefits in fibrocystic disease may be felt within 1 month. Beneficial effects on endometriosis may not be apparent for 3 – 12 months.

Duration of action
1 – 2 days.

Diet advice
None.

Storage
Keep in a closed container in a cool, dry place away from reach of children.

Missed dose
Take as soon as you remember. If your next dose is due within 4 hours, take a single dose now and skip the next.

Stopping the drug
Do not stop the drug without consulting your physician; symptoms may recur.

Exceeding the dose
An occasional unintentional extra dose is unlikely to be a cause for concern. But if you notice unusual symptoms, or if a large overdose has been taken, notify your physician.

SPECIAL PRECAUTIONS

Be sure to tell your physician if:
▼ You have impaired liver or kidney function.
▼ You have heart disease.
▼ You have had epileptic seizures.
▼ You suffer from unexplained vaginal bleeding.
▼ You are or may be pregnant.
▼ You are taking other medications.

Pregnancy
▼ Not prescribed. May cause masculine characteristics in a female baby. Pregnancy should be avoided for 3 months following cessation of treatment.

Breast feeding
▼ Discuss with your physician. The drug passes into the breast milk and may affect the baby adversely.

Infants and children
▼ Reduced dose necessary.

Over 60
▼ Unlikely to be required.

Driving and hazardous work
▼ No known problems.

Alcohol
▼ No known problems.

POSSIBLE ADVERSE EFFECTS

Danazol rarely causes adverse effects in low doses. Adverse effects from higher doses – such as acne, weight gain, and nausea – are the result of hormonal changes. Voice changes and unusual hair growth in women are largely reversed after treatment.

Symptom/effect	Frequency		Discuss with physician		Stop taking drug now	Call physician now
	Common	Rare	Only if severe	In all cases		
Swollen feet/ankles	●		■			
Weight gain	●		■			
Nausea	●		■			
Acne/oily skin	●		■			
Women only						
Unusual hair growth	●			■		
Reduced breast size		●	■			
Voice changes		●		■		

INTERACTIONS

None.

PROLONGED USE

This drug normally needs to be taken for several months before full beneficial effects are felt. There is a slight risk of liver damage. See also Possible adverse effects, left.

Monitoring Periodic liver function tests may be carried out.

DANTROLENE

Brand name Dantrium
Used in the following combined preparations None

GENERAL INFORMATION

Dantrolene acts directly in muscles to relieve the muscle spasm and rigidity caused by neurological diseases (such as multiple sclerosis and cerebral palsy), strokes, or spinal injury. It does not cure these conditions, but increases mobility and the effectiveness of other treatments, such as physical therapy. Drug treatment usually needs to continue for several weeks before there is any improvement.

Dantrolene, available since 1974, is also prescribed to relax bladder muscles in cases of urinary retention. It is sometimes injected to prevent or treat malignant hyperthermia, a reaction to general anesthetics.

Because it acts directly in the muscles and only minimally on the brain and nervous system, dantrolene causes less drowsiness than other muscle relaxants. The drug may in rare cases cause a rash when the skin is exposed to sunlight. Exposure to strong sunlight should therefore be avoided during treatment.

INFORMATION FOR USERS

Your drug prescription is tailored for you. Do not alter dosage without checking with your physician.

How taken

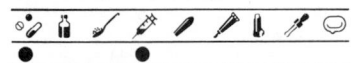

Capsules, injection.

Frequency and timing of doses
2 – 4 x daily.

Adult dosage range
25mg daily (starting dose), increased by 15mg daily until maximum effect is achieved with 50 – 100mg, 4 x daily.

Onset of effect
Within one hour. Full beneficial effect may not be felt for several weeks.

Duration of action
6 – 12 hours.

Diet advice
None.

Storage
Keep in a closed container in a cool, dry place away from reach of children.

Missed dose
Take as soon as you remember. If your next dose is due within 2 hours, take a single dose now and skip the next.

Stopping the drug
Do not stop the drug without consulting your physician. Dosage needs to be reduced gradually because abrupt cessation of treatment can lead to excessive muscle tension.

Exceeding the dose
An occasional unintentional extra dose is unlikely to cause problems. Large overdoses may cause severe muscle weakness and drowsiness. Notify your physician.

SPECIAL PRECAUTIONS

Be sure to tell your physician if:
▼ You have any form of liver disease.
▼ You have heart problems.
▼ You have a lung disorder such as asthma or bronchitis.
▼ You are taking other medications.

Pregnancy
▼ Not usually prescribed. Safety in pregnancy not established. Discuss with your physician so that you can weigh the benefits of the drug against its possible risks.

Breast feeding
▼ Discuss with your physician. The drug passes into the breast milk and may affect the baby adversely.

Infants and children
▼ Not recommended in children under 5 years. Reduced dose necessary in older children.

Over 60
▼ No special problems.

Driving and hazardous work
▼ Avoid such activities until you have learned how the drug affects you, because it can cause drowsiness and muscle weakness.

Alcohol
▼ Avoid. Alcohol may increase the sedative effects of this drug and worsen its effect on the liver.

POSSIBLE ADVERSE EFFECTS

The most common adverse effects of dantrolene are weakness and diarrhea, which may be severe. Many of the side effects diminish as your body adjusts to the drug, and they disappear when treatment with dantrolene is stopped.

Symptom/effect	Frequency		Discuss with physician		Stop taking drug now	Call physician now
	Common	Rare	Only if severe	In all cases		
Drowsiness/lethargy	●		■			
Diarrhea	●		■			
Muscle weakness	●		■			
Light-sensitive rash	●			■		
Dizziness		●	■			

PROLONGED USE

Liver damage may occasionally occur during prolonged treatment with high doses. In such cases dosage may need to be reduced.

Monitoring Blood tests to check liver function are usually required before starting treatment and at regular intervals thereafter.

INTERACTIONS

Sedatives All drugs that have a sedative effect on the central nervous system are likely to increase the sedative properties of dantrolene. Such drugs include anti-anxiety and sleeping drugs, antihistamines, antidepressants, narcotic analgesics, and antipsychotic drugs.

DAPSONE

Brand names None
Used in the following combined preparations None

GENERAL INFORMATION

Dapsone, introduced in 1957, is the most effective treatment available for leprosy. Related to the sulfonamides, it is prescribed for all forms of the disease, initially in combination with other drugs. For tuberculoid leprosy, treatment may be continued for three to five years or more. For more severe forms of leprosy, especially disfiguring lepromatous leprosy, lifelong treatment may sometimes be necessary. Dapsone may be given with another drug, such as rifampin.

Dapsone also has a depressant effect on the immune system and is prescribed for dermatitis herpetiformis. This skin condition often occurs with celiac disease, in which the bowel is abnormally sensitive to gluten (a wheat protein). In combination with a gluten-free diet, dapsone improves the skin condition.

Side effects are rare with dapsone, even during prolonged treatment. The most serious adverse effect is hemolytic anemia. Periodic blood tests are recommended to detect early signs of this disorder.

INFORMATION FOR USERS

Your drug prescription is tailored for you. Do not alter dosage without checking with your physician.

How taken

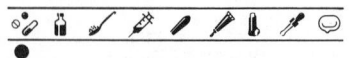

Tablets.

Frequency and timing of doses
Once daily (leprosy); 3 – 4 x daily (dermatitis herpetiformis).

Dosage range
Adults 50 – 100mg daily (leprosy); 150 – 200mg daily (dermatitis herpetiformis). *Children* Reduced dose according to age and weight.

Onset of effect
1 – 3 days (dermatitis herpetiformis); within a few weeks (leprosy).

Duration of action
30 – 150 hours.

Diet advice
A gluten-free diet may be recommended for dermatitis herpetiformis sufferers.

Storage
Keep in a closed container in a cool, dry place away from reach of children. Protect from light.

Missed dose
Take as soon as you remember. If your doses are scheduled 3– 4 times daily, and your next dose is due within 2 hours, take a single dose now and skip the next. If your doses are scheduled once daily, space the missed dose and next 10 – 12 hours apart.

Stopping the drug
Do not stop the drug without consulting your physician; symptoms may recur.

Exceeding the dose
An occasional unintentional extra dose is unlikely to cause problems. Large overdoses may cause nausea, vomiting, dizziness, and headache. Notify your physician.

SPECIAL PRECAUTIONS

Be sure to tell your physician if:
▼ You have impaired liver or kidney function.
▼ You have glucose-6-phosphate dehydrogenase (G6PD) deficiency or another blood disorder.
▼ You are allergic to sulfonamides.
▼ You are taking other medications.

Pregnancy
▼ Not usually prescribed. Safety in pregnancy not established. Discuss with your physician so that you can weigh the benefits of the drug against its possible risks.

Breast feeding
▼ Discuss with your physician. The drug passes into the breast milk and could cause hemolytic anemia in babies with glucose-6-phosphate dehydrogenase (G6PD) deficiency.

Infants and children
▼ Reduced dose necessary.

Over 60
▼ Reduced dose may be necessary.

Driving and hazardous work
▼ No known problems.

Alcohol
▼ No known problems.

POSSIBLE ADVERSE EFFECTS

Side effects are usually dose-related and rare at recommended doses. Loss of appetite and unusual tiredness or weakness may be signs of hemolytic anemia and should be reported promptly to your physician.

Symptom/effect	Frequency		Discuss with physician		Stop taking drug now	Call physician now
	Common	Rare	Only if severe	In all cases		
Nausea/vomiting	●		■			
Dizziness/headache	●		■			
Palpitations	●			■		
Loss of appetite	●			■		
Tiredness/weakness	●			■		
Jaundice	●			■		
Rash	●			■	▲	■

INTERACTIONS

Rifampin may lower the blood levels of dapsone, requiring an increase in dosage.

Probenecid reduces the excretion of dapsone by the kidneys.

PROLONGED USE

There is a risk of serious blood disorders and liver damage with prolonged use of dapsone.

Monitoring Periodic blood counts and liver function tests may be performed.

DESIPRAMINE

Brand names Norpramin, Pertofrane
Used in the following combined preparations None

GENERAL INFORMATION

Introduced in 1964, desipramine is an antidepressant of the tricyclic group. It is used in the treatment of severe, prolonged depression to elevate mood, increase physical activity, improve appetite, and restore interest in everyday activities.

Less sedating than some other antidepressants, desipramine is particularly useful for people who are withdrawn or apathetic. Another advantage of desipramine is that side effects such as dry mouth, dizziness, and blurred vision tend to be less severe than with other similar drugs.

An overdose may cause dangerous heart rhythms and coma, but in normal use serious side effects are rare.

INFORMATION FOR USERS

Your drug prescription is tailored for you. Do not alter dosage without checking with your physician.

How taken

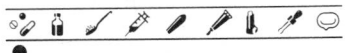

Tablets, capsules.

Frequency and timing of doses
1 – 4 x daily.

Adult dosage range
75 – 150mg daily (occasionally a higher dose is required).

Onset of effect
Some benefits and effects may appear within 14 days of starting treatment, but full benefits may not be felt for 4 weeks or more.

Duration of action
Following prolonged treatment, antidepressant effects may persist for up to 6 weeks. Adverse effects may wear off within days.

Diet advice
None.

Storage
Keep in a closed container in a cool, dry place away from reach of children. Protect from light.

Missed dose
Take as soon as you remember. If your next dose is due within 3 hours, take a single dose now and skip the next.

Stopping the drug
Do not stop the drug without consulting your physician, who may supervise a gradual reduction in dosage. Abrupt cessation may cause withdrawal symptoms.

OVERDOSE ACTION

 Seek immediate medical advice in all cases. Take emergency action if abnormal heart rhythms, seizures, or loss of consciousness occurs.

See Drug poisoning emergency guide (p.590).

SPECIAL PRECAUTIONS

Be sure to tell your physician if:
▼ You have heart problems.
▼ You have impaired kidney or liver function.
▼ You have epilepsy.
▼ You have glaucoma.
▼ You have prostate trouble.
▼ You are taking other medications.

 Pregnancy
▼ Not usually prescribed. Safety in pregnancy not established. Discuss with your physician so that you can weigh the benefits of the drug against its possible risks.

 Breast feeding
▼ Discuss with your physician. The drug passes into the breast milk and may affect the baby adversely.

 Infants and children
▼ Not recommended under 12 years. Reduced dose necessary for older children.

 Over 60
▼ Reduced dose may be necessary. Increased likelihood of adverse effects.

 Driving and hazardous work
▼ Avoid such activities until you have learned how the drug affects you, because the drug may cause drowsiness and blurred vision.

 Alcohol
▼ Avoid. Alcohol may increase the sedative effects of this drug.

PROLONGED USE

No problems expected.

POSSIBLE ADVERSE EFFECTS

The most common adverse effects of desipramine are the result of its mild anticholinergic action. These diminish if the dosage is reduced.

Symptom/effect	Frequency		Discuss with physician		Stop taking drug now	Call physician now
	Common	Rare	Only if severe	In all cases		
Sweating/flushing	●		■			
Dry mouth	●		■			
Blurred vision	●			■		
Dizziness/fainting	●			■		
Rash		●		■	▲	!
Palpitations		●		■	▲	!

INTERACTIONS

Monoamine oxidase inhibitors (MAOIs) There is a possibility of a serious interaction producing seizures and delirium. Such drugs are prescribed together only under strict supervision.

Heavy smoking This may reduce the antidepressant effect of desipramine.

Sedatives All drugs that have a sedative effect on the central nervous system are likely to increase the sedative properties of desipramine.

Antihypertensive drugs Desipramine may reduce the effect of some of these.

DEXAMETHASONE

Brand names Dalalone, Dalalone D.P., Decadron, Decadron-LA, Maxidex
Used in the following combined preparations AK-Trol, Dexacidin, Maxitrol, Neodecadron

GENERAL INFORMATION

Dexamethasone, introduced in 1958, is a long-acting corticosteroid prescribed for a variety of skin, soft tissue, and gastrointestinal conditions caused by allergy or inflammation. Dexamethasone can be injected into joints to relieve joint pain and stiffness due to rheumatoid arthritis (see p.146). It can be injected into a vein in the emergency treatment of shock.

The drug may also be prescribed to treat certain blood disorders, kidney disease, brain swelling (due to head injury, stroke, or a tumor), asthma, and emphysema. Eye drops are available to treat eye inflammation.

Low doses of dexamethasone taken for short periods rarely cause serious side effects. However, as with other corticosteroids, long-term treatment with high doses can cause unpleasant or dangerous side effects.

QUICK REFERENCE

Drug group Corticosteroid (p.169)
Overdose danger rating Low
Dependence rating Low
Prescription needed Yes
Available as generic Yes

INFORMATION FOR USERS

Your drug prescription is tailored for you. Do not alter dosage without checking with your physician.

How taken

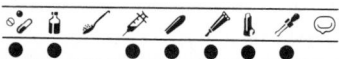

Tablets, liquid, injection, rectal suppositories, ointment, nasal spray, aerosol, eye drops.

Frequency and timing of doses
2 – 4 x daily.

Dosage range
0.75 – 9mg daily.

Onset of effect
Within 2 – 4 days.

Duration of action
Up to 4 days after last dose.

Diet advice
None.

Storage
Keep in a closed container in a cool, dry place away from reach of children.

Missed dose
Take as soon as you remember. If your next dose is within 2 hours, take a single dose now and skip the next.

Stopping the drug
Do not stop taking the drug without consulting your physician.

Exceeding the dose
An occasional unintentional extra dose is unlikely to be a cause for concern. But if you notice unusual symptoms, or if a large over-dose has been taken, notify your physician.

POSSIBLE ADVERSE EFFECTS

The more serious adverse effects only occur when dexamethasone is taken in high doses for long periods of time. These are carefully monitored during prolonged treatment. Other adverse effects tend to become less noticeable as your body adjusts to the drug.

Symptom/effect	Frequency		Discuss with physician		Stop taking drug now	Call physician now
	Common	Rare	Only if severe	In all cases		
Indigestion	●		■			
Weight gain	●		■			
Acne		●	■			
Fluid retention		●		■		
Muscle weakness		●		■		
Mood changes		●		■		

INTERACTIONS

Antidiabetic drugs Dexamethasone decreases the action of these drugs. Dosage may need to be adjusted to prevent abnormally high blood sugar.

Barbiturates These drugs may reduce the effectiveness of dexamethasone. The dosage may need to be adjusted accordingly.

Antihypertensive drugs Dexamethasone can cause fluid retention and elevate blood pressure, reducing the effects of antihypertensive drugs.

Vaccines Dexamethasone can interact dangerously with some vaccines. Vaccination should therefore be postponed until dexamethasone treatment is finished.

SPECIAL PRECAUTIONS

Be sure to tell your physician if:
▼ You have had a peptic ulcer.
▼ You have glaucoma.
▼ You have had tuberculosis.
▼ You have suffered from depression or mental illness.
▼ You have a herpes infection.
▼ You are taking other medications.

Pregnancy
▼ Not usually prescribed. May cause defects in the developing baby. Discuss with your physician so that you may weigh the benefits of the drug against its risks.

Breast feeding
▼ Discuss with your physician. The drug passes into the breast milk and may affect the baby adversely.

Infants and children
▼ Reduced dose necessary.

Over 60
▼ No known problems.

Driving and hazardous work
▼ No known problems.

Alcohol
▼ Avoid. Alcohol may increase the risk of peptic ulcer with this drug.

PROLONGED USE

Prolonged use of this drug can lead to glaucoma, cataracts, diabetes, fragile bones, and thin skin, and can retard growth in children.

DEXTROMETHORPHAN

Brand names Benylin DM, Delsym, Mediquell, Pedia Care 1, Sucrets
Used in the following combined preparations Benylin DME, Formula 44, Robitussin-DM, Tussi-Organidin DM

GENERAL INFORMATION

Dextromethorphan, introduced in 1958, is a non-narcotic cough suppressant available over the counter in a large number of cough remedies. The safest drug of its kind, it acts directly on the cough control center in the brain to relieve persistent dry cough.

It has little general sedative effect, and unlike the stronger narcotic cough suppressants it is unlikely to lead to dependence when taken as recommended.

Like other cough suppressants, it should not be used for phlegm-producing coughs because it may prolong a chest infection by preventing the normal elimination of sputum. Although the drug is less sedative than many similar drugs, drowsiness is the principal adverse effect.

QUICK REFERENCE

Drug group Cough suppressant (p.122)

Overdose danger rating Medium

Dependence rating Medium

Prescription needed No

Available as generic Yes

INFORMATION FOR USERS

Follow instructions on the label. Call your physician if symptoms worsen.

How taken

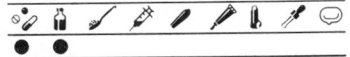

Tablets, lozenges, liquid.

Frequency and timing of doses
Up to 6 x daily as required.

Dosage range
Adults 10 – 30mg per dose up to a maximum of 120mg daily.
Children 2.5 – 7.5mg per dose up to a maximum of 30mg daily (2 – 6 years); 5 – 15mg per dose up to a maximum of 60mg daily (over 6 years).

Onset of effect
Within 30 minutes.

Duration of action
4 – 8 hours.

Diet advice
None.

Storage
Keep in a closed container in a cool, dry place away from reach of children.

Missed dose
Take as soon as you remember if needed to relieve coughing.

Stopping the drug
Can be safely stopped as soon as you no longer need it.

Exceeding the dose
An occasional unintentional extra dose is unlikely to cause problems. Large overdoses may cause nausea, vomiting, stomach pain, dizziness, and drowsiness. Notify your physician.

SPECIAL PRECAUTIONS

Be sure to tell your physician before taking this drug if:
▼ You have a liver disorder.
▼ You suffer from asthma or another serious respiratory problem.
▼ You are taking other medications.

Pregnancy
▼ Not usually prescribed. Safety in pregnancy not established. Large doses taken for a long time could cause dependence and breathing problems in the baby, but there is little or no risk with normal use in late pregnancy.

Breast feeding
▼ The drug passes into the breast milk, but at normal doses adverse effects on the baby are unlikely. Discuss with your physician.

Infants and children
▼ Not recommended under 2 years. Reduced dose necessary for older children.

Over 60
▼ Reduced dose necessary.

Driving and hazardous work
▼ Avoid such activities until you have learned how the drug affects you, because the drug may reduce alertness.

Alcohol
▼ Avoid. Alcohol may increase the sedative effects of this drug.

POSSIBLE ADVERSE EFFECTS

Adverse effects are rare when dextromethorphan is taken in recommended doses, and diminish if the dosage is reduced and as your body adjusts to the drug.

Symptom/effect	Frequency		Discuss with physician		Stop taking drug now	Call physician now
	Common	Rare	Only if severe	In all cases		
Dizziness/drowsiness		●		■		
Constipation		●		■		
Nausea/vomiting		●		■		
Abdominal pain		●		■		

INTERACTIONS

Sedatives All drugs that have a sedative effect on the central nervous system are likely to increase the sedative properties of dextromethorphan. Such drugs include antihistamines, anti-anxiety and sleeping drugs, antidepressants, narcotic analgesics, and antipsychotic drugs.

Monoamine oxidase inhibitors (MAOIs) These drugs may interact dangerously with dextromethorphan to cause excitation and fever.

PROLONGED USE

Dextromethorphan should not be taken for longer than 2 days except on the advice of a physician.

DIAZEPAM

Brand names Valium, Valrelease
Used in the following combined preparations None

GENERAL INFORMATION

Introduced in the early 1960s, diazepam is the best known and most widely used of a group of drugs known as the benzodiazepines. These drugs help relieve nervousness and tension, relax muscles, and encourage sleep. The actions and adverse effects of this group of drugs are described more fully on p.111.

Diazepam has a wide range of uses. Besides being commonly used in the treatment of anxiety and anxiety-related insomnia, it is prescribed as a muscle relaxant, in the treatment of alcohol withdrawal, and for the relief of epileptic seizures. Given intravenously, diazepam is used to sedate people undergoing certain uncomfortable medical procedures.

Diazepam can be habit-forming if taken regularly over a long period. Its effects may also diminish with time. Changing medications or tapering off diazepam for a while may restore desired effects. Treatment with diazepam is usually reviewed frequently.

QUICK REFERENCE

Drug group Benzodiazepine anti-anxiety drug (p.111), muscle-relaxant drug (p.148), and anticonvulsant drug (p.114)

Overdose danger rating Medium

Dependence rating High

Prescription needed Yes CIV

Available as generic Yes

INFORMATION FOR USERS

Your drug prescription is tailored for you. Do not alter dosage without checking with your physician.

How taken

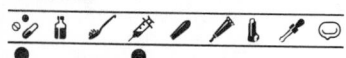

Tablets, capsules, injection, intravenously.

Frequency and timing of doses
1 – 4 x daily with food or milk.

Adult dosage range
Anxiety 4 – 40mg daily
Muscle spasm 6 – 40mg daily.

Onset of action
Immediate effect (intravenously); 30 minutes – 2 hours (other methods of administration).

Duration of action
Up to 24 hours. Some effect may last up to 4 days.

Diet advice
None.

Storage
Keep in a closed container in a cool, dry place away from reach of children.

Missed dose
No cause for concern, but take when you next feel you need the drug. If your next dose is due within 2 hours, take a single dose now and skip the next.

Stopping the drug
If you have been taking the drug continuously for less than 2 weeks, it can be safely stopped as soon as you feel you no longer need it. However, if you have been taking it for longer, consult your physician, who will supervise a gradual reduction in dosage. Stopping abruptly may lead to withdrawal symptoms (see p.111).

Exceeding the dose
An occasional unintentional extra dose is unlikely to cause problems. Larger overdoses may cause unusual drowsiness. Notify your physician.

SPECIAL PRECAUTIONS

Be sure to tell your physician if:
▼ You have severe respiratory disease.
▼ You have impaired kidney or liver function.
▼ You have had problems with alcohol or drug abuse.
▼ You are taking other medications.

Pregnancy
▼ Not usually prescribed. Safety in pregnancy not established. Discuss with your physician so that you can weigh the benefits of the drug against its possible risks.

Breast feeding
▼ Discuss with your physician. The drug passes into the breast milk. Its effects on the baby are not clearly known.

Infants and children
▼ Reduced dose necessary.

Over 60
▼ Reduced dose may be necessary. Increased likelihood of adverse effects.

Driving and hazardous work
▼ Avoid such activities until you have learned how the drug affects you, because the drug can cause reduced alertness and slowed reactions.

Alcohol
▼ Avoid. Alcohol may increase the sedative effects of this drug.

POSSIBLE ADVERSE EFFECTS

The principal adverse effects of this drug are related to its sedative properties. These effects, including drowsiness and dizziness, normally diminish after the first few days and, if troublesome, can often be reduced by adjustment of dosage.

Symptom/effect	Frequency		Discuss with physician		Stop taking drug now	Call physician now
	Common	Rare	Only if severe	In all cases		
Daytime drowsiness	●		■			
Dizziness/unsteadiness	●			■		
Headache		●	■			
Blurred vision		●		■		
Forgetfulness/confusion		●		■		
Rash		●		■		▲

INTERACTIONS

Sedatives All drugs that have a sedative effect on the central nervous system, including alcohol, are likely to increase the sedative properties of diazepam.

Cimetidine Breakdown of diazepam in the liver may be inhibited by cimetidine. This can cause a buildup of diazepam levels in the blood, which increases the likelihood of adverse effects.

PROLONGED USE

Regular use of this drug over several weeks can lead to a reduction in its effect as the body adapts. It may also be habit-forming when taken for extended periods. Severe withdrawal reactions have occurred.

DICUMAROL

Brand names None
Used in the following combined preparations None

GENERAL INFORMATION

Dicumarol is an anticoagulant used to prevent blood clots in areas where the blood flow is at its slowest, particularly in the legs and pelvis. Such clots can break off and travel through the bloodstream to lodge in the lungs, where they cause pulmonary embolism. It is also used to reduce the risk of clots forming in the heart in people with an irregular heartbeat, or after the insertion of artificial heart valves. These clots may travel via the arteries to the brain and cause a stroke.

Dicumarol is not easily absorbed by the body and so needs frequent monitoring to ensure that it is working effectively. Because full effects do not occur for 3 – 5 days after starting treatment, a faster-acting anticoagulant such as heparin is often used to complement the effects of dicumarol in the first few days of treatment.

The most serious adverse effect of dicumarol, as with all anticoagulants, is the risk of excessive bleeding, usually from overdosage.

QUICK REFERENCE

Drug group Anticoagulant drug (p.132)

Overdose danger rating High

Dependence rating Low

Prescription needed Yes

Available as generic Yes

INFORMATION FOR USERS

Your drug prescription is tailored for you. Do not alter dosage without checking with your physician.

How taken

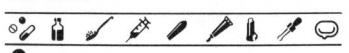

Tablets, capsules.

Frequency and timing of doses
Once daily, or less.

Dosage range
200 – 300mg on the first day, then 25 – 150mg daily.

Onset of effect
Within 24 – 48 hours, with full effect 3 – 5 days.

Duration of action
Up to 10 days after treatment is stopped.

Diet advice
High fiber foods help to prevent constipation.

Storage
Keep in a closed container in a cool, dry place away from reach of children.

Missed dose
Take as soon as you remember. If your next dose is due within 4 hours, take both doses now and return to your normal schedule for the following dose.

Stopping the drug
Do not stop the drug without consulting your physician; stopping the drug may lead to worsening of the underlying condition.

OVERDOSE ACTION

Seek immediate medical advice in all cases. Take emergency action if severe bleeding or loss of consciousness occurs.

See Drug poisoning emergency guide (p.590).

POSSIBLE ADVERSE EFFECTS

As with all anticoagulants, hemorrhaging is the most common adverse effect. Any bruising, dark stools, dark urine, or unusual bleeding should be reported to your physician.

Symptom/effect	Frequency		Discuss with physician		Stop taking drug now	Call physician now
	Common	Rare	Only if severe	In all cases		
Nausea/vomiting	●		■			
Loss of appetite	●		■			
Bleeding	●			■		▮
Abdominal pain/diarrhea		●	■			
Hair loss		●		■		
Rash		●		■		
Bruising		●		■		▮

INTERACTIONS

General note A wide variety of drugs interact with dicumarol, either by increasing or decreasing the anticlotting effect. These include barbiturates, oral contraceptives, diuretics, laxatives, and antibiotics.

Aspirin may significantly prolong or intensify the effect of dicumarol.

SPECIAL PRECAUTIONS

Be sure to tell your physician if:
▼ You have impaired kidney or liver function.
▼ You have high blood pressure.
▼ You have peptic ulcers.
▼ You are taking other medications either prescribed or over-the-counter.
▼ You bleed easily.

 Pregnancy
▼ Not usually prescribed. May cause defects in the unborn baby. Taken near the time of delivery it may also cause the mother to bleed excessively.

 Breast feeding
▼ The drug passes into the breast milk, but at normal doses adverse effects on the baby are uncommon. Discuss with your physician.

 Infants and children
▼ Reduced dose necessary.

 Over 60
▼ No special problems.

 Driving and hazardous work
▼ Avoid activities which involve a risk of even minor injury, because of the danger of bleeding.

 Alcohol
▼ Avoid. Alcohol may increase the anticoagulant effects of this drug.

Surgery and general anesthetics
▼ Dicumarol may need to be stopped before any surgery. Discuss this with your physician or dentist.

PROLONGED USE

No special problems.

Monitoring Regular monitoring of the blood is necessary to test the drug's capacity to interfere with coagulation; the dose may be adjusted accordingly.

A B C D E F G H I J K L M N O P Q R S T U V W X Y Z

DICYCLOMINE

Brand names Antispas, Bentyl, Neoquess
Used in the following combined preparations None

GENERAL INFORMATION

Available since 1950, dicyclomine is an *anticholinergic* antispasmodic drug that relieves cramping conditions caused by spasm in the gastrointestinal tract. Used to treat irritable bowel syndrome, the drug has also been prescribed to treat the condition known as "evening colic" in babies.

Because dicyclomine has anti-cholinergic properties, it is sometimes helpful in increasing bladder capacity in people with certain forms of incontinence.

Dicyclomine relieves symptoms, but does not cure the underlying condition. Additional treatment with other drugs and self-help measures may therefore be recommended by your physician.

QUICK REFERENCE

Drug group Antispasmodic antidiarrheal drug (p.138)

Overdose danger rating Medium

Dependence rating Low

Prescription needed Yes

Available as generic Yes

INFORMATION FOR USERS

Your drug prescription is tailored for you. Do not alter dosage without checking with your physician.

How taken

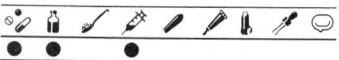

Tablets, capsules, liquid, injection.

Frequency and timing of doses
3 – 4 x daily.

Dosage range
Adults 30 – 80mg daily.
Children Reduced dose according to age and weight.

Onset of effect
Within 2 – 4 hours.

Duration of action
Approximately 6 hours.

Diet advice
None.

Storage
Keep in a closed container in a cool, dry place away from reach of children. Protect from light.

Missed dose
Take as soon as you remember. If your next dose is due within 2 hours, take a single dose now and skip the next.

Stopping the drug
Do not stop the drug without consulting your physician; symptoms may recur.

Exceeding the dose
An occasional unintentional extra dose is unlikely to cause problems. Large overdoses may cause drowsiness. Notify your physician.

SPECIAL PRECAUTIONS

Be sure to tell your physician if:
▼ You have impaired liver or kidney function.
▼ You have glaucoma.
▼ You have urinary problems.
▼ You have ulcerative colitis.
▼ You are taking other medications.

Pregnancy
▼ No evidence of risk to developing baby.

Breast feeding
▼ The drug passes into the breast milk, but at normal doses adverse effects on the baby are uncommon. Discuss with your physician.

Infants and children
▼ Reduced dose necessary.

Over 60
▼ No special problems.

Driving and hazardous work
▼ Avoid such activities until you have learned how the drug affects you, because the drug can cause drowsiness and blurred vision.

Alcohol
▼ Avoid. Alcohol may increase the sedative effects of this drug.

POSSIBLE ADVERSE EFFECTS

Most people do not notice any adverse effects when taking dicyclomine. Those that do occur are related to its anticholinergic properties and include drowsiness and dry mouth. Such symptoms may be overcome by an adjustment of dosage, or may pass off after a few days of usage as your body adjusts to the drug.

Symptom/effect	Frequency		Discuss with physician		Stop taking drug now	Call physician now
	Common	Rare	Only if severe	In all cases		
Dry mouth	●		■			
Headache		●	■			
Blurred vision		●	■			
Bloating		●	■			
Drowsiness/dizziness		●	■			
Difficulty passing urine		●		■		

INTERACTIONS

Sedatives All drugs that have a sedative effect on the central nervous system are likely to increase the sedative properties of dicyclomine.

PROLONGED USE

No problems expected.

DIETHYLSTILBESTROL

Brand names Stilbestrol, Stilphostrol
Used in the following combined preparations None

GENERAL INFORMATION

Diethylstilbestrol (DES), introduced in 1941, is a powerful synthetic estrogen preparation. It mimics the natural ovarian hormone, estradiol, and may be used in estrogen deficiency disorders such as ovarian failure, hypogonadism (underdeveloped ovaries), or menopausal symptoms. For these conditions, it is generally given with a progestin (see p.175).

In the form of vaginal suppositories, it is used to treat postmenopausal vaginal discomfort (atrophic vaginitis).

The major use of diethylstilbestrol, however, is in the treatment of advanced cancer of the prostate when it is given by mouth or by injection.

At high doses, diethylstilbestrol is effective in preventing pregnancy if started within 72 hours of intercourse. Because it causes severe nausea and vomiting at these doses, it is reserved for emergency treatment of rape and incest victims.

QUICK REFERENCE

Drug group Female sex hormone (p.175)

Overdose danger rating Low

Dependence rating Low

Prescription needed Yes

Available as generic Yes

INFORMATION FOR USERS

Your drug prescription is tailored for you. Do not alter dosage without checking with your physician.

How taken

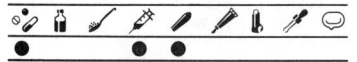

Tablets, injection, vaginal suppositories.

Frequency and timing of doses
Tablets Once daily, with food.
Vaginal suppositories Once daily.
Injections 1 – 2 x weekly (prostate cancer).

Adult dosage range
Replacement therapy 0.2 – 0.5mg daily.
Prostate cancer 1 – 3mg daily or 250 – 500mg once or twice depending on preparation.
Post-coital contraception 50mg daily for 5 days.

Onset of effect
Within 5 days (contraceptive effect); 10 – 20 days (other actions).

Duration of action
10 – 20 days.

Diet advice
None.

Storage
Keep in a closed container in a cool, dry place away from reach of children.

Missed dose
Take as soon as you remember. If your doses are scheduled once daily and your next dose is due within 12 hours, or if your doses are scheduled 2 – 3 times daily and your next dose is due within 2 hours, take a single dose now and skip the next.

Stopping the drug
Do not stop the drug without consulting your physician.

Exceeding the dose
An occasional unintentional extra dose is unlikely to be a cause for concern. But if you notice unusual symptoms, or if a large overdose has been taken, notify your physician.

SPECIAL PRECAUTIONS

Be sure to tell your physician if:
▼ You have heart failure or high blood pressure.
▼ You have had blood clots or a stroke.
▼ You have diabetes.
▼ You suffer from migraine or epilepsy.
▼ You are taking other medications.

Pregnancy
▼ Not prescribed.

Breast feeding
▼ Discuss with your physician. The drug passes into the breast milk and may affect the baby adversely.

Infants and children
▼ Not usually prescribed.

Over 60
▼ No special problems.

Driving and hazardous work
▼ No known problems.

Alcohol
▼ No known problems.

Surgery and general anesthetics
▼ Diethylstilbestrol may need to be stopped several weeks before you have major surgery. Discuss this with your physician.

POSSIBLE ADVERSE EFFECTS

The most common adverse effects are similar to symptoms in early pregnancy, but improve after 2 – 3 months of treatment.

A sudden, sharp pain in the chest, groin, or legs may indicate an abnormal blood clot and requires urgent medical attention.

Symptom/effect	Frequency		Discuss with physician		Stop taking drug now	Call physician now
	Common	Rare	Only if severe	In all cases		
Nausea/vomiting	●		■			
Tender/enlarged breasts	●		■			
Swollen feet/ankles	●		■			
Pain in chest/groin/legs		●		■	▲	∎

INTERACTIONS

Tobacco smoking Smoking increases the risk of serious adverse effects on the heart and circulation with diethylstilbestrol.

Anticonvulsant drugs, rifampin, and certain antibiotics These drugs may reduce the effectiveness of diethylstilbestrol.

Antihypertensive drugs and diuretics Diethylstilbestrol reduces the blood pressure-lowering effect of these drugs by causing fluid retention.

PROLONGED USE

Prolonged use of diethylstilbestrol without a progestin increases the risk of cancer of the uterus in women after the menopause. The risk of gallstones is also increased.

Monitoring Periodic general physical examinations and checks on blood pressure are usually required.

A B C D E F G H I J K L M N O P Q R S T U V W X Y Z

DIFLUNISAL

Brand name Dolobid
Used in the following combined preparations None

GENERAL INFORMATION

Diflunisal, introduced in 1982, is a non-steroidal anti-inflammatory drug (NSAID) with a prolonged duration of action. Like other members of this group, it reduces pain, stiffness, and inflammation.

Diflunisal is used to relieve discomfort in osteoarthritis and rheumatoid arthritis, although it does not cure the underlying disease. It is also effective for pain relief after minor operations

and dental treatment, and may also be given to treat sprains, strains, and some types of back pain.

Serious adverse effects with diflunisal are unusual, even with prolonged use. It is generally considered safer than aspirin, and rarely causes gastrointestinal bleeding, dizziness, ringing in the ears, or fluid buildup. However, diarrhea, nausea, indigestion, headache, or a skin rash may occur.

INFORMATION FOR USERS

Your drug prescription is tailored for you. Do not alter dosage without checking with your physician.

How taken

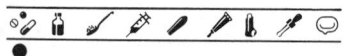

Tablets.

Frequency and timing of doses
2 x daily with food or milk (arthritis); 2 – 3 x daily (general pain relief).

Adult dosage range
500mg – 1g daily.

Onset of effect
Pain relief begins within 1 hour. Full anti-inflammatory effect in arthritic conditions may not be felt for up to 2 weeks.

Duration of action
8 – 14 hours.

Diet advice
None.

Storage
Keep in a closed container in a cool, dry place away from reach of children.

Missed dose
Take as soon as you remember. If your next dose is due within 2 – 4 hours, take a single dose now and skip the next.

Stopping the drug
When taken for short-term pain relief, diflunisal can be safely stopped as soon as you no longer need it. If prescribed for long-term treatment of arthritis, however, you should seek medical advice before stopping the drug.

Exceeding the dose
An occasional unintentional extra dose is unlikely to cause problems. Large overdoses may cause nausea, drowsiness, and disorientation. Notify your physician.

SPECIAL PRECAUTIONS

Be sure to tell your physician if:
▼ You have impaired kidney function.
▼ You have had a peptic ulcer, esophagitis, or acid indigestion.
▼ You have heart problems.
▼ You have high blood pressure.
▼ You have bleeding problems.
▼ You are allergic to aspirin.
▼ You are taking other medications.

 Pregnancy
▼ Not usually prescribed. May cause defects in the unborn baby and, taken in late pregnancy, may prolong labor. Discuss with your physician so that you may weigh the benefits of the drug against its risks.

 Breast feeding
▼ Discuss with your physician. The drug passes into the breast milk, but at normal doses adverse effects on the baby are uncommon.

 Infants and children
▼ Not recommended.

 Over 60
▼ Reduced dose may be necessary. Increased likelihood of adverse effects.

 Driving and hazardous work
▼ No known problems.

 Alcohol
▼ Avoid. Alcohol may increase the risk of stomach disorders with diflunisal.

POSSIBLE ADVERSE EFFECTS

Gastrointestinal side effects and headache are not generally serious and may diminish with continued use as your body adapts.

The occurrence of black or bloodstained bowel movements should be reported to your physician without delay.

Symptom/effect	Frequency		Discuss with physician		Stop taking drug now	Call physician now
	Common	Rare	Only if severe	In all cases		
Nausea/diarrhea	●		■			
Heartburn/indigestion	●		■			
Abdominal pain	●		■			
Rash	●			■	▲	
Headache		●	■			
Drowsiness/dizziness		●		■		
Wheezing/breathlessness		●		■	▲	▮

INTERACTIONS

General note Diflunisal interacts with a wide range of drugs to increase the risk of bleeding and/or peptic ulcers. Such drugs include oral anticoagulants, corticosteroids, other non-steroidal anti-inflammatory drugs (NSAIDs), aspirin, sulfinpyrazone, dipyridamole, some antibiotics, and valproic acid.

Antihypertensive drugs and diuretics The beneficial effects of these drugs may be reduced by diflunisal.

PROLONGED USE

There is an increased risk of bleeding from peptic ulcers and in the bowel with prolonged use of diflunisal.

DIGITOXIN

Brand names Crystodigin, Purodigin
Used in the following combined preparations None

GENERAL INFORMATION

Digitoxin is the main active ingredient in digitalis, a chemical found in the leaves of the foxglove plant. Strengthening the force of the heart's contractions, digitoxin is used in cases of heart failure. It is also effective in the treatment of abnormal heart rhythms and is particularly effective in slowing fast, irregular beats.

Because the effects of digitoxin are longer lasting than those of some other digitalis drugs, it continues to be effective even if a dose is missed. Unlike some other similar drugs, digitoxin can safely be used by people with impaired kidney function, though it must be used in these cases with caution and in reduced doses.

For digitoxin to be effective, the dose must be very close to toxic levels. The drug can accumulate in the body, and levels must be monitored regularly. Any unusual symptoms should be reported to your physician.

QUICK REFERENCE

Drug group Digitalis drug (p.124)
Overdose danger rating High
Dependence rating Low
Prescription needed Yes
Available as generic Yes

INFORMATION FOR USERS

Your drug prescription is tailored for you. Do not alter dosage without checking with your physician.

How taken

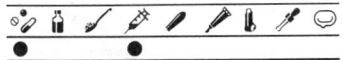

Tablets, injection.

Frequency and timing of doses
Every 6 – 8 hours for first few doses; once daily for maintenance.

Adult dosage range
0.05 – 0.2mg daily.

Onset of effect
1 – 4 hours (tablets); 25 minutes – 2 hours (injection).

Duration of action
5 – 9 days.

Diet advice
None.

Storage
Keep in a closed container in a cool, dry place away from reach of children.

Missed dose
Take the missed dose as soon as you remember. Take your next dose as usual.

Stopping the drug
Do not stop the drug without consulting your physician; symptoms may recur.

OVERDOSE ACTION

 Seek immediate medical advice in all cases. Take emergency action if severe nausea, vomiting, drowsiness, or loss of consciousness occurs.

See Drug poisoning emergency guide (p.590).

SPECIAL PRECAUTIONS

Be sure to tell your physician if:
▼ You have impaired liver function.
▼ You have thyroid disease.
▼ You are taking other medications.

 Pregnancy
▼ Not usually prescribed. Safety in pregnancy not established.

 Breast feeding
▼ Discuss with your physician. Effect on breast feeding uncertain.

 Infants and children
▼ Not usually prescribed.

 Over 60
▼ Reduced dose may be necessary. Increased likelihood of adverse effects.

 Driving and hazardous work
▼ No known problems.

 Alcohol
▼ No special problems.

PROLONGED USE

Digitoxin is toxic if it accumulates in the body over a period of time.

Monitoring Periodic checks on levels of the drug in the blood are usually performed.

POSSIBLE ADVERSE EFFECTS

Any adverse effect may be an early warning sign of an excessive buildup of digitoxin in the body. Report any symptoms to your physician without delay.

Symptom/effect	Frequency		Discuss with physician		Stop taking drug now	Call physician now
	Common	Rare	Only if severe	In all cases		
Tiredness or weakness	●			■		
Stomach pain	●			■		
Loss of appetite	●			■		
Nausea/vomiting	●			■		▮
Drowsiness/dizziness		●		■		▮
Blurred/yellow vision		●		■		▮

INTERACTIONS

Diuretics can lower levels of potassium in the body, and this increases the risk of adverse effects with digitoxin.

Quinidine and verapamil may increase the amount of digitoxin in the blood, which increases the risk of adverse effects.

Sympathomimetic drugs (ephedrine, epinephrine, isoproterenol) There is an increased risk of abnormal heart rhythms if these drugs are taken with digitoxin.

Phenobarbital and phenytoin reduce the effectiveness of digitoxin.

A
B
C
D
E
F
G
H
I
J
K
L
M
N
O
P
Q
R
S
T
U
V
W
X
Y
Z

DIGOXIN

Brand names Lanoxicaps, Lanoxin
Used in the following combined preparations None

GENERAL INFORMATION

Digoxin is the most widely used form of digitalis, a drug extracted from the leaves of the foxglove plant. It is given in the treatment of congestive heart failure and certain alterations of heart rhythm.

Digoxin slows down the rate of the heart so that each beat is more effective in pumping blood. In congestive heart failure, it also helps to control tiredness, breathlessness, and

fluid retention. Its effects are not as long-lasting as those of other digitalis drugs, and this makes any adverse reactions easier to control.

For digoxin to be effective, the dose must be very near the toxic dose, and treatment must be monitored closely. A number of adverse effects (see below) may indicate the toxic level is being reached and should be reported to your physician immediately.

QUICK REFERENCE

Drug group Digitalis drug (p.124)
Overdose danger rating High
Dependence rating Low
Prescription needed Yes
Available as generic Yes

INFORMATION FOR USERS

Your drug prescription is tailored for you. Do not alter dosage without checking with your physician.

How taken

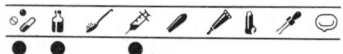

Tablets, capsules, liquid, injection.

Frequency and timing of doses
Up to 3 x daily while dosage is being established. Once daily for maintenance.

Dosage range
Adults 0.125 – 0.25mg daily (by mouth).
Children Reduced dose according to age and weight.

Onset of effect
Within a few minutes (injection); within 12 hours (by mouth).

Duration of action
Up to 4 days.

Diet advice
This drug may be more toxic if potassium

levels are depleted . Include fruit and vegetables in your diet (see p.178).

Storage
Keep in a closed container in a cool, dry place away from reach of children.

Missed dose
Take as soon as you remember. If your next dose is due within 4 hours, take both doses now and skip the next. Return to your normal schedule tomorrow.

Stopping the drug
Do not stop the drug without consulting your physician; stopping the drug may lead to worsening of the underlying condition.

OVERDOSE ACTION

 Seek immediate medical advice in all cases. Take emergency action if palpitations, severe weakness, chest pain, or loss of consciousness occurs.

See Drug poisoning emergency guide (p.590).

SPECIAL PRECAUTIONS

Be sure to tell your physician if:
▼ You have impaired kidney or liver function.
▼ You are taking other medications.

 Pregnancy
▼ Not usually prescribed. Safety in pregnancy not established. Discuss with your physician so that you can weigh the benefits of the drug against its possible risks.

 Breast feeding
▼ The drug passes into the breast milk, but at normal doses adverse effects on the baby are uncommon. Discuss with your physician.

 Infants and children
▼ Reduced dose necessary.

 Over 60
▼ Reduced dose may be necessary. Increased likelihood of adverse effects.

 Driving and hazardous work
▼ No known problems.

 Alcohol
▼ No special problems.

POSSIBLE ADVERSE EFFECTS

The possible adverse effects of digoxin are usually due to increased levels of the drug in the blood. Any symptoms should be reported to your physician without delay.

Symptom/effect	Frequency		Discuss with physician		Stop taking drug now	Call physician now
	Common	Rare	Only if severe	In all cases		
Tiredness	●		■			
Nausea/loss of appetite	●			■		
Confusion	●			■		
Visual disturbance	●			■		
Palpitations	●			■	▲	▮

PROLONGED USE

No problems expected.

Monitoring Periodic checks on blood levels of digoxin and body salts may be advised.

INTERACTIONS

General note Many drugs interact with digoxin. Do not take any medication without your physician's advice. Only the most important interactions are described below.

Diuretics may increase the risk of adverse effects from digoxin.

Anticholinergic drugs and antacids reduce the effects of digoxin. The effect of digoxin may increase when such drugs are stopped.

Anti-arrhythmic drugs may increase blood levels of digoxin.

DILTIAZEM

Brand name Cardizem
Used in the following combined preparations None

GENERAL INFORMATION

Introduced in 1984, diltiazem belongs to the group of drugs known as calcium channel blockers (p.129). These interfere with the conduction of signals in the muscles of the heart and blood vessels.

Diltiazem is mainly used in the treatment of angina and hypertension. When taken regularly for angina, it reduces the frequency of angina attacks but does not work quickly enough to reduce the pain.

Diltiazem does not adversely affect breathing and is of particular value for people who suffer from asthma, for whom other anti-angina drugs may not be suitable. Adverse effects include headache, nausea, and constipation.

INFORMATION FOR USERS

Your drug prescription is tailored for you. Do not alter dosage without checking with your physician.

How taken

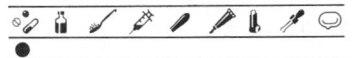

Tablets.

Frequency and timing of doses
4 x daily.

Adult dosage range
240 – 360mg daily.

Onset of effect
2 – 3 hours.

Duration of action
6 – 8 hours.

Diet advice
None.

Storage
Keep in a closed container in a cool, dry place away from reach of children.

Missed dose
Take as soon as you remember. If your next dose is due within 2 hours, take a single dose now and skip the next.

Stopping the drug
Do not stop taking the drug without consulting your physician; symptoms may recur.

Exceeding the dose
An occasional unintentional extra dose is unlikely to be a cause for concern. Large overdoses may cause dizziness. Notify your physician.

SPECIAL PRECAUTIONS

Be sure to tell your physician if:
▼ You have impaired kidney or liver function.
▼ You have heart failure.
▼ You are taking other medications.

Pregnancy
▼ Not usually prescribed. Safety in pregnancy not established. Discuss with your physician so that you can weigh the benefits of the drug against its possible risks.

Breast feeding
▼ Discuss with your physician. The drug passes into the breast milk and may affect the baby adversely.

Infants and children
▼ Not recommended.

Over 60
▼ Reduced dose may be necessary. Increased likelihood of adverse effects.

Driving and hazardous work
▼ Avoid such activities until you have learned how the drug affects you, because the drug may cause dizziness due to lowered blood pressure.

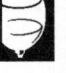
Alcohol
▼ Avoid. Alcohol may further reduce blood pressure, causing dizziness.

POSSIBLE ADVERSE EFFECTS

Diltiazem can cause a variety of minor symptoms that are common to other calcium channel blockers. These include headache, nausea, and constipation. The most serious effect is the possibility of a slowed heartbeat, which may cause tiredness or dizziness. These effects can sometimes be controlled by an adjustment in dosage.

Symptom/effect	Frequency		Discuss with physician		Stop taking drug now	Call physician now
	Common	Rare	Only if severe	In all cases		
Headache	●		■			
Loss of appetite/nausea	●		■			
Constipation	●		■			
Tiredness	●		■			
Dry mouth	●		■			
Leg and ankle swelling	●			■		
Dizziness/fainting		●		■		
Rash		●		■		▲

INTERACTIONS

Antihypertensive drugs Diltiazem increases their effects, leading to a further reduction in blood pressure.

Digoxin Blood levels and adverse effects of this drug may be increased if it is taken with diltiazem. The dosage of digoxin may need to be reduced.

PROLONGED USE

No problems expected.

Monitoring Periodic tests on liver function may be advised.

DIMENHYDRINATE

Brand name Dramamine
Used in the following combined preparations None

GENERAL INFORMATION

Introduced in 1949, dimenhydrinate is an antihistamine that is mainly used as an anti-emetic drug. It is especially effective for treating the nausea and vomiting that occur with vertigo. It is also prescribed to relieve the symptoms of inner ear disorders such as Ménière's disease and to prevent and treat motion sickness.

Dimenhydrinate is often effective in treating other forms of nausea and vomiting, including those caused by pregnancy and by drug and radiation treatments for cancer.

Like other antihistamines, dimenhydrinate has a sedative effect that can cause problems if you need to drive or operate machinery.

QUICK REFERENCE

Drug group Antihistamine (p.152) and anti-emetic drug (p.118)

Overdose danger rating Medium

Dependence rating Low

Prescription needed No

Available as generic Yes

INFORMATION FOR USERS

Follow the instructions on the label. Call your physician if symptoms worsen.

How taken

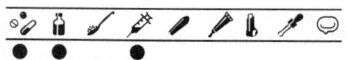

Tablets, liquid, injection.

Frequency and timing of doses
Adults every 4 hours.
Children every 6 – 8 hours. To prevent motion sickness the first dose should be taken 30 – 60 minutes before travel.

Dosage range
Adults 50 – 100mg per dose (maximum 400mg in 24 hours).
Children 2 - 6 years, 25mg per dose (maximum 75mg in 24 hours);
6 – 12 years, 25 – 50mg per dose (maximum 150mg in 24 hours).

Onset of effect
Within 30 minutes.

Duration of action
6 – 8 hours.

Diet advice
None.

Storage
Keep in a closed container in a cool, dry place away from reach of children.

Missed dose
Take when you remember. Adjust the timing of your next dose accordingly.

Stopping the drug
Can be safely stopped as soon as you no longer need it.

Exceeding the dose
An occasional unintentional extra dose is unlikely to cause problems. Larger overdoses may cause unusual drowsiness. Notify your physician.

POSSIBLE ADVERSE EFFECTS

The principal adverse effects of this drug are related to its *anticholinergic* properties and, if troublesome, can sometimes be reduced by adjustment of dosage.

Symptom/effect	Frequency		Discuss with physician		Stop taking drug now	Call physician now
	Common	Rare	Only if severe	In all cases		
Drowsiness	●		■			
Dry mouth	●		■			
Blurred vision	●			■		

INTERACTIONS

Sedatives All drugs that have a sedative effect on the central nervous system are likely to increase the sedative properties of dimenhydrinate. Such drugs include anti-anxiety and sleeping drugs, anti-depressants, narcotic analgesics, and antipsychotics.

SPECIAL PRECAUTIONS

Be sure to consult your physician before taking this drug if:
▼ You have impaired kidney or liver function.
▼ You have had glaucoma.
▼ You have prostate trouble.
▼ You are taking other medications.

Pregnancy
▼ No evidence of risk to baby.

Breast feeding
▼ Discuss with your physician. The drug passes into the breast milk. Its effects on the baby are not clearly known.

Infants and children
▼ Reduced dose necessary.

Over 60
▼ No special problems.

Driving and hazardous work
▼ Because of the possibility of drowsiness, avoid such activities until you have learned how the drug affects you.

Alcohol
▼ Avoid. Alcohol may increase the sedative effects of this drug.

PROLONGED USE

No special problems, but this drug should not be used for more than a few days except on medical advice.

DIPHENHYDRAMINE

Brand names Benadryl, Bendylate, Benylin, Valdrene
Used in the following combined preparations Benadryl Decongestant, Caladryl, Ziradryl

GENERAL INFORMATION

Diphenhydramine, introduced in 1945, is one of the oldest antihistamines and one of the most common over-the-counter sleeping preparations. It is used for treating allergies such as allergic rhinitis and urticaria (hives). Injected diphenhydramine is also used in the treatment of anaphylaxis and hypersensitivity reactions to food, drugs, or insect stings.

Because it has *anticholinergic*

properties, it is useful in the treatment of parkinsonism and movement disorders caused by antipsychotic drugs (p.113). It is also an effective anti-emetic, used to prevent and treat vertigo and motion sickness and to relieve nausea and vomiting in pregnancy. Syrup form relieves coughs.

Diphenhydramine has a marked sedative action and often causes drowsiness.

INFORMATION FOR USERS

Follow instructions on the label. Call your physician if symptoms worsen.

How taken

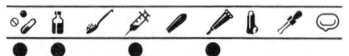

Capsules, liquid, injection, cream, lotion.

Frequency and timing of dose
By mouth 3 – 4 x daily (allergic conditions); every 4 hours (coughs); 30 minutes before travelling and before meals (motion sickness); 20 – 30 minutes before bedtime (insomnia).
Injection Every 6 hours (adults).
Cream, lotion As directed.

Dosage range
Adults 50 – 200 mg daily (by mouth) with a maximum dose of 150 mg daily for cough syrup.
Children Reduced dose according to age and weight. For cough syrup, up to 75 mg (30 ml) daily for children over 6 years.

Onset of effect
Within 60 minutes (by mouth), within 20 minutes (injection).

Duration of action
4 – 6 hours.

Diet advice
None.

Storage
Keep in a closed container in a cool, dry place away from reach of children. Do not freeze.

Missed dose
Take as soon as you remember. If your next dose is due within 2 hours, take a single dose now and skip the next.

Stopping the drug
Do not stop taking the drug without consulting your physician; symptoms may recur. Over-the-counter preparations can be stopped when you no longer need them.

Exceeding the dose
An occasional unintentional extra dose is unlikely to cause problems. Large overdoses may cause drowsiness or agitation. Notify your physician.

SPECIAL PRECAUTIONS

Be sure to consult your physician before taking this drug if:
▼ You have impaired liver function.
▼ You have had epileptic seizures.
▼ You have glaucoma.
▼ You have urinary difficulties.
▼ You are taking other medications.

Pregnancy
▼ No evidence of risk to developing baby.

Breast feeding
▼ Discuss with your physician. The drug passes into the breast milk and may make the baby drowsy or irritable. It may also inhibit milk secretion.

Infants and children
▼ Not recommended for newborn or premature infants. Reduced dose necessary for older children. Cough syrup should not be given to children under 6 years except on the advice of a physician.

Over 60
▼ Reduced dose may be necessary. Increased likelihood of adverse effects.

Driving and hazardous work
▼ Avoid such activities until you have learned how the drug affects you, because the drug can cause drowsiness.

Alcohol
▼ Avoid. Alcohol may increase the sedative effects of this drug.

POSSIBLE ADVERSE EFFECTS

Drowsiness is the commonest adverse effect of diphenhydramine. Other side effects, such as dry mouth and blurred vision, are due to its *anticholinergic* action.

Symptom/effect	Frequency		Discuss with physician		Stop taking drug now	Call physician now
	Common	Rare	Only if severe	In all cases		
Drowsiness	●		■			
Dry mouth	●		■			
Nausea/abdominal pain		●	■			
Blurred vision		●	■			
Urinary difficulties		●		■		
Disorientation/excitation		●		■		

PROLONGED USE

The effect of the drug may become weaker with prolonged use over a period of weeks or months as the body adapts. Transfer to another drug may be recommended.

INTERACTIONS

Sedatives These drugs are likely to enhance the sedative effect of this drug.

Anticholinergic drugs These are likely to increase the anticholinergic effects of diphenhydramine.

Monoamine oxidase inhibitors (MAOIs) There is a risk of a dangerous rise in blood pressure if diphenhydramine is taken within 14 days of MAOIs.

DIPHENOXYLATE

Brand names None
Used in the following combined preparation Lomotil

GENERAL INFORMATION

Diphenoxylate, introduced in 1960, is a narcotic antidiarrheal drug chemically related to the opiate analgesics. It reduces bowel contractions and consequently the frequency and fluidity of bowel movements.

Available as tablets and liquid, it is used for the relief of sudden or recurrent bouts of diarrhea.

It is not suitable for diarrhea caused by infection, antibiotics, or poisons because it may delay recovery by slowing the expulsion of harmful substances from the bowel. It is also potentially dangerous in ulcerative colitis. Diphenoxylate can cause toxic megacolon, a dangerous dilation of the bowel that shuts off the blood supply to the wall of the bowel and increases the risk of perforation.

At recommended doses, serious adverse effects are rare. To guard against addiction, atropine is added to all diphenoxylate preparations. If these are taken in excessive amounts, the atropine will cause highly unpleasant *anticholinergic* reactions. Diphenoxylate is especially dangerous for young children. Be sure to store it out of their reach.

QUICK REFERENCE

Drug group Narcotic antidiarrheal drug (p.138)

Overdose danger rating Medium

Dependence rating Medium

Prescription needed Yes

Available as generic Yes

INFORMATION FOR USERS

Your drug prescription is tailored for you. Do not alter dosage without checking with your physician.

How taken

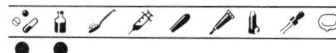

Tablets, liquid.

Frequency and timing of doses
3 – 4 x daily.

Dosage range
Adults 10 – 20mg daily.
Children Reduced dose necessary according to age and weight.

Onset of effect
Within 1 hour. Control of diarrhea may take 1 – 6 hours.

Duration of action
Up to 24 hours.

Diet advice
Ensure adequate fluid intake during an attack of diarrhea.

Storage
Keep in a closed container in a cool, dry place away from reach of children. Protect from light.

Missed dose
Take as soon as you remember. If your next dose is due within 3 hours, take a single dose now and skip the next.

Stopping the drug
Can be safely stopped as soon as you no longer need it.

Exceeding the dose
An occasional unintentional extra dose is unlikely to cause problems. Large overdoses may cause unusual drowsiness, dryness of the mouth and skin, restlessness, and in extreme cases, loss of consciousness. Notify your physician.

POSSIBLE ADVERSE EFFECTS

Side effects occur infrequently with diphenoxylate. If abdominal pain or distension, nausea, vomiting, or severe constipation occurs, notify your physician.

Symptom/effect	Frequency		Discuss with physician		Stop taking drug now	Call physician now
	Common	Rare	Only if severe	In all cases		
Drowsiness	●		■			
Restlessness		●	■			
Headache		●	■			
Blurred vision		●	■			
Constipation		●		■	▲	
Nausea/vomiting		●		■	▲	
Abdominal swelling/pain		●		■	▲	∎

INTERACTIONS

Sedatives All drugs that have a sedative effect on the central nervous system may increase the sedative effect of diphenoxylate.

Monoamine oxidase inhibitors (MAOIs) There is a risk of a dangerous rise in blood pressure if MAOIs are taken together with diphenoxylate.

SPECIAL PRECAUTIONS

Be sure to tell your physician if:
▼ You have impaired liver function.
▼ You have severe abdominal pain.
▼ You have bloodstained diarrhea.
▼ You have recently taken antibiotics.
▼ You have glaucoma.
▼ You have urinary difficulties.
▼ You are taking other medications.

Pregnancy
▼ Not usually prescribed. Safety in pregnancy not established. Discuss with your physician so that you can weigh the benefits of the drug against its possible risks.

Breast feeding
▼ The drug passes into the breast milk and may cause drowsiness in the baby. Discuss with your physician.

Infants and children
▼ Reduced dose necessary. Not recommended for children under 2 years. Tablets not recommended for children under 12 years.

Over 60
▼ Reduced dose may be necessary.

Driving and hazardous work
▼ Avoid such activities until you have learned how the drug affects you, because the drug may cause drowsiness.

Alcohol
▼ Avoid. Alcohol may increase the sedative effects of this drug.

PROLONGED USE

No problems expected at recommended doses.

DIPYRIDAMOLE

Brand name Persantine
Used in the following combined preparations None

GENERAL INFORMATION

Dipyridamole was originally introduced in the late 1970s as an anti-angina drug, theoretically improving the capacity of those with angina to exercise. Its efficacy in this regard was never demonstrated, however. With more effective drugs now available for that purpose, dipyridamole is used as an antiplatelet drug. It is usually given with aspirin to "thin" the blood of people who have just had a heart attack, coronary artery surgery, or a stroke. It is also given to reduce the frequency of transient ischemic attacks (temporary strokes). Its action reduces platelet stickiness, preventing blood clotting within arteries.

The effectiveness of dipyridamole in these conditions has not been clearly shown. However, it is believed to be particularly useful for preventing clots following heart valve replacement when used with aspirin or warfarin.

INFORMATION FOR USERS

Your drug prescription is tailored for you. Do not alter dosage without checking with your physician.

How taken

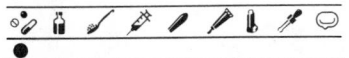

Tablets, capsules.

Frequency and timing of doses
3 – 4 x daily one hour before meals.

Adult dosage range
75 – 400mg daily.

Onset of action
Within 30 – 60 minutes. Full therapeutic effect may not be felt for 2 – 3 weeks.

Duration of action
Up to 8 hours.

Diet advice
None.

Storage
Keep in a closed container in a cool, dry place away from reach of children. Protect from light.

Missed dose
Take as soon as you remember. If your next dose is due within 2 hours, take a single dose now and skip the next.

Stopping the drug
Do not stop taking the drug without consulting your physician; withdrawal of the drug could lead to abnormal blood clotting.

Exceeding the dose
An occasional unintentional extra dose is unlikely to cause problems, but you may experience dizziness or vomiting. Notify your physician.

SPECIAL PRECAUTIONS

Be sure to tell your physician if:
▼ You have low blood pressure.
▼ You suffer from migraine.
▼ You are taking other medications.

Pregnancy
▼ Not usually prescribed. Safety in pregnancy not established. Discuss with your physician so that you can weigh the benefits of the drug against its possible risks.

Breast feeding
▼ The drug passes into the breast milk, but at normal doses adverse effects on the baby are uncommon. Discuss with your physician.

Infants and children
▼ Not recommended.

Over 60
▼ No special problems.

Driving and hazardous work
▼ Avoid such activities until you have learned how the drug affects you, because of the possibility of dizziness and faintness.

Alcohol
▼ No known problems.

POSSIBLE ADVERSE EFFECTS

Adverse effects are rare. Possible symptoms include dizziness, headache, faintness, nausea, and rash. In rare cases, it may aggravate angina.

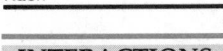

Symptom/effect	Frequency		Discuss with physician		Stop taking drug now	Call physician now
	Common	Rare	Only if severe	In all cases		
Nausea	●		■			
Headache		●	■			
Flushing		●	■			
Dizziness/faintness		●			■	
Rash		●		■		▲

PROLONGED USE

No known problems.

INTERACTIONS

Anticoagulant drugs The effects of these drugs are increased by dipyridamole, increasing the risk of uncontrolled bleeding. The dosage of the anticoagulant should be reduced accordingly.

DISOPYRAMIDE

Brand names Norpace, Norpace CR
Used in the following combined preparations None

GENERAL INFORMATION

Introduced as an anti-arrhythmic drug in 1978, disopyramide is used to treat irregular heart rhythms, particularly cases of rapid heartbeat. It has a mild *anticholinergic* action, and some of its less serious adverse effects are connected to this. Because it reduces the force of the heartbeat, it can worsen existing heart failure and low blood pressure. These effects may be more common with disopyramide than with other anti-arrhythmics. Since disopyramide can lower blood sugar levels, monitoring may be necessary, and people with diabetes must use the drug with caution.

INFORMATION FOR USERS

Your drug prescription is tailored for you. Do not alter dosage without checking with your physician.

How taken

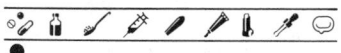

Capsules.

Frequency and timing of doses
4 x daily or every 12 hours (slow-release capsules).

Adult dosage range
Adults 400 – 800mg daily.
Children Reduced dose according to age and weight.

Onset of effect
Within 2 hours.

Duration of action
6 – 7 hours or up to 12 hours (slow-release capsules).

Diet advice
None.

Storage
Keep in a closed container in a cool, dry place away from reach of children.

Missed dose
Take as soon as you remember. If your next dose is due within 2 hours, take a single dose now and skip the next.

Stopping the drug
Do not stop the drug without consulting your physician; stopping the drug may lead to worsening of the underlying condition.

OVERDOSE ACTION

Seek immediate medical advice in all cases. Take emergency action if consciousness is lost.

See Drug poisoning emergency guide (p.590).

SPECIAL PRECAUTIONS

Be sure to tell your physician if:
▼ You have impaired kidney or liver function.
▼ You have heart failure.
▼ You have low blood pressure.
▼ You have had glaucoma.
▼ You have prostate trouble.
▼ You have diabetes.
▼ You are taking other medications.

Pregnancy
▼ Not usually prescribed. Safety in pregnancy not established. Discuss with your physician so that you can weigh the benefits of the drug against its possible risks.

Breast feeding
▼ Discuss with your physician. The drug passes into breast milk and may affect the baby adversely.

Infants and children
▼ Not usually prescribed. Reduced dose necessary.

Over 60
▼ No special problems.

Driving and hazardous work
▼ Avoid such activities until you have learned how the drug affects you, because the drug can cause dizziness and drowsiness.

Alcohol
▼ Avoid. Alcohol may increase the adverse effects of this drug.

POSSIBLE ADVERSE EFFECTS

Some of the possible adverse effects of this drug are mainly the result of its *anticholinergic* action. These include dry mouth, constipation, and blurred vision. The most serious adverse effect is the possibility of worsening existing heart failure or low blood pressure. Some of these problems can be overcome by an adjustment in dosage.

Symptom/effect	Frequency		Discuss with physician		Stop taking drug now	Call physician now
	Common	Rare	Only if severe	In all cases		
Dry mouth	●		■			
Constipation	●		■			
Blurred vision	●		■			
Nausea/vomiting		●		■		
Dizziness/fatigue		●		■		
Rash		●		■	▲	

PROLONGED USE

No problems expected.

Monitoring Periodic checks on blood sugar levels may be advised.

INTERACTIONS

Phenytoin The effect of disopyramide is reduced by this drug.

Rifampin The effect of disopyramide is reduced by this drug.

DISULFIRAM

Brand name Antabuse
Used in the following combined preparations None

GENERAL INFORMATION

Since its introduction in 1948, disulfiram has been used to help alcoholics maintain a regimen of abstinence. The drug does not cure alcoholism but provides a powerful deterrent to drinking.

If you are taking disulfiram as directed and drink even a small amount of alcohol, serious and highly unpleasant reactions follow. These can include: flushing, throbbing headache, breathlessness, nausea, thirst, palpitations, dizziness, and fainting. Such reactions may last from 30 minutes to several hours, leaving the person feeling drowsy and sleepy. Because the reactions can also include unconsciousness, it may be wise to carry a card indicating that you are taking disulfiram and listing the person to notify in an emergency.

When a person takes both disulfiram and alcohol, a toxic substance (acetaldehyde) that is manufactured in the body and ordinarily broken down rises to higher concentrations in the blood, thereby triggering the unwelcome reactions. Many physicians who prescribe disulfiram for alcoholism give a small test dose of alcohol a few days after treatment is started to give the patient an idea of what may happen. Many physicians also recommend that disulfiram treatment be combined with alcoholism counseling programs.

QUICK REFERENCE

Drug group Alcohol abuse deterrent
Overdose danger rating Medium
Dependence rating Low
Prescription needed Yes
Available as generic Yes

INFORMATION FOR USERS

Your drug prescription is tailored for you. Do not alter dosage without checking with your physician.

How taken

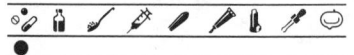

Tablets

Frequency and timing of doses
Once daily.

Adult dosage range
500mg (starting dose for first week or two), 125 – 500mg (maintenance dose).

Onset of effect
Interaction with alcohol occurs within a few minutes of dosing with alcohol.

Duration of action
Interaction with alcohol occurs for about 6 days after the last dose of disulfiram.

Diet advice
Avoid all alcoholic drinks even in very small amounts. Food, fermented vinegar, mouthwashes, medicines, and lotions containing alcohol should also be avoided.

Storage
Keep in a closed container in a cool, dry place away from reach of children.

Missed dose
Take as soon as you remember. If your next dose is due within 2 hours, take a single dose now and skip the next.

Stopping the drug
Do not stop taking the drug without consulting your physician.

Exceeding the dose
An occasional unintentional extra dose is unlikely to cause problems. Large overdoses may cause a temporary increase in adverse effects. Notify your physician.

SPECIAL PRECAUTIONS

Be sure to tell your physician if
▼ You have kidney disease, cirrhosis, or liver insufficiency.
▼ You have heart problems or coronary artery disease.
▼ You have had epileptic seizures.
▼ You have diabetes.
▼ You have an underactive thyroid.
▼ You are taking other medications.

Pregnancy
▼ Not usually prescribed. Safety in pregnancy not established. Discuss with your physician so that you can weigh the benefits of the drug against its possible risks.

Breast feeding
▼ Discuss with your physician. The drug passes into the breast milk and may affect the baby adversely.

Over 60
▼ Reduced dose necessary.

Driving and hazardous work
▼ Avoid such activities until you have learned how the drug affects you, because the drug can cause blurred vision, drowsiness, and dizziness.

Alcohol
▼ Never drink while under treatment with disulfiram. Alcohol may interact dangerously with this drug.

POSSIBLE ADVERSE EFFECTS

Adverse effects to disulfiram usually disappear when you get used to taking the drug. If they continue indefinitely or become severe, the dosage may need to be adjusted.

Symptom/effect	Frequency		Discuss with physician		Stop taking drug now	Call physician now
	Common	Rare	Only if severe	In all cases		
Headache/drowsiness	●		■			
Metallic or garlic taste	●		■			
Nausea/vomiting		●	■			
Temporary impotence		●	■			
Blurred vision		●		■		

INTERACTIONS

Phenytoin The blood levels of this drug are increased when taken with disulfiram.

Anticoagulants Disulfiram increases the anticoagulant effect of these drugs.

Isoniazid Disulfiram may markedly increase the adverse effects of this drug.

PROLONGED USE

Not usually prescribed for long-term use because of the possibility of eye damage and nerve damage. It is wise to carry a card indicating you are taking disulfiram with instructions as to who should be notified in an emergency.

DOXEPIN

Brand names Adapin, Sinequan
Used in the following combined preparations None

GENERAL INFORMATION

Introduced in 1969, doxepin belongs to a class of antidepressant drugs known as the tricyclics (see Antidepressant drugs, p.112). Used in the treatment of major depressive episodes in severe depression and manic (bipolar) depression, it elevates mood, increases physical activity, improves appetite, and renews interest in everyday activities. Doxepin has a stronger sedative effect than some of the other tricyclic antidepressants and is therefore particularly useful when depression is accompanied by anxiety and insomnia. Taken at night, it may reduce the need for sleeping drugs.

Doxepin can cause a variety of minor side effects (see below).

INFORMATION FOR USERS

Your drug prescription is tailored for you. Do not alter dosage without checking with your physician.

How taken

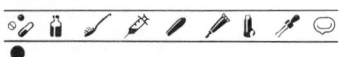

Capsules.

Frequency and timing of doses
1 – 3 x daily.

Adult dosage range
75 – 150mg daily (starting dose); gradually increased if necessary.

Onset of effect
Some benefits and effects may appear within hours, but full antidepressant effect may not be felt for 2 – 6 weeks.

Duration of action
Following prolonged treatment antidepressant effect may persist for up to 6 weeks. Adverse effects wear off within a few days.

Diet advice
None.

Storage
Keep in a closed container in a cool, dry place away from the reach of children.

Missed dose
Take as soon as you remember. If your next dose is due within 3 hours, take a single dose now and skip the next.

Stopping the drug
Do not stop the drug without consulting your physician. Stopping abruptly sometimes causes withdrawal symptoms (see p.112), and your original symptoms may recur.

OVERDOSE ACTION

 Seek immediate medical advice in all cases. Take emergency action if consciousness is lost.

See Drug poisoning emergency guide (p.590).

SPECIAL PRECAUTIONS

Be sure to tell your physician if:
▼ You have heart problems.
▼ You have had epileptic seizures.
▼ You have impaired kidney or liver function.
▼ You have had glaucoma.
▼ You have urinary difficulties.
▼ You are taking other medications.

 Pregnancy
▼ Not usually prescribed. Safety in pregnancy not established. Discuss with your physician so that you can weigh the benefits of the drug against its possible risks.

 Breast-feeding
▼ Discuss with your physician. The drug passes into the breast milk and may affect the baby adversely.

 Infants and children
▼ Not usually prescribed.

 Over 60
▼ Reduced dose may be necessary. Increased likelihood of adverse effects.

 Driving and hazardous work
▼ Avoid until you know how the drug affects you, because of the possibility of blurred vision and reduced alertness.

 Alcohol
▼ Avoid. Alcohol may increase the sedative effects of this drug.

Surgery and general anesthetics
▼ Doxepin treatment may need to be stopped before you have a general anesthetic. Discuss this with your physician or dentist before any operation.

POSSIBLE ADVERSE EFFECTS

The possible adverse effects of this drug are mainly the result of its *anticholinergic* action and its blocking action on the transmission of signals in the heart. Some problems can be overcome by medically supervised adjustment of dosage.

Symptom/effect	Frequency		Discuss with physician		Stop taking drug now	Call physician now
	Common	Rare	Only if severe	In all cases		
Drowsiness	●		■			
Sweating/flushing	●		■			
Dry mouth	●		■			
Blurred vision	●			■		
Dizziness/fainting	●			■		
Rash		●		■	▲	
Urinary difficulties		●		■	▲	
Palpitations		●		■	▲	■

INTERACTIONS

Sedatives All drugs that have a sedative effect are likely to increase the sedative properties of doxepin.

Antihypertensive drugs Doxepin counteracts some of these drugs, especially guanethidine and clonidine.

Monoamine oxidase inhibitors (MAOIs) A serious interaction between these drugs and doxepin may occur, producing seizures and delirium.

Heavy smoking This may reduce the antidepressant effect of doxepin.

PROLONGED USE

No known problems expected.

DOXORUBICIN

Brand name Adriamycin
Used in the following combined preparations None

GENERAL INFORMATION

Introduced in 1974, doxorubicin is one of the most effective anticancer drugs that has ever been developed. It is prescribed to treat a wide variety of cancers, usually in conjunction with other anticancer drugs. Doxorubicin is an effective treatment for acute leukemia and for cancer of the lymph nodes (Hodgkin's disease), lung, breast, bladder, stomach, thyroid, and reproductive organs.

Nausea and vomiting are the most common side effects of doxorubicin.

Although unpleasant, these symptoms (usually after an injection) tend to be less severe as the body adjusts to treatment. The drug may stain the urine bright red, though no harm is done. More seriously, because doxorubicin interferes with the production of blood cells, blood-clotting disorders, anemia, and infections may occur. Blood counts are carefully monitored. Hair loss is also a common side effect. Dose-dependent changes in heart rhythm and heart failure are also risks.

INFORMATION FOR USERS

This drug is given only under medical supervision and is not for self-administration.

How taken

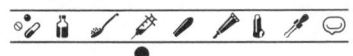

Injection.

Frequency and timing of doses
Every 3 – 4 weeks.

Adult dosage range
Dosage is determined individually according to body height, weight, and response.

Onset of effect
Some adverse effects may appear within one hour of starting treatment, but full beneficial effects may not be felt for up to 4 weeks.

Duration of action
Adverse effects can persist for up to 2 weeks after stopping treatment.

Diet advice
None.

Storage
Not applicable. The drug is not normally kept in the home.

Missed dose
The drug is administered in the hospital under close medical supervision. If for some reason you miss a dose, contact your physician as soon as you can.

Stopping the drug
Discuss with your physician. Stopping the drug prematurely may lead to a worsening of the underlying condition.

Exceeding the dose
Overdosage is unlikely since treatment is carefully monitored.

SPECIAL PRECAUTIONS

Doxorubicin is prescribed only under close medical supervision, taking account of your present condition and medical history.

Pregnancy
▼ Not usually prescribed. Doxorubicin may cause birth defects or premature birth. Discuss with your physician so that you can weigh the benefits of the drug against its risks.

Breast feeding
▼ Discontinue breast feeding. The drug passes into the breast milk and may affect the baby adversely.

Infants and children
▼ Reduced dose necessary.

Over 60
▼ Reduced dose may be necessary. Increased risk of adverse effects.

Driving and hazardous work
▼ No known problems.

Alcohol
▼ No known problems.

POSSIBLE ADVERSE EFFECTS

Nausea and vomiting generally occur within an hour or so of injection. Hair loss and loss of appetite are also experienced by many people. Palpitations may be a symptom of an adverse effect of the drug on the heart. Since treatment with this drug is closely supervised in the hospital, all adverse effects are monitored.

Symptom/effect	Frequency		Discuss with physician		Stop taking drug now	Call physician now
	Common	Rare	Only if severe	In all cases		
Nausea/vomiting	●			■		
Loss of appetite	●			■		
Hair loss	●			■		
Diarrhea		●		■		
Mouth ulcers		●		■		
Palpitations		●		■		■

INTERACTIONS

Drugs for gout Doxorubicin may increase the level of uric acid in the blood. Dosage of drugs for gout may need to be increased accordingly.

PROLONGED USE

Prolonged use of doxorubicin may reduce the activity of the bone marrow, leading to reduced production of all types of blood cell. It may also affect the heart adversely.

Monitoring Periodic checks on blood composition are usually required. Regular heart examinations are also carried out.

DOXYCYCLINE

Brand names Doryx, Vibramycin, Vibramycin IV, Vibra Tabs
Used in the following combined preparations None

GENERAL INFORMATION

Introduced in 1967, doxycycline is a member of the tetracycline group of antibiotics. Longer acting than some other drugs in this group, it is mainly used in the treatment of chronic prostatitis, pelvic inflammatory disease, and flare-ups of infection in chronic bronchitis. It is particularly effective against chlamydial infection. Doxycycline is also occasionally used to prevent and treat traveler's diarrhea.

It is less likely to cause diarrhea as a side effect than other tetracyclines, and absorption of the drug is not significantly impaired by food. It can therefore be taken with meals to reduce side effects such as nausea or indigestion. Doxycycline is also safe (unlike other tetracyclines) for people with impaired kidney function. Like other tetracyclines, doxycycline can damage developing teeth and is therefore usually not prescribed for young children or pregnant women.

QUICK REFERENCE

Drug group Tetracycline antibiotic (p.156)

Overdose danger rating Low

Dependence rating Low

Prescription needed Yes

Available as generic Yes

INFORMATION FOR USERS

Your drug prescription is tailored for you. Do not alter dosage without checking with your physician.

How taken

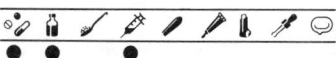

Tablets, capsules, liquid, injection.

Frequency and timing of doses
1 – 2 x daily.

Dosage range
Adults 100 – 200mg daily.
Children Reduced dose according to age and weight.

Onset of effect
1 – 2 days.

Duration of action
1 – 2 days.

Diet advice
None.

Storage
Keep in a closed container in a cool, dry place away from reach of children.

Missed dose
Take as soon as you remember. If your next dose is due within 8 hours, take a single dose now and skip the next.

Stopping the drug
Take the full course. Even if you feel better, the original infection may still be present and symptoms may recur if treatment is stopped too soon.

Exceeding the dose
An occasional unintentional extra dose is unlikely to be a cause for concern. But if you notice unusual symptoms, or if a large overdose has been taken, notify your physician.

SPECIAL PRECAUTIONS

Be sure to tell your physician if:
▼ You have previously suffered an allergic reaction to a tetracycline antibiotic.
▼ You are taking other medications.

Pregnancy
▼ Not usually prescribed. May discolor the teeth of the developing baby.

Breast feeding
▼ Discuss with your physician. The drug passes into the breast milk and may lead to damage to the baby's teeth.

Infants and children
▼ Not recommended under 8 years old. Reduced dose necessary for older children.

Over 60
▼ No special problems.

Driving and hazardous work
▼ No known problems.

Alcohol
▼ No known problems.

POSSIBLE ADVERSE EFFECTS

Adverse effects from doxycycline are rare, although some people may experience nausea, vomiting, or diarrhea. Other rare adverse effects include rash, itching, and increased sensitivity of the skin to sunlight, which may cause a rash to develop.

Symptom/effect	Frequency		Discuss with physician		Stop taking drug now	Call physician now
	Common	Rare	Only if severe	In all cases		
Nausea/vomiting		●	■			
Diarrhea		●	■			
Rash/itching		●		■	▲	▐
Light-sensitive rash		●		■	▲	▐

PROLONGED USE

No problems expected.

INTERACTIONS

Barbiturates, carbamazepine, and phenytoin All these drugs reduce the effectiveness of doxycycline. The doxycycline dosage may need to be increased accordingly.

Oral anticoagulant drugs Doxycycline increases the anticoagulant action of these drugs.

Lithium Doxycycline may increase blood levels of lithium.

Antacids, iron, and bismuth preparations may interfere with doxycycline absorption.

Penicillin Doxycycline interferes with the antibacterial action of penicillin.

Oral contraceptives Doxycycline can reduce the effectiveness of oral contraceptives.

ECONAZOLE

Brand name Spectazole
Used in the following combined preparations None

GENERAL INFORMATION

Econazole is a relatively new, effective, fast-acting antifungal drug. Since its introduction in 1983, it has been widely used in the form of a cream for the treatment of tinea (ringworm) infections of the skin such as athlete's foot and jock itch. Econazole is also prescribed for candida (thrush)

infections of the skin, including some forms of diaper rash.

Its main advantage over similar antifungal drugs is that it begins to work within two days or so. Also, serious adverse effects with econazole are rare, though local stinging, burning, and skin irritation can sometimes occur.

QUICK REFERENCE

Drug group Antifungal drug (p.166)
Overdose danger rating Low
Dependence rating Low
Prescription needed Yes
Available as generic No

INFORMATION FOR USERS

Your drug prescription is tailored for you. Do not alter dosage without checking with your physician.

How taken

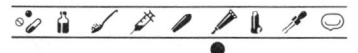

Cream.

Frequency and timing of doses
1 – 2 x daily.

Dosage range
Use a sufficient amount of cream to cover the affected and surrounding areas at each application.

Onset of effect
1 – 2 days.

Duration of action
Up to 24 hours.

Diet advice
None.

Storage
Keep in a closed container in a cool, dry place away from reach of children.

Missed dose
No cause for concern, but apply as soon as you remember.

Stopping the drug
Apply the full course. Even if symptoms disappear, the original infection may still be present and symptoms may recur if treatment is stopped too soon.

Exceeding the dose
An occasional unintentional extra dose is unlikely to be a cause for concern. But if you notice any unusual symptoms, notify your physician.

SPECIAL PRECAUTIONS

Be sure to tell your physician if:
▼ You have had a previous allergic reaction to this drug.

 Pregnancy
▼ No evidence of risk to developing baby.

 Breast feeding
▼ No evidence of risk.

 Infants and children
▼ No special problems.

 Over 60
▼ No special problems.

 Driving and hazardous work
▼ No known problems.

 Alcohol
▼ No known problems.

POSSIBLE ADVERSE EFFECTS

Local irritation may occur at the site of application, but always disappears when treatment is stopped. More serious adverse effects rarely occur with econazole.

Symptom/effect	Frequency		Discuss with physician		Stop taking drug now	Call physician now
	Common	Rare	Only if severe	In all cases		
Local burning	●		■			
Redness/itching of skin		●	■			
Rash		●		■	▲	

INTERACTIONS

None. Econazole is for topical use only; it should not be used in the eyes.

PROLONGED USE

No problems expected.

ENALAPRIL

Brand name Vasotec
Used in the following combined preparations None

GENERAL INFORMATION

Enalapril, introduced in 1986, is an ACE inhibitor (see p.126) prescribed to treat hypertension (high blood pressure) and heart failure. It is often given in conjunction with a diuretic to increase its effect.

The first dose of enalapril may cause a sudden drop in blood pressure. You should be resting at the time and able to lie down afterwards for 2 – 3 hours.

The more common adverse effects, such as dizziness and headache, usually diminish with long-term treatment. Rashes can also occur during treatment. These usually disappear when the drug is stopped. In some cases they clear up on their own despite continued treatment.

INFORMATION FOR USERS

Your drug prescription is tailored for you. Do not alter dosage without checking with your physician.

How taken

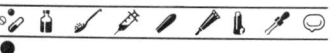

Tablets.

Frequency and timing of doses
Once daily.

Adult dosage range
10 – 40mg daily.

Onset of effect
Within 1 hour.

Duration of action
24 hours.

Diet advice
None.

Storage
Keep in a closed container in a cool, dry place away from reach of children. Protect from light.

Missed dose
Take as soon as you remember. If your next dose is due within 8 hours, do not take the skipped dose. Take your next dose as usual.

Stopping the drug
Do not stop taking the drug without consulting your physician; stopping the drug may lead to worsening of the underlying condition.

Exceeding the dose
An occasional unintentional extra dose is unlikely to cause problems. Large overdoses may cause dizziness or fainting. Notify your physician.

SPECIAL PRECAUTIONS

Be sure to tell your physician if:
▼ You have impaired kidney or liver function.
▼ You are taking other medications.

Pregnancy
▼ Not usually prescribed. Safety in pregnancy not established. Discuss with your physician so that you can weigh the benefits of the drug against its possible risks.

Breast feeding
▼ Discuss with your physician. Effect on breast feeding uncertain.

Infants and children
▼ Not recommended.

Over 60
▼ Reduced dose may be necessary.

Driving and hazardous work
▼ Avoid such activities until you have learned how the drug affects you, because it can cause dizziness and fainting.

Alcohol
▼ Avoid. Alcohol increases the likelihood of an excessive drop in blood pressure.

POSSIBLE ADVERSE EFFECTS

The more common adverse effects, such as dizziness and headache, usually diminish with long-term treatment. The less common effects may also diminish during long-term treatment, but an adjustment in dosage may be necessary.

Symptom/effect	Frequency		Discuss with physician		Stop taking drug now	Call physician now
	Common	Rare	Only if severe	In all cases		
Dizziness	●		■			
Headache	●		■			
Nausea		●		■		
Diarrhea		●		■		
Rash		●		■		
Muscle cramps		●		■		

PROLONGED USE

No problems expected.

Monitoring Periodic tests on blood and urine may be performed.

INTERACTIONS

Antihypertensive drugs are likely to add to the blood pressure-lowering effect of enalapril.

Lithium Enalapril increases the levels of lithium in the blood, and serious adverse effects from lithium excess may occur.

Potassium supplements and potassium-sparing diuretics Enalapril may add to the effect of these drugs leading to raised levels of potassium in the blood.

EPHEDRINE

Brand names None
Used in the following combined preparations Bronkolixir, Marax, Quadrinal, Tedral

GENERAL INFORMATION

By stimulating the release of the hormone norepinephrine from the nerve endings, ephedrine constricts the vessels of the nose and thus relieves congestion. In use for more than 50 years, ephedrine also serves as a bronchodilator, relaxing the bronchial muscles and easing the bronchospasm associated with asthma, bronchitis, and emphysema.

While newer and more effective drugs have considerably replaced ephedrine for those purposes, it has found a variety of other applications. Together with a vasodilator, it is occasionally used for severe congestive heart failure. With an anti-emetic drug, it is given by mouth to treat motion sickness. It is also prescribed for bedwetting in children, stress incontinence of the bladder in adults, and delayed ejaculation.

INFORMATION FOR USERS

Follow instructions on the label. Call your physician if symptoms worsen.

How taken

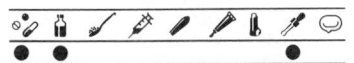

Capsules, tablets, syrup, nose drops.

Frequency and timing of doses
By mouth Every 3 – 4 hours (asthma and congestion); 4 x daily (urinary incontinence); once daily at bedtime (bedwetting); 1 – 2 hours before intercourse (delayed ejaculation).
Nose drops As required.

Dosage range
Adults 45 – 240mg daily (by mouth).
Children Reduced dose according to age and weight.

Onset of effect
Within 15 – 60 minutes.

Duration of action
3 – 6 hours.

Diet advice
None.

Storage
Keep in a closed container in a cool, dry place away from reach of children. Protect from light.

Missed dose
Do not take the missed dose. Take your next dose as usual.

Stopping the drug
Can be safely stopped as soon as you no longer need it.

Exceeding the dose
An occasional unintentional extra dose is unlikely to cause problems. Large over-doses may cause shortness of breath, high fever, seizures, or loss of consciousness. Notify your physician.

SPECIAL PRECAUTIONS

Be sure to consult your physician before taking this drug if:
▼ You have heart disease.
▼ You have high blood pressure.
▼ You have diabetes.
▼ You have an overactive thyroid gland.
▼ You have had glaucoma.
▼ You have urinary difficulties.
▼ You are taking other medications.

Pregnancy
▼ Not usually prescribed. Safety in pregnancy not established. Discuss with your physician so that you can weigh the benefits of the drug against its possible risks.

Breast feeding
▼ Discuss with your physician. The drug passes into the breast milk and may affect the baby adversely.

Infants and children
▼ Reduced dose necessary.

Over 60
▼ Not usually prescribed.

Driving and hazardous work
▼ Avoid such activities until you have learned how the drug affects you, because it may cause dizziness.

Alcohol
▼ No special problems.

Surgery and general anesthetics
▼ Ephedrine may need to be stopped before you have a general anesthetic. Discuss this with your physician or dentist before any surgery.

POSSIBLE ADVERSE EFFECTS

Its main adverse effects – palpitations, tremor, and restlessness – are caused by its stimulatory action on the heart and central nervous system, and may disappear with a reduction in dose. Taking the last dose before 4 pm may prevent insomnia.

Symptom/effect	Frequency		Discuss with physician		Stop taking drug now	Call physician now
	Common	Rare	Only if severe	In all cases		
Anxiety/restlessness	●		■			
Insomnia	●		■			
Dizziness		●	■			
Headache		●	■			
Urinary difficulties		●	■			
Palpitations/chest pain		●		■	▲	▮

INTERACTIONS

Monoamine oxidase inhibitors (MAOIs) Ephedrine may interact with these drugs to cause a dangerous rise in blood pressure.

Digitalis drugs Ephedrine increases the risk of palpitations with these drugs.

Antihypertensive drugs Ephedrine may counteract the antihypertensive effects of reserpine, methyldopa, guanethidine, and beta blockers.

PROLONGED USE

Prolonged use is not recommended except on medical advice. Decongestant effects may lessen. Adverse cardiac effects may occur with large doses.

A B C D E F G H I J K L M N O P Q R S T U V W X Y Z

EPINEPHRINE

Brand names Adrenalin, Micronefrin, Primatene, Sus-Phrine, Vaponefrin
Used in the following combined preparations None

GENERAL INFORMATION

Epinephrine is a hormone produced in the center (medulla) of the adrenal glands. Usually called adrenalin, it is the "juice" you feel when "all your juices are flowing" and your body is preparing for physical challenge. Medically, epinephrine raises cardiac output and dilates the airways to improve breathing, and narrows blood vessels in the skin and intestine.

Produced synthetically since 1900, epinephrine is injected to counteract cardiac arrest, relieve the severe allergic reactions (anaphylaxis) to drugs or insect stings, and control the symptoms of asthma.

Because it constricts blood vessels, epinephrine is used to control bleeding in surgery, to stop nosebleeds, and to slow the dispersal and thereby prolong the effect of local anesthetics. Newer drugs, with fewer side effects, have been introduced and largely replaced epinephrine in its traditional role as a nasal decongestant.

In drop form, it can lower the pressure within the eye, making it useful in some types of glaucoma and eye surgery.

INFORMATION FOR USERS

Your drug prescription is tailored for you. Do not alter dosage without checking with your physician.

How taken

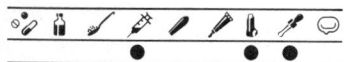

Injection, inhaler, eye and nose drops.

Frequency and timing of doses
As directed according to method of administration and underlying disorder.

Dosage range
As directed according to method of administration and underlying disorder.

Onset of effect
Within 5 minutes (injection, inhaler); within 1 hour (eye drops).

Duration of action
Up to 4 hours (inhaler); up to 4 hours (injection); up to 24 hours (eye drops).

Diet advice
None.

Storage
Keep in a closed container in a cool, dry place away from reach of children. Protect from light.

Missed dose
Do not take the missed dose. Take your next dose as usual.

Stopping the drug
Do not stop taking the drug without consulting your physician; stopping the drug may lead to worsening of the underlying condition.

OVERDOSE ACTION

 Seek immediate medical advice in all cases. Take emergency action if palpitations, breathing difficulties or loss of consciousness occur.

See Drug poisoning emergency guide (p.590).

POSSIBLE ADVERSE EFFECTS

The principal adverse effects of this drug are related to its stimulant action on the heart and central nervous system. Eye drops cause local burning or inflammation.

Symptom/effect	Frequency		Discuss with physician		Stop taking drug now	Call physician now
	Common	Rare	Only if severe	In all cases		
Dry mouth	●		■			
Nervousness/restlessness	●		■			
Palpitations	●			■		▮
Headache/blurred vision		●		■		

INTERACTIONS

General note A variety of drugs interact with epinephrine to increase the risk of palpitations and/or high blood pressure. Such drugs include digitalis drugs, guanethidine, and tricyclic antidepressants.

Beta blockers may block the effects of epinephrine and vice versa.

Antidiabetic drugs The effectiveness of such drugs may be reduced by epinephrine.

SPECIAL PRECAUTIONS

Be sure to tell your physician if:
▼ You have heart problems.
▼ You have diabetes.
▼ You have an overactive thyroid gland.
▼ You have nervous problems.
▼ You are taking other medications.

 Pregnancy
▼ Not usually prescribed. May cause defects in the unborn baby and prolong labor. Discuss with your physician so that you may weigh the benefits of the drug against its risks.

 Breast feeding
▼ Discuss with your physician. The drug passes into the breast milk and may affect the baby adversely.

 Infants and children
▼ Not usually prescribed for asthma in children. Reduced dose necessary.

 Over 60
▼ Reduced dose may be necessary. Increased likelihood of adverse effects.

 Driving and hazardous work
▼ No known problems.

Alcohol
▼ No known problems.

Surgery and general anesthetics
▼ Epinephrine may need to be stopped before you have a general anesthetic. Discuss this with your physician or dentist before any surgery.

PROLONGED USE

The bronchodilator effects of the drug may be reduced with prolonged use. With eye drops, pigment deposits on the eyeball and eyelids and hypersensitivity can occur.

ERGONOVINE

Brand name Ergotrate
Used in the following combined preparations None

GENERAL INFORMATION

Introduced in 1935, ergonovine is obtained from ergot, a fungus that grows on rye. It is used primarily to stop bleeding from the uterus after childbirth or termination of pregnancy. Occasionally, it may be given after a miscarriage to help expel the contents of the uterus. It contracts the muscles of the uterus, thereby compressing blood vessels and reducing bleeding.

Ergonovine is usually given as an intramuscular injection immediately after delivery, but may also be given by mouth. Intravenous injection is reserved for emergencies when rapid onset of effect is needed (such as excessive bleeding from the uterus). This type of injection is used with restraint because it can cause vomiting, dizziness, headache, and in rare cases, confusion and seizures, associated with a rise in blood pressure. Ergonovine is not usually given to women who have suffered from high blood pressure during pregnancy or labor.

INFORMATION FOR USERS

Your drug prescription is tailored for you. Do not alter dosage without checking with your physician.

How taken

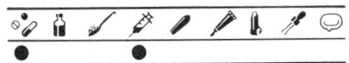

Tablets, injection.

Frequency and timing of doses
2 – 4 x daily (by mouth); single dose, repeated after 2 – 4 hours as necessary up to 5 doses (injection).

Adult dosage range
0.4 – 1.6mg daily (by mouth).

Onset of effect
Immediately (intravenous injection); 7 – 8 minutes (intramuscular injection); 10 – 20 minutes (by mouth).

Duration of action
Up to 3 hours.

Diet advice
None.

Storage
Keep in a closed container in a cool, dry place away from reach of children.

Missed dose
Do not take the missed dose. Take your next dose as usual.

Stopping the drug
Do not stop the drug without consulting your physician.

OVERDOSE ACTION

 Seek immediate medical advice in all cases. Take emergency action if seizures or loss of consciousness occurs.

See Drug poisoning emergency guide (p.590).

POSSIBLE ADVERSE EFFECTS

Adverse effects occur most frequently with intravenous injection. This often causes a temporary rise in blood pressure, which may lead to nausea, vomiting, or headache. Narrowing of the blood vessels may lead to cold hands and feet and weakness in the legs. All these effects are uncommon with intramuscular injection and tablets.

Symptom/effect	Frequency		Discuss with physician		Stop taking drug now	Call physician now
	Common	Rare	Only if severe	In all cases		
Nausea/vomiting	●			■		
Headache/blurred vision		●		■		
Dizziness/confusion		●		■		
Weakness in legs		●		■		
Cold hands or feet		●		■	▲	
Seizures		●		■	▲	∎

INTERACTIONS

Tobacco smoking may increase the risk of high blood pressure with ergonovine.

SPECIAL PRECAUTIONS

Be sure to tell your physician if:
▼ You have impaired liver or kidney function.
▼ You have heart or circulatory problems.
▼ You have high blood pressure.
▼ You are taking other medications.

 Pregnancy
▼ Not prescribed during pregnancy.

 Breast feeding
▼ No evidence of risk with normal doses. High doses may affect the baby adversely. Discuss with your physician.

 Infants and children
▼ Not prescribed.

 Over 60
▼ Not prescribed.

 Driving and hazardous work
▼ No special problems.

Alcohol
▼ No known problems.

PROLONGED USE

Not used for prolonged periods.

ERGOTAMINE

Brand names Ergomar, Eryostat, Medihaler Ergotamine, Wigrettes
Used in the following combined preparations Bellergal, Bellergal-S, Cafergot P-B, Wigraine

GENERAL INFORMATION

Ergotamine is used in the prevention and treatment of migraine headaches (p.117). It constricts blood vessels around the skull and is usually only used by people for whom analgesics such as aspirin or acetaminophen fail to provide sufficient relief. It is most effective if taken at the first sign that a migraine is going to occur. Once headache and nausea are established, ergotamine is less likely to be effective and may cause stomach upset and increase the nausea of migraine. It is more effective when taken with caffeine, and combined ergotamine and caffeine preparations are available.

Ergotamine causes temporary narrowing of blood vessels throughout the body and therefore is not prescribed for those with poor circulation. If it is taken too frequently it can dangerously reduce blood circulation to the hands and feet; ergotamine should never be taken regularly.

(p.117)

QUICK REFERENCE

Drug group Drug used for migraine (p.117)

Overdose danger rating Medium

Dependence rating Low

Prescription needed Yes

Available as generic Yes

INFORMATION FOR USERS

Your drug prescription is tailored for you. Do not alter dosage without checking with your physician.

How taken

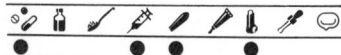

Tablets, injection, rectal suppositories, aerosol.

Frequency and timing of doses
Once at the onset of a migraine attack, repeated as necessary every 30 minutes up to the maximum dose (below).

Adult dosage range
1 – 2mg per dose. Take no more than 6mg in 24 hours or 10mg in 1 week (by mouth), or 4mg in 24 hours or 6mg in 1 week (rectally).

Onset of effect
Within 30 minutes.

Duration of action
Up to 48 hours.

Diet advice
Changes in diet are unlikely to affect the action of this drug, but certain foods may provoke migraine attacks in some people (see p.117).

Storage
Keep in a closed container in a cool, dry place away from reach of children. Protect from light. Refrigerate aerosol, but do not freeze.

Missed dose
Regular doses of this drug are not necessary and may be dangerous. Take only when you have symptoms of migraine.

Stopping the drug
Can be safely stopped as soon as you no longer need it.

Exceeding the dose
An occasional unintentional extra dose is unlikely to cause problems. Large overdoses may cause vomiting, dizziness, seizures, or coma. Notify your physician.

SPECIAL PRECAUTIONS

Be sure to tell your physician if:
▼ You have impaired kidney or liver function.
▼ You have heart problems.
▼ You have poor circulation.
▼ You have high blood pressure.
▼ You have had a recent stroke.
▼ You have asthma.
▼ You are taking other medications.

Pregnancy
▼ Not usually prescribed. Ergotamine can cause contractions of the uterus.

Breast feeding
▼ Not recommended during breast feeding. It passes into the milk and may have adverse effects on the baby. It may also reduce your milk supply.

Infants and children
▼ Not usually prescribed.

Over 60
▼ Use with caution. Hidden heart or circulatory problems may be aggravated.

Driving and hazardous work
▼ No special problems.

Alcohol
▼ No special problems, but some drinks may provoke migraine in some people (see p.117).

Surgery and general anesthetics
▼ Notify your physician if you have used ergotamine within 48 hours prior to surgery.

POSSIBLE ADVERSE EFFECTS

The more common symptoms of treatment with ergotamine are drowsiness, digestive disturbances, and nausea. An anti-emetic drug may be prescribed to relieve nausea.

Symptom/effect	Frequency		Discuss with physician		Stop taking drug now	Call physician now
	Common	Rare	Only if severe	In all cases		
Drowsiness	●		■			
Nausea and vomiting	●		■			
Diarrhea		●	■			
Muscle pain and stiffness		●		■		
Chest pain		●		■	▲	▮

INTERACTIONS

Erythromycin There is an increased likelihood of adverse effects when this drug is taken with ergotamine.

Cold remedies Some ingredients in these over-the-counter products can lead to a dangerous rise in blood pressure if taken with ergotamine.

PROLONGED USE

Headaches and reduced circulation to the hands and feet may result if doses near to the maximum are taken for a long time. Dependency may also occur. Consult your physician about a different treatment.

ERYTHROMYCIN

Brand names E-Mycin, E-Mycin 333, Eryc, Eryc 125, Ilotycin
Used in the following combined preparation Pediazole

GENERAL INFORMATION

Introduced in 1952 and one of the safest antibiotics, erythromycin is effective against a wide range of bacteria. It is a useful alternative to penicillins and tetracyclines for people who are allergic to those drugs.

Erythromycin is commonly prescribed for throat, middle ear and chest infections, including some rare types of pneumonia such as walking (myco-plasma) pneumonia and Legionnaires' disease, and in sexually transmitted diseases such as gonorrhea, chlamydial infections, and syphilis.

Sometimes given to reduce the likelihood of infecting others with whooping cough, erythromycin may also be included as part of the treatment for diphtheria. *Topical* preparations are used for skin and eye infections and acne. It is available in combination with the sulfonamide sulfisoxazole for the treatment of middle ear infections and sinusitis in children.

Erythromycin taken by mouth may sometimes cause nausea and vomiting, which can be avoided by taking the drug with food. Other possible adverse effects include rash and a rare risk of liver disorders.

QUICK REFERENCE

Drug group Antibiotic (p.156)
Overdose danger rating Low
Dependence rating Low
Prescription needed Yes
Available as generic Yes

INFORMATION FOR USERS

Your drug prescription is tailored for you. Do not alter dosage without checking with your physician.

How taken

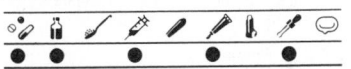

Tablets, capsules, liquid, injection, ointment, eye drops.

Frequency and timing of doses
Every 6 – 12 hours.

Dosage range
Wide variation depending on dosage form and the disorder being treated. Follow your physician's instructions.

Onset of effect
2 – 4 hours.

Duration of action
6 – 12 hours.

Diet advice
None.

Storage
Keep in a closed container in a cool, dry place away from reach of children.

Missed dose
Take as soon as you remember. If your next dose is due within 2 hours, take a single dose now and skip the next.

Stopping the drug
Take the full course. Even if you feel better, the original infection may still be present and symptoms may recur if treatment is stopped too soon.

Exceeding the dose
An occasional unintentional extra dose is unlikely to be a cause for concern. But if you notice unusual symptoms, or if a large overdose has been taken, notify your physician.

SPECIAL PRECAUTIONS

Be sure to tell your physician if:
▼ You have a liver disease or impaired liver function.
▼ You have impaired kidney function.
▼ You have had a previous allergic reaction to erythromycin.
▼ You are taking other medications.

Pregnancy
▼ Not usually prescribed. Safety in pregnancy not established. Discuss with your physician so that you can weigh the benefits of the drug against its possible risks.

Breast feeding
▼ The drug passes into the breast milk, but at normal doses adverse effects on the baby are uncommon. Discuss with your physician.

Infants and children
▼ Reduced dose necessary.

Over 60
▼ No special problems.

Driving and hazardous work
▼ No known problems.

Alcohol
▼ No known problems.

POSSIBLE ADVERSE EFFECTS

Nausea and vomiting are the most common adverse effects and are most likely to occur with large doses taken by mouth. Symptoms such as fever, rash, and jaundice may be a sign of a liver disorder and should always be reported to your physician.

Symptom/effect	Frequency		Discuss with physician		Stop taking drug now	Call physician now
	Common	Rare	Only if severe	In all cases		
Nausea/vomiting	●		■			
Diarrhea	●		■			
Rash/itching	●			■	▲	∎
Deafness		●		■		∎
Jaundice		●		■	▲	∎
Unexplained fever		●		■	▲	∎

PROLONGED USE

Courses of longer than 10 days may increase the risk of liver damage.

INTERACTIONS

Theophylline Erythromycin increases the risk of side effects with this drug.

Carbamazepine Erythromycin may increase blood levels of this drug.

Warfarin Erythromycin increases the risk of bleeding with warfarin.

Digoxin Erythromycin may increase blood levels of this drug.

A B C D E F G H I J K L M N O P Q R S T U V W X Y Z

ESTRADIOL

Brand names Delestrogen, Depo-Estradiol, Esta-L, Estrace, Valergen
Used in the following combined preparations Deladumone, Depo-Testadiol, Valertest

GENERAL INFORMATION

Estradiol is the principal and most powerful estrogen produced by the ovaries. Synthetically produced since 1940, it is used to supplement or replace the naturally occurring hormone in women with estrogen deficiency, especially at the time of the menopause.

Given by injection or by mouth, it is effective in controlling menopausal symptoms such as hot flashes and sweating. It is also used in the treatment of ovarian failure and hypogonadism (underdeveloped ovaries).

As replacement therapy, it is often taken in conjunction with a progestin (see p.175). Withdrawal bleeding resembling a menstrual period occurs on stopping the drug. It may be prescribed in the form of vaginal cream to relieve pain and dryness of the vagina or vulva after the menopause. It is also occasionally used to treat prostate cancer.

QUICK REFERENCE

Drug group Female sex hormone (p.175)

Overdose danger rating Low

Dependence rating Low

Prescription needed Yes

Available as generic Yes

INFORMATION FOR USERS

Your drug prescription is tailored for you. Do not alter dosage without checking with your physician.

How taken

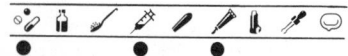

Tablets, injection, cream.

Frequency and timing of doses
Tablets 1 – 3 x daily with food.
Cream 1 – 7 x a week.
Injection Depending on formulation and condition, from 3 x daily to once every 4 – 6 weeks.

Adult dosage range
Replacement therapy 1 – 2mg daily (tablets); 2 – 4mg daily (cream).
Prostate cancer 1 – 6mg daily.

Onset of effect
10 – 20 days.

Duration of action
4 days to 4 weeks.

Diet advice
None.

Storage
Keep in a closed container in a cool, dry place away from reach of children. Protect from light.

Missed dose
Take as soon as you remember.

Stopping the drug
Do not stop the drug without consulting your physician; symptoms may recur.

Exceeding the dose
An occasional unintentional extra dose is unlikely to be a cause for concern. But if you notice unusual symptoms, or if a large overdose has been taken, notify your physician.

SPECIAL PRECAUTIONS

Be sure to tell your physician if:
▼ You have heart failure or high blood pressure.
▼ You have had blood clots or a stroke.
▼ You have impaired liver or kidney function.
▼ You have diabetes.
▼ You are a smoker.
▼ You suffer from migraine or epilepsy.
▼ You are taking other medications.

 Pregnancy
▼ Not prescribed. May adversely affect the development of the baby's sex organs.

 Breast feeding
▼ Not prescribed. The drug may inhibit the flow of milk.

 Infants and children
▼ Not usually prescribed.

 Over 60
▼ No special problems.

 Driving and hazardous work
▼ No known problems.

 Alcohol
▼ No known problems.

Surgery and general anesthetics
▼ Estradiol may need to be stopped several weeks before you have major surgery. Discuss this with your physician.

POSSIBLE ADVERSE EFFECTS

The most common adverse effects of estradiol are similar to symptoms that occur in the early stages of pregnancy, and generally diminish or disappear after 2 – 3 months of treatment. A sudden, sharp pain in the chest, groin, or legs may indicate an abnormal blood clot and requires urgent medical attention.

Symptom/effect	Frequency		Discuss with physician		Stop taking drug now	Call physician now
	Common	Rare	Only if severe	In all cases		
Nausea	●		■			
Breast swelling/tenderness	●		■			
Reduced sex drive		●	■			
Depression		●		■		
Abnormal vaginal bleeding		●		■		
Pain in chest/groin/legs		●		■	▲	■

INTERACTIONS

Tobacco smoking Smoking increases the risk of serious adverse effects on the heart and circulation with estradiol.

Oral anticoagulant drugs Estradiol reduces the anticoagulant effect of these drugs.

PROLONGED USE

Prolonged use of estradiol slightly increases the risk of cancer of the uterus after the menopause when used without a progestin. The risk of gallstones is also increased.

Monitoring Periodic checks on blood pressure and physical examinations may be performed.

ETHAMBUTOL

Brand name Myambutol
Used in the following combined preparations None

GENERAL INFORMATION

Ethambutol, introduced in 1967, is used in the treatment of tuberculosis. Given in conjunction with other antituberculous drugs, it helps to boost their effects.

Occasionally, it may be given early in treatment, when resistance to the more commonly used drugs is suspected. This may apply particularly when people may have caught the disease by contact with a recent immigrant from Africa, Asia, or South America, where resistance to other drugs is increasing.

Although the drug has few common adverse effects, it may occasionally cause optic neuritis, a sometimes permanent type of eye damage, leading to blurring and fading of vision. Ethambutol is not usually given to children under five, and older people will need periodic eye checks.

INFORMATION FOR USERS

Your drug prescription is tailored for you. Do not alter dosage without checking with your physician.

How taken

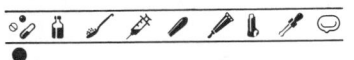

Tablets.

Frequency and timing of doses
Once daily or twice weekly.

Adult dosage range
According to body weight. 500mg – 2.5g daily.

Onset of effect
Several days.

Duration of action
Up to 96 hours.

Diet advice
None.

Storage
Keep in a closed container in a cool, dry place away from reach of children.

Missed dose
Take as soon as you remember. If your next dose is scheduled within 8 hours, take both doses now.

Stopping the drug
Take the full course. Even if you feel better the original infection may still be present and may recur if treatment is stopped too soon.

Exceeding the dose
An occasional unintentional extra dose is unlikely to cause problems. Large overdoses may cause headache and abdominal pain. Notify your physician.

POSSIBLE ADVERSE EFFECTS

Side effects are uncommon with this drug, but are more likely after prolonged treatment at high doses. Blurred vision or eye pain requires prompt medical attention.

Symptom/effect	Frequency		Discuss with physician		Stop taking drug now	Call physician now
	Common	Rare	Only if severe	In all cases		
Nausea/vomiting		●	■			
Dizziness		●	■			
Numb/tingling hands/feet		●		■		
Blurred vision		●		■	▲	
Eye pain		●		■	▲	
Loss of color vision		●		■	▲	
Rash/itching		●		■	▲	■

INTERACTIONS

Aluminum-containing antacids may reduce the effectiveness of ethambutol.

SPECIAL PRECAUTIONS

Be sure to tell your physician if:
▼ You have impaired kidney function.
▼ You have cataracts or other eye problems.
▼ You have had a previous allergic reaction to this drug.
▼ You are taking other medications.

Pregnancy
▼ Not prescribed. Safety in pregnancy not established.

Breast feeding
▼ The drug passes into the breast milk, but at normal doses adverse effects on the baby are unlikely. Discuss with your physician.

Infants and children
▼ Not prescribed for children under 5. Reduced dose necessary in older children.

Over 60
▼ Reduced dose may be necessary. Increased likelihood of adverse effects.

Driving and hazardous work
▼ No special problems unless visual disturbances occur.

Alcohol
▼ No known problems.

PROLONGED USE

Prolonged use may increase the risk of eye damage.

Monitoring Periodic eye tests may be recommended.

ETHINYL ESTRADIOL

Brand names Estinyl, Feminone
Used in the following combined preparations Lo/Ovral, Nordette, Ortho-Novum 1/35, Ortho-Novum 7 7/7, Triphasil

A B C D E F G H I J K L M N O P Q R S T U V W X Y Z

GENERAL INFORMATION

Introduced in 1944, ethinyl estradiol is a powerful synthetic estrogen similar to the natural female sex hormone estradiol. The widest use of ethinyl estradiol now is in oral contraceptive pill preparations, combined with a synthetic progesterone drug (progestin). Ethinyl estradiol is also used to supplement natural estrogen when the body's production is low. In such conditions, it is often given with a progestin. That sort of treatment relieves menopausal symptoms such as hot flashes and sweating, dryness of the vagina, and painful intercourse.

It is also used to control abnormal bleeding from the uterus and to treat delayed sexual development (hypogonadism) in females. Certain cancers of the prostate respond to ethinyl estradiol. It is sometimes given, in high doses, for post-coital contraception.

QUICK REFERENCE

Drug group Female sex hormone (p.175)

Overdose danger rating Low

Dependence rating Low

Prescription needed Yes

Available as generic Yes

INFORMATION FOR USERS

Your drug prescription is tailored for you. Do not alter dosage without checking with your physician.

How taken

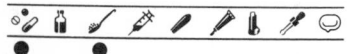

Tablets, powder.

Frequency and timing of doses
1 – 3 x daily with food.

Adult dosage range
Menopausal symptoms, abnormal bleeding from the uterus, hypogonadism 0.02 – 0.15mg daily.
Post-coital contraception 5mg daily for 5 days.
Cancer 0.15 – 3mg daily.
Combined contraceptive pills 20 – 50mcg daily depending on preparation.

Onset of effect
Within 5 days (post-coital contraception), 10 – 20 days (other actions). Contraceptive protection is not effective in under 28 days.

Duration of action
1 – 2 days.

Diet advice
None.

Storage
Keep in a closed container in a cool, dry place away from reach of children.

Missed dose
Take as soon as you remember. If your next dose is due within 4 hours, take a single dose now and skip the next. If you are taking the drug for contraceptive purposes, see p. 189.

Stopping the drug
Do not stop the drug without consulting your physician. Contraceptive protection will be lost unless alternative methods of contraception are used.

Exceeding the dose
An occasional extra dose is unlikely to be a cause for concern. But if you notice unusual symptoms, or if a large overdose has been taken, notify your physician.

SPECIAL PRECAUTIONS

Be sure to tell your physician if:
▼ You have heart failure or high blood pressure.
▼ You have had blood clots or a stroke.
▼ You have impaired liver or kidney function.
▼ You are a smoker.
▼ You have diabetes.
▼ You suffer from migraine or epilepsy.
▼ You are taking other medications.

 Pregnancy
▼ Not prescribed. May adversely affect development of the baby's sex organs.

 Breast feeding
▼ Not prescribed. The drug passes into the breast milk and may inhibit the flow of milk.

 Infants and children
▼ Not usually prescribed.

 Over 60
▼ No special problems.

 Driving and hazardous work
▼ No known problems.

 Alcohol
▼ No known problems.

Surgery and general anesthetics
▼ Ethinyl estradiol may need to be stopped several weeks before you have major surgery. Discuss this with your physician.

POSSIBLE ADVERSE EFFECTS

The most common adverse effects are similar to symptoms in the early stages of pregnancy and generally diminish with time. Sudden, sharp pain in the chest, groin, or legs may indicate an abnormal blood clot and needs immediate medical attention.

Symptom/effect	Frequency		Discuss with physician		Stop taking drug now	Call physician now
	Common	Rare	Only if severe	In all cases		
Nausea	●		■			
Breast swelling/tenderness	●		■			
Swollen feet/ankles	●		■			
Headache		●	■			
Reduced sex drive		●	■			
Depression		●		■		
Abnormal vaginal bleeding		●		■		
Pain in chest/groin/legs		●		■	▲	■

INTERACTIONS

Tobacco smoking Smoking increases the risk of serious adverse effects on the heart and circulation with ethinyl estradiol.

Oral anticoagulant drugs Ethinyl estradiol reduces the anticoagulant effect of these drugs.

PROLONGED USE

Prolonged use of ethinyl estradiol slightly increases the risk of cancer of the uterus after the menopause when used without a progestin. The risk of gallstones may also be higher.

Monitoring Periodic checks on blood pressure and physical examinations may be performed.

ETHIONAMIDE

Brand name Trecator-SC
Used in the following combined preparations None

GENERAL INFORMATION

Ethionamide, introduced in 1962, is used in the long-term treatment of tuberculosis and leprosy.

As an antituberculous drug, it is less effective than some more commonly used treatments and is generally reserved for use after other drugs have failed. It is always prescribed in conjunction with other drugs to prevent the development of resistance during prolonged use.

At the doses used to treat tuberculosis, nausea and other digestive disturbances are a common problem, and dose reduction is often necessary. In addition, ethionamide may increase the elimination of pyridoxine (vitamin B_6) from the body. Since deficiency of this vitamin can lead to irreversible nerve damage, supplements are usually advised. There is also a risk of liver damage.

QUICK REFERENCE

Drug group Antituberculous drug (p.160)

Overdose danger rating Medium

Dependence rating Low

Prescription needed Yes

Available as generic No

INFORMATION FOR USERS

Your drug prescription is tailored for you. Do not alter dosage without checking with your physician.

How taken

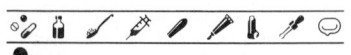

Tablets.

Frequency and timing of doses
1 – 3 x daily after meals.

Dosage range
Adults 500mg – 1g daily (tuberculosis); 250 – 375mg daily (leprosy).
Children Reduced dose according to age and weight.

Onset of effect
Several days.

Duration of action
Up to 24 hours.

Diet advice
Ethionamide may deplete pyridoxine (vitamin B_6) levels in the body; supplements are usually prescribed.

Storage
Keep in a closed container in a cool, dry place away from reach of children.

Missed dose
Take as soon as you remember. If your next dose is due within 6 hours (doses scheduled 1 – 2 times daily), or 3 hours (doses scheduled 3 times daily), take a single dose now and skip the next.

Stopping the drug
Take the full course. Even if you feel better the original infection may still be present and may recur if treatment is stopped too soon.

Exceeding the dose
An occasional unintentional extra dose is unlikely to cause problems. Large overdoses may cause nausea and vomiting. Notify your physician.

POSSIBLE ADVERSE EFFECTS

Gastrointestinal side effects, such as nausea, vomiting, and loss of appetite, are common with ethionamide and usually resolve with continued treatment at a lower dose. Serious adverse effects are rare. Numbness or tingling of the hands or feet may indicate nerve damage and should be brought to your physician's notice promptly.

Symptom/effect	Frequency		Discuss with physician		Stop taking drug now	Call physician now
	Common	Rare	Only if severe	In all cases		
Nausea/vomiting	●		■			
Loss of appetite	●		■			
Drowsiness/dizziness	●		■			
Depression/impotence		●		■		
Numbness/tingling		●		■	▲	▮
Jaundice		●		■	▲	▮
Rash		●		■	▲	▮

INTERACTIONS

None.

SPECIAL PRECAUTIONS

Be sure to tell your physician if:
▼ You have impaired liver function.
▼ You have diabetes.
▼ You are taking other medications.

Pregnancy
▼ Not usually prescribed. Safety in pregnancy not established. Discuss with your physician so that you can weigh the benefits of the drug against its possible risks.

Breast feeding
▼ The drug passes into the breast milk, but at normal doses adverse effects on the baby are uncommon. Discuss with your physician.

Infants and children
▼ Reduced dose necessary.

Over 60
▼ No special problems.

Driving and hazardous work
▼ Avoid such activities until you have learned how the drug affects you. The drug may cause drowsiness and dizziness.

Alcohol
▼ Avoid. Alcohol may increase the risk of liver damage with this drug.

PROLONGED USE

Pyridoxine (vitamin B_6) deficiency may occur with prolonged use and may lead to nerve damage. Supplements are usually prescribed. There is also a risk of liver damage.

Monitoring Periodic blood tests are usually performed to monitor liver function.

A B C D E F G H I J K L M N O P Q R S T U V W X Y Z

ETHOSUXIMIDE

Brand name Zarontin
Used in the following combined preparations None

GENERAL INFORMATION

Ethosuximide was introduced in 1960. It belongs to a group of drugs known as anticonvulsants, used in the treatment of epilepsy. Ethosuximide is most commonly prescribed for the long-term prevention of absence seizures (daydream-like episodes, also known as petit mal). Other types of epilepsy do not respond well to ethosuximide and may in some cases be made worse by it. The major drawback to the use of ethosuximide is that it can reduce production of blood cells. People on regular treatment with the drug therefore need to have blood checks at regular intervals.

QUICK REFERENCE

Drug group Anticonvulsant (p.114)
Overdose danger rating Medium
Dependence rating Low
Prescription needed Yes
Available as generic No

INFORMATION FOR USERS

Your drug prescription is tailored for you. Do not alter dosage without checking with your physician.

How taken

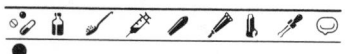

Capsules.

Frequency and timing of doses
Once daily.

Dosage range
Adults 500mg daily (starting dose), gradually increased until maximum benefit is felt.
Children Reduced dose according to age and weight.

Onset of effect
Within 30 minutes.

Duration of action
Approximately 2 days.

Diet advice
None.

Storage
Keep in a closed container in a cool, dry place away from reach of children.

Missed dose
Take as soon as you remember. If your next dose is due within 2 hours, take both doses now.

Stopping the drug
Do not stop the drug without consulting your physician; symptoms may recur.

Exceeding the dose
An occasional unintentional extra dose is unlikely to cause problems. Larger over-doses may cause unusual drowsiness. Notify your physician.

SPECIAL PRECAUTIONS

Be sure to tell your physician if:
▼ You have had a kidney or liver disorder.
▼ You have diabetes.
▼ You have porphyria.
▼ You are taking other medications.

Pregnancy
▼ Not usually prescribed. Safety in pregnancy not established. Discuss with your physician so that you can weigh the benefits of the drug against its possible risks.

Breast feeding
▼ Discuss with your physician. The drug passes into the breast milk. Its effects on the baby are not clearly known.

Infants and children
▼ Not recommended for children under 3 years. Reduced dose necessary in older children.

Over 60
▼ Reduced dose may be necessary.

Driving and hazardous work
▼ Your underlying condition, as well as the sedative effects of this drug, may make such activities inadvisable. Discuss with your physician.

Alcohol
▼ Avoid. Alcohol increases the sedative effect of this drug.

POSSIBLE ADVERSE EFFECTS

Most people experience few adverse effects with this drug, but when blood levels get too high, adverse effects are common and the dose may need to be reduced.

Symptom/effect	Frequency		Discuss with physician		Stop taking drug now	Call physician now
	Common	Rare	Only if severe	In all cases		
Drowsiness	●		■			
Loss of appetite	●		■			
Dizziness	●		■			
Digestive disturbances	●		■			
Nervousness/insomnia		●	■			
Persistent hiccups		●		■		
Paranoia		●		■		
Sore throat		●		■		
Easy bruising		●		■		
Rash		●		■		

INTERACTIONS

Sedatives All drugs that have a sedative effect on the central nervous system are likely to increase the sedative properties of ethosuximide. Such drugs include antihistamines, sleeping drugs, narcotic analgesics, antipsychotics, and anti-depressants.

Alcohol Alcohol increases the sedative effect of this drug.

PROLONGED USE

There is a slight risk of serious blood abnormalities occurring.

Monitoring Monthly blood checks are normally required.

ETRETINATE

Brand name Tegison
Used in the following combined preparations None

GENERAL INFORMATION

Etretinate is a drug chemically related to vitamin A that is used in the treatment of psoriasis. Developed in Europe and approved in the US in 1986, it is prescribed only under special hospital supervision. It is particularly useful for treating severe psoriasis when other drugs have failed to cure the condition.

Etretinate works by reducing production of the protein (keratin) that forms the hard outer layers of skin. This also makes it a useful treatment for certain other rare skin disorders that involve abnormal production of keratin, such as ichthyosis (scaly skin tissue). It also has an anti-inflammatory effect and may help to relieve the joint inflammation that is sometimes associated with psoriasis.

Symptoms generally improve after two to four weeks of treatment. Effects may last for several months after treatment has been stopped, since etretinate accumulates in fatty tissue and is eliminated slowly from the body. Courses are usually limited to short periods of up to four months, with a four-month gap before starting again. Side effects are rarely serious, but there is a risk of liver damage and a rise in blood fats.

QUICK REFERENCE

Drug group Drug for psoriasis (p.206)

Overdose danger rating Low

Dependence rating Low

Prescription needed Yes

Available as generic No

INFORMATION FOR USERS

Your drug prescription is tailored for you. Do not alter dosage without checking with your physician.

How taken

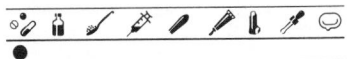

● By mouth.

Frequency and timing of doses
2 x daily.

Adult dosage range
According to individual response and condition treated.

Onset of effect
2 – 4 weeks.

Duration of action
Effects may persist for several months after the drug has been stopped.

Diet advice
None.

Storage
Keep in a closed container in a cool, dry place away from reach of children. Protect from light.

Missed dose
Take as soon as you remember. If your next dose is due within 2 hours, take a single dose now and skip the next.

Stopping the drug
Do not stop the drug without consulting your physician; symptoms may recur.

Exceeding the dose
An occasional unintentional extra dose is unlikely to be a cause for concern. But if you notice unusual symptoms, or if a large overdose has been taken, notify your physician.

POSSIBLE ADVERSE EFFECTS

Dryness and cracking of the lips occur in most people. Dryness of the mouth and nose, nosebleeds, and hair loss are also fairly common. If severe headache accompanied by nausea and vomiting occurs, consult your physician promptly.

Symptom/effect	Frequency		Discuss with physician		Stop taking drug now	Call physician now
	Common	Rare	Only if severe	In all cases		
Dry lips/skin	●		■			
Nosebleeds	●		■			
Hair loss	●		■			
Itching/peeling skin		●		■		
Inflamed nails		●		■		
Nausea/vomiting/headache		●		■	▲	■

INTERACTIONS

Tetracycline antibiotics increase the risk of high pressure in the skull, leading to headaches and nausea.

Skin-drying preparations Medicated soaps and toiletries increase the likelihood of irritation of the skin with etretinate.

Vitamin A supplements increase the risk of adverse effects with etretinate.

SPECIAL PRECAUTIONS

Be sure to tell your physician if:
▼ You have impaired liver or kidney function.
▼ You are taking other medications.

Pregnancy
▼ Not prescribed. Effective contraceptive measures must be used for 2 years after stopping the drug.

Breast feeding
▼ Discuss with your physician. The drug may pass into the breast milk and may affect the baby adversely.

Infants and children
▼ Not usually prescribed.

Over 60
▼ Reduced dose may be necessary.

Driving and hazardous work
▼ No special problems.

Alcohol
▼ Avoid. Alcohol may increase the rise in blood fat levels with etretinate, and thus increase the risk of heart and blood vessel disease.

PROLONGED USE

Prolonged use of this drug may increase the risk of liver damage. Courses of treatment are not usually continued for longer than 16 weeks, and a drug-free period of several months is usually allowed between courses.

Monitoring Periodic tests of liver function and fat levels in the blood are usually recommended.

A B C D E F G H I J K L M N O P Q R S T U V W X Y Z

FENOPROFEN

Brand names Nalfon, Nalfon 200
Used in the following combined preparations None

GENERAL INFORMATION

Fenoprofen, introduced in 1976, is one of the newer non-steroidal anti-inflammatory drugs (NSAIDs). Like other drugs of this group, it reduces pain, stiffness, and inflammation.

It is used to treat rheumatoid arthritis and osteoarthritis, and may be prescribed for ankylosing spondylitis. With prolonged treatment, it relieves pain in these conditions, but does not cure the disease.

Fenoprofen is effective in acute attacks of gout. It may also be prescribed for pain relief after childbirth, minor surgery, and minor injuries.

Adverse effects are similar to those of other NSAIDs; gastrointestinal disturbances are fairly common, including a risk of peptic ulcer. Although the risk of kidney inflammation is rare, the drug is not generally given to people with impaired kidney function.

QUICK REFERENCE

Drug group Non-steroidal anti-inflammatory drug (p.144) and drug for gout (p.147)

Overdose danger rating Low

Dependence rating Low

Prescription needed Yes

Available as generic No

INFORMATION FOR USERS

Your drug prescription is tailored for you. Do not alter dosage without checking with your physician.

How taken

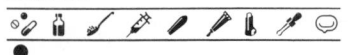

Tablets, capsules.

Frequency and timing of doses
4 x daily with food or milk (arthritis); every 4 – 6 hours (general pain relief).

Adult dosage range
1.2 – 2.4g daily (arthritis); 800mg – 1.2g daily (general pain relief).

Onset of effect
Pain relief begins in 30 – 90 minutes. Full anti-inflammatory effect in arthritis may not be felt for up to 2 weeks.

Duration of action
Up to 6 hours.

Diet advice
None.

Storage
Keep in a closed container in a cool, dry place away from reach of children.

Missed dose
Take as soon as you remember. If your next dose is due within 2 hours, take a single dose now and skip the next.

Stopping the drug
When taken for short-term pain relief, fenoprofen can be safely stopped as soon as you no longer need it. If prescribed for the long-term treatment of arthritis, however, you should seek medical advice before stopping the drug.

Exceeding the dose
An occasional unintentional extra dose is unlikely to be a cause for concern. But if you notice unusual symptoms, or if a large overdose has been taken, notify your physician.

SPECIAL PRECAUTIONS

Be sure to tell your physician if:
▼ You have impaired kidney function.
▼ You have had a peptic ulcer, esophagitis, or acid indigestion.
▼ You have heart problems.
▼ You have bleeding problems.
▼ You are allergic to aspirin.
▼ You are taking other medications.

Pregnancy
▼ Not usually prescribed. When taken in the last three months of pregnancy, may increase the risk of adverse effects on the baby's heart and may prolong labor. Discuss with your physician so that you may weigh the benefits of the drug against its risks.

Breast feeding
▼ Discuss with your physician. The drug passes into the breast milk and may affect the baby adversely.

Infants and children
▼ Not recommended.

Over 60
▼ Reduced dose may be necessary. Increased likelihood of adverse effects.

Driving and hazardous work
▼ No known problems.

Alcohol
▼ Avoid. Alcohol may increase the risk of stomach disorders with fenoprofen.

Surgery and general anesthetics
▼ Fenoprofen may prolong bleeding. Discuss this with your physician or dentist before any surgery.

POSSIBLE ADVERSE EFFECTS

Gastrointestinal disturbances and central nervous system side effects, including headache, dizziness, and drowsiness, are not usually serious. Black or bloodstained bowel movements should be reported to your physician without delay.

Symptom/effect	Frequency		Discuss with physician		Stop taking drug now	Call physician now
	Common	Rare	Only if severe	In all cases		
Nausea/vomiting	●		■			
Indigestion/heartburn	●		■			
Drowsiness/dizziness	●		■			
Headache	●		■			
Ringing in the ears		●		■		
Rash/itching		●		■	▲	
Wheezing/breathlessness		●		■	▲	▮

INTERACTIONS

General note Fenoprofen interacts with a wide range of drugs to increase the risk of bleeding and/or peptic ulcers. Such drugs include oral anticoagulants, corticosteroids, other non-steroidal anti-inflammatory drugs (NSAIDs), and aspirin.

Antihypertensive drugs and diuretics
The beneficial effects of these drugs may be reduced by fenoprofen.

Oral antidiabetic drugs Fenoprofen may increase the blood sugar lowering effect of these drugs.

PROLONGED USE

There is an increased risk of bleeding from peptic ulcers and in the bowel with prolonged use of fenoprofen.

FLAVOXATE

Brand name Urispas
Used in the following combined preparations None

GENERAL INFORMATION

Introduced in 1971, flavoxate is an antispasmodic drug with *analgesic* properties. It is used to relieve the symptoms (including painful urination) of urinary tract infections, inflammation of the bladder (cystitis), and of the prostate (prostatitis). It is also prescribed for over-frequent or uncontrollable urination.

Having no germ-killing power of its own, flavoxate is usually administered together with an antibiotic or antibacterial drug to eradicate the underlying infection.

The drug may cause nausea and vomiting, and, due to its mild *anticholinergic* action, it may lead to blurred vision and dry mouth.

QUICK REFERENCE

Drug group Urinary antispasmodic and analgesic drug (p.194)

Overdose danger rating Medium

Dependence rating Low

Prescription needed Yes

Available as generic No

INFORMATION FOR USERS

Your drug prescription is tailored for you. Do not alter dosage without checking with your physician.

How taken

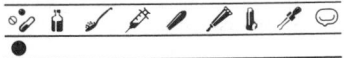

Tablets.

Frequency and timing of doses
3 – 4 x daily.

Dosage range
300 – 800mg daily.

Onset of effect
Within 2 hours.

Duration of action
6 – 8 hours.

Diet advice
None.

Storage
Keep in a closed container in a cool, dry place away from reach of children.

Missed dose
Take as soon as you remember. If your next dose is due within 2 hours, take a single dose now and skip the next.

Stopping the drug
Do not stop the drug without consulting your physician; symptoms may recur.

Exceeding the dose
An occasional unintentional extra dose is unlikely to cause problems. Large overdoses may cause dizziness, drowsiness, hallucinations, and palpitations. Notify your physician.

SPECIAL PRECAUTIONS

Be sure to tell your physician if:
▼ You have had glaucoma.
▼ You have prostate trouble.
▼ You have had epileptic seizures.

Pregnancy
▼ Not usually prescribed. Safety in pregnancy not established. Discuss with your physician so that you can weigh the benefits of the drug against its possible risks.

Breast feeding
▼ Discuss with your physician. The drug may pass into the breast milk and could affect the baby adversely.

Infants and children
▼ Not usually prescribed.

Over 60
▼ Reduced dose necessary. Increased risk of adverse effects.

Driving and hazardous work
▼ Avoid such activities until you have learned how the drug affects you, because the drug can cause drowsiness and blurred vision.

Alcohol
▼ No known problems.

POSSIBLE ADVERSE EFFECTS

Flavoxate rarely causes side effects; those that do occur are due to the drug's *anti-*

cholinergic action and can often be reduced by adjustment in dosage.

Symptom/effect	Frequency		Discuss with physician		Stop taking drug now	Call physician now
	Common	Rare	Only if severe	In all cases		
Drowsiness/lethargy		●	■			
Dry mouth		●	■			
Nausea/vomiting		●	■			
Headache		●		■		
Confusion		●		■	▲	▮
Blurred vision		●		■	▲	▮

INTERACTIONS

None.

PROLONGED USE

No problems expected.

FLUOCINOLONE

Brand names Fluonid, Flurosyn, Synalar, Synalar HP, Synemol
Used in the following combined preparation Neo-Synalar

GENERAL INFORMATION

Fluocinolone, introduced in 1969, is prescribed to relieve the redness, swelling, itching, and discomfort of many skin disorders that occur as a result of inflammation or allergy. Available as an ointment in various strengths, it can be applied directly to relieve the affected area. Fluocinolone is not an appropriate treatment for skin infections caused by bacteria, fungi, or viruses, and may make them worse. It is not prescribed for the treatment of acne, and should not normally be applied to the face.

Few people encounter side effects when they use fluocinolone for short periods of time because it acts locally and only small amounts are absorbed into the body. Excessive, prolonged use may lead to thinning of the skin.

QUICK REFERENCE

Drug group Topical corticosteroid (p.202)

Overdose danger rating Low

Dependence rating Low

Prescription needed Yes

Available as generic Yes

INFORMATION FOR USERS

Your drug prescription is tailored for you. Do not alter dosage without checking with your physician.

How taken

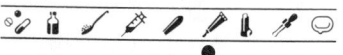

Ointment.

Frequency and timing of doses
2 – 3 x daily.

Dosage range
Sufficient ointment to cover the affected area at each application.

Onset of effect
Within a few days.

Duration of action
Up to 24 hours after each dose.

Diet advice
None.

Storage
Keep in a closed container in a cool, dry place away from reach of children.

Missed dose
No cause for concern but take as soon as you remember.

Stopping the drug
Use as directed by your physician. When symptoms improve discuss stopping the drug with your physician.

Exceeding the dose
An occasional unintentional extra dose is unlikely to be a cause for concern. But if you notice unusual symptoms, notify your physician.

POSSIBLE ADVERSE EFFECTS

Adverse effects from fluocinolone ointment are rare and are restricted to the site of application. Irritation occurs only occasionally. Thinning of the skin is unlikely and only occurs when the drug is used too frequently or for extended periods of time.

Symptom/effect	Frequency		Discuss with physician		Stop taking drug now	Call physician now
	Common	Rare	Only if severe	In all cases		
Loss of scalp hair		●		■		
Local irritation		●		■	▲	
Thinning of the skin		●		■	▲	
Reddening of the skin		●		■	▲	

INTERACTIONS

None.

SPECIAL PRECAUTIONS

Be sure to tell your physician if:
▼ You are taking other medications.

Pregnancy
▼ No evidence of risk to developing baby.

Breast feeding
▼ No evidence of risk.

Infants and children
▼ No special problems.

Over 60
▼ No special problems.

Driving and hazardous work
▼ No known problems.

Alcohol
▼ No known problems.

PROLONGED USE

Long-term treatment can cause permanent thinning of the skin.

FLUOROURACIL

Brand names Adrucil, Efudex, Fluoroplex
Used in the following combined preparations None

GENERAL INFORMATION

Introduced in 1962, this anticancer drug works by interfering with the growth of tumor cells. It is given by injection in conjunction with other anticancer drugs to limit growth of tumors in the colon, rectum, breast, and liver. Cancers of the bladder, throat, and prostate are also sometimes treated with this drug.

Fluorouracil is also available as a topical preparation to treat solar keratoses (a skin disorder caused by overexposure to sunlight). It is particularly effective against keratoses on the face, forehead, bald scalp, and ears.

When given by injection, fluorouracil affects healthy as well as cancerous cells, causing a number of side effects. Nausea, vomiting, and diarrhea are the most common symptoms, but these tend to diminish as the body adjusts to the drug. Fluorouracil by injection also interferes with the production of blood cells; this may lead to anemia, increased susceptibility to infection, and hair loss.

INFORMATION FOR USERS

Your drug prescription is tailored for you. Do not alter dosage without checking with your physician.

How taken

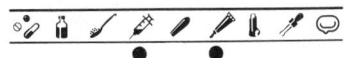

Injection, cream, solution.

Frequency and timing of doses
Once daily (injection); 2 x daily (cream or solution).

Adult dosage range
Injection Dosage is determined individually according to body weight and response.
Cream or solution Apply as directed.

Onset of effect
Some benefits and adverse effects appear within hours of injection. Full beneficial effects may not be felt for up to 4 weeks.

Duration of action
Side effects may last for several weeks.

Diet advice
None.

Storage
Keep in a closed container in a cool, dry place away from reach of children.

Missed dose
Injections are given only in the hospital under close medical supervision. If you are using cream or solution there is no cause for concern, but apply as soon as you remember.

Stopping the drug
The drug will be stopped under medical supervision (injection). Do not stop the drug without consulting your physician (cream or solution); symptoms may recur.

Exceeding the dose
An occasional unintentional extra application of cream is unlikely to be a cause for concern. But if you notice unusual symptoms, or if a large overdose has been taken, notify your physician.

SPECIAL PRECAUTIONS

Be sure to tell your physician if:
▼ You have impaired liver function.
▼ You have a history of heart disease.
▼ You have recently had chicken pox or a herpes infection.
▼ You are taking other medications.

Pregnancy
▼ Discuss treatment with your physician so that you can weigh the benefits of the drug against its possible risks.

Breast feeding
▼ Discuss with your physician. When given by injection the drug passes into the breast milk and may affect the baby adversely. When applied as a cream or solution the drug passes into the breast milk, but at normal doses adverse effects on the baby are unlikely.

Infants and children
▼ Not usually prescribed.

Over 60
▼ Reduced dose may be necessary. Increased risk of adverse effects.

Driving and hazardous work
▼ No known problems.

Alcohol
▼ No known problems.

POSSIBLE ADVERSE EFFECTS

When injected, fluorouracil often causes nausea, vomiting, and diarrhea, but these symptoms tend to diminish with time. Other adverse effects include itchy, inflamed skin, loss of hair, and anemia. Topical preparations may also occasionally cause blistering and redness of the skin that worsens following exposure to sunlight.

Symptom/effect	Frequency		Discuss with physician		Stop taking drug now	Call physician now
	Common	Rare	Only if severe	In all cases		
Nausea/vomiting	●		■			
Loss of appetite	●		■			
Hair loss/skin irritation	●			■		
Diarrhea	●			■		▮
Mouth ulcers		●		■		
Abdominal pain		●		■		▮
Bloodstained vomit		●		■		▮

INTERACTIONS

Cimetidine This drug may increase the possibility of adverse effects from fluorouracil. The fluorouracil dosage may need to be adjusted accordingly.

PROLONGED USE

Fluorouracil given by injection is likely to reduce resistance to infection and may reduce production of blood cells.

Monitoring Periodic checks on blood composition are advised.

FLUPHENAZINE

Brand names Permitil, Prolixin
Used in the following combined preparations None

GENERAL INFORMATION

Introduced in the late 1960s, fluphenazine is the most potent of a group of drugs called the phenothiazines. These are used to suppress abnormal behavior, reduce aggression, and tranquilize those who are agitated. Phenothiazines (see p.113) cannot cure mental disease, but they can control the symptoms of schizophrenia, mania, dementia, and other disorders that cause abnormal or confused behavior.

Fluphenazine's principal advantage is its long-lasting effect. It can be given in the form of a long-acting depot injection. Thus it is valuable for people who cannot remember to take daily medication. However, fluphenazine is also available in tablet or liquid form.

It is sometimes used to treat nausea and vomiting caused by drug or radiation treatment. It has also been tried in conjunction with antidepressants to relieve certain types of pain.

The main drawback to its use is that it often produces abnormal shaking, especially at the start of treatment.

QUICK REFERENCE

Drug group Phenothiazine antipsychotic (p.113) and anti-emetic drug (p.118)

Overdose danger rating Medium

Dependence rating Low

Prescription needed Yes

Available as generic Yes

INFORMATION FOR USERS

Your drug prescription is tailored for you. Do not alter dosage without checking with your physician.

How taken

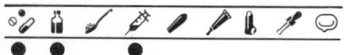

Tablets, liquid, injection.

Frequency and timing of doses
Mental illness 2 – 3 x daily (by mouth); every 2 – 4 weeks (depot injection).
Nausea and vomiting Every 6 – 8 hours.

Adult dosage range
Mental illness 2.5 – 10mg daily (starting dose), reduced to 1 – 3mg daily (maintenance dose); 25 – 100mg (depot injection).
Nausea and vomiting 1.25mg per dose.

Onset of effect
1 hour (by mouth); 24 – 72 hours (by depot injection).

Duration of action
6 – 8 hours (by mouth); 2 – 6 weeks (by depot injection, depending on formulation).

Diet advice
None.

Storage
Keep in a closed container in a cool, dry place away from reach of children. Protect from light.

Missed dose
Take as soon as you remember. If your next dose is due within 2 hours do not take the missed dose. Take the next scheduled dose as usual.

Stopping the drug
Do not stop the drug without consulting your physician; symptoms may recur.

Exceeding the dose
An occasional unintentional extra dose is unlikely to cause problems. Larger overdoses may cause unusual drowsiness, muscle rigidity, and agitation. Notify your physician.

POSSIBLE ADVERSE EFFECTS

The most marked adverse effect of this drug is stiffness and abnormal movements of the face and limbs (*parkinsonism*). This can usually be controlled by medically supervised adjustment of dosage, or a change of drug.

Symptom/effect	Frequency		Discuss with physician		Stop taking drug now	Call physician now
	Common	Rare	Only if severe	In all cases		
Drowsiness/lethargy	●		■			
Parkinsonism	●		■			
Dry mouth		●	■			
Blurred vision		●		■		
Dizziness/faintness		●		■		

INTERACTIONS

Sedatives Likely to increase the sedative properties of fluphenazine.

Anticholinergic drugs Their side effects may be increased by fluphenazine.

Antiparkinsonism drugs Fluphenazine may counter the beneficial effect of such drugs.

SPECIAL PRECAUTIONS

Be sure to tell your physician if:
▼ You have heart problems.
▼ You have had epileptic seizures.
▼ You have an overactive thyroid gland.
▼ You have impaired kidney or liver function.
▼ You have Parkinson's disease.
▼ You have had glaucoma.
▼ You have prostate trouble.
▼ You are taking other medications.

Pregnancy
▼ Not usually prescribed. Safety in pregnancy not established. Discuss with your physician so that you can weigh the benefits of the drug against its possible risks.

Breast feeding
▼ Discuss with your physician. The drug passes into the breast milk. Its effects on the baby are not clearly known.

Infants and children
▼ Not usually prescribed. Reduced dose necessary.

Over 60
▼ Reduced dose may be necessary.

Driving and hazardous work
▼ Avoid such activities until you have learned how the drug affects you, because the drug can cause drowsiness and slowed reactions.

Alcohol
▼ Avoid. Alcohol may increase the sedative effects of this drug.

PROLONGED USE

Use of this drug for more than a few months may lead to the development of *tardive dyskinesia*, and occasionally jaundice may occur.

Monitoring Periodic blood tests may be performed.

FLURAZEPAM

Brand name Dalmane
Used in the following combined preparations None

GENERAL INFORMATION

Flurazepam was introduced in 1972, one of a large group of drugs known as the benzodiazepines, generally used to quiet anxieties. The actions and adverse effects of this group of drugs are described fully on p.111. Because it has a relatively long duration of sedative action compared with other benzodiazepines, fluraze-pam is primarily used to treat insomnia, especially in sufferers with a tendency to wake early.

Taken over a long period, it can be habit-forming. For that reason, and also because the effects of this drug are likely to diminish over time, flurazepam treatment is usually reviewed every two weeks.

QUICK REFERENCE

Drug group Benzodiazepine sleeping drug (p.110)

Overdose danger rating Medium

Dependence rating High

Prescription needed Yes CIV

Available as generic Yes

INFORMATION FOR USERS

Your drug prescription is tailored for you. Do not alter dosage without checking with your physician.

How taken

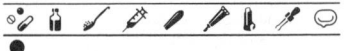

Capsules

Frequency and timing of doses
Once daily at bedtime.

Adult dosage range
15 – 30mg daily.

Onset of effect
15 – 45 minutes.

Duration of action
7 – 8 hours, but some effect can last up to 24 hours.

Diet advice
None.

Storage
Keep in a closed container in a cool, dry place away from reach of children. Protect from light.

Missed dose
If you fall asleep without having taken a dose, and wake some hours later, do not take the missed dose. If necessary, return to your normal dose schedule the following night.

Stopping the drug
If you have been taking the drug continuously for less than 2 weeks, it can be safely stopped as soon as you feel you no longer need it. However, if you have been taking the drug for longer, consult your physician, who will supervise a gradual reduction in dosage. Stopping abruptly may lead to withdrawal symptoms (see p.110).

Exceeding the dose
An occasional unintentional extra dose is unlikely to cause problems. Larger overdoses may cause unusual drowsiness. Notify your physician.

SPECIAL PRECAUTIONS

Be sure to tell your physician if:
▼ You have severe respiratory disease.
▼ You have impaired kidney or liver function.
▼ You have had problems with alcohol or drug abuse.
▼ You are taking other medications.

 Pregnancy
▼ Not usually prescribed. May cause defects in the unborn baby. Discuss with your physician so that you may weigh the benefits of the drug against its risks.

 Breast feeding
▼ Discuss with your physician. The drug passes into the breast milk and may affect the baby adversely.

 Infants and children
▼ Not usually prescribed. Reduced dose necessary.

 Over 60
▼ Reduced dose may be necessary. Increased likelihood of adverse effects.

 Driving and hazardous work
▼ Avoid such activities until you have learned how the drug affects you, because the drug can cause reduced alertness and slowed reactions.

 Alcohol
▼ Avoid. Alcohol may increase the sedative effects of this drug.

POSSIBLE ADVERSE EFFECTS

The principal adverse effects of this drug are related to its sedative and tranquilizing properties.

Symptom/effect	Frequency		Discuss with physician		Stop taking drug now	Call physician now
	Common	Rare	Only if severe	In all cases		
Daytime drowsiness	●		■			
Dizziness/unsteadiness	●			■		
Headache		●	■			
Blurred vision		●		■		
Forgetfulness/confusion		●		■		
Rash		●		■	▲	

PROLONGED USE

Regular use of this drug over several weeks can lead to a reduction in its effect as the body adapts. It may also be habit-forming when taken for extended periods, especially if larger than average doses are taken.

INTERACTIONS

Sedatives All drugs that have a sedative effect on the central nervous system are likely to increase the sedative properties of flurazepam. Such drugs include other anti-anxiety and sleeping drugs, antihistamines, antidepressants, narcotic analgesics, and antipsychotics.

Cimetidine Breakdown of flurazepam in the liver may be inhibited by cimetidine. This can cause a buildup of flurazepam levels in the blood, which increases the likelihood of adverse effects.

A B C D E F G H I J K L M N O P Q R S T U V W X Y Z

FUROSEMIDE

Brand name Lasix
Used in the following combined preparations None

GENERAL INFORMATION

Furosemide is a powerful, short-acting loop diuretic that has been in use for over 20 years. Like other diuretics, it is used to treat the edema (fluid retention) caused by heart failure, nephrotic syndrome, or liver cirrhosis. Because it is fast acting, furosemide is often used in emergencies to relieve pulmonary edema. The drug is also employed in the long-term treatment of hypertension. Furosemide is particularly useful for people with impaired kidney function because they do not respond well to thiazide diuretics.

Furosemide increases the loss of potassium, a condition which can produce a wide variety of symptoms. For that reason, supplements of potassium or a potassium-sparing diuretic are often given with the drug.

INFORMATION FOR USERS

Your drug prescription is tailored for you. Do not alter dosage without checking with your physician.

How taken

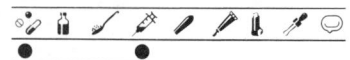

Tablets, injection.

Frequency and timing of doses
Once daily, usually in the morning.

Adult dosage range
20 – 80mg daily. Dose may be increased to a maximum of 600mg daily if kidney function is impaired.

Onset of effect
Within 1 hour (tablets); within 5 minutes (injection).

Duration of action
2 – 6 hours.

Diet advice
Use of this drug may reduce potassium in the body. Eat plenty of potassium-rich fresh fruit and vegetables (p.178).

Storage
Keep in a closed container in a cool, dry place away from reach of children.

Missed dose
No cause for concern, but take as soon as you remember. However, if it is late in the day do not take the missed dose, or you may need to get up during the night to pass urine. Take the next scheduled dose as usual.

Stopping the drug
Do not stop the drug without consulting your physician; symptoms may recur.

Exceeding the dose
An occasional unintentional extra dose is unlikely to be a cause for concern. But if you notice any unusual symptoms, or if a large overdose has been taken, notify your physician.

SPECIAL PRECAUTIONS

Be sure to tell your physician if:
▼ You have impaired kidney or liver function.
▼ You have gout.
▼ You have diabetes.
▼ You have prostate trouble.
▼ You are taking other medications.

Pregnancy
▼ Discuss with your physician.

Breast feeding
▼ Discuss with your physician. The drug may reduce milk supply.

Infants and children
▼ Not usually prescribed. Reduced dose necessary.

Over 60
▼ Increased likelihood of adverse effects.

Driving and hazardous work
▼ No special problems.

Alcohol
▼ Avoid. Furosemide increases the likelihood of dehydration and hangovers after consumption of alcohol.

POSSIBLE ADVERSE EFFECTS

Adverse effects are caused mainly by the rapid fluid loss produced by furosemide. These diminish as the body adjusts to the drug.

Symptom/effect	Frequency		Discuss with physician		Stop taking drug now	Call physician now
	Common	Rare	Only if severe	In all cases		
Dizziness	●		■			
Lethargy		●	■			
Noises in ears (high dose)		●	■			
Cramps		●	■			
Rash		●		■		

INTERACTIONS

Non-steroidal anti-inflammatory drugs (NSAIDs) may reduce the diuretic effect of furosemide.

Lithium Furosemide may increase the blood level of lithium, leading to an increased risk of lithium poisoning.

Aminoglycoside antibiotics increase the risk of hearing problems when taken with furosemide.

PROLONGED USE

Serious problems are unlikely, but levels of salts, such as potassium, sodium, and calcium, may occasionally become depleted during prolonged use.

Monitoring Periodic tests may be performed to check on kidney function and levels of body salts.

GEMFIBROZIL

Brand name Lopid
Used in the following combined preparations None

GENERAL INFORMATION

Gemfibrozil, introduced in 1982, is one of the newest lipid-lowering drugs. It is used to lower blood levels of certain types of fats in people with hyperlipidemia to reduce the risk of fatty deposits accumulating in the blood vessels (atherosclerosis). This may help to reduce the chance of heart attacks and strokes. With a continued low-fat diet, it is usually given after dietary measures alone have failed to reduce blood fat levels. It is occasionally given with niacin to treat certain types of inherited hyperlipidemia.

Like similar drugs, gemfibrozil can cause symptoms such as nausea, indigestion, and diarrhea. It is not usually prescribed for people with kidney or liver problems or those with gallstones. Gemfibrozil is prescribed with caution to diabetics because it may alter blood sugar levels.

Because this is a new drug, knowledge of its long-term effects is limited. For this reason, gemfibrozil is generally reserved for treating people who have failed to respond to more established drugs.

QUICK REFERENCE

Drug group Lipid-lowering drug (p.131)

Overdose danger rating Medium

Dependence rating Low

Prescription needed Yes

Available as generic No

INFORMATION FOR USERS

Your drug prescription is tailored for you. Do not alter dosage without checking with your physician.

How taken

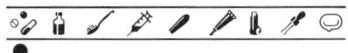

Capsules.

Frequency and timing of doses
2 x daily (morning and evening before meals).

Dosage range
1.2g daily.

Onset of effect
2 – 5 days. Full beneficial effect may not be felt for several months.

Duration of action
Some effect may last for up to 6 weeks after treatment has stopped.

Diet advice
A low-fat diet is recommended.

Storage
Keep in a closed container in a cool, dry place away from reach of children.

Missed dose
Take as soon as you remember. If your next dose is due within 2 hours, take a single dose now and skip the next.

Stopping the drug
Do not stop taking the drug without consulting your physician; stopping the drug may lead to worsening of the underlying condition.

Exceeding the dose
An occasional unintentional extra dose is unlikely to cause problems. Large overdoses may cause nausea or indigestion. Notify your physician.

SPECIAL PRECAUTIONS

Be sure to tell your physician if:
▼ You have a kidney or liver disorder.
▼ You have gallbladder disease or a history of gallstones.
▼ You have diabetes.
▼ You are taking other medications.

Pregnancy
▼ Not usually prescribed. Safety in pregnancy not established. Discuss with your physician so that you may weigh the benefits of the drug against its risks.

Breast feeding
▼ Discuss with your physician. The drug passes into the breast milk, but at normal doses adverse effects on the baby are unlikely.

Infants and children
▼ Not usually prescribed.

Over 60
▼ Reduced dose may be necessary.

Driving and hazardous work
▼ No special problems.

Alcohol
▼ Avoid. Alcohol may reduce the effect of this drug.

POSSIBLE ADVERSE EFFECTS

Gastrointestinal disturbances (especially nausea and diarrhea), and rashes are the most common side effects of gemfibrozil. These and other adverse effects are not usually serious and generally go away during treatment. If severe, prolonged abdominal pain and vomiting persist or flu-like symptoms occur, consult your physician.

Symptom/effect	Frequency		Discuss with physician		Stop taking drug now	Call physician now
	Common	Rare	Only if severe	In all cases		
Nausea/vomiting	●		■			
Abdominal pain	●		■			
Diarrhea	●		■			
Rash	●			■		▲
Flatulence		●	■			
Drowsiness		●	■			
Fever/aching muscles		●		■		▲

PROLONGED USE

The risk of gallstones is increased in people on extended gemfibrozil treatment. The drug may also affect liver function.

Monitoring Regular tests of blood fat levels and liver function may be advised.

INTERACTIONS

Antidiabetic drugs Gemfibrozil may raise blood sugar levels, thereby reducing the effect of these drugs.

Oral anticoagulant drugs The effect of these drugs may be increased with gemfibrozil.

GENTAMICIN

Brand names Garamycin injection/solution, Genoptic solution, Gentacidin
Used in the following combined preparations None

GENERAL INFORMATION

Gentamicin, introduced in 1966, is an aminoglycoside antibiotic. Given by injection, it is generally reserved for hospital treatment of serious or complicated infections. These include peritonitis, meningitis, and lung, bone, joint, wound, and urinary tract infections. It is also used with a penicillin for the prevention and treatment of heart valve infections (endocarditis). This drug combination is also used to treat severe infections in newborn babies.

Also available as drops and ointment, gentamicin is commonly given for eye and ear infections. Ointment may also occasionally be prescribed for infected burns or ulcers.

Development of resistance to the drug, however, is a common problem following treatment with skin preparations.

Gentamicin given by injection can have serious adverse effects on the kidneys and on the ears, leading to damage to the balance mechanism and deafness. Treatment is monitored with care when high doses are needed or when kidney function is poor.

QUICK REFERENCE

Drug group Aminoglycoside antibiotic (p.158)

Overdose danger rating Medium

Dependence rating Low

Prescription needed Yes

Available as generic Yes

INFORMATION FOR USERS

Your drug prescription is tailored for you. Do not alter dosage without checking with your physician.

How taken

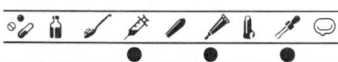

Injection, ointment, cream, eye/ear drops.

Frequency and timing of doses
Every 8 – 24 hours (injection); 3 – 4 x daily (skin preparations); every 6 – 12 hours (eye ointment); every 4 – 8 hours (eye and ear drops).

Adult dosage range
According to condition and response (injection); according to your physician's instructions (eye, ear, and skin preparations).

Onset of effect
2 – 3 days.

Duration of action
8 – 12 hours.

Diet advice
None.

Storage
Keep in a closed container in a cool, dry place away from reach of children.

Missed dose
Apply skin, eye, and ear preparations as soon as you remember.

Stopping the drug
Apply the full course. Even if you feel better, the original infection may still be present and may recur if treatment is stopped too soon.

Exceeding the dose
Overdose by injection is unlikely since treatment is carefully monitored. For other preparations, an occasional unintentional extra dose is unlikely to be a cause for concern. If you notice unusual symptoms, notify your physician.

SPECIAL PRECAUTIONS

Be sure to tell your physician if:
▼ You have impaired kidney function.
▼ You have a hearing disorder.
▼ You have myasthenia gravis.
▼ You have had a previous allergic reaction to aminoglycosides.
▼ You are taking other medications.

Pregnancy
▼ No evidence of risk with *topical* preparations. Injections are not prescribed, as they cause hearing defects in the baby.

Breast feeding
▼ No evidence of risk with eye, ear, or skin preparations. Given by injection, the drug may pass into the breast milk. Discuss with your physician.

Infants and children
▼ Reduced dose necessary for injections.

Over 60
▼ Reduced dose may be necessary. Increased likelihood of adverse effects.

Driving and hazardous work
▼ No known problems.

Alcohol
▼ No known problems.

Surgery and general anesthetics
▼ Gentamicin may need to be stopped before you have a general anesthetic.

POSSIBLE ADVERSE EFFECTS

Adverse effects are rare but those that occur with the injectable form may be serious. Dizziness, loss of balance (vertigo), impaired hearing, and changes in the urine should be reported promptly. Allergic reactions, including rash and itching, are symptoms that may occur with all preparations that contain gentamicin.

Symptom/effect	Frequency		Discuss with physician		Stop taking drug now	Call physician now
	Common	Rare	Only if severe	In all cases		
Nausea/vomiting		●	■			
Headache/lethargy		●		■	▲	▮
Dizziness/vertigo		●		■	▲	▮
Rash/itching		●		■	▲	▮
Ringing in the ears		●		■	▲	▮
Loss of hearing		●		■	▲	▮
Bloody/cloudy urine		●		■	▲	▮

INTERACTIONS

General note A wide range of drugs increase the risk of hearing loss and/or kidney failure with gentamicin. Such drugs include other aminoglycoside and polymyxin antibiotics, furosemide, and cisplatin.

PROLONGED USE

Not usually given for longer than 10 days. There is a risk of adverse effects on hearing, balance, and kidney function.

Monitoring Blood levels of the drug are usually checked during injection treatment.

GLIPIZIDE

Brand name Glucotrol
Used in the following combined preparations None

GENERAL INFORMATION

Glipizide, introduced in 1984, is one of the newest oral antidiabetic drugs. Like other drugs of this type, it stimulates the secretion of insulin from the pancreas and promotes the uptake of sugar into body cells, thereby lowering the level of sugar in the blood.

It is used in the treatment of adult (maturity-onset) diabetes mellitus, in conjunction with a diabetic diet low in refined sugar and fats. Unlike some other antidiabetic drugs, glipizide has a mild diuretic action, making it useful for people with a tendency to retain water, such as those with congestive heart failure.

In conditions of severe illness, injury, or stress, the drug may lose its effectiveness, making insulin injections necessary.

QUICK REFERENCE

Drug group Oral antidiabetic drug (p.170)

Overdose danger rating High

Dependence rating Low

Prescription needed Yes

Available as generic No

INFORMATION FOR USERS

Your drug prescription is tailored for you. Do not alter dosage without checking with your physician.

How taken

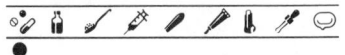

Tablets.

Frequency and timing of doses
Once daily (in the morning), or 2 x daily (in the morning and evening before meals).

Adult dosage range
5 – 40mg daily.

Onset of effect
Within 1 hour.

Duration of action
18 – 24 hours.

Diet advice
A low-sugar, low-fat diet must be maintained in order for the drug to be fully effective. Follow the advice of your physician.

Storage
Keep in a closed container in a cool, dry place away from reach of children.

Missed dose
Take before your next meal.

Stopping the drug
Do not stop the drug without consulting your physician; stopping the drug may lead to worsening of your diabetes.

OVERDOSE ACTION

Seek immediate medical advice in all cases. If early warning symptoms of excessively low blood sugar such as faintness, sweating, trembling, confusion or headache occur, eat or drink something sugary. Take emergency action if seizures or loss of consciousness occurs.

See Drug poisoning emergency guide (p.590).

SPECIAL PRECAUTIONS

Be sure to tell your physician if:
▼ You have impaired liver or kidney function.
▼ You are allergic to sulfonamide drugs.
▼ You are taking other medications.

Pregnancy
▼ Not usually prescribed. May cause abnormally low blood sugar in the newborn baby. Insulin is generally substituted in pregnancy.

Breast feeding
▼ Discuss with your physician. The drug passes into the breast milk and may cause low blood sugar in the baby.

Infants and children
▼ Not prescribed.

Over 60
▼ Signs of low blood sugar may be more difficult to recognize.

Driving and hazardous work
▼ Usually no problem. Avoid these activities if you have warning signs of low blood sugar.

Alcohol
▼ Avoid. Alcoholic drinks upset diabetic control.

Surgery and general anesthetics
▼ Surgery may alter the effect of glipizide on diabetes. Notify your physician that you are diabetic before any surgery; insulin treatment may need to be substituted.

POSSIBLE ADVERSE EFFECTS

Serious adverse effects are rare. More common symptoms, often accompanied by hunger, may be signs of low blood sugar due to lack of food or too high a dose of glipizide.

Symptom/effect	Frequency		Discuss with physician		Stop taking drug now	Call physician now
	Common	Rare	Only if severe	In all cases		
Faintness/confusion	●			■		
Weakness/tremor	●			■		
Sweating	●			■		
Nausea/vomiting		●	■			
Thirst		●		■		
Rash/itching		●		■		

INTERACTIONS

General note A variety of drugs may reduce the effect of glipizide and so raise blood sugar levels. These include corticosteroids, estrogens, diuretics, rifampin, phenobarbital, antipsychotic drugs, and phenytoin. Other drugs increase the risk of low blood sugar. These include dicumarol, sulfonamides, anabolic steroids, aspirin, and ketoconazole.

Beta blockers These mask the signs of low blood sugar.

PROLONGED USE

No problems expected.

Monitoring Regular monitoring of levels of sugar in the urine or blood is required.

GLYBURIDE

Brand names DiaBeta, Micronase
Used in the following combined preparations None

GENERAL INFORMATION

Glyburide, introduced in 1984, is one of the newest oral antidiabetic drugs. Used in the treatment of adult (maturity-onset) diabetes mellitus, it lowers blood sugar by stimulating the secretion of insulin from the pancreas and promoting the uptake of sugar into body cells.

It has a prolonged action, and one dose daily is sufficient for most people. Control of the blood sugar depends on keeping to a diet low in refined sugar and fats, and on losing excess weight.

Serious adverse effects with glyburide are rare. Unlike some antidiabetic drugs, it has a mild diuretic effect, making it useful for people with a tendency to retain water, such as those with congestive heart failure.

In conditions of severe illness, injury, or stress, the drug may lose its effectiveness in stimulating the pancreas, making insulin injections necessary.

QUICK REFERENCE

Drug group Oral antidiabetic drug (p.170)

Overdose danger rating High

Dependence rating Low

Prescription needed Yes

Available as generic No

INFORMATION FOR USERS

Your drug prescription is tailored for you. Do not alter dosage without checking with your physician.

How taken

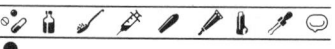

Tablets.

Frequency and timing of doses
Once daily (in the morning), or 2 x daily (in the morning and evening with meals).

Dosage range
1.25 – 20mg daily.

Onset of effect
Within 1 hour.

Duration of action
Approximately 24 hours.

Diet advice
A low-sugar, low-fat diet must be maintained in order for the drug to be fully effective. Follow your physician's advice.

Storage
Keep in a closed container in a cool, dry place away from reach of children.

Missed dose
Take before your next meal.

Stopping the drug
Do not stop the drug without consulting your physician; stopping the drug may lead to worsening of your diabetes.

OVERDOSE ACTION

 Seek immediate medical advice in all cases. If early warning symptoms of excessively low blood sugar such as faintness, sweating, trembling, confusion or headache occur, eat or drink something sugary. Take emergency action if seizures or loss of consciousness occurs.

See Drug poisoning emergency guide (p.590).

SPECIAL PRECAUTIONS

Be sure to tell your physician if:
▼ You have impaired liver or kidney function.
▼ You are allergic to sulfonamide drugs.
▼ You are taking other medications.

 Pregnancy
▼ Not usually prescribed. May cause abnormally low blood sugar in the newborn baby. Insulin is generally substituted in pregnancy.

 Breast feeding
▼ Discuss with your physician. The drug passes into the breast milk and may cause low blood sugar in the baby.

 Infants and children
▼ Not prescribed.

 Over 60
▼ Signs of low blood sugar may be more difficult to recognize.

 Driving and hazardous work
▼ Usually no problem. Avoid these activities if you have warning signs of low blood sugar.

 Alcohol
▼ Avoid. Alcoholic drinks upset diabetic control.

Surgery and general anesthetics
▼ Surgery may reduce the response to glyburide. Notify your physician that you are diabetic before any surgery; insulin treatment may need to be substituted.

POSSIBLE ADVERSE EFFECTS

Serious adverse effects are rare. Faintness, sweating, tremor, weakness, and confusion may be signs of low blood sugar due to lack of food or too high a dose of glyburide.

Symptom/effect	Frequency		Discuss with physician		Stop taking drug now	Call physician now
	Common	Rare	Only if severe	In all cases		
Faintness/confusion	●			■		
Weakness/tremor	●			■		
Sweating	●			■		
Nausea/vomiting		●	■			
Thirst		●		■		
Rash/itching		●		■		

PROLONGED USE

No problems expected.

Monitoring Regular monitoring of levels of sugar in the urine or blood is required.

INTERACTIONS

General note A variety of drugs may reduce the effect of glyburide and so raise blood sugar levels. Such drugs include corticosteroids, estrogens, diuretics, rifampin, phenobarbital, antipsychotic drugs, and phenytoin. Other drugs increase the risk of low blood sugar with glyburide. These include dicumarol, sulfonamides, anabolic steroids, aspirin, and ketoconazole.

Beta blockers These mask the signs of low blood sugar.

GRAMICIDIN

Used in the following combined preparations Cortisporin Cream, Mycolog II Cream, Neosporin Ophthalmic Solution, Spectrocin Ointment

GENERAL INFORMATION

Gramicidin, introduced in 1949, is a naturally occurring antibiotic produced by bacteria. Available only in combined preparations, it is prescribed along with other antibiotics to treat skin conditions and eye infections such as sties. Some gramicidin preparations contain a corticosteroid, such as triamcinolone, to relieve itching and inflammation. Gramicidin is also available in a combined preparation with nystatin, an antifungal drug, for the treatment of mixed bacterial and fungal infections.

Gramicidin itself rarely causes side effects. If a rash develops this may indicate an allergy to the additional ingredient in the preparation.

QUICK REFERENCE

Drug group Antibiotic (p.156)

Overdose danger rating Low

Dependence rating Low

Prescription needed Yes

Available as generic Yes

INFORMATION FOR USERS

Your drug prescription is tailored for you. **Do not alter dosage without checking with your physician.**

How taken

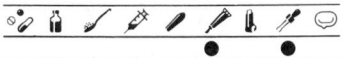

Cream, ointment, eye drops.

Frequency and timing of doses
2 – 4 x daily.

Dosage range
Skin conditions Enough cream or ointment to cover the affected area at each application.
Eye infections 1 – 2 drops per application.

Onset of effect
1 – 2 hours.

Duration of action
Up to 1 day.

Diet advice
None.

Storage
Keep in a closed container in a cool, dry place away from reach of children.

Missed dose
No cause for concern. Take as soon as you remember.

Stopping the drug
Apply the full course. Even if you feel better, the original infection may still be present and may recur if treatment is stopped too soon.

Exceeding the dose
An occasional unintentional extra dose is unlikely to be a cause for concern. But if you notice unusual symptoms, notify your physician.

POSSIBLE ADVERSE EFFECTS

Preparations containing gramicidin rarely cause side effects. If a local allergic reaction such as a rash occurs, it may be caused by one of the other ingredients.

Symptom/effect	Frequency		Discuss with physician		Stop taking drug now	Call physician now
	Common	Rare	Only if severe	In all cases		
Rash		●		■		▲
Irritation		●		■		▲

INTERACTIONS

None.

SPECIAL PRECAUTIONS

Be sure to tell your physician if:
▼ You have any allergies.

Pregnancy
▼ No evidence of risk to developing baby.

Breast feeding
▼ No evidence of risk.

Infants and children
▼ No special problems.

Over 60
▼ No special problems.

Driving and hazardous work
▼ No known problems.

Alcohol
▼ No known problems.

PROLONGED USE

No problems expected but prolonged use of gramicidin preparations is unlikely to be necessary.

GRISEOFULVIN

Brand names Fulvicin P/G, Fulvicin U/F, Grifulvin V, Gris-Peg, Grisactin Ultra
Used in the following combined preparations None

GENERAL INFORMATION

Griseofulvin, extracted from a species of penicillin bacteria, has been available since 1959 to treat forms of fungal skin infection that do not respond to creams and lotions. Given by mouth, it is claimed to be effective for tinea (ringworm) infections of the scalp, beard, palms, soles of feet, and nails.

Some of these infections are stubborn and take several months before any noticeable improvement is seen. Sometimes during this period a *topical* antifungal drug may also be prescribed. Fingernail infections usually improve after 6 to 9 months. In toenail infections there may not be any noticeable improvement until a healthy nail has grown, which may take a year.

The most common adverse effects are headache, loss of taste, dry mouth, and abdominal pain. Some people may become more sensitive to sunlight. Griseofulvin may cause damage to the liver in rare cases and may affect bone marrow activity adversely. For these reasons it is prescribed only when other treatments have failed, and never when liver function is impaired.

QUICK REFERENCE

Drug group Antifungal drug (p.166)
Overdose danger rating Low
Dependence rating Low
Prescription needed Yes
Available as generic No

INFORMATION FOR USERS

Your drug prescription is tailored for you. Do not alter dosage without checking with your physician.

How taken

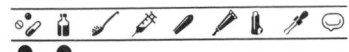

Tablets, capsules, liquid.

Frequency and timing of doses
1 – 4 x daily after meals and at bedtime.

Dosage range
Adults 330mg – 1g daily depending on preparation.
Children Reduced dose according to age and weight.

Onset of effect
Full beneficial effect may not be felt for 3 – 4 weeks (skin); 4 – 6 weeks (scalp); 6 – 9 months (fingernails); 8 – 18 months (toenails).

Duration of action
Up to 24 hours.

Diet advice
None.

Storage
Keep in a closed container in a cool, dry place away from reach of children.

Missed dose
Do not take the missed dose. Take your next dose as usual.

Stopping the drug
Take the full course. Even if symptoms disappear, the original infection may still be present and symptoms may recur if treatment is stopped too soon.

Exceeding the dose
An occasional unintentional extra dose is unlikely to be a cause for concern. But if you notice unusual symptoms, or if a large overdose has been taken, notify your physician.

POSSIBLE ADVERSE EFFECTS

Most adverse reactions are minor and diminish within a few days of treatment.

Symptom/effect	Frequency		Discuss with physician		Stop taking drug now	Call physician now
	Common	Rare	Only if severe	In all cases		
Headache	●		■			
Dry mouth/loss of taste	●		■			
Nausea/vomiting	●		■			
Diarrhea		●	■			
Painful/swollen joints		●		■		
Dizziness/confusion		●		■		
Rash		●		■	▲	▮

INTERACTIONS

Oral anticoagulant drugs Griseofulvin reduces the effect of these drugs by increasing their breakdown by the liver.

Barbiturates These drugs reduce the effect of griseofulvin.

Oral contraceptives When used with griseofulvin, breakthrough bleeding and pregnancies have occurred.

SPECIAL PRECAUTIONS

Be sure to tell your physician if:
▼ You have impaired liver function.
▼ You suffer from porphyria.
▼ You have previously had a skin rash after taking griseofulvin.
▼ You are allergic to penicillin antibiotics.
▼ You are taking other medications.

 Pregnancy
▼ Not usually prescribed. Safety in pregnancy not established. Discuss with your physician so that you may weigh the benefits of the drug against its possible risks.

 Breast feeding
▼ No evidence of risk.

 Infants and children
▼ Reduced dose necessary.

 Over 60
▼ No special problems.

 Driving and hazardous work
▼ Avoid such activities until you have learned how the drug affects you, because the drug can cause dizziness.

 Alcohol
▼ Avoid. Alcohol may increase the sedative effects of this drug.

PROLONGED USE

There is a slight risk of liver damage; there is also a risk of reduced bone marrow function, which causes low levels of white blood cells.

Monitoring Periodic blood tests may be performed to check liver function and blood composition.

GROWTH HORMONE

Brand name Protropin
Used in the following combined preparations None

GENERAL INFORMATION

Growth hormone, somatropin, is produced by the pituitary gland. In children and adolescents it promotes the normal growth and development of the body. But if it is not produced in sufficient quantities, growth is slowed and abnormally short stature results.

Replacing the once available natural hormone is a synthetic form of the compound known as somatrem. It is produced by genetic engineering techniques and has been available since 1986.

Administered regularly by injection to children who have a deficiency of the natural hormone, it promotes normal growth. Treatment is continued throughout childhood until the expected height is reached in late adolescence. The earlier treatment is started, the greater the chance of complete success. Somatrem is not effective as a means of increasing height when hormone levels are normal. In spite of condemnation by physicians and sports authorities, the drug has occasionally been abused by athletes for its muscle-building properties, which are similar to those of anabolic steroids (p.174).

Treatment with this drug rarely causes adverse effects. Careful monitoring of growth is carried out. There is a slight risk of provoking the onset of diabetes mellitus, and sometimes thyroid function may be reduced.

QUICK REFERENCE

Drug group Pituitary hormone (p.173)

Overdose danger rating Low

Dependence rating Low

Prescription needed Yes

Available as generic No

INFORMATION FOR USERS

The drug is given only under medical supervision and is not for self-administration.

How taken

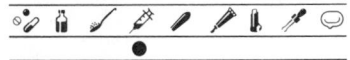

Injection.

Frequency and timing of doses
1 – 3 x weekly.

Dosage range
Dosage is adjusted according to age, weight, and individual response.

Onset of effect
1 – 2 months.

Duration of action
1 week.

Diet advice
Drug treatment for growth needs to be accompanied by a nourishing balanced diet. Excessive intake of protein may cause a buildup of nitrogen waste in the body. Your physician will give detailed advice.

Storage
Not applicable. This drug is not normally kept in the home.

Missed dose
Arrange for a missed injection to be administered as soon as possible.

Stopping the drug
Treatment can be safely stopped when the child has reached mature adult height. Stopping the drug prematurely may prevent full growth from being achieved.

Exceeding the dose
Overdosage is unlikely, since treatment is carefully monitored.

POSSIBLE ADVERSE EFFECTS

Somatrem rarely causes adverse effects if taken in normal doses. Abnormal overgrowth of bones may occur if the drug is given in too high a dosage.

Symptom/effect	Frequency		Discuss with physician		Stop taking drug now	Call physician now
	Common	Rare	Only if severe	In all cases		
Injection site pain/swelling		●		■		

INTERACTIONS

Corticosteroids These may reduce the effect of somatrem.

SPECIAL PRECAUTIONS

Be sure to tell your physician if:
▼ Your child has diabetes.
▼ Your child has a thyroid problem.
▼ Your child is taking other medications.

 Pregnancy
▼ Not prescribed.

 Breast feeding
▼ Not prescribed.

 Infants and children
▼ Safe for use throughout childhood.

 Over 60
▼ Not prescribed.

 Driving and hazardous work
▼ No special problems.

 Alcohol
▼ Not applicable.

PROLONGED USE

Rate of growth may decrease during prolonged treatment. Treatment may be stopped for a few months and then restarted.

Monitoring Regular checks on height, bone growth, thyroid function, and urine glucose levels are usually carried out.

A
B
C
D
E
F
G
H
I
J
K
L
M
N
O
P
Q
R
S
T
U
V
W
X
Y
Z

GUANETHIDINE

Brand name Ismelin
Used in the following combined preparations None

GENERAL INFORMATION

Guanethidine, in use since 1960, is an antihypertensive drug. It is powerful and therefore generally used only in severe hypertension (high blood pressure) when there has been little or no response to other drugs. Because it has a number of adverse effects, it is now rarely used. It is usually given with a diuretic to prevent fluid retention and enhance its beneficial effects.

Guanethidine also improves blood flow to the fingers and toes in Raynaud's disease. It is under investigation for the treatment of glaucoma in combination with epinephrine as eye drops.
  Adverse effects of guanethidine include a tendency for blood pressure to drop suddenly when a person rises from a sitting or lying position, resulting in dizziness and faintness.

QUICK REFERENCE

Drug group Antihypertensive drug (p.130).

Overdose danger rating High

Dependence rating Low

Prescription needed Yes

Available as generic Yes

INFORMATION FOR USERS

Your drug prescription is tailored for you. Do not alter dosage without checking with your physician.

How taken

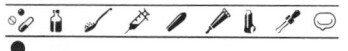

Tablets.

Frequency and timing of doses
Once daily.

Adult dosage range
10 – 12.5mg daily (starting dose), increased as necessary up to 100mg daily. In some cases larger doses may be required.

Onset of effect
Within 8 hours. Full beneficial effect on blood pressure may not occur for 1 – 3 weeks.

Duration of action
Up to 5 days. Some beneficial effects may last for 1 – 3 weeks after stopping the drug.

Diet advice
A low-sodium diet and/or weight reduction may also be recommended for hypertension treatment.

Storage
Keep in a closed container in a cool, dry place away from reach of children.

Missed dose
Take as soon as you remember. If your next dose is due within 6 hours, take a single dose now and skip the next.

Stopping the drug
Do not stop the drug without consulting your physician; stopping the drug may lead to worsening of the underlying condition.

OVERDOSE ACTION

 Seek immediate medical advice in all cases. Take emergency action if severe dizziness, faintness, or loss of consciousness occurs.

See Drug poisoning emergency guide (p.590).

SPECIAL PRECAUTIONS

Be sure to tell your physician if:
▼ You have impaired liver or kidney function.
▼ You have heart failure.
▼ You have diabetes.
▼ You have a lung disorder such as asthma or bronchitis.
▼ You have had a stomach ulcer.
▼ You have pheochromocytoma.
▼ You are taking other medications.

 Pregnancy
▼ Not usually prescribed. Safety in pregnancy not established. Discuss with your physician so that you can weigh the benefits of the drug against its possible risks.

 Breast feeding
▼ Discuss with your physician. Effect on breast feeding uncertain.

 Infants and children
▼ Not usually prescribed.

 Over 60
▼ Reduced dose may be necessary. Increased risk of dizziness on standing.

 Driving and hazardous work
▼ No known problems.

 Alcohol
▼ Avoid. Alcohol may lead to dizziness and fainting with this drug.

Surgery and general anesthetics
▼ Guanethidine may need to be stopped before you have a general anesthetic. Discuss this with your physician or dentist before any surgery.

POSSIBLE ADVERSE EFFECTS

Dizziness or faintness on standing are the most common adverse effects and can be avoided to some extent by getting up slowly; swollen feet or ankles (due to fluid retention), slowed heart rate, diarrhea, and impotence may also occur.

Symptom/effect	Frequency		Discuss with physician		Stop taking drug now	Call physician now
	Common	Rare	Only if severe	In all cases		
Dizziness/faintness	●		■			
Diarrhea	●		■			
Stuffy nose	●		■			
Swelling of feet or legs	●			■		
Impotence		●		■		
Breathlessness		●		■	▲	▮

PROLONGED USE

No problems expected.

INTERACTIONS

General note Many drugs interact with guanethidine to produce a rise in blood pressure. Such drugs include monoamine oxidase inhibitors, antipsychotics, tricyclic antidepressants, and *sympathomimetics* such as amphetamines and ephedrine.

Antidiabetic drugs Guanethidine may increase the fall in blood sugar produced by these agents.

HALOPERIDOL

Brand name Haldol
Used in the following combined preparations None

GENERAL INFORMATION

Introduced in the early 1960s, haloperidol is the most widely used of a group of drugs known as butyrophenones. They are effective in reducing the violent, aggressive manifestations of mental illnesses such as schizophrenia, mania, dementia, and other disorders where hallucinations are experienced. It does not cure the underlying disorder, but it does relieve the distressing symptoms. It is also used in the control of Tourette's syndrome and is of benefit in children with severe behavior problems where other drugs are ineffective. The main drawback to the use of haloperidol is that it produces disturbing side effects – in particular, abnormal involuntary movements and stiffness of the face and limbs.

QUICK REFERENCE

Drug group Butyrophenone antipsychotic drug (p.113)

Overdose danger rating Medium

Dependence rating Low

Prescription needed Yes

Available as generic Yes

INFORMATION FOR USERS

Your drug prescription is tailored for you. Do not alter dosage without checking with your physician.

How taken

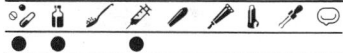

Tablets, liquid, injection.

Frequency and timing of doses
2 – 4 x daily with food or milk.

Adult dosage range
Mental illness 1.5 – 6mg (starting dose), increasing to 10 – 20mg daily (maintenance dose). Dose may be increased in cases of extreme agitation.
Nausea and vomiting 2 – 10mg daily.

Onset of effect
20 – 30 minutes (by injection); 2 – 3 hours (by mouth).

Duration of action
6 – 24 hours. Up to 4 weeks after depot injection.

Diet advice
None.

Storage
Keep in a closed container in a cool, dry place away from reach of children.

Missed dose
Take as soon as you remember. If your next dose is due within 2 hours, take a single dose now and skip the next.

Stopping the drug
Do not stop the drug without consulting your physician; symptoms may recur.

Exceeding the dose
An occasional unintentional extra dose is unlikely to cause problems. Larger overdoses may cause unusual drowsiness, muscle weakness or rigidity, and/or faintness. Notify your physician.

SPECIAL PRECAUTIONS

Be sure to tell your physician if:
▼ You have impaired liver or kidney function.
▼ You have heart or circulation problems.
▼ You have had epileptic seizures.
▼ You have an overactive thyroid gland.
▼ You have Parkinson's disease.
▼ You have had glaucoma.
▼ You have asthma, bronchitis, or another lung disorder.
▼ You are taking other medications.

Pregnancy
▼ Not usually prescribed. Safety in pregnancy not established. Discuss with your physician so that you can weigh the benefits of the drug against its possible risks.

Breast feeding
▼ Discuss with your physician. The drug passes into the breast milk. Its effects on the baby are not known.

Infants and children
▼ Rarely required. Reduced dose necessary.

Over 60
▼ Reduced dose may be necessary.

Driving and hazardous work
▼ Avoid such activities until you have learned how the drug affects you, because this drug may cause drowsiness and slowed reactions.

Alcohol
▼ Avoid. Alcohol may increase the sedative effect of this drug.

POSSIBLE ADVERSE EFFECTS

Haloperidol can cause a variety of minor *anticholinergic* symptoms that often become less marked with time. The most significant adverse effect is abnormal movements of the face and limbs (parkinsonism). This may be controlled by dosage adjustment.

Symptom/effect	Frequency		Discuss with physician		Stop taking drug now	Call physician now
	Common	Rare	Only if severe	In all cases		
Drowsiness/lethargy	●		■			
Weight gain	●		■			
Parkinsonism	●			■		
Dizziness/fainting	●			■		
Rash		●		■	▲	
High fever/confusion		●		■	▲	■

INTERACTIONS

Sedatives All drugs that have a sedative effect are likely to increase the sedative properties of haloperidol.

Antiparkinsonism drugs Haloperidol may counter the beneficial effect of such drugs.

Anticholinergic drugs The side effects of drugs with anticholinergic properties may be increased by haloperidol.

Anticonvulsant drugs Dosage may need adjustment.

PROLONGED USE

Use of this drug for more than a few months may lead to *tardive dyskinesia*, i.e., abnormal, involuntary movements of the eyes, face, and tongue. Occasionally, jaundice may occur.

Monitoring Periodic blood tests may be performed.

HEPARIN

Brand names Calciparine, Hepin Liquaemin, Lipo
Used in the following combined preparation Embolex

GENERAL INFORMATION

Heparin is an anticoagulant prescribed to prevent and aid in the dispersion of blood clots. Because it acts more quickly than other anticoagulants, it is particularly useful during emergencies – for instance, to prevent the extension of clotting when a clot has already reached the lungs or the brain. People undergoing open heart surgery and kidney dialysis are also given heparin in case the blood flow becomes sluggish. A low dose of heparin is sometimes given to elderly, bedridden people after surgery to prevent clots from forming in leg veins. Often, heparin is given in conjunction with other slower-acting anticoagulants, such as warfarin, until they reach their full beneficial effects, usually after a few days. Since it must be injected more than once daily, heparin is not usually given on its own, long-term. Its most serious adverse effect, as with all anticoagulants, is the risk of excessive bleeding, usually from overdosage, so the ability of the blood to coagulate is watched very carefully under medical supervision. Also, bruising may occur around the site of the injection.

Since heparin is a mixture of molecules of different sizes extracted from animal tissue, it is usually measured in "units" of activity rather than by weight in mg, as with other drugs.

QUICK REFERENCE

Drug group Anticoagulant drug (p.132)

Overdose danger rating High

Dependence rating Low

Prescription needed Yes

Available as generic Yes

INFORMATION FOR USERS

This drug is given only under medical supervision and is not for self-administration.

How taken

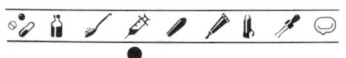

Injection.

Frequency and timing of doses
Every 4 – 6 hours.

Dosage range
Treatment 5,000 – 10,000 units initially, then 1,000 – 2,000 units per hour.
Preventive use 5,000 units subcutaneously, usually every 12 hours.

Onset of effect
Within 15 minutes.

Duration of action
4 – 8 hours after treatment is stopped.

Diet advice
None.

Storage
Not applicable. This drug is not kept in the home.

Missed dose
Call your physician.

Stopping the drug
Do not stop taking the drug without consulting your physician. Stopping the drug may lead to clotting of blood.

OVERDOSE ACTION

 Seek immediate medical advice in all cases. Take emergency action if bleeding, severe headache, or loss of consciousness occurs. Overdose can be reversed under medical supervision by a drug called protamine.

See Drug poisoning emergency guide (p.590).

POSSIBLE ADVERSE EFFECTS

As with all anticoagulants, bleeding is the most common adverse effect with heparin.

The less common effects may diminish during long-term treatment.

Symptom/effect	Frequency		Discuss with physician		Stop taking drug now	Call physician now
	Common	Rare	Only if severe	In all cases		
Bleeding/bruising	●			■		▮
Digestive disturbance		●		■		
Aching bones		●		■		
Rash		●		■	▲	

INTERACTIONS

Aspirin Do not take. Aspirin may increase the anticoagulant effect of this drug, and there is an increased risk of bleeding in the intestine or joints.

Dipyridamole The anticoagulant effect of heparin may be increased when taken along with this drug. Its dosage may need to be adjusted accordingly.

SPECIAL PRECAUTIONS

Be sure to tell your physician if:
▼ You have impaired liver or kidney function.
▼ You have high blood pressure.
▼ You bleed easily.
▼ You have any allergies.
▼ You are taking other medications.

 Pregnancy
▼ Not usually prescribed. May cause the mother to bleed excessively if taken near delivery. Discuss with your physician.

 Breast feeding
▼ No evidence of risk.

 Infants and children
▼ Reduced dose necessary according to age and weight.

 Over 60
▼ Reduced dose may be necessary.

 Driving and hazardous work
▼ Avoid risk of injury, since excessive bruising and bleeding may occur.

 Alcohol
▼ No special problems.

Surgery and general anesthetics
▼ Heparin may need to be stopped. Discuss this with your physician or dentist before any surgery.

PROLONGED USE

Osteoporosis and hair loss may occur; tolerance to heparin may develop.

Monitoring Periodic blood checks will be required.

HCG (human chorionic gonadotropin)

Brand names A.P.L., Pregnyl
Used in the following combined preparations None

GENERAL INFORMATION

Produced by the pituitary gland, chorionic gonadotropin is a hormone that stimulates the ovaries to produce two other hormones, estrogen and progesterone, that are essential to the conception and early growth of the fetus. Since 1939 the hormone, commonly called HCG, has been extracted from the urine of pregnant women and used for several purposes.

Its principal value is in the treatment of female infertility. Given by injection (usually with another hormone), HCG encourages the ovaries to release eggs (ovulation) so that they can be fertilized. Ovulation usually occurs 18 hours after injection, and intercourse should follow within 48 hours. HCG increases the likelihood of multiple births.

HCG is also given to men, improving the production of sperm after 6 – 9 months of treatment.

It is occasionally used to prevent miscarriage in women who have lost previous pregnancies. The drug is also given in rare cases to young boys to treat undescended testicles.

QUICK REFERENCE

Drug group Drug for infertility (p.192)

Overdose danger rating Low

Dependence rating Low

Prescription needed Yes

Available as generic Yes

INFORMATION FOR USERS

This drug is given only under medical supervision and is not for self-administration.

How taken

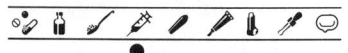

Injection.

Frequency and timing of doses
Every 2 – 3 days.

Dosage range
Dosage varies from person to person, and may need adjustment during treatment.

Onset of effect
1 – 8 days (female infertility); 6 – 9 months (male infertility).

Duration of action
2 – 3 days.

Diet advice
None.

Storage
Not applicable. This drug is not kept in the home.

Missed dose
Arrange to receive the missed dose as soon as possible. Delay of more than 24 hours may reduce the chance of conception.

Stopping the drug
Complete the course of treatment as directed. Stopping the drug prematurely will reduce the chance of conception.

Exceeding the dose
The drug is always injected under close medical supervision. Overdose is unlikely.

POSSIBLE ADVERSE EFFECTS

When taken for fertility problems, the more common adverse effects of HCG are rarely severe and tend to diminish with time. Women who take large doses of the drug may experience abdominal pain or swelling due to overstimulation of the ovaries.

Symptom/effect	Frequency		Discuss with physician		Stop taking drug now	Call physician now
	Common	Rare	Only if severe	In all cases		
Headache/tiredness	●		■			
Pain at injection site	●		■			
Mood changes	●			■		
Women only						
Swollen feet/ankles		●		■		
Abdominal pain		●		■		
Men only						
Enlarged breasts		●		■	▲	

INTERACTIONS

None.

SPECIAL PRECAUTIONS

Be sure to tell your physician if:
▼ You have had a previous allergic reaction to this drug.
▼ You have prostate trouble.

Pregnancy
▼ Not prescribed.

Breast feeding
▼ Not prescribed.

Infants and children
▼ HCG is safely prescribed to treat undescended testicles in boys.

Over 60
▼ Not usually required.

Driving and hazardous work
▼ Avoid such activities until you have learned how the drug affects you, because the drug can cause tiredness.

Alcohol
▼ Avoid. Alcohol increases the likelihood of tiredness, and taken in excess may reduce fertility.

PROLONGED USE

No special problems.

Monitoring Women taking HCG to improve fertility usually have regular pelvic examinations and checks on cervical mucus to confirm that ovulation is taking place. Men are given regular sperm counts.

HYDRALAZINE

Brand name Apresoline
Used in the following combined preparations Apresazide, Apresoline-Esidrix, Serpasil-Apresoline, Ser-Ap-Es, Unipres

GENERAL INFORMATION

Hydralazine was introduced in the 1950s for use as an antihypertensive. It is a vasodilator (see p.126), i.e., a drug that relaxes the muscles of the artery walls and dilates blood vessels. It is used most often to treat moderate to severe high blood pressure.

Although usually given orally, hydralazine has a rapid onset of action when given by injection. This makes it particularly useful in emergencies.

Hydralazine is usually given as additional medication when treatment by diuretics has failed to produce the desired antihypertensive results. Since the diuretics reduce the concentration of sodium in the body and the volume of fluid as well, they offset a tendency of hydralazine to do just the opposite. Hydralazine is sometimes taken with beta blockers to help reduce the risk of an increased heart rate. The most serious adverse effect is the possibility of drug-induced lupus erythematosus, an autoimmune illness, which occurs only with long-term treatment in high doses and disappears when the drug is withdrawn.

INFORMATION FOR USERS

Your drug prescription is tailored for you. Do not alter dosage without checking with your physician.

How taken

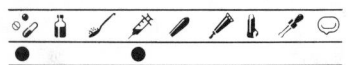

Tablets, injection.

Frequency and timing of doses
2 – 3 x daily.

Dosage range
Adults 50 – 200mg daily, up to a maximum of 300mg daily in exceptional cases.

Onset of effect
30 minutes – 2 hours (tablet), 10 – 20 minutes (injection).

Duration of action
6 – 8 hours (tablet), 2 – 4 hours (injection).

Diet advice
None.

Storage
Keep in a closed container in a cool, dry place away from reach of children.

Missed dose
Take as soon as you remember. If your next dose is due within 2 hours, take a single dose now and skip the next.

Stopping the drug
Do not stop the drug without consulting your physician; stopping the drug may lead to worsening of the underlying condition.

OVERDOSE ACTION

 Seek immediate medical advice in all cases. Take emergency action if severe nausea and vomiting, rapid heartbeat, or loss of consciousness occurs.

See Drug poisoning emergency guide (p.590).

POSSIBLE ADVERSE EFFECTS

Many of the common adverse effects diminish during long-term treatment.

Dizziness usually occurs when you get up; rising slowly will help.

Symptom/effect	Frequency		Discuss with physician		Stop taking drug now	Call physician now
	Common	Rare	Only if severe	In all cases		
Nausea/vomiting	●		■			
Headache	●		■			
Dizziness	●		■			
Irregular heartbeat	●			■		
Loss of appetite		●		■		
Rash		●		■		
Flushing		●		■		
Joint pain		●		■		

INTERACTIONS

Tricyclic antidepressants lower the blood pressure even further.

Monoamine oxidase inhibitors (MAOIs) lower the blood pressure even further.

SPECIAL PRECAUTIONS

Be sure to tell your physician if:
▼ You have impaired kidney or liver function.
▼ You have heart disease.
▼ You have had a stroke.
▼ You have had lupus erythematosus.
▼ You tend to be allergic.
▼ You are taking other medications.

 Pregnancy
▼ Not usually prescribed. Safety in pregnancy not established. Discuss with your physician so that you can weigh the benefits of the drug against its possible risks.

 Breast feeding
▼ The drug passes into the breast milk, but at normal doses adverse effects on the baby are uncommon. Discuss with your physician.

 Infants and children
▼ Not usually prescribed. Reduced dose necessary.

 Over 60
▼ No special problems.

 Driving and hazardous work
▼ Avoid such activities until you have learned how the drug affects you, because the drug can cause dizziness.

 Alcohol
▼ Avoid. Alcohol may increase the adverse effects of this drug.

PROLONGED USE

Lupus erythematosus, an autoimmune illness, may occur with prolonged use. This usually disappears when the drug is withdrawn.

Monitoring Periodic blood checks may be performed.

HYDROCHLOROTHIAZIDE

Brand names Esidrix, Hydrodiuril, Hydromal, Oretic, Thiuretic
Used in the following combined preparations Aldactazide, Aldoril, Dyazide, Maxazide, Moduretic

GENERAL INFORMATION

Hydrochlorothiazide, introduced in 1958, belongs to the thiazide group of diuretic drugs, which remove excess water from the body and reduce edema (fluid retention) in people with congestive heart failure, kidney disorders, cirrhosis of the liver, and premenstrual tension.

Hydrochlorothiazide is frequently used to treat high blood pressure (see Antihypertensive drugs, p.130), and because it reduces the amount of calcium in the urine, it may sometimes be used to prevent the recurrence of certain types of kidney stones.

As with all thiazides, hydrochlorothiazide increases the loss of potassium in the urine, which can cause a variety of symptoms (see p.127), and increases the likelihood of irregular heart rhythms, particularly if you are taking drugs such as digoxin for heart failure. Potassium supplements are often prescribed along with it.

QUICK REFERENCE

Drug group Thiazide diuretic (p.127)

Overdose danger rating Low

Dependence rating Low

Prescription needed Yes

Available as generic Yes

INFORMATION FOR USERS

Your drug prescription is tailored for you. Do not alter dosage without checking with your physician.

How taken

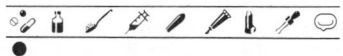

Tablets.

Frequency and timing of doses
Once daily, or every 2 days, early in the day.

Adult dosage range
25 – 100mg daily.

Onset of effect
Within 2 hours.

Duration of action
6 – 12 hours.

Diet advice
Use of this drug may reduce potassium in the body. Eat plenty of fresh fruits and vegetables. Discuss the advisability of reducing your salt intake with your physician.

Storage
Keep in a closed container in a cool, dry place away from reach of children.

Missed dose
No cause for concern, but take as soon as you remember. However, if it is late in the day do not take the missed dose, or you may need to get up during the night to pass urine. Take the next scheduled dose as usual.

Stopping the drug
Do not stop the drug without consulting your physician; symptoms may recur.

Exceeding the dose
An occasional unintentional extra dose is unlikely to be a cause for concern. But if you notice any unusual symptoms, or if a large overdose has been taken, notify your physician.

SPECIAL PRECAUTIONS

Be sure to tell your physician if:
▼ You have impaired kidney or liver function.
▼ You have had gout.
▼ You have diabetes.
▼ You have a high level of fat in your blood (hyperlipidemia).
▼ You are taking other medications.

 Pregnancy
▼ Not usually prescribed. No evidence that it harms the baby, but it may cause excessive sodium (salt) loss in the mother.

 Breast feeding
▼ The drug passes into the breast milk, but at normal doses adverse effects on the baby are uncommon. It may reduce your milk supply. Discuss with your physician.

 Infants and children
▼ Not usually prescribed. Reduced dose necessary.

 Over 60
▼ Increased likelihood of adverse effects.

 Driving and hazardous work
▼ No special problems, though morning urinary frequency can be anticipated.

 Alcohol
▼ Keep consumption low. Hydrochlorothiazide increases the likelihood of dehydration and hangovers after consumption of alcohol.

POSSIBLE ADVERSE EFFECTS

Most effects are caused by excessive loss of potassium. This can usually be put right by taking a potassium supplement. In rare cases gout may occur in susceptible people, and certain forms of diabetes may become more difficult to control.

Symptom/effect	Frequency		Discuss with physician		Stop taking drug now	Call physician now
	Common	Rare	Only if severe	In all cases		
Leg cramps	●		■			
Lethargy		●	■			
Dizziness		●	■			
Digestive disturbance		●	■			
Temporary impotence		●	■			
Rash		●		■		▲

INTERACTIONS

Non-steroidal anti-inflammatory drugs (NSAIDs) may reduce the diuretic effect of hydrochlorothiazide, whose dosage may need to be adjusted.

Digitalis drugs Their adverse effects may be increased if excessive potassium is lost.

Corticosteroids These drugs further increase the loss of potassium from the body when taken with hydrochlorothiazide.

Lithium Hydrochlorothiazide may increase lithium levels in the blood, leading to a risk of serious adverse effects.

PROLONGED USE

Excessive loss of potassium and imbalances of other salts may result.

Monitoring Blood tests may be performed periodically to check kidney function and levels of potassium and other salts.

HYDROCORTISONE

Brand names Cortaid, Cortenema, Hytone, Nutracort, Solu-Cortef
Used in the following combined preparations Anusol-HC, Coly-Mycin S Otic, Cortisporin Otic, CoSol-HC, Westcort

GENERAL INFORMATION

Hydrocortisone, introduced in 1952, is chemically identical to the hormone cortisol that is produced by the adrenal glands. One important use of the drug is the replacement of natural hormones in adrenal insufficiency (Addison's disease).

The main use of hydrocortisone, however, is palliative: it is prescribed to treat a variety of allergic and inflammatory conditions. Used in *topical* preparations, it provides prompt relief from inflammation of the skin, eye, and outer ear. It is used in oral form to relieve asthma, inflammatory bowel disease, and many other rheumatic and allergic disorders. Injected directly into the joints, it relieves pain and stiffness (see p.146). Injections may also be given to relieve severe attacks of asthma.

Overuse of hydrocortisone skin creams can lead to permanent thinning of the skin. Long-term treatment with high doses taken by mouth may cause serious side effects (see below).

QUICK REFERENCE

Drug group Corticosteroid (p.169)

Overdose danger rating Low

Dependence rating Low

Prescription needed Yes. Creams and ointments of 0.5 percent or less are available without a prescription.

Available as generic Yes

INFORMATION FOR USERS

Your drug prescription is tailored for you. Do not alter dosage without checking with your physician.

How taken

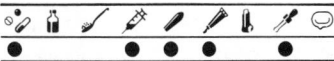

Tablets, injection, rectal suppositories, enema, lotion, ointment, cream, eye drops.

Frequency and timing of doses
Wide variation according to preparation and condition. Follow your physician's instructions.

Dosage range
Wide variation according to preparation and condition. Follow your physician's instructions.

Onset of effect
Within 2 – 4 days.

Duration of action
8 – 12 hours.

Diet advice
Salt intake may need to be restricted when the drug is taken by mouth. It may also be necessary to take potassium supplements.

Storage
Keep in a closed container in a cool, dry place away from reach of children.

Missed dose
Take as soon as you remember. If your next dose is due within 2 hours, take a single dose now and skip the next.

Stopping the drug
Do not stop taking the drug without consulting your physician. A gradual reduction in dosage is required following prolonged treatment by mouth.

Exceeding the dose
An occasional unintentional extra dose is unlikely to be a cause for concern. But if you notice unusual symptoms, or if a large overdose has been taken, notify your physician.

SPECIAL PRECAUTIONS

Be sure to tell your physician if:
▼ You have had a peptic ulcer.
▼ You have suffered from depression or a mental illness.
▼ You have glaucoma.
▼ You have had tuberculosis.
▼ You have a herpes infection.
▼ You are taking other medications.

Pregnancy
▼ No evidence of risk with topical preparations. Oral doses may adversely affect the developing baby. Discuss with your physician so that you may weigh the benefits of the drug against its risks.

Breast feeding
▼ Discuss with your physician. The drug passes into the breast milk and may affect the baby adversely.

Infants and children
▼ Reduced dose necessary.

Over 60
▼ Reduced dose may be necessary.

Driving and hazardous work
▼ No special problems, but you may suffer from blurred vision if you are using eye drops.

Alcohol
▼ Avoid. Alcohol may increase the risk of peptic ulcer when this drug is taken by mouth.

POSSIBLE ADVERSE EFFECTS

The more serious adverse effects only occur when hydrocortisone is taken by mouth in high doses for long periods of time. These are carefully monitored during treatment.

Symptom/effect	Frequency		Discuss with physician		Stop taking drug now	Call physician now
	Common	Rare	Only if severe	In all cases		
Indigestion	●		■			
Weight gain	●		■			
Acne	●		■			
Fluid retention		●			■	
Muscle weakness		●			■	
Mood changes		●			■	

PROLONGED USE

Depending on method of administration, prolonged high dosage may cause adverse effects such as diabetes, glaucoma, fragile bones, and thin skin, and may retard growth in children.

Monitoring Periodic checks on blood pressure are usually required when the drug is taken by mouth.

INTERACTIONS (by mouth only)

Barbiturates These drugs reduce the effectiveness of hydrocortisone.

Antidiabetic drugs Hydrocortisone decreases the action of these drugs: dosage may need to be adjusted to prevent abnormally high blood sugar.

Antihypertensive drugs Hydrocortisone reduces the effects of these drugs.

Vaccines Severe reactions can occur when this drug is taken with some vaccines. This does not apply to adrenal replacement therapy.

HYDROXYZINE

Brand names Atarax, Durrax, Orgatrax, Theozine, Vistaril
Used in the following combined preparations None

GENERAL INFORMATION

Hydroxyzine is an antihistamine drug. It is useful for relieving the itch from allergic skin conditions such as chronic rashes and urticaria (hives). It also has anti-emetic properties and is used to prevent motion sickness, post-operative nausea and vomiting, and sometimes vertigo (see Anti-emetic drugs, p.118). Its sedative effect also makes it useful as a sleeping aid and as a *premedication*. Hydroxyzine is occasionally prescribed as an anti-anxiety drug (p.111). However, although it is most successful in treating mild tension and agitation, long-term use of this drug is not recommended. The main side effect from treatment with hydroxyzine is mild drowsiness. This often subsides after a few days.

QUICK REFERENCE

Drug group Antihistamine (p.152)
Overdose danger rating Medium
Dependence rating Low
Prescription needed Yes
Available as generic Yes

INFORMATION FOR USERS

Your drug prescription is tailored for you. Do not alter dosage without checking with your physician.

How taken

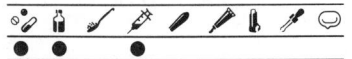

Tablets, capsules, liquid, injection.

Frequency and timing of doses
3 – 4 x daily.

Adult dosage range
75 – 400mg daily.

Onset of effect
15 – 30 minutes.

Duration of action
4 – 6 hours.

Diet advice
None.

Storage
Keep in a closed container in a cool, dry place away from reach of children.

Missed dose
Take as soon as you remember. If your next dose is due within 3 hours, take a single dose now and skip the next.

Stopping the drug
Do not stop the drug without consulting your physician; symptoms may recur.

Exceeding the dose
An occasional unintentional extra dose is unlikely to cause problems. Larger overdoses may cause unusual drowsiness. Notify your physician.

POSSIBLE ADVERSE EFFECTS

When hydroxyzine is used as an anti-emetic or anti-anxiety drug, the possibility of adverse effects is low. The most common symptoms are related to its *anticholinergic* properties and include drowsiness and dry mouth. Such symptoms may be overcome by an adjustment of dosage or may pass after a few days of usage.

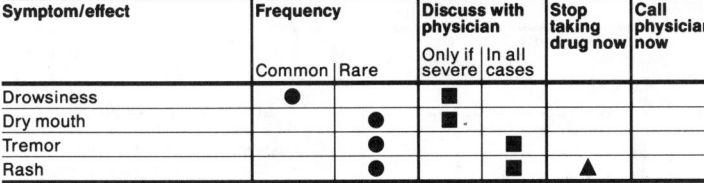

Symptom/effect	Frequency		Discuss with physician		Stop taking drug now	Call physician now
	Common	Rare	Only if severe	In all cases		
Drowsiness	●		■			
Dry mouth		●	■			
Tremor		●		■		
Rash		●		■		▲

INTERACTIONS

Sedatives All drugs that have a sedative effect are likely to increase the sedative properties of hydroxyzine. Such drugs include anti-anxiety drugs, sleeping drugs, antidepressants, and antipsychotics. This drug should not be taken with barbiturates or narcotic analgesics.

Alcohol Alcohol increases the sedative effect of hydroxyzine.

SPECIAL PRECAUTIONS

Be sure to tell your physician if:
▼ You have impaired kidney or liver function.
▼ You have had epileptic seizures.
▼ You have had glaucoma.
▼ You have Parkinson's disease.
▼ You are taking other medications.

Pregnancy
▼ Not recommended. May affect the baby adversely. Discuss with your physician so that you can weigh the benefits of the drug against its risks.

Breast feeding
▼ Discuss with your physician. Effect on breast feeding uncertain.

Infants and children
▼ Not usually prescribed. Reduced dose necessary.

Over 60
▼ Reduced dose may be necessary. Increased likelihood of adverse effects.

Driving and hazardous work
▼ Avoid such activities until you have learned how the drug affects you, because the drug can reduce alertness.

Alcohol
▼ Avoid. Alcohol increases the sedative effects of this drug.

PROLONGED USE

Hydroxyzine is not usually prescribed for prolonged periods.

IBUPROFEN

Brand names Advil, Motrin, Nuprin, Rufen
Used in the following combined preparations None

GENERAL INFORMATION

Ibuprofen, introduced in 1967, is available over the counter to relieve the pain, stiffness, and inflammation that may accompany a number of disorders. It is similar to aspirin in the way it works and in the way it can be used. Because it acts as an analgesic as well as an anti-inflammatory, it is an effective treatment for the symptoms of rheumatoid arthritis, osteoarthritis, and gout. It also relieves mild to moderate discomfort of headache, menstrual pain, soft tissue injury, and pain following an operation.

Sometimes, ibuprofen is prescribed along with slower-acting drugs in the treatment of rheumatoid arthritis.

Ibuprofen has fewer side effects than many of the other non-steroidal anti-inflammatory drugs (NSAIDs). Unlike aspirin, it rarely causes bleeding in the stomach.

QUICK REFERENCE

Drug group Non-steroidal anti-inflammatory drug (p.144)

Overdose danger rating Low

Dependence rating Low

Prescription needed No

Available as generic Yes

INFORMATION FOR USERS

Follow instructions on the label. Call your physician if symptoms worsen.

How taken

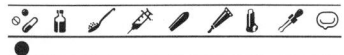

Tablets.

Frequency and timing of doses
4 – 6 x daily (general pain relief); 3 – 4 x daily with food (arthritis).

Adult dosage range
600mg – 1.2g daily (general pain relief); 1.2 – 2.4g daily (arthritis).

Onset of effect
Pain relief begins in 1 – 2 hours. Full anti-inflammatory effect in arthritic conditions may not be felt for up to 2 weeks.

Duration of action
5 – 10 hours.

Diet advice
None.

Storage
Keep in a closed container in a cool, dry place away from reach of children.

Missed dose
Take as soon as you remember. If your next dose is due within 2 hours, take a single dose now and skip the next.

Stopping the drug
When taken for short-term pain relief, ibuprofen can be safely stopped as soon as you no longer need it. If prescribed for the long-term treatment of arthritis, however, you should seek medical advice before stopping the drug.

Exceeding the dose
An occasional unintentional extra dose is unlikely to be a cause for concern. But if you notice unusual symptoms, or if a large overdose has been taken, notify your physician.

SPECIAL PRECAUTIONS

Be sure to consult your physician before taking this drug if:
▼ You have impaired kidney function.
▼ You have heart problems.
▼ You have high blood pressure.
▼ You have had a peptic ulcer, esophagitis, or acid indigestion.
▼ You are allergic to aspirin.
▼ You are taking other medications.

Pregnancy
▼ Not usually prescribed. When taken in late pregnancy may cause defects in the unborn baby and may prolong labor. Discuss with your physician so that you can weigh the benefits of the drug against its risks.

Breast feeding
▼ No evidence of risk.

Infants and children
▼ Not recommended for children under 12 years.

Over 60
▼ Reduced dose may be necessary. Increased likelihood of adverse effects.

Driving and hazardous work
▼ Avoid such activities until you have learned how the drug affects you, because the drug can cause dizziness.

Alcohol
▼ Avoid. Alcohol may increase the risk of stomach disorders with ibuprofen.

Surgery and general anesthetics
▼ Ibuprofen may prolong bleeding. Discuss with your physician or dentist before any surgery.

POSSIBLE ADVERSE EFFECTS

The most common adverse effects are the result of gastrointestinal disturbances. Black or bloodstained bowel movements should be reported to your physician without delay.

Symptom/effect	Frequency		Discuss with physician		Stop taking drug now	Call physician now
	Common	Rare	Only if severe	In all cases		
Diarrhea/constipation	●			■		
Nausea/vomiting	●		■			
Heartburn/indigestion		●	■			
Dizziness/lightheadedness		●	■			
Headache		●	■			
Rash		●		■	▲	
Wheezing/breathlessness		●		■	▲	■

INTERACTIONS

General note Ibuprofen interacts with a wide range of drugs to increase the risk of bleeding and/or peptic ulcers. Such drugs include oral anticoagulants, corticosteroids, other non-steroidal anti-inflammatory drugs (NSAIDs), and aspirin.

Lithium Ibuprofen may raise blood levels of lithium, leading to a risk of serious adverse effects.

Antihypertensive drugs and diuretics The beneficial effects of these drugs may be reduced by ibuprofen.

Oral antidiabetic drugs Ibuprofen may increase the blood sugar-lowering effect of these drugs.

PROLONGED USE

There is an increased risk of bleeding from peptic ulcers and in the bowel with prolonged use of ibuprofen.

IDOXURIDINE

Brand names Liquifilm, Stoxil
Used in the following combined preparations None

GENERAL INFORMATION

Idoxuridine, introduced in 1963, is a *topically* applied drug that is often effective against certain viral infections. Available as eye drops or ointment, it is used to treat herpes simplex infections of the inner eyelids or the cornea of the eye. It is also prescribed for infections of the cornea caused by vaccines.

In the treatment of deep herpes simplex infections of the eye, for which corticosteroids are prescribed, idoxuridine may also be given to prevent the spread of any viral growth stimulated by the corticosteroid. When high

doses of corticosteroids are administered, orally or by eye drops, for other disorders, idoxuridine is often given to prevent the flare-up of a previous herpes eye infection. Although idoxuridine can prevent and cure virus infections, it does not reverse damage to the eye resulting from an infection that has already occurred.

Serious adverse effects are rare with idoxuridine, but the risk of eye damage is increased with prolonged treatment or overuse. For this reason, courses of treatment longer than 21 days are not usually recommended.

QUICK REFERENCE

Drug group Antiviral drug (p.161)
Overdose danger rating Low
Dependence rating Low
Prescription needed Yes
Available as generic No

INFORMATION FOR USERS

Your drug prescription is tailored for you. Do not alter dosage without checking with your physician.

How taken

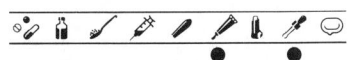

Ointment, eye drops.

Frequency and timing of doses
Every 2 – 4 hours.

Dosage range
Ointment 1cm strip every 4 hours.
Eye drops 1 drop every 2 hours during the day and if possible at night, or 1 drop every minute for 5 minutes, repeated every 4 hours, day and night.

Onset of effect
Within 3 – 4 days.

Duration of action
A few hours after each application.

Diet advice
None.

Storage
Keep in a closed container in the refrigerator or in a cool, dry place away from reach of children. Do not freeze.

Missed dose
Take as soon as you remember.

Stopping the drug
Take for 7 days after symptoms disappear, since the original infection may still be active, and symptoms may recur if treatment is stopped too soon.

Exceeding the dose
An occasional unintentional extra dose is unlikely to be a cause for concern. But if you notice unusual symptoms or if a large overdose has been taken, notify your physician.

SPECIAL PRECAUTIONS

Be sure to tell your physician if:
▼ You have ever had an allergic reaction to iodine or an iodine-containing preparation.
▼ You are taking other medications.

 Pregnancy
▼ No evidence of risk to developing baby.

 Breast feeding
▼ No evidence of risk if taken by drops or applied as ointment.

 Infants and children
▼ No special problems.

  Over 60
▼ No special problems.

 Driving and hazardous work
▼ No known problems.

 Alcohol
▼ No known problems.

POSSIBLE ADVERSE EFFECTS

Serious adverse effects are uncommon with idoxuridine. If you experience unusual sensitivity to light (photophobia), visual impairment, or allergic reactions such as itching, swelling, or pain, consult your physician promptly.

Symptom/effect	Frequency		Discuss with physician		Stop taking drug now	Call physician now
	Common	Rare	Only if severe	In all cases		
Eye irritation	●		■			
Excess flow of tears		●	■			
Unusual sensitivity to light		●		■		
Blurred vision		●		■		
Swollen lids/pain in eye		●		■		

INTERACTIONS

Boric acid eye preparations may interact with inactive ingredients or preservatives in idoxuridine preparations, increasing the risk of irritation and of eye damage.

PROLONGED USE

Rarely required. Treatment is not normally continued for longer than 21 days.

IMIPRAMINE

Brand names Janimine, SK-Pramine, Tofranil
Used in the following combined preparations None

GENERAL INFORMATION

Imipramine belongs to a class of antidepressant drugs known as the tricyclics. It is mainly used in the long-term treatment of depression to elevate mood, increase physical activity, improve appetite, and restore interest in everyday life. Less sedating than some of the other tricyclic antidepressants, it is particularly useful when a depressed person is withdrawn or apathetic, though it can aggravate insomnia if taken in the evening.

Imipramine is also given for the treatment of bedwetting in children, though proof of benefits is not conclusive. Imipramine can cause a variety of side effects. In overdose it may cause coma and dangerous heart rhythms.

QUICK REFERENCE

Drug group Tricyclic antidepressant drug (p.112)

Overdose danger rating High

Dependence rating Low

Prescription needed Yes

Available as generic Yes

INFORMATION FOR USERS

Your drug prescription is tailored for you. Do not alter dosage without checking with your physician.

How taken

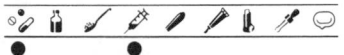

Tablets, capsules, injection.

Frequency and timing of doses
1 – 4 x daily.

Dosage range
Adults 75 – 150mg daily (dose may be increased in exceptional circumstances).
Children Reduced dose according to age and weight.

Onset of effect
Some benefits and effects may appear within hours, but full antidepressant effect may not be felt for 2 – 6 weeks.

Duration of action
Following prolonged treatment, antidepressant effect may persist for up to 6 weeks. Adverse effects may wear off within days.

Diet advice
None.

Storage
Keep in a closed container in a cool, dry place away from reach of children. Protect from light.

Missed dose
Take as soon as you remember. If your next dose is due within 3 hours, take a single dose now and skip the next.

Stopping the drug
Do not stop taking the drug without consulting your physician, who will supervise a gradual reduction in dosage. Stopping abruptly may cause withdrawal symptoms .

OVERDOSE ACTION

 Seek immediate medical advice in all cases. Take emergency action if consciousness is lost.

See Drug poisoning emergency guide (p.590).

POSSIBLE ADVERSE EFFECTS

The possible adverse effects of this drug are mainly the result of its *anticholinergic* action and its blocking action on the transmission of signals in the heart.

Symptom/effect	Frequency		Discuss with physician		Stop taking drug now	Call physician now
	Common	Rare	Only if severe	In all cases		
Sweating/flushing	●		■			
Dry mouth	●		■			
Blurred vision	●			■		
Dizziness/fainting	●			■		
Rash		●		■	▲	
Palpitations		●		■	▲	▮

INTERACTIONS

Sedatives All drugs that have a sedative effect, including anticonvulsants, are likely to increase the sedative potential of imipramine.

Antihypertensive drugs Imipramine may reduce the effect of some of these drugs.

Monoamine oxidase inhibitors (MAOIs) There is a possibility of a serious interaction, producing seizures and delirium. Such drugs are prescribed together only under strict supervision.

Heavy smoking This may reduce the antidepressant effect of imipramine.

SPECIAL PRECAUTIONS

Be sure to tell your physician if:
▼ You have had heart problems.
▼ You have impaired kidney or liver function.
▼ You have had epileptic seizures.
▼ You have had glaucoma.
▼ You have prostate trouble.
▼ You have a thyroid disorder.
▼ You are taking other medications.

 Pregnancy
▼ Not usually prescribed. Safety in pregnancy not established. Discuss with your physician so that you may weigh the benefits of the drug against its possible risks.

 Breast feeding
▼ The drug passes into the breast milk, but at normal doses adverse effects on the baby are uncommon. Discuss with your physician.

 Infants and children
▼ Not recommended for children under 6 years. Reduced dose necessary in older children.

 Over 60
▼ Reduced dose may be necessary. Increased likelihood of adverse effects.

 Driving and hazardous work
▼ Avoid such activities until you have learned how the drug affects you, because the drug may cause reduced alertness.

 Alcohol
▼ Avoid. Alcohol increases the sedative effects of this drug.

Surgery and general anesthetics
▼ Imipramine treatment may need to be stopped before you have a general anesthetic. Discuss this with your physician or dentist before any operation.

PROLONGED USE

No problems expected. Imipramine is not usually prescribed for children as a treatment for bedwetting for longer than three months.

INDOMETHACIN

Brand names Indocin, Indocin I.V., Indocin S.R.
Used in the following combined preparations None

GENERAL INFORMATION

Indomethacin, introduced in 1963, is a non-steroidal anti-inflammatory drug (NSAID). Like other drugs of this group, it reduces pain, stiffness, and inflammation.

Indomethacin is used in the treatment of many arthritic conditions, including rheumatoid arthritis, ankylosing spondylitis, osteoarthritis, acute attacks of gout, bursitis, and tendinitis. It is sometimes given to treat a heart disorder known as patent ductus arteriosus that occurs in premature infants.

Indomethacin has several potentially serious side effects, including gastrointestinal disorders, severe headache, and dizziness, and it may mask the symptoms of infections. It is not given to people with poor kidney function.

INFORMATION FOR USERS

Your drug prescription is tailored for you. Do not alter dosage without checking with your physician.

How taken

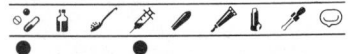

Capsules, slow-release capsules, injection.

Frequency and timing of doses
1 – 2 x daily with food (slow-release capsules); 2 – 4 x daily with food (standard capsules).

Adult dosage range
50 – 200mg daily.

Onset of effect
Some analgesic effect may be felt within 2 – 4 hours. Full anti-inflammatory effect may not be felt for up to 4 weeks.

Duration of action
5 – 10 hours. Some effect may last for up to 24 hours (slow-release capsules).

Diet advice
None.

Storage
Keep in a closed container in a cool, dry place away from reach of children.

Missed dose
Take as soon as you remember. If your next dose is due within 2 hours, take a single dose now and skip the next.

Stopping the drug
Do not stop the drug without consulting your physician; symptoms may recur.

Exceeding the dose
An occasional unintentional extra dose is unlikely to cause problems. Large overdoses may cause headache, dizziness, confusion, and nausea. Notify your physician.

SPECIAL PRECAUTIONS

Be sure to tell your physician if:
▼ You have impaired liver or kidney function.
▼ You have had a peptic ulcer, esophagitis, or acid indigestion.
▼ You have heart problems.
▼ You have high blood pressure.
▼ You have had epileptic seizures.
▼ You have Parkinson's disease.
▼ You have bleeding problems.
▼ You are allergic to aspirin.
▼ You are taking other medications.

 Pregnancy
▼ Not usually prescribed. May cause defects in the unborn baby, and taken in late pregnancy, may prolong labor.

 Breast feeding
▼ Discuss with your physician. The drug passes into the breast milk and may affect the baby adversely.

 Infants and children
▼ Not usually prescribed for children under 14. Given for juvenile arthritis only when possible benefits outweigh risks.

 Over 60
▼ Reduced dose necessary. Increased likelihood of adverse effects.

 Driving and hazardous work
▼ Avoid such activities until you have learned how the drug affects you; it can cause dizziness and drowsiness.

 Alcohol
▼ Never drink while under treatment with indomethacin. Alcohol may interact with this drug to cause peptic ulcers.

Surgery and general anesthetics
▼ Indomethacin may prolong bleeding. Discuss this with your physician or dentist before you are given a general anesthetic.

POSSIBLE ADVERSE EFFECTS

Gastrointestinal disturbances, headaches, drowsiness, and depression are common. Black or bloodstained bowel movements should be reported promptly.

Symptom/effect	Frequency		Discuss with physician		Stop taking drug now	Call physician now
	Common	Rare	Only if severe	In all cases		
Abdominal pain/indigestion	●		■			
Headache	●		■			
Dizziness/lightheadedness	●		■			
Nausea/vomiting	●			■		
Diarrhea		●		■		
Drowsiness/depression		●		■		
Rash		●		■	▲	
Wheezing/breathlessness		●		■	▲	■

INTERACTIONS

General note Indomethacin interacts with a wide range of drugs to increase the risk of bleeding and/or peptic ulcers. Such drugs include oral anticoagulants, corticosteroids, other non-steroidal anti-inflammatory drugs (NSAIDs), and aspirin.

Lithium Indomethacin may raise blood levels of lithium, leading to a risk of serious adverse effects.

Antihypertensive drugs and diuretics The beneficial effects of these drugs may be reduced by indomethacin.

Oral antidiabetic drugs Indomethacin may increase the blood sugar-lowering effect of these drugs.

PROLONGED USE

There is an increased risk of bleeding from peptic ulcers and in the bowel with prolonged use of indomethacin.

INSULIN

Brand names Humulin N, Humulin R, Lente Insulin, Novolin R, NPH Insulin
Used in the following combined preparation Mixtard

GENERAL INFORMATION

Insulin is a hormone manufactured by the pancreas and vital to the body's ability to use sugar. Introduced as a drug in 1922, it is given by injection to supplement or replace natural insulin in the treatment of diabetes mellitus. It is the only effective treatment in juvenile (insulin-dependent) diabetes and may also be prescribed in adult (maturity-onset) diabetes. It is most effective when used in conjunction with a prescribed diet. Illness, vomiting, or alterations in diet or in exercise level may necessitate dosage adjustment.

A wide variety of different insulin preparations are available. These can be short-, medium-, or long-acting. Combinations of these types are often given together. People receiving insulin should carry a warning card or tag so that in case of accident, the appropriate treatment can be given.

QUICK REFERENCE

Drug group Antidiabetic drug (p.170)
Overdose danger rating High
Dependence rating Low
Prescription needed No
Available as generic Yes

INFORMATION FOR USERS

Your drug prescription is tailored for you. Do not alter dosage without checking with your physician.

How taken

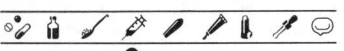

Injection, infusion pump.

Frequency and timing of doses
Varies with preparation or preparations used and individual needs. 1 – 4 x daily usually 30 – 45 minutes before meals and at bedtime.

Dosage range
The dose (and type) of insulin is determined according to the needs of the individual.

Onset of effect
30 – 60 minutes (short-acting); 1 – 4 hours (medium-acting); 4 – 6 hours (long-acting).

Duration of action
6 – 8 hours (short-acting); 18 – 26 hours (medium-acting); 28 – 36 hours (long-acting).

Diet advice
A low-sugar, low-fat diet is needed. Follow your physician's advice.

Storage
Refrigerate, but do not freeze.

Missed dose
Discuss with your physician. Appropriate action depends on dose and type of insulin .

Stopping the drug
Do not stop taking the drug without consulting your physician; stopping the drug may lead to confusion and coma.

OVERDOSE ACTION

Seek immediate medical advice in all cases. You may notice symptoms of low blood sugar such as faintness, hunger, sweating, trembling, confusion, or headache. If these occur, eat or drink something sugary. Take emergency action if seizures or loss of consciousness occurs.

See Drug poisoning emergency guide (p.590).

SPECIAL PRECAUTIONS

Be sure to tell your physician if:
▼ You have had a previous allergic reaction to insulin.
▼ You are taking other medications, or your other drug treatment is changed.

Pregnancy
▼ No evidence of risk to the developing baby from insulin, but poor control of diabetes increases the risk of birth defects. Careful monitoring is required.

Breast feeding
▼ No evidence of risk.

Infants and children
▼ Reduced dose necessary.

Over 60
▼ No special problems.

Driving and hazardous work
▼ Usually no problem, but strenuous exercise alters your insulin and sugar requirements. Avoid these activities if you have warning signs of low blood sugar.

Alcohol
▼ Avoid. Alcoholic drinks upset diabetic control.

Surgery and general anesthetics
▼ Insulin requirements may increase during surgery, and blood glucose levels will need to be monitored during and after an operation. Notify your physician or dentist that you are diabetic before any surgery.

POSSIBLE ADVERSE EFFECTS

Symptoms such as dizziness, sweating, weakness, and confusion indicate low blood sugar. Serious allergic reactions (rash, swelling, and shortness of breath) are rare.

Symptom/effect	Frequency		Discuss with physician		Stop taking drug now	Call physician now
	Common	Rare	Only if severe	In all cases		
Injection-site irritation	●			■		
Weakness/sweating	●			■		
Dimpling at injection site		●		■		
Rash/facial swelling		●		■		▮
Shortness of breath		●		■		▮

PROLONGED USE

No problems expected.

Monitoring Regular monitoring of levels of sugar in the urine and/or blood is required.

INTERACTIONS

General note Many drugs increase the risk of low blood sugar: some antibiotics, aspirin, phenylbutazone, monoamine oxidase inhibitors, oral antidiabetic drugs.

Corticosteroids oppose the effect of insulin; more insulin may be needed.

Beta blockers may mask the warning signs of low blood sugar.

INTERFERON

Brand names Intron A, Roferon-A
Used in the following combined preparations None

GENERAL INFORMATION

Interferon is the name given to a group of substances produced by cells infected by viruses or stimulated by other substances. It is thought to promote resistance to other types of viral infection. In recent years, interferon preparations have been used in clinical trials to treat various forms of cancer. One type of interferon has proved effective in the treatment of hairy cell leukemia, and investigation into its use in AIDS-related Kaposi's sarcoma (a form of skin cancer) is continuing. Research is also being carried out on the use of interferon in the treatment of life-threatening viral diseases, including those in people who have defective immune systems. The drug has significant adverse effects (see below).

INFORMATION FOR USERS

This drug is given only under medical supervision and is not for self-administration.

How taken

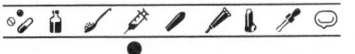

Injection.

Frequency and timing of doses
Once daily for 16 – 24 weeks, reduced to 3 x weekly for a further 6 months (hairy cell leukemia); standard dosing schedules have not yet been determined for other disorders.

Adult dosage range
3 million international units per dose (hairy cell leukemia); standard dosages have not yet been determined for other disorders.

Onset of effect
Active inside the body within 1 hour, but effects may not be noted for days or weeks.

Duration of action
Effects last for about 12 hours.

Diet advice
None.

Storage
Not applicable. The drug is not kept in the home.

Missed dose
Not applicable. This drug is given only in the hospital under close medical supervision.

Stopping the drug
Discuss with your physician.

Exceeding the dose
Overdosage is unlikely, since treatment is carefully monitored.

POSSIBLE ADVERSE EFFECTS

Because interferon has only recently been introduced, experience of adverse effects during treatment is limited. The symptoms listed below are the most common problems. All unusual symptoms should be brought to your physician's attention without delay.

Symptom/effect	Frequency		Discuss with physician		Stop taking drug now	Call physician now
	Common	Rare	Only if severe	In all cases		
Headache	●		■			
Lethargy	●		■			
Dizziness	●			■		
Digestive disturbances	●			■		
Hair loss	●			■		
Fever/chills	●			■		

INTERACTIONS

Sedatives All drugs that have a sedative effect on the nervous system are likely to increase the sedative properties of interferon. Such drugs include anti-anxiety and sleeping drugs, antihistamines, antidepressant drugs, narcotic analgesics, and antipsychotic drugs.

SPECIAL PRECAUTIONS

Be sure to tell your physician if:
▼ You have kidney or liver disease.
▼ You have heart disease.
▼ You have had epileptic seizures.
▼ You have previously suffered allergic reactions to any drugs.
▼ You have had asthma or eczema.
▼ You are taking other medications.

Pregnancy
▼ Not usually prescribed. May increase the risk of miscarriage. Discuss with your physician so that you may weigh the benefits of the drug against its risks.

Breast feeding
▼ Discuss with your physician. The drug passes into the breast milk and may affect the baby adversely.

Infants and children
▼ Not recommended.

Over 60
▼ Reduced dose may be necessary. Increased likelihood of adverse effects.

Driving and hazardous work
▼ Avoid. The drug may cause lethargy and dizziness.

Alcohol
▼ Avoid. Alcohol may increase the sedative effects of this drug.

PROLONGED USE

The long-term effects of this drug are still under investigation. There may be an increased risk of liver damage. Blood cell production in the bone marrow may be reduced.

Monitoring Periodic blood tests may be required to monitor blood composition and liver function.

A B C D E F G H I J K L M N O P Q R S T U V W X Y Z

ISOCARBOXAZID

Brand name Marplan
Used in the following combined preparations None

GENERAL INFORMATION

Isocarboxazid belongs to a group of antidepressant drugs known as the monoamine oxidase inhibitors (often abbreviated to MAOIs). These drugs help to elevate mood, improve appetite and sleep, and restore energy and interest in life in general. Isocarboxazid is used to relieve depression, especially when it is accompanied by irrational fears (phobias) or exagger-ated emotional reactions. The main drawback to the use of the drug is the risk of dangerous interactions with a wide range of other drugs and many foods. Treatment with this drug is thus usually reserved for people who have not responded to all other types of antidepressant. People taking isocarboxazid are advised to carry a warning card.

QUICK REFERENCE

Drug group MAOI antidepressant drug (p.112)

Overdose danger rating High

Dependence rating Low

Prescription needed Yes

Available as generic Yes

INFORMATION FOR USERS

Your drug prescription is tailored for you. Do not alter dosage without checking with your physician.

How taken

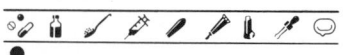

Tablets.

Frequency and timing of doses
1 – 3 x daily.

Adult dosage range
30mg daily (starting dose); 10 – 20mg daily (maintenance dose).

Onset of effect
Some benefits and effects may be felt within hours of starting treatment, but full antidepressant effect may not be felt for up to 4 weeks.

Duration of action
After prolonged treatment the antidepressant effect may persist for up to 4 weeks. Adverse effects may wear off sooner.

Diet advice
Certain foods with a high tyramine content must be avoided while taking this drug and for 14 days after treatment. When isocar-boxazid is dispensed, you should receive a card that gives full details of foods and over-the-counter medicines to avoid. These include cheese, pickled herring, red wine, meat or yeast extracts, and broad (fava) beans.

Storage
Keep in a closed container in a cool, dry place away from reach of children. Protect from light.

Missed dose
Take as soon as you remember. If your next dose is due within 4 hours, take a single dose now and skip the next.

Stopping the drug
Do not stop the drug without consulting your physician; symptoms may recur.

OVERDOSE ACTION

 Seek immediate medical advice in all cases. Take emergency action if you notice any of the symptoms described under Possible Adverse Effects below.

See Drug poisoning emergency guide (p.590).

SPECIAL PRECAUTIONS

Be sure to tell your physician if:
▼ You have impaired kidney or liver function.
▼ You have heart problems.
▼ You have had epileptic seizures.
▼ You have an adrenal gland tumor.
▼ You are taking other medications.

 Pregnancy
▼ Not usually prescribed. Safety in pregnancy not established.

 Breast feeding
▼ Discuss with your physician. The drug passes into the breast milk.

 Infants and children
▼ Not recommended.

 Over 60
▼ Increased likelihood of adverse effects. Used only when potential benefits outweigh risks.

 Driving and hazardous work
▼ Avoid such activities until you have learned how the drug affects you, because of the possibility of blurred vision and drowsiness.

 Alcohol
▼ Never drink heavy red wines, particularly chianti, when taking this drug. These may cause a dangerous reaction. Other forms of alcohol should also be avoided.

Surgery and general anesthetics
▼ Isocarboxazid treatment should be withdrawn 2 weeks before general anesthetic and some dental treatments. Discuss with your physician or dentist before any operation or dental procedure.

PROLONGED USE

No problems expected, but people taking isocarboxazid should constantly take care to avoid foods and other drugs that may interact with it because the risks do not diminish with time.

POSSIBLE ADVERSE EFFECTS

Isocarboxazid does not usually cause adverse effects. However, if you experience severe headache, nausea and/or vomiting or unexplained sweating, seek medical advice at once. Such symptoms may be a sign of rising blood pressure.

Symptom/effect	Frequency		Discuss with physician		Stop taking drug now	Call physician now
	Common	Rare	Only if severe	In all cases		
Drowsiness/insomnia	●		■			
Dizziness/fainting	●			■		▮
Dry mouth		●	■			
Blurred vision		●		■		
Jaundice		●		■		
Rash		●		■	▲	

INTERACTIONS

General note Isocarboxazid interacts with a large number of prescription drugs, over-the-counter medicines, and foods.

Do not take any type of medicine without prior consultation with your physician or pharmacist.

ISONIAZID

Brand names INH, Laniazid, Nydrazid, Teebaconin
Used in the following combined preparation Rifamate

GENERAL INFORMATION

Introduced in 1956, isoniazid remains the single most effective medicine for tuberculosis. It is given alone to prevent the disease and with other drugs for the treatment of tuberculosis. Treatment usually lasts for at least one year, although shorter courses, lasting six or nine months, may sometimes be prescribed.

One of the side effects of isoniazid is the increased loss of pyridoxine (vitamin B_6) from the body. This effect, which is more likely with high doses, is rare in children, but common among people with poor nutrition. Since pyridoxine deficiency can lead to irreversible nerve damage, supplements are usually given.

QUICK REFERENCE

Drug group Antituberculous drug (p.160)

Overdose danger rating High

Dependence rating Low

Prescription needed Yes

Available as generic Yes

INFORMATION FOR USERS

Your drug prescription is tailored for you. Do not alter dosage without checking with your physician.

How taken

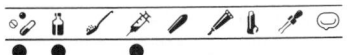

Tablets, liquid, injection.

Frequency and timing of doses
Once daily. May be given twice weekly in combination with other drugs.

Dosage range
Treatment According to body weight (adults and children).
Prevention 300mg daily (adults); according to age and weight (children).

Onset of effect
Several days.

Duration of action
Up to 96 hours.

Diet advice
Isoniazid may deplete pyridoxine (vitamin B_6) levels in the body, and supplements are usually prescribed. In some people, isoniazid may interact with cheese or fish in the diet, causing redness and itching of the skin, sweating, chills, headache, faintness, and palpitations. This rare reaction requires prompt medical attention.

Storage
Keep in a closed container in a cool, dry place away from reach of children. Protect from light.

Missed dose
Take as soon as you remember. If your next dose is scheduled within 8 hours, take both doses now.

Stopping the drug
Take the full course. Even if you feel better, the infection may still be present and may recur if treatment is stopped too soon.

OVERDOSE ACTION

Seek immediate medical advice in all cases. Take emergency action if breathing difficulties, loss of consciousness, or seizures occur.

See Drug poisoning emergency guide (p.590).

SPECIAL PRECAUTIONS

Be sure to tell your physician if:
▼ You have a liver disorder or impaired liver function.
▼ You have had liver damage following isoniazid treatment in the past.
▼ You have diabetes.
▼ You have had epileptic seizures.
▼ You are taking other medications.

Pregnancy
▼ Not usually prescribed. Safety in pregnancy not established. Discuss with your physician so that you can weigh the benefits of the drug against its possible risks.

Breast feeding
▼ The drug passes into the breast milk, but at normal doses adverse effects on the baby are uncommon. Discuss with your physician.

Infants and children
▼ Reduced dose may be necessary.

Over 60
▼ Increased likelihood of adverse effects.

Driving and hazardous work
▼ No special problems.

Alcohol
▼ Avoid. Alcohol increases the rate of breakdown of isoniazid and reduces its effectiveness.

PROLONGED USE

Pyridoxine (vitamin B_6) deficiency may occur with prolonged use and lead to nerve damage. Supplements are usually prescribed. There is also a risk of liver damage.

Monitoring Periodic blood tests are usually performed to monitor liver function.

POSSIBLE ADVERSE EFFECTS

Although serious problems are uncommon, all adverse effects of this drug should receive prompt medical attention because of the possibility of nerve or liver damage.

Symptom/effect	Frequency		Discuss with physician		Stop taking drug now	Call physician now
	Common	Rare	Only if severe	In all cases		
Nausea/vomiting		●				
Fatigue/weakness		●		■		
Numbness/tingling		●		■		
Insomnia/restlessness		●		■		
Blurred vision		●		■	▲	
Jaundice	●	●		■	▲	▮
Twitching/seizures		●		■	▲	▮

INTERACTIONS

Anticonvulsant and benzodiazepine drugs The effects of these drugs may be increased with isoniazid.

Aluminum-containing antacids These may reduce the absorption of isoniazid.

367

ISOPROTERENOL

Brand names Aerolone, Isuprel, Medihaler 150
Used in the following combined preparation Duo-Medihaler

GENERAL INFORMATION

Isoproterenol is a *sympathomimetic* drug that dilates the bronchioles (small air passages in the lungs) and improves the transmission of electrical signals in the heart. Given by aerosol inhaler, it is used as a bronchodilator to relieve the brochospasms associated with asthma, bronchitis, and emphysema. It is also given by mouth in combination with phenylephrine (a decongestant) to ease mucous congestion in the respiratory tract. In rare cases isoproterenol is given intravenously as an emergency treatment for serious heart disorders and the relief of severe asthma.

Because isoproterenol may increase the heart rate, it is not suitable for those with heart disorders such as angina. For the same reason, however, it is used in heart block as an interim treatment before an artificial pacemaker is implanted.

Occasionally, breathing difficulties may be worsened by the drug. Excessive use may cause nervousness, insomnia, headaches, and, in extreme cases, dangerous heart rhythms.

INFORMATION FOR USERS

Your drug prescription is tailored for you. Do not alter dosage without checking with your physician.

How taken

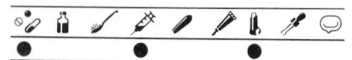

Tablets, injection, inhaler.

Frequency and timing of doses
1 – 2 puffs every 6 hours (inhaler); every 6 – 8 hours (tablets).

Dosage range
80 – 640mg daily (inhaler); 30 – 60mg daily (tablets).

Onset of effect
Within 2 – 5 minutes (inhaler).

Duration of action
Up to 6 hours.

Diet advice
None.

Storage
Keep in a closed container in a cool, dry place away from reach of children. Protect from light. Do not puncture or burn inhalers.

Missed dose
Do not take the missed dose. Take the next dose as usual.

Stopping the drug
Can be safely stopped as soon as you no longer need it.

OVERDOSE ACTION

 Seek immediate medical advice in all cases. Take emergency action if dizziness, fainting, palpitations, or loss of consciousness occurs.

See Drug poisoning emergency guide (p.590).

POSSIBLE ADVERSE EFFECTS

Many of the adverse effects go away during treatment as your body adjusts to the medicine. However, palpitations are a sign of excessive stimulation of the heart, and chest pain always requires prompt medical attention.

Symptom/effect	Frequency		Discuss with physician		Stop taking drug now	Call physician now
	Common	Rare	Only if severe	In all cases		
Dry mouth and throat	●		■			
Nervousness/insomnia	●		■			
Dizziness/fainting	●			■		❘
Chest pain/palpitations	●			■		❘
Headache		●	■			

INTERACTIONS

Diuretics The antihypertensive effect of these drugs may be reduced.

Tricyclic antidepressant drugs These may increase the adverse effects of isoproterenol.

Monoamine oxidase inhibitors (MAOIs) Isoproterenol may interact with these drugs to cause a dangerous rise in blood pressure.

SPECIAL PRECAUTIONS

Be sure to tell your physician if:
▼ You have heart problems.
▼ You have high blood pressure.
▼ You have an overactive thyroid gland.
▼ You have diabetes.
▼ You suffer from nervous problems.
▼ You are taking other medications.

 Pregnancy
▼ Not usually prescribed. May delay the onset of labor. Discuss with your physician so that you may weigh the benefits of the drug against its risks.

 Breast feeding
▼ Discuss with your physician. The drug passes into the breast milk and may affect the baby adversely.

 Infants and children
▼ Reduced dose necessary.

 Over 60
▼ Reduced dose may be necessary.

 Driving and hazardous work
▼ Avoid such activities until you have learned how the drug affects you, because the drug can cause dizziness and fainting.

 Alcohol
▼ No known problems.

PROLONGED USE

The effect of isoproterenol may wear off with prolonged use. Also, if the drug does not seem to be working as effectively, this may mean that your asthma is getting worse, and you should consult your physician.

ISOSORBIDE DINITRATE

Brand names Dilatrate-SR, Iso-Bid, Isordil, Sorbitrate, Sorbitrate SA
Used in the following combined preparations None

GENERAL INFORMATION

Isosorbide dinitrate, introduced in the late 1970s, belongs to a group of *vasodilator* drugs called nitrates. Related to nitroglycerin, it is most often used to relieve the pain and frequency of angina attacks. Isosorbide dinitrate is fast-acting, its effects lasting longer than some other nitrates. Unlike nitroglycerin, isosorbide dinitrate can also be stored for long periods of time without losing its effectiveness.

Headache and flushing, in addition to dizziness, usually occur early in treatment. These are often controlled by taking the drug in small initial doses, and they disappear after long-term treatment. The effectiveness of this drug may be reduced after a few months, and an alternative treatment may need to be substituted.

QUICK REFERENCE

Drug group Nitrate vasodilator (p.126) and anti-angina drug (p.129)

Overdose danger rating Medium

Dependence rating Low

Prescription needed Yes

Available as generic Yes

INFORMATION FOR USERS

Your drug prescription is tailored for you. Do not alter dosage without checking with your physician.

How taken

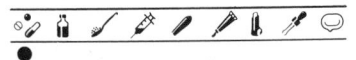

Tablets (held under the tongue, chewed, or swallowed), capsules (slow-release).

Frequency and timing of doses
Relief of angina attacks Tablets chewed or held under the tongue as needed. Dose may be repeated after 5 minutes if necessary.
Prevention of angina Every 4 hours (swallowed tablets), every 8 hours (slow-release capsules).

Adult dosage range
Relief of angina attacks 5 – 10mg per dose.
Prevention of angina 40 – 160mg daily. Larger doses are given occasionally.

Onset of action
2 – 3 minutes (chewed or held under the tongue), 30 minutes (swallowed).

Duration of effect
Up to 2 hours (chewed), up to 5 hours (swallowed), up to 10 hours (slow-release capsules).

Diet advice
None.

Storage
Keep in a closed container in a cool, dry place away from reach of children. Protect from light.

Missed dose
Take as soon as you remember. If your next dose is due within 2 hours, take a single dose now and skip the next.

Stopping the drug
Do not stop taking the drug without consulting your physician; stopping the drug may lead to worsening of the underlying condition.

Exceeding the dose
An occasional unintentional extra dose is unlikely to cause problems. Large overdoses may cause dizziness and headache. Notify your physician.

POSSIBLE ADVERSE EFFECTS

The most serious adverse effect is excessively lowered blood pressure, and this may need to be monitored on a regular basis. Other adverse effects usually improve after using isosorbide dinitrate on a regular basis; dose adjustment may help.

Symptom/effect	Frequency		Discuss with physician		Stop taking drug now	Call physician now
	Common	Rare	Only if severe	In all cases		
Headache	●		■			
Flushing	●		■			
Dizziness	●			■		
Fainting		●		■		▮

INTERACTIONS

Antihypertensive drugs A further lowering of blood pressure occurs when antihypertensives are taken with isosorbide dinitrate.

Alcohol Alcohol may be a cardiac depressant, lowering the blood pressure when taken with isosorbide dinitrate.

SPECIAL PRECAUTIONS

Be sure to tell your physician if:
▼ You have any blood disorders or anemia.
▼ You have had glaucoma.
▼ You have thyroid disease.
▼ You are taking other medications.

 Pregnancy
▼ Not usually prescribed. Effects on the developing baby are uncertain.

 Breast feeding
▼ Discuss with your physician.

 Infants and children
▼ Not usually prescribed.

 Over 60
▼ No special problems.

 Driving and hazardous work
▼ Avoid such activities until you have learned how the drug affects you, because the drug can cause dizziness.

 Alcohol
▼ Avoid. Alcohol may further lower blood pressure, depressing the heart and causing dizziness and faintness.

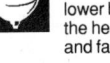

PROLONGED USE

The initial adverse effects may disappear with prolonged use. The effects of the drug become weaker as the body adapts, requiring increased dosage or other drugs.

A
B
C
D
E
F
G
H
I
J
K
L
M
N
O
P
Q
R
S
T
U
V
W
X
Y
Z

ISOTRETINOIN

Brand name Accutane
Used in the following combined preparations None

GENERAL INFORMATION

Isotretinoin, introduced in 1982, is an anti-acne drug chemically related to vitamin A. It is taken by mouth for the treatment of severe acne that has failed to respond to other treatments.

It works by reducing production of the skin's natural oil (sebum) and of the horny protein (keratin) that forms in the outer layers of the skin. This latter effect makes it useful for the treatment of some conditions in which the skin thickens abnormally, causing scaling.

A single course of isotretinoin treatment lasting about 20 weeks often clears acne completely. In the early weeks of treatment, the skin may become unusually dry, flaky, and itchy. This usually improves as treatment continues. Serious adverse effects include liver damage, visual impairment, and inflammation of the bowel. Because it can cause birth defects, women taking isotretinoin must avoid pregnancy.

INFORMATION FOR USERS

Your drug prescription is tailored for you. Do not alter dosage without checking with your physician.

How taken

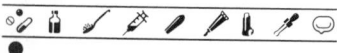

Capsules.

Frequency and timing of doses
2 x daily.

Adult dosage range
Dosage is determined individually.

Onset of effect
2 – 8 weeks. Acne may worsen during the first few weeks of treatment in some people.

Duration of action
Effects may persist for several weeks after the drug has been stopped.

Diet advice
None.

Storage
Keep in a closed container in a cool, dry place away from reach of children. Protect from light.

Missed dose
Take as soon as you remember. If your next dose is due within 2 hours, take a single dose now and skip the next.

Stopping the drug
Can be safely stopped as soon as you no longer need it, but best results are achieved when the course of treatment is completed as prescribed.

Exceeding the dose
An occasional unintentional extra dose is unlikely to cause problems. Large overdoses may cause headaches, vomiting, abdominal pain, facial flushing, dizziness, and incoordination. Notify your physician.

SPECIAL PRECAUTIONS

Be sure to tell your physician if:
▼ You have impaired liver or kidney function.
▼ You suffer from arthritis.
▼ You have diabetes.
▼ You wear contact lenses.
▼ You are taking other medications.

Pregnancy
▼ Not prescribed. May cause abnormalities in the developing baby. Pregnancy should be avoided for at least 3 months after stopping the drug.

Breast feeding
▼ Discuss with your physician. The drug passes into the breast milk and may affect the baby adversely.

Infants and children
▼ Not prescribed.

Over 60
▼ Not prescribed.

Driving and hazardous work
▼ No special problems.

Alcohol
▼ Avoid. Alcohol may increase the rise in blood fat levels with isotretinoin, and thus increase the risk of heart and blood vessel disease.

POSSIBLE ADVERSE EFFECTS

Dryness of the nose and mouth, inflammation of the lips, and drying and flaking of the skin occur in most people treated with isotretinoin. If headache accompanied by symptoms such as nausea and vomiting, abdominal pain with diarrhea, blood in bowel movements, or visual impairment occurs, consult your physician promptly.

Symptom/effect	Frequency		Discuss with physician		Stop taking drug now	Call physician now
	Common	Rare	Only if severe	In all cases		
Dry skin/nosebleeds	●		■			
Muscle/joint pain	●		■			
Inflammation of lips/eyes	●			■		
Headache/insomnia		●		■		
Impaired vision		●		■	▲	❘
Nausea/vomiting		●		■	▲	❘
Abdominal pain/diarrhea		●		■	▲	❘

INTERACTIONS

Tetracycline antibiotics These may increase the risk of high blood pressure in the skull, leading to headaches, nausea, and vomiting.

Skin-drying preparations Medicated cosmetics, soaps, toiletries, and anti-acne preparations increase the likelihood of dryness and irritation of the skin with isotretinoin.

Vitamin A Supplements of this vitamin increase the risk of adverse effects from isotretinoin.

PROLONGED USE

Prolonged use may cause a rise in fat levels in the blood, thereby increasing the risk of heart and blood-vessel disease.

Monitoring Periodic checks on fat levels in the blood and liver function tests may be recommended.

ISOXSUPRINE

Brand names Vasodilan, Voxsuprine
Used in the following combined preparations None

GENERAL INFORMATION

Introduced in 1959, isoxsuprine is a vasodilator drug used to improve blood flow through narrowed arteries, particularly in the legs and brain. It has been used to treat dementia and temporary strokes caused by a buildup of fatty deposits (atherosclerosis) in blood vessels in the brain. It has also been prescribed to relieve pain in the legs caused by peripheral vascular disease. However, although isoxsuprine is widely prescribed, there is very little evidence that it has any useful effect in these disorders.

Isoxsuprine is sometimes used to suppress contractions of the uterus in premature labor. It is used less often than other similar drugs because it is more likely to have adverse effects on heart rhythm and blood pressure.

QUICK REFERENCE

Drug group Vasodilator (p.126) and uterine muscle relaxant (p.193)

Overdose danger rating Medium

Dependence rating Low

Prescription needed Yes

Available as generic Yes

INFORMATION FOR USERS

Your drug prescription is tailored for you. Do not alter dosage without checking with your physician.

How taken

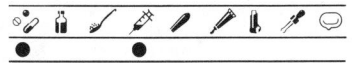

Tablets, injection.

Frequency and timing of doses
3 – 4 x daily.

Dosage range
Up to 80mg daily.

Onset of effect
Within 1 hour (tablets); within 10 – 30 minutes (injection).

Duration of action
8 – 10 hours.

Diet advice
None.

Storage
Keep in a closed container in a cool, dry place away from reach of children.

Missed dose
Take as soon as you remember. If your next dose is due within 2 hours, take a single dose now and skip the next.

Stopping the drug
Do not stop taking the drug without consulting your physician.

Exceeding the dose
An occasional unintentional extra dose is unlikely to cause problems. Large overdoses may cause palpitations or flushing. Notify your physician.

SPECIAL PRECAUTIONS

Be sure to tell your physician if:
▼ You have heart disease or high blood pressure.
▼ You have glaucoma.
▼ You have diabetes mellitus.
▼ You are taking other medications.

Pregnancy
▼ Not usually prescribed in early pregnancy. Will not harm the baby when used in late pregnancy.

Breast feeding
▼ Discuss with your physician. The drug passes into the breast milk, but at normal doses adverse effects on the baby are unlikely.

Infants and children
▼ Not usually prescribed.

Over 60
▼ Reduced dose may be necessary.

Driving and hazardous work
▼ Avoid such activities until you have learned how the drug affects you, because the drug may cause dizziness.

Alcohol
▼ No known problems.

POSSIBLE ADVERSE EFFECTS

More common adverse effects, such as dizziness resulting from low blood pressure or rapid heartbeat, can usually be controlled with an adjustment in dosage.

Symptom/effect	Frequency		Discuss with physician		Stop taking drug now	Call physician now
	Common	Rare	Only if severe	In all cases		
Dizziness	●			■		
Palpitations	●			■		
Nausea/vomiting		●		■		
Flushing		●		■		

INTERACTIONS

Antihypertensive drugs Isoxsuprine may increase the blood pressure-lowering effect of these drugs.

PROLONGED USE

No special problems.

KETOCONAZOLE

Brand name Nizoral
Used in the following combined preparations None

GENERAL INFORMATION

Ketoconazole, an antifungal drug introduced in 1981, is prescribed mainly for severe internal *systemic* fungal infections – of the lungs, brain, kidneys and lymph nodes, for example. It is also given long-term to treat serious infections of the skin and mucous membranes caused by the Candida yeast. People with rare fungal diseases (paracoccidioidomycosis, histoplasmosis, and blastomycosis)

may also be given this antifungal drug, and treatment lasts at least six months.

Investigation into the use of ketoconazole for prostate cancer and certain adrenal gland disorders is also being carried out.

The most common side effect with ketoconazole is nausea, which can be reduced by taking the drug at bedtime or with meals. Ketoconazole may also cause liver damage.

QUICK REFERENCE

Drug group Antifungal drug (p.166)
Overdose danger rating Medium
Dependence rating Low
Prescription needed Yes
Available as generic No

INFORMATION FOR USERS

Your drug prescription is tailored for you. Do not alter dosage without checking with your physician.

How taken

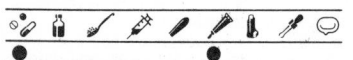

Tablets, cream.

Frequency and timing of doses
Once daily with food.

Dosage range
Adults 200 – 400mg daily. A larger dose may be given in special circumstances.
Children Reduced dose according to age and weight.

Onset of effect
Within a few weeks.

Duration of action
Up to 24 hours.

Diet advice
None.

Storage
Keep in a closed container in a cool, dry place away from reach of children.

Missed dose
Take as soon as you remember. If your next dose is due within 8 hours, take a single dose now and skip the next.

Stopping the drug
Take the full course. Even if you feel better, the original infection may still be present and symptoms may recur if treatment is stopped too soon.

Exceeding the dose
An occasional unintentional extra dose is unlikely to cause problems. Large overdoses may cause loss of consciousness. Notify your physician.

POSSIBLE ADVERSE EFFECTS

Nausea is the most common side effect of this drug. Liver damage is a rare but serious

adverse effect. It causes jaundice, and may necessitate stopping the drug.

Symptom/effect	Frequency		Discuss with physician		Stop taking drug now	Call physician now
	Common	Rare	Only if severe	In all cases		
Nausea	●		■			
Dizziness		●	■			
Headache		●	■			
Constipation/diarrhea		●	■			
Loss of interest in sex		●	■			
Rash/itching		●		■	▲	
Painful breasts (men)		●		■	▲	
Jaundice		●		■	▲	

INTERACTIONS

Antacids, cimetidine, and ranitidine These drugs may reduce the effectiveness of ketoconazole if they are taken within 4 hours before or after ketoconazole.

Rifampin reduces the effect of ketoconazole.

Warfarin Ketoconazole increases the effect of warfarin. The dosage of warfarin may need to be adjusted accordingly.

Cyclosporine Ketoconazole increases the level of cyclosporine in the blood.

SPECIAL PRECAUTIONS

Be sure to tell your physician if:
▼ You have impaired liver or kidney function.
▼ You have had stomach ulcers.
▼ You have previously had an allergic reaction to antifungal drugs.
▼ You are taking other medications.

Pregnancy
▼ Not usually prescribed. May cause defects in the developing baby. Discuss with your physician so that you may weigh the benefits of the drug against its risks.

Breast feeding
▼ Discuss with your physician. The drug passes into the breast milk and may affect the baby adversely.

Infants and children
▼ Reduced dose necessary.

Over 60
▼ No special problems.

Driving and hazardous work
▼ Avoid such activities until you have learned how the drug affects you, because the drug can cause dizziness.

Alcohol
▼ No known problems.

PROLONGED USE

The risk of liver damage increases with long-term use.

Monitoring Periodic blood tests are usually performed to check the effect of the drug on the liver.

KETOPROFEN

Brand name Orudis
Used in the following combined preparations None

GENERAL INFORMATION

Ketoprofen is one of the newer non-steroidal anti-inflammatory drugs (NSAIDs). Like other drugs of this group, it relieves pain and reduces stiffness in rheumatoid arthritis, osteoarthritis, and ankylosing spondylitis. When taken regularly, its effect does not diminish, relieving symptoms rather than curing the underlying disease. Given together with slower-acting drugs in rheumatoid arthritis, it relieves pain and inflammation while

these drugs take effect. It may also be taken for relief of mild to moderate pain, e.g., from soft-tissue injuries.

The most common adverse reactions to ketoprofen, as with all NSAIDs, are gastrointestinal disturbances such as nausea and indigestion. It is generally considered safer than aspirin, and rarely causes gastrointestinal bleeding. Switching to another NSAID may be recommended if unwanted effects are persistent or troublesome.

QUICK REFERENCE

Drug group Non-steroidal anti-inflammatory drug (p.144)

Overdose danger rating Low

Dependence rating Low

Prescription needed Yes

Available as generic No

INFORMATION FOR USERS

Your drug prescription is tailored for you. Do not alter dosage without checking with your physician.

How taken

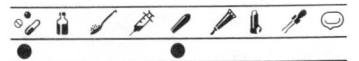

Tablets, capsules, suppositories.

Frequency and timing of doses
3 – 4 x daily with food (by mouth); 2 x daily (rectal suppositories).

Adult dosage range
150 – 200mg daily.

Onset of effect
Pain relief may be felt in 30 minutes to 2 hours. Full anti-inflammatory effect may not be felt for up to 2 weeks.

Duration of action
Up to 8 – 12 hours.

Diet advice
None.

Storage
Keep in a closed container in a cool, dry place away from reach of children.

Missed dose
Take as soon as you remember. If your next dose is due within 4 hours, take a single dose now and skip the next.

Stopping the drug
When taken for short-term pain relief, ketoprofen can be safely stopped as soon as you no longer need it. If prescribed for the long-term treatment of arthritis, however, you should seek medical advice before stopping the drug.

Exceeding the dose
An occasional unintentional extra dose is unlikely to cause problems. Large overdoses may cause vomiting, confusion, or irritability. Notify your physician.

SPECIAL PRECAUTIONS

Be sure to tell your physician if:
▼ You have impaired kidney function.
▼ You have heart problems.
▼ You have high blood pressure.
▼ You have had a peptic ulcer, esophagitis, or acid indigestion.
▼ You have bleeding problems.
▼ You are allergic to aspirin.
▼ You are taking other medications.

Pregnancy
▼ Not usually prescribed. When taken in the last three months of pregnancy, the drug may increase the risk of adverse effects on the baby's heart and may prolong labor.

Breast feeding
▼ Discuss with your physician. The drug passes into the breast milk and may affect the baby adversely.

Infants and children
▼ Not recommended.

Over 60
▼ Reduced dose may be necessary. Increased likelihood of adverse effects.

Driving and hazardous work
▼ No known problems.

Alcohol
▼ Avoid. Alcohol may increase the risk of stomach disorders with ketoprofen.

Surgery and general anesthetics
▼ Ketoprofen may prolong bleeding. Discuss this with your physician or dentist before any surgery.

POSSIBLE ADVERSE EFFECTS

Gastrointestinal disturbances such as nausea and indigestion commonly occur with ketoprofen taken by mouth. Suppositories may cause rectal irritation. Black or bloodstained bowel movements should be reported to your physician without delay.

Symptom/effect	Frequency		Discuss with physician		Stop taking drug now	Call physician now
	Common	Rare	Only if severe	In all cases		
Nausea/vomiting	●		■			
Heartburn	●		■			
Abdominal pain	●			■		
Headache		●	■			
Dizziness/lightheadedness		●	■			
Rash/itching		●		■	▲	
Wheezing/breathlessness		●		■	▲	■

INTERACTIONS

General note Ketoprofen interacts with a wide range of drugs to increase the risk of bleeding and/or stomach ulcers. Such drugs include oral anticoagulants, corticosteroids, other non-steroidal anti-inflammatory drugs (NSAIDs), and aspirin.

Oral antidiabetic drugs Ketoprofen may increase the blood sugar-lowering effect of these drugs.

Antihypertensive drugs The beneficial effects of these drugs may be reduced by ketoprofen.

PROLONGED USE

There is an increased risk of bleeding from peptic ulcers and in the bowel with prolonged use of ketoprofen.

A B C D E F G H I J K L M N O P Q R S T U V W X Y Z

LABETALOL

Brand names Normodyne, Trandate
Used in the following combined preparations None

GENERAL INFORMATION

Introduced in 1984, labetalol is a beta blocker frequently used to treat high blood pressure (hypertension). It has a twofold effect, reducing the rate and force of the heartbeat, and at the same time widening certain arteries and easing the flow of blood. For that dual action, labetalol is particularly useful for people suffering from both hypertension and angina (narrowing of the coronary arteries).

Although usually taken in tablet form, labetalol may be injected for stronger, more rapid results – in a case of hypertensive emergency, for example. The possible use of labetalol eye drops in the treatment of glaucoma is under investigation.

Nausea and indigestion are common adverse effects. Rare side effects include impotence, headache, nightmares, and depression. Like other beta blockers, labetalol may cause breathing difficulty, especially in people with lung disorders. Because it may also mask the body's response to low blood sugar, it is prescribed with caution to diabetics.

INFORMATION FOR USERS

Your drug prescription is tailored for you. Do not alter dosage without checking with your physician.

How taken

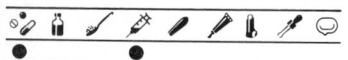

Tablets, injection.

Frequency and timing of doses
2 x daily (by mouth).

Adult dosage range
By mouth 200 – 800mg daily. Dosage may be increased for severe hypertension.
By injection 300mg daily.

Onset of effect
Within 1 – 2 hours (by mouth); within a few minutes (injection).

Duration of action
12 – 20 hours.

Diet advice
None.

Storage
Keep in a closed container in a cool, dry place away from reach of children.

Missed dose
Take as soon as you remember. If your next dose is due within 2 hours, take a single dose now and skip the next.

Stopping the drug
Do not stop the drug without consulting your physician; stopping the drug may lead to worsening of the underlying condition.

OVERDOSE ACTION

 Seek immediate medical advice in all cases. Take emergency action if breathing difficulties or loss of consciousness occurs.

See Drug poisoning emergency guide (p.590).

POSSIBLE ADVERSE EFFECTS

Common adverse effects, such as nausea and indigestion, usually diminish with long-term use. Unlike other beta blockers, labetalol may also cause temporary impotence, and, more rarely, damage to the liver, leading to jaundice.

Symptom/effect	Frequency		Discuss with physician		Stop taking drug now	Call physician now
	Common	Rare	Only if severe	In all cases		
Nausea/indigestion	●		■			
Cold hands/feet		●	■			
Temporary impotence		●	■			
Nightmares		●	■			
Dizziness		●		■		
Jaundice		●		■		
Breathing difficulties		●		■		■

INTERACTIONS

Monoamine oxidase inhibitors (MAOIs) may dangerously raise blood pressure when taken with labetalol.

Cimetidine can increase blood levels of labetalol, increasing the potential for adverse effects associated with labetalol.

SPECIAL PRECAUTIONS

Be sure to tell your physician if:
▼ You have a lung disorder such as asthma or bronchitis.
▼ You have diabetes.
▼ You are taking other medications.

 Pregnancy
▼ Not usually prescribed. Safety in pregnancy not established. Discuss with your physician so that you may weigh the benefits of the drug against its possible risks.

 Breast feeding
▼ The drug passes into the breast milk, but at normal doses adverse effects on the baby are unlikely. Discuss with your physician.

 Infants and children
▼ Not usually prescribed.

 Over 60
▼ Reduced dose may be necessary. Increased likelihood of adverse effects.

 Driving and hazardous work
▼ Avoid such activities until you have learned how the drug affects you, because labetalol may cause drowsiness.

 Alcohol
▼ No known problems.

▼ **Surgery and general anesthetics**
Labetalol may need to be stopped before you have a general anesthetic. Discuss this with your physician or dentist before any surgery.

PROLONGED USE

No problems expected.

LACTULOSE

Brand names Cephulac, Chronulac
Used in the following combined preparations None

GENERAL INFORMATION

Lactulose is an effective laxative that softens bowel movements by increasing the amount of water in the large intestine. It is useful for the relief of constipation and fecal impaction, especially in the elderly. Lactulose can also prevent and treat the brain disturbance associated with liver failure

known as hepatic encephalopathy.

Because lactulose acts locally in the large intestine and is not absorbed into the body, it is safer than many other laxatives. However, because it can cause stomach cramps and flatulence, it is often prescribed only when other laxatives have not worked.

INFORMATION FOR USERS

Your drug prescription is tailored for you. Do not alter dosage without checking with your physician.

How taken

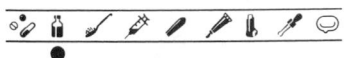

Liquid.

Frequency and timing of doses
1 – 2 x daily (chronic constipation);
3 – 4 x daily (liver failure).

Adult dosage range
15 – 60ml daily (chronic constipation);
30 – 180ml daily (liver failure).

Onset of effect
24 – 48 hours.

Duration of action
6 – 18 hours.

Diet advice
It is important to maintain an adequate intake of fluid – up to 8 glasses of water daily.

Storage
Keep in a closed container in a cool, dry place away from reach of children.

Missed dose
Take as soon as you remember. If your next dose is due within 2 hours, take a single dose now and skip the next.

Stopping the drug
Do not stop the drug without consulting your physician; symptoms may recur.

Exceeding the dose
An occasional unintentional extra dose is unlikely to be a cause for concern. But if you notice unusual symptoms, or if a large overdose has been taken, notify your physician.

POSSIBLE ADVERSE EFFECTS

Adverse effects are rarely serious and often disappear when your body adjusts to the medicine. Diarrhea indicates that the dosage of lactulose may be too high.

Symptom/effect	Frequency		Discuss with physician		Stop taking drug now	Call physician now
	Common	Rare	Only if severe	In all cases		
Flatulence/belching	●		■			
Stomach cramps	●		■			
Nausea	●		■			
Dizziness/lightheadedness		●		■		
Tiredness/weakness		●		■		
Increased thirst		●		■		
Diarrhea		●		■		

INTERACTIONS

Antibiotics Certain antibiotics such as neomycin may reduce the effectiveness of lactulose when it is used to treat liver failure.

SPECIAL PRECAUTIONS

Be sure to tell your physician if:
▼ You have severe abdominal pain.
▼ You have a kidney disorder.
▼ You have high blood pressure.
▼ You have a heart disorder.
▼ You have diabetes.
▼ You are taking other medications.

Pregnancy
▼ Not usually prescribed. May increase the risk of fluid retention; effects on the developing baby uncertain. Discuss with your physician so that you may weigh the benefits of the drug against its risks.

Breast feeding
▼ No evidence of risk.

Infants and children
▼ Not usually prescribed.

Over 60
▼ Increased likelihood of adverse effects.

Driving and hazardous work
▼ No known problems.

Alcohol
▼ No known problems.

PROLONGED USE

People on long-term treatment with this drug, especially the elderly, may develop chemical imbalances in the blood.

Monitoring Monitoring of blood levels of potassium may be advised.

LEVODOPA

Brand names Dopar, Larodopa
Used in the following combined preparation Sinemet

GENERAL INFORMATION

The treatment of Parkinson's disease underwent dramatic change in the 1960s with the introduction of levodopa. Because the body can transform levodopa into dopamine, a chemical in the brain whose absence or shortage causes Parkinson's disease (see p.115), pronounced improvements were expected. These focused not so much on a cure as on symptomatic benefits.

It was found, however, that levodopa, while effective, produced severe side effects: nausea, dizziness, palpitations. Even when levodopa treatment was initiated gradually, it was difficult to balance the benefits against the adverse reactions. What made levodopa treatment even more difficult was the need for increasingly larger dosages.

Today, when levodopa treatment is prescribed, the drug is combined with carbidopa, a substance that enhances the therapeutic effect of the levodopa. Smaller amounts of levodopa are therefore needed, reducing the adverse reactions.

QUICK REFERENCE

Drug group Antiparkinsonism drug (p.115)

Overdose danger rating Medium

Dependence rating Low

Prescription needed Yes

Available as generic Yes

INFORMATION FOR USERS

Your drug prescription is tailored for you. Do not alter dosage without checking with your physician.

How taken

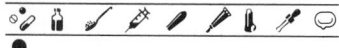

Tablets, capsules.

Frequency and timing of doses
3 – 6 x daily with food or milk.

Adult dosage range
500 – 1,000mg (starting dose), gradually increased until maximum benefit permitted by side effects is achieved.

Onset of effect
Within 30 minutes.

Duration of action
2 – 12 hours.

Diet advice
None.

Storage
Keep in a closed container in a cool, dry place away from reach of children.

Missed dose
Take as soon as you remember. If your next dose is due within 2 hours, take a single dose now and skip the next.

Stopping the drug
Do not stop taking the drug without consulting your physician; stopping the drug may lead to worsening of the underlying condition.

Exceeding the dose
An occasional unintentional extra dose is unlikely to cause problems. Larger overdoses may cause vomiting or drowsiness. Notify your physician.

SPECIAL PRECAUTIONS

Be sure to tell your physician if:
▼ You have heart problems.
▼ You have impaired kidney or liver function.
▼ You have a lung disorder such as asthma or bronchitis.
▼ You have an overactive thyroid gland.
▼ You have had glaucoma.
▼ You are taking other medications.

Pregnancy
▼ Not usually prescribed. Safety in pregnancy not established. Discuss with your physician so that you can weigh the benefits of the drug against its possible risks.

Breast feeding
▼ Discuss with your physician. The drug passes into the breast milk. Its effects on the baby are not clearly known.

Infants and children
▼ Not recommended for children under 12.

Over 60
▼ No special problems.

Driving and hazardous work
▼ Your underlying condition as well as the sedative effects of this drug may make such activities inadvisable. Discuss with your physician.

Alcohol
▼ No known problems.

POSSIBLE ADVERSE EFFECTS

Adverse effects of levodopa are closely related to dosage levels. At the start of treatment, when dosage is usually low, unwanted effects are likely to be mild. Such effects may increase in severity as dosage is increased to boost the drug's beneficial effects. All adverse effects of this drug should be discussed with your physician.

Symptom/effect	Frequency		Discuss with physician		Stop taking drug now	Call physician now
	Common	Rare	Only if severe	In all cases		
Digestive disturbance	●			■		
Nervousness/agitation	●			■		
Dizziness/fainting		●		■		
Abnormal movement		●		■		
Confusion/vivid dreams		●	●	■		
Palpitations		●		■	▲	▮

INTERACTIONS

Antidepressant drugs Levodopa may interact with MAOI antidepressants to cause a dangerous rise in blood pressure. It may also interact with tricyclic antidepressants.

Antipsychotic drugs These may counter the beneficial effects of levodopa.

Pyridoxine (vitamin B$_6$) Excessive intake of this vitamin may reduce the effect of levodopa.

PROLONGED USE

The effectiveness usually declines in time, necessitating increased dosage. The adverse effects also become more severe, to the point where ultimately the drug must be stopped altogether.

LEVOTHYROXINE

Brand names Levothroid, Synthroid
Used in the following combined preparations None

GENERAL INFORMATION

Levothyroxine, introduced in 1953, is often known as thyroxine, the major hormone produced by the thyroid gland. The drug is used primarily to replace the natural hormone when it is deficient, causing hypothyroidism and sometimes leading to myxedema, characterized by puffiness of the face. Certain types of goiter (enlarged thyroid) are helped by levothyroxine, and it may be given to prevent the development of goiter during treatment with antithyroid drugs. It is also prescribed for thyroid cancer and its prevention in people undergoing radiation therapy in the neck. Injections are reserved for myxedema coma in adults and cretinism in newborn infants.

Because adults with severe thyroid deficiency are sensitive to thyroid hormones, treatment is introduced gradually to prevent adverse effects (see below). Particular care is required in those with heart problems.

QUICK REFERENCE

Drug group Thyroid hormone (p.172)
Overdose danger rating Medium
Dependence rating Low
Prescription needed Yes
Available as generic Yes

INFORMATION FOR USERS

Your drug prescription is tailored for you. Do not alter dosage without checking with your physician.

How taken

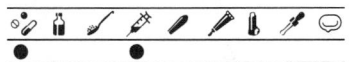

Tablets, injection.

Frequency and timing of doses
Once daily.

Dosage range
Adults Doses of 50 – 100mcg daily for mild hypothyroidism and 12.5 – 25mcg daily for severe hypothyroidism are given initially, and increased at 2 – 4 week intervals as required. The usual maintenance dose is 100 – 200mcg daily.
Children Dose according to age and weight.

Onset of effect
Within 48 hours. Full beneficial effects may not be felt for several weeks.

Duration of action
1 – 3 weeks.

Diet advice
None.

Storage
Keep tablets in a closed container in a cool, dry place away from reach of children. Protect from light.

Missed dose
Take as soon as you remember. If your next dose is due within 2 hours, take both doses now.

Stopping the drug
Do not stop the drug without consulting your physician; symptoms may recur.

Exceeding the dose
An occasional unintentional extra dose is unlikely to cause problems. Large overdoses may cause palpitations during the next few days. Notify your physician.

SPECIAL PRECAUTIONS

Be sure to tell your physician if:
▼ You have high blood pressure.
▼ You have heart problems.
▼ You are taking other medications.

Pregnancy
▼ No evidence of risk to developing baby.

Breast feeding
▼ Discuss with your physician. The drug passes into the breast milk.

Infants and children
▼ A higher dose is often necessary.

Over 60
▼ Reduced dose usually necessary.

Driving and hazardous work
▼ No known problems.

Alcohol
▼ No known problems.

POSSIBLE ADVERSE EFFECTS

Adverse effects are rare with levothyroxine and are usually the result of overdosage, causing thyroid overactivity. These effects diminish as the dose is lowered. Too low a dose of levothyroxine may cause signs of thyroid underactivity.

Symptom/effect	Frequency		Discuss with physician		Stop taking drug now	Call physician now
	Common	Rare	Only if severe	In all cases		
Anxiety/agitation		●		■		
Diarrhea		●		■		
Weight loss/gain		●		■		
Sweating/flushing		●		■		
Lethargy		●		■		
Palpitations/chest pain		●		■		■

INTERACTIONS

Oral anticoagulant drugs
Levothyroxine may increase the effect of these drugs.

Cholestyramine and colestipol These drugs reduce absorption of levothyroxine.

Antidiabetic drugs and digitalis drugs
Levothyroxine may increase requirements for these drugs.

PROLONGED USE

No special problems.

Monitoring Periodic tests of thyroid function are required.

LIDOCAINE

Brand names Xylocaine, Xylocaine IM, Xylocaine IV, Xylocaine Oral Spray, Xylocaine Viscous Solution
Used in the following combined preparation Xylocaine with Epinephrine

GENERAL INFORMATION

Lidocaine, introduced in 1949, is a powerful local anesthetic with a rapid onset of action. It penetrates tissues well, making it a useful drug for *topical* anesthesia. Available without a prescription, it is widely used to relieve pain, itching, and inflammation caused by sunburn, other minor skin disorders, and hemorrhoids. It is also used to relieve pain and discomfort during dental treatment and medical examinations in which a tube is passed down the throat or into the urethra.

Injections of lidocaine are widely used for all types of minor surgery and for epidural or spinal anesthesia during labor. It is also given by injection to treat abnormal heart rhythms after a heart attack, during heart surgery, or after overdosage with digitalis drugs.

QUICK REFERENCE

Drug group Local anesthetic (p.108) and anti-arrhythmic drug (p.128)

Overdose danger rating Medium

Dependence rating Low

Prescription needed No (ointment) Yes (other preparations)

Available as generic Yes

INFORMATION FOR USERS

Follow instructions on the label. Call your physician if symptoms worsen.

How taken

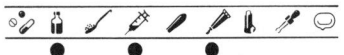

Solution, spray, injection, ointment, cream.

Frequency and timing of doses
As required for anesthesia or pain relief. For hemorrhoids, cream is applied to the anal area after bowel movement and at night. For arrhythmias, lidocaine is usually given by intravenous injection over 2 – 3 minutes, followed by continuous infusion.

Dosage range
Apply topical preparations thinly to the affected area. Do not exceed the maximum recommended dose. Doses by injection are determined individually.

Onset of effect
2 – 5 minutes (ointment, cream, solution, or spray); within 2 minutes (intravenous injection).

Duration of action
Up to 1 hour (topical preparations); 10 – 20 minutes (intravenous injection).

Diet advice
Lidocaine by mouth causes numbness of the mouth and throat and may interfere with swallowing. To avoid choking and injury to the inside of your mouth from hot food or drink, do not eat or drink anything for 1 hour after taking lidocaine.

Storage
Keep in a closed container in a cool, dry place away from reach of children.

Missed dose
Apply topical preparations as soon as you remember if still required.

Stopping the drug
Can be safely stopped as soon as you no longer need it.

Exceeding the dose
An occasional unintentional extra application is unlikely to cause problems. Regular overuse may cause anxiety, restlessness, dizziness, trembling, or drowsiness. Notify your physician.

SPECIAL PRECAUTIONS

Be sure to consult your physician before using this drug if:
▼ You have impaired liver function.
▼ You have had an allergic reaction to a local anesthetic.
▼ You have sores or broken skin at the site of application.
▼ You are taking other medications.

Pregnancy
▼ No evidence of risk with topical preparations. Given for spinal anesthesia during childbirth, it may prolong labor and increase the need for forceps-assisted delivery.

Breast feeding
▼ Creams and ointments should not be used around the nipple. No evidence of risk with topical preparations applied at other sites.

Infants and children
▼ Not recommended for children under 2 years except under medical supervision.

Over 60
▼ Reduced dose may be necessary. Increased likelihood of adverse effects.

Driving and hazardous work
▼ No special problems.

Alcohol
▼ No known problems.

POSSIBLE ADVERSE EFFECTS

Adverse effects are rare when lidocaine is used as a topical anesthetic. Central nervous system effects such as agitation, confusion, and drowsiness may occur with excessive use of topical preparations or with injections. High doses, such as those used for treating arrhythmias, may rarely cause tremors and seizures.

Symptom/effect	Frequency		Discuss with physician		Stop taking drug now	Call physician now
	Common	Rare	Only if severe	In all cases		
Anxiety/restlessness		●		■	▲	▮
Confusion/memory loss		●		■	▲	▮
Nausea/vomiting		●		■	▲	▮
Twitching/tremors		●		■	▲	▮
Shallow breathing		●		■	▲	▮
Seizures		●		■	▲	▮

INTERACTIONS

None.

PROLONGED USE

This drug should not be used for prolonged periods. If your symptoms do not improve within a few days, consult your physician.

LINCOMYCIN

Brand name Lincocin
Used in the following combined preparations None

GENERAL INFORMATION

Lincomycin, introduced in 1965, is an antibiotic used in the treatment of serious infections, particularly those that are resistant to penicillin antibiotics. These include gynecological infections, peritonitis, serious skin and lung infections, osteomyelitis, and septic arthritis. It is also useful for treating other infections in people allergic to penicillins.

When taken by mouth, lincomycin is poorly absorbed from the digestive tract, and it is therefore often given by injection. It has largely been replaced by drugs that are better absorbed when taken by mouth.

Although lincomycin can be safely used by most people, it may occasionally cause a potentially fatal disorder called pseudomembranous colitis, an intestinal inflammation causing diarrhea, fever, and painful abdominal cramps. This occurs most commonly in middle-aged and elderly women.

QUICK REFERENCE

Drug group Lincosamide antibiotic (p.156)

Overdose danger rating Low

Dependence rating Low

Prescription needed Yes

Available as generic No

INFORMATION FOR USERS

Your drug prescription is tailored for you. Do not alter dosage without checking with your physician.

How taken

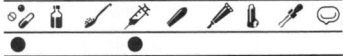

Capsules, injection.

Frequency and timing of doses
By mouth 3 – 4 x daily on an empty stomach.
Injection 1 – 3 x daily.

Dosage range
Adults 1.5 – 2.0g daily.
Children Reduced dose according to age and weight.

Onset of effect
3 – 5 days.

Duration of action
Up to 24 hours.

Diet advice
None.

Storage
Keep in a closed container in a cool, dry place away from reach of children.

Missed dose
Take as soon as you remember. If your next dose is due within 2 hours, take a single dose now and skip the next.

Stopping the drug
Take the full course. Even if you feel better, the original infection may still be present and symptoms may recur if treatment is stopped too soon.

Exceeding the dose
An occasional unintentional extra dose is unlikely to be a cause for concern. But if you notice unusual symptoms, or if a large overdose has been taken, notify your physician.

SPECIAL PRECAUTIONS

Be sure to tell your physician if:
▼ You have impaired liver or kidney function.
▼ You have recently had a bowel disorder.
▼ You have myasthenia gravis.
▼ You are taking other medications.

Pregnancy
▼ Not usually prescribed. Safety in pregnancy not established. Discuss with your physician so that you can weigh the benefits of the drug against its possible risks.

Breast feeding
▼ The drug passes into the breast milk, but at normal doses adverse effects on the baby are unlikely. Discuss with your physician.

Infants and children
▼ Not recommended for infants under 1 month. Reduced dose necessary for older children.

Over 60
▼ Reduced dose necessary. Increased likelihood of adverse effects.

Driving and hazardous work
▼ No known problems.

Alcohol
▼ No known problems.

POSSIBLE ADVERSE EFFECTS

The most common side effect of lincomycin is mild diarrhea. More severe diarrhea, especially if bloodstained or accompanied by abdominal pain or fever, may be a sign of pseudomembranous colitis and requires immediate medical attention.

Symptom/effect	Frequency		Discuss with physician		Stop taking drug now	Call physician now
	Common	Rare	Only if severe	In all cases		
Diarrhea	●		■			
Nausea/vomiting		●	■			
Fever		●		■		▌
Rash		●		■	▲	▌
Itching/hives		●		■	▲	▌
Abdominal cramps		●		■	▲	▌
Blood/mucus in stools		●		■	▲	▌

PROLONGED USE

Usually given for short courses only.

INTERACTIONS

Kaolin Kaolin reduces the absorption and hence the effectiveness of lincomycin taken by mouth. The two medicines should not be taken concurrently.

Drugs for myasthenia gravis Lincomycin may oppose the beneficial effects of these drugs on myasthenia gravis. Dosage adjustment may be necessary.

A B C D E F G H I J K L M N O P Q R S T U V W X Y Z

LINDANE

Brand names Kwell, Kwildane, Scabene, G-Well
Used in the following combined preparations None

GENERAL INFORMATION

Lindane, introduced in 1952, is an insecticide. Used in the treatment of scabies and lice infestations, it rapidly kills the parasites after being absorbed through their tough outer "skin."

A lotion or cream is used to treat scabies and body lice, while lindane shampoo is highly effective against head and pubic lice.

Adverse effects are rare when recommended doses are applied correctly, although lindane may occasionally cause irritation or a rash. Itching, due to an allergic reaction to residual mite eggs and feces, may persist for several weeks after lindane has been used to treat scabies. The drug is labeled as a poison, because excess use or accidental swallowing can cause seizures. Small children are at particular risk of accidental swallowing.

QUICK REFERENCE

Drug group Topical antiparasitic drug (p.204)

Overdose danger rating Medium

Dependence rating Low

Prescription needed Yes

Available as generic Yes

INFORMATION FOR USERS

Your drug prescription is tailored for you. Do not alter dosage without checking with your physician.

How taken

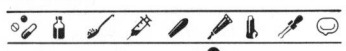

Lotion, cream, shampoo.

Frequency and timing of doses
A single dose, repeated after one week, for treatment of head lice and, where necessary, other infestations.

Dosage range
Apply as directed by your physician. For scabies, the whole body except the head and neck should be covered.

Onset of effect
Within a few minutes.

Duration of action
Active until washed off.

Diet advice
None.

Storage
Keep in a closed container in a cool, dry place away from reach of children.

Missed dose
Not applicable.

Stopping the drug
Follow the advice of your physician. A second treatment is sometimes required to clear the parasites completely.

Exceeding the dose
A single excessive application to the skin or hair is unlikely to cause problems. Frequently repeated applications of the drug may cause agitation, vomiting, muscle cramps, and seizures, requiring prompt medical attention. If the drug has been swallowed, seek immediate medical help.

See Drug poisoning emergency guide (p.590).

SPECIAL PRECAUTIONS

Be sure to tell your physician if:
▼ You have sensitive skin.
▼ You have had epileptic seizures.
▼ You are taking other medications.

 Pregnancy
▼ Not usually prescribed. Safety in pregnancy not established. Discuss with your physician so that you can weigh the benefits of the drug against its possible risks.

 Breast feeding
▼ Used as directed, adverse effects on the baby are unlikely. Discuss with your physician.

 Infants and children
▼ Not recommended for premature babies.

 Over 60
▼ No special problems.

 Driving and hazardous work
▼ No known problems.

 Alcohol
▼ No known problems.

POSSIBLE ADVERSE EFFECTS

Used correctly, lindane rarely causes adverse effects. If you develop skin irritation during treatment, wash off the drug and consult your physician.

Symptom/effect	Frequency		Discuss with physician		Stop taking drug now	Call physician now
	Common	Rare	Only if severe	In all cases		
Rash		●		■		▲
Irritation		●		■		▲

INTERACTIONS

None.

PROLONGED USE

Not given for prolonged periods.

LIOTHYRONINE

Brand names Cyronine, Cytomel
Used in the following combined preparations None

GENERAL INFORMATION

Liothyronine, introduced in 1956, is a synthetic form of triiodothyronine, a powerful hormone produced by the thyroid gland. It is used to replace natural thyroid hormones when they are deficient in hypothyroidism and myxedema; it is also given for the treatment of thyroid cancer prior to surgery.

Faster acting than other thyroid hormone preparations, it is often preferred for initial treatment of severe thyroid deficiency in adults. Injections of the drug are occasionally given for myxedema coma. Taken by mouth, it is better absorbed into the blood-stream than other thyroid drugs and may be prescribed when absorption of drugs is reduced by bowel disease.

Levels of liothyronine in the blood tend to vary widely between doses. Since this complicates monitoring of treatment, it is not generally given for prolonged periods.

Adults with severe thyroid deficiency are sensitive to thyroid hormones, and treatment needs to be introduced gradually to avoid adverse effects (see below). Since overdosage raises the blood pressure and strains the heart, this drug is given with caution to those with heart problems.

INFORMATION FOR USERS

Your drug prescription is tailored for you. Do not alter dosage without checking with your physician.

How taken

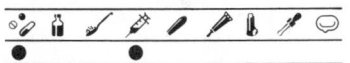

Tablets, injection.

Frequency and timing of doses
2 – 3 x daily.

Adult dosage range
Initially 25mcg daily for mild hypothyroidism and 5mcg daily for severe hypothyroidism, increased as required. The usual maintenance dose is up to 75mcg daily.

Onset of effect
Within 12 hours. Full beneficial effects may not be felt for several weeks.

Duration of action
Up to 72 hours.

Diet advice
None.

Storage
Keep in a closed container in a cool, dry place away from reach of children.

Missed dose
Take as soon as you remember. If your next dose is due within 2 hours, take a single dose now and postpone your next dose for 4 hours.

Stopping the drug
Do not stop taking the drug without consulting your physician; symptoms may recur.

Exceeding the dose
An occasional unintentional extra dose is unlikely to cause problems. Large overdoses may cause palpitations during the next few days. Notify your physician.

POSSIBLE ADVERSE EFFECTS

Serious adverse effects are rare with liothyronine. Troublesome symptoms usually indicate that the dose is too high, and generally diminish with adjustment of the dose.

Symptom/effect	Frequency		Discuss with physician		Stop taking drug now	Call physician now
	Common	Rare	Only if severe	In all cases		
Anxiety/agitation	●			■		
Headache	●			■		
Diarrhea	●			■		
Weight loss	●			■		
Sweating/flushing	●			■		
Palpitations/chest pain		●		■		▪

INTERACTIONS

Oral anticoagulant drugs Liothyronine may increase the effect of these drugs.

Cholestyramine and colestipol These drugs may reduce the absorption of liothyronine taken by mouth.

Antidiabetic drugs Liothyronine treatment may increase requirements for insulin or oral antidiabetic drugs.

SPECIAL PRECAUTIONS

Be sure to tell your physician if:
▼ You have heart problems.
▼ You have high blood pressure.
▼ You are taking other medications.

Pregnancy
▼ No evidence of risk to developing baby.

Breast feeding
▼ Discuss with your physician. The drug passes into the breast milk.

Infants and children
▼ Rarely required.

Over 60
▼ Reduced dose usually necessary.

Driving and hazardous work
▼ No known problems.

Alcohol
▼ No known problems.

PROLONGED USE

Not usually given for prolonged treatment.

Monitoring Periodic tests of thyroid function are usually required.

LITHIUM

Brand names Eskalith, Lithane, Lithobid, Lithonate, Lithotabs
Used in the following combined preparations None

GENERAL INFORMATION

A form of the lightest metal we know, the drug lithium has been used since 1949 to help those suffering from a severe mental disturbance, manic depression. Lithium decreases the intensity and frequency of the episodic swings from extreme excitement to deep depression that are characteristic of that disorder.

A preferred agent for mania alone, it is also sometimes used to prevent and treat severe depression (see p.112).

Treatment with lithium may be started in the hospital for the more seriously ill. Careful monitoring is required because high levels of lithium in the blood can cause serious adverse effects . Since it may take two to three weeks for any benefit of lithium to become apparent, an antipsychotic drug is often given with lithium until the lithium becomes effective.

(see p.112)

QUICK REFERENCE

Drug group Antimanic drug (p.113)
Overdose danger rating High
Dependence rating Low
Prescription needed Yes
Available as generic Yes

INFORMATION FOR USERS

Your drug prescription is tailored for you. Do not alter dosage without checking with your physician.

How taken

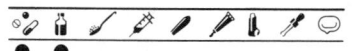

Tablets, capsules, liquid.

Frequency and timing of doses
3 x daily with meals.

Adult dosage range
900 – 2,100mg daily. Dosage may vary according to individual response.

Onset of effect
Some effects may be noticed in 3 – 5 days, but full benefits may not be felt for 3 weeks.

Duration of action
18 – 36 hours. Some effect may last for several days.

Diet advice
Lithium levels in the blood are affected by the amount of sodium (part of table salt) in the body, so you should be careful not to suddenly increase or reduce the amount of salt in your diet. Drinking large amounts of coffee and tea may also cause lithium to build up in your body, although normal consumption of these beverages is unlikely to be harmful. Be sure to drink adequate volumes of other fluids – at least 2 quarts a day, especially in hot weather.

Storage
Keep in a closed container in a cool, dry place away from reach of children.

Missed dose
Take as soon as you remember. If your next dose is due within 2 hours, take both doses now and skip the next.

Stopping the drug
Do not stop the drug without consulting your physician; symptoms may recur.

OVERDOSE ACTION

 Seek immediate medical advice in all cases. Take emergency action if consciousness is lost or if convulsions occur.

See Drug poisoning emergency guide (p.590).

See Drug poisoning emergency guide (p.590).

SPECIAL PRECAUTIONS

Be sure to tell your physician if:
▼ You have impaired kidney or liver function.
▼ You have heart or circulation problems.
▼ You have diabetes.
▼ You have had epileptic seizures.
▼ You have an overactive thyroid gland.
▼ You are taking other medications.

 Pregnancy
▼ May cause heart defects in the unborn baby. Prescribed only when benefit to mother outweighs risk to baby.

 Breast feeding
▼ Not recommended. The drug passes into the breast milk and may cause breathing difficulties and poor muscle tone in the baby. Discuss with your physician.

 Infants and children
▼ Not recommended.

 Over 60
▼ Reduced dose may be necessary. Increased likelihood of adverse effects.

 Driving and hazardous work
▼ Avoid such activities until you have learned how the drug affects you, because of the possibility of reduced alertness.

 Alcohol
▼ Avoid. Alcohol may increase the sedative effects of this drug.

POSSIBLE ADVERSE EFFECTS

Most adverse effects are related to the blood levels of the drug. Your physician will try to find a dose that is sufficient to control your condition without causing excessive adverse effects. Most of the symptoms listed below are signs of high lithium level in the blood. Stop taking the drug and seek medical advice promptly if you notice any of these.

Symptom/effect	Frequency		Discuss with physician		Stop taking drug now	Call physician now
	Common	Rare	Only if severe	In all cases		
Nausea/vomiting/diarrhea	●			■	▲	
Trembling	●			■	▲	
Drowsiness/lethargy		●		■	▲	
Blurred vision		●		■	▲	
Rash		●		■	▲	

INTERACTIONS

General note Many drugs interact with lithium. Do not take any over-the-counter or prescription drug without first consulting your physician or pharmacist.

PROLONGED USE

Prolonged use may lead to increased levels of white cells in the blood. However, this does not usually cause problems. The drug may also damage the kidneys. Treatment for periods of longer than 5 years is not normally advised unless the benefits are significant and tests show no sign of reduced kidney function.

Monitoring Regular monitoring of blood levels of the drug and the composition of the blood is usually carried out.

LOPERAMIDE

Brand name Imodium
Used in the following combined preparations None

GENERAL INFORMATION

Loperamide, introduced in 1977, is an antidiarrheal drug that is available in capsules. It reduces the loss of water and salts from the bowel and slows bowel activity, resulting in the passage of firmer bowel movements at less frequent intervals.

A fast-acting drug, it is widely prescribed for both sudden and recurrent bouts of diarrhea. However, it is not generally recommended for diarrhea caused by infection because it may delay the expulsion of harmful substances from the bowel. It is also unsuitable for acute attacks of ulcerative colitis, since it can cause massive dilation and perforation of the bowel. Loperamide is often prescribed for people who have had colostomies or ileostomies to reduce fluid loss from the stoma, or outlet.

Adverse effects from this drug are rare; unlike the opium-based antidiarrheals, there is no risk of abuse.

INFORMATION FOR USERS

Your drug prescription is tailored for you. Do not alter dosage without checking with your physician.

How taken

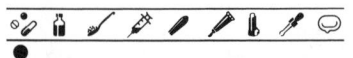

Capsules.

Frequency and timing of doses
Two capsules initially, then one after each loose bowel movement; then 1 – 2 capsules twice daily.

Adult dosage range
4 – 16mg daily.

Onset of effect
Within 1 – 2 hours.

Duration of action
6 – 18 hours.

Diet advice
None. Ensure adequate fluid, sugar, and salt intake during a diarrheal illness.

Storage
Keep in a closed container in a cool, dry place away from reach of children.

Missed dose
Do not take the missed dose. Take your next dose if needed.

Stopping the drug
Can be safely stopped as soon as you no longer need it.

Exceeding the dose
An occasional unintentional extra dose is unlikely to cause problems. Large overdoses may cause constipation, vomiting, or drowsiness. Notify your physician.

POSSIBLE ADVERSE EFFECTS

Adverse effects are rare with loperamide and often difficult to distinguish from the effects of the diarrhea it is used to treat. If symptoms such as bloating, abdominal pain, or fever persist or worsen during treatment with loperamide, consult your physician.

Symptom/effect	Frequency		Discuss with physician		Stop taking drug now	Call physician now
	Common	Rare	Only if severe	In all cases		
Constipation		●	■			
Bloating		●	■			
Abdominal pain		●	■			
Fever		●		■		
Rash		●		■	▲	

INTERACTIONS

None.

SPECIAL PRECAUTIONS

Be sure to tell your physician if:
▼ You have impaired liver or kidney function.
▼ You have had recent abdominal surgery.
▼ You are taking other medications.

Pregnancy
▼ Not usually prescribed. Safety in pregnancy not established. Discuss with your physician so that you can weigh the benefits of the drug against its possible risks.

Breast feeding
▼ Discuss with your physician. The drug passes into the breast milk and may affect the baby adversely.

Infants and children
▼ Not recommended.

Over 60
▼ No special problems.

Driving and hazardous work
▼ No known problems.

Alcohol
▼ No known problems.

PROLONGED USE

This drug is not usually taken for prolonged periods (except for persons with ileostomies), but special problems are not expected during long-term use.

LORAZEPAM

Brand name Ativan
Used in the following combined preparations None

GENERAL INFORMATION

Lorazepam, available since 1977, belongs to a group of drugs known as the benzodiazepines, which help to relieve nervousness, relax muscles, and encourage sleep. The actions and adverse effects of this group of drugs are described more fully on p.111.

Lorazepam is used to treat anxiety and insomnia. It is also used for anxiety associated with depression. Its potential as an anticonvulsant to treat epilepsy is under investigation. Lorazepam is less likely than some of the other benzodiazepines to accumulate in the body.

In common with other benzodiazepines, lorazepam can be habit-forming if taken regularly over a long period. Its effects may also diminish with time. For those reasons, treatment with lorazepam is usually reviewed every two weeks.

INFORMATION FOR USERS

Your drug prescription is tailored for you. Do not alter dosage without checking with your physician.

How taken

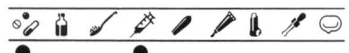

Tablets, injection.

Frequency and timing of doses
Anxiety 1 – 4 x daily.
Insomnia Once daily at bedtime.

Adult dosage range
Anxiety 1 – 10mg daily.
Insomnia 1 – 4mg daily.

Onset of action
Within 45 minutes.

Duration of action
4 – 6 hours.

Diet advice
None.

Storage
Keep in a closed container in a cool, dry place away from reach of children. Protect from light.

Missed dose
If you are taking the drug once daily for insomnia, a missed dose is no cause for concern. Return to your normal dose schedule the following night, if necessary. On a daytime schedule, take the missed dose when you remember. If your next dose is due within 2 hours, take a single dose now and skip the next.

Stopping the drug
If you have been taking the drug continuously for less than 2 weeks, it can be safely stopped as soon as you feel you no longer need it. However, if you have been taking the drug for longer, consult your physician, who will supervise a gradual reduction in dosage. Stopping abruptly may lead to withdrawal symptoms (see p.110).

Exceeding the dose
An occasional unintentional extra dose is unlikely to cause problems. Larger overdoses may cause unusual drowsiness. Notify your physician.

SPECIAL PRECAUTIONS

Be sure to tell your physician if:
▼ You have severe respiratory disease.
▼ You have impaired kidney or liver function.
▼ You have problems with alcohol or drug abuse.
▼ You are taking other medications.

 Pregnancy
▼ Not usually prescribed. May cause congenital abnormalities. Discuss with your physician so that you may weigh the benefits of the drug against its risks.

 Breast feeding
▼ Discuss with your physician. The drug passes into the breast milk. Its effects on the baby are not clearly known.

 Infants and children
▼ Not recommended for children under 12 years. Reduced dose necessary for older children.

 Over 60
▼ Reduced dose may be necessary. Increased likelihood of adverse effects.

 Driving and hazardous work
▼ Avoid such activities until you have learned how the drug affects you, because the drug can cause reduced alertness and slowed reactions.

 Alcohol
▼ Avoid. Alcohol increases the sedative effects of this drug.

POSSIBLE ADVERSE EFFECTS

The principal adverse effects of this drug are related to its sedative and tranquilizing properties. These effects normally diminish after the first few days of treatment and, if troublesome, can often be reduced by adjustment of dosage.

Symptom/effect	Frequency		Discuss with physician		Stop taking drug now	Call physician now
	Common	Rare	Only if severe	In all cases		
Drowsiness/unsteadiness	●		■			
Dizziness/weakness	●		■			
Confusion		●		■		
Headache		●		■		
Nausea		●		■		
Rash		●		■	▲	

PROLONGED USE

Regular use of this drug over several weeks can lead to a reduction in its effect as the body adapts. It may also be habit-forming when taken for extended periods, especially if large doses are taken.

INTERACTIONS

Sedatives All drugs that have a sedative effect on the central nervous system are likely to increase the sedative properties of lorazepam. Such drugs include other anti-anxiety and sleeping drugs, antihistamines, antidepressants, narcotic analgesics, and antipsychotics.

Alcohol The sedative effect of lorazepam is increased by alcohol.

LYPRESSIN

Brand name Diapid
Used in the following combined preparations None

GENERAL INFORMATION

Introduced in 1967, lypressin is a synthetic form of a hormone called vasopressin, which regulates an important kidney function. A vasopressin deficiency causes diabetes insipidus, a water imbalance arising from the kidneys' inability to concentrate the urine. Frequent urination occurs, and continued thirst.

Taken as a nasal spray, it helps correct the hormonal deficiency.

Lypressin is short-acting, and is most helpful for people with milder forms of the disease. In more severely affected individuals, it may not give adequate control of urine production, and longer-acting treatments are usually prescribed.

Side effects are rare. Nasal congestion reduces absorption of the drug, making larger doses necessary to maintain its beneficial effect.

QUICK REFERENCE

Drug group Drug for diabetes insipidus (p.173)

Overdose danger rating Medium

Dependence rating High

Prescription needed Yes

Available as generic No

INFORMATION FOR USERS

Your drug prescription is tailored for you. Do not alter dosage without checking with your physician.

How taken

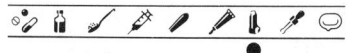

Nasal spray.

Frequency and timing of doses
3 – 7 x daily.

Dosage range
1 – 4 sprays in each nostril per dose.

Onset of effect
Within a few minutes.

Duration of action
3 – 6 hours.

Diet advice
Your physician may advise you to reduce your fluid intake at the start of treatment.

Storage
Keep in a closed container in a cool, dry place away from reach of children.

Missed dose
Take as soon as you remember. Space subsequent doses at equal intervals throughout the day.

Stopping the drug
Do not stop the drug without consulting your physician; symptoms may recur.

Exceeding the dose
An occasional unintentional overdose is unlikely to cause problems. Large overdoses may cause abdominal cramps. Notify your physician.

SPECIAL PRECAUTIONS

Be sure to tell your physician if:
▼ You have heart problems.
▼ You have high blood pressure.
▼ You suffer from allergic rhinitis.
▼ You are taking other medications.

Pregnancy
▼ Has been used in pregnancy without ill effect on the baby. Discuss with your physician so that you may weigh the benefits of the drug against its possible risks.

Breast feeding
▼ The drug passes into the breast milk, but at normal doses adverse effects on the baby are uncommon. Discuss with your physician.

Infants and children
▼ No special problems.

Over 60
▼ No special problems.

Driving and hazardous work
▼ No known problems.

Alcohol
▼ No known problems.

Surgery and general anesthetics
▼ Your treatment may need to be changed before you have a general anesthetic. Discuss this with your physician or dentist before any surgery.

POSSIBLE ADVERSE EFFECTS

Adverse effects are rare. The drug may occasionally cause nasal congestion or ulceration. It may also stimulate contraction of the bowel, leading to abdominal cramps and an increased urge to defecate. Coughing and breathing difficulty may be caused by inadvertent inhalation of the spray into the lungs.

Symptom/effect	Frequency		Discuss with physician		Stop taking drug now	Call physician now
	Common	Rare	Only if severe	In all cases		
Abdominal cramps	●		■			
Urge to defecate	●		■			
Chest tightness		●	■			
Coughing		●	■			
Shortness of breath		●	■			
Runny/stuffy nose		●		■		
Irritation/sores in nose		●		■		

INTERACTIONS

Chlorpropamide, clofibrate, and carbamazepine may increase the effect of lypressin.

Lithium and norepinephrine These drugs may reduce or eliminate the effect of lypressin.

PROLONGED USE

No problems expected.

A
B
C
D
E
F
G
H
I
J
K
L
M
N
O
P
Q
R
S
T
U
V
W
X
Y
Z

MAGNESIUM HYDROXIDE

Brand names Milk of Magnesia, Milk of Magnesia Concentrate
Used in the following combined preparations Aludrox, Camalox, Gelusil, Maalox, Mylanta

GENERAL INFORMATION

Magnesium hydroxide is a fast-acting antacid used to neutralize stomach acid. It is available in a number of over-the-counter preparations for the treatment of indigestion and heartburn. Magnesium hydroxide is also useful for preventing pain due to stomach and duodenal ulcers, gastritis, and reflux esophagitis. It also acts as a laxative by pulling water into the intestine from surrounding blood vessels to increase the fluidity of feces.

Magnesium hydroxide is not often used alone as an antacid because of this laxative effect. However, this is countered when the drug is combined with aluminum hydroxide, which tends to be constipating.

QUICK REFERENCE

Drug group Antacid (p.136) and laxative (p.139)

Overdose danger rating Low

Dependence rating Low

Prescription needed No

Available as generic Yes

INFORMATION FOR USERS

Follow instructions on the label. Call your physician if symptoms worsen.

How taken

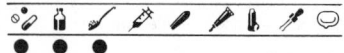

Tablets, liquid, powder.

Frequency and timing of doses
4 x daily with water.

Adult dosage range
Antacid 5 – 10ml per dose (liquid); 600mg – 1.2g per dose (tablets).
Laxative 30 – 45ml per dose (liquid); 2 – 4g per dose (tablets).

Onset of effect
Within 15 minutes (antacid); 2 – 8 hours (laxative).

Duration of action
2 – 4 hours.

Diet advice
None.

Storage
Keep in a closed container in a cool, dry place away from reach of children. Discard liquid within 6 months of opening.

Missed dose
Take as soon as you remember.

Stopping the drug
When used as an antacid, can be safely stopped as soon as you no longer need it. When given as ulcer treatment, follow your physician's advice.

Exceeding the dose
An occasional unintentional extra dose is unlikely to be a cause for concern. But if you notice unusual symptoms, or if a large over-dose has been taken, notify your physician.

SPECIAL PRECAUTIONS

Be sure to consult your physician before taking this drug if:
▼ You have impaired kidney function.
▼ You have a bowel disorder.
▼ You are taking other medications.

Pregnancy
▼ No evidence of risk to developing baby in normal doses.

Breast feeding
▼ No evidence of risk.

Infants and children
▼ Not recommended under 6 years except on the advice of a physician. Reduced dose necessary for older children.

Over 60
▼ No special problems.

Driving and hazardous work
▼ No known problems.

Alcohol
▼ Avoid excess alcohol as it irritates the stomach and may reduce the benefits of this drug.

POSSIBLE ADVERSE EFFECTS

Diarrhea is the most common adverse effect of this drug. Dizziness and muscle weakness due to absorption of excess magnesium in the body are likely to occur only in people with poor kidney function.

Symptom/effect	Frequency		Discuss with physician		Stop taking drug now	Call physician now
	Common	Rare	Only if severe	In all cases		
Diarrhea	●		■			
Nausea	●		■			
Vomiting		●		■		
Dizziness		●		■		

PROLONGED USE

Magnesium hydroxide should not be used for longer than four weeks without consulting your physician. Prolonged use in people with kidney damage may cause nausea, dizziness, and weakness, due to accumulation of magnesium in the body.

INTERACTIONS

General note Magnesium hydroxide interferes with the absorption or excretion of a wide range of drugs taken by mouth, including tetracycline antibiotics, phenothiazine antipsychotics, anti-emetics and iron supplements.

Enteric-coated tablets As with other antacids, magnesium hydroxide may allow breakup of the enteric coating of tablets such as bisacodyl, causing stomach irritation.

MAPROTILINE

Brand name Ludiomil
Used in the following combined preparations None

GENERAL INFORMATION

Maprotiline, introduced in 1981, was the first of a group of antidepressant drugs known as the tetracyclics to be approved in the U.S. Tetracyclics help to lift mood, restore appetite, and renew interest in everyday activities. Maprotiline is used to treat many types of depression and is claimed to be effective for manic depression and depression with neurosis and anxiety. It is somewhat sedative in effect.

In common with the tricyclic antidepressants, maprotiline can cause abnormal heart rhythms. It is therefore used with caution in those with heart problems or thyroid disorders. It is not usually prescribed for epileptics because it may provoke seizures.

INFORMATION FOR USERS

Your drug prescription is tailored for you. Do not alter dosage without checking with your physician.

How taken

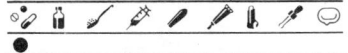

Tablets.

Frequency and timing of doses
2 x daily or once at bedtime.

Adult dosage range
75 – 150mg daily. Dose may be increased in exceptional circumstances.

Onset of effect
Some effects may appear within a couple of days, but full antidepressant effect may not be felt for 2 – 6 weeks.

Duration of action
Beneficial effects may persist, sometimes in diminishing degrees, for up to 6 weeks. Adverse effects may wear off within days.

Diet advice
None.

Storage
Keep in a closed container in a cool, dry place away from reach of children. Protect from light.

Missed dose
Take as soon as you remember. If your next dose is due within 3 hours, take a single dose now and skip the next.

Stopping the drug
Do not stop the drug without consulting your physician. Stopping abruptly may cause withdrawal symptoms (see p.112) and symptoms of the original illness may recur.

OVERDOSE ACTION

Seek immediate medical advice in all cases. Take emergency action if consciousness is lost.

See Drug poisoning emergency guide (p.590).

POSSIBLE ADVERSE EFFECTS

The possible adverse effects of this drug are mainly the result of its *anticholinergic* action and its blocking action on the transmission of signals in the heart.

Symptom/effect	Frequency		Discuss with physician		Stop taking drug now	Call physician now
	Common	Rare	Only if severe	In all cases		
Drowsiness	●		■			
Rash	●			■	▲	
Sweating/flushing		●	■			
Dizziness/fainting		●		■		
Difficulty passing urine		●		■	▲	
Palpitations		●		■	▲	▮
Seizures		●		■	▲	▮

INTERACTIONS

Sedatives All drugs that have a sedative effect on the central nervous system are likely to increase the sedative properties of maprotiline.

Antihypertensive drugs Maprotiline reduces the beneficial effects of some of these drugs.

Monoamine oxidase inhibitors (MAOIs) There is a possibility of a serious interaction, producing seizures and delirium. Two weeks should elapse between maprotiline and MAOI treatments.

SPECIAL PRECAUTIONS

Be sure to tell your physician if:
▼ You have heart problems.
▼ You have had epileptic seizures.
▼ You have impaired kidney or liver function.
▼ You have had glaucoma.
▼ You have had prostate trouble.
▼ You are pregnant or breast feeding.
▼ You are taking other medications.

 Pregnancy
▼ Not usually prescribed. Safety in pregnancy not established. Discuss with your physician so that you can weigh the benefits of the drug against its possible risks.

 Breast feeding
▼ The drug passes into the breast milk and may affect the baby adversely. Discuss with your physician.

 Infants and children
▼ Not usually prescribed.

 Over 60
▼ Reduced dose may be necessary. Increased likelihood of adverse effects, particularly dizziness or unsteadiness on standing.

 Driving and hazardous work
▼ Avoid such activities until you have learned how the drug affects you, because the drug may cause blurred vision and reduced alertness.

 Alcohol
▼ Avoid. Alcohol may increase the sedative effects of this drug.

Surgery and general anesthetics
▼ Maprotiline treatment may need to be stopped before you have a general anesthetic. Discuss this with your physician or dentist before any operation.

PROLONGED USE

No problems expected.

MEBENDAZOLE

Brand name Vermox
Used in the following combined preparations None

GENERAL INFORMATION

Mebendazole, introduced in 1975, is an anthelmintic drug, used to treat a variety of worm infestations, particularly whipworm, pinworm, and hookworm infections of the bowel. Because it has a wide range of activity, it is sometimes prescribed for multiple worm infections and may be useful when the worm cannot be identified.

Taken as tablets, mebendazole kills worms by blocking their energy supply. Pinworm infections are usually cleared up by a single dose, while other worm infections of the bowel require treatment for three consecutive days. Treatment may be repeated after 2 to 3 weeks if the infection is not completely cleared up. For pinworms, which are highly infectious, all members of a household are usually treated.

Because mebendazole is absorbed into the bloodstream only in small amounts, it rarely causes side effects other than diarrhea and abdominal pain. It is under investigation as a treatment for certain types of worm infections not located in the intestine, namely trichinosis and hydatid disease. In these conditions, high doses are given for prolonged periods, and blood levels of the drug are further increased by taking it with meals.

QUICK REFERENCE

Drug group Anthelmintic drug (p.167)

Overdose danger rating Medium

Dependence rating Low

Prescription needed Yes

Available as generic No

INFORMATION FOR USERS

Your drug prescription is tailored for you. Do not alter dosage without checking with your physician.

How taken

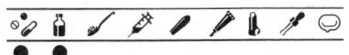

Tablets, liquid.

Frequency and timing of doses
2 x daily morning and evening for 3 days (hookworm, common roundworm, whipworm); single dose (pinworm).

Dosage range
200mg daily (hookworm, common roundworm, whipworm); one 100mg dose (pinworm).

Onset of effect
2 – 4 hours.

Duration of action
2 – 3 days.

Diet advice
None.

Storage
Keep in a closed container in a cool, dry place away from reach of children.

Missed dose
Take as soon as you remember. If your next dose is due at this time, take the two doses together. Return to your normal schedule thereafter.

Stopping the drug
Take the full course. Even if you feel better, the original infection may still be present and may recur if treatment is stopped too soon.

Exceeding the dose
An occasional unintentional extra dose is unlikely to cause problems. Large overdoses may cause abdominal cramps, nausea, vomiting, and diarrhea. Notify your physician.

SPECIAL PRECAUTIONS

Be sure to tell your physician if:
▼ You have impaired liver function.
▼ You have a bowel disorder.
▼ You are taking other medications.

 Pregnancy
▼ Not usually prescribed. Safety in pregnancy not established. Discuss with your physician so that you can weigh the benefits of the drug against its possible risks.

 Breast feeding
▼ No evidence of risk.

 Infants and children
▼ Not recommended for children under 2 years.

 Over 60
▼ No special problems.

 Driving and hazardous work
▼ No known problems.

 Alcohol
▼ No known problems.

POSSIBLE ADVERSE EFFECTS

Abdominal pain and diarrhea may occur occasionally with mebendazole, but are rarely serious and generally disappear as treatment continues.

Symptom/effect	Frequency		Discuss with physician		Stop taking drug now	Call physician now
	Common	Rare	Only if severe	In all cases		
Diarrhea		●	■			
Abdominal pain		●	■			
Fever		●		■	▲	
Rash/itching		●		■	▲	

INTERACTIONS

Antidiabetic drugs Mebendazole may increase the blood sugar-lowering effects of these drugs.

PROLONGED USE

High-dose therapy may increase the risk of a blood disorder.

Monitoring Periodic white blood cell counts are usually performed.

MECLIZINE

Brand names Antivert, Bonine, Ru-Vert-M
Used in the following combined preparations None

GENERAL INFORMATION

Meclizine is an antihistamine that is used as an anti-emetic drug (see p.118). It is effective in preventing and treating motion sickness. Meclizine has a slower onset of action and its effects last longer than those of many similar drugs; therefore it needs to be taken less frequently.

Meclizine is used to treat the vertigo, vomiting, and nausea caused by inner-ear disorders. It is also occasionally used to relieve nausea and vomiting caused by drug or radiation therapy for cancer.

Meclizine has adverse effects similar to those of other antihistamines and *anticholinergic* drugs, including drowsiness, dry mouth, and blurred vision.

INFORMATION FOR USERS

Your drug prescription is tailored for you. Do not alter dosage without checking with your physician.

How taken

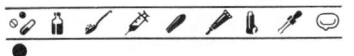

Tablets.

Frequency and timing of doses
Nausea and vertigo 1 – 2 x daily.
Motion sickness Once daily 2 hours before travel.

Adult dosage range
25 – 100mg daily.

Onset of effect
Within 1 hour.

Duration of action
12 – 24 hours.

Diet advice
None.

Storage
Keep in a closed container in a cool, dry place away from reach of children. Protect from light.

Missed dose
Take as soon as you remember. If your next dose is due within 2 hours, take a single dose now and skip the next.

Stopping the drug
Can be safely stopped as soon as you no longer need it.

Exceeding the dose
An occasional unintentional extra dose is unlikely to cause problems. Large overdoses may cause drowsiness or agitation. Notify your physician.

SPECIAL PRECAUTIONS

Be sure to tell your physician if:
▼ You have impaired kidney or liver function.
▼ You have had epileptic seizures.
▼ You have urinary difficulties.
▼ You are taking other medications.

Pregnancy
▼ Not recommended. May cause defects in the unborn baby.

Breast feeding
▼ Discuss with your physician. The drug passes into the breast milk in small amounts.

Infants and children
▼ Not recommended for children under 5 years. Reduced dose necessary for older children.

Over 60
▼ No special problems.

Driving and hazardous work
▼ Avoid such activities until you have learned how the drug affects you, because the drug can cause drowsiness.

Alcohol
▼ Avoid. Alcohol increases the sedative effects of this drug.

POSSIBLE ADVERSE EFFECTS

The adverse effects of meclizine are similar to those of other antihistamines. The most common effect, drowsiness, may be controlled by an adjustment in dosage.

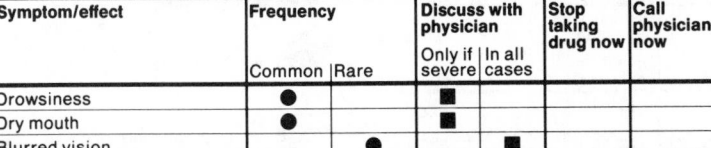

Symptom/effect	Frequency		Discuss with physician		Stop taking drug now	Call physician now
	Common	Rare	Only if severe	In all cases		
Drowsiness	●		■			
Dry mouth	●		■			
Blurred vision		●		■		

PROLONGED USE

Continuous use of this drug for more than a few days is unlikely to be necessary.

INTERACTIONS

Sedatives All drugs that have a sedative effect on the central nervous system are likely to increase the sedative effect of meclizine. Such drugs include anti-anxiety drugs, sleeping drugs, narcotic analgesics, antihistamines, and antidepressants.

Anticonvulsant drugs Taking meclizine in conjunction with anticonvulsants may increase its sedation.

Alcohol Alcohol increases the sedative effect of meclizine.

MECLOFENAMATE

Brand name Meclomen
Used in the following combined preparations None

GENERAL INFORMATION

Introduced in the 1950s, meclofenamate is a non-steroidal anti-inflammatory drug (NSAID) often prescribed for people suffering from rheumatoid arthritis and osteoarthritis because it relieves the pain, swelling, inflammation, and redness associated with these disorders. Meclofenamate does not cure the disease; it only relieves the symptoms. Improvement in these symptoms may begin within a few days, but the drug may not become fully effective until it has been taken continuously for 2 to 3 weeks.

Meclofenamate is normally prescribed only when other NSAIDs have not worked because diarrhea is a common and sometimes severe side effect.

QUICK REFERENCE

Drug group Non-steroidal anti-inflammatory drug (p.144)

Overdose danger rating Medium

Dependence rating Low

Prescription needed Yes

Available as generic No

INFORMATION FOR USERS

Your drug prescription is tailored for you. Do not alter dosage without checking with your physician.

How taken

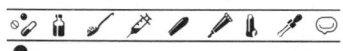

Capsules.

Frequency and timing of doses
3 – 4 x daily with food or milk.

Adult dosage range
500mg – 1500mg daily.

Onset of effect
The drug starts to act within an hour, but the full benefits may not be felt for 2 – 3 weeks.

Duration of action
6 – 8 hours.

Diet advice
None.

Storage
Keep in a closed container in a cool, dry place away from reach of children. Protect from light.

Missed dose
Take as soon as you remember if required for pain. If your next dose is due within 2 hours, take a single dose now and skip the next, then return to your normal dose schedule if necessary.

Stopping the drug
Can be safely stopped as soon as you no longer need it.

Exceeding the dose
An occasional unintentional extra dose is unlikely to cause problems. Large over-doses may cause drowsiness, bloody diarrhea, and vomiting. Notify your physician.

POSSIBLE ADVERSE EFFECTS

Adverse effects of meclofenamate are fairly common and in some cases are severe enough to make continued use of the drug unwise. Some adverse effects are worse if this drug is taken in conjunction with other analgesics.

Symptom/effect	Frequency		Discuss with physician		Stop taking drug now	Call physician now
	Common	Rare	Only if severe	In all cases		
Indigestion	●		■			
Nausea/vomiting	●			■		
Headache		●	■			
Dizziness		●		■		
Rash		●		■	▲	▮

INTERACTIONS

Acetaminophen Taking acetaminophen for an extended period while you are taking meclofenamate may cause kidney damage. Regular medical checks are necessary.

Anticoagulant drugs The effects of these drugs may be increased when they are taken along with meclofenamate. The anticoagulant dosage may need to be adjusted.

Aspirin There is an increased likelihood of digestive problems when aspirin is taken with meclofenamate.

SPECIAL PRECAUTIONS

Be sure to tell your physician if:
▼ You have impaired kidney or liver function.
▼ You have heart problems.
▼ You have a stomach ulcer or other digestive problems.
▼ You are allergic to aspirin.
▼ You are taking other medications.

Pregnancy
▼ Not usually prescribed. Safety in pregnancy not established. Taken near the time of delivery, it may prolong labor.

Breast feeding
▼ At normal doses adverse effects on the baby are uncommon. Discuss with your physician.

Infants and children
▼ Not recommended.

Over 60
▼ Reduced dose may be necessary. Increased likelihood of adverse effects.

Driving and hazardous work
▼ Avoid such activities until you have learned how the drug affects you, because the drug can cause dizziness:

Alcohol
▼ Avoid. Alcohol may increase the adverse effects of this drug on the digestive system.

PROLONGED USE

Prolonged use of this drug may lead to anemia. Gastric or duodenal ulcers may occur if meclofenamate is taken for an extended period.

Monitoring Blood tests may be performed at regular intervals.

MEDROXYPROGESTERONE

Brand names Amen, Curretab, Depo-Provera, Provera
Used in the following combined preparations None

GENERAL INFORMATION

Medroxyprogesterone, introduced in 1959, is a progestin, a synthetic female sex hormone similar to the natural hormone progesterone. It is used to treat menstrual disorders such as mid-cycle bleeding and amenorrhea (absence of menstruation).

The drug may also be given in conjunction with estrogen replacement therapy for menopausal symptoms or underdeveloped ovaries. This reduces the risk of cancer of the uterus with estrogen treatment.

Medroxyprogesterone is often used to treat endometriosis, a condition in which there is abnormal growth of uterine-lining tissue in the pelvic cavity. Occasionally, it may be prescribed for hirsutism (abnormal hairiness).

Depot injections of the drug are widely used as a contraceptive in developing countries. However, since it may cause serious side effects including persistent bleeding from the uterus, amenorrhea, and prolonged infertility, this use remains controversial. It is not approved for general use as a contraceptive in the US.

Medroxyprogesterone may be used to treat some types of cancer.

QUICK REFERENCE

Drug group Female sex hormone (p.175)

Overdose danger rating Low

Dependence rating Low

Prescription needed Yes

Available as generic Yes

INFORMATION FOR USERS

Your drug prescription is tailored for you. Do not alter dosage without checking with your physician.

How taken

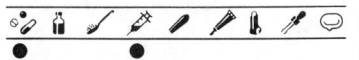

Tablets, injection.

Frequency and timing of doses
Once daily with food.

Adult dosage range
Cancer 200 – 400mg daily.
Other conditions 5 – 30mg daily.

Onset of effect
1 – 2 months (cancer); 1 – 2 weeks (other conditions).

Duration of action
1 – 2 days (by mouth); 1 week – 1 month (injected as cancer therapy).

Diet advice
None.

Storage
Keep in a closed container in a cool, dry place away from reach of children.

Missed dose
Take as soon as you remember. If your next dose is due within 12 hours, take a single dose now and skip the next.

Stopping the drug
Do not stop the drug without consulting your physician; symptoms may recur.

Exceeding the dose
An occasional unintentional extra dose is unlikely to be a cause for concern. But if you notice unusual symptoms, or if a large overdose has been taken, notify your physician.

SPECIAL PRECAUTIONS

Be sure to tell your physician if:
▼ You have high blood pressure.
▼ You have diabetes.
▼ You have had blood clots or a stroke.
▼ You have impaired liver or kidney function.
▼ You are taking other medications.

 Pregnancy
▼ Not prescribed.

 Breast feeding
▼ Discuss with your physician. The drug passes into the breast milk and may affect the baby adversely.

 Infants and children
▼ Not usually prescribed.

 Over 60
▼ No special problems.

 Driving and hazardous work
▼ No known problems.

 Alcohol
▼ No known problems.

POSSIBLE ADVERSE EFFECTS

Medroxyprogesterone rarely causes serious adverse effects. Fluid retention may lead to weight gain, swollen feet or ankles, and breast tenderness. Long-term treatment may cause irregular menstrual bleeding or spotting between periods.

Symptom/effect	Frequency		Discuss with physician		Stop taking drug now	Call physician now
	Common	Rare	Only if severe	In all cases		
Weight gain	●		■			
Swollen ankles	●		■			
Breast tenderness		●	■			
Acne		●	■			
Numb fingers		●		■		
Irregular menstruation		●		■		
Rash/itching/jaundice		●		■	▲	

INTERACTIONS

Bromocriptine Medroxyprogesterone may interfere with the beneficial effects of bromocriptine.

Insulin The blood sugar-lowering effect of insulin may be reduced by medroxyprogesterone.

PROLONGED USE

Long-term use of this drug may slightly increase the risk of blood clots in the leg veins.

Monitoring Periodic checks on blood pressure, yearly cervical smear tests, and breast examinations are usually required.

A B C D E F G H I J K L M N O P Q R S T U V W X Y Z

MEFENAMIC ACID

Brand name Ponstel
Used in the following combined preparations None

GENERAL INFORMATION

Mefenamic acid, introduced in 1967, is a non-steroidal anti-inflammatory drug (NSAID). Like other NSAIDs, it relieves pain and inflammation. It is an effective analgesic, and is used to treat menstrual pains (dysmenorrhea) and excessive menstrual bleeding (menorrhagia). It is often used for the relief of pain after minor operations.

Mefenamic acid is also used for long-term relief of pain and stiffness in rheumatoid arthritis and osteoarthritis.
The most common side effects of mefenamic acid are gastrointestinal: abdominal pain, indigestion, nausea, and vomiting. Other more serious adverse effects include kidney problems and blood disorders.

QUICK REFERENCE

Drug group Non-steroidal anti-inflammatory drug (p.144)

Overdose danger rating Medium

Dependence rating Low

Prescription needed Yes

Available as generic No

INFORMATION FOR USERS

Your drug prescription is tailored for you. Do not alter dosage without checking with your physician.

How taken

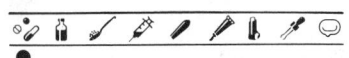

Capsules.

Frequency and timing of doses
Every 6 hours with food.

Adult dosage range
500mg (starting dose), then 250mg per dose as required.

Onset of effect
1 – 2 hours.

Duration of action
Up to 6 hours.

Diet advice
None.

Storage
Keep in a closed container in a cool, dry place away from reach of children.

Missed dose
Take as soon as you remember. If your next dose is due within 2 hours, take a single dose now and skip the next.

Stopping the drug
Can be safely stopped as soon as you no longer need it.

Exceeding the dose
An occasional unintentional extra dose is unlikely to cause problems. Large over-doses may cause muscle twitching, poor coordination, or seizures.

POSSIBLE ADVERSE EFFECTS

Gastrointestinal disturbances are the most common side effects of mefenamic acid. The drug should be stopped if diarrhea or a rash occurs, and not used thereafter. Black or bloodstained bowel movements should be reported to your physician without delay.

Symptom/effect	Frequency		Discuss with physician		Stop taking drug now	Call physician now
	Common	Rare	Only if severe	In all cases		
Indigestion	●		■			
Dizziness/drowsiness	●		■			
Abdominal pain	●			■		
Diarrhea	●			■	▲	
Nausea/vomiting		●	■			
Headache		●	■			
Rash		●		■	▲	
Wheezing/breathlessness		●		■	▲	∎

INTERACTIONS

General note Mefenamic acid interacts with a wide range of drugs to increase the risk of bleeding and/or peptic ulcers. Such drugs include oral anticoagulants, corticosteroids, other non-steroidal anti-inflammatory drugs (NSAIDs), aspirin, some antibiotics, sulfinpyrazone, dipyridamole, and valproic acid.

Lithium Mefenamic acid may raise blood levels of lithium, leading to a risk of serious adverse effects.

Antihypertensive drugs and diuretics
The beneficial effects of these drugs may be reduced by mefenamic acid.

Oral antidiabetic drugs Mefenamic acid may increase the blood sugar-lowering effect of these drugs.

SPECIAL PRECAUTIONS

Be sure to tell your physician if:
▼ You have impaired liver or kidney function.
▼ You have had a peptic ulcer, esophagitis, or acid indigestion.
▼ You have heart problems.
▼ You have high blood pressure.
▼ You are allergic to aspirin.
▼ You are taking other medications.

Pregnancy
▼ Not usually prescribed. May cause defects in the unborn baby and, taken in late pregnancy, may prolong labor. Discuss with your physician so that you may weigh the benefits of the drug against its risks.

Breast feeding
▼ Discuss with your physician. The drug passes into the breast milk, but at normal doses adverse effects on the baby are uncommon.

Infants and children
▼ Not recommended for children under 14 years.

Over 60
▼ Reduced dose may be necessary. Increased likelihood of adverse effects.

Driving and hazardous work
▼ No known problems.

Alcohol
▼ Avoid. Alcohol may increase the risk of stomach irritation with mefenamic acid.

Surgery and general anesthetics
▼ Mefenamic acid may prolong bleeding. Discuss this with your physician or dentist before any surgery.

PROLONGED USE

There is an increased risk of bleeding from peptic ulcers and in the bowel during long-term use.

MEGESTROL

Brand name Megace
Used in the following combined preparations None

GENERAL INFORMATION

Megestrol, introduced in 1972, is a synthetic female sex hormone similar to the natural hormone progesterone. Available as tablets, it is used in the treatment of certain types of advanced cancer of the breast and uterus that are sensitive to hormones. It is often prescribed when the tumor cannot be removed by surgery, when the disease has recurred after surgery, or when other anticancer drugs or radiation treatment have failed.

Successful treatment reduces the size of the tumor; it may also cause secondary growths to disappear. Improvement usually occurs within two months of treatment. Because the drug does not eradicate the cancer completely, megestrol treatment may need to be continued indefinitely.

INFORMATION FOR USERS

Your drug prescription is tailored for you. Do not alter dosage without checking with your physician.

How taken

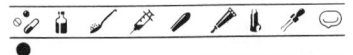

Tablets.

Frequency and timing of doses
2 – 4 x daily.

Adult dosage range
Breast cancer 160mg daily.
Cancer of the uterus 40 – 320mg daily.

Onset of effect
Within 2 months.

Duration of action
1 – 2 days.

Diet advice
None.

Storage
Keep in a closed container in a cool, dry place away from reach of children.

Missed dose
Take as soon as you remember. If your next dose is due within 2 hours, take a single dose now and skip the next.

Stopping the drug
Do not stop the drug without consulting your physician. Stopping the drug may lead to worsening of your underlying condition.

Exceeding the dose
An occasional unintentional extra dose is unlikely to be a cause for concern. But if you notice unusual symptoms, or if a large overdose has been taken, notify your physician.

SPECIAL PRECAUTIONS

Be sure to tell your physician if:
▼ You have impaired liver or kidney function.
▼ You have diabetes.
▼ You have high blood pressure.
▼ You have heart problems.
▼ You are taking other medications.

 Pregnancy
▼ Not usually prescribed.

 Breast feeding
▼ Discuss with your physician. Breast feeding is usually discontinued.

 Infants and children
▼ Not usually required.

 Over 60
▼ No special problems.

 Driving and hazardous work
▼ No known problems.

 Alcohol
▼ No known problems.

POSSIBLE ADVERSE EFFECTS

Adverse effects are rare. Megestrol may cause loss of appetite, and fluid retention may lead to swollen feet and ankles, but these symptoms are not usually severe.

Symptom/effect	Frequency		Discuss with physician		Stop taking drug now	Call physician now
	Common	Rare	Only if severe	In all cases		
Swollen feet/ankles	●		■			
Loss of appetite	●		■			
Migraine headache	●			■		
Dizziness	●			■		
Rash	●			■	▲	▮
Blurred vision	●			■	▲	▮

PROLONGED USE

Long-term use of this drug may increase the risk of blood clots in the leg veins.

Monitoring Periodic checks on blood pressure may be performed.

INTERACTIONS

None.

MELPHALAN

Brand name Alkeran
Used in the following combined preparations None

GENERAL INFORMATION

Introduced in 1964, melphalan is an anticancer drug that is mainly used to treat multiple myeloma, a cancer that affects bone marrow cell production and causes bone and kidney damage. Melphalan is also prescribed to treat cancer of the ovary and breast. It is given in short courses that are usually repeated at six-week intervals.

Melphalan has a number of potentially serious adverse effects. It inter-

feres with production of blood cells, leading to anemia, reduced blood clotting, and increased susceptibility to infection. Careful monitoring of blood count is therefore necessary during treatment. Other side effects such as nausea and vomiting, sore throat, and loss of appetite are less common than those of other anticancer drugs, and they tend to diminish as treatment continues.

QUICK REFERENCE

Drug group Anticancer drug (p.182)
Overdose danger rating Medium
Dependence rating Low
Prescription needed Yes
Available as generic No

INFORMATION FOR USERS

Your drug prescription is tailored for you. Do not alter dosage without checking with your physician.

How taken

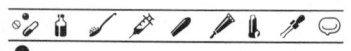

Tablets.

Frequency and timing of doses
3 x daily with food for 4 days every 6 weeks.

Adult dosage range
Dosage is determined individually according to body height, weight, and response.

Onset of effect
Some adverse effects such as nausea and vomiting may appear within hours of treatment. Full beneficial effects may not be felt for up to 4 weeks.

Duration of action
Side effects may last for several weeks after treatment is stopped.

Diet advice
None.

Storage
Keep in a closed container in a cool, dry place away from reach of children.

Missed dose
Take as soon as you remember. If your next dose is due within 6 hours, take a single dose now and skip the next. Tell your physician that you missed a dose.

Stopping the drug
Discuss with your physician. Failure to complete a course of treatment may lead to a worsening of the underlying condition.

Exceeding the dose
An occasional unintentional extra dose is unlikely to cause problems. Large overdoses may cause nausea and vomiting. Notify your physician.

SPECIAL PRECAUTIONS

Melphalan is prescribed only under close medical supervision, taking account of your present condition and medical history.

Pregnancy
▼ Not usually prescribed. May cause birth defects or premature birth. Discuss with your physician.

Breast feeding
▼ Discontinue breast feeding. The drug passes into the breast milk and may affect the baby adversely.

Infants and children
▼ Not usually prescribed.

Over 60
▼ Reduced dose may be necessary. Increased risk of adverse effects.

Driving and hazardous work
▼ No known problems.

Alcohol
▼ No known problems.

POSSIBLE ADVERSE EFFECTS

Nausea and vomiting generally occur within a few hours of taking melphalan, but these tend to diminish as your body adjusts to the

drug. Also, some people may experience a temporary loss of appetite, but this tends not to be severe.

Symptom/effect	Frequency		Discuss with physician		Stop taking drug now	Call physician now
	Common	Rare	Only if severe	In all cases		
Nausea/vomiting	●		■			
Fever	●			■		
Sore throat	●			■		
Loss of appetite		●	■			
Loss of hair		●		■		
Mouth ulcers		●		■		
Diarrhea		●		■		

INTERACTIONS

General note A number of drugs increase the adverse effects of melphalan. Because melphalan is given only under

close medical supervision, these interactions are carefully monitored and the dosage is adjusted accordingly.

PROLONGED USE

Each four-day course of treatment is followed by a recovery period of 6 weeks. Over several months there is an increased risk of damage to the blood cell-forming tissue in the bone marrow.

Monitoring Periodic checks on numbers of blood cells are carried out.

MENOTROPINS

Brand name Pergonal
Used in the following combined preparations None

GENERAL INFORMATION

Introduced in 1970 as a treatment for infertility, menotropins, also known as human menopausal gonadotropin (HMG), is a hormone preparation obtained from the urine of women who have passed the menopause. It is given under medical supervision when there is a deficiency of the hormones normally produced by the pituitary gland that stimulate ovulation (release of an egg) in women. Since these same hormones are involved in sperm production, menotropins can also be used as a treatment for some types of male infertility.

The main effect of menotropins in women is to prepare the ovary for ovulation. Ovulation itself is triggered by injection of another hormone, human chorionic gonadotropin (HCG), which is usually given 24 hours after a course of menotropins. Courses of treatment are repeated during each menstrual cycle. In men, the drug is given continuously.

Regular measurement of blood or urine levels of the female hormone estrogen are performed to monitor the dose of menotropins and prevent over-stimulation of the ovaries. Multiple pregnancy occurs in one of five pregnancies after menotropins treatment.

QUICK REFERENCE

Drug group Drug for infertility (p.192)

Overdose danger rating Medium

Dependence rating Low

Prescription needed Yes

Available as generic No

INFORMATION FOR USERS

This drug is given only under medical supervision and is not for self-administration.

How taken

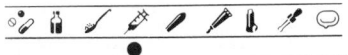

●

Injection.

Frequency and timing of doses
Women Once daily for 9 – 12 days.
Men As directed.

Dosage range
Dosage is determined according to individual response.

Onset of effect
Within a few hours.

Duration of action
48 – 72 hours.

Diet advice
None.

Storage
Not applicable. The drug is not kept in the home.

Missed dose
Contact your physician and arrange to receive the missed dose as soon as possible. Delay of more than 24 hours may reduce the chance of conception.

Stopping the drug
Complete the course of treatment as directed by your physician. Stopping the drug prematurely will reduce the chance of conception.

Exceeding the dose
The drug is always injected under close medical supervision. Overdose is extremely unlikely.

SPECIAL PRECAUTIONS

Be sure to tell your physician if:
▼ You are taking other medications.

Pregnancy
▼ Not prescribed. The drug is stopped as soon as pregnancy occurs.

Breast feeding
▼ Not prescribed.

Infants and children
▼ Not prescribed.

Over 60
▼ Not prescribed.

Driving and hazardous work
▼ No known problems.

Alcohol
▼ Keep consumption low. Alcohol does not interact directly with menotropins but taken in excess may reduce the chance of conception.

PROLONGED USE

No problems expected.

POSSIBLE ADVERSE EFFECTS

In women, abdominal pain due to enlargement of the ovaries is fairly common. If these effects occur after treatment has stopped, or if you experience dizziness, reduced frequency of urination, or breathing difficulties, notify your physician promptly.

Symptom/effect	Frequency		Discuss with physician		Stop taking drug now	Call physician now
	Common	Rare	Only if severe	In all cases		
Women						
Abdominal pain/bloating	●		■			
Weight gain	●			■		
Reduced urination		●		■		
Dizziness		●		■		
Fever		●		■		
Shortness of breath		●		■		■
Men						
Breast enlargement		●	■			

INTERACTIONS

None.

MEPERIDINE

Brand name Demerol
Used in the following combined preparations Demerol APAP, Fortis, Mepergan

GENERAL INFORMATION

Similar to morphine, meperidine is a strong *narcotic* analgesic that was introduced in 1939. It is used almost exclusively in hospitals to relieve the severe pain felt during labor, and to relieve and sedate people before an operation. It takes effect quickly but its effect lasts for a short time compared to other analgesics. This means that doses can be timed during labor to minimize adverse effects on the baby.

Meperidine is habit-forming. Both *tolerance* and dependence can develop if the drug is used inappropriately or excessively. When taken for pain relief of the appropriate conditions for brief periods of time, it is unlikely that drug dependence will occur.

QUICK REFERENCE

Drug group Narcotic analgesic (see p.108 and p.193)

Overdose danger rating High

Dependence rating High

Prescription needed Yes CII

Available as generic Yes

INFORMATION FOR USERS

Your drug prescription is tailored for you. Do not alter dosage without checking with your physician.

How taken

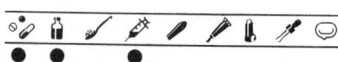

Tablets, liquid, injection.

Frequency and timing of doses
Every 3 – 4 hours as needed for pain.

Adult dosage range
50 – 150mg per dose.

Onset of effect
Within 1 hour (by mouth); within 15 minutes (by injection).

Duration of action
2 – 4 hours.

Diet advice
None.

Storage
Keep in a closed container in a cool, dry place away from reach of children. Protect from light.

Missed dose
Take only if required for pain relief.

Stopping the drug
If you have been given the drug for pain relief, it can be safely stopped as soon as you no longer need it.

OVERDOSE ACTION

 Seek immediate medical advice in all cases. Take emergency action if there are symptoms such as muscle twitching, nervousness, shallow breathing, severe drowsiness, or loss of consciousness.

See Drug poisoning emergency guide (p.590).

SPECIAL PRECAUTIONS

Be sure to tell your physician if:
▼ You have impaired kidney or liver function.
▼ You have heart problems.
▼ You have had epileptic seizures.
▼ You have a lung disorder such as asthma or bronchitis.
▼ You have a thyroid disorder.
▼ You have urinary difficulties.
▼ You are taking other medications.

 Pregnancy
▼ Not usually prescribed before the onset of labor. Safety in pregnancy not established. Meperidine is often used to relieve pain during labor, but is given with care as it may cause breathing difficulties in the newborn baby.

 Breast feeding
▼ Discuss with your physician. The drug passes into the breast milk.

 Infants and children
▼ Reduced dose necessary.

 Over 60
▼ Reduced dose may be necessary. Increased likelihood of adverse effects.

 Driving and hazardous work
▼ It is unlikely that someone requiring this drug will be engaging in these activities.

 Alcohol
▼ Avoid. Alcohol may increase the sedative effects of this drug.

POSSIBLE ADVERSE EFFECTS

Adverse effects of meperidine are common but may wear off with continued use of the drug as your body adjusts. Discuss any symptoms with your physician.

Symptom/effect	Frequency		Discuss with physician		Stop taking drug now	Call physician now
	Common	Rare	Only if severe	In all cases		
Dizziness	●		■			
Nausea/vomiting	●		■			
Drowsiness	●		■			
Constipation	●			■		
Confusion	●			■		
Shortness of breath		●		■	▲	■

INTERACTIONS

Monoamine oxidase inhibitors (MAOIs) If meperidine is taken within 14 days of MAOIs, it may cause dangerous toxic reactions.

Alcohol The sedative effect of meperidine is reinforced by alcohol.

Sedatives All drugs that have a sedative effect on the central nervous system may dangerously increase the sedative properties of meperidine.

PROLONGED USE

The effects of the drug usually become weaker during prolonged use as the body adapts. It may also be habit-forming if taken for extended periods.

MEPROBAMATE

Brand names Equanil, Miltown
Used in the following combined preparations Deprol, Equagesic, Micrainin, Milprem, Pathibamate

GENERAL INFORMATION

Introduced in the 1950s, meprobamate was first used as a muscle relaxant, but soon became popular as a short-term treatment for the symptoms associated with anxiety and stress (see Anti-anxiety drugs, p.111).

In addition to its use in anxiety, meprobamate has been combined with aspirin for the treatment of pain, anxiety, and tension that may accompany injuries and arthritic conditions affecting the muscles, bones, and joints.

Since the 1960s meprobamate has largely been replaced in the treatment of anxiety by the benzodiazepines (p. 111), which have proven to be safer and more effective.

QUICK REFERENCE

Drug group Non-benzodiazepine anti-anxiety drug (p.111)

Overdose danger rating Medium

Dependence rating Medium

Prescription needed Yes CIV

Available as generic Yes

INFORMATION FOR USERS

Your drug prescription is tailored for you. Do not alter dosage without checking with your physician.

How taken

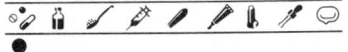

Capsules, tablets.

Frequency and timing of doses
3 – 4 x daily.

Adult dosage range
1200 – 1600mg daily.

Onset of effect
Within 1 hour.

Duration of action
8 hours.

Diet advice
None.

Storage
Keep in a closed container in a cool, dry place away from reach of children.

Missed dose
Take as soon as you remember. If your next dose is due within 2 hours, take a single dose now and skip the next.

Stopping the drug
If you have been taking the drug for less than 2 weeks, it can be safely stopped as soon as you feel you no longer need it. If you have been taking it regularly for longer than 2 weeks, sudden discontinuation may be accompanied by severe withdrawal reactions. Consult your physician, who will supervise a gradual reduction in dosage.

Exceeding the dose
An occasional unintentional extra dose is unlikely to cause problems. Large overdoses may cause unusual drowsiness. Notify your physician.

SPECIAL PRECAUTIONS

Be sure to tell your physician if:
▼ You have impaired kidney or liver function.
▼ You suffer from porphyria.
▼ You have had problems with alcohol or drug abuse.
▼ You are taking other medications.

Pregnancy
▼ Not usually prescribed. May cause defects in the unborn baby. Discuss with your physician so that you may weigh the benefits of the drug against its risks.

Breast feeding
▼ Discuss with your physician. The drug passes into the breast milk and may affect the baby adversely.

Infants and children
▼ Not usually prescribed. Reduced dose necessary.

Over 60
▼ Reduced dose may be necessary.

Driving and hazardous work
▼ Avoid such activities until you have learned how the drug affects you, because the drug can cause drowsiness.

Alcohol
▼ Avoid. Alcohol increases the sedative effects of this drug.

POSSIBLE ADVERSE EFFECTS

The main adverse effects of this drug are related to its sedative properties. Drowsiness and dizziness normally diminish after the first few days of treatment, and can often be reduced by medically supervised adjustment of dosage.

Symptom/effect	Frequency		Discuss with physician		Stop taking drug now	Call physician now
	Common	Rare	Only if severe	In all cases		
Drowsiness/dizziness	●		■			
Unusual excitement		●		■		
Rash		●		■	▲	

INTERACTIONS

Anticoagulant drugs Meprobamate may reduce the effect of anticoagulant drugs. The anticoagulant dose may need to be adjusted accordingly.

Oral contraceptives Meprobamate may reduce the effectiveness of oral contraceptives. Discuss with your physician.

Alcohol Alcohol increases the sedative effect of meprobamate, and may reduce its anti-anxiety effect.

PROLONGED USE

Regular use of this drug may lead to dependence and severe withdrawal reactions if suddenly discontinued. Courses of longer than 2 weeks are not usually recommended.

A B C D E F G H I J K L M N O P Q R S T U V W X Y Z

MERCAPTOPURINE

Brand name Purinethol
Used in the following combined preparations None

GENERAL INFORMATION

Introduced in 1953, mercaptopurine is widely used to prevent the recurrence of certain forms of leukemia; it is more effective among children than adults. Prescribed with other anticancer drugs, it is also given to leukemia victims who have not responded well to other treatment.

Recent research indicates that mercaptopurine may be effective in treating cancer of the lymph nodes in children and valuable as an immuno-suppressant drug (p. 184) in certain inflammatory diseases of the intestine.

Nausea and vomiting, mouth ulcers, and loss of appetite are the most common side effects of mercaptopurine. Such symptoms tend to be milder than those of other cytotoxic drugs, and they often disappear as the body adjusts to the drug. More seriously, mercaptopurine can cause liver damage and interfere with the production of blood cells, causing blood-clotting disorders and anemia. Also, there is an increased likelihood of infections.

QUICK REFERENCE

Drug group Anticancer drug (p.182)
Overdose danger rating Medium
Dependence rating Low
Prescription needed Yes
Available as generic No

INFORMATION FOR USERS

Your drug prescription is tailored for you. Do not alter dosage without checking with your physician.

How taken

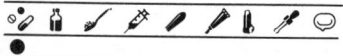

Tablets.

Frequency and timing of doses
Once daily.

Dosage range
Dosage is determined individually according to body weight and response.

Onset of effect
1 – 2 weeks.

Duration of action
Side effects may persist for several weeks after treatment is stopped.

Diet advice
None.

Storage
Keep in a closed container in a cool, dry place away from reach of children.

Missed dose
If your next dose is due within 6 hours, take a single dose now and skip the next. Tell your physician that you missed a dose.

Stopping the drug
Do not stop taking the drug without consulting your physician; stopping the drug may lead to worsening of your underlying condition.

Exceeding the dose
An occasional unintentional extra dose is unlikely to cause problems. Large overdoses may cause nausea and vomiting. Notify your physician.

SPECIAL PRECAUTIONS

Be sure to tell your physician if:
▼ You have impaired liver or kidney function.
▼ You suffer from gout.
▼ You have recently had chicken pox or a herpes infection.
▼ You are taking other medications.

Pregnancy
▼ Not usually prescribed. May cause miscarriage. Discuss with your physician so that you may weigh the benefits of the drug against its risks.

Breast feeding
▼ Discontinue breast feeding. The drug passes into the breast milk and may affect the baby adversely.

Infants and children
▼ Not recommended for children under 5 years. Increased risk of liver damage or jaundice in older children.

Over 60
▼ Reduced dose may be necessary. Increased risk of adverse effects.

Driving and hazardous work
▼ No known problems.

Alcohol
▼ Avoid. Alcohol may increase the adverse effects of this drug.

POSSIBLE ADVERSE EFFECTS

The most common adverse effects with mercaptopurine are nausea, vomiting, and loss of appetite. Jaundice is also a common side effect, which is reversible on stopping the drug. Because mercaptopurine interferes with the production of blood cells, anemia, blood-clotting disorders, and infections are more likely.

Symptom/effect	Frequency		Discuss with physician		Stop taking drug now	Call physician now
	Common	Rare	Only if severe	In all cases		
Nausea/vomiting	●		■			
Loss of appetite	●		■			
Mouth ulcers	●			■		▮
Jaundice		●		■		
Black bowel movements		●		■		▮
Bloodstained vomit		●		■		▮

INTERACTIONS

Allopurinol This drug increases blood levels of mercaptopurine, so the dose of mercaptopurine has to be reduced considerably.

PROLONGED USE

Prolonged use of this drug may reduce bone marrow activity, leading to reduced production of blood cells.

Monitoring Periodic blood checks are required.

METAPROTERENOL

Brand names Alupent, Metaprel
Used in the following combined preparations None

GENERAL INFORMATION

Metaproterenol, introduced in 1973, is a *sympathomimetic* bronchodilator that acts selectively to dilate the airways in the lungs while having little stimulant effect on the heart.

Used in the prevention and treatment of attacks of bronchospasm occurring in asthma, bronchitis, and emphysema, it is generally given by aerosol inhaler or nebulizer, and sometimes by mouth.

Anxiety and restlessness may occur, as with all other sympathomimetics. Fine tremor of the hands is common, although it may be controlled by reducing the dose. Heart palpitations as well as tolerance to its beneficial effects occur less often with metaproterenol than with similar drugs.

INFORMATION FOR USERS

Your drug prescription is tailored for you. Do not alter dosage without checking with your physician.

How taken

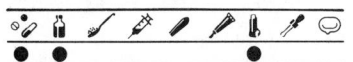

Tablets, liquid, inhaler, nebulizer.

Frequency and timing of doses
3 – 4 x daily (tablets, liquid); every 4 – 6 hours (inhaler, nebulizer).

Adult dosage range
60 – 80mg daily (tablets); 1.3mg (2 puffs) per dose (inhaler); according to instructions depending on preparation and equipment (nebulizer).

Onset of effect
Within 15 minutes (inhaler, nebulizer); within 30 – 60 minutes (tablets).

Duration of action
Up to 4 hours.

Diet advice
None.

Storage
Keep in a closed container in a cool, dry place away from reach of children. Protect from light. Do not puncture or burn aerosol container.

Missed dose
Do not take the missed dose. Take your next dose as usual.

Stopping the drug
People with mild or infrequent attacks should take metaproterenol as needed. If you have severe asthma, do not stop your treatment without consulting your physician.

Exceeding the dose
An occasional unintentional extra dose is unlikely to be a cause for concern. But if you notice any unusual symptoms, or if a large overdose has been taken, notify your physician.

SPECIAL PRECAUTIONS

Be sure to tell your physician if:
▼ You have heart problems.
▼ You have high blood pressure.
▼ You have an overactive thyroid.
▼ You have diabetes.
▼ You have urinary difficulties.
▼ You are taking other medications.

Pregnancy
▼ Not usually prescribed, especially during the first 3 months. Safety in pregnancy not established. Taken near the time of delivery, the drug may delay labor.

Breast feeding
▼ Discuss with your physician. Effect on breast feeding unknown.

Infants and children
▼ Not usually prescribed for inhalation under the age of 12 years. Reduced dose necessary.

Over 60
▼ Reduced dose may be necessary. Increased likelihood of adverse effects.

Driving and hazardous work
▼ Avoid such activities until you have learned how the drug affects you, because it can cause trembling.

Alcohol
▼ No special problems.

POSSIBLE ADVERSE EFFECTS

Muscle tremor, anxiety, and restlessness are the most common adverse effects.

Palpitations and headache due to stimulation of the heart are rare.

Symptom/effect	Frequency		Discuss with physician		Stop taking drug now	Call physician now
	Common	Rare	Only if severe	In all cases		
Nausea	●		■			
Tremor	●		■			
Anxiety/restlessness	●		■			
Headache		●	■			
Bad taste in mouth		●	■			
Palpitations		●		■		

PROLONGED USE

Prolonged use may result in tolerance to the effects of metaproterenol. However, failure to respond can also be a sign of worsening asthma, requiring urgent medical treatment.

INTERACTIONS

Beta blockers may inhibit the effect of metaproterenol and vice versa.

Other sympathomimetic drugs, such as those listed on p.120, may increase the effects of metaproterenol, thus increasing the risk of adverse effects.

Monoamine oxidase inhibitors (MAOIs) can interact with metaproterenol to produce a dangerous rise in blood pressure. Allow 14 days after last MAOI dose before taking metaproterenol.

METHIMAZOLE

Brand name Tapazole
Used in the following combined preparations None

GENERAL INFORMATION

Methimazole, introduced in 1951, is an antithyroid drug; it is used to suppress the creation of thyroid hormones in people with an overactive thyroid gland (thyrotoxicosis). In some people, particularly those with Graves' disease (the most common form of thyrotoxicosis), drug treatment alone may relieve the disorder.

Methimazole is also used in more serious cases to restore the normal function of the thyroid before its partial removal by surgery, to intensify its absorption of radioactive iodine when that cell-destroying drug is used, or to prevent a harmful release of hormones that sometimes follows the use of radioactive iodine.

Because the full benefits of this medicine are not felt for several weeks, beta blockers may be given during this period for control of symptoms.

Longer-acting than many similar drugs, methimazole may be effective in single daily doses for some people, making it convenient for prolonged use. Methimazole may occasionally reduce the bone marrow's production of white blood cells, creating an increased risk of infection.

QUICK REFERENCE

Drug group Antithyroid drug (p.172)
Overdose danger rating Medium
Dependence rating Low
Prescription needed Yes
Available as generic No

INFORMATION FOR USERS

Your drug prescription is tailored for you. Do not alter dosage without checking with your physician.

How taken

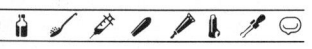

Tablets.

Frequency and timing of doses
Every 6 – 8 hours (initial treatment); 1 – 3 x daily (maintenance treatment); may be given every 4 hours for thyrotoxic crisis.

Dosage range
Adults 15 – 60mg daily (initial dose); 10 – 30mg daily (maintenance dose); 60 – 120mg daily (thyrotoxic crisis).

Onset of effect
10 – 20 days. Full beneficial effects may not be felt for 6 – 10 weeks.

Duration of action
12 – 24 hours.

Diet advice
Your physician may advise you to avoid foods that are high in iodine (see p.538).

Storage
Keep in a closed container in a cool, dry place away from reach of children.

Missed dose
Take as soon as you remember. If your next dose is due, take the missed dose and the next scheduled dose together.

Stopping the drug
Do not stop the drug without consulting your physician; stopping the drug may lead to worsening of your underlying condition.

Exceeding the dose
An occasional unintentional extra dose is unlikely to cause problems. Large overdoses may cause nausea, vomiting, and headache. Notify your physician.

POSSIBLE ADVERSE EFFECTS

Serious side effects are rare. Skin rashes, itching, and nausea are fairly common, although itching may sometimes be caused by overactivity of the thyroid. Sore throat or fever may indicate reduced white blood cell production.

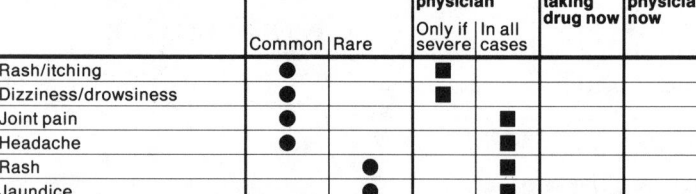

Symptom/effect	Frequency		Discuss with physician		Stop taking drug now	Call physician now
	Common	Rare	Only if severe	In all cases		
Rash/itching	●		■			
Dizziness/drowsiness	●		■			
Joint pain	●			■		
Headache	●			■		
Rash		●		■		
Jaundice		●		■		
Sore throat/fever		●		■		

INTERACTIONS

Anticoagulant drugs Methimazole may enhance the effects of these drugs. The dosage of anticoagulant drugs may need to be adjusted.

SPECIAL PRECAUTIONS

Be sure to tell your physician if:
▼ You have impaired liver or kidney function.
▼ You are taking other medications.

Pregnancy
▼ Not usually prescribed. May cause goiter and thyroid hormone deficiency (hypothyroidism) in the newborn infant. Discuss with your physician so that you may weigh the benefits of the drug against its risks.

Breast feeding
▼ The drug passes into the breast milk, but at normal doses adverse effects on the baby are uncommon. Discuss with your physician.

Infants and children
▼ Reduced dose necessary.

Over 60
▼ No special problems.

Driving and hazardous work
▼ Avoid such activities until you have learned how the drug affects you, because the drug may cause dizziness and drowsiness.

Alcohol
▼ No known problems.

PROLONGED USE

High doses of methimazole over a prolonged period may reduce the body's production of white blood cells.

Monitoring Periodic tests of thyroid function are usually required, and blood cell counts may also be carried out.

METHOCARBAMOL

Brand names Delaxin, Marbaxin-750, Robaxin
Used in the following combined preparation Robaxisal

GENERAL INFORMATION

Methocarbamol, introduced in 1957, acts on nerve cells in the central nervous system to relieve muscle spasm, rigidity, and pain arising from muscle injury. Because the drug does not help the underlying damage, treatment usually includes rest and physical therapy. Methocarbamol is also sometimes injected to relieve the symptoms of tetanus. Muscle spasm from other serious causes, such as disease of or injury to the spinal cord, or multiple sclerosis, rarely responds effectively to treatment by methocarbamol.

Drowsiness is the most common adverse effect, but there is also a slight risk of liver damage.

INFORMATION FOR USERS

Your drug prescription is tailored for you. Do not alter dosage without checking with your physician.

How taken

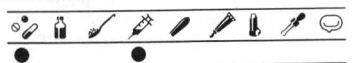

Tablets, injection.

Frequency and timing of doses
4 x daily.

Adult dosage range
6 – 8g daily for 2 – 3 days, then 4g daily.

Onset of effect
Within 30 minutes.

Duration of action
Up to 8 hours.

Diet advice
None.

Storage
Keep in a closed container in a cool, dry place away from reach of children.

Missed dose
Take as soon as you remember. If your next dose is due within 2 hours, take a single dose now and skip the next.

Stopping the drug
If you have been taking the drug for less than 6 weeks, it can be safely stopped as soon as you feel that you no longer need it. However, if you have been taking the drug for longer, consult your physician.

Exceeding the dose
An occasional unintentional extra dose is unlikely to cause problems. Large over-doses may cause severe drowsiness and muscle weakness. Notify your physician.

SPECIAL PRECAUTIONS

Be sure to tell your physician if:
▼ You have impaired liver or kidney function.
▼ You have had epileptic seizures.
▼ You have a history of allergies.
▼ You are taking other medications.

Pregnancy
▼ Not usually prescribed. Safety in pregnancy not established. Discuss with your physician so that you can weigh the benefits of the drug against its possible risks.

Breast feeding
▼ Discuss with your physician. The drug passes into the breast milk and may affect the baby adversely.

Infants and children
▼ Not recommended.

Over 60
▼ Reduced dose may be necessary. Increased likelihood of adverse effects.

Driving and hazardous work
▼ Avoid such activities until you have learned how the drug affects you, because the drug can cause drowsiness.

Alcohol
▼ Avoid. Alcohol may increase the sedative effects of this drug.

Surgery and general anesthetics
▼ Methocarbamol may need to be stopped before you have a general anesthetic. Discuss this with your physician or dentist before any surgery.

POSSIBLE ADVERSE EFFECTS

The most common adverse effects of methocarbamol are due to the drug's action on the central nervous system. These usually diminish as your body adjusts to the drug, and they disappear when treatment with methocarbamol is stopped.

Symptom/effect	Frequency		Discuss with physician		Stop taking drug now	Call physician now
	Common	Rare	Only if severe	In all cases		
Drowsiness	●			■		
Dizziness	●			■		
Nausea		●		■		
Headache		●		■		
Loss of appetite		●		■		
Flushing		●		■		
Metallic taste		●		■		
Rash		●			■	

INTERACTIONS

Sedatives All drugs that have a sedative effect on the central nervous system are likely to increase the sedative properties of methocarbamol. Such drugs include anti-anxiety and sleeping drugs, antihistamines, antidepressants, narcotic analgesics, and antipsychotic drugs.

PROLONGED USE

There is a slight risk of liver damage during long-term treatment.

Monitoring Periodic blood tests to check liver function are usually required.

METHOTREXATE

Brand names Folex, Mexate, Mexate AQ
Used in the following combined preparations None

GENERAL INFORMATION

Methotrexate, introduced in 1955, is effective against a wide range of cancers. Used with other anticancer drugs, it is particularly effective against a certain cancer of the uterus (choriocarcinoma), certain forms of leukemia (cancer of the blood), and lymph node cancer (lymphoma).

This drug is also sometimes given to treat cancer of the testicle, ovary, breast, neck, bone, bladder, and lung. In addition, methotrexate is prescribed cautiously for people with severe psoriasis. It may also be used for rheumatoid arthritis that has not responded to other treatment.

As with other anticancer drugs, methotrexate affects healthy as well as cancerous cells, creating a number of side effects. Nausea and vomiting, diarrhea, and mouth ulcers are common.

The drug may also increase the risk of anemia and disorders of blood clotting. There may also be an increased susceptibility to infection.

INFORMATION FOR USERS

Your drug prescription is tailored for you. Do not alter dosage without checking with your physician.

How taken

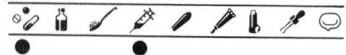

Tablets, injection.

Frequency and timing of doses
Once daily (tablets); 2 x daily (injection).

Adult dosage range
Dosage is determined individually according to body weight and response.

Onset of effect
Some effects such as nausea and vomiting may appear within hours of starting drug treatment. Full beneficial effects may not be felt for up to 6 weeks.

Duration of action
Adverse effects may last for several weeks after stopping treatment.

Diet advice
Drink at least 2 quarts of water daily.

Storage
Keep in a closed container in a cool, dry place away from reach of children.

Missed dose
Take as soon as you remember. If your next dose is due within 6 hours, take a single dose now and skip the next. Tell your physician that you missed a dose.

Stopping the drug
Do not stop taking the drug without consulting your physician; stopping the drug may lead to worsening of the underlying condition.

OVERDOSE ACTION

 Seek immediate medical advice in all cases.

See Drug poisoning emergency guide (p.590).

SPECIAL PRECAUTIONS

Methotrexate is prescribed only under close medical supervision, taking account of your present condition and medical history.

 Pregnancy
▼ Not usually prescribed. Methotrexate may cause birth defects or premature birth. Discuss with your physician so that you may weigh the benefits of the drug against its risks.

 Breast feeding
▼ Discontinue breast feeding. The drug passes into the breast milk and may affect the baby adversely.

 Infants and children
▼ Not usually prescribed.

 Over 60
▼ Reduced dose may be necessary. Increased risk of adverse effects.

 Driving and hazardous work
▼ No special problems.

 Alcohol
▼ Avoid. Alcohol may increase the adverse effects of this drug.

POSSIBLE ADVERSE EFFECTS

Nausea and vomiting generally occur within a few hours of taking methotrexate.

Diarrhea and mouth ulcers are also common side effects of methotrexate.

Symptom/effect	Frequency		Discuss with physician		Stop taking drug now	Call physician now
	Common	Rare	Only if severe	In all cases		
Nausea/vomiting	●		■			
Diarrhea	●		■			
Mouth ulcers	●			■		
Wheezing		●		■		
Hair loss		●		■		
Rash		●		■	▲	
Jaundice		●		■	▲	∎

PROLONGED USE

Prolonged use of this drug may lead to an increased risk of damage to the liver, kidneys, and bone marrow.

Monitoring Periodic checks on liver and kidney function are required.

INTERACTIONS

General note A number of drugs increase the adverse effects of methotrexate. Because methotrexate is given only under close medical supervision, these interactions are carefully monitored and the dosage is adjusted accordingly.

METHOXSALEN

Brand name Oxsoralen
Used in the following combined preparations None

GENERAL INFORMATION

Methoxsalen, introduced in 1953, belongs to a group of substances called psoralens. These occur naturally in plants and have been used historically to correct vitiligo, a condition in which patches of skin lose their color, or pigmentation. Nowadays, methoxsalen is more often given for severe psoriasis that has failed to improve with other treatments.

Used in conjunction with ultraviolet light treatment (UVA), it stimulates the production of skin pigment and, in psoriasis, halts the accelerated growth of skin cells. Methoxsalen lotion is used for small areas of vitiligo, while capsules are given for widespread depigmentation and severe psoriasis.

The pigment-promoting effect of methoxsalen has led to its inclusion in some countries in preparations for the promotion of suntanning. This use is prohibited in the United States because of the risk of burns. After taking methoxsalen, a person should limit his or her exposure to sunlight; sunglasses and sun-screening lipstick are recommended for 48 hours.

QUICK REFERENCE

Drug group Psoriasis drug (p.206)
Overdose danger rating Medium
Dependence rating Low
Prescription needed Yes
Available as generic No

INFORMATION FOR USERS

This drug is given only under medical supervision and is not for self-administration.

How taken

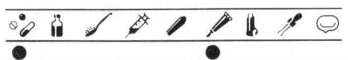

Capsules, lotion.

Frequency and timing of doses
By mouth 2 – 3 x weekly 2½ hours before UVA treatment.
Lotion Once weekly or every 3 – 5 days, 30 – 45 minutes before UVA treatment.

Dosage range
By mouth 20 – 40mg per dose depending on skin color (vitiligo); according to body weight (psoriasis).
Lotion Applied to the affected area under medical supervision.

Onset of effect
Within 1 hour (by mouth); within 15 minutes (lotion). Full beneficial effects may not be seen for 10 weeks (psoriasis) or 6 months (vitiligo).

Duration of action
Sensitivity of the skin to sunlight is increased for 24 – 48 hours after drug is taken.

Diet advice
Certain foods, such as limes, figs, parsley, parsnips, mustard, carrots, and celery may increase the sensitivity of the skin to light with methoxsalen.

Storage
Not applicable. The drug is not kept in the home.

Missed dose
No cause for concern. Attend your next scheduled treatment as usual.

Stopping the drug
Can be safely stopped as soon as you no longer need it.

Exceeding the dose
Overdose is unlikely, since treatment is carried out under medical supervision.

SPECIAL PRECAUTIONS

Be sure to tell your physician if:
▼ You have impaired liver function.
▼ You are regularly exposed to intense sunlight, X-rays, or industrial or laboratory chemicals.
▼ You have porphyria or systemic lupus erythematosus.
▼ You have had skin cancer.
▼ You have recently received anticancer drugs or radiation therapy.
▼ You are taking other medications.

 Pregnancy
▼ Not usually prescribed. Safety in pregnancy not established. Discuss with your physician so that you can weigh the benefits of the drug against its possible risks.

 Breast feeding
▼ Discuss with your physician. The effects of this drug during breast feeding are not established.

 Infants and children
▼ Not recommended for children under 12 years.

 Over 60
▼ No special problems.

 Driving and hazardous work
▼ No known problems.

 Alcohol
▼ No known problems.

POSSIBLE ADVERSE EFFECTS

Slight redness of the skin normally occurs for a day or two after treatment. High doses of methoxsalen or overexposure to ultraviolet light may cause severe redness, soreness, blistering, or peeling of the skin and swelling of the feet or lower legs.

Symptom/effect	Frequency		Discuss with physician		Stop taking drug now	Call physician now
	Common	Rare	Only if severe	In all cases		
Redness/soreness	●				■	
Nausea		●	■			
Dizziness/headache		●	■			
Depression/insomnia		●	■			
Blistering/peeling		●			■	
Swollen feet/ankles		●			■	

INTERACTIONS

General note Any drug that increases the sensitivity of the skin to light may increase the risk of redness, blistering, and peeling. Such drugs include griseofulvin, coal tar, thiazide diuretics, phenothiazines, sulfonamides, and tetracyclines.

PROLONGED USE

Prolonged use may increase the risk of premature aging of the skin and skin cancer in fair-skinned people, and cataracts are a risk of ultraviolet light treatment.

A B C D E F G H I J K L M N O P Q R S T U V W X Y Z

METHYLCELLULOSE

Brand name Cologel
Used in the following combined preparation Murocel

GENERAL INFORMATION

Methylcellulose, introduced in 1947, is a laxative commonly used to treat constipation, diverticular disease, and irritable bowel syndrome. Taken by mouth, it is not absorbed into the bloodstream but remains in the gastro-intestinal tract. It absorbs up to 25 times its volume of water, thereby softening and increasing the volume of stools. It is also used to reduce the frequency and increase the firmness of stools in chronic watery diarrhea, and to control the consistency of bowel movements after colostomies and ileostomies.

Believed in the past to assist weight loss by swelling the stomach to produce a feeling of fullness, it is now generally regarded as ineffective for this purpose. Although it fills the stomach, it does not stop hunger pangs or reduce food intake.

Artificial tear preparations of methyl-cellulose that include an antiseptic/preservative are used as eye drops to relieve discomfort and dryness caused by wind, sun, and other irritants. It is also found in contact lens irrigation solutions and in a variety of lotions, creams, ointments, and pastes.

QUICK REFERENCE

Drug group Laxative (p.139), antidiarrheal drug (p.138), and artificial tear preparation (p.198)

Overdose danger rating Low

Dependence rating Low

Prescription needed No

Available as generic Yes

INFORMATION FOR USERS

Follow instructions on the label. Call your physician if symptoms worsen.

How taken

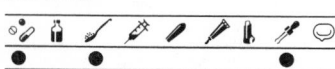

Capsules, powder, eye drops.

Frequency and timing of doses
By mouth 3 x daily (first day), then 1 – 2 x daily with water, preferably after meals.
Eye drops As required.

Dosage range
Adults 4 – 6g daily.
Children over 6 years 1 – 1.5g daily.

Onset of effect
1 – 3 days.

Duration of action
5 – 7 days.

Diet advice
If taken as a laxative, drink plenty of fluid, at least 6 – 8 glasses daily.

Storage
Keep in a closed container in a cool, dry place away from reach of children.

Missed dose
Take as soon as you remember. Resume normal dosing thereafter.

Stopping the drug
Can be safely stopped as soon as you no longer need it.

Exceeding the dose
An occasional unintentional extra dose is unlikely to be a cause for concern. But if you notice unusual symptoms, or if a large over-dose has been taken, notify your physician.

SPECIAL PRECAUTIONS

Be sure to consult your physician before taking this drug if:
▼ You have severe constipation and/or abdominal pain.
▼ You have unexplained rectal bleeding.
▼ You have difficulty swallowing.
▼ You vomit readily.
▼ You are taking other medications.

Pregnancy
▼ No evidence of risk to developing baby.

Breast feeding
▼ No evidence of risk.

Infants and children
▼ Not recommended as a laxative or antidiarrheal drug for children under 6 years. Reduced dose necessary for older children.

Over 60
▼ No special problems.

Driving and hazardous work
▼ No known problems.

Alcohol
▼ No known problems.

POSSIBLE ADVERSE EFFECTS

There are no adverse effects of eye drops. When taken by mouth, methylcellulose may cause bloating and excess gas. Insufficient fluid intake may rarely cause blockage of the esophagus (gullet) or intestine. Consult your physician if you experience severe abdominal pain or if you have no bowel movement for 2 days after taking methylcellulose.

Symptom/effect	Frequency		Discuss with physician		Stop taking drug now	Call physician now
	Common	Rare	Only if severe	In all cases		
Abdominal distension		●	■			
Flatulence		●	■			
Abdominal pain		●		■		
Difficulty in swallowing		●		■		

PROLONGED USE

No problems expected.

INTERACTIONS

General note Methylcellulose may reduce the absorption of oral anticoag-ulants, digitalis drugs, salicylates, and nitrofurantoin. Spacing of doses may be recommended.

METHYLDOPA

Brand name Aldomet
Used in the following combined preparations Aldoclor, Aldoril

A
B
C
D
E
F
G
H
I
J
K
L
M
N
O
P
Q
R
S
T
U
V
W
X
Y
Z

GENERAL INFORMATION

Methyldopa, introduced in the 1960s, is one of the most well known and widely used antihypertensive drugs. People take this drug to deal with varying degrees of high blood pressure. A diuretic is usually prescribed along with methyldopa in order to enhance its effect and to reduce fluid retention. Other antihypertensive drugs, such as hydralazine, and beta blockers (p.125) are also often prescribed to lower blood pressure more effectively.

Women with high blood pressure during late pregnancy often take methyldopa, as it will not affect the unborn child.

The most common adverse effect of methyldopa is that it often causes drowsiness, and sometimes depression. Methyldopa does not add to the fall in blood pressure that occurs on standing, so there is less likelihood of dizziness. Also, because this drug does not reduce blood flow to the kidneys, it is particularly useful for people with kidney disorders.

QUICK REFERENCE

Drug group Antihypertensive drug (p.130)

Overdose danger rating Medium

Dependence rating Low

Prescription needed Yes

Available as generic Yes

INFORMATION FOR USERS

Your drug prescription is tailored for you. Do not alter dosage without checking with your physician.

How taken

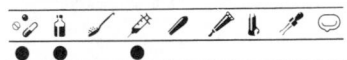

Tablets, liquid, injection.

Frequency and timing of doses
3 – 4 x daily.

Dosage range
Adults 750mg – 2g daily.
Children Reduced dose necessary according to age and weight.

Onset of effect
3 – 6 hours. Full effect begins after 2 – 3 days.

Duration of action
6 – 12 hours. Some effect may last for 1 – 2 days after stopping the drug.

Diet advice
None.

Storage
Keep in a closed container in a cool, dry place away from reach of children.

Missed dose
Take as soon as you remember. If your next dose is due within 2 hours, take a single dose now and skip the next.

Stopping the drug
Do not stop the drug without consulting your physician, who will gradually reduce your dose. Suddenly stopping methyldopa may lead to an increase in blood pressure.

Exceeding the dose
An occasional unintentional extra dose is unlikely to cause problems. Large overdoses may cause drowsiness or palpitations. Notify your physician.

SPECIAL PRECAUTIONS

Be sure to tell your physician if:
▼ You have impaired liver function.
▼ You have anemia.
▼ You have angina.
▼ You suffer from depression.
▼ You are taking other medications.

 Pregnancy
▼ Effects on the developing baby are uncertain. It is taken during late pregnancy to treat high blood pressure with no serious effects on the baby.

 Breast feeding
▼ The drug passes into the breast milk, but at normal doses adverse effects on the baby are uncommon. Discuss with your physician.

 Infants and children
▼ Reduced dose necessary.

 Over 60
▼ No special problems.

 Driving and hazardous work
▼ Avoid such activities until you have learned how the drug affects you, because the drug can cause drowsiness.

 Alcohol
▼ Avoid. Alcohol may increase the sedative effects of this drug.

Surgery and general anesthetics
▼ Discuss the possibility of stopping methyldopa with your physician or dentist before any surgery.

POSSIBLE ADVERSE EFFECTS

Most adverse effects are uncommon and diminish in time. The fluid retention that occurs during treatment with methyldopa is counteracted by taking a diuretic.

Symptom/effect	Frequency		Discuss with physician		Stop taking drug now	Call physician now
	Common	Rare	Only if severe	In all cases		
Drowsiness	●		■			
Depression	●			■		
Fever	●			■		
Stuffy nose		●		■		
Dizziness/fainting		●		■		
Nausea/vomiting		●		■		
Rash		●		■	▲	
Jaundice		●		■	▲	■

INTERACTIONS

Monoamine oxidase inhibitors (MAOIs) may lead to serious adverse effects when taken with methyldopa.

Tricyclic antidepressants may reduce the effect of methyldopa.

Levodopa Methyldopa reduces its antiparkinsonism effect and may not be able to reduce blood pressure as effectively.

Phenothiazines may make methyldopa reduce blood pressure less effectively.

PROLONGED USE

Liver and blood problems may occur in rare cases.

Monitoring Periodic checks on blood and urine are usually required.

METHYLPREDNISOLONE

Brand names Depo-Medrol, Medrol, Medrol Enpak, Solu-Medrol
Used in the following combined preparations None

GENERAL INFORMATION

Methylprednisolone, introduced in 1957, is a synthetic corticosteroid drug derived from prednisolone. It is prescribed as an ointment to relieve skin conditions such as dermatitis, eczema, and psoriasis. Given as an enema, it provides relief of inflammatory bowel disease (p.140). Methylprednisolone can be injected into joints to relieve rheumatoid arthritis and other types of joint inflammation (see p.146). It is also prescribed by mouth to replace hormones in pituitary or adrenal gland disorders that reduce the body's natural corticosteroid production. Occasionally, methylprednisolone tablets are given for the long-term control of severe asthma.

Side effects are rare when the drug is administered short-term. However, long-term treatment by mouth can cause adverse effects such as fluid retention, indigestion, fragile bones, and muscle weakness. It may induce diabetes.

INFORMATION FOR USERS

Your drug prescription is tailored for you. Do not alter dosage without checking with your physician.

How taken

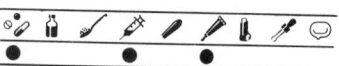

Tablets, injection, enema, ointment.

Frequency and timing of doses
1 – 2 x daily or alternate days (by mouth); 1 – 4 x daily (ointment).

Dosage range
Considerable variation. Follow the instructions given.

Onset of effect
2 – 4 days.

Duration of action
12 – 36 hours.

Diet advice
A low-sodium, high-potassium diet is recommended when the oral or injectable form of the drug is prescribed for extended periods. Follow the advice of your physician.

Storage
Keep in a closed container in a cool, dry place away from reach of children.

Missed dose
Take tablets or apply ointment as soon as you remember. If your next dose is due within 6 hours, take a single dose now and skip the next.

Stopping the drug
Do not stop tablets without consulting your physician, who may supervise a gradual reduction in dosage. Abrupt cessation may cause adrenal collapse.

Exceeding the dose
An occasional unintentional extra dose is unlikely to be a cause for concern. But if you notice unusual symptoms, or if a large overdose has been taken, notify your physician.

SPECIAL PRECAUTIONS

Be sure to tell your physician if:
▼ You have had glaucoma.
▼ You have high blood pressure.
▼ You have diabetes.
▼ You have had a peptic ulcer.
▼ You have suffered from depression.
▼ You have a herpes infection.
▼ You are taking other medications.

Pregnancy
▼ No evidence of risk with ointment or joint injections. Prescribed in tablet form in low doses, harm to baby is unlikely. Discuss with your physician so that you may weigh the benefits of the drug against its possible risks.

Breast feeding
▼ No evidence of risk with ointment or joint injections. Taken regularly by mouth, the drug may adversely affect the baby's growth. Discuss with your physician.

Infants and children
▼ Reduced dose necessary.

Over 60
▼ Reduced dose may be necessary.

Driving and hazardous work
▼ No known problems.

Alcohol
▼ Alcohol may increase the risk of peptic ulcers with methylprednisolone tablets. No special problems with other dosage forms.

POSSIBLE ADVERSE EFFECTS

The rare, but more serious, adverse effects occur only when methylprednisolone is taken by mouth in high doses or for long periods of time.

Symptom/effect	Frequency		Discuss with physician		Stop taking drug now	Call physician now
	Common	Rare	Only if severe	In all cases		
Indigestion/weight gain	●		■			
Muscle weakness		●		■		
Mood changes		●		■		
Seizures		●		■	▲	▮
Black/bloody stools		●		■	▲	▮

INTERACTIONS

Digoxin Methylprednisolone may increase the risk of adverse effects from digoxin.

Oral anticoagulant drugs Methylprednisolone increases blood clotting.

Vaccines Serious reactions can occur when vaccinations are given with methylprednisolone. Discuss with your physician.

Insulin and antidiabetic drugs Methylprednisolone by mouth or injection reduces the actions of these drugs.

Antihypertensive drugs Methylprednisolone by mouth or injection may reduce the effect of antihypertensive drugs.

PROLONGED USE

Prolonged use of methylprednisolone by mouth can lead to serious adverse effects, such as diabetes, glaucoma, muscle weakness, cataracts, and fragile bones. The drug may retard growth in children.

METHYSERGIDE

Brand name Sansert
Used in the following combined preparations None

GENERAL INFORMATION

Methysergide, introduced in 1962, is used in the prevention of migraine and cluster headaches. It is one of the most effective treatments for the prevention of migraine, abolishing attacks in 25 percent of people and markedly reducing their frequency in a further 50 percent. It is usually reserved for those with severe, recurrent attacks that have failed to respond to other treatments, since prolonged use may cause rare but serious adverse effects (see below). Episodic cluster headaches may be treated initially with a short course of methysergide.

Minor adverse effects include dizziness, drowsiness, nausea, and diarrhea, and usually disappear as treatment continues. Long-term use may occasionally lead to abnormal growth of fibrous tissue in the lungs, chest, urinary tract or blood vessels, causing chest pain, loin pain and urinary difficulties; reduced blood supply to the limbs can lead to leg cramps and cold fingers and toes. Frequent checks are therefore necessary.

INFORMATION FOR USERS

Your drug prescription is tailored for you. Do not alter dosage without checking with your physician.

How taken

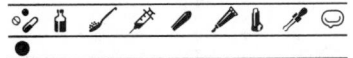

Tablets.

Frequency and timing of doses
2 – 4 x daily with meals.

Adult dosage range
Prevention of migraine 2mg daily (starting dose), increased to 6mg daily (maintenance dose).
Prevention of cluster headaches 2mg daily (starting dose), increased to 8mg daily (maintenance dose).

Onset of effect
1 – 2 days.

Duration of action
1 – 2 days.

Diet advice
None.

Storage
Keep in a closed container in a cool, dry place away from reach of children.

Missed dose
Do not take the missed dose. Take your next dose as usual.

Stopping the drug
Do not stop taking the drug without consulting your physician, who may supervise a gradual reduction in dosage. Abrupt withdrawal may cause rebound headache.

Exceeding the dose
An occasional unintentional extra dose is unlikely to cause problems. Large over-doses may cause nausea, vomiting, abdominal pain, diarrhea, and incoordination. Notify your physician.

SPECIAL PRECAUTIONS

Be sure to tell your physician if:
▼ You have impaired liver or kidney function.
▼ You have heart or circulation problems.
▼ You have high blood pressure.
▼ You have rheumatoid arthritis.
▼ You are taking other medications.

Pregnancy
▼ Not usually prescribed. Safety in pregnancy not established. Discuss with your physician so that you can weigh the benefits of the drug against its possible risks.

Breast feeding
▼ Discuss with your physician. The drug passes into the breast milk and may cause vomiting, diarrhea, and seizures in the baby.

Infants and children
▼ Not recommended.

Over 60
▼ Not usually prescribed. Increased likelihood of adverse effects.

Driving and hazardous work
▼ Avoid such activities until you have learned how the drug affects you, because the drug can cause dizziness, lightheadedness, and drowsiness.

Alcohol
▼ No known problems.

POSSIBLE ADVERSE EFFECTS

Dizziness, drowsiness, nausea, vomiting, abdominal pain, and diarrhea are common and may diminish with time. Cold, numb or tingling fingers or toes, chest pain, leg cramps, and pain on urination should be reported without delay.

Symptom/effect	Frequency		Discuss with physician		Stop taking drug now	Call physician now
	Common	Rare	Only if severe	In all cases		
Nausea/vomiting/diarrhea	●		■			
Dizziness/drowsiness	●		■			
Insomnia/nightmares	●			■		
Cold/numb fingers/toes		●		■		▮
Leg/groin pain		●		■	▲	▮
Difficult/painful urination		●		■	▲	▮
Chest pain		●		■	▲	▮

INTERACTIONS

Tobacco smoking Heavy smoking may reduce blood flow to the limbs and increase the risk of leg cramps, cold or numb hands and feet, and swollen hands or ankles when methysergide is used.

PROLONGED USE

There is an increased risk of abnormal changes in the heart, lungs, urinary tract, and blood vessels. For this reason, treatment is continued for no longer than 6 months, with a drug-free period of at least 4 weeks between courses.

Monitoring Regular X-rays of the urinary tract may be recommended.

METOCLOPRAMIDE

Brand name Reglan
Used in the following combined preparations None

GENERAL INFORMATION

The only drug of its kind, metoclopramide stimulates an integrated, propulsive action within the entire gastrointestinal tract, with its strongest effect at the upper end, where the stomach empties into the duodenum.

Available since 1986, metoclopramide is used to relieve retention of food and acid in the stomach and the inflammation of the esophagus that can result from reflux of the stomach contents. Persons with diabetes are among those most likely to experience such gastric retention.

Metoclopramide has a number of other uses. It may be given to help the nausea experienced by cancer sufferers undergoing radiation or treatment with anticancer drugs. It is sometimes administered as *premedication* before surgery to avoid the vomiting caused by anesthetics.

Adverse effects include sedation, muscle spasms in the face, parkinsonian symptoms, and increased secretion of the hormone prolactin, which may induce the discharge of a milky fluid by the breasts.

QUICK REFERENCE

Drug group Gastrointestinal motility regulator and anti-emetic drug (p.118)

Overdose danger rating Medium

Dependence rating Low

Prescription needed Yes

Available as generic Yes

INFORMATION FOR USERS

Your drug prescription is tailored for you. Do not alter dosage without checking with your physician.

How taken

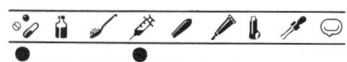

Tablets, injection.

Frequency and timing of doses
3 x daily, 15 minutes – 1 hour before meals.

Adult dosage range
10 – 30mg daily, occasionally higher.

Onset of effect
Within 1 hour.

Duration of action
6 – 8 hours.

Diet advice
Fatty and spicy foods and alcohol are best avoided if nausea is a problem.

Storage
Keep in a closed container in a cool, dry place away from reach of children.

Missed dose
Take as soon as you remember. If your next dose is due within 2 hours, take a single dose now and skip the next.

Stopping the drug
Can be safely stopped as soon as you no longer need it.

Exceeding the dose
An occasional unintentional extra dose is unlikely to be a cause for concern. Large overdoses may cause drowsiness and muscle spasms. Notify your physician.

SPECIAL PRECAUTIONS

Be sure to tell your physician if:
▼ You have impaired kidney or liver function.
▼ You are taking other medications.

Pregnancy
▼ Not usually prescribed. Safety in pregnancy not established. Discuss with your physician so that you may weigh the benefits of the drug against its possible risks.

Breast feeding
▼ Discuss with your physician. The drug passes into the breast milk but in normal doses adverse effects on the baby are unlikely.

Infants and children
▼ Reduced dose necessary.

Over 60
▼ No special problems.

Driving and hazardous work
▼ No special problems.

Alcohol
▼ Avoid. Alcohol may oppose the beneficial effects and increase the sedative effects of this drug.

POSSIBLE ADVERSE EFFECTS

The main adverse effects of metoclopramide are drowsiness and, less commonly, uncontrolled muscle spasm. Other symptoms rarely occur.

Symptom/effect	Frequency		Discuss with physician		Stop taking drug now	Call physician now
	Common	Rare	Only if severe	In all cases		
Drowsiness/lethargy	●		■			
Constipation		●		■		
Diarrhea		●		■		
Muscle spasm of face		●		■		
Parkinsonism		●		■		

PROLONGED USE

No special problems.

INTERACTIONS

Sedatives All drugs that have a sedative effect on the central nervous system are likely to increase the sedative properties of metoclopramide. Such drugs include anti-anxiety and sleeping drugs, antidepressants, antihistamines, narcotic analgesics, and antipsychotics.

Antipsychotic and anti-emetic drugs Metoclopramide increases the likelihood of adverse effects from these drugs.

METOLAZONE

Brand names Diulo, Zaroxolyn
Used in the following combined preparations None

GENERAL INFORMATION

Metolazone, introduced in 1973, is similar in action and effects to the group of drugs known as the thiazide diuretics. It is, however, longer-acting than most. Diuretics remove excess water from the body, reducing edema (fluid retention) in people with congestive heart failure, kidney disorders, cirrhosis of the liver, and premenstrual tension.

Metolazone is most frequently used to treat high blood pressure (see Antihypertensive drugs, p.130), and because it reduces the amount of calcium in the urine, it is sometimes used to prevent the recurrence of certain types of kidney stones.

As with all thiazides, metolazone increases the loss of potassium, magnesium, and bicarbonate in the urine. Loss of potassium can cause a variety of symptoms (see p.540) and increases the likelihood of irregular heart rhythms, particularly if you are taking drugs such as digoxin for heart failure. For this reason potassium supplements are often prescribed along with metolazone.

QUICK REFERENCE

Drug group Thiazide diuretic (p.127).

Overdose danger rating Low

Dependence rating Low

Prescription needed Yes

Available as generic Yes

INFORMATION FOR USERS

Your drug prescription is tailored for you. Do not alter dosage without checking with your physician.

How taken

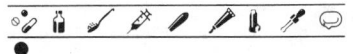

Tablets.

Frequency and timing of doses
Once a day, early in the day.

Adult dosage range
2.5 – 20 mg daily.

Onset of effect
Within 1 hour.

Duration of action
24 – 48 hours.

Diet advice
Use of this drug may reduce potassium in the body. Eat plenty of fresh fruit and vegetables. Discuss the advisability of reducing your salt intake with your physician.

Storage
Keep in a closed container in a cool, dry place away from reach of children.

Missed dose
No cause for concern, but take as soon as you remember. However, if it is late in the day, do not take the missed dose, or you may need to get up during the night to pass urine. Take the next scheduled dose as usual.

Stopping the drug
Do not stop the drug without consulting your physician; symptoms may recur.

Exceeding the dose
An occasional unintentional extra dose is unlikely to be a cause for concern. But if you notice unusual symptoms, or if a large overdose has been taken, notify your physician.

SPECIAL PRECAUTIONS

Be sure to tell your physician if:
▼ You have impaired kidney or liver function.
▼ You have gout.
▼ You have diabetes.
▼ You have a high level of fat in your blood (hyperlipidemia).
▼ You are taking other medications.

Pregnancy
▼ Not usually prescribed. No evidence that it harms the baby, but it may cause excessive sodium (salt) loss in the mother.

Breast feeding
▼ The drug passes into the breast milk and may reduce your milk supply. Discuss with your physician.

Infants and children
▼ Not usually prescribed. Reduced dose necessary.

Over 60
▼ Increased likelihood of adverse effects.

Driving and hazardous work
▼ No special problems.

Alcohol
▼ Keep consumption low. Metolazone increases the likelihood of dehydration and hangovers after consumption of alcohol.

POSSIBLE ADVERSE EFFECTS

Most effects are caused by excessive loss of potassium. This can usually be put right by taking a potassium supplement. In rare cases gout may occur in susceptible people, and certain forms of diabetes may become more difficult to control.

Symptom/effect	Frequency		Discuss with physician		Stop taking drug now	Call physician now
	Common	Rare	Only if severe	In all cases		
Lethargy		●	■			
Dizziness		●	■			
Rash		●	■			
Digestive disturbance		●	■			
Temporary impotence		●	■			

INTERACTIONS

Non-steroidal anti-inflammatory drugs (NSAIDs) These may reduce the diuretic effect of metolazone. The dosage of metolazone may need to be adjusted.

Digitalis drugs The adverse effects of such drugs may be increased if excessive amounts of potassium are lost.

Corticosteroids These drugs further increase the loss of potassium from the body when taken with metolazone.

Lithium Metolazone may increase lithium levels in the blood, leading to a risk of serious adverse effects.

PROLONGED USE

Prolonged use of this drug can lead to excessive loss of potassium and imbalances of other salts.

Monitoring Blood tests may be performed periodically to check kidney function and levels of blood sugar, potassium, and other salts.

METOPROLOL

Brand name Lopressor
Used in the following combined preparation Lopressor HCT

GENERAL INFORMATION

Introduced in 1978, metoprolol is a beta blocker used in the treatment of angina and, in combination with a diuretic, hypertension. It is also prescribed to relieve palpitations and tremor caused by overactivity of the thyroid gland. Metoprolol may be given following a heart attack to prevent further damage.

Unlike similar drugs that act on the heart and lungs, metoprolol is cardio-selective, acting mainly on the heart. This makes it especially valuable for people with asthma, bronchitis, or other lung problems, although caution is still required. Metoprolol masks the body's response to low blood sugar, a problem in diabetics.

It can also bring on an attack of Raynaud's phenomenon or reduce circulation to the hands and feet, making them feel cold.

INFORMATION FOR USERS

Your drug prescription is tailored for you. Do not alter dosage without checking with your physician.

How taken

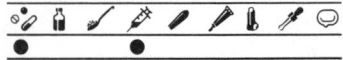

Tablets, injection.

Frequency and timing of doses
1 – 3 x daily.

Dosage range
Angina 50 – 100mg daily.
Hypertension 100 – 450mg daily.

Onset of effect
Within 2 hours.

Duration of action
Up to 4 weeks (hypertension); up to 12 hours (angina).

Diet advice
None.

Storage
Keep in a closed container in a cool, dry place away from reach of children. Protect from light.

Missed dose
Take as soon as you remember. If your next dose is due within 2 hours (if you take the drug 2 – 3 times daily), or 5 hours (if you take the drug once daily), take a single dose now and skip the next.

Stopping the drug
Do not stop the drug without consulting your physician; stopping the drug suddenly may lead to worsening of the underlying condition or precipitate a heart attack.

OVERDOSE ACTION

Seek immediate medical advice in all cases. Take emergency action if breathing difficulties, collapse, or loss of consciousness occurs.

See Drug poisoning emergency guide (p.590).

POSSIBLE ADVERSE EFFECTS

Metoprolol has adverse effects that are common to most beta blockers. Symptoms such as fatigue and nausea are usually temporary and diminish with long-term use. Metoprolol can occasionally provoke or worsen asthma and some heart problems.

Symptom/effect	Frequency		Discuss with physician		Stop taking drug now	Call physician now
	Common	Rare	Only if severe	In all cases		
Lethargy	●		■			
Cold hands and feet	●		■			
Nausea/nightmares/dreams		●	■			
Rash		●		■	▲	
Breathing difficulties		●		■	▲	▮
Fainting		●		■	▲	▮

INTERACTIONS

Indomethacin reduces the antihypertensive effect of metoprolol.

Cimetidine can increase the levels of metoprolol in the blood.

Nifedipine can lower the blood pressure excessively if taken with metoprolol.

Ergotamine can aggravate circulation problems in hands and feet if taken with metoprolol.

SPECIAL PRECAUTIONS

Be sure to tell your physician if:
▼ You have impaired liver or kidney function.
▼ You have heart failure.
▼ You have a lung disorder such as asthma or bronchitis.
▼ You have diabetes.
▼ You are taking other medications.

 Pregnancy
▼ No evidence of risk to baby when taken in early pregnancy. If taken in late pregnancy, the baby's heart may be affected. Discuss with your physician so that you can weigh the benefits of the drug against its possible risks.

 Breast feeding
▼ Discuss with your physician. The drug passes into the breast milk and may affect the baby adversely.

 Infants and children
▼ Not usually prescribed.

 Over 60
▼ Increased likelihood of adverse effects.

 Driving and hazardous work
▼ Avoid such activities until you have learned how the drug affects you, because the drug can cause dizziness and tiredness.

 Alcohol
▼ No known problems.

Surgery and general anesthetics
▼ Metoprolol may need to be stopped before you have a general anesthetic. Discuss this with your physician or dentist before any surgery.

PROLONGED USE

No special problems.

METRONIDAZOLE

Brand names Flagyl, Flagyl IV, Metryl 500, Protostat, Satric 500
Used in the following combined preparations None

GENERAL INFORMATION

Metronidazole, introduced in 1960, is prescribed to fight protozoal infections and a variety of bacterial infections.

Its main use is in the treatment of trichomonas infection of the vagina. Because the organism responsible for this disorder is sexually transmitted and may not cause any symptoms, a simultaneous course of treatment is usually advised for sexual partners.

Certain infections of the heart (endocarditis), abdomen, pelvis, and skin also respond well to metronidazole, usually given in combination with other drugs. Metronidazole may be given to prevent infection before bowel surgery or to treat bowel infection that has occurred as a side effect of antibiotics. Because metronidazole in high doses is capable of penetrating the brain, it is also used to treat abscesses occurring there.

The drug is also prescribed for amebic dysentery and giardiasis, a protozoal infection.

The most common adverse effects that occur with metronidazole are nausea, abdominal pain, and diarrhea.

QUICK REFERENCE

Drug group Antibacterial (p.159) and antiprotozoal drug (p.164)

Overdose danger rating Low

Dependence rating Low

Prescription needed Yes

Available as generic Yes

INFORMATION FOR USERS

Your drug prescription is tailored for you. Do not alter dosage without checking with your physician.

How taken

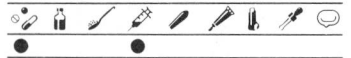

Tablets, injection.

Frequency and timing of doses
Usually 3 x daily for 5 – 10 days, depending on condition being treated. Occasionally a single large dose may be prescribed.

Adult dosage range
750mg daily (trichomonas); 750mg – 1.5g daily (giardiasis); 1.5 – 2.25g daily (amebic infections); according to body weight (other infections).

Onset of effect
Within minutes (injection); 1 – 3 hours (by mouth).

Duration of action
6 – 12 hours.

Diet advice
Avoid alcohol.

Storage
Keep in a closed container in a cool, dry place away from reach of children. Protect from light.

Missed dose
Take as soon as you remember. If your next dose is due within 2 hours, take a single dose now and skip the next.

Stopping the drug
Take the full course. Even if you feel better, the infection may still be present and symptoms may recur if treatment is stopped too soon.

Exceeding the dose
An occasional unintentional extra dose is unlikely to be a cause for concern. But if you notice unusual symptoms, especially numbness or tingling, or if a large overdose has been taken, notify your physician.

SPECIAL PRECAUTIONS

Be sure to tell your physician if:
- ▼ You have impaired liver or kidney function.
- ▼ You have a blood disorder.
- ▼ You have a disorder of the central nervous system, such as epilepsy.
- ▼ You are taking other medications.

Pregnancy
▼ Not usually prescribed. Safety in pregnancy not established. Discuss with your physician so that you can weigh the benefits of the drug against its possible risks.

Breast feeding
▼ The drug passes into the breast milk, but at normal doses adverse effects on the baby are unlikely. Discuss with your physician.

Infants and children
▼ Reduced dose necessary.

Over 60
▼ No special problems.

Driving and hazardous work
▼ No known problems.

Alcohol
▼ Avoid. Taken with metronidazole, alcohol may cause flushing, nausea, vomiting, abdominal pain, and headache.

PROLONGED USE

Not usually prescribed for longer than 10 days. Prolonged treatment may cause temporary loss of sensation in the hands and feet, and may also reduce production of white blood cells.

POSSIBLE ADVERSE EFFECTS

The most common problems are minor gastrointestinal disturbances that tend to diminish as your body adjusts to the drug. It commonly causes a darkening of the urine, which is of no concern. More serious adverse effects affecting the central nervous system, causing numbness or tingling, are extremely rare.

Symptom/effect	Frequency		Discuss with physician		Stop taking drug now	Call physician now
	Common	Rare	Only if severe	In all cases		
Nausea/loss of appetite	●		■			
Abdominal pain/dark urine	●		■			
Dry mouth/metallic taste		●	■			
Headache/dizziness		●	■			
Numbness/tingling		●		■		

INTERACTIONS

Oral anticoagulant drugs Metronidazole may increase the effect of oral anticoag- ulants, and the anticoagulant dose may need to be adjusted accordingly.

MICONAZOLE

Brand names Micatin, Monistat 3, Monistat 7, Monistat-Derm, Monistat I.V.
Used in the following combined preparations None

GENERAL INFORMATION

A widely used antifungal drug dating from the 1970s, miconazole is used in creams and suppositories to treat candida (thrush) infection of the vagina and tinea (ringworm) infections of the skin, such as athlete's foot and jock itch. Miconazole given by injection can also be used in severe internal (*systemic*) fungal infections that have occurred in the lungs, brain, kidney, and lymph nodes.

Minor adverse effects, such as nausea and vomiting, are common when miconazole is given by injection. Applied to the skin, adverse effects are uncommon.

INFORMATION FOR USERS

Your drug prescription is tailored for you. Do not alter dosage without checking with your physician.

How taken

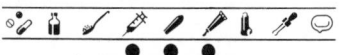

Injection, vaginal suppositories, cream.

Frequency and timing of doses
2 x daily (skin infections); once daily at bedtime (vaginal infections); 2 – 3 x daily (systemic infections).

Adult dosage range
Skin infections Sufficient cream to cover the affected skin and surrounding area at each application.
Vaginal infections 100mg or 200mg daily (vaginal suppository), one applicatorful daily (cream).
Systemic infections 600 – 3,600mg daily (injection) according to condition.

Onset of effect
2 – 7 days.

Duration of action
Up to 24 hours after each dose.

Diet advice
None.

Storage
Keep in a closed container in a cool, dry place away from reach of children.

Missed dose
No cause for concern, but make up the missed dose or application as soon as you remember.

Stopping the drug
Take the full course. Even if symptoms disappear, the original infection may still be present and symptoms may recur if treatment is stopped too soon.

Exceeding the dose
An occasional unintentional extra dose when using cream or vaginal suppositories is unlikely to be a cause for concern. But if you notice unusual symptoms, or if a large overdose has been taken by mouth, consult your physician.

SPECIAL PRECAUTIONS

Be sure to tell your physician if:
▼ You have previously had an allergic reaction to this drug.
▼ You are taking other medications.

Pregnancy
▼ No evidence of risk to developing baby from cream or vaginal suppositories. Injections not usually prescribed. Safety in pregnancy not established. Discuss with your physician so that you can weigh the benefits of the drug against its possible risks.

Breast feeding
▼ No evidence of risk from cream or vaginal suppositories. Given by injection the drug passes into the breast milk and may affect the baby adversely. Discuss with your physician.

Infants and children
▼ Reduced dose necessary.

Over 60
▼ No special problems.

Driving and hazardous work
▼ No known problems.

Alcohol
▼ No known problems.

POSSIBLE ADVERSE EFFECTS

Miconazole given in the form of cream or vaginal suppositories rarely causes troublesome adverse effects. Irritation at the site of application is unusual. When the drug is injected, it may cause a variety of more serious symptoms, but these are always closely monitored in the hospital, and the dosage is adjusted accordingly.

Symptom/effect	Frequency		Discuss with physician		Stop taking drug now	Call physician now
	Common	Rare	Only if severe	In all cases		
Injection						
Nausea/vomiting	●			■		
Fever/chills	●			■		
Pain at injection site	●			■	▲	
Cream						
Irritation/burning		●	■			
Rash		●		■	▲	

INTERACTIONS (injection only)

Anticoagulant drugs Miconazole increases the anticoagulant effect of these drugs.

Oral antidiabetic drugs Miconazole increases the effect of these drugs, so that blood sugar levels may fall too low.

Phenytoin Miconazole increases the blood levels of phenytoin, which may increase the risk of adverse effects.

Amphotericin B The antifungal action of this drug is reduced by miconazole.

PROLONGED USE

Given by injection for long periods, the drug may alter the composition of the blood, leading to anemia.

Monitoring Periodic blood tests are usually required to check for anemia.

MINOXIDIL

Brand name Loniten
Used in the following combined preparations None

GENERAL INFORMATION

Minoxidil, an antihypertensive introduced in 1979, is a vasodilator drug (see p.126). These relax the muscles of artery walls and dilate blood vessels. It is effective in controlling dangerously high blood pressure or pressure that is rising very rapidly. Because it is stronger acting than many other antihypertensive drugs, it is particularly useful for people whose blood pressure has not been controlled by other treatment. Because minoxidil, like other vasodilators, can cause fluid retention and

increased heart rate, it is always prescribed with a diuretic and a beta blocker to increase effectiveness and counteract side effects. Unlike many other antihypertensives, minoxidil does not cause dizziness and fainting, although those side effects do occur occasionally. Its major drawback is that, if taken for longer than two months, it increases hair growth, especially on the face. Although this can be controlled by shaving or depilatories, some find the abnormal growth distressing.

INFORMATION FOR USERS

Your drug prescription is tailored for you. Do not alter dosage without checking with your physician.

How taken

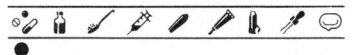

Tablets.

Frequency and timing of doses
Once or twice daily.

Adult dosage range
5 – 40mg daily. Dose may be increased in exceptional circumstances.

Onset of effect
Within 1 hour.

Duration of action
Up to 24 hours. Some effect may last for 2 – 5 days after the drug is stopped.

Diet advice
None.

Storage
Keep in a closed container in a cool, dry place away from reach of children.

Missed dose
Take as soon as you remember. If your next dose is due within 6 hours, take a single dose now and skip the next.

Stopping the drug
Do not stop the drug without consulting your physician; stopping the drug may lead to worsening of the underlying condition.

OVERDOSE ACTION

 Seek immediate medical advice in all cases. Take emergency action if palpitations, nausea, vomiting, dizziness, or loss of consciousness occurs.

See Drug poisoning emergency guide (p.590).

POSSIBLE ADVERSE EFFECTS

Fluid retention is a common adverse effect of this drug, which may lead to an increase in weight. Diuretics are often prescribed to control this.

Symptom/effect	Frequency		Discuss with physician		Stop taking drug now	Call physician now
	Common	Rare	Only if severe	In all cases		
Increased hair growth	●					
Fluid retention	●			■		
Shortness of breath	●			■		
Tiredness		●		■		
Headache		●		■		
Rash		●		■		
Dizziness/lightheadedness		●		■		▮
Nausea		●		■		▮

INTERACTIONS

Guanethidine increases the risk of dizziness and lightheadedness when taken with minoxidil. Whenever possible, guanethidine will be discontinued before treatment with minoxidil begins.

SPECIAL PRECAUTIONS

Be sure to tell your physician if:
▼ You have impaired kidney or liver function.
▼ You have heart problems.
▼ You retain fluid.
▼ You are taking other medications.

 Pregnancy
▼ Not usually prescribed. Safety in pregnancy not established. Discuss with your physician so that you can weigh the benefits of the drug against its possible risks.

 Breast feeding
▼ The drug passes into the breast milk, but at normal doses adverse effects on the baby are uncommon. Discuss with your physician.

 Infants and children
▼ Not usually prescribed. Reduced dose necessary.

 Over 60
▼ Reduced dose may be necessary.

 Driving and hazardous work
▼ Avoid such activities until you have learned how the drug affects you, because the drug can cause dizziness and lightheadedness.

 Alcohol
▼ No known problems.

PROLONGED USE

Prolonged use of this drug may lead to swelling of the ankles and increased hair growth. It is being investigated for long-term application on the scalp as a treatment for male-pattern baldness.

MORPHINE

Brand names Duromorph, Roxanol
Used in the following combined preparations None

GENERAL INFORMATION

A classic analgesic since the 19th century, morphine takes its name from Morpheus, the god of dreams and sleep in Greek mythology. It belongs to a group of drugs called the narcotic analgesics (see p.108) that are derived from opium, which in turn is prepared from the unripe seed capsules of the opium poppy.

Morphine relieves the severe pain that can be caused by injury, surgery, heart attack, or such chronic diseases as cancer. Additionally, to make a patient feel sleepy and less anxious, morphine may be administered as *premedication* before surgery.

Its painkilling effect wears off quickly, in contrast to some other narcotic analgesics, and it may be given as tablets to relieve continuous, severe pain.

It is habit-forming; dependence and addiction do occur. However, most patients taking morphine for pain relief over brief periods of time do not become dependent and are able to stop taking the drug without difficulty.

QUICK REFERENCE

Drug group Narcotic analgesic (p.108)

Overdose danger rating High

Dependence rating High

Prescription needed Yes CII

Available as generic Yes

INFORMATION FOR USERS

Your drug prescription is tailored for you. Do not alter dosage without checking with your physician.

How taken

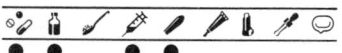

Tablets, liquid, injection, rectal suppositories.

Frequency and timing of doses
Every 4 hours, when necessary.

Adult dosage range
5 – 25mg per dose; however, some patients may need 75mg or more per dose. Doses vary considerably for each individual.

Onset of effect
Within 1 hour.

Duration of action
4 hours.

Diet advice
None.

Storage
Keep in a closed container in a cool, dry place away from reach of children.

Missed dose
Take as soon as you need for recurrent pain. If you are not in pain, do not take the missed dose but return to your normal dosing schedule when necessary.

Stopping the drug
If the reason for taking the drug no longer exists, you may stop the drug and notify your physician.

OVERDOSE ACTION

Seek immediate medical advice in all cases. Take emergency action if there are symptoms such as slow or irregular breathing, severe drowsiness, or loss of consciousness.

See **Drug poisoning emergency guide (p.590).**

POSSIBLE ADVERSE EFFECTS

Adverse effects of morphine are common with continued use of the drug.

Symptom/effect	Frequency		Discuss with physician		Stop taking drug now	Call physician now
	Common	Rare	Only if severe	In all cases		
Drowsiness	●			■		
Nausea/vomiting	●			■		
Constipation	●			■		
Dizziness	●			■		
Slow heartbeat	●			■		
Confusion		●		■		

INTERACTIONS

Sedatives Morphine increases the sedative properties of all drugs that have a sedative effect. Such drugs include alcohol, antidepressants, antipsychotics, sleeping drugs, and antihistamines.

Monoamine oxidase inhibitors (MAOIs) These drugs may produce a severe rise in blood pressure when taken with morphine.

SPECIAL PRECAUTIONS

Be sure to tell your physician if:
▼ You have impaired kidney or liver function.
▼ You have heart or circulatory problems.
▼ You have a lung disorder such as asthma or bronchitis.
▼ You have thyroid disease.
▼ You are taking other medications.

 Pregnancy
▼ Not usually prescribed. Taken near the time of delivery may cause breathing difficulties in the newborn baby.

 Breast feeding
▼ The drug passes into the breast milk in small amounts and may affect the baby adversely. Discuss with your physician.

 Infants and children
▼ Reduced dose necessary.

 Over 60
▼ Reduced dose may be necessary. Increased likelihood of adverse effects.

 Driving and hazardous work
▼ People on morphine treatment are unlikely to be well enough to undertake such activities.

 Alcohol
▼ Avoid. Alcohol may increase the sedative effects of this drug.

PROLONGED USE

The effects of the drug usually become weaker during prolonged use as the body adapts. But it is likely to be addictive if taken for extended periods, causing (among other things) impotence and loss of libido.

NADOLOL

Brand name Corgard
Used in the following combined preparation Corzide

GENERAL INFORMATION

Nadolol, introduced in 1980, is a beta blocker prescribed for hypertension (high blood pressure), angina, and arrhythmias (abnormal heart rhythms). It is used as an adjunct in the treatment of overactive thyroid gland and the prevention of migraine headaches. When prescribed for hypertension, nadolol is often prescribed in a combined preparation containing a diuretic. One advantage it has over some other beta blockers is that it needs to be taken only once daily.

Because it can cause breathing difficulties, nadolol should not be taken by asthmatics or people suffering from chronic bronchitis. In common with all beta blockers, nadolol has a slowing effect on the heart rate, and masks the body's response to low blood sugar; it should be used with caution by diabetics.

QUICK REFERENCE

Drug group Beta blocker (p.125)
Overdose danger rating High
Dependence rating Low
Prescription needed Yes
Available as generic No

INFORMATION FOR USERS

Your drug prescription is tailored for you. Do not alter dosage without checking with your physician.

How taken

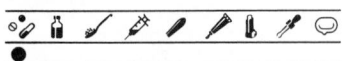

Tablets.

Frequency and timing of doses
Once daily.

Dosage range
Hypertension 40 – 320mg daily; larger doses may be prescribed.
Angina 40 – 240mg daily.
Arrhythmia 60 – 160mg daily.

Onset of effect
2 – 4 hours. For high blood pressure, it may be several weeks before full benefit is felt.

Duration of action
Over 24 hours.

Diet advice
None.

Storage
Keep in a closed container in a cool, dry place away from reach of children. Protect from light.

Missed dose
Take as soon as you remember. If your next dose is due within 6 hours, take a single dose now and skip the next.

Stopping the drug
Do not stop the drug without consulting your physician; stopping the drug may lead to worsening of your underlying condition.

OVERDOSE ACTION

Seek immediate medical advice in all cases. Take emergency action if collapse or loss of consciousness occurs.

See Drug poisoning emergency guide (p.590).

SPECIAL PRECAUTIONS

Be sure to tell your physician if:
▼ You have impaired kidney function.
▼ You have a lung disorder such as asthma or bronchitis.
▼ You have diabetes.
▼ You are taking other medications.

Pregnancy
▼ Discuss with physician. Other beta blockers may be safer.

Breast feeding
▼ The drug passes into the breast milk, but at normal doses adverse effects are uncommon. Discuss with your physician.

Infants and children
▼ Not usually prescribed.

Over 60
▼ No special problems.

Driving and hazardous work
▼ No special problems.

Alcohol
▼ No special problems.

Surgery and general anesthetics
▼ Nadolol may need to be stopped before you have a general anesthetic. Discuss this with your physician or dentist before any surgery.

PROLONGED USE

No special problems.

POSSIBLE ADVERSE EFFECTS

Nadolol has a number of adverse effects which are usually temporary and diminish with long-term use. Breathing difficulties, fainting, and rash require medical attention.

Symptom/effect	Frequency		Discuss with physician		Stop taking drug now	Call physician now
	Common	Rare	Only if severe	In all cases		
Cold hands and feet	●		■			
Lethargy		●	■			
Insomnia		●	■			
Dry eyes		●	■			
Breathing difficulties		●		■		▮
Fainting		●		■		▮
Rash		●		■		▮

INTERACTIONS

Indomethacin reduces the antihypertensive effect of nadolol.

NALIDIXIC ACID

Brand name NegGram
Used in the following combined preparations None

GENERAL INFORMATION

Nalidixic acid, introduced in 1963, is one of the oldest synthetic antibiotics. It is used in the treatment of lower urinary tract infections (cystitis). It is also sometimes given for the prevention of recurrent urinary tract infections.

Taken by mouth, it does not accumulate in the body tissues but is concentrated in the urine. It is effective against almost all the species of bacteria that commonly infect the urinary tract, including some that are resistant to other antibiotics. However, because some organisms rapidly develop resistance, a second course of treatment is less likely to be as effective.

Nalidixic acid is fast-acting and usually clears acute outbreaks of infection completely within a few days.

Though generally safe, nalidixic acid sometimes causes serious side effects. The drug may interfere with some urine tests and can give a false high reading of blood sugar level.

QUICK REFERENCE

Drug group Antibiotic (p.156)
Overdose danger rating Medium
Dependence rating Low
Prescription needed Yes
Available as generic No

INFORMATION FOR USERS

Your drug prescription is tailored for you. Do not alter dosage without checking with your physician.

How taken

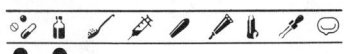

Tablets, liquid.

Frequency and timing of doses
4 x daily.

Dosage range
Adults 4g daily for one week for acute infections, reduced to 2g daily during longer courses of treatment.
Children Reduced dose according to age and weight.

Onset of effect
2 – 3 days.

Duration of action
Up to 12 hours.

Diet advice
None.

Storage
Keep in a closed container in a cool, dry place away from reach of children.

Missed dose
Take as soon as you remember. If your next dose is due within 2 hours, take a single dose now and skip the next.

Stopping the drug
Take the full course. Even if you feel better, the infection may still be present and symptoms may recur if treatment is stopped too soon.

Exceeding the dose
An occasional unintentional extra dose is unlikely to cause problems. Large overdoses may cause nausea, vomiting, lethargy, mental disturbance (psychosis), and seizures. Notify your physician.

SPECIAL PRECAUTIONS

Be sure to tell your physician if:
▼ You have impaired liver or kidney function.
▼ You have had epileptic seizures.
▼ You have Parkinson's disease.
▼ You are taking other medications.

Pregnancy
▼ Not usually prescribed. May cause birth defects in the developing baby. Discuss with your physician so that you may weigh the benefits of the drug against its risks.

Breast feeding
▼ Discuss with your physician. The drug passes into the breast milk and may affect the baby adversely.

Infants and children
▼ Reduced dose necessary. Generally, not recommended for children.

Over 60
▼ Reduced dose may be necessary.

Driving and hazardous work
▼ Avoid such activities until you have learned how the drug affects you, because the drug may cause dizziness, drowsiness, and blurred vision.

Alcohol
▼ Avoid. Alcohol may increase the sedative effects of this drug.

POSSIBLE ADVERSE EFFECTS

Nalidixic acid does not usually cause adverse effects. The most common side effects are nausea or vomiting and rashes. In some people it increases the sensitivity of the skin to sunlight. It can also cause visual disturbances, drowsiness, and dizziness.

Symptom/effect	Frequency		Discuss with physician		Stop taking drug now	Call physician now
	Common	Rare	Only if severe	In all cases		
Nausea/vomiting	●		■			
Rash/itching	●			■		
Dizziness/drowsiness		●	■			
Diarrhea		●	■			
Light-sensitive rash		●		■		
Blurred vision		●		■		

PROLONGED USE

No problems expected.

INTERACTIONS

Oral anticoagulant drugs Nalidixic acid may increase the anticoagulant effect of these drugs; dosage adjustment may be necessary.

Nitrofurantoin Nitrofurantoin interferes with the effectiveness of nalidixic acid.

Antacids Antacids decrease the absorption of nalidixic acid.

NALOXONE

Brand name Narcan
Used in the following combined preparations None

GENERAL INFORMATION

Naloxone, introduced in 1971, is a semi-synthetic drug that blocks the action of narcotics (opium-based drugs). Given by injection, it rapidly reverses the effects of a narcotics overdose. Within a minute it improves the rate and volume of breathing and improves the level of consciousness.

Naloxone is occasionally given to improve breathing in newborn babies who have been affected by narcotic analgesics given to the mother during labor. It is also used to enhance breathing in some people who have been given these drugs during surgery. Since naloxone reverses all narcotic effect, the analgesic and sedative actions are also lost.

When given to narcotics addicts, the injection of naloxone may trigger severe but short-lived withdrawal symptoms, including stomach cramps, nausea, vomiting, diarrhea, and tremors. Particular care is therefore exercised in using naloxone in known or suspected narcotics addicts.

QUICK REFERENCE

Drug group Antidote to narcotic drug poisoning

Overdose danger rating Low

Dependence rating Low

Prescription needed Yes

Available as generic Yes

INFORMATION FOR USERS

This drug is given only under medical supervision and is not for self-administration.

How taken

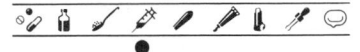

Injection.

Frequency and timing of doses
Adults and children A single injection, repeated at 2- to 3-minute intervals as needed. Further doses may be given at 20- to 60-minute intervals. The drug is sometimes given by continuous infusion. *Newborn infants* A single injection repeated if necessary after 3 – 5 minutes and after 30 – 90 minutes.

Dosage range
Adults and children Dosage is determined according to individual condition and response.

Onset of effect
30 seconds – 3 minutes.

Duration of action
Approximately 30 minutes.

Diet advice
None.

Storage
Not applicable. The drug is not kept in the home.

Missed dose
Not applicable. The drug is given only in a hospital under medical supervision.

Stopping the drug
Not applicable. The drug is stopped when breathing is satisfactory or when other symptoms of narcotic poisoning have resolved.

Exceeding the dose
This drug is always injected by a trained nurse or physician, and overdose is unlikely.

SPECIAL PRECAUTIONS

Naloxone is administered only under close medical supervision, taking account of the patient's present condition and medical history.

Pregnancy
▼ This drug is administered only when the life of the mother is at risk.

Breast feeding
▼ The drug is used only when the life of the mother is at risk, and is unlikely to have lasting adverse effects on breast feeding.

Infants and children
▼ Reduced dose necessary.

Over 60
▼ No special problems.

Driving and hazardous work
▼ Not applicable.

Alcohol
▼ Not applicable.

POSSIBLE ADVERSE EFFECTS

Adverse effects are rare with naloxone. Nausea, vomiting, agitation, and increased sweating may occur with high doses. Palpitations have been known to occur only in critically ill people treated with multiple doses of the drug.

Symptom/effect	Frequency		Discuss with physician		Stop taking drug now	Call physician now
	Common	Rare	Only if severe	In all cases		
Nausea/vomiting		●	■			
Agitation		●	■			
Unusual sweating		●	■			
Palpitations		●			■	

INTERACTIONS

None.

PROLONGED USE

Not applicable. Naloxone is not used for prolonged periods.

NANDROLONE

Brand names Decadurabolin, Durabolin, Nandrolin
Used in the following combined preparations None

GENERAL INFORMATION

Nandrolone, introduced in 1959, is an anabolic steroid, a synthetic hormone related to the male sex hormone testosterone. Given by injection, it encourages growth in boys whose development has been slowed because of hormone disturbances. It has been claimed to help people gain weight after a serious illness or injury. It has also been used to treat certain types of anemia.

Violating the rules of most athletic organizations, athletes have taken nandrolone and other anabolic steroids to increase body weight and muscle strength. But scientific studies indicate that the weight gain may be caused by fluid retention; the evidence of increased strength is equivocal.

Because the testosterone-like properties cannot be completely separated from the anabolic effects, women taking nandrolone are likely to suffer from excessive hair growth and disturbed menstrual periods. An advantage of nandrolone, for men as well as women, is that this drug rarely causes damage to the liver.

INFORMATION FOR USERS

This drug is given only under medical supervision and is not for self-administration.

How taken

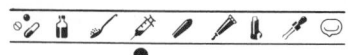

Injection.

Frequency and timing of doses
Once every 3 – 4 weeks.

Dosage range
Dosage varies according to preparation and the condition being treated.

Onset of effect
Within a few hours.

Duration of action
1 – 4 weeks.

Diet advice
Drug treatment for weight gain and growth needs to be accompanied by a nourishing balanced diet. Excessive intake of protein may cause a buildup of nitrogen waste in the body. Your physician will give detailed advice.

Storage
Not applicable. This drug is not normally kept in the home.

Missed dose
Arrange for a missed injection to be administered as soon as possible.

Stopping the drug
Treatment can be safely stopped when it has effectively dealt with the disorder.

Exceeding the dose
Overdosage is unlikely, since treatment is carefully monitored.

POSSIBLE ADVERSE EFFECTS

Most of the more serious adverse effects are likely to occur only with long-term treatment with nandrolone, and may be helped by a reduction in dosage.

Symptom/effect	Frequency		Discuss with physician		Stop taking drug now	Call physician now
	Common	Rare	Only if severe	In all cases		
Swollen feet/ankles	●		■			
Nausea/vomiting		●	■			
Aggressive behavior		●		■		
Jaundice		●		■	▲	
Men only						
Difficulty passing urine		●		■	▲	
Women only						
Irregular menstruation	●			■		
Unusual hair growth		●		■		

INTERACTIONS

Anticoagulant drugs Nandrolone increases the effects of these drugs. Anticoagulant dosage may need to be adjusted accordingly.

Antidiabetic drugs Because nandrolone lowers blood sugar levels, dosage of these drugs may need to be reduced.

SPECIAL PRECAUTIONS

Be sure to tell your physician if:
▼ You have impaired kidney or liver function.
▼ You have heart problems.
▼ You have urinary difficulties.
▼ You have diabetes.
▼ You are taking other medications.

Pregnancy
▼ Not prescribed.

Breast feeding
▼ Not prescribed.

Infants and children
▼ Reduced dose necessary.

Over 60
▼ Reduced dose may be necessary. Increased risk of prostate problems in men.

Driving and hazardous work
▼ No known problems.

Alcohol
▼ No known problems.

PROLONGED USE

Prolonged use of this drug may lead to early stopping of growth in children and masculinization in women. Long-term use may also raise blood cholesterol levels, thereby increasing the chances of coronary heart disease. Because the benefits are doubtful, athletes taking anabolic steroids over long periods of time run a needless risk.

Monitoring Periodic checks on the level of salts in the blood are usually needed.

NAPHAZOLINE

Brand names Albalon Liquifilm, Naphcon, Opcon, VasoClear, Vasocon
Used in the following combined preparations Albalon-A, Naphcon-A, Opcon-A, Vasocon-A

GENERAL INFORMATION

Naphazoline, introduced in 1942, is a *sympathomimetic* decongestant available over the counter in a variety of single-ingredient and combined-drug preparations.

Taken in the form of nose drops or spray, it is used for temporary relief of stuffiness in common colds, sinusitis, and allergic rhinitis. Naphazoline reduces nasal congestion by narrowing blood vessels. Eye drop preparations of naphazoline act in a similar way to relieve redness caused by minor irritations. They are widely used to clear bloodshot eyes.

Adverse effects are rare if naphazoline is used for short periods at recommended doses. Excessive or prolonged use can lead to local irritation and worsening of congestion after the drug is stopped. Dilation of the pupils, leading to blurred vision and oversensitivity to light, may occur occasionally, particularly in people with light-colored eyes and those who wear contact lenses. They may also cause an attack of glaucoma in susceptible people.

QUICK REFERENCE

Drug group Sympathomimetic decongestant (p.121)

Overdose danger rating Medium

Dependence rating Low

Prescription needed No

Available as generic Yes

INFORMATION FOR USERS

Follow instructions on the label. Call your physician if symptoms worsen.

How taken

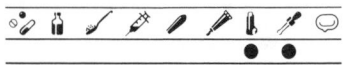

Nasal spray, nose drops, eye drops.

Frequency and timing of doses
Every 3 – 8 hours (nose drops); every 4 – 6 hours (nasal spray); up to 4 x daily (eye drops).

Dosage range
Nose drops, nasal spray 2 – 4 drops, or 2 sprays in each nostril per application (adults and children over 6 years).
Eye drops 1 – 2 drops in each eye per application (adults only).

Onset of effect
Within 10 minutes.

Duration of action
4 – 8 hours.

Diet advice
None.

Storage
Keep in a closed container in a cool, dry place away from reach of children.

Missed dose
Take as soon as you remember if required. Do not use more than once in 3 hours.

Stopping the drug
Can be safely stopped as soon as you no longer need it.

Exceeding the dose
An occasional unintentional extra dose is unlikely to cause problems. Large overdoses or accidental swallowing of the drug may cause severe drowsiness with sweating, weakness, headache, dizziness, or palpitations. Notify your physician.

POSSIBLE ADVERSE EFFECTS

Naphazoline rarely causes side effects at recommended doses. Overuse, however, may lead to local irritation and to adverse effects on the heart and central nervous system, such as palpitations, headache, drowsiness, and restlessness.

Symptom/effect	Frequency		Discuss with physician		Stop taking drug now	Call physician now
	Common	Rare	Only if severe	In all cases		
Burning/stinging/rash		●		■	▲	
Headache		●		■	▲	
Restlessness		●		■	▲	
Palpitations		●		■	▲	
Eye drops only						
Blurred vision		●		■		
Oversensitivity to light		●		■		

INTERACTIONS

Monoamine oxidase inhibitors (MAOIs) These drugs may interact dangerously with naphazoline to raise blood pressure.

Antihypertensives Naphazoline may reduce the blood pressure-lowering effect of these drugs, and is best avoided by people under treatment for high blood pressure.

SPECIAL PRECAUTIONS

Be sure to consult your physician before using this drug if:
▼ You have heart problems.
▼ You have high blood pressure.
▼ You have glaucoma.
▼ You have an eye infection or other eye disease.
▼ You are taking other medications.

Pregnancy
▼ Not recommended, since the possible adverse effects, although uncommon, include a rise in blood pressure that could harm the developing baby.

Breast feeding
▼ Not recommended. The drug may pass into the breast milk, although at normal doses adverse effects on the baby are unlikely.

Infants and children
▼ Eye drops should not be used in children of any age. Nose drops are not recommended for those under 2 years, and should be used in children under 6 years only under medical supervision.

Over 60
▼ Reduced dose may be necessary. Increased likelihood of adverse effects.

Driving and hazardous work
▼ No known problems.

Alcohol
▼ No known problems.

PROLONGED USE

Naphazoline should not be used for longer than 5 days except on the advice of a physician.

NAPROXEN

Brand names Anaprox, Naprosyn
Used in the following combined preparations None

GENERAL INFORMATION

Naproxen was introduced in 1970. Like other non-steroidal anti-inflammatory drugs (NSAIDs), it reduces pain, stiffness, and inflammation.

It is used to relieve symptoms of adult and juvenile rheumatoid arthritis, osteoarthritis, and ankylosing spondylitis, although it does not cure the underlying disease. Taken in combination with antirheumatic drugs, it relieves pain and inflammation while these drugs take effect.

Naproxen is also used to treat acute attacks of gout, and it may sometimes be prescribed short-term for pain relief after childbirth, orthopedic surgery, dental treatment, strains, and sprains. It is also effective for treating headaches and painful menstrual cramps. Gastrointestinal side effects are fairly common, and there is an increased risk of bleeding. It is safer than aspirin, and in long-term use it needs to be taken only twice daily.

INFORMATION FOR USERS

Your drug prescription is tailored for you. Do not alter dosage without checking with your physician.

How taken

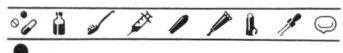

Tablets.

Frequency and timing of doses
2 x daily with food (arthritis); every 6 – 8 hours as required (general pain relief); 2 x daily (muscular pain); every 8 hours (gout). All doses should be taken with food.

Adult dosage range
Mild to moderate pain, menstrual cramps 500mg (starting dose), then 250mg every 6 – 8 hours as required up to 1.25g daily. *Muscular pain* 500mg – 825mg daily. *Arthritis* 500 – 750mg daily. *Gout* 750mg (starting dose), then 250mg every 8 hours until attack has subsided.

Onset of effect
Pain relief begins within 1 hour. Full anti-inflammatory effect may take 2 weeks.

Duration of action
Up to 12 hours.

Diet advice
None.

Storage
Keep in a closed container in a cool, dry place away from reach of children.

Missed dose
Take as soon as you remember. If your next dose is due within 6 hours, take a single dose now and skip the next.

Stopping the drug
When taken for short-term pain relief, naproxen can be safely stopped as soon as you no longer need it. If prescribed for long-term treatment, however, you should seek medical advice before stopping the drug.

Exceeding the dose
An occasional unintentional extra dose is unlikely to be a cause for concern. But if you notice any unusual symptoms, or if a large overdose has been taken, notify your physician.

SPECIAL PRECAUTIONS

Be sure to tell your physician if:
▼ You have impaired kidney function.
▼ You have heart problems.
▼ You have a bleeding disorder.
▼ You have high blood pressure.
▼ You have had a peptic ulcer, esophagitis, or acid indigestion.
▼ You are allergic to aspirin.
▼ You are taking other medications.

Pregnancy
▼ Not usually prescribed. When taken in the last three months of pregnancy, the drug may increase the risk of adverse effects on the baby's heart and may prolong labor. Discuss with your physician so that you may weigh the benefits of the drug against its risks.

Breast feeding
▼ Discuss with your physician. The drug passes into the breast milk and may affect the baby adversely.

Infants and children
▼ Reduced dose necessary.

Over 60
▼ Reduced dose may be necessary. Increased likelihood of adverse effects.

Driving and hazardous work
▼ No known problems.

Alcohol
▼ Avoid. Alcohol may increase the risk of stomach irritation with naproxen.

Surgery and general anesthetics
▼ Naproxen may prolong bleeding. Discuss with your physician or dentist before any surgery.

POSSIBLE ADVERSE EFFECTS

Most adverse effects are not serious and may diminish with time. Black or blood-stained bowel movements should be reported to your physician without delay.

Symptom/effect	Frequency		Discuss with physician		Stop taking drug now	Call physician now
	Common	Rare	Only if severe	In all cases		
Gastrointestinal disorders	●		■			
Headache		●	■			
Dizziness/drowsiness		●	■			
Ringing in the ears		●		■		
Swollen feet/ankles		●		■		
Rash/itching		●		■	▲	
Wheezing/breathlessness		●		■	▲	∎

INTERACTIONS

General note Naproxen interacts with a wide range of drugs to increase the risk of bleeding and/or peptic ulcers.

Antihypertensive drugs and diuretics The beneficial effects of these drugs may be reduced by naproxen.

PROLONGED USE

There is an increased risk of bleeding from peptic ulcers and in the bowel with prolonged use of naproxen.

NEOMYCIN

Brand names Mycifradin, Myciguent
Used in the following combined preparations Cortisporin, Mycitracin, Neo-Synalar, Neosporin, triple antibiotic

GENERAL INFORMATION

Neomycin, introduced in 1951, is one of the oldest aminoglycoside antibiotics. It is most commonly prescribed in the form of drops, cream, or ointment, often in combination with other drugs for ear and skin infections. It is not given by injection because it is more damaging to the kidneys than other aminoglycosides.

Given by mouth, neomycin is effective in killing bacteria inside the intestine and is used together with erythromycin prior to bowel surgery to prevent infections. It is prescribed in the treatment of hepatic coma caused by high blood levels of ammonia in people with liver failure. It may also be given for some types of bowel infection. Because neomycin has a lipid-lowering effect, it may be given to those with high levels of fat in the blood (hyperlipidemia).

QUICK REFERENCE

Drug group Aminoglycoside antibiotic (p.158) and lipid-lowering drug (p.131)

Overdose danger rating Low

Dependence rating Low

Prescription needed Yes

Available as generic Yes

INFORMATION FOR USERS

Your drug prescription is tailored for you. Do not alter dosage without checking with your physician.

How taken

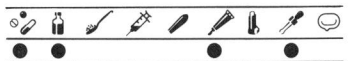

Tablets, liquid, cream, ointment, eye/ear drops.

Frequency and timing of doses
By mouth 4 x daily (diarrhea, hepatic coma); 3 x daily (bowel sterilization).
Skin preparations 1 – 3 x daily.
Eye preparations Every 3 – 4 hours.
Ear drops Every 6 – 8 hours.

Adult dosage range
By mouth 0.5 – 2g daily (hyperlipidemia); 3g daily (bowel sterilization); 4 – 12g daily initially, then 2 – 3 g daily (hepatic coma); according to weight (diarrhea).
Skin, eye and ear preparations As directed.

Onset of effect
1 – 2 days.

Duration of action
6 – 8 hours (by mouth); up to 24 hours (on skin).

Diet advice
A low-protein diet is usually recommended in hepatic coma, and a low-fat diet is recommended in hyperlipidemia.

Storage
Keep in a closed container in a cool, dry place away from reach of children. Protect liquid preparations from light.

Missed dose
Take as soon as you remember. If your next dose is due within 2 hours, take a single dose now and skip the next.

Stopping the drug
Do not stop the drug without consulting your physician.

Exceeding the dose
An occasional unintentional extra dose is unlikely to be a cause for concern. But if you notice unusual symptoms, or if a large overdose has been taken, notify your physician.

SPECIAL PRECAUTIONS

Be sure to tell your physician if:
▼ You have impaired kidney function.
▼ You have a hearing disorder.
▼ You have myasthenia gravis or Parkinson's disease.
▼ You are taking other medications.

 Pregnancy
▼ Not usually prescribed. Safety in pregnancy of oral forms not established. Discuss with your physician so that you can weigh the benefits of the drug against its possible risks.

 Breast feeding
▼ Taken by mouth, the drug passes into the breast milk, but at normal doses adverse effects on the baby are uncommon. Discuss with your physician.

 Infants and children
▼ Reduced dose necessary.

 Over 60
▼ Increased likelihood of adverse effects.

 Driving and hazardous work
▼ No special problems.

 Alcohol
▼ No known problems.

Surgery and general anesthetics
▼ Neomycin may need to be stopped before you have a general anesthetic. Discuss this with your physician or dentist before any surgery.

POSSIBLE ADVERSE EFFECTS

Allergic reactions including rash and itching occur commonly with skin, eye, and ear preparations. Taken by mouth, the drug may cause diarrhea and abdominal cramps. Dizziness, loss of balance, or ringing in the ears should be reported promptly.

Symptom/effect	Frequency		Discuss with physician		Stop taking drug now	Call physician now
	Common	Rare	Only if severe	In all cases		
Mild diarrhea	●		■			
Nausea/vomiting	●		■			
Rash/itching	●			■	▲	
Loss of hearing		●		■	▲	
Ringing in the ears		●		■	▲	
Dizziness/vertigo		●		■	▲	
Severe/bloody diarrhea		●		■	▲	▮

INTERACTIONS

General note Any drug that has adverse effects on hearing and/or kidney function increases the risk of such effects with neomycin. Such drugs include other aminoglycosides, furosemide, polymyxin antibiotics, and cisplatin.

Oral anticoagulant drugs Neomycin by mouth may increase the effect of these drugs.

Digitalis drugs and penicillin V Neomycin taken by mouth may reduce the absorption of these drugs.

PROLONGED USE

There is a rare risk of adverse effects on hearing, balance, and kidney function with prolonged high-dose neomycin therapy.

A
B
C
D
E
F
G
H
I
J
K
L
M
N
O
P
Q
R
S
T
U
V
W
X
Y
Z

NEOSTIGMINE

Brand name Prostigmin
Used in the following combined preparations None

GENERAL INFORMATION

Shorter acting and more potent than some other drugs in its field, neostigmine has been used for over 50 years to treat myasthenia gravis, a rare autoimmune condition (see p. 149). The disorder involves muscle weakness caused by faulty transmission of nerve impulses. By prolonging them, neostigmine improves muscle strength, though it does not cure the disease. In severe cases it may be prescribed in conjunction with corticosteroids.

The response to neostigmine is so predictable that it is also used to help diagnose the disease: lack of a response to an injection indicates that myasthenia gravis is not the problem.

The injectable form of neostigmine is also used to relieve urinary retention or temporary paralysis of the bowel (paralytic ileus).

see p. 149

QUICK REFERENCE

Drug group Drug for myasthenia gravis (p.149)

Overdose danger rating High

Dependence rating Low

Prescription needed Yes

Available as generic Yes

(p.149)

INFORMATION FOR USERS

Your drug prescription is tailored for you. Do not alter dosage without checking with your physician.

How taken

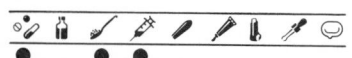

Tablets, powder, injection.

Frequency and timing of doses
Every 3 – 4 hours initially. Thereafter according to the needs of the individual.

Dosage range
Adults 45 – 300mg daily (by mouth); 1 – 15mg daily (injection).
Children Reduced dose necessary according to age and weight.

Onset of effect
45 – 75 minutes (by mouth); within 20 minutes (injection).

Duration of action
2 – 4 hours.

Diet advice
None.

Storage
Keep in a closed container in a cool, dry place away from reach of children. Protect from light.

Missed dose
Take as soon as you remember. If your next dose is due within 2 hours, take a single dose now and skip the next.

Stopping the drug
Do not stop the drug without consulting your physician; symptoms may recur.

OVERDOSE ACTION

Seek immediate medical advice in all cases. You may experience severe abdominal cramps, diarrhea, vomiting, increased salivation, weakness, and tremor. Take emergency action if unusually slow heartbeat, troubled breathing, seizures, or loss of consciousness occurs.

See Drug poisoning emergency guide (p.590).

(p.590)

POSSIBLE ADVERSE EFFECTS

Most of the common adverse effects of neostigmine are dose-related and due to overstimulation of the parasympathetic nervous system (see p.107).

see p.107

Symptom/effect	Frequency		Discuss with physician		Stop taking drug now	Call physician now
	Common	Rare	Only if severe	In all cases		
Increased salivation	●		■			
Diarrhea	●			■		
Abdominal cramps	●			■		
Nausea/vomiting	●			■		
Blurred vision/sweating	●			■		
Muscle cramps/twitching	●			■		
Rash		●		■	▲	▮

SPECIAL PRECAUTIONS

Be sure to tell your physician if:
▼ You have heart problems.
▼ You have had epileptic seizures.
▼ You have asthma.
▼ You have difficulty passing urine.
▼ You have Parkinson's disease.
▼ You are taking other medications.

Pregnancy
▼ No evidence of risk to developing baby with neostigmine taken in the first 6 months of pregnancy. Large doses near the time of delivery may cause premature labor and lead to temporary muscle weakness (lasting 1 week to 1 month) in the newborn baby.

Breast feeding
▼ Discuss with your physician. The drug may pass into the breast milk.

Infants and children
▼ Reduced dose necessary.

Over 60
▼ No special problems.

Driving and hazardous work
▼ Your underlying condition may make such activities inadvisable. Discuss with your physician.

Alcohol
▼ Avoid. Alcohol may cause breathing difficulties in myasthenia gravis sufferers.

Surgery and general anesthetics
▼ Neostigmine may interact with some anesthetics. Make sure your treatment is known to your physician or dentist before any surgery.

INTERACTIONS

General note Drugs that suppress the transmission of nerve signals in muscles may aggravate myasthenia gravis and oppose the effect of neostigmine. Such drugs include digoxin, quinidine, procainamide, phenytoin, lithium, aminoglycoside antibiotics, and thyroid hormones.

PROLONGED USE

Reduced effectiveness may occur during prolonged use. This may be restored by stopping the drug for a few days or by adjusting the dose.

NETILMICIN

Brand name Netromycin
Used in the following combined preparations None

GENERAL INFORMATION

Netilmicin, introduced in 1983, is one of the newest aminoglycoside antibiotics. Given by injection into a muscle or vein, it is rapidly absorbed into the body and is effective against a wide range of bacteria.

Netilmicin is reserved for the treatment of serious or complicated infections in the hospital. These include peritonitis, internal abscesses, septicemia, and severe infections of the lungs, skin, bones, joints, and urinary tract. It is often used when such conditions have failed to respond to other antibiotics, or when tests have shown resistance to other antibacterial drugs. It is frequently given in combination with other antibiotics to enhance their effects.

Like other aminoglycoside antibiotics, netilmicin can have serious adverse effects on the nerves to the ears – leading to damage to the balance mechanism and deafness – and on the kidneys. Treatment is monitored with particular care when high doses are needed or when kidney function is poor. The elderly and very young are also at particular risk from adverse effects when taking high doses.

INFORMATION FOR USERS

The drug is given only under medical supervision and is not for self-administration.

How taken

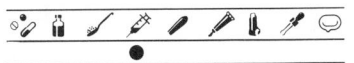

Injection.

Frequency and timing of doses
Every 8 – 12 hours.

Dosage range
Dosage is determined according to the individual's condition and response.

Onset of effect
1 – 2 days.

Duration of action
Up to 24 hours.

Diet advice
None.

Storage
Not applicable. The drug is not kept in the home.

Missed dose
Not applicable. The drug is given only under close medical supervision.

Stopping the drug
Not applicable. The drug will be stopped under medical supervision.

Exceeding the dose
Overdosage is unlikely, since treatment is carefully monitored.

SPECIAL PRECAUTIONS

Be sure to tell your physician if:
▼ You have impaired kidney function.
▼ You have a hearing disorder.
▼ You have myasthenia gravis or Parkinson's disease.
▼ You are taking other medications.

Pregnancy
▼ Not usually prescribed. Safety in pregnancy not established. Discuss with your physician so that you can weigh the benefits of the drug against its possible risks.

Breast feeding
▼ Discuss with your physician. The drug passes into the breast milk and may affect the baby adversely.

Infants and children
▼ Reduced dose necessary.

Over 60
▼ Reduced dose may be necessary. Increased likelihood of adverse effects.

Driving and hazardous work
▼ Not usually applicable but no known problems.

Alcohol
▼ No known problems.

Surgery and general anesthetics
▼ Netilmicin may need to be stopped before you have a general anesthetic. Discuss with your physician or dentist before any surgery.

POSSIBLE ADVERSE EFFECTS

Adverse effects are uncommon, but those that do occur may be serious. Such effects include damage to hearing or to the kidneys during treatment or after treatment is stopped. Dizziness, vertigo, or ringing in the ears, and any change in the frequency of urination or the appearance of the urine, should be reported without delay.

Symptom/effect	Frequency		Discuss with physician		Stop taking drug now	Call physician now
	Common	Rare	Only if severe	In all cases		
Vomiting/diarrhea	●		■			▮
Rash/itching	●			■		▮
Dizziness/vertigo	●			■		▮
Ringing in the ears	●			■		▮
Loss of hearing	●			■		▮
Bloody/cloudy urine	●			■		▮

INTERACTIONS

General note Many drugs increase the risk of hearing loss and/or kidney failure with netilmicin. Such drugs include other aminoglycosides, furosemide, polymyxin antibiotics, amphotericin B, cisplatin, and cyclosporine.

PROLONGED USE

Not usually given for longer than 14 days. There is a rare risk of adverse effects on hearing, balance, and kidney function.

Monitoring Kidney, hearing, and blood tests are needed.

NICLOSAMIDE

Brand name Niclocide
Used in the following combined preparations None

GENERAL INFORMATION

Niclosamide, introduced in 1982, is an anthelmintic used in the treatment of tapeworm infections of the intestine. Taken as chewable tablets, it kills the worms on contact, loosening their grip on the bowel wall so they can be passed in the bowel movements.

The dosage schedule prescribed depends on the type of infection. For beef, pork, and fish tapeworms, caused by eating raw or undercooked food, and for dog tapeworms, which infect mainly children via dog fleas, one dose only is generally sufficient.

In pork tapeworm infections, an antiemetic drug and a laxative may also be given to prevent any risk of cysticercosis, a potentially serious infection of many organs with immature, larval forms of the worm.

Dwarf tapeworm infections – the commonest type of tapeworm infections in the US, caused by fecal contamination of hands or food or contact with contaminated soil – are more resistant to the drug. Repeated courses of treatment may be necessary.

QUICK REFERENCE

Drug group Anthelmintic drug (p.167)

Overdose danger rating Low

Dependence rating Low

Prescription needed Yes

Available as generic No

INFORMATION FOR USERS

Your drug prescription is tailored for you. Do not alter dosage without checking with your physician.

How taken

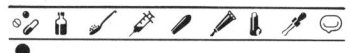

●

Tablets (to be chewed thoroughly).

Frequency and timing of doses
A single dose on an empty stomach before breakfast. Do not eat for 2 hours after.

Dosage range
Adults Usually 2g per dose. For multiple-day therapy, 1g may be given on the second or subsequent days.
Children over 2 years Reduced dose according to weight.

Onset of effect
2 – 4 hours.

Duration of action
2 – 3 days.

Diet advice
None.

Storage
Keep in a closed container in a cool, dry place away from reach of children.

Missed dose
If you are taking multiple-day therapy, take as soon as you remember, spacing the missed dose and the next dose 10 – 12 hours apart.

Stopping the drug
Complete the course of treatment as directed.

Exceeding the dose
An occasional unintentional extra dose is unlikely to be a cause for concern. But if you notice unusual symptoms, or if a large overdose has been taken, notify your physician.

POSSIBLE ADVERSE EFFECTS

Absorption of niclosamide is very slight, and serious side effects are unknown. Gastrointestinal upset, including loss of appetite, abdominal pain, and nausea, may occur on the day or days of treatment, but is usually short-lived.

Symptom/effect	Frequency		Discuss with physician		Stop taking drug now	Call physician now
	Common	Rare	Only if severe	In all cases		
Gastrointestinal upset	●		■			
Dizziness/lightheadedness		●	■			
Drowsiness		●	■			
Headache		●	■			
Anal itching		●	■			
Rash		●		■	▲	▮

INTERACTIONS

None.

SPECIAL PRECAUTIONS

Pregnancy
▼ Not usually prescribed. Safety in pregnancy not established. Discuss with your physician so that you can weigh the benefits of the drug against its possible risks.

Breast feeding
▼ No evidence of risk.

Infants and children
▼ Not recommended for children under 2 years. Reduced dose necessary for older children.

Over 60
▼ No special problems.

Driving and hazardous work
▼ Avoid such activities until you have learned how the drug affects you, because the drug can cause drowsiness and lightheadedness.

Alcohol
▼ No known problems.

PROLONGED USE

Not taken for prolonged periods.

NIFEDIPINE

Brand names Adalat, Procardia
Used in the following combined preparations None

GENERAL INFORMATION

Nifedipine, introduced in 1982, belongs to a group of drugs known as calcium channel blockers (p.130), which interfere with the conduction of signals in the muscles of the heart and blood vessels.

Nifedipine is used mainly in the treatment of angina, both as a regular medication to help prevent attacks and for the immediate relief of pain during an attack (see p.129). Unlike some other anti-angina drugs (i.e., beta blockers), it can be used safely by asthmatics and is often successful when other treatments have failed. Nifedipine is also widely used to reduce raised blood pressure, and is often helpful in improving circulation to the limbs (e.g., in Raynaud's disease).

In common with other drugs of its class, nifedipine may cause blood pressure to fall too low and may occasionally cause disturbances of heart rhythm. In rare cases, as a result of taking nifedipine, angina worsens, and the drug may increase susceptibility to heart failure and lead to the retention of fluid in body tissues.

QUICK REFERENCE

Drug group Anti-angina drug (p.129), antihypertensive drug (p.130)

Overdose danger rating Medium

Dependence rating Low

Prescription needed Yes

Available as generic No

INFORMATION FOR USERS

Your drug prescription is tailored for you. Do not alter dosage without checking with your physician.

How taken

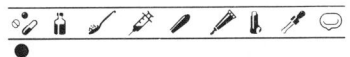

Capsules.

Frequency and timing of doses
Angina 3 x daily. For rapid relief of pain an additional capsule may be bitten open and the contents held in the mouth for a few moments.
High blood pressure 2 x daily.

Adult dosage range
30 – 60mg daily. Larger doses are sometimes prescribed.

Onset of effect
30 – 60 minutes. When capsules are bitten, beneficial effects may be felt within minutes.

Duration of action
8 – 12 hours.

Diet advice
None.

Storage
Keep in a closed container in a cool, dry place away from reach of children. Protect from light.

Missed dose
Take as soon as you remember, or when needed. If your next dose is due within 2 hours, take a single dose now and skip the next.

Stopping the drug
Do not stop the drug without consulting your physician; symptoms may recur.

Exceeding the dose
An occasional unintentional extra dose is unlikely to cause problems. Large over-doses may cause dizziness. Notify your physician.

SPECIAL PRECAUTIONS

Be sure to tell your physician if:
▼ You have impaired kidney or liver function.
▼ You have heart failure.
▼ You have diabetes.
▼ You are taking other medications.

 Pregnancy
▼ Not usually prescribed. Safety in pregnancy not established. Discuss with your physician so that you can weigh the benefits of the drug against its possible risks.

 Breast feeding
▼ Discuss with your physician. The drug passes into the breast milk and may affect the baby adversely.

 Infants and children
▼ Not recommended.

 Over 60
▼ Reduced dose may be necessary. Increased likelihood of adverse effects.

 Driving and hazardous work
▼ Avoid such activities until you have learned how the drug affects you, because the drug can cause dizziness owing to lowered blood pressure.

 Alcohol
▼ Avoid. Alcohol may further reduce blood pressure, causing dizziness or other symptoms.

PROLONGED USE

No problems expected.

POSSIBLE ADVERSE EFFECTS

Nifedipine can cause a variety of minor symptoms, including headache, dizziness, fatigue, and nausea. Dizziness, especially on rising, may be caused by an excessive reduction in blood pressure. The most serious effect is the rare possibility of angina becoming worse. An increase in the severity or frequency of attacks after starting nifedipine treatment should always be reported to your physician. This can sometimes be controlled by an adjustment in dosage, or a change of drug may be necessary.

Symptom/effect	Frequency		Discuss with physician		Stop taking drug now	Call physician now
	Common	Rare	Only if severe	In all cases		
Headache	●		■			
Dizziness/fatigue	●		■			
Flushing	●		■			
Leg cramps		●	■			
Nausea		●		■		
Increased angina		●		■	▲	▮

INTERACTIONS

Antihypertensive drugs Nifedipine may increase the effects of these drugs.

Digoxin Blood levels of digoxin may be increased when it is taken with nifedipine.

NITROFURANTOIN

Brand names Furadantin, Macrodantin
Used in the following combined preparations None

GENERAL INFORMATION

Nitrofurantoin, introduced in 1953, is a fast-acting antibacterial prescribed to treat urinary tract infections such as cystitis. It does not have any *systemic* effect, but reaches high levels in the urinary tract, where the bacteria are concentrated. Nitrofurantoin usually cures an infection within days.

Unfortunately, this drug produces adverse effects in about 10 percent of people taking it, the most common of

which is irritation of the stomach. This can be alleviated to a certain extent by taking the drug with food. Nitrofurantoin occasionally causes inflammation of the lungs and/or nervous system; it may also affect liver function, leading to jaundice. Serious adverse effects are much more likely in people with reduced kidney function, causing drug levels to build up in the body.

QUICK REFERENCE

Drug group Antibacterial drug (p.159)

Overdose danger rating Low

Dependence rating Low

Prescription needed Yes

Available as generic Yes

INFORMATION FOR USERS

Your drug prescription is tailored for you. Do not alter dosage without checking with your physician.

How taken

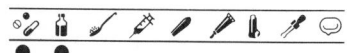

Tablets, capsules, liquid.

Frequency and timing of doses
3 – 4 x daily with food.

Dosage range
Adults 50 – 100mg daily at bedtime (prevention); 150 – 400mg daily (treatment).
Children Reduced dose necessary according to age and weight.

Onset of effect
20 – 30 minutes.

Duration of action
6 – 8 hours.

Diet advice
None.

Storage
Keep in a closed container in a cool, dry place away from reach of children. Protect from light.

Missed dose
Take as soon as you remember. If your next dose is due within 2 hours, take a single dose now and skip the next.

Stopping the drug
Take the full course. Even if you feel better the original infection may still be present, and symptoms may recur if treatment is stopped too soon.

Exceeding the dose
An occasional unintentional extra dose is unlikely to be a cause for concern. But if you notice unusual symptoms, or if a large overdose has been taken, notify your physician.

SPECIAL PRECAUTIONS

Be sure to tell your physician if:
▼ You have impaired kidney function.
▼ You have diabetes.
▼ You have anemia.
▼ You have a lung disorder.
▼ You have glucose-6-phosphate dehydrogenase (G6PD) deficiency.
▼ You are taking other medications.

Pregnancy
▼ Not usually prescribed. May cause blood disorders in the baby. Discuss with your physician so that you may weigh the benefits of the drug against its risks.

Breast feeding
▼ Discuss with your physician. The drug passes into the breast milk and may cause anemia in the baby.

Infants and children
▼ Not usually prescribed for infants. Reduced dose necessary in older children.

Over 60
▼ No special problems.

Driving and hazardous work
▼ No known problems.

Alcohol
▼ No known problems.

POSSIBLE ADVERSE EFFECTS

Nitrofurantoin has a number of serious adverse effects that may make it necessary to stop taking the drug. The more common adverse effects, such as loss of appetite, nausea, and vomiting, tend to diminish as your body adjusts to the drug.

Symptom/effect	Frequency		Discuss with physician		Stop taking drug now	Call physician now
	Common	Rare	Only if severe	In all cases		
Loss of appetite	●		■			
Nausea/vomiting	●		■			
Shortness of breath	●			■	▲	▮
Diarrhea		●	■			
Headache/dizziness		●		■		
Dark urine		●		■	▲	
Numb/tingling face		●		■	▲	
Unexplained fever		●		■	▲	

PROLONGED USE

Nitrofurantoin is not usually prescribed for long periods; it may produce changes in the lungs when taken over extended periods.

INTERACTIONS

Probenecid Probenecid may increase the risk of adverse effects when taken in conjunction with nitrofurantoin.

Nalidixic acid This reduces the antibacterial effect of nitrofurantoin.

NITROGLYCERIN

Brand names Nitro-bid, Nitrodisc, Nitro-Dur, Nitrostat, Transderm-Nitro
Used in the following combined preparations None

GENERAL INFORMATION

Introduced in the late 1800s, nitroglycerin (trinitrin) is one of the oldest drugs in continual use. It belongs to a group of vasodilator drugs called nitrates, which are used to relieve the pain of angina attacks. Nitroglycerin is not a cure for heart disease; it can only relieve symptoms, and it may have to be taken for long periods of time. Vasodilator drugs are sometimes used to lower blood pressure during surgery and in treatment for heart failure or shock.

Nitroglycerin acts very quickly but for a short time only. It may cause a variety of minor symptoms, such as flushing and headache, most of which can be controlled by adjusting the dosage. Nitroglycerin is best taken for the first time while you are sitting. Fainting may follow the drop in blood pressure.

QUICK REFERENCE

Drug group Anti-angina drug (p.129)
Overdose danger rating Medium
Dependence rating Low
Prescription needed Yes
Available as generic Yes

INFORMATION FOR USERS

Your drug prescription is tailored for you. Do not alter dosage without checking with your physician.

How taken

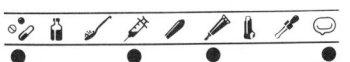

Tablets, capsules, injection, ointment, skin patches, sublingual spray.

Frequency and timing of doses
Angina attacks Use when necessary up to every 1 – 2 minutes until relief is obtained (sublingual tablets), but no more than 3 in 15 minutes, and no more than every 2 hours (buccal tablets).
To prevent angina attacks 3 x daily (buccal tablets), 2 – 3 x daily before meals (oral tablets), once daily (skin patches), 4 – 6 x hourly on chest, back, stomach, or thighs (ointment).

Adult dosage range
2.6 – 27mg daily (oral tablets), 0.15 – 0.6 mg per dose (sublingual), 1– 2 mg per dose (buccal), 1 – 2 inches of 2 percent ointment per dose (ointment), 1 patch daily (skin patches).

Onset of action
2 – 3 minutes (sublingual/buccal), 60 – 90 minutes (oral), 1 hour (ointment), 1 – 2 hours (patches).

Duration of effect
3 – 5 minutes (sublingual/buccal), 60 – 90 minutes (oral tablets), 1 hour (ointment), 1 – 2 hours (patches).

Diet advice
None.

Storage
Keep in a tightly closed container fitted with a metal screw-on cap in a cool, dry place away from reach of children. Protect from light. Do not expose to heat.

Missed dose
Take as soon as you remember, or when needed. If your next dose is due within 2 hours, take a single dose now and skip the next.

Stopping the drug
Do not stop taking the drug without consulting your physician.

Exceeding the dose
An occasional unintentional extra dose is unlikely to cause problems. Large overdoses may cause dizziness, vomiting, severe headache, seizures, or loss of consciousness. Notify your physician.

SPECIAL PRECAUTIONS

Be sure to tell your physician if:
▼ You have any blood disorders.
▼ You have had glaucoma.
▼ You have thyroid disease.
▼ You are taking other medications.

Pregnancy
▼ Not usually prescribed. Safety in pregnancy not established. Discuss with your physician so that you can weigh the benefits of the drug against its possible risks.

Breast feeding
▼ Discuss with your physician. Effects on breast milk are uncertain.

Infants and children
▼ Not usually prescribed.

Over 60
▼ No special problems.

Driving and hazardous work
▼ Avoid such activities until you have learned how the drug affects you, because the drug can cause dizziness.

Alcohol
▼ Never drink while under treatment with nitroglycerin. Alcohol may increase dizziness due to lowered blood pressure.

POSSIBLE ADVERSE EFFECTS

The most serious adverse effect is lowered blood pressure, and this should be monitored on a regular basis. Other adverse effects usually disappear after use on a regular basis, and they can also be controlled by an adjustment in dosage.

Symptom/effect	Frequency		Discuss with physician		Stop taking drug now	Call physician now
	Common	Rare	Only if severe	In all cases		
Headache	●		■			
Flushing	●		■			
Dizziness	●			■		

PROLONGED USE

The effects of the drug usually become slightly weaker during prolonged use as the body adapts.

Monitoring Periodic checks on blood pressure are usually required.

INTERACTIONS

Antihypertensive drugs These drugs increase the possibility of lowered blood pressure when taken with nitroglycerin.

Sympathomimetics Because of their effect on the central nervous system, these drugs reduce the effect of nitroglycerin.

NORGESTREL

Brand name Ovrette
Used in the following combined preparations Lo/Ovral, Ovral

GENERAL INFORMATION

Introduced in 1968 and an active ingredient in many oral contraceptives, norgestrel is a progestin, a synthetic hormone similar to a natural female sex hormone, progesterone. Its contraceptive action is to thicken the mucus at the neck of the uterus (cervix), thereby preventing sperm from entering the uterus and reaching the fallopian tubes, where the egg is fertilized.

Norgestrel is available in progestin-only preparations and in combined oral contraceptives with an estrogen drug.

Norgestrel is occasionally given with an estrogen for emergency, post-coital contraception to rape victims. Nausea and vomiting are less likely than with estrogen alone in such cases, and treatment is completed in one day rather than five.

Norgestrel rarely causes serious adverse effects, although menstrual irregularities – particularly mid-cycle or "breakthrough" bleeding – are common.

INFORMATION FOR USERS

Your drug prescription is tailored for you. Do not alter dosage without checking with your physician.

How taken

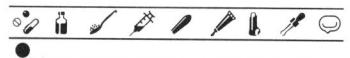

Tablets.

Frequency and timing of doses
Once daily, at the same time each day. For post-coital contraception, 2 doses are taken 12 hours apart.

Adult dosage range
Progestin-only pills 75 mcg daily.

Onset of effect
Norgestrel starts to act within 4 hours, but contraceptive protection may not be fully effective for 14 days.

Duration of action
24 hours. Some effects may persist for up to 3 months after norgestrel is stopped.

Diet advice
None.

Storage
Keep in a closed container in a cool, dry place away from reach of children.

Missed dose
See What to do if you miss a pill, p.191.

Stopping the drug
The drug can be safely stopped as soon as contraceptive protection is no longer required.

Exceeding the dose
An occasional unintentional extra dose is unlikely to be a cause for concern. But if you notice unusual symptoms, or if a large overdose has been taken, notify your physician.

POSSIBLE ADVERSE EFFECTS

Menstrual irregularities (blood spotting between menstrual periods or absence of menstruation) are the most common side effects of norgestrel alone. Other adverse effects, such as nausea and fluid retention (leading to weight gain or swollen feet and ankles), occur more frequently with combined contraceptive pills.

Symptom/effect	Frequency		Discuss with physician		Stop taking drug now	Call physician now
	Common	Rare	Only if severe	In all cases		
Swollen feet/ankles	●		■			
Weight gain	●		■			
Irregular vaginal bleeding	●			■		
Nausea/vomiting		●	■			
Breast tenderness		●	■			
Depression		●		■		
Headache		●		■		

INTERACTIONS

General note Norgestrel may interfere with the beneficial effects of many drugs, including bromocriptine, oral anticoagulant, anticonvulsant, antihypertensive, and antidiabetic drugs. Many other drugs may affect the action of oral contraceptives, possibly leading to reduction of contraceptive protection. These include certain anticonvulsant and antituberculous drugs, antibiotics, and migraine preparations. Be sure to inform your physician that you are taking this drug before taking additional prescribed medication.

SPECIAL PRECAUTIONS

Be sure to tell your physician if:
▼ You have impaired liver function.
▼ You have heart failure or high blood pressure.
▼ You have diabetes.
▼ You have had blood clots or a stroke.
▼ You are taking other medications.

 Pregnancy
▼ Not prescribed. May cause abnormalities in the developing baby.

 Breast feeding
▼ The drug passes into the breast milk, but at normal doses adverse effects on the baby are uncommon. Discuss with your physician.

 Infants and children
▼ Not prescribed.

 Over 60
▼ Not prescribed.

 Driving and hazardous work
▼ No known problems.

 Alcohol
▼ No known problems.

PROLONGED USE

Problems are rare.

NYSTATIN

Brand names Mycostatin, Mykinac, Nilstat, Nystex, O-V Statin
Used in the following combined preparation Mycolog II

GENERAL INFORMATION

Introduced in 1954, the antifungal drug nystatin was named after the New York State Institute of Health, where it was developed.

It is effective against candidiasis (thrush), an infection caused by the Candida yeast. Available in a variety of dosage forms, it is used to treat infections of the skin, mouth, throat, esophagus, and vagina. Poorly absorbed from the digestive tract into the bloodstream, it is of little use against *systemic* infections. It is not given by injection.

In the form of eye drops, ointment, or powder, it is also used to combat eye infections caused by Candida and another organism, Aspergillus. Resistance to nystatin is unknown. It rarely causes adverse effects and can be safely used during pregnancy to treat vaginal candidiasis.

QUICK REFERENCE

Drug group Antifungal drug (p.166)
Overdose danger rating Low
Dependence rating Low
Prescription needed Yes
Available as generic Yes

INFORMATION FOR USERS

Your drug prescription is tailored for you. Do not alter dosage without checking with your physician.

How taken

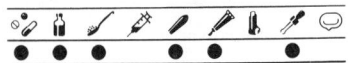

● ● ● ● ● ●

Tablets, liquid, powder, vaginal suppositories, cream, ointment, eye drops.

Frequency and timing of doses
Mouth or throat infections 3 – 4 x daily for 2 weeks. Tablets or liquid should be held in the mouth for several minutes before swallowing.
Skin and nail infections 2 – 4 x daily for 2 – 4 weeks.
Vaginal infections 1 – 2 x daily for 2 weeks, then once at night for 2 – 3 weeks.
Eye infections Every 15 minutes or 4 x daily (as directed).

Adult dosage range
1.5 million – 3 million units daily (by mouth); 100,000 – 200,000 units daily (vaginal suppositories); as directed (skin and eye preparations).

Onset of effect
1 – 3 days. Full beneficial effect may not be felt for 7 – 14 days.

Duration of action
Up to 6 hours.

Diet advice
None.

Storage
Keep in a closed container in a cool, dry place away from reach of children. Protect from light.

Missed dose
Take as soon as you remember. Take your next dose as usual.

Stopping the drug
Take the full course. Even if the affected area seems to be cured, the original infection may still be present, and symptoms may recur if treatment is stopped too soon.

Exceeding the dose
An occasional unintentional extra dose is unlikely to be a cause for concern. But if you notice unusual symptoms, or if a large overdose has been taken, notify your physician.

SPECIAL PRECAUTIONS

Pregnancy
▼ No evidence of risk to developing baby.

Breast feeding
▼ No evidence of risk.

Infants and children
▼ Reduced dose necessary.

Over 60
▼ No special problems.

Driving and hazardous work
▼ No known problems.

Alcohol
▼ No known problems.

POSSIBLE ADVERSE EFFECTS

Adverse effects are uncommon, and are usually mild and transient. Nausea, vomiting, and abdominal pain may occur with high doses of nystatin taken by mouth.

Symptom/effect	Frequency		Discuss with physician		Stop taking drug now	Call physician now
	Common	Rare	Only if severe	In all cases		
Diarrhea		●	■			
Nausea/vomiting		●	■			
Abdominal pain		●	■			
Local irritation		●		■	▲	▮

INTERACTIONS

None.

PROLONGED USE

No problems expected.

ORPHENADRINE

Brand names Disipal, Flexoject, Marflex, Norflex, X-Otag
Used in the following combined preparations Norgesic, Norgesic Forte

GENERAL INFORMATION

Orphenadrine, introduced in 1957, is a muscle relaxant chemically related to the antihistamines. It is used primarily to relieve the pain and discomfort of muscle spasm, sprains, and strains. In these conditions, drug treatment is usually accompanied by rest and some form of heat, such as an electric pad. Its mechanism of action is not clearly known but may be related to its sedative and analgesic properties, since orphenadrine does not affect muscle directly.

By its *anticholinergic* action, orphenadrine is also used to reduce muscle rigidity in Parkinson's disease. However, it has little effect on the slowing of movement or tremor that are prominent features of this condition; they are usually treated with other drugs.

INFORMATION FOR USERS

Your drug prescription is tailored for you. Do not alter dosage without checking with your physician.

How taken

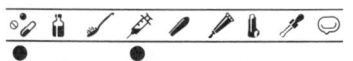

Tablets, slow-release tablets, injection.

Frequency and timing of doses
2 – 3 x daily.

Dosage range
120 – 200mg daily.

Onset of effect
Within 60 minutes (tablets); within 5 minutes (injection).

Duration of action
8 – 12 hours.

Diet advice
None.

Storage
Keep in a closed container in a cool, dry place away from reach of children. Protect from light.

Missed dose
Take as soon as you remember. If your next dose is due within 2 hours, take a single dose now and skip the next.

Stopping the drug
Do not stop the drug without consulting your physician; symptoms may recur.

OVERDOSE ACTION

Seek immediate medical advice in all cases. Take emergency action if palpitations, seizures, or loss of consciousness occurs.

See Drug poisoning emergency guide (p.590).

SPECIAL PRECAUTIONS

Be sure to tell your physician if:
▼ You have impaired kidney or liver function.
▼ You have heart problems.
▼ You have had glaucoma.
▼ You have difficulty passing urine.
▼ You have had peptic ulcers.
▼ You have myasthenia gravis.
▼ You are taking other medications.

Pregnancy
▼ Not usually prescribed. Safety in pregnancy not established. Discuss with your physician so that you can weigh the benefits of the drug against its possible risks.

Breast feeding
▼ Discuss with your physician. The drug may pass into the breast milk and may affect the baby adversely.

Infants and children
▼ Not recommended.

Over 60
▼ Reduced dose may be necessary. Increased likelihood of adverse effects.

Driving and hazardous work
▼ Avoid such activities until you have learned how the drug affects you, because the drug can cause dizziness and lightheadedness.

Alcohol
▼ Avoid. Alcohol may increase the sedative effects of this drug.

Surgery and general anesthetics
▼ Orphenadrine may need to be stopped before you have a general anesthetic. Discuss this with your physician or dentist before any surgery.

POSSIBLE ADVERSE EFFECTS

The adverse effects of orphenadrine are similar to those of other anticholinergic drugs. The more common symptoms, such as dryness of the mouth and blurred vision, can often be overcome by an adjustment in dosage.

Symptom/effect	Frequency		Discuss with physician		Stop taking drug now	Call physician now
	Common	Rare	Only if severe	In all cases		
Dry mouth/skin	●		■			
Difficulty passing urine	●		■			
Constipation	●		■			
Dizziness	●		■			
Blurred vision	●			■		
Confusion/agitation		●		■		
Rash/itching		●		■	▲	
Palpitations		●		■	▲	∎

INTERACTIONS

Anticholinergic drugs The anticholinergic effects of orphenadrine are likely to be increased by these drugs.

Propoxyphene Confusion, anxiety, and tremors may occur if this drug is given together with orphenadrine.

Sedatives The effects of all drugs that have a sedative effect on the central nervous system are likely to be increased with orphenadrine.

PROLONGED USE

No problems expected. Effectiveness in treating Parkinson's disease may diminish with time.

OXANDROLONE

Brand name Anavar
Used in the following combined preparations None

GENERAL INFORMATION

Introduced in 1964, oxandrolone is an anabolic steroid, a synthetic hormone related to the male sex hormone testosterone. It has a number of uses. It is prescribed to encourage growth in children whose development has been delayed by male hormone disturbances. Some claim its usefulness in helping people who have lost weight after a major illness or injury. Oxandrolone is also sometimes prescribed to reduce the levels of fat in the blood in a hereditary blood disorder called hypertriglyceridemia.

Risking suspension or disqualification by leading athletic organizations, some athletes have taken oxandrolone or other anabolic steroids to increase body weight and muscle strength. Authoritative medical studies have, however, raised questions about the validity of such results.

The main advantage that oxandrolone has over some other anabolic steroids is that it can be taken by mouth.

Most side effects of oxandrolone occur only rarely. However, swollen feet and ankles and, in women, irregular periods, are fairly common.

QUICK REFERENCE

Drug group Anabolic steroid (p.174)
Overdose danger rating Low
Dependence rating Low
Prescription needed Yes
Available as generic No

INFORMATION FOR USERS

Your drug prescription is tailored for you. Do not alter dosage without checking with your physician.

How taken

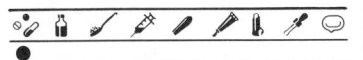

Tablets.

Frequency and timing of doses
2 – 4 x daily.

Dosage range
Adults 5 – 10 mg daily.
Children Reduced dose according to age and weight.

Onset of effect
Within 4 hours.

Duration of action
Several days.

Diet advice
Drug treatment needs to be accompanied by a nourishing diet. Excessive protein intake may cause a buildup of nitrogen waste in the body. Your physician will give detailed advice.

Storage
Keep in a closed container in a cool, dry place away from reach of children.

Missed dose
No cause for concern, but take as soon as you remember. If your next dose is due within 3 hours, take a single dose now and skip the next.

Stopping the drug
There are no harmful effects if the drug is suddenly stopped.

Exceeding the dose
An occasional unintentional extra dose is unlikely to be a cause for concern. But if you notice unusual symptoms, or if a large overdose has been taken, notify your physician.

SPECIAL PRECAUTIONS

Be sure to tell your physician if:
▼ You have impaired kidney or liver function.
▼ You have prostate trouble.
▼ You have diabetes.
▼ You are taking other medications.

Pregnancy
▼ Not prescribed.

Breast feeding
▼ Not prescribed.

Infants and children
▼ Reduced dose necessary.

Over 60
▼ Reduced dose may be necessary. Increased risk of prostate problems.

Driving and hazardous work
▼ No known problems.

Alcohol
▼ No known problems.

POSSIBLE ADVERSE EFFECTS

Most of the more serious adverse effects are likely to occur only with long-term treatment with oxandrolone, and may be helped by a reduction in dosage.

Symptom/effect	Frequency		Discuss with physician		Stop taking drug now	Call physician now
	Common	Rare	Only if severe	In all cases		
Swollen feet/ankles	●		■			
Nausea/vomiting		●	■			
Jaundice		●		■	▲	▮
Men only						
Difficulty passing urine		●		■	▲	▮
Women only						
Irregular menstruation	●			■		

INTERACTIONS

Anticoagulant drugs Oxandrolone increases the effects of these drugs. Anticoagulant dosage may need to be adjusted.

Antidiabetic drugs Because oxandrolone lowers the sugar level in the blood, the dosage of antidiabetic drugs may need to be reduced.

PROLONGED USE

Prolonged use of this drug may lead to early stopping of growth in children and menstrual disorders in women. Long-term use may also raise cholesterol levels, thereby increasing the chances of coronary heart disease. Because the benefits are doubtful, athletes taking anabolic steroids over long periods of time run a needless risk.

Monitoring Periodic checks on the level of salts and calcium in the blood are usually needed.

OXAZEPAM

Brand name Serax
Used in the following combined preparations None

GENERAL INFORMATION

Introduced in 1965, oxazepam belongs to a group of drugs known as the benzodiazepines. These drugs help to relieve nervousness and tension, relax muscles, and encourage sleep. Their actions and adverse effects are described more fully on p.111.

Oxazepam is used to treat anxiety and insomnia. Although it does not have a rapid onset of effect, it is relatively long-acting. For this reason, it is more effective for treating early

waking than for difficulty falling asleep. Oxazepam is less likely than similar drugs to accumulate in the body, making it especially useful for people with impaired liver function.

In common with other benzodiazepines, oxazepam can be habit-forming if taken regularly over a long period. Its effects may also become weaker with time. For these reasons, treatment with oxazepam should be limited to a few weeks and then reviewed.

QUICK REFERENCE

Drug group Benzodiazepine anti-anxiety drug (p.111)

Overdose danger rating Medium

Dependence rating High

Prescription needed Yes CIV

Available as generic Yes

INFORMATION FOR USERS

Your drug prescription is tailored for you. Do not alter dosage without checking with your physician.

How taken

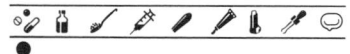

Tablets, capsules.

Frequency and timing of doses
3 – 4 x daily with food or milk.

Adult dosage range
Anxiety 30 – 120mg daily.
Insomnia 45 – 120mg daily.

Onset of effect
1 – 2 hours.

Duration of action
Up to 12 hours.

Diet advice
None.

Storage
Keep in a closed container in a cool, dry place away from reach of children.

Missed dose
If you are taking the drug once daily for insomnia, a missed dose is no cause for concern. Return to your normal dose schedule the following night, if necessary. Otherwise, take the missed dose when you remember. If your next dose is due within 2 hours, take a single dose now and skip the next.

Stopping the drug
If you have been taking the drug continuously for less than 2 weeks, it can be safely stopped as soon as you feel you no longer need it. However, if you have been taking it for longer, consult your physician, who will supervise a gradual reduction in dosage. Stopping abruptly may lead to withdrawal symptoms.

Exceeding the dose
An occasional unintentional extra dose is unlikely to cause problems. Larger over-doses may cause unusual drowsiness. Notify your physician.

SPECIAL PRECAUTIONS

Be sure to tell your physician if:
▼ You have impaired kidney function.
▼ You have had problems with alcohol or drug abuse.
▼ You are taking other medications.

 Pregnancy
▼ Not usually prescribed. Safety in pregnancy not established. Discuss with your physician so that you can weigh the benefits of the drug against its possible risks.

 Breast feeding
▼ Discuss with your physician. The drug passes into the breast milk and may affect the baby adversely.

 Infants and children
▼ Not prescribed for children under 6 years. Dosage uncertain for older children.

 Over 60
▼ Reduced dose may be necessary. Increased likelihood of adverse effects.

 Driving and hazardous work
▼ Avoid such activities until you have learned how the drug affects you, because the drug can cause reduced alertness and slowed reactions.

 Alcohol
▼ Avoid. Alcohol increases the sedative effects of this drug.

POSSIBLE ADVERSE EFFECTS

The principal adverse effects of this drug are related to its sedative and tranquilizing properties. These effects normally diminish after the first few days of treatment.

Symptom/effect	Frequency		Discuss with physician		Stop taking drug now	Call physician now
	Common	Rare	Only if severe	In all cases		
Daytime drowsiness	●		■			
Dizziness/unsteadiness	●		■			
Headache		●	■			
Blurred vision		●	■			
Forgetfulness/confusion		●		■		▍
Rash		●		■	▲	▍

INTERACTIONS

Sedatives All drugs that have a sedative effect on the central nervous system are likely to increase the sedative properties of oxazepam.

Alcohol Alcohol should be avoided because it increases the sedative effect of oxazepam, making you feel drowsy.

PROLONGED USE

Regular use of this drug over several weeks can lead to a reduction in its effect as the body adapts. It may also be habit-forming when taken for extended periods, especially if larger than average doses are taken.

432

OXTRIPHYLLINE

Brand names Choledyl, Choledyl SA
Used in the following combined preparation Brondecon

GENERAL INFORMATION

Introduced in 1954, oxtriphylline belongs to the xanthine group of bronchodilating drugs that widen the airways to the lungs. It is closely related to theophylline, and breaks down into theophylline in the body.

Oxtriphylline is mainly used to ease breathing in bronchial disease, especially asthma. It is available as tablets or liquid medicine, and is included in a combined preparation with guaifenesin, an expectorant (see Drugs to treat coughs, p.122).

Since there is a relatively narrow margin between the dose required for a beneficial effect and that producing a *toxic* effect, careful monitoring of blood levels of theophylline is usually required. The likelihood of adverse effects such as nausea, vomiting, and headache can be reduced by checking blood levels and correcting the dose.

QUICK REFERENCE

Drug group Bronchodilator (p.120)
Overdose danger rating High
Dependence rating Low
Prescription needed Yes
Available as generic Yes

INFORMATION FOR USERS

Your drug prescription is tailored for you. Do not alter dosage without checking with your physician.

How taken

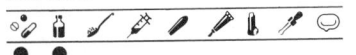

Tablets, syrup.

Frequency and timing of doses
Every 6 – 8 hours during or after meals; or every 12 or 24 hours if taken as timed-release tablets.

Dosage range
Adults 400 – 1600mg daily.
Children Reduced dose necessary according to age and weight.

Onset of effect
Within 1 – 2 hours.

Duration of action
About 8 hours; 12 – 24 hours (timed-release tablets).

Diet advice
Avoid charcoal-broiled foods, because these may reduce the effectiveness of the drug.

Storage
Keep in a closed container in a cool, dry place away from reach of children. Protect from light.

Missed dose
Take as soon as you remember. If your next dose is due within 2 hours, take half the dose (short-acting preparations) or forget about the missed dose and take your next dose now (long-acting preparations). Return to your normal dose schedule thereafter.

Stopping the drug
Do not stop the drug without consulting your physician; stopping the drug may lead to worsening of the underlying condition.

OVERDOSE ACTION

Seek immediate medical advice in all cases. Take emergency action if confusion, chest pains, palpitations, seizures, or loss of consciousness occurs.

See Drug poisoning emergency guide (p.590).

SPECIAL PRECAUTIONS

Be sure to tell your physician if:
▼ You have impaired liver function.
▼ You have angina or irregular heartbeat.
▼ You have peptic ulcers.
▼ You smoke.
▼ You are taking other medications.

Pregnancy
▼ Not usually prescribed. Safety in pregnancy not established. Discuss with your physician so that you can weigh the benefits of the drug against its possible risks.

Breast feeding
▼ Discuss with your physician. The drug passes into the breast milk and may cause irritability in the baby.

Infants and children
▼ Reduced dose necessary.

Over 60
▼ Reduced dose may be necessary. Increased risk of adverse effects.

Driving and hazardous work
▼ Avoid such activities until you have learned how the drug affects you, because the drug can cause dizziness.

Alcohol
▼ No known problems.

PROLONGED USE

No problems expected.

Monitoring Periodic checks on blood levels of theophylline are usually required.

POSSIBLE ADVERSE EFFECTS

The common adverse effects usually indicate that the dosage is too high. They usually diminish when dosage is reduced, although nausea may remain a problem.

Symptom/effect	Frequency		Discuss with physician		Stop taking drug now	Call physician now
	Common	Rare	Only if severe	In all cases		
Nausea/vomiting	●		■			
Agitation	●			■		
Dizziness	●			■		
Palpitations		●		■	▲	▮
Seizures		●		■	▲	▮

INTERACTIONS

Erythromycin, cimetidine, influenza vaccine, some antibiotics, allopurinol, beta blockers These drugs increase the effects of oxtriphylline.

Carbamazepine, phenytoin, rifampin, sulfinpyrazone, phenobarbital, nicotine These reduce the effects of oxtriphylline.

OXYMETAZOLINE

Brand names Afrin, Afrin Pediatric, Dristan Long Lasting, Neo Synephrine 12 Hour, Nostrilla
Used in the following combined preparations None

GENERAL INFORMATION

Oxymetazoline is an over-the-counter decongestant that relieves the symptoms of hay fever, sinusitis, and head colds. By constricting the small blood vessels in the nose, it reduces swelling and congestion in the nasal passages.

Because oxymetazoline has a longer-lasting effect than other decongestants, it needs to be taken only twice daily. However, it should not be used for more than a few days at a time, since prolonged use can lead to a rebound of nasal congestion and stuffiness.

Although side effects are milder than with some other decongestants, care should be taken not to exceed the recommended dose; this may cause discomfort in the nasal passages.

QUICK REFERENCE

Drug group Decongestant (p.121)
Overdose danger rating Medium
Dependence rating Low
Prescription needed No
Available as generic No

INFORMATION FOR USERS

Follow instructions on the label. Call your physician if symptoms worsen.

How taken

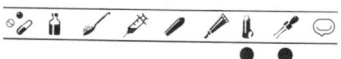

Spray, nose drops.

Frequency and timing of doses
2 x daily, early in the morning and at bedtime.

Dosage range
Adults and children over 6 years 2 – 4 drops or 1 – 2 sprays in each nostril.
Children 2 –5 years 2 – 3 drops in each nostril.

Onset of effect
Within 5 – 10 minutes.

Duration of action
Up to 12 hours.

Diet advice
None.

Storage
Keep in a closed container in a cool, dry place away from reach of children.

Missed dose
No cause for concern. If still needed, take your next dose as usual.

Stopping the drug
Can be safely stopped as soon as you no longer need it. Seek medical advice if symptoms persist for more than a few days.

Exceeding the dose
An occasional unintentional extra dose is unlikely to cause problems. Large overdoses may cause palpitations, headache, or sleeplessness. Notify your physician.

SPECIAL PRECAUTIONS

Be sure to consult your physician before using this drug if:
▼ You have high blood pressure.
▼ You have an overactive thyroid.
▼ You are taking other medications.

Pregnancy
▼ No evidence of risk to developing baby.

Breast feeding
▼ The drug passes into the breast milk, but at normal doses adverse effects on the baby are uncommon. Discuss with your physician.

Infants and children
▼ Reduced dose necessary in older children. Not recommended for children under 2 years.

Over 60
▼ No special problems.

Driving and hazardous work
▼ No special problems.

Alcohol
▼ No known problems.

POSSIBLE ADVERSE EFFECTS

The adverse effects of oxymetazoline are milder than those of many other drugs of the same group. Also, this drug does not have any effect on the central nervous system.

Symptom/effect	Frequency		Discuss with physician		Stop taking drug now	Call physician now
	Common	Rare	Only if severe	In all cases		
Nasal congestion	●		■			
Sneezing		●	■			
Dizziness		●		■		
Lightheadedness		●		■		
Palpitations		●		■	▲	
Headache		●		■	▲	
Sleeplessness		●		■	▲	

INTERACTIONS

Antihypertensive drugs Oxymetazoline may interact with these drugs to reverse their effect.

Monoamine oxidase inhibitors (MAOIs) These drugs may interact with oxymetazoline to raise the blood pressure level.

PROLONGED USE

Prolonged use of this drug may lead to worsening of the condition. Courses of longer than a few days are not recommended.

OXYTETRACYCLINE

Brand name Terramycin
Used in the following combined preparations Terra-Cortril Ophthalmic, Terramycin with Polymyxin, Urobiotic

GENERAL INFORMATION

Introduced in 1950, oxytetracycline, a member of the tetracycline group of drugs, is among the most commonly prescribed antibiotics.

Like other tetracyclines, it is effective for certain types of pneumonia, including those caused by psittacosis or Mycoplasma bacteria. Several sexually transmitted diseases such as syphilis, gonorrhea, and non-specific urethritis are also treated with oxytetracycline. Some people with chronic bronchitis are given oxytetracycline to control or prevent chest infections. One of the most common uses for

oxytetracycline is in the long-term treatment of acne.

Such rare infections as certain types of septic arthritis, cholera, trachoma, Rocky Mountain spotted fever, relapsing fever, and brucellosis may also be treated with oxytetracycline.

The most frequent side effects are nausea, vomiting, and diarrhea. Oxytetracycline may discolor developing teeth if taken by children or by the mother during pregnancy. The drug is not prescribed for people with poor kidney function because it can worsen the condition.

QUICK REFERENCE

Drug group Tetracycline antibiotic (p.158)

Overdose danger rating Low

Dependence rating Low

Prescription needed Yes

Available as generic Yes

INFORMATION FOR USERS

Your drug prescription is tailored for you. Do not alter dosage without checking with your physician.

How taken

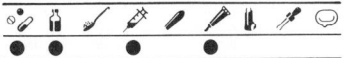

Tablets, capsules, liquid, injection, ointment.

Frequency and timing of doses
2 – 4 x daily, at least 1 hour before or 2 hours after meals. Long-term treatment of acne may require only a single dose every 2 days.

Adult dosage range
1 – 2g daily (by mouth).

Onset of effect
2 – 5 days (infections); 4 weeks (acne).

Duration of action
Up to 12 hours.

Diet advice
Milk products and antacids may impair absorption. Avoid from one hour before to one hour after dosage.

Storage
Keep in a closed container in a cool, dry place away from reach of children.

Missed dose
Take as soon as you remember. If your next dose is due within 2 hours, take a single dose now and skip the next.

Stopping the drug
Take the full course. Even if you feel better, the original infection may still be present and symptoms may recur if treatment is stopped too soon.

Exceeding the dose
An occasional unintentional extra dose is unlikely to be a cause for concern. But if you notice unusual symptoms, or if a large overdose has been taken, notify your physician.

SPECIAL PRECAUTIONS

Be sure to tell your physician if:
▼ You have impaired kidney function.
▼ You have previously suffered an allergic reaction to a tetracycline antibiotic.
▼ You are taking other medications.

 Pregnancy
▼ Not usually prescribed. May discolor the teeth of the developing baby. Discuss with your physician so that you may weigh the benefits of the drug against its risks.

 Breast feeding
▼ Discuss with your physician. The drug passes into the breast milk and may lead to discoloration of the baby's teeth.

 Infants and children
▼ Not recommended for children under 8 years. Reduced dose necessary for older children.

 Over 60
▼ No special problems.

 Driving and hazardous work
▼ No known problems.

 Alcohol
▼ No known problems.

POSSIBLE ADVERSE EFFECTS

Oxytetracycline may occasionally cause nausea, vomiting, or diarrhea. Other less common adverse effects are rashes and increased sensitivity of the skin to sunlight.

Symptom/effect	Frequency		Discuss with physician		Stop taking drug now	Call physician now
	Common	Rare	Only if severe	In all cases		
Nausea/vomiting	●		■			
Diarrhea	●		■			
Light-sensitive rash		●		■	▲	❙
Rash/itching		●		■	▲	❙

PROLONGED USE

No problems expected.

INTERACTIONS

Oral anticoagulant drugs Oxytetracycline increases anticoagulant action.

Oral contraceptives Oxytetracycline can reduce the effectiveness of oral contraceptives.

Iron may reduce the effectiveness of oxytetracycline.

Lithium Oxytetracycline may increase blood levels of lithium, leading to a risk of serious adverse effects.

Penicillins Oxytetracycline interferes with the antibacterial action of penicillins.

Antacids Antacids interfere with the absorption of oxytetracycline.

A B C D E F G H I J K L M N O P Q R S T U V W X Y Z

OXYTOCIN

Brand names Pitocin, Syntocinon
Used in the following combined preparations None

GENERAL INFORMATION

Oxytocin is a hormone secreted by the pituitary gland. It causes contraction of the uterus during labor and stimulates the flow of milk in nursing mothers. Introduced as a drug in 1957, it is used to induce labor when this is overdue or when other medical problems make early delivery necessary. It may also be given to stimulate labor when contractions are weak or absent and to help expel the placenta after birth. It is also given to expel the contents of the uterus after an incomplete miscarriage or a fetal death. Given after delivery, it makes the uterine muscles contract, thereby controlling bleeding. A nasal spray is occasionally prescribed to stimulate the flow of milk (the "let down" reflex) at

the start of breast feeding.

Though the procedure has been largely superseded by electronic monitoring, oxytocin is still sometimes used to test the well-being of the fetus of a mother at high risk because of diabetes or high blood pressure. In such cases the response of the baby's heart rate to the drug-induced contractions is monitored. If there are difficulties, labor may be induced or a cesarean section performed.

Oxytocin does not usually cause troublesome side effects for mother or baby. However, induced labor may be more painful because the contractions are more powerful. For that reason, dosage is carefully controlled to avoid excessively strong contractions.

QUICK REFERENCE

Drug group Uterine stimulant used in labor (p.193)

Overdose danger rating Medium

Dependence rating Low

Prescription needed Yes

Available as generic Yes

INFORMATION FOR USERS

Your drug prescription is tailored for you. Do not alter dosage without checking with your physician.

How taken

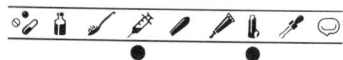

Injection, nasal spray.

Frequency and timing of doses
Continuously during labor (injection); 2 – 3 minutes before nursing to stimulate milk flow (nasal spray).

Adult dosage range
Dosage is determined by individual response (injection); spray in one or both nostrils before nursing (nasal spray).

Onset of effect
Within 10 minutes.

Duration of action
20 minutes (nasal spray); up to 1 hour (injection).

Diet advice
None.

Storage
Not applicable. The drug is not kept in the home.

Missed dose
Not applicable. The drug is given only in the hospital under medical supervision.

Stopping the drug
Not applicable. The drug is stopped as soon as regular strong contractions of the uterus are established.

Exceeding the dose
Overdosage by injection is unlikely, since treatment is carefully monitored. An occasional unintentional extra dose of nasal spray is no cause for concern.

SPECIAL PRECAUTIONS

Be sure to tell your physician if:
▼ You have high blood pressure.
▼ You have heart disease.
▼ You have had a previous difficult delivery or a cesarean section.
▼ You have had an operation on the uterus.
▼ You are taking other medications.

 Pregnancy
▼ Not usually prescribed in early or mid-pregnancy. Used for induction of labor and for testing the well-being of the baby under medical supervision.

 Breast feeding
▼ No evidence of risk.

 Infants and children
▼ Not prescribed.

 Over 60
▼ Not prescribed.

 Driving and hazardous work
▼ Not applicable.

 Alcohol
▼ Not applicable.

POSSIBLE ADVERSE EFFECTS

Oxytocin does not usually cause lasting adverse effects on mother or baby. The major adverse effect is an increase in the strength and frequency of contractions of

the uterus. Additional pain relief may be needed. Since the drug is only given in the hospital, all adverse effects are closely monitored and quickly dealt with.

Symptom/effect	Frequency		Discuss with physician		Stop taking drug now	Call physician now
	Common	Rare	Only if severe	In all cases		
Nausea/vomiting		●	■			
Painful spasm of the uterus		●		■		
Palpitations		●		■		
Seizures/coma		●		■		■

INTERACTIONS

None.

PROLONGED USE

Not used for prolonged periods.

PAPAVERINE

Brand names Cerespan, Myobid, Pavabid, Pavabid - HP, Pavagen
Used in the following combined preparations None

GENERAL INFORMATION

Introduced in 1937, papaverine is sometimes prescribed as a vasodilator to widen blood vessels and improve the circulation. Papaverine has been prescribed to treat peripheral vascular disease (reduced blood supply to the lower limbs) and transient ischemic attacks (temporarily reduced blood flow to the brain), although there is no conclusive evidence for its effectiveness. In higher doses, papaverine has been used to correct certain types of irregular heartbeat (arrhythmias).

Papaverine has largely been superseded by more effective drugs and is only rarely prescribed nowadays. It may cause side effects such as nausea, loss of appetite, and abdominal pain. Drowsiness, rash, and jaundice may also occur. More seriously, when taken in large doses papaverine may also interfere with the pumping action of the heart and cause heart failure.

QUICK REFERENCE

Drug group Vasodilator (p.126)

Overdose danger rating Low

Dependence rating Low

Prescription needed Yes

Available as generic Yes

INFORMATION FOR USERS

Your drug prescription is tailored for you. Do not alter dosage without checking with your physician.

How taken

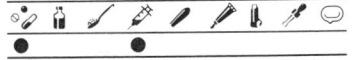

Tablets, capsules, injection.

Frequency and timing of doses
2 – 5 x daily.

Dosage range
100 – 1500mg daily.

Onset of effect
Within 1 hour.

Duration of action
8 – 12 hours.

Diet advice
None.

Storage
Keep in a closed container in a cool, dry place away from reach of children.

Missed dose
Take as soon as you remember. If your next dose is due within 2 hours, take a single dose now and skip the next.

Stopping the drug
Do not stop the drug without consulting your physician; stopping the drug may lead to worsening of the underlying condition.

Exceeding the dose
An occasional unintentional extra dose is unlikely to be a cause for concern. But if you notice unusual symptoms, or if a large overdose has been taken, notify your physician.

SPECIAL PRECAUTIONS

Be sure to tell your physician if:
▼ You have impaired liver function.
▼ You suffer from migraine.
▼ You have heart problems.
▼ You have Parkinson's disease.
▼ You are taking other medications.

Pregnancy
▼ Not usually prescribed. Safety in pregnancy not established. Discuss with your physician so that you can weigh the benefits of the drug against its possible risks.

Breast feeding
▼ Discuss with your physician. The drug passes into the breast milk and may affect the baby adversely.

Infants and children
▼ Not usually prescribed.

Over 60
▼ Reduced dose may be necessary. Increased likelihood of adverse effects.

Driving and hazardous work
▼ Avoid such activities until you have learned how the drug affects you, because the drug may cause drowsiness.

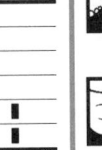

Alcohol
▼ Avoid. Alcohol may increase the sedative effects of this drug.

POSSIBLE ADVERSE EFFECTS

The common adverse effects tend to diminish as your body adjusts to the drug.

The rarer adverse effects usually occur only when the drug is given in high dosages.

Symptom/effect	Frequency		Discuss with physician		Stop taking drug now	Call physician now
	Common	Rare	Only if severe	In all cases		
Nausea/loss of appetite	●		■			
Flushing	●		■			
Drowsiness	●		■			
Sweating		●	■			
Jaundice		●		■	▲	!
Rash		●		■	▲	!

INTERACTIONS

Levodopa Papaverine reduces the effect of this drug. The levodopa dosage may need to be adjusted accordingly.

PROLONGED USE

No problems expected.

PENICILLAMINE

Brand names Cuprimine, Depen
Used in the following combined preparations None

GENERAL INFORMATION

Available since 1963, penicillamine has two principal uses. It is an antirheumatic drug, given to adults and juveniles to slow or even halt the progression of rheumatoid arthritis. Because of its potentially serious side effects on the blood and kidneys, it is used only when the inflammation of the joints is disabling or when other drugs have proven ineffective.

Penicillamine is also a *chelating* agent, used in cases of metal poison-ing to eliminate copper, mercury, lead, or arsenic from the body. Penicilla-mine binds (i.e., combines) with those substances, forming a chemical compound that the body can excrete. It is also prescribed in Wilson's disease, a rare disorder involving copper deposits in the liver and brain, and prevents a certain rare type of urinary stone (cystine). Penicillamine has sometimes been used in the treatment of primary biliary cirrhosis.

INFORMATION FOR USERS

Your drug prescription is tailored for you. Do not alter dosage without checking with your physician.

How taken

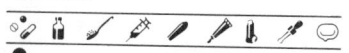

Tablets, capsules.

Frequency and timing of doses
Once daily one hour before meals (rheumatoid arthritis); 4 x daily one hour before meals (Wilson's disease, kidney stones, metal poisoning).

Dosage range
Adults 125 – 250mg daily (starting dose) increasing to 500 – 750mg over 6 –12 months (rheumatoid arthritis); 125 – 250mg daily (starting dose), increasing to up to 1g daily over 4 – 8 weeks (Wilson's disease); 1– 4g daily (kidney stones); according to size or weight (metal poisoning).
Children Reduced dose necessary according to age and weight.

Onset of effect
Full effect may not be felt for 2 – 3 months.

Duration of action
Some effect may last for 1 – 3 months after the drug has been stopped.

Diet advice
People with Wilson's disease may be advised to follow a low-copper diet. Discuss with your physician.

Storage
Keep in a closed container in a cool, dry place away from reach of children.

Missed dose
Take as soon as you remember.

Stopping the drug
Do not stop the drug without consulting your physician; symptoms may recur.

Exceeding the dose
An occasional unintentional extra dose is unlikely to cause problems. Large over-doses may cause joint pain, fever, or a rash. Consult your physician.

POSSIBLE ADVERSE EFFECTS

Adverse effects are frequent. Allergic rashes and itching, gastrointestinal disturbances (nausea, vomiting, abdominal pain) and loss of taste are common and often dose-related. More serious, life-threatening reactions may occur.

Symptom/effect	Frequency		Discuss with physician		Stop taking drug now	Call physician now
	Common	Rare	Only if severe	In all cases		
Digestive disturbance	●		■			
Loss of taste	●		■			
Rash/itching	●			■	▲	▮
Fever		●		■		
Weakness		●		■		

INTERACTIONS

Iron preparations These may interfere with the effects of penicillamine.

Digoxin Penicillamine may reduce the effect of digoxin.

SPECIAL PRECAUTIONS

Be sure to tell your physician if:
▼ You have impaired liver or kidney function.
▼ You have a blood disorder.
▼ You have a skin disorder.
▼ You are taking other medications.

 Pregnancy
▼ Not usually prescribed. May cause defects in the baby. Discuss with your physician so that you may weigh the benefits of the drug against its risks.

 Breast feeding
▼ Discuss with your physician. The drug may pass into the breast milk and may affect the baby adversely.

 Infants and children
▼ Reduced dose necessary.

 Over 60
▼ Increased likelihood of adverse effects.

 Driving and hazardous work
▼ No known problems.

 Alcohol
▼ No known problems.

PROLONGED USE

Prolonged use may deplete pyridoxine (vitamin B6) and iron; supplements may be advised. In rare cases, blood disorders or impaired kidney function may develop.

Monitoring Blood and urine are regularly tested for kidney damage or blood abnormalities.

PENICILLIN G

Brand names Bicillin, Bicillin L-A, Crysticillin, Pentids, Wycillin
Used in the following combined preparation Bicillin C-R

GENERAL INFORMATION

Also known as benzylpenicillin, penicillin G (introduced in 1943) was one of the first antibiotics to be discovered, purified, and used in medicine. Because it is broken down in the digestive tract, penicillin G has a variable effect when taken by mouth. Usually given by injection, it is used to treat a variety of bacterial infections when the organisms are shown to be susceptible. These infections include certain types of tonsillitis, bronchitis, and pneumonia. It is effective in a gum infection known as Vincent's gingivitis,

and may be used to treat certain sexually transmitted diseases, including gonorrhea and syphilis.

Penicillin G is also prescribed for less common conditions caused by streptococcal infections, such as scarlet fever and erysipelas (a skin infection). The drug is also used to treat bacterial endocarditis.

As with other penicillin antibiotics, the most serious possible adverse effect of this drug is an allergic reaction that can cause a rash, wheezing, or, in extreme cases, shock.

INFORMATION FOR USERS

Your drug prescription is tailored for you. Do not alter dosage without checking with your physician.

How taken

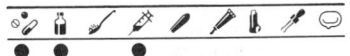

Tablets, liquid, injection.

Frequency and timing of doses
3 – 4 x daily on an empty stomach (by mouth); up to 6 x daily depending on preparation (by injection).

Dosage range
Adults 1 – 2g daily (by mouth).
Children Reduced dose according to age and weight.

Onset of effect
2 – 3 days.

Duration of action
Up to 12 hours.

Diet advice
Do not eat one hour before to one hour after dosage.

Storage
Keep in a closed container in a cool, dry place away from reach of children.

Missed dose
Take as soon as you remember. If your next dose is due within 2 hours, take a single dose now and skip the next.

Stopping the drug
Take the full course. Even if you feel better, the original infection may still be present and may recur if treatment is stopped too soon.

Exceeding the dose
An occasional unintentional extra dose is unlikely to be a cause for concern. But if you notice unusual symptoms, or if a large overdose has been taken, notify your physician.

POSSIBLE ADVERSE EFFECTS

Most people do not experience any adverse effects with penicillin G. Allergic reactions that produce a rash are uncommon, but necessitate stopping the drug.

Symptom/effect	Frequency		Discuss with physician		Stop taking drug now	Call physician now
	Common	Rare	Only if severe	In all cases		
Nausea/vomiting	●			■		
Diarrhea	●			■		
Breathing difficulties	●		■	▲		▮
Rash	●		■	▲		▮

INTERACTIONS

Probenecid increases the level of penicillin G in the blood.

SPECIAL PRECAUTIONS

Be sure to tell your physician if:
▼ You have impaired kidney function.
▼ You have an allergic disorder such as asthma or urticaria.
▼ You have had a previous allergic reaction to a penicillin or cephalosporin antibiotic.
▼ You are taking other medications.

Pregnancy
▼ No evidence of risk to developing baby.

Breast feeding
▼ Discuss with your physician. The drug passes into the milk and may sensitize the child to the drug, possibly creating a lifelong allergy.

Infants and children
▼ Reduced dose necessary.

Over 60
▼ Reduced dose may be necessary. Increased likelihood of adverse effects.

Driving and hazardous work
▼ No known problems.

Alcohol
▼ May reduce effect of the drug.

PROLONGED USE

Prolonged use may increase the risk of diarrhea and yeast infections of the mouth or vagina.

PENICILLIN V

Brand names Ledercillin-VK, Pen-Vee-K, SK-Penicillin-VK, V-Cillin-K, Veetids
Used in the following combined preparations None

GENERAL INFORMATION

Penicillin V, introduced in 1955, is a synthetic antibiotic prescribed for a wide range of infections. It is readily absorbed and when taken with food its effects are more reliable than those of other oral penicillins.

Various commonly occurring respiratory tract infections – some types of tonsillitis, bronchitis, and pharyngitis, for example – often respond well to treatment with penicillin V. It is also effective against the gum disease

known as Vincent's gingivitis.

Less common infections caused by the Streptococcus bacterium, such as scarlet fever and erysipelas (a skin infection), may also be treated with penicillin V. It is also prescribed to prevent the recurrence of rheumatic fever, a rare though potentially serious condition.

As with other penicillin antibiotics, one possible adverse effect is an allergic reaction that can cause a rash or breathing difficulties among other symptoms.

QUICK REFERENCE

Drug group Penicillin antibiotic (p.158)

Overdose danger rating Low

Dependence rating Low

Prescription needed Yes

Available as generic Yes

INFORMATION FOR USERS

Your drug prescription is tailored for you. Do not alter dosage without checking with your physician.

How taken

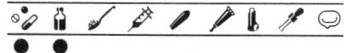

Tablets, capsules, liquid.

Frequency and timing of doses
2 – 4 x daily.

Dosage range
Adults 500mg – 2g daily.
Children Reduced dose according to age and weight.

Onset of effect
2 – 3 days.

Duration of action
Up to 12 hours.

Diet advice
None.

Storage
Keep in a closed container in a cool, dry place away from reach of children.

Missed dose
Take as soon as you remember. If your next dose is due within 2 hours, take a single dose now and skip the next.

Stopping the drug
Take the full course. Even if you feel better the original infection may still be present and may recur if treatment is stopped too soon.

Exceeding the dose
An occasional unintentional extra dose is unlikely to be a cause for concern. But if you notice unusual symptoms, or if a large overdose has been taken, notify your physician.

SPECIAL PRECAUTIONS

Be sure to tell your physician if:
▼ You have impaired kidney function.
▼ You have had a previous allergic reaction to a penicillin or cephalosporin antibiotic.
▼ You have an allergic disorder such as asthma or urticaria.
▼ You are taking other medications.

Pregnancy
▼ No evidence of risk to the developing baby.

Breast feeding
▼ Discuss with your physician. The drug passes into the breast milk and may sensitize your child to the drug, possibly creating lifelong allergy.

Infants and children
▼ Reduced dose necessary.

Over 60
▼ Reduced dose may be necessary. Increased likelihood of adverse effects.

Driving and hazardous work
▼ No known problems.

Alcohol
▼ No known problems.

POSSIBLE ADVERSE EFFECTS

Most people do not feel any serious adverse effects when taking penicillin V. However, this drug may occasionally provoke an allergic rash in susceptible people.

Symptom/effect	Frequency		Discuss with physician		Stop taking drug now	Call physician now
	Common	Rare	Only if severe	In all cases		
Nausea/vomiting	●		■			
Diarrhea	●		■			
Rash	●			■	▲	▮
Breathing difficulties	●			■	▲	▮

INTERACTIONS

Probenecid increases the level of penicillin V in the blood.

PROLONGED USE

Prolonged use may increase the risk of yeast infections and diarrhea.

PENTOXIFYLLINE

Brand name Trental
Used in the following combined preparations None

GENERAL INFORMATION

Pentoxifylline is a drug related to caffeine that has been recently introduced in the US for the treatment of peripheral vascular disease. This is a group of conditions, including Raynaud's disease and intermittent claudication (pain in the legs during exercise), caused by poor circulation to the limbs. It is not, however, recommended for the treatment of severe arterial obstructive disease, including conditions such as gangrene or ischemic skin ulcers.

Pentoxifylline, it is claimed, makes the red blood cells more flexible and improves their ability to pass through the smallest capillaries. This enables the blood to flow through narrowed arteries and increases the supply of blood and oxygen to all parts of the body.

Adverse effects from this drug are uncommon, but dizziness, headaches, and nausea may occur. It may not be suitable for people who react adversely to caffeine or related drugs.

QUICK REFERENCE

Drug group Vasodilator (p.126)
Overdose danger rating Medium
Dependence rating Low
Prescription needed Yes
Available as generic No

INFORMATION FOR USERS

Your drug prescription is tailored for you. Do not alter dosage without checking with your physician.

How taken

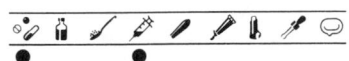

Slow-release tablets, injection.

Frequency and timing of doses
3 x daily with meals.

Dosage range
800 – 1200mg daily.

Onset of effect
Some effects may occur within a few hours, but full benefits may not be felt for 2 – 4 weeks.

Duration of action
8 – 12 hours.

Diet advice
None.

Storage
Keep in a closed container in a cool, dry place away from reach of children.

Missed dose
Take as soon as you remember. If your next dose is due within 2 hours, take a single dose now and skip the next.

Stopping the drug
Do not stop taking the drug without consulting your physician; symptoms may recur.

Exceeding the dose
An occasional unintentional extra dose is unlikely to cause problems. Large overdoses may cause severe drowsiness, flushing, and faintness. Notify your physician.

SPECIAL PRECAUTIONS

Be sure to tell your physician if:
▼ You have impaired kidney function.
▼ You have heart problems.
▼ You have diabetes.
▼ You have low blood pressure.
▼ You are taking other medications.

Pregnancy
▼ Not usually prescribed. Safety in pregnancy not established. Discuss with your physician so that you can weigh the benefits of the drug against its possible risks.

Breast feeding
▼ Discuss with your physician. The drug passes into the breast milk and may affect the baby adversely.

Infants and children
▼ Not recommended.

Over 60
▼ Increased likelihood of adverse effects.

Driving and hazardous work
▼ Avoid such activities until you have learned how the drug affects you, because the drug can cause dizziness.

Alcohol
▼ No known problems.

POSSIBLE ADVERSE EFFECTS

Severe adverse effects are rare with pentoxifylline. Dizziness, headaches, and gastrointestinal disturbances may be controlled by reducing the dose. If chest pain or palpitations occur, consult your physician at once.

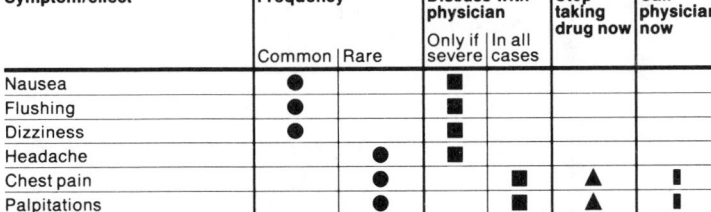

Symptom/effect	Frequency		Discuss with physician		Stop taking drug now	Call physician now
	Common	Rare	Only if severe	In all cases		
Nausea	●		■			
Flushing	●		■			
Dizziness	●		■			
Headache		●	■			
Chest pain		●		■	▲	▌
Palpitations		●		■	▲	▌

PROLONGED USE

No known problems.

INTERACTIONS

Antihypertensive drugs Pentoxifylline may increase the effect of antihypertensive drugs, and the dosages of both may need to be adjusted accordingly.

Tobacco smoking This may worsen the underlying condition and interfere with the beneficial effect of pentoxifylline.

PERPHENAZINE

Brand name Trilafon
Used in the following combined preparations Etrafon, Triavil

GENERAL INFORMATION

Perphenazine was introduced in 1958 and belongs to a group of drugs called the phenothiazines. These drugs act on the brain to modify abnormal behavior (see Antipsychotic drugs, p.113).

Perphenazine is used in the treatment of schizophrenia, mania, dementia and other disorders where confused or agitated behavior may occur. It does not cure the disorders but does relieve some of the distressing symptoms of these illnesses.

Another use of perphenazine is in the treatment of nausea and vomiting, especially if caused by drug treatment, radiation therapy, or anesthetics.

The main drawback to the use of this drug is that it often produces drowsiness and may cause abnormal shaking movements (*parkinsonism*).

INFORMATION FOR USERS

Your drug prescription is tailored for you. Do not alter dosage without checking with your physician.

How taken

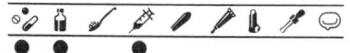

Tablets, liquid, injection.

Frequency and timing of doses
2 – 6 x daily.

Adult dosage range
4 – 8mg (non-hospitalized persons); 16 – 64mg daily (mental illness); 8 – 24mg daily (nausea and vomiting).

Onset of effect
30 minutes – 1 hour; full effect in mental illness may not be felt for several weeks.

Duration of action
6 – 8 hours; up to 12 hours in slow-release capsules.

Diet advice
None.

Storage
Keep in a closed container in a cool, dry place away from reach of children. Protect from light.

Missed dose
Take as soon as you remember. If your next dose is due within 2 hours, take a single dose now and skip the next.

Stopping the drug
Do not stop the drug without consulting your physician; symptoms may recur.

Exceeding the dose
An occasional unintentional extra dose is unlikely to cause problems. Large overdoses may cause drowsiness, muscle stiffness, or trembling. Notify your physician.

SPECIAL PRECAUTIONS

Be sure to tell your physician if:
▼ You have impaired kidney or liver function.
▼ You have heart problems.
▼ You have poor circulation.
▼ You have had epileptic seizures.
▼ You have thyroid disease.
▼ You have had glaucoma.
▼ You have urinary difficulties.
▼ You have Parkinson's disease.
▼ You are taking other medications.

Pregnancy
▼ Not usually prescribed. Effects on the developing baby uncertain. Discuss with your physician so that you can weigh the benefits of the drug against its possible risks.

Breast feeding
▼ Discuss with your physician. The drug passes into the breast milk. Its effects on the baby are not known.

Infants and children
▼ Not recommended.

Over 60
▼ Reduced dose may be necessary. Increased likelihood of adverse effects.

Driving and hazardous work
▼ Avoid such activities until you have learned how the drug affects you, because the drug can cause drowsiness and slowed reactions.

Alcohol
▼ Avoid. Alcohol may increase the sedative effects of this drug.

POSSIBLE ADVERSE EFFECTS

When used as an antipsychotic, drowsiness is the most common adverse effect of perphenazine. This effect usually weakens after long-term treatment, and adjusting the dosage often helps. Other adverse effects, such as blurred vision, stuffy nose, and headache, are more common when the drug is used as an anti-emetic.

Symptom/effect	Frequency		Discuss with physician		Stop taking drug now	Call physician now
	Common	Rare	Only if severe	In all cases		
Drowsiness	●		■			
Stuffy nose	●		■			
Constipation	●		■			
Parkinsonism	●			■		
Dizziness	●			■		
Blurred vision	●			■		
Muscle rigidity and stupor		●		■	▲	▮

PROLONGED USE

Use of this drug for more than a few months may lead to the development of abnormal movements of the face and limbs (*tardive dyskinesia*), and occasionally jaundice may occur. Sometimes a reduction in dosage may be recommended.

INTERACTIONS

Sedatives All drugs that have a sedative effect are likely to increase the sedative effect of perphenazine.

Antacids reduce the effect of perphenazine if the two drugs are taken less than 1 hour apart.

Cold and cough remedies There is an increased likelihood of adverse effects from perphenazine if taken in conjunction with cold and cough remedies containing antihistamines or codeine.

PHENAZOPYRIDINE

Brand names Pyridiate, Pyridium, Urodine, Urogesic
Used in the following combined preparations Azo Gantanol, Azo Gantrisin, Pyridium Plus, Urobiotic 250

GENERAL INFORMATION

Introduced in 1927, phenazopyridine is an analgesic that passes quickly into the urine and relieves pain or discomfort in the urinary tract. Such symptoms can result from infection, injury, surgery, catheterization, and cystoscopy.

With urinary tract infection, other drugs are given to cure the infection. Phenazopyridine is an analgesic only, its effectiveness limited to 48 hours. It is available in combination with antibac-terial drugs, but most physicians prefer separate prescriptions.

Abdominal pain is a fairly common side effect of phenazopyridine, but it is usually not severe enough to necessitate stopping the treatment. Because this drug is a dye, it colors the urine orange or red, and this may stain clothing. Headache, dizziness, and skin discoloration occur only occasionally. Diabetics may have false readings of urine sugar tests.

QUICK REFERENCE

Drug group Urinary analgesic (p.194)

Overdose danger rating Low

Dependence rating Low

Prescription needed Yes

Available as generic Yes

INFORMATION FOR USERS

Your drug prescription is tailored for you. Do not alter dosage without checking with your physician.

How taken

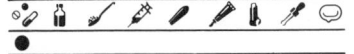

●

Tablets.

Frequency and timing of doses
3 x daily after meals.

Dosage range
Adults 600mg daily.
Children Reduced dose necessary according to age and weight.

Onset of effect
Within 4 hours.

Duration of action
8 – 12 hours.

Diet advice
None.

Storage
Keep in a closed container in a cool, dry place away from reach of children.

Missed dose
Take as soon as you remember. If your next dose is due within 2 hours, take a single dose now and skip the next.

Stopping the drug
Can be safely stopped as soon as you no longer need it.

Exceeding the dose
An occasional unintentional extra dose is unlikely to be a cause for concern. But if you notice unusual symptoms, or if a large overdose has been taken, notify your physician.

SPECIAL PRECAUTIONS

Be sure to tell your physician if:
▼ You have impaired liver or kidney function.
▼ You are taking other medications.

Pregnancy
▼ Not usually prescribed. Safety in pregnancy not established. Discuss with your physician so that you may weigh the benefits of the drug against its risks.

Breast feeding
▼ No evidence of risk.

Infants and children
▼ Not recommended for children under 6 years. Reduced dose necessary for older children.

Over 60
▼ No special problems.

Driving and hazardous work
▼ No known problems.

Alcohol
▼ No known problems.

Abdominal pain is the most common adverse effect. Discoloration of the urine may be inconvenient, but is no cause for concern. Other adverse effects are rare.

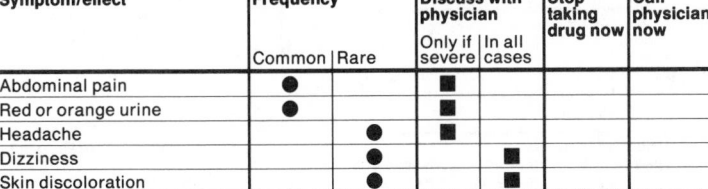

Symptom/effect	Frequency		Discuss with physician		Stop taking drug now	Call physician now
	Common	Rare	Only if severe	In all cases		
Abdominal pain	●			■		
Red or orange urine	●			■		
Headache		●		■		
Dizziness		●			■	
Skin discoloration		●			■	

INTERACTIONS

None.

PROLONGED USE

No problems expected. Phenazopyridine is not usually prescribed for long periods because it tends to lose its effect after 48 hours when used for urinary tract infections.

PHENELZINE

Brand name Nardil
Used in the following combined preparations None

GENERAL INFORMATION

Phenelzine belongs to a group of antidepressant drugs known as the monoamine oxidase inhibitors (often abbreviated to MAOIs). These drugs help to elevate mood, improve appetite and sleep, and restore energy, and interest in life in general. Phenelzine is most commonly used to relieve depression, especially when accompanied by irrational fears (phobias) or exaggerated emotional reactions.

The main problem associated with the use of phenelzine is the risk of dangerous interactions with a wide range of other drugs and many foods. Since these interactions can be life-threatening, treatment with this drug is usually reserved for people who have not responded to all other types of antidepressant. People on phenelzine treatment are advised to carry a warning card.

INFORMATION FOR USERS

Your drug prescription is tailored for you. Do not alter dosage without checking with your physician.

How taken

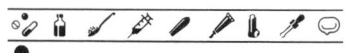

Tablets.

Frequency and timing of doses
2 – 3 x daily initially. Once treatment is established, frequency may be reduced.

Adult dosage range
45 – 90mg daily (starting dose). When full benefit is felt, dosage is gradually reduced to a lower maintenance dose.

Onset of effect
1 – 4 weeks.

Duration of action
Up to 14 days after treatment is begun or discontinued.

Diet advice
Certain foods with a high tyramine content must be avoided while taking this drug and for at least 14 days after treatment finishes. When phenelzine is dispensed, the pharmacist should provide a card listing foods and medicines to avoid. These include cheese, pickled herring, red wine, meat and yeast extracts, and broad (fava) beans.

Storage
Keep in a closed container in a cool, dry place away from reach of children.

Missed dose
Take as soon as you remember. If your next dose is due within 3 hours, take a single dose now and skip the next.

Stopping the drug
Do not stop the drug without consulting your physician; symptoms may recur.

OVERDOSE ACTION

 Seek immediate medical advice in all cases. Take emergency action if you notice any of the symptoms described under Possible adverse effects below.

See Drug poisoning emergency guide (p.590).

SPECIAL PRECAUTIONS

Be sure to tell your physician if:
▼ You have impaired kidney or liver function.
▼ You have heart problems.
▼ You have had epileptic seizures.
▼ You have celiac disease or gluten enteropathy (the tablets contain gluten).
▼ You are taking other medications.

 Pregnancy
▼ Not usually prescribed. Safety in pregnancy not established. Discuss with your physician.

 Breast feeding
▼ The drug passes into the breast milk, but at normal doses adverse effects on the baby are uncommon. Discuss with your physician.

 Infants and children
▼ Not recommended.

 Over 60
▼ Used only when potential benefits outweigh risks. Increased likelihood of adverse effects.

 Driving and hazardous work
▼ Avoid such activities until you have learned how the drug affects you, because of the possibility of loss of concentration and dizziness.

 Alcohol
▼ Never drink heavy red wines, particularly chianti, when taking this drug. These may cause a dangerous reaction. Other forms of alcohol should also be avoided.

Surgery and general anesthetics
▼ Phenelzine treatment should be withdrawn at least 2 weeks before general anesthetics and before some dental treatments are given. Discuss this with your physician or dentist before any operation or dental procedure.

POSSIBLE ADVERSE EFFECTS

Phenelzine does not usually cause adverse effects. However, if you experience severe headache, nausea and/or vomiting, or unexplained sweating, seek medical advice at once. Such symptoms may be a sign of rising blood pressure.

Symptom/effect	Frequency		Discuss with physician		Stop taking drug now	Call physician now
	Common	Rare	Only if severe	In all cases		
Dizziness/fainting	●		■			▌
Digestive disturbances		●	■			▌
Jaundice		●	■			▌
Rash		●	■	▲		▌

INTERACTIONS

General note Phenelzine interacts with a large number of prescription drugs, over-the-counter medicines, and foods. Do not take any type of medicine without prior consultation with your physician or pharmacist.

PROLONGED USE

No problems expected, but people taking phenelzine should constantly take care to avoid interactions with food or other drugs, as the risk does not diminish with time.

PHENOBARBITAL

Brand names Barbita, Luminal, Solfoton
Used in the following combined preparations Barbidonna, Bronkotab, Donnatal, Quadrinal

GENERAL INFORMATION

Introduced over 75 years ago, phenobarbital is one of the most widely employed and useful of the anticonvulsants. It is a barbiturate, a group of drugs prescribed primarily for sleep (see p.110). But the principal use of phenobarbital is in the prevention and treatment of epileptic seizures (see Anticonvulsant drugs, p.114).

It is also prescribed by some physicians for daytime sedation and is found in a large number of combination products for irritable bowel.

Although it has to some extent been replaced by newer anticonvulsant drugs, phenobarbital remains widely used in conjunction with phenytoin to treat epilepsy in young children for whom other drugs may not be suitable. The main drawback is its sedative effect. In children and the elderly it may also cause excitement.

QUICK REFERENCE

Drug group Barbiturate anticonvulsant drug (p.114)

Overdose danger rating High

Dependence rating High

Prescription needed Yes CIV

Available as generic Yes

INFORMATION FOR USERS

Your drug prescription is tailored for you. Do not alter dosage without checking with your physician.

How taken

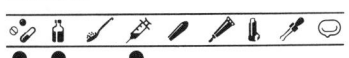

Tablets, liquid, injection.

Frequency and timing of doses
1 – 4 x daily.

Dosage range
Adults 15 – 120mg daily; up to 300mg daily may be used to control seizures.
Children Reduced dose according to age and weight.

Onset of effect
30 – 60 minutes (by mouth).

Duration of action
24 – 48 hours (some effect may persist for up to 6 days).

Diet advice
None.

Storage
Keep in a closed container in a cool, dry place away from reach of children.

Missed dose
Take as soon as you remember for seizure control. If your next dose is due within 2 hours, do not take the missed dose. Take the next dose as usual. For other purposes take a dose at the next scheduled time.

Stopping the drug
Do not stop taking the drug without consulting your physician, who may supervise a gradual reduction in dosage. Abrupt cessation may cause seizures or lead to restlessness, trembling, and insomnia.

OVERDOSE ACTION

 Seek immediate medical advice in all cases. Take emergency action if unsteadiness, severe weakness, confusion, or loss of consciousness occurs.

See Drug poisoning emergency guide (p.590).

POSSIBLE ADVERSE EFFECTS

Most of the adverse effects of phenobarbital are the result of its sedative effect on the brain. They can sometimes be minimized by medically supervised reduction of dosage.

Symptom/effect	Frequency		Discuss with physician		Stop taking drug now	Call physician now
	Common	Rare	Only if severe	In all cases		
Drowsiness	●		■			
Dizziness/faintness	●		■			
Clumsiness/unsteadiness	●			■		▮
Rash		●		■	▲	
Confusion		●		■		▮

INTERACTIONS

Sedatives All drugs that have a sedative effect on the central nervous system are likely to increase the sedative properties of phenobarbital.

Corticosteroids Phenobarbital may reduce the effect of corticosteroid drugs.

Anticoagulant drugs The effect of these drugs may be reduced when they are taken with phenobarbital.

Oral contraceptives Phenobarbital may reduce the effectiveness of oral contraceptives. Discuss with your physician.

SPECIAL PRECAUTIONS

Be sure to tell your physician if:
▼ You have impaired kidney or liver function.
▼ You have heart problems.
▼ You have poor circulation.
▼ You have porphyria.
▼ You have persistent pain.
▼ You are taking other medications.

 Pregnancy
▼ Not usually prescribed. May cause abnormalities in the unborn baby. Discuss with your physician so that you can weigh the benefits of the drug against its possible risks.

 Breast feeding
▼ Discuss with your physician. The drug passes into the breast milk and may affect the baby adversely.

 Infants and children
▼ Reduced dose necessary.

 Over 60
▼ Reduced dose may be necessary. May, surprisingly, cause excitement in the elderly.

 Driving and hazardous work
▼ Your underlying condition as well as the possibility of reduced alertness while taking this drug may make such activities inadvisable. Discuss with your physician.

 Alcohol
▼ Never drink while under treatment with phenobarbital. Alcohol may interact dangerously with this drug.

PROLONGED USE

The sedative effect of phenobarbital can build up during prolonged use, causing excessive drowsiness and lethargy. However, *tolerance* may develop and reduce these effects. In rare cases it may cause deficiency of vitamin D.

Monitoring Blood samples are taken periodically to test blood levels of the drug.

PHENYLBUTAZONE

Brand names Azolid, Butazolidin
Used in the following combined preparation Azolid-A

GENERAL INFORMATION

Phenylbutazone, introduced in 1949, is one of the oldest non-steroidal anti-inflammatory drugs (NSAIDs), and a strong one; it was allegedly once used illegally to dope lame racehorses.

It is effective for reducing pain, stiffness, and inflammation in the treatment of ankylosing spondylitis and acute attacks of gouty arthritis. Although it may also relieve symptoms of other types of arthritis, including severe rheumatoid arthritis, it does not cure the underlying disease.

Phenylbutazone has several potentially serious adverse effects, including a rare risk of blood disorders. For this reason it is prescribed only when other drugs have failed and is not usually prescribed for prolonged periods. If treatment is continued for longer than 2 weeks, regular blood tests are required.

INFORMATION FOR USERS

Your drug prescription is tailored for you. Do not alter dosage without checking with your physician.

How taken

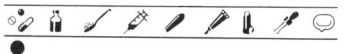

Tablets, capsules.

Frequency and timing of doses
1 – 4 x daily with food (arthritis). Every 4 hours with food (gout).

Adult dosage range
Arthritis 300 – 600mg daily (first week), then 100 – 400mg daily (maintenance).
Gout 400mg (starting dose), then 100mg every 4 hours for several days.

Onset of effect
Pain relief may be noticed after 2 hours. Full effect may not be felt for 3 – 4 days.

Duration of action
Some effect may last for 3 – 4 days.

Diet advice
None.

Storage
Keep in a closed container in a cool, dry place away from reach of children.

Missed dose
Take as soon as you remember. If your next dose is due within 2 hours, take a single dose now and skip the next.

Stopping the drug
Can be safely stopped as soon as you no longer need it.

OVERDOSE ACTION

 Seek immediate medical advice in all cases. Take emergency action if seizures or loss of consciousness occurs.

See Drug poisoning emergency guide (p.590).

POSSIBLE ADVERSE EFFECTS

Nausea, water retention, and rashes occur commonly. Black or bloodstained bowel movements, sore throat, or fever should be reported to your physician without delay.

Symptom/effect	Frequency		Discuss with physician		Stop taking drug now	Call physician now
	Common	Rare	Only if severe	In all cases		
Nausea/vomiting	●		■			
Abdominal pain	●			■		
Swollen feet/ankles	●			■		
Rash	●			■	▲	
Drowsiness/confusion		●	■	■		
Wheezing/breathlessness		●		■	▲	■

INTERACTIONS

General note Phenylbutazone interacts with a wide range of drugs to increase the risk of bleeding and/or peptic ulcers. Such drugs include oral anticoagulants, corticosteroids, and aspirin.

Lithium Phenylbutazone may raise blood levels of lithium, leading to a risk of serious adverse effects.

Antihypertensive drugs and diuretics The beneficial effects of these drugs may be reduced by phenylbutazone.

Oral antidiabetic drugs Phenylbutazone may increase the blood sugar-lowering effect of these drugs.

SPECIAL PRECAUTIONS

Be sure to tell your physician if:
▼ You have impaired liver or kidney function.
▼ You have heart problems.
▼ You have high blood pressure.
▼ You have had a blood disorder.
▼ You have had a peptic ulcer, esophagitis, or acid indigestion.
▼ You are allergic to aspirin.
▼ You are taking other medications.

 Pregnancy
▼ Not usually prescribed. When taken in the last 3 months of pregnancy, the drug may cause adverse effects on the baby's heart and prolong labor. Discuss with your physician.

 Breast feeding
▼ Discuss with your physician. The drug passes into the breast milk and may affect the baby adversely.

 Infants and children
▼ Not recommended for children under 15 years.

 Over 60
▼ Reduced dose necessary. Increased likelihood of adverse effects.

 Driving and hazardous work
▼ No special problems.

 Alcohol
▼ Avoid. Alcohol may increase the risk of stomach irritation with phenylbutazone.

Surgery and general anesthetics
▼ Phenylbutazone may prolong bleeding. Discuss this with your physician or dentist before any surgery.

PROLONGED USE

Phenylbutazone is not usually prescribed for prolonged periods except in ankylosing spondylitis.

PHENYLEPHRINE

Brand names Alconefrin, Allerest Nasal, Coricidin Nasal Mist, Mydfrin
Used in the following combined preparations Comhist LA, Phenergan VC Syrup, Phenergan with codeine, Rynatan

GENERAL INFORMATION

Phenylephrine is one of the most common nasal decongestants, and as an ingredient in a variety of topical preparations, it relieves the symptoms of hay fever and head colds. It is less potent but longer acting than other nasal decongestants, with fewer adverse effects.

By constricting blood vessels in the lining of the eye, small doses of the drug can also reduce the pain of conjunctivitis. Combined with local anesthetics, it constricts the blood vessels around an injection site,

prolonging the anesthetic's effect by delaying its absorption. Phenylephrine is also used to dilate the pupil during eye examinations and eye surgery.

Care should be taken not to exceed the dose, because this may cause increased eye irritation and produce congestion and swelling in the nasal passages. High or prolonged doses of phenylephrine are liable to cause a rebound of nasal stuffiness and a rise in blood pressure and heart rate, and should be avoided by people with heart trouble or high blood pressure.

QUICK REFERENCE

Drug group Decongestant (p.121)
Overdose danger rating Medium
Dependence rating Low
Prescription needed Yes
Available as generic Yes

INFORMATION FOR USERS

Your drug prescription is tailored for you. Do not alter dosage without checking with your physician.

How taken

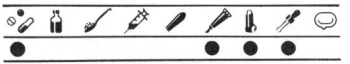

Tablets, jelly, nasal drops, spray, eye drops.

Frequency and timing of doses
Up to 4 x daily (eye drops); every 3 – 6 hours (nasal drops, spray, jelly).

Dosage range
Adults 0.25% – 1% (nasal drops, spray); 1 – 2 drops (eye drops).
Children 0.125% (nasal drops, spray); 0.5% (jelly).

Onset of effect
Within a few minutes.

Duration of action
4 – 6 hours.

Diet advice
None.

Storage
Keep in a closed container in a cool, dry place away from reach of children. Protect from light.

Missed dose
Take as soon as you remember. If your next dose is due within 2 hours, take a single dose now and skip the next.

Stopping the drug
Can be safely stopped as soon as you no longer need it.

Exceeding the dose
An occasional unintentional extra dose is unlikely to cause problems. Large overdoses may cause irritation of the eyes or palpitations. Notify your physician.

SPECIAL PRECAUTIONS

Be sure to tell your physician if:
▼ You have angina.
▼ You have high blood pressure.
▼ You have had glaucoma.
▼ You are taking other medications.

Pregnancy
▼ Not usually prescribed. May cause heart defects in the unborn baby. Discuss with your physician so that you can weigh the benefits of the drug against its risks.

Breast feeding
▼ Discuss with your physician. The drug passes into the breast milk, but at normal doses adverse effects on the baby are unlikely.

Infants and children
▼ Reduced dose necessary.

Over 60
▼ Reduced dose necessary. Increased likelihood of adverse effects.

Driving and hazardous work
▼ Avoid such activities until you have learned how the drug affects you, because when used in the eye the drug can cause blurred vision.

Alcohol
▼ No known problems.

POSSIBLE ADVERSE EFFECTS

Phenylephrine has fewer adverse effects than many other drugs of the same group because it has little stimulating effect on the central nervous system. Most of the symptoms are related to frequent use, and should be reported promptly.

Symptom/effect	Frequency		Discuss with physician		Stop taking drug now	Call physician now
	Common	Rare	Only if severe	In all cases		
Blurred vision	●			■		
Headache	●			■		
Rebound nasal stuffiness	●			■		
Eye pain		●		■	▲	
Chest pain		●		■	▲	
Palpitations		●		■	▲	

INTERACTIONS

Monoamine oxidase inhibitors (MAOIs) There is a risk of a dangerous rise in blood pressure if phenylephrine is taken with these drugs. It should not be taken during or within 14 days of MAOI treatment.

Antihypertensive drugs Phenylephrine may interact with these drugs to reverse their effect.

PROLONGED USE

Prolonged continuous use may lead to worsening of the underlying condition.

Monitoring Periodic eye examinations may be required.

A B C D E F G H I J K L M N O P Q R S T U V W X Y Z

PHENYLPROPANOLAMINE

Brand names Dexatrim, Prolamine, Propadrine, Sucrets
Used in the following combined preparations Dimetapp, Entex, Entex-LA, Naldecon, Ornade

GENERAL INFORMATION

Phenylpropanolamine, a popular decongestant used in many over-the-counter preparations, belongs to a group of drugs known as *sympathomimetics*. By reducing inflammation and swelling of blood vessels, it relieves stuffiness and nasal congestion in colds, hay fever, and sinusitis.

But because it mimics some of the actions of the sympathetic (i.e., autonomic) nervous system, phenylpropanolamine can produce undesirable side effects. It may raise the heart rate and severely elevate blood pressure; it can cause palpitations and wakefulness.

Together with caffeine and a low-calorie regimen, phenylpropanolamine has been prescribed to help people lose weight, although its effectiveness for this purpose has not been proved. It is sometimes prescribed to relieve mild to moderate stress incontinence.

INFORMATION FOR USERS

Follow instructions on the label. Call your physician if symptoms worsen.

How taken

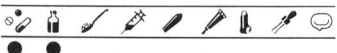

Tablets, capsules, liquid.

Frequency and timing of doses
3 – 6 x daily. With a glass of water before meals for weight loss.

Dosage range
Adults and children over 8 years 150 – 200mg daily (colds, hay fever); 75mg daily (weight loss); 150 – 225mg daily (incontinence).

Onset of effect
Within 15 – 30 minutes.

Duration of action
4 – 6 hours. Up to 12 hours (slow-release preparations).

Diet advice
When the drug is being used to help weight loss, a calorie-controlled diet may be advised by your physician.

Storage
Keep in a closed container in a cool, dry place away from reach of children. Protect from light.

Missed dose
Take as soon as you remember. If your next dose is due within 2 hours, take a single dose now and skip the next.

Stopping the drug
Can be safely stopped as soon as you no longer need it.

OVERDOSE ACTION

 Seek immediate medical advice in all cases. Take emergency action if delirium, seizures, or loss of consciousness occurs.

See Drug poisoning emergency guide (p.590).

SPECIAL PRECAUTIONS

Be sure to consult your physician before taking this drug if:
▼ You have high blood pressure.
▼ You have heart problems.
▼ You have had glaucoma.
▼ You have an overactive thyroid gland.
▼ You have diabetes.
▼ You have urinary difficulties.
▼ You are taking other medications.

 Pregnancy
▼ Not usually prescribed. Safety in pregnancy not established. Discuss with your physician so that you can weigh the benefits of the drug against its possible risks.

 Breast feeding
▼ Discuss with your physician. The drug passes into the breast milk in small amounts and may make the baby irritable.

 Infants and children
▼ Not recommended for children under 8 years, and should not be used as an appetite regulator by children under 12.

 Over 60
▼ Reduced dose may be necessary. Increased likelihood of adverse effects.

 Driving and hazardous work
▼ No known problems.

 Alcohol
▼ No known problems.

POSSIBLE ADVERSE EFFECTS

High doses may be associated with anxiety, nausea, dizziness, and, rarely, with a marked rise in blood pressure, causing palpitations, headache, and breathlessness.

Symptom/effect	Frequency		Discuss with physician		Stop taking drug now	Call physician now
	Common	Rare	Only if severe	In all cases		
Nausea/vomiting		●	■			
Dizziness/lightheadedness		●	■			
Nervousness/insomnia		●	■			
Hallucinations		●		■		
Rash		●		■	▲	
Palpitations/breathlessness		●		■		▮
Headache		●		■		▮

INTERACTIONS

Other sympathomimetic drugs increase the risk of adverse effects with this drug.

Antihypertensives Phenylpropanolamine reduces the blood pressure-lowering effect of antihypertensive drugs.

Monoamine oxidase inhibitors (MAOIs) dangerously increase the risk of high blood pressure with phenylpropanolamine. It should not be taken during or within 14 days following MAOI treatment.

PROLONGED USE

Phenylpropanolamine should not be taken for long periods without medical supervision because it may raise the blood pressure and put a strain on the heart.

PHENYTOIN

Brand names Dilantin, Dilantin Infatabs, Dilantin 30, Dyphenylan
Used in the following combined preparation Dilantin with phenobarbital

GENERAL INFORMATION

By reducing electrical discharges within the brain, phenytoin reduces the likelihood of convulsions (see Anticonvulsant drugs, p.114). Introduced in 1938, it has been widely prescribed for the long-term treatment of several types of epilepsy, including grand mal and temporal lobe seizures.

Over the years other uses for phenytoin have been found: for migraine and some other types of pain, and for correction of certain types of abnormal heart rhythms.

Because some adverse effects of phenytoin (such as overgrowth of the gums) are more pronounced in children, it is prescribed for children only when other drugs are unsuitable. However, careful dental hygiene can delay or minimize the gum problems.

INFORMATION FOR USERS

Your drug prescription is tailored for you. Do not alter dosage without checking with your physician.

How taken

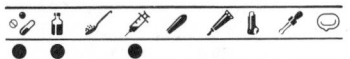

Tablets, capsules, liquid, injection.

Frequency and timing of doses
Once or 3 x daily (depending on preparation) with food or water.

Dosage range
Adults 300 – 400mg daily. The dose may be increased if blood levels so dictate. *Children* According to age and weight.

Onset of effect
Full anticonvulsant effect may not be felt for 7 – 10 days.

Duration of action
24 hours.

Diet advice
Folic acid deficiency may occasionally occur while phenytoin is taken. Folic acid is found in some multivitamin preparations. Make sure you eat a balanced diet containing fresh green vegetables.

Storage
Keep in a tightly closed container in a cool, dry place away from reach of children.

Missed dose
Take as soon as you remember. If your next dose is due within 2 hours, take two doses now and skip the next.

Stopping the drug
Do not stop the drug without consulting your physician; symptoms may recur.

Exceeding the dose
An occasional unintentional extra dose is unlikely to cause problems. You may notice unusual drowsiness or confusion. Notify your physician.

SPECIAL PRECAUTIONS

Be sure to tell your physician if:
▼ You have impaired kidney or liver function.
▼ You have diabetes.
▼ You are taking other medications.

Pregnancy
▼ Not usually prescribed. May cause heart defects in the unborn baby. Discuss with your physician so that you may weigh the benefits of the drug against its risks.

Breast feeding
▼ Discuss with your physician. The drug passes into the breast milk. Its effects on the baby are not known.

Infants and children
▼ Reduced dose necessary. Increased likelihood of overgrowth of the gums and excessive growth of body hair.

Over 60
▼ Reduced dose may be necessary.

Driving and hazardous work
▼ Your underlying condition, as well as the sedative effects of this drug, may make such activities inadvisable. Discuss with your physician.

Alcohol
▼ Avoid. Alcohol increases the sedative effects of this drug.

POSSIBLE ADVERSE EFFECTS

Phenytoin has a number of adverse effects, many of which appear only after prolonged use. If they become severe, your physician may prescribe a different anticonvulsant.

Symptom/effect	Frequency		Discuss with physician		Stop taking drug now	Call physician now
	Common	Rare	Only if severe	In all cases		
Slurred speech	●		■			
Dizziness	●		■			
Confusion	●		■			
Overgrowth of gums	●			■		
Increased body hair		●	■			
Rash		●		■		▲

INTERACTIONS

General note Many drugs may interact with phenytoin, causing either an increase or a reduction in the blood level of phenytoin. The dosage of phenytoin may need to be adjusted while you are taking other medications. Consult your physician.

Oral contraceptives Phenytoin may reduce the effectiveness of oral contraceptives.

Sedatives All drugs that have a sedative effect are likely to increase the sedative properties of phenytoin.

Alcohol Alcohol increases the sedative effect of phenytoin. Chronic alcohol abuse may reduce phenytoin's beneficial anticonvulsant effect.

PROLONGED USE

There is a slight risk of blood abnormalities occurring. Prolonged use may also lead to adverse effects on skin, gums, and bones. It may also disrupt control of diabetes.

Monitoring Periodic blood tests may be performed to monitor levels of the drug in the body and composition of the blood cells and blood chemistry.

PHYTONADIONE

Brand names Aquamephyton, Konakion, Mephyton
Used in the following combined preparations None

GENERAL INFORMATION

A hemostatic drug, phytonadione is actually a synthetic form of vitamin K, which is found in leafy green vegetables, is produced by bacteria in the intestine, and which is essential to the production of substances required for blood clotting. Phytonadione is therefore used to treat bleeding and other disorders caused by vitamin K deficiency – a condition that may result from poor nutrition, liver disease, drug treatment, or from the body's failure to produce or absorb the vitamin.

Phytonadione is the only drug that can reverse bleeding induced by oral anticoagulants such as warfarin and dicumarol.

Since it is stronger, faster-acting and longer-lasting than other vitamin K preparations, it is preferred when large doses or long-term therapy is needed. Phytonadione is also used for the prevention of bleeding in newborn babies, since it carries little risk of anemia and jaundice. It rarely causes adverse effects.

INFORMATION FOR USERS

Your drug prescription is tailored for you. Do not alter dosage without checking with your physician.

How taken

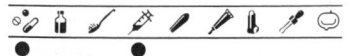

Tablets, injection.

Frequency and timing of doses
As required.

Adult dosage range
2.5 – 10mg daily. Occasionally, larger doses may be needed.

Onset of effect
6 – 12 hours (tablets); 6 – 24 hours (injection).

Duration of action
Up to 14 hours.

Diet advice
If bleeding is due to vitamin K deficiency, your physician may advise you to include more green vegetables in your diet.

Storage
Keep in a closed container in a cool, dry place away from reach of children. Protect from light.

Missed dose
Not applicable, since phytonadione is rarely taken on a regular basis.

Stopping the drug
Do not stop the drug without consulting your physician; symptoms may recur.

Exceeding the dose
An occasional unintentional extra dose is unlikely to be a cause for concern. But if you notice unusual symptoms, or if a large overdose has been taken, notify your physician.

POSSIBLE ADVERSE EFFECTS

There is a rare risk of serious allergic-type reactions following the intravenous injection of phytonadione. Common side effects include dizziness and flushing.

Symptom/effect	Frequency		Discuss with physician		Stop taking drug now	Call physician now
	Common	Rare	Only if severe	In all cases		
Flushing	●			■		
Dizziness	●			■		
Bad taste in mouth		●	■			
Chest pain/tightness		●		■		▮
Palpitations		●		■		▮

INTERACTIONS

Oral anticoagulant drugs Phytonadione reverses the action of oral anticoagulants, so they are not given together unless this action is required, for example, to treat bleeding due to warfarin overdose. Phytonadione does not affect heparin.

SPECIAL PRECAUTIONS

Be sure to tell your physician if:
▼ You have impaired liver or kidney function.
▼ You have heart problems.
▼ You are taking other medications.

Pregnancy
▼ It may be safely given to the mother 12 – 24 hours before delivery to prevent bleeding in a baby who is at special risk.

Breast feeding
▼ No evidence of risk.

Infants and children
▼ Not usually prescribed except for bleeding in the newborn.

Over 60
▼ No known problems.

Driving and hazardous work
▼ No known problems.

Alcohol
▼ No known problems.

PROLONGED USE

Phytonadione is not used for long periods.

PILOCARPINE

Brand names Adsorbocarpine, Isopto Carpine, Ocusert Pilo, Pilocarpine HS
Used in the following combined preparations E-Pilo, Isopto P-ES

GENERAL INFORMATION

Pilocarpine, in use since 1875, is a pupil-constricting drug (miotic) used to treat glaucoma. Obtained from the leaves of an American plant, *Pilocarpus*, it is frequently prescribed for chronic glaucoma and, less often, for emergency treatment of severe glaucoma prior to surgery. It may also be given to counteract the dilation of the pupil induced by drugs given during surgery or eye examination.

It is prescribed most frequently in the form of eye drops. These are quick-acting but have to be re-applied every six to eight hours in chronic glaucoma. A long-acting gel formulation, applied once daily, and a slow-release formulation (Ocusert) inserted under the eyelid once weekly, may be more convenient for long-term use.

Like other similar drugs, pilocarpine frequently causes blurred vision. Excessive spasm of eye muscles may cause headaches, particularly at the start of treatment. However, serious adverse effects are rare.

INFORMATION FOR USERS

Your drug prescription is tailored for you. Do not alter dosage without checking with your physician.

How taken

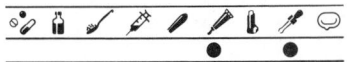

Gel, eye drops, slow-release inserts (Ocuserts).

Frequency and timing of doses
Eye drops 3 – 4 x daily (chronic glaucoma). In acute glaucoma, pilocarpine is given at 5-minute intervals until the condition is controlled.
Gel Once daily at bedtime.
Ocusert Once every 7 days at bedtime.

Dosage range
According to formulation and condition. In general, one eye drop is used per application. Gel is applied as a 1.5cm strip daily.

Onset of effect
15 – 30 minutes.

Duration of action
6 – 14 hours (eye drops); 18 – 24 hours (gel); about 7 days (Ocusert).

Diet advice
None.

Storage
Keep in a closed container in a cool, dry place away from reach of children (eye drops). Refrigerate but do not freeze (gel, Ocusert).

Missed dose
Take as soon as you remember. If not remembered until the next day (gel) or until 2 hours before your next dose (eye drops), skip the missed dose and take your next dose now.

Stopping the drug
Do not stop the drug without consulting your physician; symptoms may recur.

Exceeding the dose
An occasional unintentional extra application is unlikely to cause problems. Excessive use may cause facial flushing, an increase in the flow of saliva, and sweating. If accidentally swallowed, seek medical attention immediately.

SPECIAL PRECAUTIONS

Be sure to tell your physician if:
▼ You have asthma.
▼ You have inflamed eyes.
▼ You are taking other medications.

Pregnancy
▼ No evidence of risk at the doses used for chronic glaucoma.

Breast feeding
▼ The drug passes into the breast milk, but at normal doses adverse effects on the baby are unlikely. Discuss with your physician.

Infants and children
▼ Not usually prescribed.

Over 60
▼ No special problems.

Driving and hazardous work
▼ Avoid such activities, especially in poor light, until you have learned how the drug affects you, because the drug may cause nearsightedness and poor night vision.

Alcohol
▼ No known problems.

POSSIBLE ADVERSE EFFECTS

Gel applied overnight may cause sticking of the eyelids the following morning. The Ocuserts may cause irritation if they move out of position. Brow ache and eye pain are common at the start of treatment, but effects usually wear off after a few days.

Symptom/effect	Frequency		Discuss with physician		Stop taking drug now	Call physician now
	Common	Rare	Only if severe	In all cases		
Blurred vision	●		■			
Poor night vision	●		■			
Headache/brow ache	●		■			
Eye pain/irritation	●			■		■
Twitching eyelids		●	■			
Red/watery eyes		●	■			

PROLONGED USE

The effect of the drug may occasionally wear off with prolonged use as the body adapts, but may be restored by temporary substitution of another antiglaucoma drug.

INTERACTIONS

None.

PIROXICAM

Brand name Feldene
Used in the following combined preparations None

GENERAL INFORMATION

Piroxicam is one of the newer (1982) non-steroidal anti-inflammatory drugs (NSAIDs). Like other drugs of this group, it reduces pain, stiffness, and inflammation. Blood levels of the drug remain high for many hours after a dose, so that it need be taken only once daily and may be considered particularly suitable for prolonged use.

It is prescribed for rheumatoid arthritis, osteoarthritis, ankylosing spondylitis, and acute attacks of gout.

Although piroxicam gives lasting relief of the symptoms of arthritis, it does not cure the disease. It is sometimes prescribed in conjunction with the slow-acting drugs in rheumatoid arthritis to relieve pain and inflammation while these drugs take effect. It may be given for pain relief in bursitis and tendinitis or after minor surgery.

It is less likely than aspirin to cause stomach ulcers and is generally considered safer for long-term use.

INFORMATION FOR USERS

Your drug prescription is tailored for you. Do not alter dosage without checking with your physician.

How taken

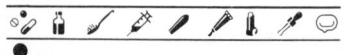

Capsules.

Frequency and timing of doses
Once daily with food.

Adult dosage range
10 – 40mg daily.

Onset of effect
Pain relief begins in 3 – 4 hours. Used for arthritis, the full anti-inflammatory effect develops over 2 – 4 weeks. Used for gout, this effect develops over 4 – 5 days.

Duration of action
Up to 2 days. Some effect may last for 7 – 10 days after treatment has been stopped.

Diet advice
None.

Storage
Keep in a closed container in a cool, dry place away from reach of children. Protect from light.

Missed dose
Take as soon as you remember. If your next dose is due within 6 hours, take a single dose now and skip the next.

Stopping the drug
When taken for short-term pain relief, piroxicam can be safely stopped as soon as you no longer need it. If prescribed for the long-term treatment of arthritis, however, you should seek medical advice before stopping the drug.

Exceeding the dose
An occasional unintentional extra dose is unlikely to cause problems. Large overdoses may cause nausea and vomiting. Notify your physician.

SPECIAL PRECAUTIONS

Be sure to tell your physician if:
▼ You have impaired liver or kidney function.
▼ You have heart problems.
▼ You have high blood pressure.
▼ You have had a peptic ulcer, esophagitis, or acid indigestion.
▼ You have asthma.
▼ You are allergic to aspirin.
▼ You are taking other medications.

 Pregnancy
▼ Not usually prescribed. When taken in the last three months of pregnancy, piroxicam may increase the risk of adverse effects on the baby's heart and may prolong labor. Discuss with your physician.

 Breast feeding
▼ Discuss with your physician. The drug passes into the breast milk but at normal doses adverse effects are uncommon.

 Infants and children
▼ Not recommended.

 Over 60
▼ Reduced dose may be necessary. Increased likelihood of adverse effects.

 Driving and hazardous work
▼ No known problems.

 Alcohol
▼ Avoid. Alcohol may increase the risk of stomach disorders with piroxicam.

Surgery and general anesthetics
▼ Piroxicam may prolong bleeding. Discuss this with your physician or dentist before any surgery.

POSSIBLE ADVERSE EFFECTS

Gastrointestinal side effects, dizziness, and headache are not generally serious. Black or bloodstained bowel movements should be reported to your physician promptly.

Symptom/effect	Frequency		Discuss with physician		Stop taking drug now	Call physician now
	Common	Rare	Only if severe	In all cases		
Nausea/indigestion	●		■			
Abdominal pain	●			■		
Dizziness/headache		●	■			
Swollen feet/ankles		●		■		
Rash/itching		●		■	▲	
Wheezing/breathlessness		●		■	▲	■

INTERACTIONS

General note Piroxicam interacts with a wide range of drugs to increase the risk of bleeding and/or peptic ulcers. Such drugs include oral anticoagulants, corticosteroids, other NSAIDs, and aspirin.

Lithium Piroxicam may raise blood levels of lithium, leading to a risk of serious adverse effects.

Antihypertensive drugs and diuretics The beneficial effects of these drugs may be reduced by piroxicam.

Oral antidiabetic drugs Piroxicam may increase the blood sugar-lowering effect of these drugs.

PROLONGED USE

There is an increased risk of bleeding from peptic ulcers and in the bowel with prolonged use of piroxicam.

PRAZEPAM

Brand name Centrax
Used in the following combined preparations None

GENERAL INFORMATION

Prazepam, introduced in 1977, belongs to the benzodiazepine group of drugs. These help relieve nervousness and tension, relax muscles, and encourage sleep.

A long-acting drug, prazepam is used primarily to treat anxiety disorders. Occasionally, it is given to control the symptoms of withdrawal (restlessness, tremors, delirium, and hallucinations) in alcoholics who are undergoing detoxification.

As with other benzodiazepines, prazepam can be habit-forming if taken at high doses over long periods. Its beneficial effects may also diminish with prolonged use. For these reasons, it is generally prescribed in short courses. The need for treatment is usually reviewed every two weeks.

INFORMATION FOR USERS

Your drug prescription is tailored for you. Do not alter dosage without checking with your physician.

How taken

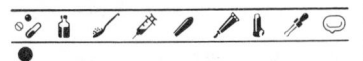

Tablets, capsules.

Frequency and timing of doses
3 x daily or once daily, usually at bedtime.

Adult dosage range
20 – 60mg daily.

Onset of effect
1 hour. Full beneficial effect may not be felt for 5 – 7 days.

Duration of action
36 hours. Some effect may persist for several days.

Diet advice
None.

Storage
Keep in a closed container in a cool, dry place away from reach of children. Protect from light.

Missed dose
Take as soon as you remember. If your next dose is due within 4 hours, take a single dose now and skip the next.

Stopping the drug
If you have been taking the drug continuously for less than 2 weeks, it can be safely stopped as soon as you feel you no longer need it. However, if you have been taking it for longer, consult your physician, who will supervise a gradual reduction in dosage. Stopping abruptly may lead to withdrawal symptoms (see p.111).

Exceeding the dose
An occasional unintentional extra dose is unlikely to cause problems. Large overdoses may cause lethargy and unsteadiness or loss of consciousness. Notify your physician.

SPECIAL PRECAUTIONS

Be sure to tell your physician if:
▼ You have impaired liver or kidney function.
▼ You have severe respiratory disease.
▼ You are taking other medications.

Pregnancy
▼ Not usually prescribed. Safety in pregnancy not established. Discuss with your physician so that you may weigh the benefits of the drug against its risks.

Breast feeding
▼ Discuss with your physician. The drug passes into the breast milk and may make the baby drowsy.

Infants and children
▼ Not recommended.

Over 60
▼ Reduced dose usually necessary. Increased likelihood of adverse effects.

Driving and hazardous work
▼ Avoid such activities until you have learned how the drug affects you, because prazepam may reduce alertness and slow reactions.

Alcohol
▼ Avoid. Alcohol may increase the sedative effects of this drug.

POSSIBLE ADVERSE EFFECTS

The principal adverse effects of this drug are related to its sedative properties. These usually diminish within a few days, and can be reduced by an adjustment in the dose.

Symptom/effect	Frequency		Discuss with physician		Stop taking drug now	Call physician now
	Common	Rare	Only if severe	In all cases		
Daytime drowsiness	●		■			
Dizziness/unsteadiness	●		■			
Forgetfulness/confusion		●	■			
Headache		●	■			
Rash		●		■		

PROLONGED USE

Regular use of this drug over several weeks can lead to a reduction in its effect as the body adapts. It may also be habit-forming when taken for extended periods, especially if larger than average doses are taken.

INTERACTIONS

Sedatives All drugs that have a sedative effect on the central nervous system are likely to increase the sedative properties of prazepam. Such drugs include other anti-anxiety and sleeping drugs, antihistamines, antidepressant drugs, narcotic analgesics, and antipsychotic drugs.

PRAZIQUANTEL

Brand name Biltricide
Used in the following combined preparations None

GENERAL INFORMATION

Praziquantel, an anthelmintic introduced in 1983, is active against flatworms, such as tapeworms and flukes. Ingested by the parasites, it causes calcium loss, leading to muscle paralysis, disintegration of the outer skin, and death.

In the United States, praziquantel is used mainly to treat beef, fish, pork, and dwarf tapeworm infections. Given for cysticercosis, in which pork tapeworm larvae invade muscle, it can clear cysts within one to two weeks.

The drug is particularly useful in the treatment of blood fluke infections (bilharzia), in which immature fluke larvae penetrate the skin and make their way into the blood vessels. Such infections are, however, rare in the United States.

Praziquantel may also be prescribed for a variety of other fluke infestations. These include Chinese and Oriental liver fluke infections (common in Southeast Asia), and infection with lung flukes, giant intestinal flukes, and sheep liver flukes.

Serious adverse effects are rare with this drug. Chemically related to the benzodiazepine tranquilizers, it commonly causes drowsiness, which may impair driving ability. Tablets are bitter-tasting and should be swallowed whole with liquid.

QUICK REFERENCE

Drug group Anthelmintic drug (p.167)

Overdose danger rating Low

Dependence rating Low

Prescription needed Yes

Available as generic No

INFORMATION FOR USERS

Your drug prescription is tailored for you. Do not alter dosage without checking with your physician.

How taken

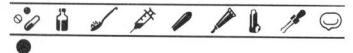

Tablets.

Frequency and timing of doses
Blood fluke infections A single dose or 1 – 3 x daily (4 – 6 hours apart).
Other fluke infections 3 x daily for 1 – 3 days.
Tapeworm infections A single dose.
Cysticercosis 3 x daily for 14 days.

Dosage range
According to body weight and type of worm.

Onset of effect
Within 1 hour.

Duration of action
About 24 hours.

Diet advice
None.

Storage
Keep in a closed container in a cool, dry place away from reach of children.

Missed dose
Take as soon as you remember. If your doses are scheduled 3 times daily, space missed dose and remaining dose(s) 4 hours apart.

Stopping the drug
Take the full course as instructed. This is necessary to eliminate the parasite.

Exceeding the dose
An occasional unintentional extra dose is unlikely to be a cause for concern. If you notice unusual symptoms, or if a large overdose has been taken, notify your physician.

SPECIAL PRECAUTIONS

Be sure to tell your physician if:
▼ You have severe diarrhea.
▼ You are taking other medications.

Pregnancy
▼ Not usually prescribed. Safety in pregnancy not established. Discuss with your physician so that you can weigh the benefits of the drug against its possible risks.

Breast feeding
▼ Discuss with your physician. The drug passes into the breast milk and may affect the baby adversely.

Infants and children
▼ Not recommended for children under 4 years. Reduced dose necessary for older children.

Over 60
▼ No special problems.

Driving and hazardous work
▼ Avoid such activities on the day(s) of treatment and for 24 hours after treatment ends, because the drug may cause dizziness and drowsiness.

Alcohol
▼ Sedative effect may be intensified.

PROLONGED USE

No problems expected.

POSSIBLE ADVERSE EFFECTS

Serious adverse effects are rare with this drug. Dizziness, headache and abdominal pain or nausea are more common with high doses but are usually short-lasting.

Symptom/effect	Frequency		Discuss with physician		Stop taking drug now	Call physician now
	Common	Rare	Only if severe	In all cases		
Dizziness/drowsiness	●		■			
Headache	●		■			
Abdominal pain	●		■			
Nausea	●		■			
Diarrhea	●		■			
Rash/itching		●		■		▮
Fever/sweating		●		■		▮

INTERACTIONS

None.

PRAZOSIN

Brand name Minipress
Used in the following combined preparation Minizide

GENERAL INFORMATION

Available since 1975, prazosin relieves high blood pressure by relaxing the muscles in the walls of the blood vessels, dilating them and easing the flow of blood. For the same reason, it is also sometimes given to those suffering from heart failure or Raynaud's disease, characterized by poor circulation to the hands and feet.

Unlike some other antihypertensives, prazosin does not slow the heart rate, making it useful in the treatment of several varieties of raised blood pressure. It is usually prescribed with a diuretic; in moderate to severe high blood pressure, it may be given with beta blockers or other antihypertensive drugs.

Dizziness and fainting are common at the onset of treatment with prazosin because of the dramatic drop in blood pressure or elevated pulse rate. For this reason, the initial dose is usually low and given when the person is lying down. Dosage levels may later be increased as necessary.

QUICK REFERENCE

Drug group Antihypertensive drug (p.130)

Overdose danger rating Medium

Dependence rating Low

Prescription needed Yes

Available as generic No

INFORMATION FOR USERS

Your drug prescription is tailored for you. Do not alter dosage without checking with your physician.

How taken

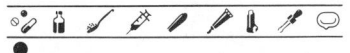

Capsules.

Frequency and timing of doses
2 – 3 x daily.

Adult dosage range
1mg (starting dose), increased as necessary to 20mg daily (maintenance dose). Larger doses may occasionally be prescribed.

Onset of effect
Within 2 hours.

Duration of action
7 – 8 hours.

Diet advice
None.

Storage
Keep in a closed container in a cool, dry place away from reach of children.

Missed dose
Take as soon as you remember. If your next dose is due within 2 hours, take a single dose now and skip the next.

Stopping the drug
Do not stop taking the drug without consulting your physician; stopping the drug may lead to a rise in blood pressure.

Exceeding the dose
An occasional unintentional extra dose is unlikely to cause problems. Large overdoses may cause dizziness or fainting. Notify your physician.

SPECIAL PRECAUTIONS

Be sure to tell your physician if:
▼ You have impaired kidney or liver function.
▼ You have heart failure.
▼ You are taking other medications.

 Pregnancy
▼ Not usually prescribed. Safety in pregnancy not established. Discuss with your physician so that you can weigh the benefits of the drug against its possible risks.

 Breast feeding
▼ Discuss with your physician. Effect on breast milk uncertain.

 Infants and children
▼ Not recommended.

 Over 60
▼ Reduced dose may be necessary.

 Driving and hazardous work
▼ Avoid such activities until you have learned how the drug affects you, because the drug can cause dizziness and fainting.

 Alcohol
▼ Avoid. Alcohol may increase the adverse effects of this drug.

POSSIBLE ADVERSE EFFECTS

Prazosin may cause dizziness and fainting on rising, so it is important that the first dose is taken at bedtime. You should remain in bed for at least 3 hours after taking the drug.

Some of the minor symptoms, such as headache and nausea, will diminish after long-term therapy, although this may take up to 3 months.

Symptom/effect	Frequency		Discuss with physician		Stop taking drug now	Call physician now
	Common	Rare	Only if severe	In all cases		
Nausea	●		■			
Headache	●		■			
Dizziness/faintness	●		■			
Dry mouth	●		■			
Stuffy nose	●		■			
Joint pains		●		■		
Rash		●		■		■

PROLONGED USE

No problems expected.

INTERACTIONS

Diuretics Diuretics increase the blood-pressure-lowering effect of prazosin.

PREDNISOLONE

Brand names AK-Tate, Hydeltra TBA, Inflamase Forte, Inflamase Mild, Pred Forte
Used in the following combined preparations AK-Cide, Blephamide, Metimyd, Poly-Pred, Vasocidin

GENERAL INFORMATION

Introduced in 1955, prednisolone is a powerful corticosteroid. It is available as a *topical* preparation for a variety of skin conditions such as dermatitis, eczema, and psoriasis (see p.202). Given as eye drops, it reduces eye inflammation in conjunctivitis or iritis. Prednisolone enemas may be given to treat inflammatory bowel disease. The drug can be injected into joints to relieve rheumatoid and other forms of arthritis. Blood disorders such as thrombocytopenia and leukemia are also treated with prednisolone. With fludrocortisone, prednisolone is also prescribed for pituitary or adrenal gland disorders.

Low doses taken by mouth over a short term or topical applications rarely cause serious side effects. However, long-term treatment with large doses can cause fluid retention, indigestion, acne, and hypertension. Prednisolone may also induce diabetes.

QUICK REFERENCE

Drug group Corticosteroid (p.169)
Overdose danger rating Low
Dependence rating Low
Prescription needed Yes
Available as generic Yes

INFORMATION FOR USERS

Your drug prescription is tailored for you. Do not alter dosage without checking with your physician.

How taken

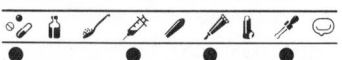

Tablets, injection, cream, eye drops, enema.

Frequency and timing of doses
2 – 4 x daily (eye drops); 3 – 4 x daily (cream); 1 – 2 x daily or on alternate days (by mouth or injection).

Adult dosage range
Considerable variation. Follow your physician's instructions.

Onset of effect
2 – 4 days.

Duration of action
12 – 72 hours.

Diet advice
A low-sodium, high-potassium diet is recommended when the oral or injected form of the drug is prescribed for extended periods. Follow the advice of your physician.

Storage
Keep in a closed container in a cool, dry place away from reach of children.

Missed dose
Take as soon as you remember. If your next dose is due within 6 hours, take a single dose now and skip the next.

Stopping the drug
Do not stop the drug without consulting your physician. Abrupt cessation of long-term treatment by mouth or injection may cause hormonal imbalance.

Exceeding the dose
An occasional unintentional extra dose is unlikely to be a cause for concern. But if you notice unusual symptoms, or if a large overdose has been taken, notify your physician.

POSSIBLE ADVERSE EFFECTS

The rare but more serious adverse effects occur only when prednisolone is taken by mouth or injection in high doses or for long periods of time.

Symptom/effect	Frequency		Discuss with physician		Stop taking drug now	Call physician now
	Common	Rare	Only if severe	In all cases		
Indigestion	●			■		
Acne	●			■		
Weight gain		●		■		
Muscle weakness		●		■		
Mood changes		●		■		
Bloody/black stools		●		■	▲	▮

INTERACTIONS

Oral anticoagulant drugs Prednisolone by mouth or injection increases blood clotting.

Digoxin Prednisolone may increase the risk of adverse effects from digoxin.

Vaccines Serious reactions can occur when vaccinations are given with this drug. Discuss with your physician.

Insulin and antidiabetic drugs Prednisolone by mouth or injection reduces the actions of these drugs.

Antihypertensive drugs Prednisolone by mouth or injection may reduce the effect of antihypertensive drugs.

SPECIAL PRECAUTIONS

Be sure to tell your physician if:
▼ You have had a peptic ulcer.
▼ You have had glaucoma.
▼ You have had tuberculosis.
▼ You suffer from depression.
▼ You have a herpes infection.
▼ You have diabetes.
▼ You are taking other medications.

Pregnancy
▼ No evidence of risk with ointment or joint injections. Given by tablets in low doses, harm to the baby is unlikely. Discuss with your physician so that you can weigh the benefits of the drug against its possible risks.

Breast feeding
▼ No evidence of risk with ointment or joint injections. Taken by mouth, the drug passes into the breast milk and if taken regularly may adversely affect the baby. Discuss with your physician.

Infants and children
▼ Reduced dose may be necessary.

Over 60
▼ Reduced dose may be necessary. Increased likelihood of adverse effects.

Driving and hazardous work
▼ No known problems.

Alcohol
▼ Alcohol may increase the risk of peptic ulcers with prednisolone by mouth or injection. No special problems with other dosage forms.

PROLONGED USE

Prolonged use of prednisolone by mouth or injection is recommended only when essential because it can lead to adverse effects such as diabetes, glaucoma, cataracts, and fragile bones, and may retard growth in children.

PREDNISONE

Brand names Deltasone, Liquid Pred, Meticorten, Orasone, Pred-5
Used in the following combined preparations None

GENERAL INFORMATION

Prednisone, introduced in 1955, is a long-acting, synthetic corticosteroid drug used in the treatment of a variety of inflammatory disorders, including inflammatory bowel disease, and connective tissue diseases and joint disorders such as rheumatoid arthritis. Severe asthma may also be controlled by regular administration of prednisone.

Less common uses of the drug include the prevention of organ transplant rejection, replacement therapy in Addison's disease, and treatment of blood disorders such as thrombocytopenia and leukemia, when it is often used in conjunction with other drugs.

Used in low doses, prednisone seldom causes troublesome side effects. However, large doses taken over a prolonged period can cause adverse effects such as indigestion, mood changes, weakness and bone damage, fluid retention, acne, diabetes mellitus, facial rounding, excessive hair, and hypertension.

INFORMATION FOR USERS

Your drug prescription is tailored for you. Do not alter dosage without checking with your physician.

How taken

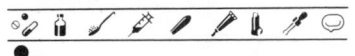

Tablets.

Frequency and timing of doses
2 x daily with food.

Dosage range
Adults 5 – 10mg daily (Addison's disease); 5 – 60mg daily (inflammatory and other disorders).
Children Dosage is adjusted according to the condition and the child's response.

Onset of effect
2 – 4 days.

Duration of action
Up to 24 hours.

Diet advice
Salt intake may need to be restricted when the drug is taken by mouth. Potassium levels may be depleted, so you may need to take supplements.

Storage
Keep in a closed container in a cool, dry place away from reach of children.

Missed dose
Take as soon as you remember. If your next dose is scheduled within 4 hours, take both doses now.

Stopping the drug
Do not stop the drug without consulting your physician. A gradual reduction in dose is required following prolonged treatment.

Exceeding the dose
An occasional unintentional extra dose is unlikely to be a cause for concern. But if you notice unusual symptoms, or if a large overdose has been taken, notify your physician.

SPECIAL PRECAUTIONS

Be sure to tell your physician if:
▼ You have had a peptic ulcer.
▼ You have glaucoma.
▼ You have a herpes infection.
▼ You have suffered from depression or psychotic illness.
▼ You have had tuberculosis.
▼ You are taking other medications.

Pregnancy
▼ Not usually prescribed. Safety in pregnancy not established. Discuss with your physician so that you can weigh the benefits of the drug against its possible risks.

Breast feeding
▼ Discuss with your physician. The drug passes into the breast milk and may affect the baby adversely.

Infants and children
▼ Reduced dose necessary.

Over 60
▼ Reduced dose may be necessary. Increased likelihood of adverse effects.

Driving and hazardous work
▼ No known problems.

Alcohol
▼ Avoid. Alcohol may increase the risk of developing peptic ulcers.

POSSIBLE ADVERSE EFFECTS

Adverse effects are uncommon at low doses; serious adverse effects occur only when prednisone is taken in high doses or for long periods.

Symptom/effect	Frequency		Discuss with physician		Stop taking drug now	Call physician now
	Common	Rare	Only if severe	In all cases		
Indigestion	●		■			
Acne	●		■			
Weight gain		●		■		
Muscle weakness		●		■		
Mood changes		●		■		
Bloody/black stools		●		■	▲	∎

INTERACTIONS

Insulin and antidiabetic drugs Prednisone reduces the actions of these drugs.

Antihypertensive drugs Prednisone may reduce the effect of antihypertensives.

Oral anticoagulant drugs Prednisone increases blood clotting.

Digoxin Prednisone may increase the risk of adverse effects from digoxin.

Vaccines Serious reactions can occur when vaccinations are given with this drug. Discuss with your physician.

PROLONGED USE

Prolonged use of this drug is recommended only when essential because it can lead to adverse effects such as diabetes, glaucoma, cataracts, and fragile bones and may retard growth in children.

PRIMAQUINE

Brand names None
Used in the following combined preparation Aralen Phosphate with Primaquine Phosphate

GENERAL INFORMATION

Primaquine, introduced in 1952, is highly effective against certain types of malaria, eliminating the parasite from all parts of the body, including the latent infestations of the liver and spleen. It is often used after initial treatment by chloroquine, a faster-acting antimalarial drug that suppresses the chills and fever of malaria in its symptomatic form. Because its onset of effect is slow and its duration of action short, primaquine is not effective as a preventive treatment. The drug is also given for South American trypanosomiasis, or Chagas' disease.

Serious side effects are rare with primaquine, although it may occasionally cause breakdown of red blood cells (hemolysis). The risk of this condition is particularly high in those with glucose-6-phosphate dehydrogenase (G6PD) deficiency.

QUICK REFERENCE

Drug group Antimalarial drug (p.165)
Overdose danger rating Medium
Dependence rating Low
Prescription needed Yes
Available as generic Yes

INFORMATION FOR USERS

Your drug prescription is tailored for you. Do not alter dosage without checking with your physician.

How taken

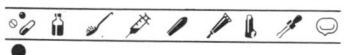

Tablets.

Frequency and timing of doses
Once daily.

Dosage range
Adults 15mg (daily) or 30 – 45mg (weekly).
Children Reduced dose according to age and weight.

Onset of effect
2 – 3 days.

Duration of action
Up to 24 hours.

Diet advice
Take with food.

Storage
Keep in a closed container in a cool, dry place away from reach of children. Protect from light.

Missed dose
Take as soon as you remember. If your next dose is due within 6 hours (once daily schedule) or within 2 days (once weekly schedule), take both doses now.

Stopping the drug
Take the full course. Even if you feel better, the original infection may still be present and symptoms may recur if treatment is stopped too soon.

Exceeding the dose
An occasional unintentional extra dose is unlikely to cause problems. Large overdoses may cause vomiting, dizziness, breathlessness, and fatigue. Notify your physician.

SPECIAL PRECAUTIONS

Be sure to tell your physician if:
▼ You or a member of your family has glucose-6-phosphate dehydrogenase (G6PD) deficiency or another blood disorder.
▼ You have rheumatoid arthritis.
▼ You have lupus erythematosus.
▼ You are taking other medications.

Pregnancy
▼ Not usually prescribed. Safety in pregnancy not established. Discuss with your physician so that you can weigh the benefits of the drug against its possible risks.

Breast feeding
▼ The drug passes into the breast milk and may affect the baby adversely. Discuss with your physician.

Infants and children
▼ Reduced dose necessary.

Over 60
▼ No special problems.

Driving and hazardous work
▼ No known problems.

Alcohol
▼ No known problems.

POSSIBLE ADVERSE EFFECTS

Primaquine may occasionally cause serious adverse effects on the blood, including hemolytic anemia leading to dark/cloudy urine and unusual tiredness or weakness.

Gastrointestinal side effects that may occur while taking this drug – including nausea, vomiting, and abdominal pain – can be minimized by taking the drug with food.

Symptom/effect	Frequency		Discuss with physician		Stop taking drug now	Call physician now
	Common	Rare	Only if severe	In all cases		
Nausea/vomiting	●		■			
Abdominal pain	●		■			
Blurred vision		●		■		
Itching		●		■		
Dizziness/headache		●		■		
Dark/cloudy urine		●		■	▲	▮

INTERACTIONS

General note Any drug that suppresses bone marrow activity or may cause hemolytic anemia may increase the risk of adverse effects with primaquine.

Such drugs include immunosuppressants, anticancer drugs, antirheumatic drugs, sulfonamides, chloramphenicol, and trimethoprim.

PROLONGED USE

Prolonged use of primaquine may increase the risk of hemolytic anemia in those with glucose-6-phosphate dehydrogenase (G6PD) deficiency.

Monitoring Periodic counts of blood cells may be performed.

PRIMIDONE

Brand names Myidone, Mysoline
Used in the following combined preparations None

GENERAL INFORMATION

Introduced in 1954, primidone belongs to a group of drugs known as the anticonvulsants. It is chemically related to the barbiturates (see Sleeping drugs, p.110) and is partially converted to phenobarbital in the body. Primidone is mainly used for its effect in suppressing epileptic seizures.

However, it is also occasionally prescribed to treat people who suffer from benign tremors.

Though it may be prescribed on its own, it is more frequently taken with another anticonvulsant. Its major adverse effects are due to its sedative action on the central nervous system.

INFORMATION FOR USERS

Your drug prescription is tailored for you. Do not alter dosage without checking with your physician.

How taken

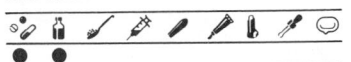

Tablets, liquid.

Frequency and timing of doses
2 – 4 x daily.

Adult dosage range
750mg – 2g daily.

Onset of effect
Within 30 minutes.

Duration of action
24 hours.

Diet advice
None.

Storage
Keep in a closed container in a cool, dry place away from reach of children.

Missed dose
Take as soon as you remember. If your next dose is due within 2 hours, wait for 6 hours to take it.

Stopping the drug
Do not stop the drug without consulting your physician; symptoms may recur.

OVERDOSE ACTION

 Seek immediate medical advice in all cases. Take emergency action if consciousness is lost.

See Drug poisoning emergency guide (p.590).

POSSIBLE ADVERSE EFFECTS

Most people experience very few adverse effects with this drug, but when blood levels get too high, adverse effects are common and the dose may need to be reduced.

Symptom/effect	Frequency		Discuss with physician		Stop taking drug now	Call physician now
	Common	Rare	Only if severe	In all cases		
Drowsiness	●		■			
Clumsiness/unsteadiness	●		■			
Dizziness/faintness	●		■			
Confusion	●		■			
Excitement		●	■			
Rash		●		■	▲	

INTERACTIONS

Sedatives All drugs that have a sedative effect on the central nervous system are likely to increase the sedative properties of primidone. Such drugs include antihistamines, sleeping drugs, narcotic analgesics, antipsychotics, and antidepressants.

Anticoagulant drugs Primidone may reduce the effect of anticoagulant drugs. The anticoagulant dose may need to be adjusted accordingly.

Tricyclic antidepressants Use of tricyclic antidepressants may counteract the effect of primidone.

Oral contraceptives Primidone may reduce the effectiveness of oral contraceptives. An alternative form of contraception may need to be used. Discuss with your physician.

Corticosteroids Primidone opposes the action of some of these drugs. The corticosteroid dose may need to be adjusted accordingly.

SPECIAL PRECAUTIONS

Be sure to tell your physician if:
▼ You have impaired kidney or liver function.
▼ You have heart problems.
▼ You have poor circulation.
▼ You have a lung disorder such as asthma or bronchitis.
▼ You have porphyria.
▼ You have persistent pain.
▼ You are taking other medications.

 Pregnancy
▼ Not usually prescribed. May cause abnormalities in the unborn baby. Discuss with your physician so that you may weigh the benefits of the drug against its risks.

 Breast feeding
▼ Discuss with your physician. The drug passes into the breast milk and may affect the baby adversely.

 Infants and children
▼ Not usually prescribed. Reduced dose necessary.

 Over 60
▼ Reduced dose may be necessary. May cause unusual excitement in the elderly.

 Driving and hazardous work
▼ Your underlying condition, as well as the possibility of reduced alertness while taking this drug, may make such activities inadvisable. Discuss with your physician.

 Alcohol
▼ Avoid. Alcohol may dangerously increase the sedative effects of this drug.

PROLONGED USE

Continued use of this drug may sometimes lead to dependence.

Monitoring Regular blood tests may be performed to measure blood levels of primidone.

PROBENECID

Brand names Benemid, Proban
Used in the following combined preparations ColBenemid, Polycillin-PRB

GENERAL INFORMATION

Since 1951 probenecid has been pre-scribed for people who suffer from recurrent attacks of gout. It reduces the level of uric acid in the body by increasing the amount excreted in the urine. It is used for the long-term prevention of gout attacks, not for the inflammation and pain once an attack has begun. During the first six months of treatment, attacks may even be more frequent, and colchicine may be given in addition during this period. Probenecid is occasionally prescribed to boost the effect of penicillin or cephalosporin antibiotics in the treatment of certain infections, since it blocks their secretion by the kidneys, thereby increasing their levels in the blood.

Serious adverse reactions are rare, though by increasing uric acid secretion by the kidneys, probenecid can increase the risk of uric acid kidney stones. It is therefore mainly used for those who secrete little or no uric acid.

QUICK REFERENCE

Drug group Drug for gout (p.147)
Overdose danger rating Medium
Dependence rating Low
Prescription needed Yes
Available as generic Yes

INFORMATION FOR USERS

Your drug prescription is tailored for you. Do not alter dosage without checking with your physician.

How taken

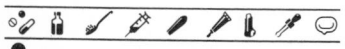

Tablets.

Frequency and timing of doses
1 – 2 x daily with water (gout), 4 x daily (with penicillin).

Dosage range
Gout 0.5g daily for 1 week then 1 – 1.5g daily. Dose may be increased in exceptional circumstances.
With penicillin 1 – 2g daily.

Onset of effect
Within 3 – 6 months (gout), within 2 hours (with penicillin).

Duration of action
4 – 17 hours.

Diet advice
None.

Storage
Keep in a closed container in a cool, dry place away from reach of children.

Missed dose
Take as soon as you remember. If your next dose is due within 4 hours, take a single dose now and skip the next.

Stopping the drug
Do not stop the drug without consulting your physician; symptoms may recur.

Exceeding the dose
An occasional unintentional extra dose is unlikely to cause problems. Large over-doses may cause nausea, vomiting, or tremors. Notify your physician.

SPECIAL PRECAUTIONS

Be sure to tell your physician if:
▼ You have impaired kidney function.
▼ You have had a blood disorder.
▼ You have had kidney stones.
▼ You have had a peptic ulcer.
▼ You are taking other medications.

Pregnancy
▼ Not usually prescribed. Safety in pregnancy not established. Discuss with your physician so that you can weigh the benefits of the drug against its possible risks.

Breast feeding
▼ Discuss with your physician. The drug passes into the breast milk and may affect the baby adversely.

Infants and children
▼ Not recommended for children under 2 years. Reduced dose necessary in older children.

Over 60
▼ No special problems.

Driving and hazardous work
▼ No known problems.

Alcohol
▼ Avoid. Alcohol may reduce the beneficial effects of this drug.

POSSIBLE ADVERSE EFFECTS

Most people do not feel any severe adverse effects when taking probenecid. The more common ones usually diminish as your body adjusts to the medicine. However, excretion of uric acid crystals can lead to the passing of blood and painful urination.

Symptom/effect	Frequency		Discuss with physician		Stop taking drug now	Call physician now
	Common	Rare	Only if severe	In all cases		
Nausea/vomiting	●		■			
Headache	●		■			
Flushing		●		■		
Blood in urine		●		■		▮
Painful urination		●		■		▮
Rash/itching		●		■	▲	▮

PROLONGED USE

No problems expected.

Monitoring Periodic blood tests may be carried out to ensure that blood levels of uric acid are not excessively reduced.

INTERACTIONS

General note Many drugs affect the action of probenecid and may require an adjustment of dosage. Some may reduce the effect of probenecid (for example, thiazide diuretics, aspirin, and alcohol).

The action of other drugs may be increased by probenecid. Such drugs include oral antidiabetic drugs, indomethacin, sulfonamides, and methotrexate.

PROBUCOL

Brand name Lorelco
Used in the following combined preparations None

GENERAL INFORMATION

Because it can reduce the level of certain fats (lipids) in the blood, probucol is given to people threatened with coronary artery disease and other conditions arising from the clogging caused by the buildup of fatty deposits on the interior of the arteries. In most such cases, a low-fat diet is also prescribed.

Introduced in 1977 and sometimes less effective than other lipid-lowering drugs, probucol is usually prescribed only when other drugs have failed or proved to be unsuitable. It is often given with such drugs as cholestyramine or colestipol to boost their effect.

Regular monitoring of the effects of probucol is required because the drug can upset the balance of different fats in the blood. If no improvement is evident after three to four months, the drug is usually withdrawn.

QUICK REFERENCE

Drug group Lipid-lowering drug (p.131)

Overdose danger rating Low

Dependence rating Low

Prescription needed Yes

Available as generic No

INFORMATION FOR USERS

Your drug prescription is tailored for you. Do not alter dosage without checking with your physician.

How taken

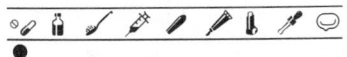

Tablets.

Frequency and timing of doses
2 x daily (morning and evening) with meals.

Adult dosage range
1g daily.

Onset of effect
1 – 3 months.

Duration of action
12 – 24 hours. Some effects may last for up to 6 months after drug treatment is stopped.

Diet advice
A low-fat diet is recommended with this drug.

Storage
Keep in a closed container in a cool, dry place away from reach of children. Protect from light.

Missed dose
Take as soon as you remember. If your next dose is due within 4 hours, take a single dose with your next meal and resume your usual dose schedule thereafter.

Stopping the drug
Do not stop the drug without consulting your physician; stopping the drug may lead to worsening of the underlying condition.

Exceeding the dose
An occasional unintentional extra dose is unlikely to be a cause for concern. But if you notice unusual symptoms, or if a large overdose has been taken, notify your physician.

SPECIAL PRECAUTIONS

Be sure to tell your physician if:
▼ You have impaired liver function.
▼ You have abnormal heart rhythms or other heart problems.
▼ You have diabetes.
▼ You have gallstones.
▼ You are taking other medications.

Pregnancy
▼ Not usually prescribed. Safety in pregnancy not established. Discuss with your physician so that you can weigh the benefits of the drug against its possible risks.

Breast feeding
▼ Discuss with your physician. The drug passes into the breast milk and may affect the baby adversely.

Infants and children
▼ Not recommended.

Over 60
▼ No special problems.

Driving and hazardous work
▼ No known problems.

Alcohol
▼ Follow your physician's diet instructions with respect to alcohol.

POSSIBLE ADVERSE EFFECTS

Gastrointestinal disturbances such as indigestion, diarrhea, and abdominal pain occur in some people but are usually temporary. Less common adverse effects include headache, dizziness, numbness or tingling of the toes and fingers, and swellings of the hands, feet, face, or in the mouth (angioedema).

Symptom/effect	Frequency		Discuss with physician		Stop taking drug now	Call physician now
	Common	Rare	Only if severe	In all cases		
Diarrhea/flatulence	●		■			
Nausea/vomiting	●		■			
Abdominal pain	●		■			
Dizziness and headache		●		■		
Numb toes or fingers		●		■		
Palpitations		●		■		
Swollen hands and feet		●		■	▲	▌
Swollen face and mouth		●		■	▲	▌

INTERACTIONS

None.

PROLONGED USE

Probucol may alter the ratio of certain fats in the bloodstream, leading to an excessive buildup of fat in the arteries.

Monitoring Periodic checks on fat levels in the blood are usually desired to monitor the drug's effectiveness and to guard against adverse effects on blood fats.

A B C D E F G H I J K L M N O P Q R S T U V W X Y Z

PROCAINAMIDE

Brand names Procan SR, Pronestyl, Pronestyl-SR
Used in the following combined preparations None

GENERAL INFORMATION

Procainamide was introduced in the 1940s as an anti-arrhythmic drug. It is used to treat abnormal heart rhythms (tachycardia), especially the too rapid heartbeats in the ventricles. It may be administered when lidocaine, a more commonly used anti-arrhythmic, is unsuccessful.

Procainamide is sometimes used in the treatment of Wolff-Parkinson-White syndrome, a congenital heart abnormality characterized by episodes of rapid or irregular rhythms (tachyarrhythmias). Procainamide is often given in the hospital, where its effect on the heartbeat can be carefully monitored.

Many of the adverse effects common to anti-arrhythmics occur less often with procainamide. However, when taken over a long period, a drug-induced lupus erythematosus may occur in some people, thus limiting procainamide's usefulness.

INFORMATION FOR USERS

Your drug prescription is tailored for you. Do not alter dosage without checking with your physician.

How taken

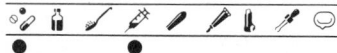

Tablets, capsules, injection.

Frequency and timing of doses
Every 3 – 6 hours (tablets); every 6 – 8 hours (slow-release capsules).

Adult dosage range
1 – 4g daily (tablets, capsules).

Onset of effect
30 – 60 minutes.

Duration of action
3 – 6 hours (tablets); 6 – 8 hours (slow-release capsules).

Diet advice
No special problems.

Storage
Keep in a closed container in a cool, dry place away from reach of children.

Missed dose
Take as soon as you remember. If your next dose is due within 2 hours, take a single dose now and skip the next.

Stopping the drug
Do not stop the drug without consulting your physician; symptoms may recur.

Exceeding the drug
An occasional unintentional extra dose is unlikely to cause problems. Large overdoses may cause palpitations, lethargy, confusion, nausea, and vomiting. Notify your physician.

SPECIAL PRECAUTIONS

Be sure to tell your physician if:
▼ You have impaired kidney or liver function.
▼ You have a lung disorder such as asthma or bronchitis.
▼ You have myasthenia gravis.
▼ You have had lupus erythematosus.
▼ You are taking other medications.

Pregnancy
▼ Not usually prescribed. Safety in pregnancy not established. Discuss with your physician so that you can weigh the benefits of the drug against its possible risks.

Breast feeding
▼ Discuss with your physician. Effect on breast milk uncertain.

Infants and children
▼ Not usually prescribed. Reduced dose necessary.

Over 60
▼ Reduced dose may be necessary.

Driving and hazardous work
▼ No special problems.

Alcohol
▼ No special problems.

POSSIBLE ADVERSE EFFECTS

Some of the minor symptoms, such as loss of appetite, nausea, and vomiting are common to many anti-arrhythmic drugs.

The more serious effects occur much less frequently with procainamide than with other similar drugs (see also Prolonged Use).

Symptom/effect	Frequency		Discuss with physician		Stop taking drug now	Call physician now
	Common	Rare	Only if severe	In all cases		
Nausea/vomiting	●		■			
Loss of appetite	●		■			
Fever		●		■		
Joint pain and swelling		●		■		
Confusion/lethargy		●		■		
Rash		●		■		

INTERACTIONS

Antihypertensive drugs These drugs increase the likelihood of excessively lowered blood pressure.

Anticholinergic drugs Procainamide reduces the effect of anticholinergic drugs.

PROLONGED USE

Prolonged use of this drug may lead to lupus erythematosus, including fever, joint pain, swelling, and rash. These effects disappear when the drug is withdrawn.

PROCAINE

Brand name Novocain
Used in the following combined preparations Anuject, Durathesia

GENERAL INFORMATION

In use since 1905, procaine was for years the most effective and widely used local anesthetic. Given by injection, it provides relief of pain prior to surgery or dental treatment and, occasionally, during childbirth. It is often given in combination with epinephrine to prolong its action and reduce the risk of side effects.

Procaine has now been largely replaced by drugs that are quicker- or longer-acting when given by injection. It is ineffective as a *topical* anesthetic, since it is poorly absorbed through the skin or mucous membranes.

Adverse effects are rare, although allergic rashes may occur occasionally in susceptible people.

INFORMATION FOR USERS

This drug is given only under medical supervision and is not for self-administration.

How taken

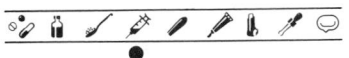

Injection.

Frequency and timing of doses
Shortly before surgery or other procedure.

Dosage range
According to site of injection and individual response.

Onset of effect
Varies according to the type of injection, the injection site, and the individual. Usually 10 – 15 minutes.

Duration of action
40 – 60 minutes.

Diet advice
Given for dental treatment, procaine injection causes numbness and may interfere with swallowing. To avoid choking and injury to the inside of your mouth from hot food or drink, do not eat or drink anything for 1 hour.

Storage
Not applicable. The drug is not kept in the home.

Missed dose
Not applicable. The drug is given only under medical supervision.

Stopping the drug
Not applicable.

Exceeding the dose
Procaine is always injected by a physician or other trained professional and overdose is extremely rare.

SPECIAL PRECAUTIONS

Be sure to tell your physician if:
▼ You have impaired liver or kidney function.
▼ You have heart problems.
▼ You have had epileptic seizures.
▼ You have myasthenia gravis.
▼ You have had an allergic reaction to a local anesthetic.
▼ You are taking other medications.

Pregnancy
▼ Not usually prescribed. Given for spinal anesthesia during childbirth, procaine may prolong labor and increase the need for forceps-assisted delivery.

Breast feeding
▼ No evidence of risk.

Infants and children
▼ Not usually prescribed.

Over 60
▼ No special problems.

Driving and hazardous work
▼ No known problems.

Alcohol
▼ No known problems.

POSSIBLE ADVERSE EFFECTS

Allergic reactions such as rash, hives, or swelling of the face, lips, mouth, or throat may occur occasionally with procaine.

Other symptoms such as anxiety, drowsiness, and ringing in the ears are very rarely experienced with this drug.

Symptom/effect	Frequency		Discuss with physician		Stop taking drug now	Call physician now
	Common	Rare	Only if severe	In all cases		
Rash		●		■	▲	▮
Swelling		●		■	▲	▮
Dizziness/drowsiness		●		■	▲	▮
Anxiety/restlessness		●		■	▲	▮
Ringing in the ears		●		■	▲	▮
Blurred vision		●		■	▲	▮

INTERACTIONS

Sulfonamides Procaine may reduce the antibacterial effect of these drugs.

PROLONGED USE

This drug is not used for prolonged periods.

PROCARBAZINE

Brand name Matulane
Used in the following combined preparations None

GENERAL INFORMATION

Introduced in 1967, procarbazine is taken by mouth for certain kinds of cancer. Its main use is in the treatment of lymphatic cancers, such as Hodgkin's disease, when it is usually given with other drugs. It has also been used to treat brain tumors and certain forms of cancer of the skin, lungs, and bone marrow.

Nausea and vomiting are the most common side effects of procarbazine.

If nausea and vomiting are particularly serious, an anti-emetic drug (p.118) may be prescribed.

Use of procarbazine may increase the risk of anemia and blood clotting disorders. There may also be increased susceptibility to infection. Since procarbazine is related to the MAOI antidepressants, it is important to avoid certain foods that can cause a sudden rise in blood pressure.

QUICK REFERENCE

Drug group Anticancer drug (p.182)
Overdose danger rating Medium
Dependence rating Low
Prescription needed Yes
Available as generic No

INFORMATION FOR USERS

Your drug prescription is tailored for you. Do not alter dosage without checking with your physician.

How taken

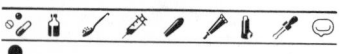

Tablets.

Frequency and timing of doses
2 – 3 x daily.

Adult dosage range
Dosage is determined individually according to body weight and response.

Onset of effect
Some adverse effects such as nausea and vomiting may appear within hours of starting treatment. Full beneficial effects may not occur for up to 12 weeks.

Duration of action
Several weeks after stopping treatment.

Diet advice
Certain foods with a high tyramine content must be avoided while taking this drug and for at least 14 days after treatment finishes. When procarbazine is dispensed, the pharmacist should provide a card listing foods and medicines to avoid. These include cheese, pickled herring, red wine, meat and yeast extracts, and broad (fava) beans.

Storage
Keep in a closed container in a cool, dry place away from reach of children. Protect from light.

Missed dose
Take as soon as you remember. If your next dose is due within 4 hours, take a single dose now and skip the next.

Stopping the drug
Treatment is stopped under medical supervision.

Exceeding the dose
An occasional unintentional extra dose is unlikely to cause problems. Large overdoses may cause severe nausea and vomiting. Notify your physician.

SPECIAL PRECAUTIONS

Procarbazine is prescribed only under close medical supervision, taking account of your present condition and medical history.

Pregnancy
▼ Not usually prescribed. Drugs such as procarbazine may cause birth defects or premature birth. Discuss with your physician.

Breast feeding
▼ Discuss with your physician. The drug passes into the breast milk and may affect the baby adversely.

Infants and children
▼ Not usually prescribed.

Over 60
▼ Not usually prescribed.

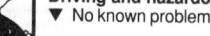

Driving and hazardous work
▼ No known problems.

Alcohol
▼ Never drink heavy red wines, particularly chianti, when taking this drug, because they may cause a particularly dangerous reaction. Other forms of alcohol should also be avoided.

POSSIBLE ADVERSE EFFECTS

All adverse effects are carefully monitored because procarbazine is given only under close medical supervision. Nausea and vomiting are experienced by most people taking this drug; other adverse effects are less common.

Symptom/effect	Frequency		Discuss with physician		Stop taking drug now	Call physician now
	Common	Rare	Only if severe	In all cases		
Nausea/vomiting	●		■			
Fatigue/weakness	●		■			
Depression	●			■		
Diarrhea		●	■			
Muscle pain		●	■			
Mouth ulcers		●		■		▮
Jaundice/rash		●		■		▮

PROLONGED USE

Prolonged use of this drug may lead to damage to the nervous system with numbness of the hands and feet.

Monitoring Periodic blood tests are advised.

INTERACTIONS

Tricyclic antidepressant drugs, phenothiazine drugs and levodopa Procarbazine increases the effects of these drugs, and their dosage may need to be reduced accordingly.

Antidiabetic drugs Procarbazine may increase the effects of these drugs on blood sugar.

PROCHLORPERAZINE

Brand names Compazine, Prochlor-Iso, Pro-Iso
Used in the following combined preparation Combid

GENERAL INFORMATION

Prochlorperazine, introduced in the late 1950s, belongs to a group of drugs called the phenothiazines, which act on the central nervous system.

In small doses, it will control nausea and vomiting, especially when they occur as the aftereffects of medical treatment by drugs, radiation, or anesthesia. It does not, however, prevent vertigo or motion sickness. In large doses, it is effective as an antipsychotic, suppressing abnormal behavior, reducing aggressiveness, and producing a generally tranquilizing effect (see p. 113). It thus minimizes and controls the abnormal behavior associated with schizophrenia, mania, dementia, and other mental disorders. It does not cure these diseases but helps relieve symptoms.

QUICK REFERENCE

Drug group Phenothiazine anti-emetic (p.118) and antipsychotic drug (p.113)

Overdose danger rating Medium

Dependence rating Low

Prescription needed Yes

Available as generic Yes

INFORMATION FOR USERS

Your drug prescription is tailored for you. Do not alter dosage without checking with your physician.

How taken

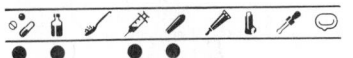

Tablets, slow-release capsules, liquid, injection, rectal suppositories.

Frequency and timing of doses
3 – 4 x daily (tablets); 2 x daily (rectal suppositories); 1 – 2 x daily (slow-release capsules); every 2 – 4 hours (injection).

Adult dosage range
Nausea and vomiting 5 – 10mg per dose (tablets); 25mg per dose (rectal suppositories); 15mg per dose (slow-release capsules).
Mental illness 15 – 40mg daily. Larger doses may be given in exceptional circumstances.

Onset of effect
Within 60 minutes by suppository, 30 – 40 minutes by mouth, 10 – 20 minutes by injection.

Duration of action
3 – 4 hours (up to 12 hours in slow-release form).

Diet advice
None.

Storage
Keep in a closed container in a cool, dry place away from reach of children. Protect from light.

Missed dose
Take as soon as you remember. If your next dose is due within 2 hours, do not take the missed dose; take the next scheduled dose as usual.

Stopping the drug
Do not stop the drug without consulting your physician; symptoms may recur.

Exceeding the dose
An occasional unintentional extra dose is unlikely to cause problems. Large overdoses may cause unusual drowsiness. Notify your physician.

POSSIBLE ADVERSE EFFECTS

Prochlorperazine has a strong *anticholinergic* effect, which can cause a variety of minor symptoms. These often become less marked with time. The most significant adverse effect is abnormal movements of the face and limbs (parkinsonism) caused by changes in the balance of chemicals in the brain.

Symptom/effect	Frequency		Discuss with physician		Stop taking drug now	Call physician now
	Common	Rare	Only if severe	In all cases		
Drowsiness/lethargy	●		■			
Dry mouth	●		■			
Blurred vision	●			■		
Dizziness/fainting	●			■		
Parkinsonism	●			■		
Rash		●		■	▲	

INTERACTIONS

Antiparkinsonism drugs Prochlorperazine may block their beneficial effect.

Anticholinergic drugs The side effects of these drugs may be increased by prochlorperazine.

Sedatives All drugs that have a sedative effect on the central nervous system are likely to increase the sedative properties of prochlorperazine.

SPECIAL PRECAUTIONS

Be sure to tell your physician if:
▼ You have heart problems.
▼ You have impaired kidney or liver function.
▼ You have a lung disorder such as asthma or bronchitis.
▼ You have had epileptic seizures.
▼ You have Parkinson's disease.
▼ You have an overactive thyroid gland.
▼ You are taking other medications.

 Pregnancy
▼ Not usually prescribed. Safety in pregnancy not established. Discuss with your physician so that you can weigh the benefits of the drug against its possible risks.

 Breast feeding
▼ Discuss with your physician. The drug passes into the breast milk and may affect the baby adversely.

 Infants and children
▼ Not recommended for children under 2 years. Reduced dose necessary in older children.

 Over 60
▼ Reduced dose necessary. Increased likelihood of adverse effects.

 Driving and hazardous work
▼ Avoid such activities until you have learned how the drug affects you, because the drug may cause drowsiness and reduced alertness.

 Alcohol
▼ Avoid. Alcohol may increase and prolong the sedative effects of this drug.

PROLONGED USE

Use of this drug for more than a few months may lead to the development of involuntary, potentially irreversible movements of the eyes, mouth, and tongue (*tardive dyskinesia*). Occasionally jaundice may occur.

Monitoring Periodic blood tests may be performed.

PROCYCLIDINE

Brand name Kemadrin
Used in the following combined preparations None

GENERAL INFORMATION

Introduced in 1956, procyclidine is an *anticholinergic* drug that is used to treat Parkinson's disease. It is particularly helpful in the early stages of the disorder for treating muscle rigidity . It also helps to reduce excess salivation and to some extent the tremor. However, it has little effect on the shuffling gait and slow muscular movements that are also characteristic of Parkinson's disease.

Procyclidine is also frequently used to treat parkinsonism resulting from treatment with antipsychotic drugs.

The drug may cause a number of minor adverse effects (see below), but these are rarely sufficiently serious to warrant stopping treatment.

INFORMATION FOR USERS

Your drug prescription is tailored for you. Do not alter dosage without checking with your physician.

How taken

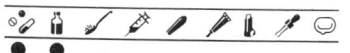

Tablets, liquid.

Frequency and timing of doses
2 – 3 x daily.

Adult dosage range
5 – 30mg daily. Dosage with this drug has to be determined individually in order to find the best balance between effective relief of symptoms and the occurrence of adverse effects.

Onset of effect
Within 30 minutes.

Duration of action
8 – 12 hours.

Diet advice
None.

Storage
Keep in a closed container in a cool, dry place away from reach of children.

Missed dose
Take as soon as you remember. If your next dose is due within 2 hours, take a single dose now and skip the next.

Stopping the drug
Do not stop the drug without consulting your physician; symptoms may recur.

OVERDOSE ACTION

Seek immediate medical advice in all cases. Take emergency action if palpitations, seizures, or unconsciousness occurs.

See Drug poisoning emergency guide (p.590).

SPECIAL PRECAUTIONS

Be sure to tell your physician if:
▼ You have impaired kidney or liver function.
▼ You have had glaucoma.
▼ You have high blood pressure.
▼ You suffer from constipation.
▼ You have prostate trouble.
▼ You have had peptic ulcers.
▼ You are taking other medications.

Pregnancy
▼ Not usually prescribed. Safety in pregnancy not established. Discuss with your physician so that you may weigh the benefits of the drug against its possible risks.

Breast feeding
▼ The drug passes into the breast milk, but at normal doses adverse effects on the baby are uncommon. Discuss with your physician.

Infants and children
▼ Not recommended.

Over 60
▼ Reduced dose may be necessary. Increased likelihood of adverse effects.

Driving and hazardous work
▼ Avoid such activities until you have learned how the drug affects you, because the drug can cause blurred vision and mild confusion.

Alcohol
▼ Avoid. Alcohol increases the adverse effects of this drug.

POSSIBLE ADVERSE EFFECTS

The possible adverse effects of procyclidine are mainly the result of its *anticholinergic* action. Some of the more common symptoms, such as dry eyes and mouth, constipation, and blurred vision, may be overcome by adjustment of dosage.

Symptom/effect	Frequency		Discuss with physician		Stop taking drug now	Call physician now
	Common	Rare	Only if severe	In all cases		
Dry mouth/eyes	●		■			
Difficulty in passing urine	●		■			
Constipation	●		■			
Nervousness	●		■			
Blurred vision	●			■		
Confusion		●		■		
Nausea/vomiting		●		■		
Rash		●		■	▲	
Palpitations		●		■	▲	▮

INTERACTIONS

Anticholinergic drugs and antihistamines These drugs may increase the adverse effects of procyclidine.

Alcohol Alcohol increases the sedative effect of procyclidine.

PROLONGED USE

Prolonged use of this drug may provoke the onset of glaucoma.

Monitoring Periodic eye examinations are usually required.

PROMAZINE

Brand name Sparine
Used in the following combined preparations None

GENERAL INFORMATION

Promazine was introduced in the late 1950s and is a member of a group of drugs called phenothiazines. These drugs act on the brain to regulate abnormal behavior (see Antipsychotic drugs, p.113), and also have a calming effect on the part of the brain that controls nausea and vomiting (see Antiemetic drugs, p.118). Promazine has some beneficial effect on agitated and restless behavior and can be used as a sedative, especially in the elderly.

It is also used for its anti-emetic effect, and is especially valuable in preventing and treating the nausea and vomiting caused by anesthetics or drug or radiation treatment.

In theory, promazine may cause the unpleasant side effects common to other phenothiazine drugs, particularly abnormal movements of arms and legs (parkinsonism). In practice, the drug is rarely used for long enough to cause these problems.

INFORMATION FOR USERS

Your drug prescription is tailored for you. Do not alter dosage without checking with your physician.

How taken

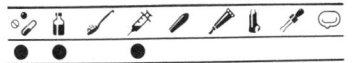

Tablets, liquid, injection.

Frequency and timing of doses
4 – 6 x daily.

Adult dosage range
100mg – 300mg daily.

Onset of effect
30 minutes – 1 hour.

Duration of action
4 – 6 hours.

Diet advice
None.

Storage
Keep in a closed container in a cool, dry place away from reach of children.

Missed dose
Take as soon as you remember. If your next dose is due within 2 hours, do not take the missed dose. Take the next scheduled dose as usual.

Stopping the drug
Do not stop the drug without consulting your physician; symptoms may recur.

Exceeding the dose
An occasional unintentional extra dose is unlikely to cause problems. Large overdoses may cause drowsiness, dizziness, and unsteadiness. Notify your physician.

SPECIAL PRECAUTIONS

Be sure to tell your physician if:
▼ You have heart problems.
▼ You have impaired kidney or liver function.
▼ You have had epileptic seizures.
▼ You have had glaucoma.
▼ You have an overactive thyroid gland.
▼ You have Parkinson's disease.
▼ You are taking other medications.

 Pregnancy
▼ Not usually prescribed. Safety in pregnancy not established. Discuss with your physician so that you can weigh the benefits of the drug against its possible risks.

 Breast feeding
▼ The drug passes into the breast milk, but at normal doses adverse effects on the baby are uncommon. Discuss with your physician.

 Infants and children
▼ Not recommended.

 Over 60
▼ Reduced dose may be necessary. Increased likelihood of adverse effects.

Driving and hazardous work
▼ Avoid such activities until you have learned how the drug affects you, because the drug may cause drowsiness and reduced alertness.

Alcohol
▼ Avoid. Alcohol may increase the sedative effect of this drug.

POSSIBLE ADVERSE EFFECTS

The more common adverse effects of promazine, such as drowsiness, dry mouth, and blurred vision, may be helped by an adjustment of dosage. Parkinsonism is rare.

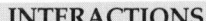

Symptom/effect	Frequency		Discuss with physician		Stop taking drug now	Call physician now
	Common	Rare	Only if severe	In all cases		
Drowsiness/lethargy	●		■			
Dry mouth	●		■			
Constipation	●		■			
Blurred vision	●			■		
Parkinsonism		●		■		
Jaundice		●		■		
Rash		●		■	▲	

INTERACTIONS

Sedatives All drugs that have a sedative effect are likely to increase the sedative properties of promazine.

Anticonvulsant drugs These preparations may increase the likelihood of adverse effects from promazine.

Antacids These drugs may reduce the absorption of promazine from the stomach, so preventing its full effect from being felt. Antacids and promazine should be taken at least 1 hour apart.

PROLONGED USE

Use of this drug for more than a few months may be associated with *jaundice*. Abnormal movements of the face and limbs may also occur. Sometimes a reduction in dosage may be recommended.

Monitoring Periodic blood tests may be performed.

PROMETHAZINE

Brand names Anergan, Phenazine, Phenergan, Prorex, Remsed
Used in the following combined preparations Mepergan, Phenergan D, Phenergan with codeine

GENERAL INFORMATION

Promethazine is one of the pheno-thiazines, a class of drugs developed in the 1950s for their beneficial effect on abnormal behavior arising from mental illnesses (see Antipsychotic drugs, p.113). Promethazine was, however, found to have effects more like the antihistamines used to treat allergies (see p.152) and some types of nausea and vomiting (see Anti-emetic drugs, p.118). It is primarily used for such conditions, though it is sometimes combined with certain narcotics to increase their effect.

Promethazine is widely used to reduce itching in a variety of skin conditions including urticaria (hives), chicken pox, and eczema. It can also relieve the nausea and vomiting caused by inner ear disturbances such as motion sickness and Ménière's disease. Because of its sedative effect, promethazine is sometimes used as a sleeping medicine for children for short periods, and is given as *premedication* before surgery. Occasionally it is administered to produce sedation during labor.

Promethazine is sometimes com-bined with codeine or other ingredients for the relief of allergy-related coughs and nasal congestion.

QUICK REFERENCE

Drug group Antihistamine (p.152) and anti-emetic drug (p.118)

Overdose danger rating Medium

Dependence rating Low

Prescription needed Yes

Available as generic Yes

INFORMATION FOR USERS

Your drug prescription is tailored for you. Do not alter dosage without checking with your physician.

How taken

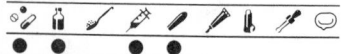

Tablets, liquid, injection, rectal suppository.

Frequency and timing of doses
Allergic symptoms 1 – 3 x daily before meals.
Motion sickness 30 – 60 minutes before travel, then every 6 – 8 hours as necessary.
Nausea and vomiting Every 4 – 6 hours as necessary.

Dosage range
Adults 25mg per dose.
Children Reduced dose according to age and weight.

Onset of effect
Within 1 hour. If dose is taken after nausea has started, the onset of effect is delayed.

Duration of action
12 – 24 hours.

Diet advice
None.

Storage
Keep in a closed container in a cool, dry place away from reach of children.

Missed dose
No cause for concern, but take as soon as you remember. Adjust the timing of your next dose accordingly.

Stopping the drug
Can be safely stopped as soon as symptoms disappear.

Exceeding the dose
An occasional unintentional extra dose is unlikely to cause problems. Large over-doses may cause drowsiness, unsteadiness, or agitation. Notify your physician.

SPECIAL PRECAUTIONS

Be sure to tell your physician if:
▼ You have impaired kidney or liver function.
▼ You have had epileptic seizures.
▼ You have heart disease.
▼ You have Parkinson's disease.
▼ You have urinary difficulties.
▼ You are taking other medications.

Pregnancy
▼ Discuss with your physician. No evidence of risk to baby, but all drugs should be used with caution during pregnancy.

Breast feeding
▼ The drug passes into the breast milk, but at normal doses adverse effects on the baby are uncommon. Discuss with your physician.

Infants and children
▼ Not recommended for children under 2 years. Reduced dose necessary for older children.

Over 60
▼ No special problems.

Driving and hazardous work
▼ Avoid such activities until you have learned how the drug affects you, because the drug can cause drowsiness.

Alcohol
▼ Avoid. Alcohol may increase the sedative effects of this drug.

POSSIBLE ADVERSE EFFECTS

Promethazine usually causes only minor *anti-cholinergic* effects. More serious adverse effects generally occur only during long-term use or with abnormally high doses.

Symptom/effect	Frequency		Discuss with physician		Stop taking drug now	Call physician now
	Common	Rare	Only if severe	In all cases		
Drowsiness/lethargy	●		■			
Dry mouth	●		■			
Blurred vision	●		■			
Light-sensitive rash		●		■	▲	

INTERACTIONS

Sedatives All drugs that have a sedative effect are likely to increase the sedative properties of promethazine. Such drugs include antihistamines, sleeping drugs, and antipsychotics.

Antacids These drugs may reduce the absorption of promethazine from the stomach, thus preventing its full effect from being felt. Antacids and promethazine should be taken at least 1 hour apart.

PROLONGED USE

Use of this drug for extended periods is rarely necessary, but may sometimes cause abnormal movements of the face and limbs (parkinsonism). The problem normally disappears when the drug is stopped.

PROPOXYPHENE

Brand names Darvon, Darvon-N, Dolene, Doxaphene, Prophene 65
Used in the following combined preparations Darvocet N-50 and N-100, Darvon Compound 65, Lorcet, Wygesic

GENERAL INFORMATION

Propoxyphene, introduced in 1957, is a weak narcotic analgesic used to relieve mild or moderate pain. It is not useful for severe pain. Longer-lasting than many other drugs of this class, it may be more convenient for relief of chronic pain. It may sometimes be given in combination with another analgesic, such as aspirin or acetaminophen, to boost its effect.

High doses of propoxyphene taken for prolonged periods may lead to physical dependence on the drug. However, it is less addictive than other similar drugs, and most people are able to stop treatment without difficulty.
Side effects such as dizziness, drowsiness, and nausea are more common in active people, and can often be overcome by rest.

INFORMATION FOR USERS

Your drug prescription is tailored for you. Do not alter dosage without checking with your physician.

How taken

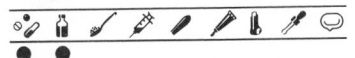

Tablets, capsules, liquid.

Frequency and timing of doses
Every 3 – 4 hours.

Adult dosage range
65mg or 100mg per dose depending on preparation, up to a maximum of 6 doses in 24 hours.

Onset of effect
15 – 60 minutes.

Duration of action
4 – 12 hours.

Diet advice
None.

Storage
Keep in a closed container in a cool, dry place away from reach of children. Protect from light.

Missed dose
Take as soon as you remember if required for pain.

Stopping the drug
If you have been taking the drug for less than 2 weeks, it can be safely stopped as soon as you no longer need it. However, if you have been regularly taking it for longer than this, consult your physician, who may supervise a gradual reduction in dosage.

OVERDOSE ACTION

Seek immediate medical advice in all cases. Take emergency action if breathing difficulties, seizures, or loss of consciousness occurs.

See Drug poisoning emergency guide (p.590).

SPECIAL PRECAUTIONS

Be sure to tell your physician if:
▼ You have impaired liver or kidney function.
▼ You have a lung disorder such as asthma or bronchitis.
▼ You are taking other medications.

Pregnancy
▼ Not usually prescribed. Safety in pregnancy not established. Discuss with your physician so that you may weigh the benefits of the drug against its possible risks.

Breast feeding
▼ The drug passes into the breast milk, but at normal doses adverse effects on the baby are unlikely. Discuss with your physician.

Infants and children
▼ Not recommended.

Over 60
▼ Reduced dose may be necessary.

Driving and hazardous work
▼ Avoid such activities until you have learned how the drug affects you, because the drug can cause drowsiness and dizziness.

Alcohol
▼ Avoid. Alcohol may increase the sedative effects of this drug.

POSSIBLE ADVERSE EFFECTS

Minor side effects are common with propoxyphene, but often wear off with continued use. Dizziness, drowsiness, and nausea are often relieved by lying down and resting. Serious adverse effects are rare except in overdose.

Symptom/effect	Frequency		Discuss with physician		Stop taking drug now	Call physician now
	Common	Rare	Only if severe	In all cases		
Dizziness/drowsiness	●		■			
Nausea/vomiting	●		■			
Headache		●	■			
Constipation		●	■			
Confusion		●		■		▮
Rash		●		■	▲	▮

INTERACTIONS

Sedatives All drugs that have a sedative effect on the central nervous system are likely to increase sedation with propoxyphene.

Monoamine oxidase inhibitors (MAOIs) Propoxyphene may interact with these drugs to cause a dangerous rise in blood pressure.

PROLONGED USE

The effects of the drug may become weaker during prolonged use as the body adapts. It may also be habit-forming if taken for extended periods.

PROPRANOLOL

Brand names Inderal, Inderal-LA
Used in the following combined preparations Inderide, Inderide-LA

GENERAL INFORMATION

Propranolol, introduced in 1968, was the first of the beta blockers to be available in the US. Most often used to treat hypertension, angina, and abnormal heart rhythms, it is also helpful in controlling the fast heart rate and other symptoms caused by overactivity of the thyroid gland and in reducing the palpitations, sweating, and tremor caused by anxiety that goes with stage fright. It is also effective in the prevention of migraine headaches.

Because propranolol can cause breathing difficulties, it is not prescribed to anyone suffering from asthma, chronic bronchitis, or emphysema. Like all beta blockers, propranolol affects the body's response to low blood sugar; it should be used with caution by diabetics.

QUICK REFERENCE

Drug group Beta blocker (p.125)
Overdose danger rating High
Dependence rating Low
Prescription needed Yes
Available as generic Yes

INFORMATION FOR USERS

Your drug prescription is tailored for you. Do not alter dosage without checking with your physician.

How taken

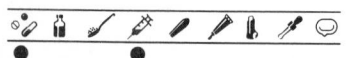

Tablets, capsules, injection.

Frequency and timing of doses
2 – 4 x daily; once daily (slow-release capsules).

Adult dosage range
Abnormal heart rhythms 30 – 320mg daily.
Angina 30 – 80mg daily (starting dose); 160 – 240mg daily (maintenance dose).
Hypertension 80 – 160mg daily. Larger doses may be prescribed.
Migraine prevention and anxiety 60mg daily.

Onset of effect
1 – 2 hours (tablets); after 6 hours (slow-release capsules). In hypertension and migraine, it may be several weeks before full benefits of this drug are felt.

Duration of action
6 – 12 hours (tablets); 24 – 30 hours (slow-release capsules).

Diet advice
None.

Storage
Keep in a closed container in a cool, dry place away from reach of children. Protect from light.

Missed dose
Take as soon as you remember. If your next dose is due within 2 hours (tablets) or 12 hours (slow-release capsules), take a single dose now and skip the next.

Stopping the drug
Do not stop the drug without consulting your physician. Abrupt cessation may lead to worsening of the underlying condition.

OVERDOSE ACTION

 Seek immediate medical advice in all cases. Take emergency action if breathing difficulties, collapse, or loss of consciousness occurs.

See Drug poisoning emergency guide (p.590).

SPECIAL PRECAUTIONS

Be sure to tell your physician if:
▼ You have a lung disorder such as asthma, bronchitis, or emphysema.
▼ You have heart failure.
▼ You have diabetes.
▼ You have poor circulation in the legs.
▼ You are taking other medications.

 Pregnancy
▼ Not usually prescribed. Safety in pregnancy not established. Discuss with your physician so that you can weigh the benefits of the drug against its possible risks.

 Breast feeding
▼ The drug passes into breast milk, but at normal doses adverse effects on the baby are uncommon. Discuss with your physician.

 Infants and children
▼ Reduced dose necessary.

 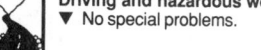 **Over 60**
▼ No special problems.

Driving and hazardous work
▼ No special problems.

 Alcohol
▼ No special problems.

Surgery and general anesthetics
▼ Propranolol may need to be stopped before you have a general anesthetic. Discuss this with your physician or dentist before any surgery.

PROLONGED USE

No problems expected.

POSSIBLE ADVERSE EFFECTS

Propranolol has adverse effects that are common to most beta blockers. Symptoms such as fatigue and nausea are usually temporary and diminish with long-term use. Fainting may be a sign that the drug has slowed the heartbeat excessively.

Symptom/effect	Frequency		Discuss with physician		Stop taking drug now	Call physician now
	Common	Rare	Only if severe	In all cases		
Lethargy	●		■			
Cold hands and feet	●		■			
Nausea		●	■			
Nightmares/vivid dreams		●		■	▲	▮
Rash		●		■	▲	▮
Fainting/breathlessness		●		■	▲	▮

INTERACTIONS

Indomethacin reduces the antihypertensive effect of propranolol.

Cimetidine can increase the levels of propranolol in the blood.

A B C D E F G H I J K L M N O P Q R S T U V W X Y Z

PROPYLTHIOURACIL

Brand names None
Used in the following combined preparations None

GENERAL INFORMATION

Propylthiouracil, introduced in 1947, is an antithyroid drug used to manage an overactive thyroid gland (thyrotoxicosis). In some people, particularly those with Graves' disease (the commonest form of the disorder), drug treatment alone may bring on a remission. It may also be prescribed for long-term treatment of the disease in those who may be at special risk from surgery, such as children and pregnant women.

When more radical treatments for overactive thyroid are undertaken, propylthiouracil is also employed: to restore the normal functioning of the gland before its partial removal by surgery, to intensify its absorption of radioactive iodine when that cell-destroying drug is used, or to prevent a harmful release of hormones that can sometimes follow the use of radioactive iodine. More effective than other antithyroid drugs in the treatment of thyrotoxic crisis (thyroid storm), propyl-thiouracil is also thought to cross the placenta less readily than similar drugs do, and it is preferred when treatment is essential during pregnancy.

The major possible adverse effect of this drug is a reduction in white blood cells, leading to risk of infection.

QUICK REFERENCE

Drug group Antithyroid drug (p.172)
Overdose danger rating Medium
Dependence rating Low
Prescription needed Yes
Available as generic Yes

INFORMATION FOR USERS

Your drug prescription is tailored for you. Do not alter dosage without checking with your physician.

How taken

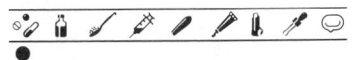

Tablets.

Frequency and timing of doses
Every 6 – 8 hours. May be given every 4 hours for treatment of thyrotoxic crisis.

Dosage range
Adults 300 – 1200mg daily (starting dose); 100 – 300mg daily (maintenance dose).
Children Reduced dose necessary according to age and weight.

Onset of effect
10 – 20 days. Full beneficial effects may not be felt for 6 – 10 weeks.

Duration of action
24 – 36 hours.

Diet advice
Your physician may advise you to avoid foods that are high in iodine (see p.538).

Storage
Keep in a closed container in a cool, dry place away from reach of children.

Missed dose
Take as soon as you remember. If your next dose is due, take the missed dose and the next scheduled dose together.

Stopping the drug
Do not stop the drug without consulting your physician; stopping the drug may lead to recurrence of thyrotoxicosis.

Exceeding the dose
An occasional unintentional extra dose is unlikely to cause problems. Large overdoses may cause nausea, vomiting, and headache. Notify your physician.

POSSIBLE ADVERSE EFFECTS

Serious side effects are rare with propylthiouracil. Skin rashes and itching are fairly common, although itching may sometimes be caused by overactivity of the thyroid gland. Sore throat or fever may indicate reduced white blood cell production.

Symptom/effect	Frequency		Discuss with physician		Stop taking drug now	Call physician now
	Common	Rare	Only if severe	In all cases		
Rash/itching	●		■			
Dizziness/drowsiness	●		■			
Joint pain	●			■		
Headache	●			■		
Rash		●		■		
Jaundice		●		■	▲	▮
Sore throat/fever		●		■	▲	▮

INTERACTIONS

Anticoagulant drugs Propylthiouracil may enhance the effects of these drugs.

SPECIAL PRECAUTIONS

Be sure to tell your physician if:
▼ You have impaired liver or kidney function.
▼ You are taking other medications.

Pregnancy
▼ Prescribed with caution. May cause goiter and thyroid hormone deficiency (hypothyroidism) in the newborn infant if too high a dose is used. Discuss with your physician so that you may weigh the benefit of the drug against its possible risks.

Breast feeding
▼ The drug passes into the breast milk, but at normal doses adverse effects on the baby are rare. Discuss with your physician.

Infants and children
▼ Reduced dose necessary.

Over 60
▼ No special problems.

Driving and hazardous work
▼ Avoid such activities until you have learned how the drug affects you, because the drug may cause dizziness and drowsiness.

Alcohol
▼ No known problems.

PROLONGED USE

High doses of propylthiouracil over a prolonged period may reduce the number of white blood cells.

Monitoring Periodic tests of thyroid function are usually required, and blood cell counts may also be carried out.

A B C D E F G H I J K L M N O P Q R S T U V W X Y Z

PSEUDOEPHEDRINE

Brand names Afrinol, Novafed, Sudafed
Used in the following combined preparations Actifed, Deconamine, Novahistine-DH, Rondec-DM, Trinalin

GENERAL INFORMATION

Pseudoephedrine, a component of many non-prescription remedies, is a *sympathomimetic* nasal decongestant. It reduces congestion of the nasal passages and sinuses by narrowing blood vessels in the nose.

Apart from its use in nasal congestion, it is also useful for reducing congestion of the eustachian tube (the tube connecting the middle ear with the cavity at the back of the nose). This often occurs with inflammation and infection of the middle ear.

Pseudoephedrine is less likely than other decongestants to cause anxiety, tremor, and restlessness by stimulating the central nervous system. But in common with other drugs in this group, it may cause rebound congestion (worsening of congestion after prolonged use).

Pseudoephedrine is also occasionally used to control urinary incontinence (see p. 194).

QUICK REFERENCE

Drug group Decongestant (p.121)
Overdose danger rating High
Dependence rating Low
Prescription needed No
Available as generic Yes

INFORMATION FOR USERS

Follow instructions on the label. Call your physician if symptoms worsen.

How taken

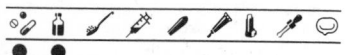

Tablets, capsules, liquid.

Frequency and timing of doses
Every 6 – 8 hours.

Dosage range
Adults Up to 240mg daily.
Children Up to 60 – 120mg daily (6 – 12 years). (120mg slow-release preparations are not recommended under 12 years).

Onset of effect
15 – 30 minutes.

Duration of action
4 – 6 hours (tablets and liquid); 8 – 12 hours (slow-release preparations).

Diet advice
None.

Storage
Keep in a closed container in a cool, dry place away from reach of children. Protect from light.

Missed dose
Take as soon as you remember. If your next dose is due within 2 hours, take a single dose now and skip the next.

Stopping the drug
Can be safely stopped as soon as you no longer need it.

OVERDOSE ACTION

Seek immediate medical advice in all cases. Take emergency action if delirium, seizures, or loss of consciousness occurs.

See Drug poisoning emergency guide (p.590).

SPECIAL PRECAUTIONS

Be sure to consult your physician before taking this drug if:
▼ You have heart problems.
▼ You have high blood pressure.
▼ You have had glaucoma.
▼ You have diabetes.
▼ You have an overactive thyroid.
▼ You have urinary difficulties.
▼ You are taking other medications.

Pregnancy
▼ Not usually prescribed. Safety in pregnancy not established. Discuss with your physician so that you can weigh the benefits of the drug against its possible risks.

Breast feeding
▼ Discuss with your physician. The drug passes into the breast milk, but at normal doses adverse effects on the baby are unlikely.

Infants and children
▼ Not recommended for children under 6 years. Reduced dose necessary in older children.

Over 60
▼ Reduced dose may be necessary. Increased likelihood of adverse effects.

Driving and hazardous work
▼ No known problems.

Alcohol
▼ No known problems.

POSSIBLE ADVERSE EFFECTS

High doses may cause anxiety, nausea, dizziness, and, rarely, a marked rise in blood pressure, causing palpitations, headache, and breathlessness.

Symptom/effect	Frequency		Discuss with physician		Stop taking drug now	Call physician now
	Common	Rare	Only if severe	In all cases		
Nausea/vomiting		●	■			
Dizziness/lightheadedness		●	■			
Nervousness/insomnia		●	■			
Hallucinations		●		■		
Rash	●	●		■	▲	
Palpitations/breathlessness		●		■		▮
Headache		●		■		▮

INTERACTIONS

Other sympathomimetic drugs increase the risk of adverse effects with this drug.

Monoamine oxidase inhibitors (MAOIs) There is a risk of a dangerous rise in blood pressure if pseudoephedrine is taken with these drugs.

Antihypertensive drugs Pseudoephedrine counteracts the lowered blood pressure from antihypertensive drugs such as methyldopa and guanethidine.

PROLONGED USE

Pseudoephedrine is not normally taken for prolonged periods. It should not be taken for longer than 5 days except on the advice of your physician.

PSYLLIUM

Brand names Effersyllium, Hydrocil, Konsyl, Metamucil, Naturacil
Used in the following combined preparations Fiberall, Perdiem

GENERAL INFORMATION

This bulk-forming laxative has been extracted from the seeds of Plantago plants since 1934. It is used in the treatment of constipation, diverticular disease, and irritable bowel syndrome. Taken by mouth, usually as powder or granules dissolved in water, psyllium passes through the stomach to the intestines, where it continues to absorb up to 25 times its volume in water, softening and increasing the volume of bowel movements. It may take up to two weeks for improved bowel habits to be established.

Psyllium is also used to reduce the frequency and increase the firmness of bowel movements of people with persistent watery diarrhea or those who have had intestinal surgery such as colostomies or ileostomies. Psyllium may dry up and plug the bowel if the intake of fluids is insufficient.

Side effects are rare, but the drug may cause bloating and excess gas in some people, especially at the start of treatment. It should not be taken without medical advice for constipation that is accompanied by severe abdominal pain because of the risk of obstructing the bowel.

QUICK REFERENCE

Drug group Bulk-forming laxative (p.139) and antidiarrheal drug (p.138)

Overdose danger rating Low

Dependence rating Low

Prescription needed No

Available as generic No

INFORMATION FOR USERS

Follow instructions on the label. Call your physician if symptoms worsen.

How taken

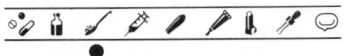

Powder, granules.

Frequency and timing of doses
1 – 3 x daily with water or fruit juice, preferably after meals.

Dosage range
Adults 2.5g – 30g daily.
Children over 6 years 1.25g – 15g daily.

Onset of effect
12 – 24 hours.

Duration of action
Up to 24 hours.

Diet advice
Drink plenty of fluids, at least 6 – 8 glasses daily.

Storage
Keep in a closed container in a cool, dry place away from reach of children.

Missed dose
Take as soon as you remember. Resume normal dosing thereafter.

Stopping the drug
Can be safely stopped as soon as you no longer need it.

Exceeding the dose
An occasional unintentional extra dose is unlikely to be a cause for concern. But if you notice unusual symptoms, or if a large overdose has been taken, notify your physician.

SPECIAL PRECAUTIONS

Be sure to consult your physician before taking this drug if:
▼ You have severe constipation and/or abdominal pain.
▼ You have unexplained rectal bleeding.
▼ You have difficulty swallowing.
▼ You have diabetes.
▼ You have a known narrowing of the bowel.
▼ You are taking other medications.

Pregnancy
▼ No evidence of risk to developing baby.

Breast feeding
▼ No evidence of risk.

Infants and children
▼ Given to children over 6 only on medical advice.

Over 60
▼ No special problems.

Driving and hazardous work
▼ No known problems.

Alcohol
▼ No known problems.

POSSIBLE ADVERSE EFFECTS

Serious adverse effects are rare, but persistent or severe abdominal pain following the use of this (or any) laxative should always receive medical attention.

Symptom/effect	Frequency		Discuss with physician		Stop taking drug now	Call physician now
	Common	Rare	Only if severe	In all cases		
Excess gas		●	■			
Bloating		●	■			
Abdominal pain		●		■		

INTERACTIONS

General note Psyllium may reduce the absorption of oral anticoagulant drugs, digitalis drugs, and nitrofurantoin. Spacing of doses may be recommended.

PROLONGED USE

No problems expected.

PYRANTEL

Brand name Antiminth
Used in the following combined preparations None

GENERAL INFORMATION

Pyrantel, introduced in 1972, is an anthelmintic used in the treatment of worm infection of the bowel. Available as a flavored oral suspension, pyrantel works by paralyzing the worms so that they let go and pass in the bowel movements.

Common roundworm or pinworm infections, which are caused by fecal contamination of hands or food or by eating contaminated soil (on raw vegetables, for example), are usually cleared with a single dose. Since pinworms are highly infectious, all members of a household are usually treated at the same time. Dosing may be repeated after two to three weeks if the infection is not completely cleared.

For hookworm infection, which is less common in the US and occurs only in certain southern areas, the drug may be prescribed for three consecutive days. Iron supplements may also be given to treat any anemia resulting from the infection.

Occasionally, pyrantel may be used to treat pork roundworm infections, which are caused by infected meat.

QUICK REFERENCE

Drug group Anthelmintic drug (p.167)

Overdose danger rating Low

Dependence rating Low

Prescription needed Yes

Available as generic No

INFORMATION FOR USERS

Your drug prescription is tailored for you. Do not alter dosage without checking with your physician.

How taken

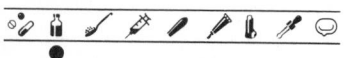

Liquid.

Frequency and timing of doses
A single dose that may be repeated after 2–3 weeks.

Dosage range
According to body weight up to a maximum dose of 1g daily.

Onset of effect
2–4 hours.

Duration of action
2–3 days.

Diet advice
None.

Storage
Keep in a closed container in a cool, dry place away from reach of children. Protect from light. Do not freeze.

Missed dose
If you are taking multiple-day therapy, take as soon as you remember, spacing the missed dose and the next dose 10–12 hours apart.

Stopping the drug
If multiple-day therapy is required, complete the course of treatment. If the drug is stopped prematurely, the infection may recur.

Exceeding the dose
An occasional unintentional extra dose is unlikely to be a cause for concern. But if you notice unusual symptoms, or if a large overdose has been taken, notify your physician.

SPECIAL PRECAUTIONS

Be sure to tell your physician if:
▼ You have impaired liver function.
▼ You are taking other medications.

Pregnancy
▼ Not usually prescribed. Safety in pregnancy not established. Discuss with your physician so that you can weigh the benefits of the drug against its possible risks.

Breast feeding
▼ No evidence of risk.

Infants and children
▼ Not usually prescribed in children under 2 years.

Over 60
▼ No known problems.

Driving and hazardous work
▼ Avoid such activities until you have learned how the drug affects you, because the drug can cause drowsiness and dizziness.

Alcohol
▼ No known problems.

POSSIBLE ADVERSE EFFECTS

Side effects are rarely serious with pyrantel. Gastrointestinal disturbances, including nausea, loss of appetite, and abdominal pain, are the most common problems.

Symptom/effect	Frequency		Discuss with physician		Stop taking drug now	Call physician now
	Common	Rare	Only if severe	In all cases		
Nausea/vomiting	●		■			
Diarrhea	●		■			
Abdominal cramps	●		■			
Drowsiness/dizziness	●		■			
Headache	●		■			
Rash		●		■	▲	▮

PROLONGED USE

Not taken for prolonged periods.

INTERACTIONS

Piperazine may reduce the effect of pyrantel.

PYRAZINAMIDE

Brand names None
Used in the following combined preparations None

GENERAL INFORMATION

Pyrazinamide, introduced in 1955, is used in the treatment of tuberculosis. Commonly used when other treatments have failed, pyrazinamide is usually given along with other drugs to prevent the development of resistance and maximize the effectiveness of the treatment.

Prolonged treatment, for up to two years or more, is usually necessary. Short courses, lasting six to nine months, are sometimes prescribed for initial treatment, particularly when resistance to the more commonly used

drugs is suspected. In some cases, pyrazinamide may then be discontinued after laboratory tests have shown sensitivity to the other drugs.

The major drawback of this drug is its possible effect on the liver. Although the damage (if it occurs) is usually slight, it may in rare cases be fatal. For that reason monitoring of liver function is usually recommended every two to four weeks throughout treatment. Pyrazinamide also blocks excretion of uric acid and may cause gout.

QUICK REFERENCE

Drug group Antituberculous drug (p.160)

Overdose danger rating Medium

Dependence rating Low

Prescription needed Yes

Available as generic Yes

INFORMATION FOR USERS

Your drug prescription is tailored for you. Do not alter dosage without checking with your physician.

How taken

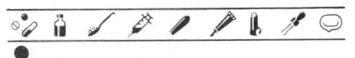

Tablets.

Frequency and timing of doses
3 – 4 x daily.

Adult dosage range
According to body weight, up to a maximum of 3g daily.

Onset of effect
Several days.

Duration of action
Up to 24 hours.

Diet advice
None.

Storage
Keep in a closed container in a cool, dry place away from reach of children.

Missed dose
Take as soon as you remember. If your next dose is due within 2 hours, take a single dose now and skip the next.

Stopping the drug
Take the full course. Even if you feel better, the original infection may still be present and may recur if treatment is stopped too soon.

Exceeding the dose
An occasional unintentional extra dose is unlikely to cause problems. Large overdoses may cause nausea, vomiting, and marked lethargy. Notify your physician.

SPECIAL PRECAUTIONS

Be sure to tell your physician if:
▼ You have impaired liver or kidney function.
▼ You have diabetes.
▼ You have had attacks of gout.
▼ You have porphyria.
▼ You are taking other medications.

Pregnancy
▼ Not usually prescribed. Safety in pregnancy not established. Discuss with your physician so that you can weigh the benefits of the drug against its possible risks.

Breast feeding
▼ No evidence of risk.

Infants and children
▼ Not recommended.

Over 60
▼ No special problems.

Driving and hazardous work
▼ No known problems.

Alcohol
▼ Avoid. Alcohol may increase the risk of liver damage with this drug.

POSSIBLE ADVERSE EFFECTS

The main possible adverse effect of pyrazinamide is liver damage. Nausea and loss of appetite may be the first signs of this.

Later symptoms include weakness, fatigue, fever, and jaundice. Joint pain and swelling are rare and may be due to gout.

Symptom/effect	Frequency		Discuss with physician		Stop taking drug now	Call physician now
	Common	Rare	Only if severe	In all cases		
Loss of appetite	●			■		
Jaundice	●			■	▲	▮
Nausea/vomiting		●		■		
Weakness/fatigue/fever		●		■		
Joint pain/swelling		●		■		
Rash/itching		●		■	▲	

INTERACTIONS

Drugs used for gout Pyrazinamide may reduce the beneficial effect of these drugs. Dosage adjustment may be necessary.

Ethionamide may increase the risk of adverse effects with pyrazinamide.

PROLONGED USE

There is a risk of liver damage with prolonged use of pyrazinamide.

Monitoring Periodic blood tests are usually performed to monitor liver function and to measure blood levels of uric acid.

A
B
C
D
E
F
G
H
I
J
K
L
M
N
O
P
Q
R
S
T
U
V
W
X
Y
Z

PYRIDOSTIGMINE

Brand names Mestinon, Regonol
Used in the following combined preparations None

GENERAL INFORMATION

Pyridostigmine has been used since 1955 for myasthenia gravis, a rare auto-immmune condition involving the faulty transmission of nerve impulses to the muscles (p.149). By prolonging nerve signals, pyridostigmine improves muscle strength, though it does not cure the disease. In severe cases it may be prescribed with corticosteroids. Because the response to pyridostigmine is predictable, it may also be used to help diagnose the disease: lack of a response rules out myasthenia gravis. Pyridostigmine may also be given to reverse temporary paralysis of the bowel.

Side effects such as abdominal cramps, nausea, and diarrhea generally disappear when the dose of pyridostigmine is reduced.

INFORMATION FOR USERS

Your drug prescription is tailored for you. Do not alter dosage without checking with your physician.

How taken

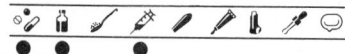

Tablets, slow-release tablets, syrup, injection.

Frequency and timing of doses
Tablets Every 3 – 4 hours initially. Thereafter, according to the needs of the individual.
Slow-release tablets 1 – 2 x daily.

Adult dosage range
Adults 60mg – 1.5g daily (by mouth); 2mg every 2 – 3 hours (injection).
Children Reduced dose necessary according to age and weight.

Onset of effect
30 – 60 minutes (by mouth); within 15 minutes (injection).

Duration of action
3 – 6 hours (tablets, syrup); 2 – 4 hours (injection); 6 – 12 hours (slow-release tablets).

Diet advice
None.

Storage
Keep in a closed container in a cool, dry place away from reach of children. Protect from light.

Missed dose
Take as soon as you remember. If your next dose is due within 2 hours, take a single dose now and skip the next.

Stopping the drug
Do not stop the drug without consulting your physician; symptoms may recur.

OVERDOSE ACTION

 Seek immediate medical advice in all cases. You may experience severe abdominal cramps, vomiting, weakness and tremor. Take emergency action if unusually slow heartbeat, troubled breathing, seizures, or loss of consciousness occurs.

See Drug poisoning emergency guide (p.590).

SPECIAL PRECAUTIONS

Be sure to tell your physician if:
▼ You have heart problems.
▼ You have had epileptic seizures.
▼ You have asthma.
▼ You have difficulty passing urine.
▼ You are taking other medications.

 Pregnancy
▼ No evidence of risk to developing baby in the first 6 months of pregnancy. Large doses near the time of delivery may cause premature labor and lead to temporary muscle weakness in the newborn baby.

 Breast feeding
▼ No evidence of risk.

 Infants and children
▼ Reduced dose necessary.

 Over 60
▼ Increased likelihood of adverse effects.

 Driving and hazardous work
▼ Your underlying condition may make such activities inadvisable. Discuss with your physician.

 Alcohol
▼ Avoid. Alcohol may cause breathing difficulties in myasthenia gravis sufferers.

Surgery and general anesthetics
▼ Pyridostigmine may interact with some anesthetic agents. Make sure your treatment is known to your physician, dentist, and anesthesiologist before any surgery.

PROLONGED USE

The effects of the drug may diminish with time. Benefits may be restored by stopping the drug for a few days or by adjusting the dose.

POSSIBLE ADVERSE EFFECTS

Adverse effects of pyridostigmine are usually dose-related. In rare cases, hypersensitivity may occur, leading to an allergic skin rash.

Symptom/effect	Frequency		Discuss with physician		Stop taking drug now	Call physician now
	Common	Rare	Only if severe	In all cases		
Nausea/vomiting	●		■			
Increased salivation	●		■			
Sweating	●		■			
Abdominal cramps/diarrhea	●		■			
Watering eyes/small pupils		●	■			
Injection-site pain/swelling		●		■		
Rash		●		■		▲

INTERACTIONS

General note Drugs that suppress transmission of nerve signals may oppose the effect of pyridostigmine. Such drugs include digoxin, aminoglycoside antibiotics, chlorpromazine, and thyroid hormones.

PYRIMETHAMINE

Brand name Daraprim
Used in the following combined preparation Fansidar

GENERAL INFORMATION

Pyrimethamine, introduced in 1953, is an antimalarial drug generally used against types of malaria resistant to other drugs. Though it does not cure malaria, pyrimethamine is valuable as a preventive, and it effectively relieves the chills-and-fever symptoms of malaria attacks.

Because malaria parasites can readily develop resistance to pyrimethamine, the drug is usually given with sulfadoxine, an antibacterial drug. The activity of the two greatly exceeds that of either drug alone.

Pyrimethamine is prescribed with other sulfonamides to treat toxoplasmosis, which is a much rarer protozoal infection. Because blood disorders can arise during prolonged use, regular blood counts are made and vitamin supplements are given.

INFORMATION FOR USERS

Your drug prescription is tailored for you. Do not alter dosage without checking with your physician.

How taken

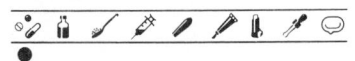

Tablets.

Frequency and timing of doses
Once weekly starting 2 weeks before travel and continuing for 6 weeks after leaving malarial area (prevention of malaria); 2 – 3 x daily for 3 days (treatment of malaria); 1 – 2 x daily (toxoplasmosis). Doses are best taken with food.

Dosage range
Adults 25mg per dose (prevention of malaria); 50 – 100mg daily for 1 – 3 days, then 25mg daily for 4 – 6 weeks (toxoplasmosis).
Children Reduced dose necessary according to age and weight.

Onset of effect
24 hours.

Duration of action
Up to 1 week.

Diet advice
None.

Storage
Keep in a closed container in a cool, dry place away from reach of children. Protect from light.

Missed dose
Take as soon as you remember. If your next dose is due within 24 hours (once weekly schedule), 12 hours (once daily schedule), or 2 hours (more than once daily schedule), take a single dose now and skip the next.

Stopping the drug
Take the full course. If stopped too soon treatment may fail.

Exceeding the dose
An occasional unintentional extra dose is unlikely to cause problems. Large overdoses may cause trembling, clumsiness, unsteadiness, and seizures. Notify your physician.

SPECIAL PRECAUTIONS

Be sure to tell your physician if:
▼ You have impaired liver or kidney function.
▼ You have had epileptic seizures.
▼ You have anemia.
▼ You have glucose-6-phosphate dehydrogenase (G6PD) deficiency.
▼ You are taking other medications.

Pregnancy
▼ Not prescribed. May cause defects in the unborn baby. Discuss with your physician so that you may weigh the benefits of the drug against its risks.

Breast feeding
▼ The drug passes into the breast milk. Although adverse effects on the baby are uncommon, the drug may cause hemolytic anemia in glucose-6-phosphate dehydrogenase (G6PD) deficient infants.

Infants and children
▼ Reduced dose necessary.

Over 60
▼ No special problems.

Driving and hazardous work
▼ No special problems.

Alcohol
▼ No known problems.

POSSIBLE ADVERSE EFFECTS

Side effects of pyrimethamine occur only rarely with the low doses given for prevention of malaria. Vomiting may be prevented by taking the drug with food.

Unusual tiredness, weakness, bleeding, bruising, and sore throat may be signs of a blood disorder. Notify your physician promptly if they occur.

Symptom/effect	Frequency		Discuss with physician		Stop taking drug now	Call physician now
	Common	Rare	Only if severe	In all cases		
Loss of appetite	●		■			
Vomiting	●		■			
Weakness/fatigue		●		■		
Rash		●		■		▮
Unusual bleeding/bruising		●		■		▮
Sore throat/fever		●		■		▮

PROLONGED USE

Prolonged use of this drug in high doses may cause folic acid deficiency, leading to serious blood disorders. Supplements of folic acid may be recommended.

Monitoring Regular blood cell counts may be required during high-dose treatment for toxoplasmosis.

INTERACTIONS

General note Drugs that suppress the bone marrow or cause folic acid deficiency may increase the risk of serious blood disorders. Such drugs include anticancer and antirheumatic drugs, phenylbutazone, sulfasalazine, and trimethoprim.

QUINACRINE

Brand name Atabrine
Used in the following combined preparations None

GENERAL INFORMATION

Quinacrine was first developed during World War II and widely used by US servicemen to prevent malaria. Later supplanted by more effective antimalarial drugs, quinacrine is now used to treat another protozoal infection, giardiasis. That disease is characterized by diarrhea, gas (flatulence), and abdominal pain.

Quinacrine commonly causes nausea and vomiting, symptoms that can be minimized by taking the drug with meals. The bright yellow color of quinacrine may lead to a similar discoloration of the skin or to a deep yellow colored urine, side effects which are harmless. Cases of mental derangement or blood disorders have been reported following prolonged use of the drug. The treatment of giardiasis, however, involves only four to seven days of treatment.

QUICK REFERENCE

Drug group Antiprotozoal drug (p.164)

Overdose danger rating Medium

Dependence rating Low

Prescription needed Yes

Available as generic No

INFORMATION FOR USERS

Your drug prescription is tailored for you. Do not alter dosage without checking with your physician.

How taken

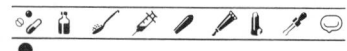

Tablets.

Frequency and timing of doses
3 x daily with meals for up to 7 days.

Dosage range
Adults 300mg daily.
Children Reduced dose necessary according to age and weight.

Onset of effect
2 – 3 days.

Duration of action
8 – 12 hours.

Diet advice
None.

Storage
Keep in a closed container in a cool, dry place away from reach of children. Protect from light.

Missed dose
Take as soon as you remember. If your next dose is due within 2 hours, take a single dose now and skip the next.

Stopping the drug
Take the full course. Even if you feel better, the original infection may still be present and symptoms may recur if treatment is stopped too soon.

Exceeding the dose
An occasional unintentional extra dose is unlikely to cause problems. Large overdoses may cause nausea, vomiting, and abdominal cramps. Notify your physician.

SPECIAL PRECAUTIONS

Be sure to tell your physician if:
▼ You have impaired liver or kidney function.
▼ You have glucose-6-phosphate dehydrogenase (G6PD) deficiency.
▼ You have psoriasis.
▼ You have had a mental disorder.
▼ You are taking other medications.

Pregnancy
▼ Not usually prescribed. May cause defects in the unborn baby. Treatment is usually postponed until after delivery.

Breast feeding
▼ No problems expected.

Infants and children
▼ Not usually prescribed. Reduced dose necessary.

Over 60
▼ Increased likelihood of adverse effects.

Driving and hazardous work
▼ Avoid such activities until you have learned how the drug affects you, because it can cause dizziness.

Alcohol
▼ Avoid. Taken with quinacrine, alcohol may cause flushing, nausea, vomiting, abdominal pain, and headache.

POSSIBLE ADVERSE EFFECTS

Nausea and vomiting are the most common side effects of quinacrine. Headache, dizziness, and yellow discoloration of the skin and urine may also occur. Serious adverse effects are rare when the drug is taken for short periods.

Symptom/effect	Frequency		Discuss with physician		Stop taking drug now	Call physician now
	Common	Rare	Only if severe	In all cases		
Headache	●		■			
Dizziness	●		■			
Nausea/vomiting	●		■			
Yellow skin/urine	●		■			
Mental disturbance		●		■	▲	
Rash		●		■	▲	■

INTERACTIONS

Primaquine Quinacrine reduces the breakdown of primaquine, and so increases its blood levels and the risk of adverse effects.

PROLONGED USE

Prolonged use of this drug may lead to skin rashes and rarely to serious blood disorders. Courses of longer than 7 days are not usually recommended.

QUINIDINE

Brand names Cardioquin, Duraquin, Quinaglute, Quinidex, Quinora
Used in the following combined preparations None

GENERAL INFORMATION

Introduced in the 1920s, quinidine is one of the oldest of the anti-arrhythmic drugs. It is used to treat many different abnormal heart rhythms, particularly in cases where the heartbeat is irregular or too rapid.

When taken by mouth, the onset of action is slow. It is given by injection in emergencies, in the hospital, when rapid control of an abnormal heart rhythm is required.

Quinidine has a number of adverse effects. Diarrhea, nausea, and vomiting, which are common, may be due to its irritant effect. Serious allergic reactions have also occurred. The most serious adverse effect is the possibility of further abnormal heart rhythms.

INFORMATION FOR USERS

Your drug prescription is tailored for you. Do not alter dosage without checking with your physician.

How taken

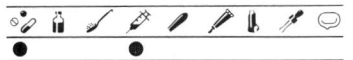

Tablets, slow-release capsules, injection.

Frequency and timing of doses
Every 6 hours (tablets); every 8 – 12 hours (slow-release capsules).

Dosage range
Adults 500mg – 3g daily.
Children Reduced dose necessary according to age and weight.

Onset of effect
Within 3 hours.

Duration of action
6 – 8 hours (tablets), up to 12 hours (slow-release capsules).

Diet advice
None.

Storage
Keep in a closed container in a cool, dry place away from reach of children. Protect from light.

Missed dose
Take as soon as you remember. If your next dose is due within 2 hours, take a single dose now and skip the next.

Stopping the drug
Do not stop the drug without consulting your physician; symptoms may recur.

OVERDOSE ACTION

Seek immediate medical advice in all cases. Take emergency action if breathing difficulties, seizures, or loss of consciousness occurs.

See Drug poisoning emergency guide (p.590).

SPECIAL PRECAUTIONS

Be sure to tell your physician if:
▼ You have impaired kidney or liver function.
▼ You have heart failure.
▼ You have myasthenia gravis.
▼ You have had a rash following quinidine on a previous occasion.
▼ You are taking other medications.

Pregnancy
▼ Not usually prescribed. Safety in pregnancy not established. Discuss with your physician so that you can weigh the benefits of the drug against its possible risks.

Breast feeding
▼ Discuss with your physician. The drug passes into the breast milk and may affect the baby adversely.

Infants and children
▼ Not usually prescribed.

Over 60
▼ Reduced dose necessary.

Driving and hazardous work
▼ No known problems.

Alcohol
▼ No known problems.

POSSIBLE ADVERSE EFFECTS

The most common adverse effects are diarrhea, nausea, and vomiting. If they become severe, a change of drug may be necessary. Vertigo or palpitations may indicate the dose is too high; notify your physician promptly.

Symptom/effect	Frequency		Discuss with physician		Stop taking drug now	Call physician now
	Common	Rare	Only if severe	In all cases		
Diarrhea	●		■			
Nausea/vomiting	●		■			
Dizziness	●		■			
Ringing in the ears		●		■		
Blurred vision		●		■		
Headache/vertigo		●		■		▮
Palpitations		●		■	▮	▮
Rash		●		■	▮	▮

PROLONGED USE

Sudden onset of abnormal heart rhythms or abnormalities of the blood may be encountered.

Monitoring Periodic checks on blood levels of the drug may be required.

INTERACTIONS

Digoxin Quinidine increases the effects of digoxin, requiring that blood levels be checked.

Anticoagulant drugs Quinidine increases the effect of these drugs.

Phenobarbital and rifampin reduce the effect of quinidine.

QUININE

Brand names Quinamm, Quindan, Quine, Quiphile
Used in the following combined preparations None

GENERAL INFORMATION

Quinine, obtained from the bark of the cinchona tree, is the earliest antimalarial drug. Introduced in 1888, it is no longer widely used because it frequently causes side effects (see below). However, it is still occasionally given for malaria that is resistant to safer treatments. In some of these cases, it is administered by mouth in conjunction with other drugs. Quinine is also prescribed in low doses for prevention of painful nighttime leg cramps, and this is now its most common use in many countries.

At the high doses used to treat malaria, quinine may cause ringing in the ears, headaches, nausea, hearing loss, and blurred vision, a group of symptoms known as cinchonism. In rare cases, the drug may also cause *subcutaneous* bleeding due to a reduction in blood platelets.

QUICK REFERENCE

Drug group Antimalarial drug (p.165)
Overdose danger rating High
Dependence rating Low
Prescription needed Yes
Available as generic Yes

INFORMATION FOR USERS

Your drug prescription is tailored for you. Do not alter dosage without checking with your physician.

How taken

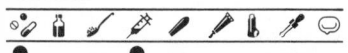

Tablets, capsules, injection.

Frequency and timing of doses
Malaria Every 8 hours (by mouth); every 6 – 8 hours (injection).
Muscle cramps Once daily at bedtime or 2 x daily after evening meal and at bedtime.

Dosage range
Adults 1,950mg daily (malaria); 200 – 600mg daily (cramps).
Children Reduced dose according to age and weight.

Onset of effect
2 – 3 hours (cramps); 1 – 2 days (malaria).

Duration of action
Up to 24 hours.

Diet advice
None.

Storage
Keep in a closed container in a cool, dry place away from reach of children. Protect from light.

Missed dose
Take as soon as you remember. If your next dose is due within 4 hours, skip the missed dose and resume your normal dosing schedule thereafter.

Stopping the drug
If prescribed for malaria, take the full course. Even if you feel better, the original infection may still be present and may recur if treatment is stopped too soon. If taken for muscle cramps, the drug can safely be stopped as soon as you no longer need it.

OVERDOSE ACTION

 Seek immediate medical advice in all cases. Take emergency action if breathing problems, seizures, or loss of consciousness occurs.

See Drug poisoning emergency guide (p.590).

SPECIAL PRECAUTIONS

Be sure to tell your physician if:
▼ You have impaired kidney function.
▼ You have tinnitus (ringing in the ears).
▼ You have optic neuritis.
▼ You have myasthenia gravis.
▼ You have glucose-6-phosphate dehydrogenase (G6PD) deficiency.
▼ You have heart problems.
▼ You are taking other medications.

 Pregnancy
▼ Not prescribed. May cause miscarriage and could cause defects in the unborn baby.

 Breast feeding
▼ Discuss with your physician. The drug passes into the breast milk, but at normal doses adverse effects on the baby are rare.

 Infants and children
▼ Reduced dose necessary.

 Over 60
▼ No special problems.

 Driving and hazardous work
▼ Blurring of vision, an uncommon side effect, may impair these activities.

 Alcohol
▼ No known problems.

PROLONGED USE

No problems expected.

POSSIBLE ADVERSE EFFECTS

Adverse effects are unlikely with low doses. At antimalarial doses, hearing disturbances, headache, and blurred vision are more common. Nausea and diarrhea may occur.

Symptom/effect	Frequency		Discuss with physician		Stop taking drug now	Call physician now
	Common	Rare	Only if severe	In all cases		
Nausea/diarrhea	●		■			
Headache	●			■		
Ringing in the ears	●			■		
Loss of hearing	●			■		
Blurred vision		●		■	▲	
Rash/itching		●		■	▲	

INTERACTIONS

Digoxin Quinine increases the blood level of digoxin.

Aluminum-containing antacids reduce the absorption of quinine.

Oral anticoagulant drugs Quinine may enhance the action of oral anticoagulants.

Antimyasthenia drugs Quinine may oppose the beneficial effects of these drugs.

RANITIDINE

Brand name Zantac
Used in the following combined preparations None

GENERAL INFORMATION

Ranitidine, a drug similar to cimetidine, was introduced in 1983 and is mainly used in the prevention and treatment of stomach and duodenal ulcers. It acts by reducing the amount of acid produced by the stomach, allowing the ulcers time to heal. Ranitidine also reduces discomfort and inflammation from reflux esophagitis.

Treatment is usually given in courses lasting from four to eight weeks, with further short courses if symptoms recur.

Unlike cimetidine, this drug does not affect the actions of certain enzymes in the liver, where many drugs are broken down before being absorbed into the body. This means that ranitidine can be taken with other drugs, like anticoagulants and anticonvulsants, without causing an interaction that may reduce the effectiveness of either treatment.

Most people do not experience any serious effects during a course of treatment with ranitidine. As ranitidine promotes healing of the stomach lining, there is a risk that it may mask stomach cancer, delaying diagnosis. It is therefore usually prescribed only when the possibility of stomach cancer has been ruled out.

QUICK REFERENCE

Drug group Anti-ulcer drug (p.137)
Overdose danger rating Low
Dependence rating Low
Prescription needed Yes
Available as generic No

INFORMATION FOR USERS

Your drug prescription is tailored for you. Do not alter dosage without checking with your physician.

How taken

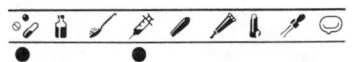

Tablets, injection.

Frequency and timing of doses
Once daily at bedtime or 2 x daily.

Adult dosage range
300mg daily (active ulcer); 150mg daily (ulcer prevention).

Onset of effect
Within 1 hour.

Duration of action
12 hours.

Diet advice
None.

Storage
Keep in a closed container in a cool, dry place away from reach of children.

Missed dose
Take as soon as you remember. If your next dose is due within 3 hours, take a single dose now and skip the next.

Stopping the drug
Do not stop the drug without consulting your physician; symptoms may recur.

Exceeding the dose
An occasional unintentional extra dose is unlikely to be a cause for concern. But if you notice unusual symptoms, or if a large overdose has been taken, notify your physician.

SPECIAL PRECAUTIONS

Be sure to tell your physician if:
▼ You have impaired liver or kidney function.

Pregnancy
▼ Not usually prescribed. Safety in pregnancy not established. Discuss with your physician so that you can weigh the benefits of the drug against its possible risks.

Breast feeding
▼ Discuss with your physician. The drug passes into the breast milk and may affect the baby adversely.

Infants and children
▼ Not usually prescribed. Reduced dose necessary.

Over 60
▼ No special problems.

Driving and hazardous work
▼ No known problems.

Alcohol
▼ Avoid. Alcohol may aggravate your underlying condition and reduce the beneficial effects of this drug.

POSSIBLE ADVERSE EFFECTS

The adverse effects of ranitidine, of which headache is the most common, are usually related to dosage level and almost always disappear when treatment finishes.

Symptom/effect	Frequency		Discuss with physician		Stop taking drug now	Call physician now
	Common	Rare	Only if severe	In all cases		
Headache	●		■			
Nausea		●	■			
Constipation		●	■			
Lethargy/weakness		●	■			

INTERACTIONS

None.

PROLONGED USE

Courses of longer than 6 months are not usually necessary, although repeat courses may be required in cases of relapse. Continuous use of the drug for longer than 1 year is not recommended except in exceptional circumstances, because the safety of this drug for prolonged use has not yet been confirmed.

RIFAMPIN

Brand names Rifadin, Rimactane
Used in the following combined preparation Rifamate

GENERAL INFORMATION

Rifampin, introduced in 1971, is an antibacterial drug that is highly effective in the treatment of tuberculosis. Taken by mouth, it is well absorbed in the intestines and widely distributed throughout the body, including the brain, and it is therefore especially useful in tuberculous meningitis.

It is always prescribed with other antituberculous drugs; this enhances its effect and prevents drug resistance.

Treatment may continue for six months to two years or more.

Rifampin is also used for leprosy and other serious infections, including artificial heart valve infections, osteomyelitis, and certain types of boils. Rifampin is never used alone to treat such infections because of the rapid emergence of resistance in the organisms responsible for the condition under treatment.

QUICK REFERENCE

Drug group Antituberculous drug (p.160)

Overdose danger rating Medium

Dependence rating Low

Prescription needed Yes

Available as generic No

INFORMATION FOR USERS

Your drug prescription is tailored for you. Do not alter dosage without checking with your physician.

How taken

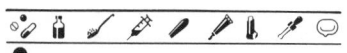

Capsules.

Frequency and timing of doses
Once daily in the morning 30 minutes before food (tuberculosis); 1 – 2 x daily (prevention of meningitis, treatment of endocarditis); once daily or once monthly (leprosy).

Adult dosage range
According to weight, usually 450 – 600mg daily (tuberculosis); 600mg – 1.2g daily (prevention of meningitis, treatment of endocarditis); 600mg per dose (leprosy).

Onset of effect
Several days.

Duration of action
Up to 72 hours.

Diet advice
None.

Storage
Keep in a closed container in a cool, dry place away from reach of children. Protect from light.

Missed dose
Take as soon as you remember. If your next dose is due within 6 hours, take both doses now and return to normal dosing thereafter.

Stopping the drug
Take the full course. Even if you feel better, the original infection may still be present and symptoms may recur if treatment is stopped too soon. In rare cases stopping the drug suddenly after high-dose treatment can lead to a severe flu-like illness.

Exceeding the dose
An occasional unintentional extra dose is unlikely to cause problems. Large overdoses may cause nausea, vomiting, and lethargy. Notify your physician.

SPECIAL PRECAUTIONS

Be sure to tell your physician if:
▼ You have impaired liver function.
▼ You are taking other medications.

Pregnancy
▼ Not usually prescribed. Safety in pregnancy not established. Discuss with your physician so that you can weigh the benefits of the drug against its possible risks.

Breast feeding
▼ The drug passes into the breast milk, but at normal doses adverse effects on the baby are uncommon. Discuss with your physician.

Infants and children
▼ Reduced dose necessary.

Over 60
▼ Reduced dose may be necessary. Increased risk of adverse effects.

Driving and hazardous work
▼ Avoid such activities until you have learned how the drug affects you, because the drug may cause dizziness.

Alcohol
▼ No special problems.

POSSIBLE ADVERSE EFFECTS

Rifampin normally causes a harmless orange-red discoloration of the urine and other body fluids. Serious adverse effects are rare. Jaundice usually improves during treatment but should nevertheless be reported to your physician. Symptoms such as headache and breathing difficulties may occur after stopping high-dose treatment.

Symptom/effect	Frequency		Discuss with physician		Stop taking drug now	Call physician now
	Common	Rare	Only if severe	In all cases		
Muscle cramps/aches		●	■			
Nausea/vomiting/diarrhea		●	■			
Jaundice		●		■	▲	▮
Flu-like illness		●		■	▲	▮
Rash/itching		●		■	▲	▮

INTERACTIONS

General note Rifampin may reduce the effectiveness of a wide variety of drugs. Such drugs include digitoxin, oral contraceptives, corticosteroids, oral antidiabetics, disopyramide, and oral anticoagulants.

Aminosalicylic acid may impair the absorption of rifampin. Spacing of doses may be recommended.

PROLONGED USE

Prolonged use of rifampin may cause liver damage.

Monitoring Periodic blood tests may be performed to monitor liver function.

RITODRINE

Brand name Yutopar
Used in the following combined preparations None

GENERAL INFORMATION

Ritodrine, introduced in 1980, is a *sympathomimetic* drug that relaxes the muscles of the uterus. It is used to prevent premature labor. After contractions are initially stopped by intravenous infusion of the drug, tablets are substituted. These continue to be administered until the physician considers it safe for the baby to be born, usually at or before 36 weeks.

Ritodrine may also be used to halt labor temporarily while corticosteroid drugs are given to help development of the baby's lungs and lessen the risk of breathing problems after delivery.

Stimulation of the heart leading to palpitations is the commonest side effect of ritodrine. Given by injection, it may also increase blood sugar levels and aggravate diabetes.

INFORMATION FOR USERS

Your drug prescription is tailored for you. Do not alter dosage without checking with your physician.

How taken

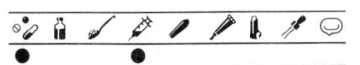

Tablets, injection.

Frequency and timing of doses
By continuous infusion until contractions stop. Then by mouth every 2 hours for 24 hours, and every 4 – 6 hours thereafter.

Dosage range
Up to 120mg daily (by mouth).

Onset of effect
Within a few minutes (injection); 30 – 60 minutes (by mouth).

Duration of action
6 – 8 hours.

Diet advice
Eat nothing and drink only clear fluids until drug treatment has halted contractions.

Storage
Keep in a closed container in a cool, dry place away from reach of children.

Missed dose
Take as soon as you remember. If your doses are scheduled every 4 – 6 hours and your next dose is due within 2 hours, take a single dose now and skip the next.

Stopping the drug
Do not stop taking the drug without consulting your physician; stopping the drug may lead to the onset of labor.

Exceeding the dose
An occasional unintentional extra dose is unlikely to cause problems. Large overdoses may cause palpitations and breathing difficulty. Notify your physician.

SPECIAL PRECAUTIONS

Be sure to tell your physician if:
▼ You have heart problems.
▼ You suffer from migraine headaches.
▼ You have pre-eclampsia (high blood pressure, swollen ankles, protein in urine).
▼ You have an overactive thyroid.
▼ You have diabetes.
▼ You are taking other medications.

Pregnancy
▼ Used in pregnancy of over 20 weeks, there is no proven risk to the health of the baby. Ritodrine is not prescribed in pregnancies of less than 20 weeks, since its safety is not established.

Breast feeding
▼ Not applicable. Ritodrine is not used during breast feeding.

Infants and children
▼ Not prescribed.

Over 60
▼ Not prescribed.

Driving and hazardous work
▼ Your underlying condition may make such activities inadvisable. Discuss with your physician.

Alcohol
▼ Not advisable during pregnancy.

Surgery and general anesthetics
▼ Ritodrine may increase the risk of low blood pressure and palpitations with a general anesthetic. Discuss with your physician before any surgery.

POSSIBLE ADVERSE EFFECTS

Adverse effects are dose-related and are more severe when ritodrine is given by injection. By mouth, adverse effects other than palpitations are rare. Breathlessness due to fluid in the lungs may occasionally occur after the drug is stopped.

Symptom/effect	Frequency		Discuss with physician		Stop taking drug now	Call physician now
	Common	Rare	Only if severe	In all cases		
Trembling/agitation	●		■			
Palpitations	●			■		
Nausea/vomiting		●		■		
Chest pain/breathlessness		●		■	▲	!
Rash		●		■	▲	!

INTERACTIONS

Diuretics Ritodrine may increase the risk of side effects with some diuretics.

Beta blockers These drugs reduce the effect of ritodrine.

Other sympathomimetic drugs Ritodrine may increase the effects of these drugs.

Corticosteroids There is an increased risk of high blood sugar and shortness of breath when ritodrine is taken with corticosteroids.

Antidiabetic drugs Ritodrine may increase blood sugar. Antidiabetic drug dosage may need to be increased.

PROLONGED USE

No special problems.

SECOBARBITAL

Brand name Seconal
Used in the following combined preparation Tuinal

GENERAL INFORMATION

Secobarbital is a barbiturate drug that has been in use since the 1930s. It has many actions similar to those of the other drugs in this group (see Sleeping drugs, p.110), but its onset of action is more rapid and its duration of action more brief.

Secobarbital and similar drugs were once commonly prescribed as sleeping drugs but are now seldom prescribed because of their adverse effects and the danger of paralysis of the breathing mechanism when taken in overdose. Secobarbital and similar drugs have a high habit-forming potential. This drug is sometimes given as *premedication* to help relieve anxiety before surgery.

INFORMATION FOR USERS

Your drug prescription is tailored for you. Do not alter dosage without checking with your physician.

How taken

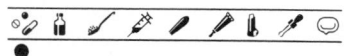

Tablets.

Frequency and timing of doses
Once daily 15 minutes before bedtime.

Adult dosage range
100 – 200mg daily.

Onset of effect
Within 15 minutes.

Duration of action
3 – 5 hours.

Storage
Keep in a closed container in a cool, dry place away from reach of children.

Missed dose
If you fall asleep without having taken a dose and wake some hours later, do not take the missed dose. Return to your normal dose schedule the following night if necessary.

Stopping the drug
If you have been taking the drug for a short period only, it can be safely stopped as soon as you feel that you no longer need it. However, if you have been taking the drug every night for more than two weeks, consult your physician, who may supervise a gradual reduction in dosage. Stopping abruptly may lead to withdrawal symptoms (see p.110).

OVERDOSE ACTION

 Seek immediate medical advice in all cases. Take emergency action if unsteadiness, severe weakness, confusion, or loss of consciousness occurs.

See Drug poisoning emergency guide (p.590).

POSSIBLE ADVERSE EFFECTS

Most of the adverse effects of secobarbital are the result of its sedative effect on the brain. They can sometimes be minimized by medically supervised reduction of dosage.

Symptom/effect	Frequency		Discuss with physician		Stop taking drug now	Call physician now
	Common	Rare	Only if severe	In all cases		
Dizziness/lightheadedness	●		■			
Daytime drowsiness	●		■			
Clumsiness/unsteadiness	●		■			▪
Rash		●		■	▲	
Confusion		●		■	▲	▪

INTERACTIONS

Sedatives All drugs that have a sedative effect on the central nervous system are likely to increase the sedative properties of secobarbital.

Oral contraceptives Secobarbital may reduce the effectiveness of oral contraceptives. Discuss with your physician.

Anticonvulsant drugs Secobarbital reduces the effect of some of these drugs.

Alcohol Alcohol dangerously increases the sedative effect of secobarbital.

Anticoagulant drugs The effects of these drugs may be reduced if secobarbital is taken regularly with them.

SPECIAL PRECAUTIONS

Be sure to tell your physician if:
▼ You have impaired kidney or liver function.
▼ You have heart problems.
▼ You have poor circulation.
▼ You have a lung disorder such as asthma or bronchitis.
▼ You suffer from persistent pain.
▼ You suffer from porphyria.
▼ You have had problems with alcohol or drug abuse.
▼ You are taking other medications.

 Pregnancy
▼ Prescribed only when benefit to mother outweighs risk to baby. May cause breathing difficulties in the newborn baby, and use throughout pregnancy may cause withdrawal reactions in the baby.

 Breast feeding
▼ Discuss with your physician. The drug passes into the breast milk and may affect the baby adversely.

 Infants and children
▼ Not recommended.

 Over 60
▼ Reduced dose necessary. Increased likelihood of adverse effects.

 Driving and hazardous work
▼ Avoid such activities until you have learned how the drug affects you, because secobarbital may cause daytime drowsiness even when taken at night.

 Alcohol
▼ Never drink while under treatment with secobarbital. Alcohol may interact dangerously with this drug.

PROLONGED USE

The effects of the drug usually become weaker after two weeks as the body adapts. It may also be habit-forming if taken regularly for longer than this.

SILVER SULFADIAZINE

Brand name Silvadene
Used in the following combined preparations None

GENERAL INFORMATION

Silver sulfadiazine, introduced in 1974, is an antibacterial agent applied as cream to prevent infections in burns. The silver in the drug contributes to its antibacterial action, and it is effective against a wide range of bacteria and yeasts. It is sometimes prescribed to prevent the infection of a skin graft.

Poorly absorbed from the wound surface, the drug has a long-lasting effect, one daily application generally being sufficient. The most common adverse effect of silver sulfadiazine is a local hypersensitivity reaction that may be difficult to distinguish from the effects of the burn itself. When treatment is prolonged or involves large areas of skin, more of the drug may be absorbed, increasing the risk of adverse effects to the kidneys. Monitoring of blood levels of the drug may be advised in those cases.

QUICK REFERENCE

Drug group Anti-infective skin preparation (p.203)

Overdose danger rating Low

Dependence rating Low

Prescription needed Yes

Available as generic Yes

INFORMATION FOR USERS

Your drug prescription is tailored for you. Do not alter dosage without checking with your physician.

How taken

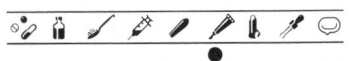

Cream.

Frequency and timing of doses
Usually once daily.

Dosage range
Apply to the affected area to a depth of 1 – 3mm.

Onset of effect
Immediately.

Duration of action
24 hours or more.

Diet advice
None.

Storage
Keep in a closed container in a cool, dry place away from reach of children. Protect from light.

Missed dose
Apply as soon as you remember, then return to your once-daily routine.

Stopping the drug
Do not stop using the drug without consulting your physician. If treatment is stopped before the affected area has healed, infection may occur.

Exceeding the dose
An occasional extra application is unlikely to be a cause for concern. If you notice unusual symptoms, notify your physician.

SPECIAL PRECAUTIONS

Be sure to tell your physician if:
▼ You have impaired liver or kidney function.
▼ You have previously had an allergic reaction to a sulfonamide drug.
▼ You have glucose-6-phosphate dehydrogenase (G6PD) deficiency.

 Pregnancy
▼ No evidence of risk to the developing baby.

 Breast feeding
▼ No evidence of risk.

 Infants and children
▼ Not recommended for infants under 2 months.

 Over 60
▼ No special problems.

 Driving and hazardous work
▼ No known problems.

 Alcohol
▼ No known problems.

POSSIBLE ADVERSE EFFECTS

Adverse effects occur rarely with silver sulfadiazine and are more likely in those being treated for extensive burns. Sore throat, fever, or jaundice may be early signs of a serious blood disorder, and blood in the urine may indicate kidney problems.

Symptom/effect	Frequency		Discuss with physician		Stop taking drug now	Call physician now
	Common	Rare	Only if severe	In all cases		
Burning sensation		●		■		▮
Rash/itching		●		■		▮
Jaundice		●		■		▮
Blood in urine		●		■		▮
Sore throat/fever		●		■		▮

PROLONGED USE

May increase the risk of serious blood disorders and kidney problems.

Monitoring In treatment of extensive burns, blood levels of the drug and kidney function may be monitored.

INTERACTIONS

None.

SODIUM BICARBONATE

Brand names None
Used in the following combined preparations Alka Seltzer, Citrocarbonate, Gaviscon, Gaviscon 2, Infalyte

GENERAL INFORMATION

Sodium bicarbonate is available without prescription on its own or in multi-ingredient preparations for the relief of occasional episodes of indigestion and heartburn. It may also relieve discomfort caused by peptic ulcers. It is seldom recommended by physicians because other drugs are safer and more effective.

Because sodium bicarbonate makes the urine more alkaline, it is used to prevent the formation of kidney stones in people suffering from gout. Given by injection, it is effective in reducing the acidity of the blood and body tissues in metabolic acidosis, a potentially fatal condition that may occur in life-threatening illnesses or cardiac arrest. Sodium bicarbonate should be avoided by people with heart failure or any condition that requires restriction of sodium intake.

QUICK REFERENCE

Drug group Antacid (p.136)
Overdose danger rating Medium
Dependence rating Low
Prescription needed No
Available as generic Yes

INFORMATION FOR USERS

Follow instructions on the label. Call your physician if symptoms worsen.

How taken

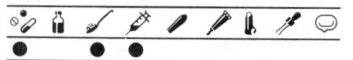

Tablets, powder (dissolved in water), injection.

Frequency and timing of doses
Indigestion As required (orally).
Gout 4 x daily.

Adult dosage range
1 – 16g daily (for short periods of time if kidney function is normal).

Onset of effect
Within 15 minutes.

Duration of action
30 – 60 minutes.

Diet advice
None.

Storage
Keep in a closed container in a cool, dry place away from reach of children.

Missed dose
No cause for concern.

Stopping the drug
When taken for indigestion, it can be safely stopped. When taken for other disorders, consult your physician.

Exceeding the dose
An occasional unintentional extra dose is unlikely to cause problems. Large overdoses may cause unusual weakness, dizziness, or headache. Notify your physician.

POSSIBLE ADVERSE EFFECTS

Belching and stomach pain may arise from the carbon dioxide produced as sodium bicarbonate neutralizes stomach acid, and can be caused by a single dose. The other effects result from the long-term regular use of sodium bicarbonate.

Symptom/effect	Frequency		Discuss with physician		Stop taking drug now	Call physician now
	Common	Rare	Only if severe	In all cases		
Belching	●		■			
Abdominal pain		●	■			
Swollen feet/ankles		●		■	▲	
Muscle cramps		●		■	▲	
Tiredness/weakness		●		■	▲	▮
Nausea/vomiting		●		■	▲	▮

INTERACTIONS

General note Sodium bicarbonate interferes with the absorption or excretion of a wide range of drugs taken by mouth. Consult your physician if you are taking oral anticoagulants, tetracycline antibiotics, phenothiazine antipsychotics, oral iron preparations, or lithium and wish to take more than an occasional dose of sodium bicarbonate.

Diuretics The sodium- and water-losing and blood pressure-reducing properties are reduced by use of sodium bicarbonate.

Corticosteroids Large amounts of sodium bicarbonate may hasten potassium loss, and increase fluid retention and high blood pressure.

SPECIAL PRECAUTIONS

Be sure to consult your physician before taking this drug if:
▼ You have impaired liver or kidney function.
▼ You have heart problems.
▼ You have high blood pressure.
▼ You have severe abdominal pain or vomiting.
▼ You are on a low-sodium diet.
▼ You are taking other medications.

Pregnancy
▼ Not usually prescribed. It is not likely to help morning sickness, and can encourage fluid retention.

Breast feeding
▼ The drug passes into the breast milk, but at normal doses adverse effects on the baby are uncommon. Discuss with your physician.

Infants and children
▼ Not usually prescribed. Not recommended for children under 6 years except on the advice of a physician. Reduced dose necessary.

Over 60
▼ Reduced dose may be necessary.

Driving and hazardous work
▼ Do not take if you are flying. The gas produced expands and may increase stomach distension and belching.

Alcohol
▼ Avoid. Alcohol irritates the stomach and may counter the beneficial effects of this drug.

PROLONGED USE

Severe weakness, fatigue, irritability, and muscle cramps may occur when this drug is taken regularly for extended periods. It should not be used daily for longer than 4 weeks without consulting your physician.

Monitoring Blood and urine tests may be performed during prolonged use.

SPIRONOLACTONE

Brand names Alatone, Aldactone
Used in the following combined preparations Alazide, Aldactazide, Spiromazide, Spirozide

GENERAL INFORMATION

Spironolactone, introduced in 1959, belongs to the class of drugs known as potassium-sparing diuretics. Combined with thiazide or loop diuretics, it is used in the treatment of hypertension and edema (fluid retention) resulting from congestive heart failure. On its own or, more commonly, in combination with a thiazide diuretic, it may be used to treat edema associated with cirrhosis of the liver, nephrotic syndrome (a kidney disorder), and a rare disease called Conn's syndrome, caused by a tumor in one of the adrenal glands.

Spironolactone is relatively slow to act, and its effects may appear only after several days of treatment. As with other potassium-sparing diuretics, there is a risk of unusually high levels of potassium in the blood if the kidneys are functioning abnormally. For that reason spironolactone is prescribed with caution for people with kidney failure. The drug does not worsen diabetes or gout, as do some other diuretics. The major side effect is nausea; abnormal breast enlargement may sometimes occur in men if high doses are given.

QUICK REFERENCE

Drug group Potassium-sparing diuretic (p.127)

Overdose danger rating Low

Dependence rating Low

Prescription needed Yes

Available as generic Yes

INFORMATION FOR USERS

Your drug prescription is tailored for you. Do not alter dosage without checking with your physician.

How taken

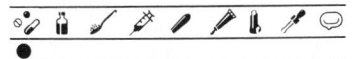

Tablets.

Frequency and timing of doses
Once daily, usually in the morning.

Dosage range
50 – 200mg daily.

Onset of effect
Within 1 – 3 days, but full effect may take up to 2 weeks.

Duration of action
2 – 3 days.

Diet advice
Avoid foods that are high in potassium, e.g. dried fruit, low-sodium milk, and salt substitutes.

Storage
Keep in a closed container in a cool, dry place away from reach of children.

Missed dose
Take as soon as you remember.

Stopping the drug
Do not stop the drug without consulting your physician; symptoms may recur.

Exceeding the dose
An occasional unintentional extra dose is unlikely to be a cause for concern. But if you notice unusual symptoms, or if a large overdose has been taken, notify your physician.

SPECIAL PRECAUTIONS

Be sure to tell your physician if:
▼ You have impaired kidney or liver function.
▼ You have a metabolic disorder.
▼ You have diabetes.
▼ You are taking other medications.

Pregnancy
▼ Not usually prescribed. May cause a reduction in the blood supply to the developing baby. Discuss with your physician so that you can weigh the benefits of the drug against its risks.

Breast feeding
▼ The drug passes into the breast milk but is not known to be harmful.

Infants and children
▼ Not usually prescribed. Reduced dose necessary.

Over 60
▼ Reduced dose may be necessary. Increased likelihood of adverse effects.

Driving and hazardous work
▼ No special problems.

Alcohol
▼ No known problems.

POSSIBLE ADVERSE EFFECTS

Spironolactone has few adverse effects; the main problem is the possibility that potassium may be retained by the body, causing muscle weakness and numbness.

Symptom/effect	Frequency		Discuss with physician		Stop taking drug now	Call physician now
	Common	Rare	Only if severe	In all cases		
Nausea/vomiting	●		■			
Diarrhea		●	■			
Lethargy		●	■			
Irregular menstruation		●	■			
Breast enlargement (men)		●		■		
Impotence		●		■		
Rash		●		■		■

INTERACTIONS

Lithium Spironolactone may increase the blood levels of lithium, leading to an increased risk of lithium poisoning.

Digoxin Adverse effects may result from increased digoxin levels.

PROLONGED USE

Serious problems are unlikely.

Monitoring Blood tests may be performed to check on kidney function and levels of body salts.

A B C D E F G H I J K L M N O P Q R S T U V W X Y Z

STREPTOKINASE

Brand names Kabikinase, Streptase
Used in the following combined preparations None

GENERAL INFORMATION

Streptokinase, an enzyme produced by streptococcus bacteria, has been used in hospitals to dissolve the fibrin (see p.133) of blood clots, especially those in the arteries of the heart and lungs. It is also used on the clots formed in shunts during kidney dialysis.

A fast-acting drug, streptokinase is most effective in dissolving newly formed clots, and it is often released at the site of the clot via a catheter inserted into an artery. Administered in the early stages of a heart attack to dissolve a clot in the coronary arteries (thrombosis), it can reduce the amount of damage to heart muscle.

Because excessive bleeding is a common side effect, treatment is closely supervised. Since streptokinase is a protein, it can cause allergic reactions. To reduce this risk it is given in highly purified form, with antihistamines also administered at the start of treatment.

QUICK REFERENCE

Drug group Thrombolytic agent (p.133)

Overdose danger rating Medium

Dependence rating Low

Prescription needed Yes

Available as generic No

INFORMATION FOR USERS

The drug is given only under medical supervision and is not for self-administration.

How taken

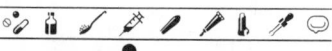

Injection.

Frequency and timing of doses
Continuously over a period of 12 – 72 hours.

Dosage range
Dosage is determined individually by the condition and response.

Onset of effect
As soon as streptokinase reaches the blood clot, which begins to dissolve within minutes. Most of the clot will be dissolved within 1 – 2 hours.

Duration of action
Effect disappears within a few minutes of stopping the drug.

Diet advice
None.

Storage
Not applicable. This drug is not normally kept in the home.

Missed dose
Not applicable. This drug is given only in a hospital under close medical supervision.

Stopping the drug
This drug is stopped as soon as the clot is dissolved.

Exceeding the dose
Overdosage is unlikely, since treatment is carefully monitored.

SPECIAL PRECAUTIONS

Streptokinase is prescribed only under close medical supervision, usually only in life-threatening circumstances.

Pregnancy
▼ Not usually prescribed. If used during the first 18 weeks of pregnancy there is a risk that the placenta may separate from the wall of the uterus.

Breast feeding
▼ No evidence of risk.

Infants and children
▼ Not recommended.

Over 60
▼ Increased likelihood of bleeding.

Driving and hazardous work
▼ Not applicable.

Alcohol
▼ Not applicable.

POSSIBLE ADVERSE EFFECTS

Streptokinase is given only under strict supervision and all adverse effects are closely monitored so that any of the symptoms below can be quickly dealt with.

Symptom/effect	Frequency		Discuss with physician		Stop taking drug now	Call physician now
	Common	Rare	Only if severe	In all cases		
Excessive bleeding	●			■		
Rash		●		■		
Fever		●		■		
Wheezing		●		■		
Abnormal heart rhythms		●		■		
Collapse		●		■		

PROLONGED USE

Streptokinase is never used long-term.

INTERACTIONS

Anticoagulant drugs There is an increased risk of bleeding when these are taken at the same time as streptokinase.

Antiplatelet drugs increase the risk of bleeding if given with streptokinase.

STREPTOMYCIN

Brand names None
Used in the following combined preparations None

GENERAL INFORMATION

Although it is one of the oldest amino-glycoside antibiotics, streptomycin is used with considerable restraint. For one thing, many bacteria have developed resistance to it since its introduction in 1946. It can also damage the nerves in the ear, upsetting the human balance system and even causing deafness. It is generally reserved for serious infections that do not respond to other antibiotics. Its greatest value is in the early treatment of tuberculosis. Given by injection, it rapidly reaches effective blood levels and enhances the antibacterial effects of other antituberculous drugs. With some people, it may be given twice weekly on an outpatient basis, but it is given only for about two months, after which other drugs are used.

In shorter courses, streptomycin is effective in the treatment of such rare diseases as tularemia, plague, severe brucellosis, and glanders. It is also given for the sexually transmitted diseases granuloma inguinale and chancroid, and occasionally for rat bite fever. With a penicillin antibiotic it is used to treat bacterial infection of the heart valves (endocarditis).

QUICK REFERENCE

Drug group Aminoglycoside antibiotic (p.158) and antituberculous drug (p.160)

Overdose danger rating Medium

Dependence rating Low

Prescription needed Yes

Available as generic Yes

INFORMATION FOR USERS

The drug is given only under medical supervision and is not for self-administration.

How taken

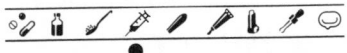

Injection.

Frequency and timing of doses
Once daily for 2 – 3 weeks, then every alternate day or 3 x weekly, reduced to 2 x weekly (tuberculosis); 2 x daily (tularemia, plague, brucellosis); 2 x daily for 7 – 10 days, then once daily (other bacterial infections).

Dosage range
Dosage is determined according to the individual's condition and response.

Onset of effect
2 – 3 days.

Duration of action
Up to 24 hours. Some beneficial effect may last for several days.

Diet advice
None.

Storage
Not applicable. The drug is not kept in the home.

Missed dose
If you miss a streptomycin injection, contact your physician as soon as possible to arrange for the missed dose to be made up.

Stopping the drug
Take the full course. Even if you feel better, the original infection may still be present and may recur if treatment is stopped too soon.

Exceeding the dose
Overdosage is unlikely, since treatment is carefully monitored.

POSSIBLE ADVERSE EFFECTS

The most common side effect of streptomycin is transient facial numbness, sometimes accompanied by tingling in the hands. Headache or malaise also occur occasionally after injection. Dizziness, loss of balance (vertigo), ringing in the ears, and any loss of hearing should be reported to your physician promptly.

Symptom/effect	Frequency		Discuss with physician		Stop taking drug now	Call physician now
	Common	Rare	Only if severe	In all cases		
Headache/malaise	●		■			
Numbness/tingling	●		■			
Nausea/vomiting		●		■		
Dizziness/vertigo		●		■	▲	▮
Ringing in the ears		●		■	▲	▮
Loss of hearing		●		■	▲	▮

INTERACTIONS

General note A wide range of drugs increase the risk of hearing loss and/or kidney failure with streptomycin. Such drugs include other aminoglycosides, furosemide, polymyxin antibiotics, amphotericin B, cisplatin, and cyclosporine.

SPECIAL PRECAUTIONS

Be sure to tell your physician if:
▼ You have impaired kidney function.
▼ You have a hearing disorder.
▼ You have myasthenia gravis or Parkinson's disease.
▼ You are taking other medications.

Pregnancy
▼ Not prescribed. May cause hearing defects in the baby.

Breast feeding
▼ The drug passes into the breast milk in small amounts, but at normal doses adverse effects on the baby are uncommon.

Infants and children
▼ Not usually prescribed. Reduced dose necessary.

Over 60
▼ Reduced dose may be necessary. Increased likelihood of adverse effects.

Driving and hazardous work
▼ No known problems.

Alcohol
▼ No known problems.

Surgery and general anesthetics
▼ Streptomycin may need to be stopped before you have a general anesthetic. Discuss this with your physician or dentist before any surgery.

PROLONGED USE

There is a risk of adverse effects on hearing and balance with prolonged use.

Monitoring Blood levels of the drug may be measured. Periodic hearing and balance tests are usually needed.

SUCRALFATE

Brand name Carafate
Used in the following combined preparations None

GENERAL INFORMATION

Sucralfate, a drug made available in 1981, is prescribed to treat gastric and duodenal ulcers. It does not neutralize stomach acid, but sucralfate forms a protective barrier over the ulcer that prevents it from being attacked by digestive juices, thus giving the ulcer time to heal.

If it is necessary during treatment to take antacids to relieve pain, they should be taken at least one hour before or an hour after sucralfate, or they will reduce its effectiveness.

Apart from constipation, sucralfate does not have any common adverse effects. However, it interferes with the absorption of fats and may therefore reduce absorption of vitamins that are dissolved in fat – notably vitamins A, D, E, and K. During prolonged treatment it may be necessary to take supplements of these.

QUICK REFERENCE

Drug group Ulcer-healing drug (p.137)

Overdose danger rating Low

Dependence rating Low

Prescription needed Yes

Available as generic No

INFORMATION FOR USERS

Your drug prescription is tailored for you. Do not alter dosage without checking with your physician.

How taken

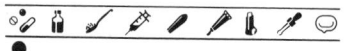

Tablets.

Frequency and timing of doses
4 x daily, one hour before each meal and at bedtime.

Dosage range
4 – 8g daily.

Onset of effect
Some improvement may be noted after one or two doses, but it takes a few weeks for an ulcer to heal.

Duration of action
Up to 5 hours.

Diet advice
During prolonged treatment make sure your diet includes foods containing vitamins A, D, E, and K (see pp.543 – 6). Your physician will advise you if supplements are necessary.

Storage
Keep in a closed container in a cool, dry place away from reach of children.

Missed dose
Do not make up the dose you missed. Take your next dose on your original schedule.

Stopping the drug
Do not stop the drug without consulting your physician; symptoms may recur.

Exceeding the dose
An occasional unintentional extra dose is unlikely to be a cause for concern. But if you notice any unusual symptoms, or if a large overdose has been taken, notify your physician.

SPECIAL PRECAUTIONS

Be sure to tell your physician if:
▼ You have impaired kidney function.
▼ You have had epileptic seizures.
▼ You are taking other medications.

Pregnancy
▼ Not usually prescribed. Safety in pregnancy not established. Discuss with your physician so that you can weigh the benefits of the drug against its possible risks.

Breast feeding
▼ No evidence of risk.

Infants and children
▼ Not usually prescribed. Reduced dose necessary.

Over 60
▼ No special problems.

Driving and hazardous work
▼ No known problems.

Alcohol
▼ Avoid. Alcohol may counteract the beneficial effect of this drug.

POSSIBLE ADVERSE EFFECTS

Most people do not feel any adverse effects while they are taking sucralfate. The most common is constipation, which diminishes as your body adjusts to the drug.

Symptom/effect	Frequency		Discuss with physician		Stop taking drug now	Call physician now
	Common	Rare	Only if severe	In all cases		
Constipation	●		■			
Diarrhea		●	■			
Abdominal pain		●	■			
Dizziness/lightheadedness		●	■			
Nausea		●	■			
Dry mouth		●	■			

PROLONGED USE

Not usually prescribed for periods longer than 8 weeks at a time. Prolonged use may lead to deficiencies of vitamins A, D, E, and K.

INTERACTIONS

Phenytoin The effect of this drug may be reduced if taken with sucralfate.

Tetracycline antibiotics Sucralfate may reduce the effect of such drugs.

Antacids and other ulcer-healing drugs These reduce the effectiveness of sucralfate and should be taken 60 minutes before or after sucralfate.

SULFACETAMIDE

Brand names AK-Sulf, Bleph, Cetamide, Isopto-Cetamide, Sodium Sulamyd
Used in the following combined preparations Blephamide, Metimyd, Sulfacet-R, Sultrin, Vasocidin

GENERAL INFORMATION

Sulfacetamide, an antibacterial drug, is a derivative of the sulfonamide drugs developed in the late 1930s. Available as eye drops or ointment, it is used to treat bacterial conjunctivitis. It is also sometimes prescribed to prevent infection after an eye injury or the removal of a foreign body.

Although it is effective against a wide range of bacteria, the development of resistance to the drug during prolonged treatment is a common problem. Sulfacetamide is therefore most useful for short courses of treatment. Given for chronic blepharitis (inflammation of the eyelids) and conjunctivitis, it is not always effective, and other treatments may be preferred. One reason for this is that pus contains an acid that inactivates sulfonamides.

Fixed-dose combinations of sulfacetamide and a corticosteroid, sometimes with a decongestant, may be used to treat conditions in which there is inflammation or allergy.

QUICK REFERENCE

Drug group Sulfonamide antibacterial drug (p.159)

Overdose danger rating Low

Dependence rating Low

Prescription needed Yes

Available as generic Yes

INFORMATION FOR USERS

Your drug prescription is tailored for you. Do not alter dosage without checking with your physician.

How taken

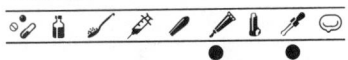

Ointment, eye drops.

Frequency and timing of doses
Every 1 – 3 hours (eye drops); every 6 hours and at bedtime (ointment).

Dosage range
1 – 2 drops per application (eye drops), 0.5 – 1 inch (1.25 – 2.5cm) per application (ointment).

Onset of effect
12 – 24 hours.

Duration of action
2 – 3 hours (drops); up to 6 hours (ointment).

Diet advice
None.

Storage
Keep in a closed container in a cool, dry place away from reach of children. Protect from light. Discard 4 weeks after opening.

Missed dose
Take as soon as you remember. If your next dose is due within 1 hour (eye drops) or within 2 hours (ointment), take a single dose now and skip the next.

Stopping the drug
Use the full course. Even if the affected area seems cured, the original infection may still be present and may recur if treatment is stopped too soon.

Exceeding the dose
An occasional unintentional extra dose is unlikely to be a cause for concern. But if you notice unusual symptoms, or if a large overdose has been taken, notify your physician.

SPECIAL PRECAUTIONS

Be sure to tell your physician if:
▼ You have had a previous allergic reaction to sulfonamides.
▼ You wear contact lenses.
▼ You are taking other medications.

 Pregnancy
▼ No evidence of risk to developing baby when the drug is used in the manner prescribed.

 Breast feeding
▼ No evidence of risk when the drug is used in the manner prescribed.

 Infants and children
▼ No special problems.

 Over 60
▼ No special problems.

 Driving and hazardous work
▼ No known problems.

 Alcohol
▼ No known problems.

POSSIBLE ADVERSE EFFECTS

Eye drops may cause stinging or burning on application. Itching, redness, or other signs of irritation may be symptoms of an allergic reaction to the drug.

Symptom/effect	Frequency		Discuss with physician		Stop taking drug now	Call physician now
	Common	Rare	Only if severe	In all cases		
Stinging/burning	●		■			
Itching/redness		●		■	▲	▮
Swelling of eyelids		●		■	▲	▮

PROLONGED USE

Not usually given for longer than 10 days.

INTERACTIONS

Silver eye preparations Sulfacetamide is incompatible with these preparations and they should not be used together.

Zinc sulfate Sulfacetamide interacts with zinc sulfate eye drops and the two should not be used together.

SULFAMETHOXAZOLE

Brand names Gantanol, Gantanol DS
Used in the following combined preparations Azo-Gantanol, Bactrim, Bactrim DS, Septra, Septra DS

GENERAL INFORMATION

Sulfamethoxazole, a sulfonamide drug introduced in 1961, is prescribed for many bacterial infections. It is available by itself or in combination with trimethoprim, another antibacterial drug.

Alone, sulfamethoxazole is used to treat urinary tract infections, conjunctivitis, and ear infections. Combined with trimethoprim, and thought by some physicians to be less likely to produce drug-resistant infections, it is widely used for bacterial infections of the respiratory and urinary tracts, gastroenteritis, gonorrhea, typhoid fever, and pneumocystis pneumonia.

A long-acting drug, sulfamethoxazole does not have to be taken as often as many other sulfonamides. Its side effects are similar to those of most antibacterials, rash and digestive upset being among the most common. An adequate fluid intake must be maintained to prevent the damaging formation of crystals in the urine.

INFORMATION FOR USERS

Your drug prescription is tailored for you. Do not alter dosage without checking with your physician.

How taken

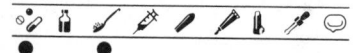

Tablets, powder.

Frequency and timing of doses
2 – 4 x daily with water.

Dosage range
Adults 2 – 3g daily.
Children Reduced dose necessary according to age and weight.

Onset of effect
Within 2 hours.

Duration of action
10 – 12 hours.

Diet advice
It is important to drink plenty of fluids (at least 1.5 quarts a day) during treatment.

Storage
Keep in a closed container in a cool, dry place away from reach of children. Protect from light.

Missed dose
Take as soon as you remember. If your next dose is due at this time, double the usual dose to make up the missed dose.

Stopping the drug
Take the full course. Even if you feel better, the original infection may still be present and symptoms may recur if treatment is stopped too soon.

Exceeding the dose
An occasional unintentional extra dose is unlikely to be a cause for concern. But if you notice unusual symptoms, or if a large overdose has been taken, notify your physician.

POSSIBLE ADVERSE EFFECTS

Sulfamethoxazole has a number of common adverse effects. When taken with trimethoprim, these effects may become slightly more severe.

Symptom/effect	Frequency		Discuss with physician		Stop taking drug now	Call physician now
	Common	Rare	Only if severe	In all cases		
Nausea/vomiting	●		■			
Loss of appetite	●		■			
Diarrhea		●	■			
Headache/dizziness		●	■			
Fever		●		■		▮
Aching joints/muscles		●		■		▮
Rash		●		■	▲	▮

SPECIAL PRECAUTIONS

Be sure to tell your physician if:
▼ You have impaired liver or kidney function.
▼ You have a blood disorder.
▼ You suffer from porphyria.
▼ You are allergic to sulfonamide.
▼ You have glucose-6-phosphate dehydrogenase (G6PD) deficiency.
▼ You are taking other medications.

Pregnancy
▼ No evidence of risk in early pregnancy, but if taken in late pregnancy it may cause jaundice and liver problems in the newborn baby. Discuss with your physician so that you may weigh the benefits of the drug against its risks.

Breast feeding
▼ Discuss with your physician. The drug passes into the breast milk and may affect the baby adversely.

Infants and children
▼ Not usually prescribed for infants under 2 months. Reduced dose necessary for older children.

Over 60
▼ Reduced dose may be necessary.

Driving and hazardous work
▼ No known problems.

Alcohol
▼ No known problems.

INTERACTIONS

Oral antidiabetic drugs Sulfamethoxazole may increase the blood sugar-lowering effect of these drugs.

Oral anticoagulant drugs Sulfamethoxazole may increase the effect of these drugs.

Phenytoin Sulfamethoxazole may cause a buildup of phenytoin in the body.

Salicylates, probenecid, and phenylbutazone These increase the likelihood of adverse effects from sulfamethoxazole.

PROLONGED USE

Use of this drug over an extended period can lead to blood disorders in rare cases.

Monitoring Periodic blood samples may be taken to check blood composition during prolonged treatment.

SULFASALAZINE

Brand names Azulfidine, Azulfidine EN-tabs, SAS 500
Used in the following combined preparations None

GENERAL INFORMATION

Sulfasalazine, introduced in 1949 and chemically related to the sulfonamide antibacterial drugs, is used to treat two inflammatory disorders of the bowel. One is ulcerative colitis (which mainly affects the large intestine); the other is Crohn's disease (which typically affects the small intestine). In recent years, sulfasalazine has also been found to be effective in the treatment of rheumatoid arthritis.

Adverse effects such as nausea, loss of appetite, and general discomfort are more likely when higher doses are taken. Side effects caused by stomach irritation may be avoided by a change to a specially coated formulation of the drug. Allergic reactions such as fever and skin rash may be avoided or minimized by low initial doses that are gradually increased. Adequate fluid intake is important. In rare cases, temporary sterility in men may occur.

INFORMATION FOR USERS

Your drug prescription is tailored for you. Do not alter dosage without checking with your physician.

How taken

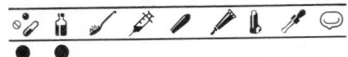

Tablets, liquid.

Frequency and timing of doses
3 – 4 x daily after meals with a glass of water.

Adult dosage range
0.5g daily (starting dose), increased as necessary by 0.5g per day. The usual maintenance dose is 2 – 4g daily.

Onset of effect
Adverse effects may be noticed within a few days, but full beneficial effects may not be felt for 1 – 3 weeks, depending on the severity of the condition.

Duration of action
About 24 hours.

Diet advice
It is important to drink plenty of fluids (at least 1.5 quarts a day) during treatment. Sulfasalazine may reduce the absorption of folic acid from the intestine, leading to a deficiency of this vitamin. Eat plenty of green vegetables.

Storage
Keep in a closed container in a cool, dry place away from reach of children.

Missed dose
Take as soon as you remember. If your next dose is due within 2 hours, take a single dose now and skip the next.

Stopping the drug
Do not stop the drug without consulting your physician; symptoms may recur.

Exceeding the dose
An occasional unintentional extra dose is unlikely to be a cause for concern. But if you notice unusual symptoms, or if a large overdose has been taken, notify your physician.

SPECIAL PRECAUTIONS

Be sure to tell your physician if:
▼ You have impaired liver or kidney function.
▼ You have glucose-6-phosphate dehydrogenase (G6PD) deficiency.
▼ You have a blood disorder.
▼ You suffer from porphyria.
▼ You are allergic to sulfonamides or salicylates.
▼ You are taking other medications.

Pregnancy
▼ No evidence of risk to the developing baby.

Breast feeding
▼ The drug passes into the breast milk, but at normal doses adverse effects on the baby are unlikely. Discuss with your physician.

Infants and children
▼ Not recommended for children under 2 years. Reduced dose necessary for older children.

Over 60
▼ No special problems.

Driving and hazardous work
▼ No special problems.

Alcohol
▼ No known problems.

POSSIBLE ADVERSE EFFECTS

Adverse effects are common with high doses, but may disappear with a reduction in the dose. Symptoms such as nausea, vomiting, and diarrhea may be helped by taking the drug with food. Orange or yellow discoloration of the urine is no cause for alarm.

Symptom/effect	Frequency		Discuss with physician		Stop taking drug now	Call physician now
	Common	Rare	Only if severe	In all cases		
Nausea/vomiting	●		■			
Malaise/loss of appetite	●		■			
Diarrhea	●		■			
Headache	●			■		
Joint pain	●			■		▮
Fever/rash		●		■		▮

PROLONGED USE

Prolonged use of this drug may lead to blood disorders.

Monitoring Periodic tests of blood composition are usually required.

INTERACTIONS

General note Sulfasalazine may increase the effects of a variety of drugs, including oral anticoagulant, oral antidiabetic, and anticonvulsant drugs, methotrexate, phenylbutazone, and sulfonamide antibacterial drugs.

Digitalis drugs Sulfasalazine may reduce the absorption of these drugs if they are taken at the same time.

Probenecid may slow the rate of elimination of sulfasalazine and increase the risk of side effects.

SULFINPYRAZONE

Brand name Anturane
Used in the following combined preparations None

GENERAL INFORMATION

Sulfinpyrazone, in use since 1959, is a powerful drug prescribed for people who suffer from frequent attacks of gout. It reduces the amount of uric acid in the body by increasing the amount excreted in the urine.

Prescribed for the long-term prevention of gout attacks, it is not helpful for relieving the pain and inflammation of gout once an attack has started.

During the first months of treatment attacks may be more frequent, and another drug, colchicine, may be pre-scribed to reduce the frequency and severity of gout attacks during this period.

Sulfinpyrazone is also prescribed to reduce blood levels of uric acid (hyper-uricemia) caused by other drugs, notably thiazide diuretics.

Recent research has shown that sulfinpyrazone has an anticoagulant effect, which may make it useful in the prevention and treatment of blood clots. Serious adverse effects of this drug are rare.

INFORMATION FOR USERS

Your drug prescription is tailored for you. Do not alter dosage without checking with your physician.

How taken

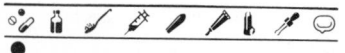

Tablets, capsules.

Frequency and timing of doses
2 x daily with meals, or with milk at bedtime.

Adult dosage range
200 – 400mg daily. Dosage may be gradually increased.

Onset of effect
Full beneficial effect may not be felt for 3 – 6 months.

Duration of action
Up to 10 hours.

Diet advice
A high fluid intake is recommended.

Storage
Keep in a closed container in a cool, dry place away from reach of children.

Missed dose
Take as soon as you remember. If your next dose is due within 3 hours, take a single dose now and skip the next.

Stopping the drug
Do not stop the drug without consulting your physician; symptoms may recur.

Exceeding the dose
An occasional unintentional extra dose is unlikely to cause problems. Large over-doses may cause nausea, vomiting, or unsteadiness. Notify your physician.

SPECIAL PRECAUTIONS

Be sure to tell your physician if:
▼ You have impaired liver or kidney function.
▼ You have kidney stones.
▼ You have asthma.
▼ You have had a peptic ulcer.
▼ You have a blood disorder.
▼ You are taking other medications.

Pregnancy
▼ Not usually prescribed. Safety in pregnancy not established. Discuss with your physician so that you can weigh the benefits of the drug against its possible risks.

Breast feeding
▼ Discuss with your physician. The drug passes into the breast milk and may affect the baby adversely.

Infants and children
▼ Not recommended.

Over 60
▼ No special problems.

Driving and hazardous work
▼ No known problems.

Alcohol
▼ Avoid. Alcohol may reduce the effect of this drug.

POSSIBLE ADVERSE EFFECTS

Most people do not notice any severe adverse effects when taking sulfinpyrazone. The more common adverse effects usually diminish during treatment as your body adjusts to the drug. A peptic ulcer may be reactivated.

Symptom/effect	Frequency		Discuss with physician		Stop taking drug now	Call physician now
	Common	Rare	Only if severe	In all cases		
Nausea/vomiting	●			■		
Headache		●		■		
Flushing		●		■		
Bloodstained/cloudy urine		●		■		
Rash/itching		●		■		
Wheezing/breathlessness		●		■		

INTERACTIONS

General note Many drugs affect the action of sulfinpyrazone and may require an adjustment of dosage. Some may reduce the effect of sulfinpyrazone (for example, thiazide diuretics, aspirin, and alcohol). Others may have their effects increased by sulfinpyrazone (for example, oral diabetic drugs, insulin, indomethacin, sulfonamides, and oral anticoagulant drugs).

PROLONGED USE

In rare cases blood disorders may occur.

Monitoring Periodic checks on blood cells and uric acid levels in the blood are usually required.

SULFISOXAZOLE

Brand name Gantrisin
Used in the following combined preparations Azo-Gantrisin, Pediazole, Vagila

GENERAL INFORMATION

Sulfisoxazole, introduced in 1949, is prescribed to treat a variety of bacterial infections. When taken by mouth, it is rapidly and efficiently absorbed from the intestine. Unlike many other sulfonamide antibacterial drugs, it does not build up in the body in excessive amounts.

The main use of sulfisoxazole is in the short-term treatment of lower urinary tract infections which do not affect the kidneys. The drug is also given with penicillin or erythromycin to treat ear and chest infections that are resistant to penicillins alone. Eye drops containing sulfisoxazole are used to prevent eye infections.

Although serious adverse effects are uncommon, sulfisoxazole sometimes causes nausea, vomiting, and loss of appetite. Allergic rashes can also occur.

QUICK REFERENCE

Drug group Sulfonamide anti-bacterial drug (p.159)

Overdose danger rating Low

Dependence rating Low

Prescription needed Yes

Available as generic Yes

INFORMATION FOR USERS

Your drug prescription is tailored for you. Do not alter dosage without checking with your physician.

How taken

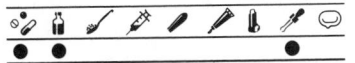

Tablets, liquid, eye drops.

Frequency and timing of doses
4 – 6 x daily with water.

Dosage range
Adult 2 – 4g (starting dose), then 4 – 8g daily (maintenance dose).
Children Reduced dose according to age and weight.

Onset of effect
1 – 2 hours.

Duration of action
4 – 6 hours.

Diet advice
It is important to drink plenty of fluids (at least 1.5 quarts a day) during sulfisoxazole treatment.

Storage
Keep in a closed container in a cool, dry place away from reach of children. Protect from light.

Missed dose
Take as soon as you remember. If your next dose is due at this time, double the usual dose to make up the missed dose.

Stopping the drug
Take the full course. Even if you feel better, the original infection may still be present and may recur if treatment is stopped too soon.

Exceeding the dose
An occasional unintentional extra dose is unlikely to be a cause for concern. But if you notice unusual symptoms, or if a large overdose has been taken, notify your physician.

SPECIAL PRECAUTIONS

Be sure to tell your physician if:
▼ You have impaired kidney function.
▼ You have a blood disorder.
▼ You suffer from porphyria.
▼ You have glucose-6-phosphate dehydrogenase (G6PD) deficiency.
▼ You are allergic to sulfonamides.
▼ You are taking other medications.

Pregnancy
▼ If taken in late pregnancy, it may cause jaundice and liver problems in the newborn baby. Discuss with your physician so that you may weigh the benefits of the drug against its risks.

Breast feeding
▼ Discuss with your physician. The drug passes into the breast milk and may affect the baby adversely.

Infants and children
▼ Not prescribed for infants under 2 months. Reduced dose necessary for older children.

Over 60
▼ Reduced dose may be necessary.

Driving and hazardous work
▼ No known problems.

Alcohol
▼ No known problems.

POSSIBLE ADVERSE EFFECTS

Sulfisoxazole commonly causes digestive upsets such as nausea and loss of appetite. If more serious adverse reactions such as rash occur, the drug may have to be stopped.

Symptom/effect	Frequency		Discuss with physician		Stop taking drug now	Call physician now
	Common	Rare	Only if severe	In all cases		
Nausea/vomiting	●		■			
Loss of appetite	●		■			
Diarrhea		●	■			
Headache/dizziness		●	■			
Rash		●		■	▲	▮

INTERACTIONS

Oral antidiabetic drugs Sulfisoxazole may increase the blood sugar-lowering effect of these drugs.

Oral anticoagulant drugs Sulfisoxazole may increase the effect of oral anti-coagulants.

Phenytoin Sulfisoxazole may cause a build-up of phenytoin in the body.

Salicylates, probenecid, and phenyl-butazone These drugs increase the likelihood of adverse effects from sulfisoxazole.

PROLONGED USE

Can lead to blood disorders in rare cases.

A B C D E F G H I J K L M N O P Q R S T U V W X Y Z

SULINDAC

Brand name Clinoril
Used in the following preparations None

GENERAL INFORMATION

Sulindac, introduced in 1978, is a non-steroidal anti-inflammatory drug (NSAID) that reduces pain, stiffness, and inflammation.

It is used in the treatment of many arthritic conditions, including rheumatoid arthritis, osteoarthritis, and chronic, low back pain. It is sometimes prescribed for psoriatic arthritis and Reiter's syndrome, a disorder that affects the joints, urinary tract, and eyes. Acute attacks of gout and bursitis or tendinitis of the shoulder usually respond to one or two weeks of treatment.

Indigestion, nausea, diarrhea, and constipation are fairly common with this drug. There is also a risk of stomach bleeding or peptic ulcer. Sulindac may be preferred to certain other NSAIDs for long-term use because it requires only two doses per day.

INFORMATION FOR USERS

Your drug prescription is tailored for you. Do not alter dosage without checking with your physician.

How taken

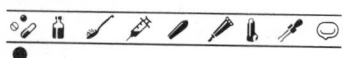

Tablets.

Frequency and timing of doses
2 x daily with food.

Adult dosage range
300 – 400mg daily.

Onset of effect
Pain relief begins within 2 hours. Full anti-inflammatory effect may not be felt for 2 – 3 weeks.

Duration of action
12 – 24 hours.

Diet advice
None.

Storage
Keep in a closed container in a cool, dry place away from reach of children.

Missed dose
Take as soon as you remember. If your next dose is due within 2 hours, take a single dose now and skip the next.

Stopping the drug
For short-term pain relief, the drug can be safely stopped when you no longer need it. For rheumatoid arthritis, do not stop the drug without consulting your physician.

Exceeding the dose
An occasional unintentional extra dose is unlikely to be a cause for concern. But if you notice unusual symptoms, or if a large overdose has been taken, notify your physician.

SPECIAL PRECAUTIONS

Be sure to tell your physician if:
▼ You have high blood pressure.
▼ You have a bleeding disorder.
▼ You have impaired liver or kidney function.
▼ You have had a peptic ulcer, esophagitis, or gastritis.
▼ You are allergic to aspirin.
▼ You are taking other medications.

Pregnancy
▼ Not usually prescribed. Safety in pregnancy not established. Discuss with your physician so that you can weigh the benefits of the drug against its possible risks.

Breast feeding
▼ Discuss with your physician. The drug passes into the breast milk and may affect the baby adversely.

Infants and children
▼ Not usually prescribed.

Over 60
▼ Reduced dose may be necessary. Increased likelihood of adverse effects.

Driving and hazardous work
▼ Avoid such activities until you have learned how the drug affects you, because the drug may occasionally cause dizziness and drowsiness.

Alcohol
▼ Avoid. Alcohol increases the risk of peptic ulcers with this drug.

Surgery and general anesthetics
▼ Sulindac may prolong bleeding. Discuss with your physician or dentist before any surgery.

POSSIBLE ADVERSE EFFECTS

Most adverse effects are not serious and may disappear as treatment continues.

Black or bloodstained bowel movements should be reported without delay.

Symptom/effect	Frequency		Discuss with physician		Stop taking drug now	Call physician now
	Common	Rare	Only if severe	In all cases		
Nausea/vomiting	●		■			
Constipation/diarrhea	●		■			
Abdominal pain/indigestion	●			■		
Dizziness/drowsiness		●		■		
Rash/itching		●		■	▲	❚
Black/bloodstained feces		●	■		▲	❚
Wheezing/breathlessness		●		■	▲	❚

INTERACTIONS

General note Sulindac interacts with a wide range of drugs to increase the risk of bleeding and/or peptic ulcers. Such drugs include oral anticoagulants, corticosteroids, other non-steroidal anti-inflammatory drugs (NSAIDs) and aspirin.

Antihypertensive and diuretic drugs The beneficial effects of these drugs may be reduced by sulindac.

Oral antidiabetic drugs Concurrent use of sulindac may increase the blood sugar-lowering effect of these drugs. Dosage adjustment may be necessary.

PROLONGED USE

There is an increased risk of bleeding from peptic ulcers and in the bowel with prolonged use of sulindac.

SUPROFEN

Brand name Suprol (not available in US)
Used in the following combined preparations None

GENERAL INFORMATION

Suprofen, introduced in 1986 but withdrawn from sale in the US by the manufacturer in 1987, is a non-steroidal anti-inflammatory drug (NSAID). It reduces pain, stiffness, and inflammation. It was used in the treatment of osteoarthritis and rheumatoid arthritis. Taken long-term, it provided relief of symptoms, but did not cure these diseases.

It was also prescribed over short periods for relief of pain due to minor injuries such as sprains, ligament strains, and low back pain.

Gastrointestinal disturbances, including indigestion, heartburn, and abdominal pain, were common adverse effects. Long-term treatment sometimes caused fluid buildup and weight gain. Suprofen was withdrawn because of evidence that it had caused kidney problems in some people.

INFORMATION FOR USERS

Your drug prescription is tailored for you. Do not alter dosage without checking with your physician.

How taken

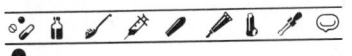

Capsules.

Frequency and timing of doses
3 – 4 x daily with food.

Adult dosage range
600 – 800mg daily.

Onset of effect
30 – 60 minutes.

Duration of action
8 hours.

Diet advice
None.

Storage
Keep in a closed container in a cool, dry place away from reach of children.

Missed dose
Take as soon as you remember. If your next dose is due within 2 hours, take a single dose now and skip the next.

Stopping the drug
When taken for short-term pain relief, suprofen can be safely stopped as soon as you no longer need it. If prescribed for arthritis, however, you should seek medical advice before stopping the drug.

Exceeding the dose
An occasional unintentional extra dose is unlikely to cause problems. Large overdoses may cause severe nausea, vomiting, and drowsiness. Notify your physician.

POSSIBLE ADVERSE EFFECTS

Gastrointestinal disturbances (such as indigestion) and central nervous system side effects (such as headache) may diminish as treatment continues. Black or bloodstained bowel movements should be reported to your physician promptly.

Symptom/effect	Frequency		Discuss with physician		Stop taking drug now	Call physician now
	Common	Rare	Only if severe	In all cases		
Heartburn/indigestion	●		■			
Headache	●		■			
Abdominal pain	●			■		
Dizziness/lightheadedness		●	■			
Vomiting		●		■		
Swollen feet/ankles		●		■		
Rash		●		■	▲	
Wheezing		●		■	▲	■

INTERACTIONS

General note Suprofen interacts with a wide range of drugs to increase the risk of bleeding and/or peptic ulcers. Such drugs include oral anticoagulants, corticosteroids, aspirin, some antibiotics, sulfinpyrazone, dipyridamole, and valproic acid.

Antihypertensive drugs and diuretics
The beneficial effects of these drugs may be reduced by suprofen.

SPECIAL PRECAUTIONS

Be sure to tell your physician if:
▼ You have impaired kidney function.
▼ You have heart problems.
▼ You have had a peptic ulcer, esophagitis, or acid indigestion.
▼ You have high blood pressure.
▼ You are allergic to aspirin.
▼ You have bleeding problems.
▼ You are taking other medications.

Pregnancy
▼ Not usually prescribed. Taken in the last 3 months of pregnancy, may have adverse effects on the baby's heart and may prolong labor. Discuss with your physician so that you may weigh the benefits of the drug against its risks.

Breast feeding
▼ Discuss with your physician. The drug passes into the breast milk and may affect the baby adversely.

Infants and children
▼ Not recommended.

Over 60
▼ Reduced dose may be necessary. Increased likelihood of adverse effects.

Driving and hazardous work
▼ No known problems.

Alcohol
▼ Avoid. Alcohol may increase the risk of stomach disorders with suprofen.

Surgery and general anesthetics
▼ Suprofen may prolong bleeding. Discuss this with your physician or dentist before any surgery.

PROLONGED USE

There is an increased risk of bleeding from peptic ulcers and in the bowel with prolonged use of suprofen.

TAMOXIFEN

Brand name Nolvadex
Used in the following combined preparations None

GENERAL INFORMATION

Tamoxifen, introduced in 1978, is an anticancer drug used in the treatment of advanced breast cancer, before and after the menopause. It works only against cancers whose growth is stimulated by female sex hormones called estrogens. By latching on to cells that recognize these hormones, it can slow the growth of the tumor and even shrink it.

For reasons that are less clear, it is also effective in treating some cases of other cancers, such as those of the prostate, kidney, and skin. In women of childbearing age, tamoxifen stimulates egg release (ovulation) and is therefore under investigation as a treatment for certain types of infertility.

Because its effect is specific, tamoxifen has fewer adverse effects than most other anticancer drugs. However, it may cause eye damage if high doses are taken for long periods.

QUICK REFERENCE

Drug group Anticancer drug (p.182)
Overdose danger rating Low
Dependence rating Low
Prescription needed Yes
Available as generic No

INFORMATION FOR USERS

Your drug prescription is tailored for you. Do not alter dosage without checking with your physician.

How taken

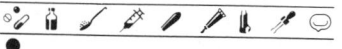

Tablets.

Frequency and timing of doses
2 x daily.

Adult dosage range
20 – 40mg daily. Dosage may occasionally be increased.

Onset of effect
Side effects may be felt within days, but beneficial effects may take 4 – 10 weeks.

Duration of action
Effects may be felt for several weeks after stopping the drug.

Diet advice
None.

Storage
Keep in a closed container in a cool, dry place away from reach of children. Protect from light.

Missed dose
Take as soon as you remember. If your next dose is due within 2 hours, take a single dose now and skip the next.

Stopping the drug
Do not stop the drug without consulting your physician; stopping the drug may lead to worsening of your underlying condition.

Exceeding the dose
An occasional unintentional extra dose is unlikely to be a cause for concern. But if you notice unusual symptoms, or if a large overdose has been taken, notify your physician.

SPECIAL PRECAUTIONS

Be sure to tell your physician if:
▼ You have cataracts or poor eyesight.
▼ You are taking other medications.

Pregnancy
▼ Not usually prescribed.

Breast feeding
▼ Discuss with your physician. Breast feeding is usually discontinued.

Infants and children
▼ Not prescribed.

Over 60
▼ No special problems.

Driving and hazardous work
▼ No known problems.

Alcohol
▼ No known problems.

POSSIBLE ADVERSE EFFECTS

These are rarely serious and do not usually require treatment to be stopped. Nausea, vomiting, and hot flashes are the most common reactions.

Symptom/effect	Frequency		Discuss with physician		Stop taking drug now	Call physician now
	Common	Rare	Only if severe	In all cases		
Hot flashes	●		■			
Swollen feet/ankles	●		■			
Irregular vaginal bleeding	●			■		
Nausea/vomiting		●	■			
Bone and tumor pain		●		■		
Rash		●		■		
Blurred vision		●		■		

INTERACTIONS

None.

PROLONGED USE

There is a risk of damage to the eyes with long-term high dose treatment.

Monitoring Eyesight may be tested periodically.

TEMAZEPAM

Brand name Restoril
Used in the following combined preparations None

GENERAL INFORMATION

Temazepam was introduced in 1972 and belongs to a group of drugs known as the benzodiazepines. The actions and adverse effects of this group of drugs are described more fully under Anti-anxiety drugs (p.111).

Temazepam is used in the short-term treatment of insomnia. Because it is moderately long-acting compared with some other benzodiazepines, it is more likely to cause a hangover, making the person using the drug feel drowsy and/or lightheaded the following day. However, the drug may be useful for people who wake early.

Like other benzodiazepines, temazepam can be habit-forming if taken regularly over a long period. Its effects may also grow weaker with time. For those reasons treatment with temazepam is usually reviewed every two weeks.

INFORMATION FOR USERS

Your drug prescription is tailored for you. Do not alter dosage without checking with your physician.

How taken

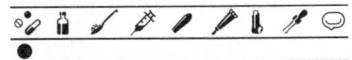

Capsules.

Frequency and timing of doses
Once daily 30 minutes before bedtime with food or milk.

Adult dosage range
15 – 30mg.

Onset of effect
20 – 40 minutes.

Duration of action
6 – 8 hours.

Diet advice
None.

Storage
Keep in a closed container in a cool, dry place away from reach of children. Protect from light.

Missed dose
If you are taking the drug once daily for insomnia, a missed dose is no cause for concern. Return to your normal dose schedule the following night, if necessary. Otherwise, for daytime use take the missed dose when you remember. If your next dose is due within 2 hours, take a single dose now and skip the next.

Stopping the drug
If you have been taking the drug continuously for less than 2 weeks, it can be safely stopped as soon as you feel you no longer need it. However, if you have been taking the drug for longer, consult your physician, who may supervise a gradual reduction in dosage. Stopping abruptly may lead to withdrawal symptoms (see p.110).

Exceeding the dose
An occasional unintentional extra dose is unlikely to cause problems. Large overdoses may cause unusual drowsiness. Notify your physician.

SPECIAL PRECAUTIONS

Be sure to tell your physician if
▼ You have severe respiratory disease.
▼ You have impaired kidney or liver function.
▼ You have had problems with alcohol or drug abuse.
▼ You are taking other medications.

Pregnancy
▼ Not usually prescribed. Safety in pregnancy not established. Taken near the time of delivery may cause drowsiness and reluctance to feed in the newborn baby.

Breast feeding
▼ The drug passes into the breast milk, but at normal doses adverse effects on the baby are uncommon. Discuss with your physician.

Infants and children
▼ Not usually prescribed. Reduced dose necessary.

Over 60
▼ Reduced dose may be necessary. Increased likelihood of adverse effects.

Driving and hazardous work
▼ Avoid such activities until you have learned how the drug affects you, because the drug can cause reduced alertness and slowed reactions.

Alcohol
▼ Avoid. Alcohol increases the sedative effects of this drug.

POSSIBLE ADVERSE EFFECTS

The principal adverse effects of this drug are related to its sedative and tranquilizing properties. These effects normally diminish after the first few days of treatment.

Symptom/effect	Frequency		Discuss with physician		Stop taking drug now	Call physician now
	Common	Rare	Only if severe	In all cases		
Daytime/drowsiness	●		■			
Dizziness/unsteadiness	●		■			
Headache		●	■			
Blurred vision		●		■		
Forgetfulness/confusion		●		■		
Rash		●		■	▲	

INTERACTIONS

Sedatives All drugs that have a sedative effect on the central nervous system are likely to increase the sedative properties of temazepam.

Alcohol The sedative effect of temazepam is increased by alcohol.

PROLONGED USE

Regular use of this drug over several weeks can lead to a reduction in its effect as the body adapts. It may also be habit-forming when taken for extended periods, especially if larger than average doses are taken.

A
B
C
D
E
F
G
H
I
J
K
L
M
N
O
P
Q
R
S
T
U
V
W
X
Y
Z

TERBUTALINE

Brand names Brethaire, Brethine, Bricanyl
Used in the following combined preparations None

GENERAL INFORMATION

Terbutaline, introduced in 1974, is a *sympathomimetic* bronchodilator that dilates the small airways in the lungs. It is used in the treatment and prevention of the bronchospasm occurring with asthma, chronic bronchitis, and emphysema. It may be given orally, by inhaler, or by injection when rapid relief of breathlessness is required. Terbutaline also relaxes the muscles of the uterus, making it useful for the prevention and arrest of premature labor. It is under investigational use as an additional medication for congestive heart failure.

Muscle tremor, especially of the hands, is common with terbutaline and usually disappears on reduction of the dosage or with continued use as the body adapts. In common with other sympathomimetics, it may produce nervousness and restlessness.

QUICK REFERENCE

Drug group Bronchodilator (p.120)
Overdose danger rating Low
Dependence rating Low
Prescription needed Yes
Available as generic No

INFORMATION FOR USERS

Your drug prescription is tailored for you. Do not alter dosage without checking with your physician.

How taken

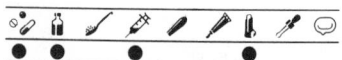

Tablets, liquid, injection, inhaler.

Frequency and timing of doses
3 x daily (tablets, liquid); as necessary (inhaler).

Dosage range
Adults 7.5 – 15mg daily (tablets).
Children Reduced dose according to age and weight.

Onset of effect
Within a few minutes (inhaler); within 15 minutes (injection); within 1 – 2 hours (tablets, capsules).

Duration of action
Up to 4 hours (injection); 4 – 8 hours (tablets, capsules).

Diet advice
None.

Storage
Keep in a closed container in a cool, dry place away from reach of children. Protect from light. Do not puncture or burn aerosol containers.

Missed dose
Do not take the missed dose. Take your next dose as usual.

Stopping the drug
Do not stop the drug without consulting your physician; symptoms may recur.

Exceeding the dose
An occasional unintentional extra dose is unlikely to be a cause for concern. But if you notice any unusual symptoms, or if a large overdose has been taken, notify your physician.

SPECIAL PRECAUTIONS

Be sure to tell your physician if:
▼ You have heart problems.
▼ You have high blood pressure.
▼ You have diabetes.
▼ You have an overactive thyroid.
▼ You are taking other medications.

Pregnancy
▼ Not usually prescribed. Safety in pregnancy not established. Discuss with your physician so that you can weigh the benefits of the drug against its possible risks.

Breast feeding
▼ Discuss with your physician. The drug passes into the breast milk and may affect the baby adversely.

Infants and children
▼ Reduced dose necessary.

Over 60
▼ Reduced dose may be necessary.

Driving and hazardous work
▼ Avoid such activities until you have learned how the drug affects you, because the drug can cause tremor of the hands.

Alcohol
▼ No special problems.

POSSIBLE ADVERSE EFFECTS

Possible adverse effects include tremor, nervousness, restlessness, and nausea. These may be reduced by adjustment of dosage. Palpitations and headache, resulting from stimulation of the heart and narrowing of the blood vessels, are rare.

Symptom/effect	Frequency		Discuss with physician		Stop taking drug now	Call physician now
	Common	Rare	Only if severe	In all cases		
Anxiety	●		■			
Nausea	●		■			
Tremor	●		■			
Restlessness	●		■			
Headache		●	■			
Palpitations		●		■		

INTERACTIONS

Other sympathomimetic drugs These may add to the effects of terbutaline and vice versa, so increasing the risk of adverse effects.

Beta blockers These may inhibit the effect of terbutaline and vice versa.

Antidepressant drugs Terbutaline may cause severe hypertension to occur.

PROLONGED USE

Prolonged use may result in tolerance to the effects of terbutaline. However, failure to respond to the drug may be a result of worsening asthma, requiring prompt medical attention.

TERFENADINE

Brand name Seldane
Used in the following combined preparations None

GENERAL INFORMATION

Terfenadine is a recently introduced antihistamine with a prolonged duration of action. Its main use is in the treatment of allergic rhinitis, particularly hay fever. Taken as tablets, it reduces sneezing and irritation of the eyes and nose. Allergic skin conditions such as urticaria (hives) may also be helped by terfenadine.

The main difference between this drug and the older, traditional antihistamines is that it has little or no sedative effect on the central nervous system. It is therefore particularly suitable for people who need to avoid drowsiness – for example, at work. It also has fewer *anticholinergic* effects than other drugs of the same group.

INFORMATION FOR USERS

Your drug prescription is tailored for you. Do not alter dosage without checking with your physician.

How taken

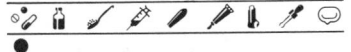

Tablets.

Frequency and timing of doses
2 x daily with food or milk.

Dosage range
Adults 120mg daily.
Children Reduced dose according to age and weight.

Onset of effect
1 – 3 hours.

Duration of action
Up to 12 hours.

Diet advice
None.

Storage
Keep in a closed container in a cool, dry place away from reach of children.

Missed dose
No cause for concern, but take as soon as you remember. If your next dose is due within 2 hours, take a single dose now and skip the next.

Stopping the drug
Can be safely stopped as soon as you no longer need it.

Exceeding the dose
An occasional unintentional extra dose is unlikely to cause problems. Large overdoses may cause nausea or drowsiness. Notify your physician.

SPECIAL PRECAUTIONS

Be sure to tell your physician if:
▼ You have impaired liver function.
▼ You have had epileptic seizures.
▼ You have glaucoma.
▼ You have urinary difficulties.
▼ You are taking other medications.

Pregnancy
▼ Not usually prescribed. Safety in pregnancy not established. Discuss with your physician so that you can weigh the benefits of the drug against its possible risks.

Breast feeding
▼ No evidence of risk.

Infants and children
▼ Not recommended for children under 3 years old. Reduced dose necessary in older children.

Over 60
▼ Reduced dose may be necessary.

Driving and hazardous work
▼ No known problems. Unlike the older antihistamines, terfenadine does not cause drowsiness.

Alcohol
▼ No known problems.

POSSIBLE ADVERSE EFFECTS

Nausea and loss of appetite occur occasionally with terfenadine; other side effects are very rare. A rash may be a sign of an unusual allergic reaction.

Symptom/effect	Frequency		Discuss with physician		Stop taking drug now	Call physician now
	Common	Rare	Only if severe	In all cases		
Nausea/loss of appetite	●		■			
Headache		●	■			
Rash		●			■	▲

INTERACTIONS

Sedatives Terfenadine may increase the sedative effects on the central nervous system of anti-anxiety drugs, sleeping drugs, antidepressants, and antipsychotic drugs.

Anticholinergic drugs The anticholinergic effects of terfenadine are likely to be increased by all drugs that have anticholinergic effects, including antipsychotic and tricyclic antidepressant drugs.

Monoamine oxidase inhibitors (MAOIs) There is a risk of a dangerous rise in blood pressure if terfenadine is taken within 14 days of MAOIs.

PROLONGED USE

No problems expected.

TESTOSTERONE

Brand names Delatestryl, Depo-Testosterone
Used in the following combined preparations Deladumone, Depo-Testadiol, Valertest

GENERAL INFORMATION

Testosterone is a male sex hormone produced by the testicles; it is produced in small quantities by the ovaries in women. It encourages bone and muscle growth in both men and women and stimulates sexual development in men. A shortage of testosterone may be caused by a disorder of the testicles or pituitary gland. When this happens, synthetic or animal testosterone supplements may be given by injection or by mouth.

Testosterone is used to initiate puberty in male adolescents if it has been delayed because of a demonstrable hormone deficiency. The drug may help to increase fertility in men who suffer from pituitary or testicular disorders. It does not, however, increase sperm production in men with normally developed testicles. Rarely, testosterone is still used for breast cancer.

Testosterone has a number of adverse effects. Dosages for treating delayed puberty in adolescents need to be controlled with particular care because it can interfere with growth or cause over-rapid sexual development. High doses may cause voice changes, excessive hair growth, or hair loss in women.

QUICK REFERENCE

Drug group Male sex hormone (p.174).

Overdose danger rating Low

Dependence rating Low

Prescription needed Yes

Available as generic Yes

INFORMATION FOR USERS

Your drug prescription is tailored for you. Do not alter dosage without checking with your physician.

How taken

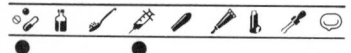

Sublingual tablets, implanted pellets, injection.

Frequency and timing of doses
1 – 3 x daily (tablets); once every 2 – 4 weeks (injection).

Dosage range
Adults 10 – 25mg daily.
Adolescents Reduced dose according to age and weight.

Onset of effect
2 – 3 days.

Duration of action
3 – 4 days (tablets); 3 – 4 weeks (injection).

Diet advice
None.

Storage
Keep in a closed container in a cool, dry place away from reach of children.

Missed dose
No cause for concern but take as soon as you remember. If your next dose is due within 3 hours, take a single dose now and skip the next.

Stopping the drug
Do not stop taking tablets without consulting your physician.

Exceeding the dose
An occasional unintentional extra dose is unlikely to be a cause for concern. But if you notice unusual symptoms, or if a large overdose has been taken, notify your physician.

SPECIAL PRECAUTIONS

Be sure to tell your physician if:
▼ You have impaired liver function.
▼ You have heart problems.
▼ You have prostate trouble.
▼ You have diabetes.
▼ You are taking other medications.

 Pregnancy
▼ Not prescribed.

 **Breast feeding**
▼ Not prescribed.

 Infants and children
▼ Not prescribed for young children. Reduced dose necessary in adolescents.

 Over 60
▼ Rarely required. Increased risk of prostate problems.

 Driving and hazardous work
▼ No special problems.

Alcohol
▼ No special problems.

POSSIBLE ADVERSE EFFECTS

Most of the more serious adverse effects are likely to occur only with long-term treatment with testosterone, and may be helped by a reduction in dosage.

Symptom/effect	Frequency		Discuss with physician		Stop taking drug now	Call physician now
	Common	Rare	Only if severe	In all cases		
Jaundice		●		■	▲	
Men only						
Difficulty passing urine		●		■	▲	
Abnormal erection		●		■	▲	■
Women only						
Unusual hair growth	●			■		
Voice changes	●			■		
Enlarged clitoris		●		■	▲	

INTERACTIONS

Anticoagulant drugs Testosterone increases the effect of these drugs. Dosage of anticoagulant drugs may need to be adjusted accordingly.

Antidiabetic drugs Because testosterone lowers the blood sugar, dosage of antidiabetic drugs may need to be reduced.

PROLONGED USE

Prolonged use of this drug may lead to reduced growth in adolescents.

Monitoring Regular checks of the effects of testosterone treatment are required.

TETRACAINE

Brand name Pontocaine
Used in the following combined preparations Cetacaine, Y-itch

GENERAL INFORMATION

Introduced in 1932, tetracaine is a powerful local anesthetic. It acts rapidly after local application, and its effects generally wear off quickly.

Widely used in non-prescription creams and ointments, tetracaine relieves the pain, itching, and inflammation associated with hemorrhoids and other painful anal disorders. Liquid forms of the drug are frequently given to ease pain and prevent gagging during dental treatment, throat examinations, and procedures requiring a tube to be passed down the throat. Eye drops and ointment are also commonly used to anesthetize the eye prior to examinations and other minor procedures such as removal of foreign bodies. Occasionally, it is given by injection for spinal and epidural anesthesia in childbirth. Injections may occasionally have adverse effects on the nervous system, causing nervousness, restlessness, and dizziness. Those problems can also occur following excessive local application.

QUICK REFERENCE

Drug group Local anesthetic (p.108)

Overdose danger rating Medium

Dependence rating Low

Prescription needed Yes (eye drops and liquid)
No (skin preparations)

Available as generic Yes

INFORMATION FOR USERS

Follow instructions on the label. Call your physician if symptoms worsen.

How taken

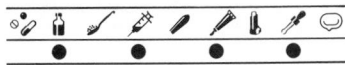

Liquid, injection, ointment, cream, eye drops, spray.

Frequency and timing of doses
Ointment or cream is applied to the anal area after bowel movements and at night for hemorrhoids; as required for other disorders. Other forms of tetracaine are given under medical supervision.

Dosage range
Apply ointment or cream thinly to the affected area.

Onset of effect
Within 1 minute (eye preparations); 3 – 10 minutes (skin or rectal ointment or cream, oral liquid or spray); 10 – 15 minutes (injection).

Duration of action
10 – 20 minutes (eye preparations); 30 – 60 minutes (skin or rectal ointment or cream, oral liquid or spray); 2 – 3 hours (injection).

Diet advice
Tetracaine by mouth causes numbness of the mouth and throat and may interfere with swallowing. To avoid choking and injury to the inside of your mouth from hot food or drink, do not eat or drink anything for 1 hour afterwards.

Storage
Keep in a closed container in a cool, dry place away from reach of children. Protect from light.

Missed dose
Take as soon as you remember if required.

Stopping the drug
Can be safely stopped as soon as you no longer need it.

Exceeding the dose
An occasional unintentional extra dose applied to the skin or rectal area is unlikely to cause problems. Regular overuse may cause anxiety, restlessness, dizziness, trembling, or drowsiness. Notify your physician.

SPECIAL PRECAUTIONS

Be sure to consult your physician before using this drug if:
▼ You have impaired liver or kidney function.
▼ You have heart problems.
▼ You suffer from epilepsy.
▼ You have had an allergic reaction to a local anesthetic.
▼ You have myasthenia gravis.
▼ You have sores or broken skin at the site of application.
▼ You are taking other medications.

 Pregnancy
▼ No evidence of risk with topical preparations. Given for spinal anesthesia during childbirth, it may prolong labor and increase the need for forceps-assisted delivery.

 Breast feeding
▼ Creams and ointments should not be used around the nipple. No evidence of risk for other sites of application.

 Infants and children
▼ No special problems.

 Over 60
▼ No special problems.

 Driving and hazardous work
▼ No special problems.

 Alcohol
▼ No known problems.

POSSIBLE ADVERSE EFFECTS

Adverse effects are rare with short-term use of tetracaine ointments. Allergic reactions – burning, redness, itching, and sometimes swelling – are the most common. Eye preparations may cause dryness or watering of the eyes. Anxiety, dizziness, and drowsiness may occur with excessive use of topical preparations or with injections.

Symptom/effect	Frequency		Discuss with physician		Stop taking drug now	Call physician now
	Common	Rare	Only if severe	In all cases		
Burning/itching/redness		●		■		
Swelling		●		■	▲	!
Dizziness/drowsiness		●		■	▲	!
Anxiety/restlessness		●		■	▲	!
Eye preparations only						
Dryness of eyes	●		■			
Watering of eyes	●			■		

PROLONGED USE

This drug should not be used for prolonged periods. If your symptoms do not improve within a few days, consult your physician.

INTERACTIONS

None.

TETRACYCLINE

Brand names Achromycin-V, Panmycin, Robitet, Sumycin, Topicycline
Used in the following combined preparation Mysteclin-F Syrup

GENERAL INFORMATION

Introduced in 1953, tetracycline is among the most widely prescribed antibiotics. Its most frequent use is probably in the long-term treatment of acne. To control this condition, tetracycline may be taken by mouth or applied *topically*.

The drug is effective in the treatment of certain types of pneumonia, including that caused by psittacosis or Mycoplasma bacteria. Syphilis, gonorrhea, and non-specific urethritis are also treated with tetracycline. It may be given to chronic bronchitis sufferers to control or prevent chest infections.

Less common infections, such as some types of septic arthritis, cholera, trachoma, Rocky Mountain spotted fever, relapsing fever, and brucellosis, may also be treated with tetracycline.

Common side effects are nausea, vomiting, and diarrhea. Rashes may also occur. Tetracycline may discolor developing teeth if taken by children or by the mother during pregnancy. It is not prescribed for people with poor kidney function, as it can cause further deterioration.

QUICK REFERENCE

Drug group Tetracycline antibiotic (p.158)

Overdose danger rating Low

Dependence rating Low

Prescription needed Yes

Available as generic Yes

INFORMATION FOR USERS

Your drug prescription is tailored for you. Do not alter dosage without checking with your physician.

How taken

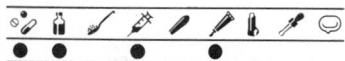

Tablets, capsules, syrup, injection, ointment.

Frequency and timing of doses
By mouth 2 – 4 x daily, at least 1 hour before or 2 hours after meals. Long-term treatment of acne may require only a single dose every 2 days.
Ointment As directed.

Adult dosage range
Infections 1 – 2g daily.
Acne (by mouth) 500mg – 2g daily (starting dose), reduced to 125 – 100mg daily (maintenance dose).

Onset of effect
2 – 5 days (infections); 4 weeks (acne).

Duration of action
Up to 12 hours.

Diet advice
Milk products and antacids may impair absorption. Avoid from one hour before to one hour after dosage.

Storage
Keep in a closed container in a cool, dry place away from reach of children.

Missed dose
Take as soon as you remember. If your next dose is due within 2 hours, take a single dose now and skip the next.

Stopping the drug
Take the full course. Even if you feel better, the original infection may still be present and may recur if treatment is stopped too soon.

Exceeding the dose
An occasional unintentional extra dose is unlikely to be a cause for concern. But if you notice unusual symptoms, or if a large overdose has been taken, notify your physician.

SPECIAL PRECAUTIONS

Be sure to tell your physician if:
▼ You have impaired kidney function.
▼ You have previously suffered an allergic reaction to a tetracycline antibiotic.
▼ You are taking other medications.

Pregnancy
▼ Not usually prescribed. May discolor the teeth of the developing baby. Discuss with your physician so that you may weigh the benefits of the drug against its risks.

Breast feeding
▼ Discuss with your physician. The drug passes into the breast milk and may lead to discoloration of the baby's teeth.

Infants and children
▼ Not recommended for children under 8 years. Reduced dose necessary for older children.

Over 60
▼ No special problems.

Driving and hazardous work
▼ No known problems.

Alcohol
▼ No known problems.

POSSIBLE ADVERSE EFFECTS

Adverse effects from tetracycline skin preparations are rare. Taken *systemically* the drug may occasionally cause nausea, vomiting, or diarrhea.

Symptom/effect	Frequency		Discuss with physician		Stop taking drug now	Call physician now
	Common	Rare	Only if severe	In all cases		
Nausea/vomiting	●		■			
Diarrhea	●		■			
Light-sensitive rash		●		■	▲	❙
Rash/itching		●		■	▲	❙

INTERACTIONS

Oral contraceptives Tetracycline can reduce the effectiveness of oral contraceptives.

Iron may reduce the effectiveness of tetracycline.

Penicillins Tetracycline interferes with the antibacterial action of penicillins.

Antacids Antacids interfere with the absorption of tetracycline and may reduce its effectiveness.

Oral anticoagulant drugs Tetracycline increases the action of these drugs.

Lithium Tetracycline may increase blood levels of lithium, leading to lithium overdose.

PROLONGED USE

No problems expected.

TETRAHYDROZOLINE

Brand names Murine Plus, Optigene 3, Soothe Eye Drops, Tyzine, Visine
Used in the following combined preparations Collyrium 2, Visine A.C.

GENERAL INFORMATION

Tetrahydrozoline, introduced in 1954, is a *sympathomimetic* decongestant. Taken as nose drops, it relieves the stuffiness of common colds, sinusitis, and allergic rhinitis. It reduces congestion of the nasal passages by narrowing blood vessels in the nose.

Tetrahydrozoline is also available without prescription in eye drops. Again by narrowing blood vessels, it relieves the redness caused by minor irritations; it is widely used for clearing bloodshot eyes.

Adverse effects are rare when tetrahydrozoline is used for short periods at recommended doses. However, prolonged use can lead to increased ("rebound") congestion when the drug is stopped. Eye drops may occasionally lead to dilation of the pupils, causing blurred vision and sensitivity to light. This occurs more frequently among people with light-colored eyes and those who wear contact lenses.

INFORMATION FOR USERS

Follow instructions on the label. Call your physician if symptoms worsen.

How taken

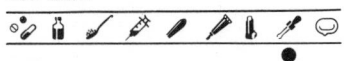

Nose drops, eye drops.

Frequency and timing of doses
Every 3 – 8 hours (nose drops); up to 4 x daily (eye drops).

Dosage range
Nose drops 2 – 4 drops in each nostril per application (adults and children over 6 years).
Eye drops 1 – 2 drops in each eye per application.

Onset of effect
Within 10 minutes.

Duration of action
4 – 8 hours.

Diet advice
None.

Storage
Keep in a closed container in a cool, dry place away from reach of children.

Missed dose
Take as soon as you remember if required. Do not use more than once in 3 hours.

Stopping the drug
Can be safely stopped as soon as you no longer need it.

Exceeding the dose
An occasional unintentional extra dose is unlikely to cause problems. Large overdoses or accidental swallowing of the drug may cause severe drowsiness with sweating, weakness, headache, dizziness, or palpitations. Notify your physician.

SPECIAL PRECAUTIONS

Be sure to consult your physician before using this drug if:
▼ You have heart problems.
▼ You have high blood pressure.
▼ You have glaucoma.
▼ You have an eye infection or other eye disease.
▼ You are taking other medications.

Pregnancy
▼ Not recommended, since the possible adverse effects, although uncommon, include a rise in blood pressure that could harm the developing baby.

Breast feeding
▼ Not recommended. The drug may pass into the breast milk, although at normal doses adverse effects on the baby are unlikely.

Infants and children
▼ Eye drops should not be used in children of any age. Nose drops are not recommended for children under 2 years, and should be used in children under 6 years only under medical supervision.

Over 60
▼ Reduced dose may be necessary. Increased likelihood of adverse effects.

Driving and hazardous work
▼ No known problems.

Alcohol
▼ No known problems.

POSSIBLE ADVERSE EFFECTS

Tetrahydrozoline rarely causes side effects at recommended doses. Overuse, however, may lead to local irritation and to adverse effects on the heart and central nervous system such as palpitations, headache, drowsiness, and restlessness.

Symptom/effect	Frequency		Discuss with physician		Stop taking drug now	Call physician now
	Common	Rare	Only if severe	In all cases		
Burning/stinging/rash		●		■		▲
Headache		●		■		▲
Restlessness		●		■		▲
Palpitations		●		■		▲
Eye drops only						
Blurred vision		●	■			
Oversensitivity to light		●	■			

INTERACTIONS

Antihypertensive drugs Tetrahydrozoline may reduce the blood pressure-lowering effect of these drugs, and is best avoided by people under treatment for high blood pressure.

Monoamine oxidase inhibitors (MAOIs) These drugs may interact dangerously with tetrahydrozoline to raise blood pressure.

PROLONGED USE

Tetrahydrozoline should not be used for longer than 5 days except on the advice of a physician.

THEOPHYLLINE

Brand names Slo-Bid, Slo-Phyllin, Theo-24, Theo-Dur, Theo-Dur Sprinkle
Used in the following combined preparations Bronkolixir, Marax, Quibron, Tedral, Theo-Organidin

A B C D E F G H I J K L M N O P Q R S T U V W X Y Z

GENERAL INFORMATION

Theophylline has two main actions: it relaxes and dilates the airways in the lungs; it stimulates breathing and the heart rate. It is used mainly in the treatment of asthma. Because it dilates the blood vessels – making the heart beat more forcefully – and increases urine flow, it is helpful in acute heart failure. It is also sometimes given to premature infants who are prone to attacks of apnea (stopped breathing).

Treatment with theophylline must be monitored because the effective dose is very close to the toxic dose. A number of its adverse effects, such as indigestion, nausea, headache, and agitation, can be controlled by regulating the dosage in accordance with the individual's weight and by following this up with checks on blood levels of the drug.

QUICK REFERENCE

Drug group Bronchodilator (p.120)
Overdose danger rating High
Dependence rating Low
Prescription needed Yes
Available as generic Yes

INFORMATION FOR USERS

Your drug prescription is tailored for you. Do not alter dosage without checking with your physician.

How taken

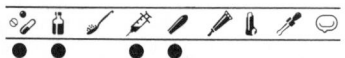

Tablets, timed-release capsules, liquid, syrup, injection, rectal suppositories.

Frequency and timing of doses
Every 6 hours (tablets, liquid, syrup); every 12 or 24 hours (timed-release capsules).

Dosage range
Adults 400 – 600mg daily (approximately).
Children Reduced dose according to age and weight.

Onset of effect
Within a few minutes (intravenous injection); within 30 minutes (oral or rectal); within one and a half hours (timed-release capsules).

Duration of action
8 hours (oral or rectal); 12 – 24 hours (timed-release capsules).

Diet advice
Avoid charcoal-broiled foods.

Storage
Keep in a closed container in a cool, dry place away from reach of children.

Missed dose
Take as soon as you remember. If your next dose is due within 2 hours, take half the dose now (short-acting preparations) or forget about the missed dose and take your next dose now (long-acting preparations). Return to your normal dose schedule thereafter.

Stopping the drug
Do not stop taking the drug without consulting your physician; stopping the drug may lead to worsening of the underlying condition.

OVERDOSE ACTION

Seek immediate medical advice in all cases. Take emergency action if confusion, chest pains, or loss of consciousness occurs.

See Drug poisoning emergency guide (p.590).

SPECIAL PRECAUTIONS

Be sure to tell your physician if:
▼ You have impaired liver function.
▼ You have angina or irregular heartbeat.
▼ You have gastrointestinal ulcers.
▼ You smoke.
▼ You have had epileptic seizures.
▼ You are taking other medications.

Pregnancy
▼ Not usually prescribed. Safety in pregnancy not established. Discuss with your physician so that you can weigh the benefits of the drug against its possible risks.

Breast feeding
▼ Discuss with your physician. The drug passes into the breast milk and may affect the baby adversely.

Infants and children
▼ Reduced dose necessary according to age and weight.

Over 60
▼ Reduced dose may be necessary.

Driving and hazardous work
▼ No known problems.

Alcohol
▼ No known problems.

POSSIBLE ADVERSE EFFECTS

Most adverse effects of this drug are related to dosage. Other effects are related to the drug's action on the central nervous system.

Symptom/effect	Frequency		Discuss with physician		Stop taking drug now	Call physician now
	Common	Rare	Only if severe	In all cases		
Agitation	●			■		
Dizziness	●			■		
Nausea/vomiting	●		■			
Diarrhea		●	■			
Palpitations		●		■	▲	▍
Seizures		●		■	▲	▍

PROLONGED USE

No problems expected.

Monitoring Periodic checks on blood levels of this drug are usually required.

INTERACTIONS

Among other drugs, erythromycin, cimetidine, some antibiotics, allopurinol, and beta blockers increase the level of theophylline in the blood.

Carbamazepine, phenytoin, rifampin, sulfinpyrazone, phenobarbital, nicotine These drugs reduce the level of theophylline in the blood.

THIABENDAZOLE

Brand name Mintezol
Used in the following combined preparations None

GENERAL INFORMATION

Thiabendazole, introduced in 1967, is an anthelmintic drug prescribed for a variety of worm infestations. Its major uses are in the treatment of pinworm infections and larva migrans affecting the skin or the internal organs. It may also be given for trichinosis, common roundworm, whipworm, and hookworm infections.

Taken by mouth as chewable tablets or as a liquid, thiabendazole generally clears infections within five days. The drug may be applied *topically* for mild cases of larva migrans of the skin.

In some cases, corticosteroids may be given in conjunction with the drug to prevent severe reactions to the dying worms.

Adverse effects with thiabendazole are not usually serious, but there is a rare risk of hypersensitivity reactions, including skin rashes and chills or fever. For this reason, the drug is not generally used unless other drugs are ineffective. Given for common round-worm infections, it may sometimes cause the worms to migrate and appear in the mouth and nose.

QUICK REFERENCE

Drug group Anthelmintic drug (p.167)

Overdose danger rating Medium

Dependence rating Low

Prescription needed Yes

Available as generic No

INFORMATION FOR USERS

Your drug prescription is tailored for you. Do not alter dosage without checking with your physician.

How taken

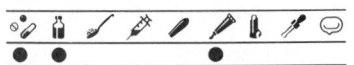

Tablets, liquid, skin lotion.

Frequency and timing of doses
By mouth 2 x daily after meals for 2 – 5 days. Tablets to be chewed thoroughly.
Skin lotion 2 – 4 x daily.

Dosage range
By mouth According to body weight (maximum 3g daily).
Skin lotion Apply around each burrow.

Onset of effect
2 – 4 hours.

Duration of action
2 – 3 days.

Diet advice
None.

Storage
Keep in a closed container in a cool, dry place away from reach of children.

Missed dose
Take as soon as you remember. If your next dose is due at this time, take a dose now and another 4 – 5 hours later (by mouth) or skip missed dose (skin lotion). Continue your normal schedule therafter.

Stopping the drug
Take the full course. Even if you feel better, the original infection may still be present and may recur if treatment is stopped too soon.

Exceeding the dose
An occasional unintentional extra dose is unlikely to cause problems. Large over-doses may cause anxiety, hallucinations, and blurred vision. Notify your physician.

POSSIBLE ADVERSE EFFECTS

Taken by mouth, thiabendazole may cause digestive disturbances, central nervous system side effects such as dizziness, and hypersensitivity reactions, including fever and skin rashes. If you notice an asparagus-like urinary odor, this is no cause for alarm. Adverse effects are rare with thiabendazole skin lotion.

Symptom/effect	Frequency		Discuss with physician		Stop taking drug now	Call physician now
	Common	Rare	Only if severe	In all cases		
Dizziness	●		■			
Loss of appetite	●		■			
Nausea/vomiting	●		■			
Headache/drowsiness		●	■			
Diarrhea		●	■			
Fever/chills		●		■	▲	
Rash/itching		●		■	▲	

INTERACTIONS

Theophylline Thiabendazole may interfere with the breakdown of theophylline and similar drugs, leading to increased blood levels.

SPECIAL PRECAUTIONS

Be sure to tell your physician if:
▼ You have impaired liver or kidney function.
▼ You are taking other medications.

 Pregnancy
▼ Not usually prescribed. Safety in pregnancy not established. Discuss with your physician so that you can weigh the benefits of the drug against its possible risks.

 Breast feeding
▼ Discuss with your physician. The drug passes into the breast milk and may affect the baby adversely.

 Infants and children
▼ Not recommended for children under 2 years. Reduced dose necessary for older children.

 Over 60
▼ No special problems.

 Driving and hazardous work
▼ Avoid such activities until you have learned how the drug affects you, because the drug may cause dizziness and blurred vision.

 Alcohol
▼ No known problems.

PROLONGED USE

No problems expected.

THIORIDAZINE

Brand names Mellaril, Mellaril-S
Used in the following combined preparations None

GENERAL INFORMATION

Thioridazine was introduced in 1959. It belongs to the phenothiazine antipsychotic group of drugs (see p.113).

Thioridazine is a very important tranquilizer widely used to treat a variety of psychotic conditions. Its tranquilizing effect suppresses abnormal behavior and reduces aggression. It is used in the treatment of schizophrenia, mania, dementia, and other disorders where confused or abnormal behavior may occur. Thioridazine does not cure the underlying disorder, but it does relieve the distressing symptoms. It also helps to relieve the anxiety and depression associated with serious mental disorders.

Thioridazine is particularly suitable for treating the elderly because it is less likely to cause abnormal shaking movements than some of the other drugs in this group.

The main drawback to the use of thioridazine is that when given in high doses it can cause eye problems. If large doses are required for long periods, another antipsychotic drug is usually substituted.

INFORMATION FOR USERS

Your drug prescription is tailored for you. Do not alter dosage without checking with your physician.

How taken

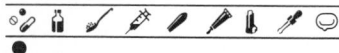

Tablets.

Frequency and timing of doses
2 – 4 x daily.

Adult dosage range
50 – 800mg daily.

Onset of effect
2 – 3 hours.

Duration of action
4 – 10 hours. Some effects may last up to 36 hours.

Diet advice
None.

Storage
Keep in a closed container in a cool, dry place away from reach of children.

Missed dose
Take as soon as you remember. If your next dose is due within 2 hours, do not take the missed dose. Take your next scheduled dose as usual.

Stopping the drug
Do not stop the drug without consulting your physician; symptoms may recur.

Exceeding the dose
An occasional unintentional extra dose is unlikely to cause problems. Large overdoses may cause unusual drowsiness, fainting, muscle rigidity, and agitation. Notify your physician.

POSSIBLE ADVERSE EFFECTS

Thioridazine has a strong *anticholinergic* effect that can cause a variety of minor symptoms (see p.107). These often become less marked with time. The most significant adverse effect is eye problems. This can occasionally be controlled by medically supervised adjustment of dosage, or a change of drug.

Symptom/effect	Frequency		Discuss with physician		Stop taking drug now	Call physician now
	Common	Rare	Only if severe	In all cases		
Drowsiness	●		■			
Dry mouth	●		■			
Stuffy nose	●			■		
Blurred vision		●		■		
Muscle stiffness		●		■		
Unsteadiness		●		■		
Dizziness/fainting		●		■	▲	

INTERACTIONS

Sedatives All drugs that have a sedative effect are likely to increase the sedative properties of thioridazine.

Antiparkinsonism drugs Thioridazine may counter the benefits of these drugs.

Anticholinergic drugs The side effects of drugs with *anticholinergic* properties may be increased by thioridazine. Such drugs include certain antiparkinsonism drugs and some over-the-counter decongestants.

SPECIAL PRECAUTIONS

Be sure to tell your physician if:
▼ You have impaired kidney or liver function.
▼ You have had epileptic seizures.
▼ You have had glaucoma.
▼ You have an overactive thyroid gland.
▼ You have Parkinson's disease.
▼ You are taking other medications.

Pregnancy
▼ Not usually prescribed. Taken near the time of delivery it can prolong labor.

Breast feeding
▼ Discuss with your physician. The drug passes into the breast milk and may affect the baby adversely.

Infants and children
▼ Not recommended for children under one year. Reduced dose is necessary for older children.

Over 60
▼ Reduced dose may be necessary. There is an increased likelihood of adverse effects.

Driving and hazardous work
▼ Avoid such activities until you have learned how the drug affects you, because of the possibility of drowsiness and blurred vision.

Alcohol
▼ Avoid. Alcohol may increase the sedative effects of this drug.

Surgery and general anesthetics
▼ Thioridazine treatment may need to be stopped before you have a general anesthetic. Discuss this with your physician or dentist before any operation.

PROLONGED USE

Use of this drug for more than a few months may lead to the development of eye problems and abnormal movements of the face and limbs known as *tardive dyskinesia*. Occasionally jaundice may occur.

THYROID

Brand names Armour Thyroid, S-P-T, Thyrar, Thyroid Strong
Used in the following combined preparations None

GENERAL INFORMATION

Introduced in 1957, the drug thyroid is prepared from the thyroid glands of domesticated animals. Like other similar thyroid hormone preparations, it may be given as replacement therapy in hypothyroidism, when naturally occurring thyroid hormones are deficient. It may also be used to treat thyroid cancer and certain forms of goiter (enlarged thyroid gland).

This drug is no longer widely used because its effect tends to vary from batch to batch and even from tablet to tablet due to variations in concentration of the active drug present. For this reason, it is now prescribed only for people who have been using it for years without problems. Others are usually treated with the more predictable synthetic hormones.

Adverse effects, which are generally due to overdosage (see below), are more likely in the elderly and those with heart disease.

INFORMATION FOR USERS

Your drug prescription is tailored for you. Do not alter dosage without checking with your physician.

How taken

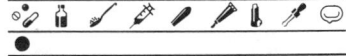

Tablets, capsules.

Frequency and timing of doses
Once daily on an empty stomach.

Adult dosage range
Thyroid replacement therapy 12 – 30mg daily (starting dose), increased at 2-week intervals as required to 60 – 120mg daily (maintenance dose).
Goiter and thyroid cancer 60mg daily (starting dose), increased as required to 90 – 180mg daily (maintenance dose).

Onset of effect
Within 48 hours. Full beneficial effect may not be felt for several weeks.

Duration of action
1 – 3 weeks.

Diet advice
None.

Storage
Keep in a closed container in a cool, dry place away from reach of children.

Missed dose
Take as soon as you remember. If your next dose is due within 2 hours, take both doses now.

Stopping the drug
Do not stop the drug without consulting your physician; symptoms may recur.

Exceeding the dose
An occasional unintentional extra dose is unlikely to cause problems. Large overdoses may cause palpitations during the next few days. Notify your physician.

SPECIAL PRECAUTIONS

Be sure to tell your physician if:
▼ You have high blood pressure.
▼ You have heart problems.
▼ You are taking other medications.

Pregnancy
▼ No evidence of risk to developing baby.

Breast feeding
▼ Discuss with your physician. The drug passes into the breast milk.

Infants and children
▼ Rarely required.

Over 60
▼ Reduced dose usually necessary.

Driving and hazardous work
▼ No known problems.

Alcohol
▼ No known problems.

POSSIBLE ADVERSE EFFECTS

Adverse effects are rare with thyroid and are usually the result of overdosage, causing thyroid overactivity. These effects diminish as the dose is lowered, but may take several weeks to disappear. Too low a dose may cause signs of thyroid underactivity.

Symptom/effect	Frequency		Discuss with physician		Stop taking drug now	Call physician now
	Common	Rare	Only if severe	In all cases		
Anxiety/agitation		●		■		
Diarrhea		●		■		
Weight loss/gain		●		■		
Sweating/flushing		●		■		
Lethargy		●		■		
Palpitations/chest pain	●			■		■

INTERACTIONS

Oral anticoagulant drugs The effect of these drugs may be increased by thyroid.

Antidiabetic drugs Thyroid hormone treatment may increase requirements for insulin or oral antidiabetic drugs. Dosage adjustment may be necessary.

Cholestyramine and colestipol Oral doses of these drugs may reduce the absorption of thyroid. They should be spaced 4 – 5 hours apart from a dose of thyroid.

PROLONGED USE

No special problems.

Monitoring Periodic tests of thyroid function are usually required.

TIMOLOL

Brand names Blocadren, Timoptic
Used in the following combined preparation Timolide

GENERAL INFORMATION

Introduced in 1972, timolol is a beta blocker prescribed to treat hypertension (high blood pressure) and angina. It may also be given to a person after a heart attack to prevent further damage. When used for hypertension, timolol may be given with a diuretic. Timolol is also administered in the form of eye drops to people suffering from certain types of glaucoma. It lowers the pressure in the eye by reducing the formation of fluid in the eye.

Taken *systemically*, timolol can cause breathing difficulties, especially in individuals with asthma, chronic bronchitis, or emphysema. As with other beta blockers, timolol masks the body's response to low blood sugar and, for that reason, is prescribed with caution to diabetics.

Serious side effects are unusual with timolol eye drops; some people may experience eye irritation, blurring of vision, and headache.

QUICK REFERENCE

Drug group Beta blocker (p.125) drug for glaucoma (p.196)

Overdose danger rating High

Dependence rating Low

Prescription needed Yes

Available as generic No

INFORMATION FOR USERS

Your drug prescription is tailored for you. Do not alter dosage without checking with your physician.

How taken

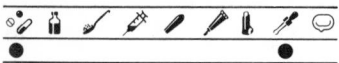

Tablets, eye drops.

Frequency and timing of doses
2 x daily.

Adult dosage range
By mouth 20 – 60mg daily (angina/hypertension); 20mg daily (after a heart attack). *Eye drops* 2 drops daily.

Onset of effect
1 – 2 hours (by mouth); within minutes (eye drops).

Duration of action
12 – 36 hours.

Diet advice
None.

Storage
Keep in a closed container in a cool, dry place away from reach of children.

Missed dose
Take as soon as you remember. If your next dose is due within 2 hours, take a single dose now and skip the next.

Stopping the drug
Do not stop the drug without consulting your physician; stopping the drug may lead to worsening of the underlying condition.

OVERDOSE ACTION

Seek immediate medical advice in all cases of overdose by mouth. Take emergency action if palpitations, breathing difficulties, or loss of consciousness occurs.

See Drug poisoning emergency guide (p.590).

SPECIAL PRECAUTIONS

Be sure to tell your physician if:
▼ You have a lung disorder such as bronchitis or emphysema.
▼ You have diabetes.
▼ You have poor circulation.
▼ You are taking other medications.

Pregnancy
▼ Not usually prescribed. Safety in pregnancy not established. Discuss with your physician so that you can weigh the benefits of the drug against its possible risks.

Breast feeding
▼ Discuss with your physician. The drug passes into the breast milk, but at normal doses adverse effects on the baby are unlikely.

Infants and children
▼ Not usually prescribed.

Over 60
▼ No special problems.

Driving and hazardous work
▼ Avoid such activities until you have learned how the drug affects you, because tablets may cause drowsiness and eye drops may cause blurred vision.

Alcohol
▼ No known problems.

Surgery and general anesthetics
▼ Timolol by mouth may need to be stopped before you have a general anesthetic. Discuss this with your physician or dentist before any surgery.

POSSIBLE ADVERSE EFFECTS

Timolol taken by mouth can occasionally provoke or worsen asthma and heart problems. Fainting may be a sign that the drug has slowed the heartbeat excessively. Eye drops cause these problems only rarely. Headache or blurred vision is more likely.

Symptom/effect	Frequency		Discuss with physician		Stop taking drug now	Call physician now
	Common	Rare	Only if severe	In all cases		
Lethargy	●		■			
Blurred vision/headache	●		■			
Cold hands/feet		●	■			
Eye irritation		●	■			
Nightmares/vivid dreams		●		■		
Fainting/breathlessness		●		■	▲	▮

INTERACTIONS

Monoamine oxidase inhibitors (MAOIs) may dangerously raise blood pressure when taken with timolol.

Cimetidine can increase the blood levels of timolol.

PROLONGED USE

No problems expected.

TPA (tissue-type plasminogen activator)

Brand name Activase
Used in the following combined preparations None

GENERAL INFORMATION

Tissue-type plasminogen activator (TPA) is an enzyme involved in the breakdown of blood clots. Manufactured or cloned by genetic engineering techniques, it is an investigational drug, being tested for the treatment of heart attacks in which a blood clot (thrombus) forms in one of the blood vessels of the heart muscle, cutting off its blood supply.

Given by infusion into a vein or directly into the coronary artery, TPA acts quickly to dissolve the clot and restore the blood supply to the heart muscle. Used within a few hours of an attack, it can dramatically reduce the amount of damage to the heart muscle. Infusion is usually continued for a few hours after the clot has dissolved to prevent further clot formation.

As with other thrombolytic drugs, there is a risk of internal bleeding with TPA, and bleeding or bruising at the injection site is common. As a naturally occurring substance, however, it is less likely to produce an allergic reaction than other thrombolytic drugs, such as streptokinase.

QUICK REFERENCE

Drug group Thrombolytic drug (p.133)

Overdose danger rating Medium

Dependence rating Low

Prescription needed Yes

Available as generic No

INFORMATION FOR USERS

This drug is given only under medical supervision and is not for self-administration.

How taken

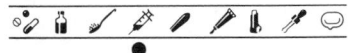

Injection.

Frequency and timing of doses
By continuous infusion over several hours.

Dosage range
Dosage is determined individually by condition and response.

Onset of effect
The blood clot begins to dissolve as soon as the drug reaches it. Most of the clot is dissolved within 1 hour.

Duration of action
The effect of the drug disappears a few minutes after it is stopped.

Diet advice
None.

Storage
Not applicable. This drug is not kept in the home.

Missed dose
Not applicable. This drug is given only in a hospital under close medical supervision.

Stopping the drug
The drug is stopped under medical supervision a few hours after the clot has dispersed.

Exceeding the dose
Overdosage is unlikely, since treatment is carefully monitored in the hospital.

POSSIBLE ADVERSE EFFECTS

There is a risk of internal bleeding with TPA, particularly in the stomach and intestinal tract. All adverse effects are closely monitored under strict medical supervision.

Symptom/effect	Frequency		Discuss with physician		Stop taking drug now	Call physician now
	Common	Rare	Only if severe	In all cases		
Bruising	●			■		▮
Abnormal bleeding	●			■		▮

INTERACTIONS

Anticoagulant drugs There is an increased risk of bleeding when these are taken at the same time as TPA.

Antiplatelet drugs increase the risk of bleeding if given with TPA.

SPECIAL PRECAUTIONS

TPA is only prescribed under close medical supervision, taking account of your present condition and medical history.

Pregnancy
▼ Used only when the life of the mother is at risk.

Breast feeding
▼ Used only when the life of the mother is at risk.

Infants and children
▼ Not recommended.

Over 60
▼ Increased likelihood of bruising at injection site.

Driving and hazardous work
▼ Not applicable.

Alcohol
▼ Not applicable.

PROLONGED USE

TPA is not used long-term.

TOBRAMYCIN

Brand names Nebcin, Tobrex Ophthalmic
Used in the following combined preparations None

GENERAL INFORMATION

Tobramycin, introduced in 1975, is an aminoglycoside antibiotic. Given by injection, it is generally reserved for serious, complicated infections among hospitalized persons. These include peritonitis and meningitis; severe infections of the lungs, skin, bones, and joints; and burn and wound infections. It is frequently used together with a penicillin, since combined treatment maximizes the antibacterial effect of both drugs.

Tobramycin eye drops and ointment are sometimes prescribed for super-ficial eye infections such as conjunctivitis and blepharitis (inflammation of the eyelids).

Tobramycin given by injection may have serious adverse effects on the kidneys and on the inner ear, leading to permanent damage to the balance mechanism and deafness. However, the risk of kidney problems is thought to be lower than with other aminoglycoside antibiotics, and tobramycin is preferred when kidney function is poor. Blood levels of the drug are usually monitored during injection treatment.

INFORMATION FOR USERS

Your drug prescription is tailored for you. Do not alter dosage without checking with your physician.

How taken

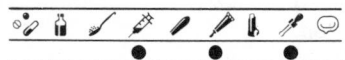

Injection, ointment, eye drops.

Frequency and timing of doses
Every 8 – 24 hours (injection); as directed between 2 x daily and once hourly (eye drops or ointment).

Adult dosage range
According to condition and response (injection); according to your physician's instructions (eye drops or ointment).

Onset of effect
2 – 3 days.

Duration of action
8 hours.

Diet advice
None.

Storage
Keep ointment in a closed container in a cool, dry place away from reach of children.

Missed dose
Apply eye drops or ointment as soon as you remember.

Stopping the drug
Apply the full course of ointment. Even if you feel better, the original infection may still be present and may recur if treatment is stopped too soon.

Exceeding the dose
Overdose by injection is unlikely, since treatment is carefully monitored. For eye preparations, an occasional unintentional extra dose is unlikely to be a cause for concern. If you notice unusual symptoms, notify your physician.

SPECIAL PRECAUTIONS

Be sure to tell your physician if:
▼ You have impaired kidney function.
▼ You have a hearing disorder.
▼ You have myasthenia gravis.
▼ You have had a previous allergic reaction to aminoglycosides.
▼ You are taking other medications.

Pregnancy
▼ Injections are not prescribed, as they may cause deafness in the baby. No evidence of risk with topical preparations.

Breast feeding
▼ No evidence of risk with topical preparations. Given by injection, the drug passes into the breast milk, but at normal doses adverse effects on the baby are uncommon. Discuss with your physician.

Infants and children
▼ Reduced dose necessary.

Over 60
▼ Reduced dose may be necessary. Increased likelihood of adverse effects.

Driving and hazardous work
▼ No known problems.

Alcohol
▼ No known problems.

POSSIBLE ADVERSE EFFECTS

Adverse effects are rare, but those that occur with the injectable form may be serious. Dizziness, loss of balance (vertigo), impaired hearing, and changes in the urine should be reported promptly. Rash and itching may occur with all preparations.

Symptom/effect	Frequency		Discuss with physician		Stop taking drug now	Call physician now
	Common	Rare	Only if severe	In all cases		
Nausea/vomiting	●		■			
Headache/lethargy	●			■	▲	▌
Dizziness/vertigo	●			■	▲	▌
Ringing in the ears	●			■	▲	▌
Rash/itching	●			■	▲	▌
Bloody/cloudy urine	●			■	▲	▌
Loss of hearing	●			■	▲	▌

PROLONGED USE

Not usually given for longer than 10 days. There is a risk of adverse effects on hearing, balance, and kidney function.

Monitoring Blood levels of the drug are usually checked during injection treatment.

INTERACTIONS

General note A wide range of drugs increases the risk of hearing loss and/or kidney failure with tobramycin. Such drugs include other aminoglycosides, furosemide, polymyxin antibiotics, amphotericin B, cisplatin, and cyclosporine.

TOLAZAMIDE

Brand name Tolinase
Used in the following combined preparations None

GENERAL INFORMATION

Tolazamide, introduced in 1966, is an oral antidiabetic drug. Like other drugs of this type, it lowers blood sugar by stimulating insulin secretion from the pancreas and promoting the uptake of sugar into body cells.

Taken by mouth, it is used in the treatment of adult (maturity-onset) diabetes mellitus, in conjunction with a special diabetic diet low in refined sugar and fats. Loss of excess weight is usually necessary for the drug to be fully effective. Since it has a pro-longed action, one dose a day is sufficient for most people.

Serious side effects occur only rarely with tolazamide. Unlike some of the older antidiabetic drugs, it has a mild diuretic action, making it useful for diabetics with a tendency to retain water, such as those with congestive heart failure.

In conditions of severe illness, injury, or stress, the drug may lose its effectiveness, making insulin injections necessary.

QUICK REFERENCE

Drug group Oral antidiabetic drug (p.170)

Overdose danger rating High

Dependence rating Low

Prescription needed Yes

Available as generic Yes

INFORMATION FOR USERS

Your drug prescription is tailored for you. Do not alter dosage without checking with your physician.

How taken

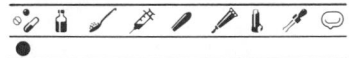

Tablets.

Frequency and timing of doses
Once daily (in the morning), or 2 x daily (in the morning and evening with meals).

Dosage range
100mg – 1g daily.

Onset of effect
Within 1 hour.

Duration of action
12 – 24 hours.

Diet advice
A low-sugar, low-fat diet must be maintained in order for the drug to be fully effective. Follow your physician's advice.

Storage
Keep in a closed container in a cool, dry place away from reach of children.

Missed dose
Take before your next meal.

Stopping the drug
Do not stop taking the drug without consulting your physician; stopping the drug may lead to worsening of your diabetes.

OVERDOSE ACTION

Seek immediate medical advice in all cases. You may notice symptoms of low blood sugar such as faintness, confusion, sweating, trembling, or head-ache. If these occur, eat or drink something sugary. Take emergency action if seizures or loss of consciousness occurs.

See Drug poisoning emergency guide (p.590).

POSSIBLE ADVERSE EFFECTS

Serious adverse effects are rare. Faintness, sweating, tremor, weakness, and confusion may be signs of low blood sugar due to lack of food or too high a dose.

Symptom/effect	Frequency		Discuss with physician		Stop taking drug now	Call physician now
	Common	Rare	Only if severe	In all cases		
Faintness/confusion	●			■		
Weakness/tremor	●			■		
Sweating	●			■		
Nausea/vomiting		●	■			
Thirst/rash/itching		●		■		

INTERACTIONS

General note Many drugs may oppose the effect of tolazamide and so may raise blood sugar levels. Such drugs include corticosteroids, estrogens, diuretics, anti-psychotics, and anticonvulsants. Other drugs increase the risk of low blood sugar.

These include dicumarol, sulfonamides, anabolic steroids, and aspirin.

Beta blockers By reducing palpitations and tremors, these mask the signs of low blood sugar.

SPECIAL PRECAUTIONS

Be sure to tell your physician if:
▼ You have impaired liver or kidney function.
▼ You are allergic to sulfonamide drugs.
▼ You are taking other medications.

 Pregnancy
▼ Not usually prescribed. May cause severe low blood sugar in the newborn baby. Insulin is generally substituted in pregnancy.

 Breast feeding
▼ Discuss with your physician. The drug passes into the breast milk and may cause low blood sugar in the baby.

 Infants and children
▼ Not prescribed.

 Over 60
▼ Signs of low blood sugar may be more difficult to recognize.

 Driving and hazardous work
▼ Usually no problem. Avoid these activities if you have warning signs of low blood sugar.

 Alcohol
▼ Avoid. Alcoholic drinks upset diabetic control.

Surgery and general anesthetics
▼ Surgery may reduce the beneficial effect of tolazamide on diabetes. Notify your physician that you are diabetic before any surgery; insulin treatment may need to be substituted.

PROLONGED USE

No problems expected.

Monitoring Regular monitoring of urine or blood sugar is required.

TOLBUTAMIDE

Brand names Oramide, Orinase
Used in the following combined preparations None

GENERAL INFORMATION

Tolbutamide, introduced in 1956, is an antidiabetic agent that lowers blood sugar by stimulating insulin secretion from the pancreas. Taken by mouth, it is used to treat adult (maturity onset) diabetes in which active insulin-secreting cells are still present. Where these are lacking, as in juvenile diabetes, the drug is ineffective.

Tolbutamide does not work in isolation, but is given in conjunction with a special diabetic diet that limits intake of sugar and fats.

Shorter acting than many oral antidiabetic drugs, tolbutamide may help in the initial control of diabetes. It may also be used in those with impaired kidney function because it is less likely to build up in the body and cause excessive lowering of blood sugar. As with other oral antidiabetic drugs, it may need to be discontinued during serious illnesses, injury, or surgery, when diabetic control is lost.

QUICK REFERENCE

Drug group Antidiabetic drug (p.170)
Overdose danger rating High
Dependence rating Low
Prescription needed Yes
Available as generic Yes

INFORMATION FOR USERS

Your drug prescription is tailored for you. Do not alter dosage without checking with your physician.

How taken

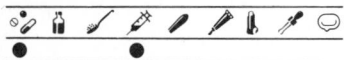

Tablets, injection.

Frequency and timing of doses
Once daily in the morning, or 2 x daily in the morning and evening before meals.

Adult dosage range
500mg – 3g daily.

Onset of effect
Within 1 hour.

Duration of action
6 – 12 hours.

Diet advice
An individualized low-fat, low-sugar diet must be maintained for the drug to be fully effective. Follow the advice of your physician.

Storage
Keep in a closed container in a cool, dry place away from reach of children.

Missed dose
Take as soon as you remember. If your next dose is due within 2 hours, take a single dose now and skip the next.

Stopping the drug
Do not stop the drug without consulting your physician; stopping the drug may lead to worsening of the underlying condition.

OVERDOSE ACTION

Seek immediate medical advice in all cases. You may notice symptoms of low blood sugar such as faintness, confusion, or headache. If these occur, eat something sugary. Take emergency action if seizures, or loss of consciousness occurs.

See Drug poisoning emergency guide (p.590).

SPECIAL PRECAUTIONS

Be sure to tell your physician if:
▼ You have impaired liver function.
▼ You are allergic to sulfonamides.
▼ You are taking other medications.

Pregnancy
▼ Not recommended. May cause birth defects if taken in the first 3 months of pregnancy. Taken near the time of delivery, may cause abnormally low blood sugar in the newborn baby.

Breast feeding
▼ Discuss with your physician. The drug passes into the breast milk and may cause low blood sugar in the baby.

Infants and children
▼ Not prescribed.

Over 60
▼ Reduced dose usually necessary. Increased likelihood of adverse effects.

Driving and hazardous work
▼ Usually no problem. Avoid these activities if you have warning signs of low blood sugar.

Alcohol
▼ Avoid. Alcohol may increase the risk of low blood sugar with this drug.

Surgery and general anesthetics
▼ Surgery may reduce the beneficial effect of tolbutamide on diabetes. Notify your physician that you are diabetic before any surgery; insulin treatment may need to be substituted.

POSSIBLE ADVERSE EFFECTS

Serious adverse effects are rare with tolbutamide. Symptoms such as dizziness, sweating, weakness, and confusion, indicate low blood sugar levels.

Symptom/effect	Frequency		Discuss with physician		Stop taking drug now	Call physician now
	Common	Rare	Only if severe	In all cases		
Dizziness/confusion	●			■		
Weakness/sweating	●			■		
Headache		●	■			
Nausea		●		■		
Vomiting		●		■		
Rash/itching		●		■		▲

INTERACTIONS

General note A variety of drugs may oppose the effect of tolbutamide. Such drugs include corticosteroids, estrogens, diuretics, phenobarbital, phenothiazine antipsychotics, and phenytoin. Other drugs increase the effects: sulfonamides, non-steroidal anti-inflammatory drugs (NSAIDs), beta blockers, probenecid, monoamine oxidase inhibitors (MAOIs), aspirin, salicylates, and acetaminophen.

PROLONGED USE

No problems expected.

Monitoring Regular monitoring of urine and/or blood sugar is required.

TOLMETIN

Brand names Tolectin, Tolectin DS
Used in the following combined preparations None

GENERAL INFORMATION

Tolmetin, introduced in 1976, is a non-steroidal anti-inflammatory drug (NSAID). Used in the treatment of osteoarthritis, rheumatoid arthritis, and ankylosing spondylitis, it does not cure the underlying disease but helps to relieve pain, stiffness, and inflammation. In rheumatoid arthritis, it may be given in conjunction with the slow-acting drugs to reduce symptoms while these drugs take effect.

Tolmetin is effective for the relief of pain from minor injuries – e.g., muscle and ligament strain in sports injuries.

Adverse effects occur less frequently with tolmetin than with certain other NSAIDs, and are rarely serious. The drug can cause fluid retention, leading to swelling of the ankles, and is therefore used with caution in those with heart failure or high blood pressure, and in the elderly.

INFORMATION FOR USERS

Your drug prescription is tailored for you. Do not alter dosage without checking with your physician.

How taken

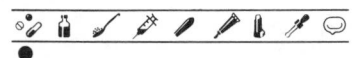

Tablets, capsules.

Frequency and timing of doses
3 x daily with food or milk.

Dosage range
Adults 1.2g daily (starting dose), then 1.8g – 2.4g daily (maintenance dose).
Children (over 2 years) Reduced dose according to age and weight.

Onset of effect
Pain relief begins in 30 – 60 minutes. Full anti-inflammatory effect may not be felt for up to 2 weeks.

Duration of action
Up to 8 hours.

Diet advice
None.

Storage
Keep in a closed container in a cool, dry place away from reach of children.

Missed dose
Take as soon as you remember. If your next dose is due within 2 hours, take a single dose now and skip the next.

Stopping the drug
When taken for short-term pain relief, tolmetin can be safely stopped as soon as you no longer need it. If prescribed for the long-term treatment of arthritis, however, you should seek medical advice before stopping the drug.

Exceeding the dose
An occasional unintentional extra dose is unlikely to be a cause for concern. But if you notice unusual symptoms, or if a large overdose has been taken, notify your physician.

SPECIAL PRECAUTIONS

Be sure to tell your physician if:
▼ You have impaired kidney function.
▼ You have heart problems.
▼ You have had a peptic ulcer, esophagitis, or acid indigestion.
▼ You have high blood pressure.
▼ You are allergic to aspirin.
▼ You have bleeding problems.
▼ You are taking other medications.

Pregnancy
▼ Not usually prescribed. Taken in the last 3 months of pregnancy, may have adverse effects on the baby's heart and may prolong labor. Discuss with your physician so that you may weigh the benefits of the drug against its risks.

Breast feeding
▼ No evidence of risk.

Infants and children
▼ Not recommended for children under 2 years. Reduced dose necessary for older children.

Over 60
▼ Reduced dose may be necessary. Increased likelihood of adverse effects.

Driving and hazardous work
▼ No known problems.

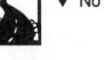

Alcohol
▼ Avoid. Alcohol may increase the risk of stomach disorders with tolmetin.

Surgery and general anesthetics
▼ Tolmetin may prolong bleeding. Discuss this with your physician or dentist before any surgery.

POSSIBLE ADVERSE EFFECTS

Adverse effects are not usually serious and may diminish during treatment. Black or bloodstained bowel movements should be reported to your physician promptly.

Symptom/effect	Frequency		Discuss with physician		Stop taking drug now	Call physician now
	Common	Rare	Only if severe	In all cases		
Indigestion	●		■			
Headache	●		■			
Abdominal pain	●			■		
Dizziness/lightheadedness		●	■			
Vomiting		●		■		
Swollen feet/ankles		●		■		
Rash		●		■	▲	
Wheezing/breathlessness		●		■	▲	■

INTERACTIONS

General note Tolmetin interacts with a wide range of drugs to increase the risk of bleeding and/or peptic ulcers. Such drugs include oral anticoagulants, corticosteroids, and aspirin.

Antihypertensive drugs and diuretics The beneficial effects of these drugs may be reduced when taken along with tolmetin.

PROLONGED USE

There is an increased risk of bleeding from peptic ulcers and in the bowel with prolonged use of tolmetin.

TOLNAFTATE

Brand names Tinactin, Tinactin Cream, Zeasorb - AF
Used in the following combined preparations None

GENERAL INFORMATION

Tolnaftate, introduced in 1965, was the first antifungal drug found to be effective when applied topically. Available over the counter as a cream, powder, or aerosol, it is used to treat tinea (ringworm) infections of the skin, although it may not work as well as some other antifungal drugs that are taken by mouth. However, its effectiveness as a cream is increased if it is used in conjunction with salicylic acid ointment, which improves its absorption. Though useful for athlete's foot, it does not help fungal infections of the scalp, nails, palms, and soles. Tolnaftate can be used long-term to prevent recurrence of infections in susceptible people.

Side effects are rare, and unlike other antifungal drugs, tolnaftate does not generally cause skin irritation or rash. Occasionally, stinging may occur when this drug is sprayed onto the skin.

INFORMATION FOR USERS

Follow instructions on the label. Call your physician if symptoms worsen.

How taken

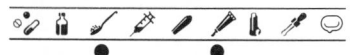

Powder, cream, gel, aerosol.

Frequency and timing of doses
2 x daily.

Dosage range
Follow manufacturer's instructions.

Onset of effect
Within 1 – 2 days. Full beneficial effects may not be felt for 2 – 6 weeks.

Duration of action
Up to 12 hours.

Diet advice
None.

Storage
Keep in a closed container in a cool, dry place away from reach of children.

Missed dose
No cause for concern, but take as soon as you remember.

Stopping the drug
Take the full course. Even if symptoms disappear, the original infection may still be present and may recur if treatment is stopped too soon.

Exceeding the dose
An occasional unintentional extra dose is unlikely to be a cause for concern. But if you notice unusual symptoms, or if a large overdose has been taken, notify your physician.

SPECIAL PRECAUTIONS

Be sure to consult your physician before using this drug if:
▼ You have had a rash when using this drug in the past.

Pregnancy
▼ No evidence of risk to developing baby.

Breast feeding
▼ No evidence of risk.

Infants and children
▼ Not usually prescribed for infants. No special problems in older children.

Over 60
▼ No known problems.

Driving and hazardous work
▼ No known problems.

Alcohol
▼ No known problems.

POSSIBLE ADVERSE EFFECTS

Adverse effects occur rarely with tolnaftate. If this antifungal drug irritates the skin, discontinue use and consult your physician about these symptoms.

Symptom/effect	Frequency		Discuss with physician		Stop taking drug now	Call physician now
	Common	Rare	Only if severe	In all cases		
Itching/irritation		●		■	▲	
Rash		●		■	▲	

INTERACTIONS

None.

PROLONGED USE

No problems expected.

TRAZODONE

Brand name Desyrel
Used in the following combined preparations None

GENERAL INFORMATION

Trazodone is one of many drugs used to treat depression. It helps to elevate mood, improve appetite, and restore interest in everyday activities. But because it has a strong sedative effect, it is particularly useful when the depression is accompanied by anxiety or insomnia or both. Taken at night, it helps to reduce the need for additional sleeping drugs.

Trazodone is less likely to cause adverse effects than the tricyclic antidepressants. It is also somewhat safer for people with heart problems and is therefore commonly used to treat depression among the elderly.

QUICK REFERENCE

Drug group Antidepressant (p.112)
Overdose danger rating Medium
Dependence rating Low
Prescription needed Yes
Available as generic No

INFORMATION FOR USERS

Your drug prescription is tailored for you. Do not alter the dosage without checking with your physician.

How taken

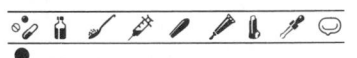

Tablets.

Frequency and timing of doses
3 x daily with food.

Adult dosage range
75 – 300mg daily. Dose may be increased in exceptional circumstances.

Onset of effect
Some benefits and adverse effects may appear within hours of starting treatment, but full antidepressant effect may not be felt for 2 – 4 weeks.

Duration of action
Adverse effects may last up to 24 hours after stopping the drug. Following cessation of prolonged treatment, the antidepressant effect may persist for up to 6 weeks.

Diet advice
None.

Storage
Keep in a closed container in a cool, dry place away from reach of children.

Missed dose
Take as soon as you remember. If your next dose is due within 3 hours, take a single dose now and skip the next.

Stopping the drug
Do not stop the drug without consulting your physician; symptoms may recur.

Exceeding the dose
An occasional unintentional extra dose is unlikely to cause problems. Large doses may cause unusual drowsiness. Notify your physician.

SPECIAL PRECAUTIONS

Be sure to tell your physician if:
▼ You have had epileptic seizures.
▼ You have impaired kidney or liver function.
▼ You have heart disease or are recovering from a recent heart attack.
▼ You are taking other medications.

Pregnancy
▼ Not usually prescribed. Safety in pregnancy not established. Discuss with your physician so that you may weigh the benefits of the drug against its possible risks.

Breast feeding
▼ The drug passes into the breast milk but at normal doses adverse effects on the baby are uncommon. Discuss with your physician.

Infants and children
▼ Not recommended.

Over 60
▼ Reduced dose necessary. Increased likelihood of adverse effects.

Driving and hazardous work
▼ Avoid such activities until you have learned how the drug affects you, because the drug can cause drowsiness.

Alcohol
▼ Avoid. Alcohol may increase the sedative effects of this drug.

POSSIBLE ADVERSE EFFECTS

Trazodone has fewer common adverse effects than some of the other antidepressants, mainly because it has a much weaker *anticholinergic* action.

Symptom/effect	Frequency		Discuss with physician		Stop taking drug now	Call physician now
	Common	Rare	Only if severe	In all cases		
Drowsiness	●		■			
Constipation		●	■			
Dry mouth		●	■			
Dizziness/fainting		●		■		
Headache		●		■		
Rash		●		■	▲	
Painful/prolonged erection		●		■	▲	■

INTERACTIONS

Antihypertensive drugs Trazodone opposes the actions of some of these drugs, especially guanethidine and clonidine, resulting in a reduction in their antihypertensive effect.

Alcohol The sedative and toxic effects of trazodone may be increased by alcohol.

Sedatives All drugs that have a sedative effect on the central nervous system are likely to increase the sedative properties of trazodone. Such drugs include antihistamines, sleeping drugs, narcotic analgesics, and antipsychotics.

PROLONGED USE

No problems expected.

TRETINOIN

Brand name Retin-A
Used in the following combined preparations None

GENERAL INFORMATION

Introduced in 1973, tretinoin is an anti-acne drug that is chemically related to vitamin A. It is available in various skin preparations. Tretinoin works by loosening the outer layers of skin, speeding up the process of skin renewal. This also makes it a useful treatment for certain other skin disorders in which the skin thickens abnormally, causing scaling.

Given for acne, tretinoin generally produces an improvement within three to four months, although there may be apparent worsening of the condition in the first few weeks of treatment.

Serious adverse *systemic* effects do not occur with tretinoin, but it sometimes causes skin irritation and peeling, particularly if overused. Excessive washing and exposure to sunlight may aggravate any irritation and lead to sunburn.

If excessive irritation occurs, a reduction in the frequency of application or strength of formulation may be advised.

INFORMATION FOR USERS

Your drug prescription is tailored for you. Do not alter dosage without checking with your physician.

How taken

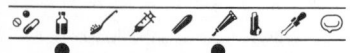

Liquid, gel, cream.

Frequency and timing of doses
Apply to dry, clean skin once daily at bedtime, 15 – 30 minutes after washing.

Dosage range
Apply to cover affected area lightly. Avoid contact with eyes, lips and nostril area.

Onset of effect
2 – 3 weeks. Maximum improvement may not be apparent for 8 – 12 weeks. Acne may worsen during the first 2 – 3 weeks of treatment in some people.

Duration of action
Effects may persist for several weeks after the drug has been stopped.

Diet advice
None.

Storage
Keep in a closed container in a cool, dry place away from reach of children. Protect from light.

Missed dose
Do not apply the missed dose. Apply your next dose as usual.

Stopping the drug
The drug can be safely stopped as soon as you no longer need it.

Exceeding the dose
A single extra application is unlikely to cause problems. Regular overuse may cause redness, stinging, or peeling of skin.

POSSIBLE ADVERSE EFFECTS

Application of tretinoin may cause temporary burning or stinging. Redness, peeling of the skin, and sometimes blistering, crusting, or swelling may occur with overuse, but generally clear up if the treatment is stopped temporarily or its use is reduced. Bleaching or darkening of the skin occurs rarely, and usually disappears when the drug is stopped.

Symptom/effect	Frequency		Discuss with physician		Stop taking drug now	Call physician now
	Common	Rare	Only if severe	In all cases		
Stinging/redness	●		■			
Peeling of the skin	●		■			
Sensitivity of skin to sunlight	●		■			
Bleaching or darkening of skin	●			■		
Blistering/crusting/swelling	●			■	▲	■

INTERACTIONS

Skin-drying preparations Medicated cosmetics, soaps, toiletries, and anti-acne preparations increase the likelihood of dryness and irritation of the skin with tretinoin.

SPECIAL PRECAUTIONS

Be sure to tell your physician if:
▼ You have eczema.
▼ Your skin is sensitive to sunlight.
▼ You have sunburn.
▼ You are taking other medications.

Pregnancy
▼ Not usually prescribed. Safety in pregnancy not established. Discuss with your physician so that you may weigh the benefits of the drug against its possible risks.

Breast feeding
▼ No evidence of risk.

Infants and children
▼ Not usually prescribed.

Over 60
▼ Not usually required.

Driving and hazardous work
▼ No known problems.

Alcohol
▼ No known problems.

PROLONGED USE

No special problems.

TRIAMCINOLONE

Brand names Aristocort , Aristocort Forte, Aristospan, Azmacort, Kenalog
Used in the following combined preparations Mycolog II, Myco-Triacet

GENERAL INFORMATION

Triamcinolone, introduced in 1958, is a corticosteroid with a wide variety of uses and forms. It comes in *topical* preparations for dermatitis, eczema, and psoriasis. There is a dental paste for mouth and gum inflammation, an inhalant for asthmatics. Taken orally, it can correct corticosteroid hormone deficiency caused by pituitary or adrenal gland disorders. Injected into the affected joints, it relieves rheumatoid arthritis and other forms of inflamma-

tion. Triamcinolone is also prescribed for certain blood disorders, such as thrombocytopenia and leukemia.

As with other corticosteroids, low doses taken by mouth over a short term or topical applications rarely cause side effects. However, long-term treatment, or large doses by mouth or injection, can cause indigestion, fluid retention, mood changes, acne, and muscle weakness. The drug may also induce diabetes.

QUICK REFERENCE

Drug group Corticosteroid (p.169)
Overdose danger rating Low
Dependence rating Low
Prescription needed Yes
Available as generic Yes

INFORMATION FOR USERS

Your drug prescription is tailored for you. Do not alter dosage without checking with your physician.

How taken

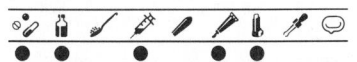

Tablets, syrup, injection, cream, ointment, dental paste, aerosol, inhaler.

Frequency and timing of doses
1 – 4 x daily (by mouth); 3 – 4 x daily (inhaler); 2 – 4 x daily (topically); 2 – 3 x daily after meals and at bedtime (dental paste); every 3 – 4 weeks (injection).

Dosage range
Considerable variation. Follow your physician's instructions.

Onset of effect
This may vary between a day and several weeks, depending on the condition.

Duration of action
Several days.

Diet advice
A low-sodium, high-potassium diet is recommended when the oral form of the drug is prescribed for extended periods. Follow the advice of your physician.

Storage
Keep in a closed container in a cool, dry place away from reach of children. Protect from light.

Missed dose
Take as soon as you remember. If your next dose is due at this time, double the usual dose to make up the missed dose.

Stopping the drug
Do not stop tablets without consulting your physician. Abrupt cessation after long-term treatment may cause adrenal collapse.

Exceeding the dose
An occasional unintentional extra dose is unlikely to be a cause for concern. But if you notice unusual symptoms, or if a large overdose has been taken, notify your physician.

SPECIAL PRECAUTIONS

Be sure to tell your physician if:
▼ You suffer from depression.
▼ You have or have had a herpes infection.
▼ You have a peptic ulcer.
▼ You have had tuberculosis.
▼ You have high blood pressure.
▼ You have diabetes.
▼ You have had glaucoma.
▼ You are taking other medications.

Pregnancy
▼ No evidence of risk with ointment, aerosol, or joint injections. Prescribed by mouth in low doses, harm to the baby is unlikely. Discuss with your physician so that you may weigh the benefits of the drug against its possible risks.

Breast feeding
▼ No evidence of risk with ointment, aerosol, or joint injections. Taken by mouth, the drug passes into the breast milk. Discuss with your physician.

Infants and children
▼ Reduced dose necessary.

Over 60
▼ Reduced dose may be necessary. Increased likelihood of adverse effects.

Driving and hazardous work
▼ Avoid such activities until you have learned how the drug affects you, because high doses by mouth can cause euphoria and make these activities unsafe.

Alcohol
▼ No known problems.

POSSIBLE ADVERSE EFFECTS

The more serious adverse effects usually occur only when triamcinolone is taken by mouth. *Topical* preparations are highly unlikely to cause any problems.

Symptom/effect	Frequency		Discuss with physician		Stop taking drug now	Call physician now
	Common	Rare	Only if severe	In all cases		
Indigestion	●		■			
Weight gain/acne	●		■			
Muscle weakness		●			■	
Mood changes		●			■	

INTERACTIONS

Digoxin Triamcinolone may increase the risk of adverse effects from digoxin.

Oral anticoagulant drugs Triamcinolone increases blood clotting.

Vaccines Serious reactions can occur when vaccinations are given during triamcinolone treatment. Discuss with your physician.

Insulin and antidiabetic drugs Triamcinolone by mouth or injection reduces the actions of these drugs.

Antihypertensive drugs Triamcinolone by mouth or injection may reduce the effect of antihypertensive drugs.

PROLONGED USE

Prolonged use of triamcinolone by mouth or injection can lead to adverse effects such as diabetes, glaucoma, cataracts, and bone damage, and may retard growth in children.

A
B
C
D
E
F
G
H
I
J
K
L
M
N
O
P
Q
R
S
T
U
V
W
X
Y
Z

TRIAMTERENE

Brand name Dyrenium
Used in the following combined preparations Dyazide, Maxzide

GENERAL INFORMATION

Triamterene, introduced in 1964, belongs to the class of drugs known as potassium-sparing diuretics. In combination with thiazide or loop diuretics, it is used in the treatment of hypertension and edema (fluid retention). On its own, or more commonly in combination with a thiazide diuretic, it may be used to treat edema as a complication of heart failure, nephrotic syndrome, or cirrhosis of the liver.

Triamterene is quick to act; its effect on urine flow is apparent within two hours. For this reason, avoid taking it after about 4 p.m. As with other potassium-sparing diuretics, there is a risk of unusually high levels of potassium building up in the blood if the kidneys are functioning abnormally. Consequently, triamterene is prescribed with caution for people with kidney failure.

QUICK REFERENCE

Drug group Potassium-sparing diuretic (p.127)

Overdose danger rating Low

Dependence rating Low

Prescription needed Yes

Available as generic No

INFORMATION FOR USERS

Your drug prescription is tailored for you. Do not alter dosage without checking with your physician.

How taken

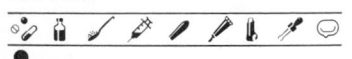

Tablets.

Frequency and timing of doses
1 – 2 x daily after meals.

Dosage range
100 – 300mg daily.

Onset of effect
Within 2 hours.

Duration of action
9 – 12 hours.

Diet advice
Avoid foods that are high in potassium, e.g. dried fruit, low-sodium milk, and salt substitutes.

Storage
Keep in a closed container in a cool, dry place away from reach of children.

Missed dose
Take as soon as you remember. However, if it is late in the day, do not take the missed dose, or you may need to get up at night to pass urine. Take the next scheduled dose as usual.

Stopping the drug
Do not stop the drug without consulting your physician; symptoms may recur.

Exceeding the dose
An occasional unintentional extra dose is unlikely to be a cause for concern. But if you notice unusual symptoms, or if a large overdose has been taken, notify your physician.

SPECIAL PRECAUTIONS

Be sure to tell your physician if:
▼ You have impaired kidney or liver function.
▼ You have had kidney stones.
▼ You are taking other medications.

Pregnancy
▼ Not usually prescribed. May cause a reduction in the blood supply to the developing baby. Discuss with your physician so that you may weigh the benefits of the drug against its risks.

Breast feeding
▼ Discuss with your physician. The drug passes into the breast milk and could also reduce your milk supply.

Infants and children
▼ Not usually prescribed. Reduced dose necessary.

Over 60
▼ Reduced dose may be necessary. Increased likelihood of adverse effects.

Driving and hazardous work
▼ No special problems.

Alcohol
▼ No known problems.

POSSIBLE ADVERSE EFFECTS

Triamterene has few adverse effects; the main problem is the possibility that potassium may be retained by the body, causing muscle weakness and numbness.

Symptom/effect	Frequency		Discuss with physician		Stop taking drug now	Call physician now
	Common	Rare	Only if severe	In all cases		
Digestive disturbance		●	■			
Lethargy		●	■			
Muscle weakness		●		■		
Rash		●		■		

INTERACTIONS

Lithium Triamterene may increase the blood levels of lithium, leading to an increased risk of lithium poisoning.

PROLONGED USE

Serious problems are unlikely, but levels of salts such as sodium and potassium may occasionally become disrupted during prolonged use.

Monitoring Blood tests may be performed to check on kidney function and levels of body salts.

TRIAZOLAM

Brand name Halcion
Used in the following combined preparations None

GENERAL INFORMATION

Triazolam was introduced in 1983, a member of a group of drugs known as the benzodiazepines. These drugs help to relieve nervousness and tension, relax muscles, and encourage sleep. Their actions and effects are described more fully on p.111.

Triazolam is used in the short-term treatment of insomnia. Because it has a relatively rapid onset and a short duration of action, it is less likely than some of the other benzodiazepines to cause drowsiness the following day. This makes it especially useful for people who need to drive or operate dangerous machinery.

In common with other benzodiazepines, triazolam can be habit-forming if taken regularly over a long period. Its effects may also become weaker with time. For these reasons, treatment with triazolam is regularly reviewed.

QUICK REFERENCE

Drug group Benzodiazepine sleeping drug (p.110)

Overdose danger rating Medium

Dependence rating Medium

Prescription needed Yes CIV

Available as generic No

INFORMATION FOR USERS

Your drug prescription is tailored for you. Do not alter dosage without checking with your physician.

How taken

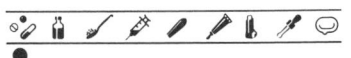

Tablets.

Frequency and timing of doses
Once daily 30 minutes before bedtime.

Adult dosage range
0.25 – 0.5mg daily.

Onset of effect
20 – 30 minutes.

Duration of action
4 – 6 hours.

Diet advice
None.

Storage
Keep in a closed container in a cool, dry place away from reach of children.

Missed dose
If you fall asleep without having taken a dose and wake some hours later, do not take the missed dose. If necessary, return to your normal dose schedule the next night.

Stopping the drug
If you have been taking the drug continuously for less than 2 weeks, it can be safely stopped as soon as you feel you no longer need it. However, if you have been taking the drug for longer, consult your physician, who may supervise a gradual reduction in dosage. Stopping abruptly may lead to withdrawal symptoms (see p.110).

Exceeding the dose
An occasional, unintentional extra dose is unlikely to cause problems. Large overdoses may cause unusual drowsiness. Notify your physician.

SPECIAL PRECAUTIONS

Be sure to tell your physician if
▼ You have impaired kidney or liver function.
▼ You have had problems with alcohol or drug abuse.
▼ You are taking other medications.

Pregnancy
▼ Not usually prescribed. Safety in pregnancy not established. Discuss with your physician so that you can weigh the benefits of the drug against its possible risks.

Breast feeding
▼ Discuss with your physician. The drug passes into the breast milk and may affect the baby adversely.

Infants and children
▼ Not usually prescribed. Reduced dose necessary.

Over 60
▼ Reduced dose may be necessary. Increased likelihood of adverse effects.

Driving and hazardous work
▼ Avoid such activities until you have learned how the drug affects you, because the drug can cause reduced alertness and slowed reactions.

Alcohol
▼ Avoid. Alcohol increases the sedative effects of this drug.

POSSIBLE ADVERSE EFFECTS

The principal adverse effects of this drug are related to its sedative and tranquilizing properties. These effects normally diminish after the first few days of treatment.

Symptom/effect	Frequency		Discuss with physician		Stop taking drug now	Call physician now
	Common	Rare	Only if severe	In all cases		
Daytime/drowsiness	●		■			
Dizziness/unsteadiness	●		■			
Blurred vision		●	■			
Forgetfulness/confusion		●	■			
Headache		●	■			
Rash		●		■	▲	

PROLONGED USE

Regular use of this drug over several weeks can lead to a reduction in its effect as the body adapts. It may also be habit-forming when taken for extended periods, especially if larger than average doses are taken.

INTERACTIONS

Sedatives All drugs that have a sedative effect on the central nervous system are likely to increase the sedative properties of triazolam. Such drugs include other anti-anxiety and sleeping drugs, antihistamines, antidepressants, narcotic analgesics, and antipsychotics.

Alcohol The sedative effect of triazolam is increased by alcohol.

TRIFLURIDINE

Brand name Viroptic
Used in the following combined preparations None

GENERAL INFORMATION

Trifluridine is a relatively recent antiviral eye medicine, administered in the form of eye drops. It is effective against superficial infections of the conjunctiva and cornea caused by the herpes simplex virus, types I and II. It may be prescribed for infections that have failed to clear up after treatment with other antiviral agents.

Dendritic keratitis, a spreading ulceration of the cornea, may heal more quickly with trifluridine than with other similar drugs. Given together with corticosteroids, trifluridine may also be used to treat deep herpes simplex eye infections and to prevent herpes virus infections activated by corticosteroid treatment for other diseases of the eye.

Serious toxicity is rare with trifluridine, but the risk is increased with prolonged treatment, overuse, and use in people with dry-eye syndromes. Courses of treatment are usually less than 21 days, and the prescribed dose should not be exceeded.

QUICK REFERENCE

Drug group Antiviral drug (p.161)
Overdose danger rating Low
Dependence rating Low
Prescription needed Yes
Available as generic No

INFORMATION FOR USERS

Your drug prescription is tailored for you. Do not alter dosage without checking with your physician.

How taken

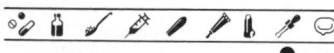

Eye drops.

Frequency and timing of doses
Every 2 – 4 hours.

Dosage range
1 drop every 2 hours while awake, up to 9 drops daily (starting dose). After complete healing, 1 drop every 4 hours while awake (minimum, 5 drops daily) for a further 7 days.

Onset of effect
Within 5 days.

Duration of action
A few hours after each application.

Diet advice
None.

Storage
Keep under refrigeration in a closed container away from reach of children.

Missed dose
Do not take the missed dose. Take your next dose as usual.

Stopping the drug
Take for 7 days after symptoms disappear, since the original infection may still be active, and symptoms may recur if treatment is stopped too soon.

Exceeding the dose
An occasional unintentional extra dose is unlikely to be a cause for concern. But if you notice unusual symptoms, or if a large overdose has been taken, notify your physician.

SPECIAL PRECAUTIONS

Pregnancy
▼ No evidence of risk to developing baby if used as eye drops.

Breast feeding
▼ No evidence of risk if used as eye drops.

Infants and children
▼ No special problems.

Over 60
▼ No special problems.

Driving and hazardous work
▼ No known problems.

Alcohol
▼ No known problems.

POSSIBLE ADVERSE EFFECTS

Stinging or burning may occur, but usually diminish as treatment continues. If swelling or signs of allergy such as itching or redness occur, consult your physician.

Symptom/effect	Frequency		Discuss with physician		Stop taking drug now	Call physician now
	Common	Rare	Only if severe	In all cases		
Burning/stinging eyes	●		■			
Swollen/painful eyelids		●		■		
Dry eyes		●		■		
Itching/redness		●		■	▲	

INTERACTIONS

None.

PROLONGED USE

Rarely required. Treatment should not be continued for more than 21 days except on the advice of your physician.

TRIHEXYPHENIDYL

Brand names Artane, Tremin, Trihexane
Used in the following combined preparations None

GENERAL INFORMATION

Trihexyphenidyl is an *anticholinergic* drug that was introduced for the treatment of Parkinson's disease in the 1940s. It continues to be widely used, especially in the early stages of the disease. It is particularly effective for relieving rigidity and tremor, but has little effect on the shuffling gait and slow muscular movements that are also characteristic of Parkinson's disease. For further information on antiparkinsonism drugs, see p.115. Trihexyphenidyl is also occasionally used to counter the adverse effects of antipsychotic drugs (p.113).

Like all anticholinergic drugs, trihexyphenidyl can cause a variety of adverse effects (see below). These symptoms have to be balanced against the benefits of the drug.

QUICK REFERENCE

Drug group Anticholinergic antiparkinsonism drug (p.115)

Overdose danger rating Medium

Dependence rating Low

Prescription needed Yes

Available as generic Yes

INFORMATION FOR USERS

Your drug prescription is tailored for you. Do not alter dosage without checking with your physician.

How taken

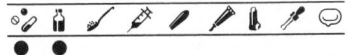

● ●

Tablets, capsules, liquid.

Frequency and timing of doses
2 – 3 x daily.

Adult dosage range
4 – 15mg daily. Larger doses may occasionally be needed.

Onset of effect
Within 30 minutes.

Duration of action
3 – 8 hours.

Diet advice
None.

Storage
Keep in a closed container in a cool, dry place away from reach of children.

Missed dose
Take as soon as you remember. If your next dose is due within 2 hours, take a single dose now and skip the next.

Stopping the drug
Do not stop taking the drug without consulting your physician; symptoms may recur. A gradual reduction in dosage is usually necessary.

Exceeding the dose
An occasional unintentional extra dose is unlikely to cause problems. Large overdoses may cause an increase in heart rate and agitation. Notify your physician.

SPECIAL PRECAUTIONS

Be sure to tell your physician if:
▼ You have high blood pressure.
▼ You have had glaucoma.
▼ You have heart problems.
▼ You have had prostate trouble.
▼ You have impaired liver or kidney function.
▼ You are taking other medications.

 Pregnancy
▼ Not usually prescribed. Safety in pregnancy not established.

 Breast feeding
▼ Unlikely to be required.

 Infants and children
▼ Not recommended.

 Over 60
▼ Sensitivity to this drug is likely to increase with age, requiring lower dosages. Regular monitoring is necessary.

 Driving and hazardous work
▼ Avoid such activities until you have learned how the drug affects you, because the drug can cause blurred vision and confusion.

 Alcohol
▼ Avoid. Alcohol may increase the sedative effects of this drug.

POSSIBLE ADVERSE EFFECTS

Most of the adverse effects of this drug are the result of its *anticholinergic* action. The severity of such effects can sometimes be reduced by adjustment of dosage.

Symptom/effect	Frequency		Discuss with physician		Stop taking drug now	Call physician now
	Common	Rare	Only if severe	In all cases		
Dry mouth/eyes	●		■			
Difficulty in passing urine	●		■			
Constipation	●		■			
Nervousness	●		■			
Blurred vision	●			■		
Confusion		●		■		
Nausea/vomiting		●		■		
Rash		●		■		
Palpitations		●		■		

PROLONGED USE

Sensitivity to this drug can develop during prolonged use, especially in the elderly, and dosage may need to be reduced periodically. Occasionally prolonged trihexyphenidyl treatment may cause abnormal movements of the face and limbs, or provoke the onset of glaucoma.

Monitoring Regular eye examinations are usually carried out to ensure that glaucoma is not developing.

INTERACTIONS

Antihistamines and anticholinergic drugs The effects of such drugs are likely to be increased by trihexyphenidyl.

Alcohol The effects of alcohol are increased when taken with this drug.

Phenothiazine antipsychotic drugs Trihexyphenidyl may increase some of the adverse effects of these drugs.

A B C D E F G H I J K L M N O P Q R S T U V W X Y Z

TRIMEPRAZINE

Brand name Temaril
Used in the following combined preparations None

GENERAL INFORMATION

Trimeprazine, an antihistamine introduced in 1958, is chemically similar to the phenothiazine antipsychotic drugs (p.113). Like other antihistamines, it prevents or reduces the response to histamine, a substance released from cells during an allergic reaction. It also causes more marked drowsiness than many other antihistamines.

Taken by mouth, it is used mainly to relieve itching in urticaria (hives) and other allergic skin conditions, such as eczema. The sedative effect of the drug is often helpful in severe itching, particularly when it is taken at bedtime. It is also sometimes used to sedate children before undergoing surgery or other medical procedures.

INFORMATION FOR USERS

Your drug prescription is tailored for you. Do not alter dosage without checking with your physician.

How taken

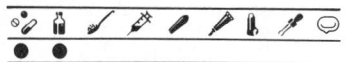

Tablets, slow-release capsules, liquid.

Frequency and timing of doses
3 – 4 x daily (tablets, liquid); 2 x daily (slow-release capsules).

Dosage range
Adults 10mg daily.
Children Reduced dose according to age and weight.

Onset of effect
15 – 60 minutes.

Duration of action
Up to 8 hours (tablets, liquid); up to 12 hours (slow-release capsules).

Diet advice
None.

Storage
Keep in a closed container in a cool, dry place away from reach of children.

Missed dose
Take as soon as you remember. If your next dose is due within 2 hours, take a single dose now and skip the next.

Stopping the drug
Can be safely stopped as soon as you no longer need it.

Exceeding the dose
An occasional unintentional extra dose is unlikely to cause problems. Large overdoses may cause drowsiness or agitation. Notify your physician.

POSSIBLE ADVERSE EFFECTS

Adverse effects are rarely serious and often wear off after a few days of continued use. Drowsiness is relatively common. Some side effects, such as dryness of the mouth, blurred vision, and urinary retention, are due to the *anticholinergic* effects of trimeprazine, and others such as shaking, tremor, and rigidity are parkinsonian side effects.

Symptom/effect	Frequency		Discuss with physician		Stop taking drug now	Call physician now
	Common	Rare	Only if severe	In all cases		
Drowsiness	●		■			
Digestive disturbances		●		■		
Urinary difficulties		●		■		
Dry mouth		●		■		
Blurred vision		●		■		
Excitation (in children)		●		■		
Shaking/tremor/rigidity		●		■		
Rash		●		■	▲	

INTERACTIONS

Sedatives All drugs having a sedative effect on the central nervous system are likely to enhance the sedative effect of trimeprazine.

Monoamine oxidase inhibitors (MAOIs) There is a risk of a dangerous rise in blood pressure if trimeprazine is taken with MAOIs.

Anticholinergic drugs The anticholinergic effects of trimeprazine are likely to be increased by all drugs that have anticholinergic effects.

SPECIAL PRECAUTIONS

Be sure to tell your physician if:
▼ You have impaired liver function.
▼ You have had epileptic seizures.
▼ You have urinary difficulties.
▼ You have Parkinson's disease.
▼ You have had glaucoma.
▼ You are taking other medications.

Pregnancy
▼ Not usually prescribed. Taken in late pregnancy, may cause jaundice in the newborn infant. Discuss with your physician so that you may weigh the benefits of the drug against its risks.

Breast feeding
▼ No evidence of risk to the baby.

Infants and children
▼ Not recommended in newborn or premature infants, children with sleep apnea (stopped breathing), or those from families with a history of sudden infant death syndrome (SIDS).

Over 60
▼ Reduced dose may be necessary. Increased likelihood of adverse effects.

Driving and hazardous work
▼ Avoid such activities until you have learned how the drug affects you, because the drug can cause drowsiness.

Alcohol
▼ Avoid. Alcohol may increase the sedative effects of this drug.

Surgery and general anesthetics
▼ If you have used the drug in the previous few hours and require an anesthetic, inform the anesthetist.

PROLONGED USE

No known problems.

TRIMETHOBENZAMIDE

Brand name Tigan
Used in the following combined preparations None

GENERAL INFORMATION

Trimethobenzamide, introduced in 1959, is chemically related to the anti-histamines and belongs to the group of drugs known as anti-emetics (p.118) that are used to suppress nausea and vomiting. It is thought to inhibit signals in the vomiting center of the brain.

It may be given after surgery and to suppress vomiting from gastroenteritis or from the side effects of radiation treatment. It has very limited effectiveness in the treatment of motion sickness, dizziness, and the vomiting produced by anticancer drugs.

Trimethobenzamide is not normally given to children with suspected viral infections, since it may contribute to the development of Reye's syndrome, a potentially fatal disorder of the brain and liver.

QUICK REFERENCE

Drug group Anti-emetic drug (p.118)
Overdose danger rating Medium
Dependence rating Low
Prescription needed Yes
Available as generic Yes

INFORMATION FOR USERS

Your drug prescription is tailored for you. Do not alter dosage without checking with your physician.

How taken

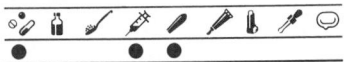

Capsules, injection, suppositories.

Frequency and timing of doses
3 – 4 x daily.

Dosage range
750mg – 1g daily (capsules); 600 – 800mg daily (suppositories, injection).

Onset of effect
Within 10 – 40 minutes.

Duration of action
2 – 4 hours.

Diet advice
None.

Storage
Keep in a closed container in a cool, dry place away from reach of children.

Missed dose
Take as soon as you remember. If your next dose is due within 2 hours, take a single dose now and skip the next.

Stopping the drug
Can be safely stopped as soon as you no longer need it.

Exceeding the dose
An occasional unintentional extra dose is unlikely to cause problems. Large overdoses may cause unusual drowsiness, agitation, dizziness, diarrhea, or muscle spasms. Notify your physician.

SPECIAL PRECAUTIONS

Be sure to tell your physician if:
▼ You have had a flu-like illness in the past week.
▼ You have a high fever.
▼ You have Parkinson's disease.
▼ You have prostate trouble.
▼ You have had glaucoma.
▼ You are taking other medications.

Pregnancy
▼ Not usually prescribed. Safety in pregnancy not established. Discuss with your physician so that you can weigh the benefits of the drug against its possible risks.

Breast feeding
▼ Discuss with your physician. The drug passes into the breast milk and may affect the baby adversely.

Infants and children
▼ Reduced dose necessary.

Over 60
▼ Increased likelihood of adverse effects.

Driving and hazardous work
▼ Avoid such activities until you have learned how the drug affects you, because the drug can cause drowsiness and blurred vision.

Alcohol
▼ Avoid. Alcohol may increase the adverse effects of this drug.

POSSIBLE ADVERSE EFFECTS

Adverse effects other than drowsiness are uncommon when trimethobenzamide is used at normal doses.

Symptom/effect	Frequency		Discuss with physician		Stop taking drug now	Call physician now
	Common	Rare	Only if severe	In all cases		
Drowsiness	●		■			
Blurred vision		●	■			
Muscle cramps		●	■			
Diarrhea		●	■			
Tremor		●		■	▲	
Rash		●		■	▲	
Jaundice		●		■	▲	

INTERACTIONS

Sedatives Trimethobenzamide may add to the effect of drugs that have a sedative effect on the central nervous system. Such drugs include sleeping drugs, narcotic analgesics, anti-anxiety drugs, antidepressants, and antipsychotics.

Drugs that may impair hearing Trimethobenzamide may mask hearing loss caused by drugs such as cisplatin, aspirin, and aspirin-related drugs.

PROLONGED USE

No special problems.

TRIMETHOPRIM

Brand names Proloprim, Trimpex
Used in the following combined preparations Bactrim, Septra

GENERAL INFORMATION

Trimethoprim, introduced in 1967, is an antibacterial drug prescribed for a wide variety of infections. On its own, trimethoprim is most commonly prescribed for the prevention and treatment of urinary tract infections. It is also effective in prostatitis and is occasionally used to treat certain types of gastroenteritis.

Trimethoprim is often prescribed in a combined preparation with another antibacterial drug, sulfamethoxazole. In addition to the infections mentioned, the combination is used for a variety of infections of the respiratory tract, gastrointestinal tract, and ear. Pneumocystis infections and gonorrhea may also be treated with this combined preparation.

The main advantage of trimethoprim alone is that it causes fewer side effects than when combined with sulfamethoxazole. It can also be taken safely by people with poor kidney function. The most common side effects of trimethoprim are rash and itching.

QUICK REFERENCE

Drug group Antibacterial drug (p.159)

Overdose danger rating Low

Dependence rating Low

Prescription needed Yes

Available as generic Yes

INFORMATION FOR USERS

Your drug prescription is tailored for you. Do not alter dosage without checking with your physician.

How taken

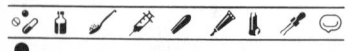

Tablets.

Frequency and timing of doses
1 – 2 x daily.

Adult dosage range
Urinary tract infections 100 – 200mg daily (treatment).
Prostatitis 400mg daily.
Gastroenteritis 400mg daily (treatment); 200mg daily (prevention).

Onset of effect
1 – 4 hours.

Duration of action
12 hours.

Diet advice
None.

Storage
Keep in a closed container in a cool, dry place away from reach of children. Protect from light.

Missed dose
Take as soon as you remember. If your next dose is due at this time, double the usual dose to make up the missed dose.

Stopping the drug
Take the full course. Even if you feel better, the original infection may still be present and symptoms may recur if treatment is stopped too soon.

Exceeding the dose
An occasional unintentional extra dose is unlikely to be a cause for concern. But if you notice unusual symptoms, or if a large overdose has been taken, notify your physician.

SPECIAL PRECAUTIONS

Be sure to tell your physician if:
▼ You have impaired liver or kidney function.
▼ You have a blood disorder.

Pregnancy
▼ Not usually prescribed. Safety in pregnancy not established. Discuss with your physician so that you can weigh the benefits of the drug against its possible risks.

Breast feeding
▼ Discuss with your physician. The drug passes into the breast milk and may affect the baby adversely.

Infants and children
▼ Not recommended for infants under 2 months old. Reduced dose necessary for older children.

Over 60
▼ No special problems.

Driving and hazardous work
▼ No known problems.

Alcohol
▼ No known problems.

POSSIBLE ADVERSE EFFECTS

Trimethoprim taken on its own rarely causes side effects, the most common being rash and itching. However, additional adverse effects of the drug sulfamethoxazole may occur when trimethoprim is taken in combination with this drug.

Symptom/effect	Frequency		Discuss with physician		Stop taking drug now	Call physician now
	Common	Rare	Only if severe	In all cases		
Rash/itching	●			■		
Nausea/vomiting		●	■			
Diarrhea		●	■			
Sore tongue		●	■			

INTERACTIONS

None.

PROLONGED USE

Long-term use of this drug may lead to folate deficiency, which in turn may lead to blood abnormalities. Folate supplements may be prescribed.

Monitoring Periodic blood tests to monitor blood composition are usually required.

TRIPROLIDINE

Brand names Actidil, Myidil
Used in the following combined preparations Actifed, Actifed with Codeine, Allerfrin, Triphed

GENERAL INFORMATION

Triprolidine, introduced in 1958, is an antihistamine used in the treatment of allergies such as hay fever and urticaria (hives). It is also a common ingredient of cough and cold remedies.

Like other antihistamines, it reduces sneezing, itching, runny eyes and nose, and other nasal discomforts. Its effect on the nose is enhanced by a mild *anticholinergic* drying action that helps relieve congestion by suppressing mucous secretion.

Taken for allergic skin conditions, it relieves itching, swelling, and redness. If itching is severe, however, an antihistamine with a stronger sedative effect may be more helpful.

Occasionally, the drug may be used to treat or prevent allergic reactions to blood transfusions or certain foods.

QUICK REFERENCE

Drug group Antihistamine (p.152)
Overdose danger rating Medium
Dependence rating Low
Prescription needed No
Available as generic Yes

INFORMATION FOR USERS

Follow instructions on the label. Call your physician if symptoms worsen.

How taken

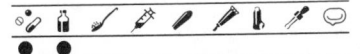

Tablets, liquid.

Frequency and timing of doses
3 – 4 x daily.

Dosage range
Adults 7.5 – 10mg daily.
Children 6 –12 years 3.75 – 5mg daily; *under 6 years* 0.9 – 2.4mg daily (liquid), depending on age.

Onset of effect
Within 1 hour.

Duration of action
6 – 8 hours.

Diet advice
None.

Storage
Keep in a closed container in a cool, dry place away from reach of children. Protect from light.

Missed dose
Take as soon as you remember. If your next dose is due within 4 hours, take a single dose now and skip the next.

Stopping the drug
Can be safely stopped as soon as you no longer need it.

Exceeding the dose
An occasional unintentional extra dose is unlikely to cause problems. Large overdoses may cause drowsiness or agitation. Notify your physician.

POSSIBLE ADVERSE EFFECTS

Drowsiness is the most common effect. Other side effects are rare. Some of these, such as dry mouth and blurred vision, are due to its anticholinergic action.

Symptom/effect	Frequency		Discuss with physician		Stop taking drug now	Call physician now
	Common	Rare	Only if severe	In all cases		
Drowsiness	●		■			
Dry mouth		●	■			
Dizziness/incoordination		●	■			
Difficulty passing urine		●	■			
Hyperactivity (children)		●		■		▲

INTERACTIONS

Sedatives All drugs that have a sedative effect on the central nervous system are likely to enhance the sedative effect of triprolidine.

Monoamine oxidase inhibitors (MAOIs) There is a risk of a dangerous rise in blood pressure if triprolidine is taken within 14 days of MAOI treatment.

Anticholinergic drugs The anticholinergic effects of triprolidine are likely to be increased by all drugs that have anticholinergic effects, including antispasmodics, antipsychotics, tricyclic antidepressants and some antiparkinsonism drugs.

SPECIAL PRECAUTIONS

Be sure to tell your physician before taking this drug if:
▼ You have impaired liver function.
▼ You have glaucoma.
▼ You have had epileptic seizures.
▼ You have difficulty passing urine.
▼ You are taking other medications.

Pregnancy
▼ No evidence of risk to developing baby.

Breast feeding
▼ Discuss with your physician. The drug passes into the breast milk and may affect the baby adversely.

Infants and children
▼ Not recommended for newborn or premature infants. Reduced dose necessary for older children.

Over 60
▼ Reduced dose necessary. Increased likelihood of adverse effects.

Driving and hazardous work
▼ Avoid such activities until you have learned how the drug affects you, because the drug can cause drowsiness.

Alcohol
▼ Avoid. Alcohol may increase the sedative effects of this drug.

PROLONGED USE

The effect of the drug may become weaker with prolonged use over a period of weeks or months as the body adapts. Transfer to a different antihistamine may be recommended.

VALPROIC ACID

Brand names Depakene, Depakote
Used in the following combined preparations None

GENERAL INFORMATION

Valproic acid was introduced in 1967. It is often used along with other anticonvulsant drugs for epilepsy when standard treatments have not been successful. Its action, however, is similar to that of other anticonvulsant drugs (see p. 114), reducing electrical discharges in the brain.

Beneficial in long-term treatment, it does not have a sedative effect. That makes it particularly suitable for children who suffer from atonic epilepsy (a sudden relaxing of the muscles throughout the body) or absence seizures (during which the person appears to be daydreaming).

QUICK REFERENCE

Drug group Anticonvulsant (p.114)
Overdose danger rating Medium
Dependency rating Low
Prescription needed Yes
Available as generic No

INFORMATION FOR USERS

Your drug prescription is tailored for you. Do not alter dosage without checking with your physician.

How taken

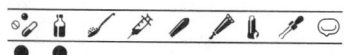

Tablets, liquid.

Frequency and timing of doses
2 x daily.

Dosage range
Dosage is calculated on an individual basis according to age and weight.

Onset of effect
Within 30 minutes.

Duration of action
12 hours or more.

Diet advice
None.

Storage
Keep in a tightly closed container in a cool, dry place away from reach of children.

Missed dose
Take as soon as you remember. If your next dose is due within 2 hours, take a single dose now and skip the next.

Stopping the drug
Do not stop the drug without consulting your physician; symptoms may recur.

Exceeding the dose
An occasional unintentional extra dose is unlikely to cause problems. Large overdoses may lead to coma. Notify your physician.

SPECIAL PRECAUTIONS

Be sure to tell your physician if:
▼ You have impaired kidney or liver function.
▼ You are taking other medications.

Pregnancy
▼ Not usually prescribed. May cause abnormalities in the unborn baby. Discuss with your physician so that you may weigh the benefits of the drug against its risks.

Breast feeding
▼ The drug passes into the breast milk, but at normal doses adverse effects on the baby are uncommon.

Infants and children
▼ Reduced dose necessary.

Over 60
▼ Reduced dose may be necessary

Driving and hazardous work
▼ Your underlying condition, as well as the possibility of reduced alertness while taking this drug, may make such activities inadvisable. Discuss with your physician.

Alcohol
▼ Avoid. Alcohol may reduce the effect of this drug and may cause deep sedation.

POSSIBLE ADVERSE EFFECTS

Most serious adverse effects of valproic acid are rare. They include liver failure, and platelet and bleeding abnormalities.

Symptom/effect	Frequency		Discuss with physician		Stop taking drug now	Call physician now
	Common	Rare	Only if severe	In all cases		
Abdominal discomfort		●	■			
Temporary loss of hair		●	■			
Weight gain		●	■			
Vomiting		●		■		
Drowsiness		●		■		
Jaundice		●		■	▲	
Rash		●		■	▲	

INTERACTIONS

Anticoagulant drugs Valproic acid can increase the effect of such drugs as warfarin and aspirin. The dose of the anticoagulant drug may need to be reduced.

Alcohol Alcohol may increase the level of the drug in the blood and produce heavy sedation.

Monoamine oxidase inhibitors (MAOIs) These may depress the central nervous system when taken with valproic acid. Dosage of the monoamine oxidase inhibitors should be adjusted accordingly.

PROLONGED USE

Use of this drug may cause liver damage, which is more likely in the first six months of use.

Monitoring Periodic checks on blood levels of the drug are usually required. Blood tests of liver function and blood composition may also be carried out.

VASOPRESSIN

Brand name Pitressin
Used in the following combined preparations None

GENERAL INFORMATION

Vasopressin, an antidiuretic hormone produced in the pituitary gland, controls the body's water balance. Synthesized and introduced as a drug in 1941, it is given for the treatment of diabetes insipidus, a disease caused by a deficiency of the natural diuretic hormone. It acts on the kidneys to increase water reabsorption, thereby reducing the volume of urine produced.

A long-acting form of the drug that can be given by injection every one to three days is usually most convenient for long-term treatment of the disease.

Short-acting vasopressin may be used for initial therapy and for close control of the water balance. Vasopressin is also given to try to control bleeding in the esophagus in people with cirrhosis of the liver.

At high doses, vasopressin may narrow the blood vessels and raise blood pressure. It may also stimulate contraction of muscles in the bowel wall, leading to colicky abdominal pain and diarrhea. Side effects are more likely to occur with the long-acting form of vasopressin.

QUICK REFERENCE

Drug group Drug for diabetes insipidus (p.173)

Overdose danger rating High

Dependence rating Low

Prescription needed Yes

Available as generic No

INFORMATION FOR USERS

Your drug prescription is tailored for you. Do not alter dosage without checking with your physician.

How taken

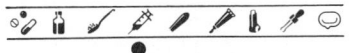

Injection.

Frequency and timing of doses
3 – 4 x daily (short-acting injection); every 1 – 3 days (long-acting injection).

Dosage range
Adults 5 – 10 units per dose (short-acting injection); 1.25 – 5 units per dose (long-acting injection).
Children Reduced dose necessary according to age and weight.

Onset of effect
Within a few minutes.

Duration of action
2 – 8 hours (short-acting injection); 24 – 72 hours (long-acting injection).

Diet advice
Your physician may advise you to reduce your fluid intake at the start of treatment.

Storage
Keep in a closed container in a cool, dry place away from reach of children.

Missed dose
Take as soon as you remember. Space your subsequent doses at equal intervals throughout the day.

Stopping the drug
Do not stop the drug without consulting your physician; symptoms may recur.

OVERDOSE ACTION

Seek immediate medical advice in all cases. Take emergency action if palpitations, vomiting, seizures, or loss of consciousness occurs.

See Drug poisoning emergency guide (p.590).

POSSIBLE ADVERSE EFFECTS

The drug may stimulate contractions of the bowel wall, causing nausea, abdominal cramps, and an increased urge to defecate.

Headache, drowsiness, and confusion may be signs of water retention. Chest pain may be due to angina.

Symptom/effect	Frequency		Discuss with physician		Stop taking drug now	Call physician now
	Common	Rare	Only if severe	In all cases		
Injection-site pain	●		■			
Nausea/abdominal pain	●		■			
Urge to defecate		●	■			
Headache		●		■	▲	∎
Drowsiness/confusion		●		■	▲	∎
Chest pain		●		■	▲	∎

INTERACTIONS

Lithium and norepinephrine These drugs may reduce the effect of vasopressin.

Chlorpropamide, clofibrate, and carbamazepine may increase the effect of vasopressin.

SPECIAL PRECAUTIONS

Be sure to tell your physician if:
▼ You have high blood pressure.
▼ You have heart problems.
▼ You have impaired kidney function.
▼ You have had seizures.
▼ You suffer from migraine.
▼ You suffer from asthma.
▼ You are taking other medications.

Pregnancy
▼ Not usually prescribed. Safety in pregnancy not established. Discuss with your physician so that you can weigh the benefits of the drug against its possible risks.

Breast feeding
▼ The drug may pass into the breast milk, but at normal doses adverse effects on the baby are uncommon. Discuss with your physician.

Infants and children
▼ Reduced dose necessary.

Over 60
▼ No special problems.

Driving and hazardous work
▼ No known problems.

Alcohol
▼ No known problems.

Surgery and general anesthetics
▼ Your treatment may need to be changed before you have a general anesthetic. Discuss this with your physician or dentist before any surgery.

PROLONGED USE

The duration of effect of the long-acting preparation of vasopressin may diminish with prolonged use in some people.

VERAPAMIL

Brand names Calan, Isoptin
Used in the following combined preparations None

GENERAL INFORMATION

Verapamil, introduced in 1981, belongs to a group of drugs known as calcium channel blockers, which interfere with the conduction of signals in the muscles of the heart and blood vessels. Used in the treatment of hypertension and arrhythmias, verapamil is also frequently given for angina. It reduces the frequency of attacks but does not, as other calcium channel blockers can, work quickly enough to help relieve pain while an attack is in progress. Verapamil increases your ability to tolerate physical exertion, and since it does not affect breathing, it can be used safely by asthmatics.

Because of its effects on the heart, verapamil is also prescribed for certain types of abnormal heart rhythm. For such disorders it can be given by injection as well as in tablet form.

It is not generally prescribed for people with low blood pressure, slow heartbeat, or heart failure, because it may make these conditions worse. It may be constipating.

INFORMATION FOR USERS

Your drug prescription is tailored for you. Do not alter dosage without checking with your physician.

How taken

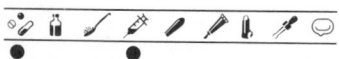

Tablets, injection.

Frequency and timing of doses
3 – 4 x daily. Slow-release tablets are taken 1 – 2 x daily.

Adult dosage range
240 – 480mg daily.

Onset of effect
1 – 2 hours (tablets); 2 – 3 minutes (injection).

Duration of action
6 – 8 hours. During prolonged treatment some beneficial effects may last for up to 12 hours. Slow-release tablets act for 12 – 24 hours.

Diet advice
None.

Storage
Keep in a closed container in a cool, dry place away from reach of children.

Missed dose
Take as soon as you remember. If your next dose is due within 2 hours, take a single dose now and skip the next.

Stopping the drug
Do not stop the drug without consulting your physician; symptoms may recur.

Exceeding the dose
An occasional unintentional extra dose is unlikely to be a cause for concern. Large overdoses may cause dizziness. Notify your physician.

SPECIAL PRECAUTIONS

Be sure to tell your physician if:
▼ You have impaired kidney or liver function.
▼ You have heart failure.
▼ You are taking beta blockers.
▼ You are taking other medications.

Pregnancy
▼ Not usually prescribed. Safety in pregnancy not established. Discuss with your physician so that you can weigh the benefits of the drug against its possible risks.

Breast feeding
▼ Discuss with your physician. The drug passes into the breast milk and may affect the baby adversely.

Infants and children
▼ Not recommended.

Over 60
▼ Reduced dose may be necessary. Increased likelihood of adverse effects.

Driving and hazardous work
▼ Avoid such activities until you have learned how the drug affects you, because the drug can cause dizziness.

Alcohol
▼ Avoid. Alcohol may further reduce blood pressure, causing dizziness or other symptoms.

POSSIBLE ADVERSE EFFECTS

Verapamil has fewer adverse effects than other calcium channel blockers, but it can still cause a variety of minor symptoms, such as constipation and headache.

Symptom/effect	Frequency		Discuss with physician		Stop taking drug now	Call physician now
	Common	Rare	Only if severe	In all cases		
Constipation	●		■			
Headache	●		■			
Nausea	●		■			
Ankle swelling	●		■			
Flushing		●	■			
Dizziness		●		■		

PROLONGED USE

No problems expected.

INTERACTIONS

Beta blockers When verapamil is taken with these drugs, there is a slight risk of abnormal heartbeats and heart failure. If these drugs are prescribed together, reduced doses are necessary.

Cimetidine Cimetidine increases the effects of verapamil.

Digoxin Blood levels and adverse effects of this drug may be increased if it is taken with verapamil. The dosage of digoxin may need to be reduced.

Antihypertensive drugs Blood pressure may be further lowered when these drugs are taken with verapamil.

WARFARIN

Brand names Coumadin, Panwarfin
Used in the following combined preparations None

GENERAL INFORMATION

Warfarin is an anticoagulant used to prevent blood clots, mainly in areas where the blood flow is at its slowest, particularly in the leg and pelvic veins. Such clots can break off and travel through the bloodstream to lodge in the lungs, where they cause pulmonary embolism. Warfarin is also used to reduce the risk of clots forming in the heart in people with atrial fibrillation, or after the insertion of artificial heart valves. These clots may travel in the arteries to the brain, where they could cause a stroke.

A widely used oral anticoagulant, warfarin requires regular monitoring to assure proper maintenance dosage. Because full beneficial effects of warfarin are not felt for 2 – 3 days, a faster-acting anticoagulant such as heparin is often used to complement its effects at the start of treatment.

Its most serious adverse effect, as with all anticoagulants, is the risk of excessive bleeding, usually from overdosage.

QUICK REFERENCE

Drug group Anticoagulant drug (p.132)

Overdose danger rating High

Dependence rating Low

Prescription needed Yes

Available as generic Yes

INFORMATION FOR USERS

Your drug prescription is tailored for you. Do not alter dosage without checking with your physician.

How taken

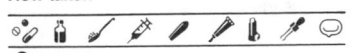

Tablets.

Frequency and timing of doses
Once daily, or less often.

Dosage range
Usually 15mg on the first day of treatment, 10mg on the second and third, and 2.5 – 7.5mg thereafter.

Onset of effect
Within 24 – 48 hours, with full effect after several days.

Duration of action
3 – 5 days.

Diet advice
A high-fiber diet helps to avoid constipation.

Storage
Keep in a closed container in a cool, dry place away from reach of children.

Missed dose
Take as soon as you remember. If your next dose is due within 4 hours, take both doses now and take the following dose on your original schedule.

Stopping the drug
Do not stop the drug without consulting your physician; stopping the drug may lead to worsening of the underlying condition.

OVERDOSE ACTION

 Seek immediate medical advice in all cases. Take emergency action if severe bleeding or loss of consciousness occurs.

See Drug poisoning emergency guide (p.590).

SPECIAL PRECAUTIONS

Be sure to tell your physician if:
▼ You have impaired kidney or liver function.
▼ You have high blood pressure.
▼ You have peptic ulcers.
▼ You bleed easily.
▼ You are taking other medications.

 Pregnancy
▼ Not usually prescribed. Given in early pregnancy the drug can cause malformations in the unborn child. Taken near the time of delivery, it may cause the mother to bleed excessively.

 Breast feeding
▼ Discuss with your physician. The drug passes into the breast milk and may affect the baby adversely.

 Infants and children
▼ Reduced dose necessary.

 Over 60
▼ No special problems.

 Driving and hazardous work
▼ Use caution. Even minor bumps can cause bad bruises and excessive bleeding.

 Alcohol
▼ Avoid. Alcohol may increase or decrease the effects of this drug.

Surgery and general anesthetics
▼ Warfarin may need to be stopped before surgery. Discuss with your physician or dentist. In an emergency, its effect can be reversed by giving vitamin K by injection or by giving fresh plasma.

POSSIBLE ADVERSE EFFECTS

Hemorrhaging is the most common adverse effect with warfarin. Any bruising, dark stools, dark urine, or unusual bleeding should be reported to your physician.

Symptom/effect	Frequency		Discuss with physician		Stop taking drug now	Call physician now
	Common	Rare	Only if severe	In all cases		
Nausea/vomiting	●		■			
Loss of appetite	●		■			
Bleeding	●			■	▲	▮
Abdominal pain/diarrhea		●		■		
Rash/bruising		●		■		
Hair loss		●		■		

INTERACTIONS

General note A wide variety of drugs interact with warfarin, either by increasing or decreasing the anticlotting effect. These include barbiturates, oral contraceptives, diuretics, laxatives, and antibiotics.

Aspirin When taken with warfarin, large daily doses of aspirin may significantly prolong or intensify its effect.

PROLONGED USE

No special problems.

XYLOMETAZOLINE

Brand names Neo-Synephrine II, Otrivin
Used in the following combined preparations None

GENERAL INFORMATION

Xylometazoline is a *sympathomimetic* nasal decongestant that can be bought over the counter to relieve a stuffy nose caused by colds, hay fever, or sinusitis. It works by constricting the small blood vessels in the nose, thereby reducing inflammation and swelling.

Because the effect of xylometazoline lasts for 4 to 6 hours, it needs to be used only two or three times daily. Using the drug more often than this will increase the likelihood of adverse effects such as headache, palpitations, and drowsiness. Nor should xylometazoline be taken for more than a few days at a time; this will make nasal congestion worse.

QUICK REFERENCE

Drug group Decongestant (p.121)
Overdose danger rating Medium
Dependence rating Low
Prescription needed No
Available as generic Yes

INFORMATION FOR USERS

Follow instructions on the label. Call your physician if symptoms worsen.

How taken

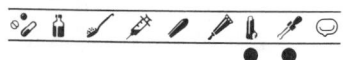

Spray, nose drops.

Frequency and timing of doses
As needed up to 3 x daily.

Dosage range
Adults and children over 12 years 2 – 3 drops or 1 – 2 sprays in each nostril (0.1 percent solution).
Children under 12 years 2 – 3 drops in each nostril (0.05 percent solution).

Onset of effect
Within 10 minutes.

Duration of action
Up to 6 hours.

Diet advice
None.

Storage
Keep in a closed container in a cool, dry place away from reach of children. Protect from light.

Missed dose
No cause for concern. Take only when needed.

Stopping the drug
Can be safely stopped as soon as you no longer need it.

Exceeding the dose
An occasional unintentional extra dose is unlikely to cause problems. Large overdoses may cause headaches, insomnia, and drowsiness. Notify your physician.

SPECIAL PRECAUTIONS

Be sure to consult your physician before using this drug if:
▼ You have glaucoma.
▼ You have high blood pressure.
▼ You have an overactive thyroid.
▼ You are taking other medications.

 Pregnancy
▼ No evidence of risk to developing baby.

 Breast feeding
▼ The drug passes into the breast milk, but at normal doses adverse effects on the baby are uncommon. Discuss with your physician.

 Infants and children
▼ Reduced dose necessary.

 Over 60
▼ No special problems.

 Driving and hazardous work
▼ No special problems.

  Alcohol
▼ No special problems.

POSSIBLE ADVERSE EFFECTS

The adverse effects of xylometazoline are mild and infrequent when the medication is taken for short periods of time. When they do occur it is usually a signal that too much of the drug is being absorbed into the body, and this can be helped by reducing the dose.

Symptom/effect	Frequency		Discuss with physician		Stop taking drug now	Call physician now
	Common	Rare	Only if severe	In all cases		
Headache	●		■			
Nasal discomfort	●		■			
Insomnia	●		■			
Drowsiness	●		■			
Excessive sneezing	●		■			
Palpitations		●		■		

PROLONGED USE

Long-term use of this drug may lead to worsening of the condition. Also, it may lead to a rise in blood pressure. The drug increases the risk of dizziness, sleeplessness, and palpitations. Courses of longer than a few days are not recommended.

INTERACTIONS

Sympathomimetic drugs There is an increased risk of adverse effects when drugs such as ephedrine, pseudoephedrine, and phenylpropanolamine are taken with xylometazoline.

Monoamine oxidase inhibitors (MAOIs) These increase the risk of high blood pressure with xylometazoline, with potentially serious effects. Xylometazoline should not be taken during or within 14 days following MAOI treatment.

Antihypertensive drugs Xylometazoline reduces the blood pressure-lowering effect of antihypertensive drugs such as methyldopa and guanethidine.

ZIDOVUDINE (AZT)

Brand name Retrovir
Used in the following combined preparations None

GENERAL INFORMATION

Zidovudine, formerly known as azido-thymidine (AZT), is an antiviral agent used in the treatment of people with AIDS (acquired immune deficiency syndrome). It is a new drug, approved for use in April 1987.

Zidovudine is used at present only for people with serious AIDS-related illnesses such as *Pneumocystis carinii* pneumonia and AIDS-virus infection of the brain cells. It reduces the frequency and severity of infections. It also pro-motes weight gain and reduces gland swelling.

The most common adverse effect of zidovudine is reduction in bone marrow activity, leading to serious blood disorders that may necessitate stopping the drug. For this reason, regular blood checks are performed.

Zidovudine has not so far provided a lasting cure for AIDS, but it has dramatically improved the prospects for many of those treated.

INFORMATION FOR USERS

Your drug prescription is tailored for you. Do not alter dosage without checking with your physician.

How taken

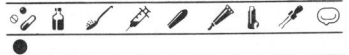

Capsules.

Frequency and timing of doses
Every 4 hours.

Adult dosage range
1.2 – 1.8g daily.

Onset of effect
Within 48 hours.

Duration of action
About 4 hours.

Diet advice
None.

Storage
Keep in a cool, dry place away from reach of children. Protect from light.

Missed dose
Take as soon as you remember. If your next dose is due within 2 hours, take a single dose now and skip the next.

Stopping the drug
Do not stop taking the drug without consulting your physician; symptoms may recur.

Exceeding the dose
An occasional unintentional extra dose is unlikely to cause problems. The effects of large overdoses are unknown. Notify your physician.

SPECIAL PRECAUTIONS

Be sure to tell your physician if:
▼ You have impaired liver or kidney function.
▼ You have had a previous allergic reaction to zidovudine.
▼ You are taking other medications.

Pregnancy
▼ Not usually prescribed. Safety in pregnancy not established. Discuss with your physician.

Breast feeding
▼ Not recommended. The drug may pass into the breast milk and may affect the baby adversely.

Infants and children
▼ Not usually prescribed.

Over 60
▼ Reduced dose may be necessary. Increased likelihood of adverse effects.

Driving and hazardous work
▼ No special problems.

Alcohol
▼ No known problems.

POSSIBLE ADVERSE EFFECTS

The most common adverse effect of zidovudine is anemia. Symptoms include pallor, fatigue, and shortness of breath; sore throat and fever are less frequent effects.

Restlessness, insomnia, and fever may occur with too high a dose. These effects may be overcome by reducing the frequency of dosing.

Symptom/effect	Frequency		Discuss with physician		Stop taking drug now	Call physician now
	Common	Rare	Only if severe	In all cases		
Nausea/vomiting	●		■			
Headache	●		■			
Breathlessness	●			■		∎
Pallor/fatigue	●			■		
Insomnia		●		■		
Restlessness		●		■		
Aching muscles		●		■		
Sore throat/fever		●		■		

INTERACTIONS

General note A wide range of drugs may increase the risk of harmful effects with zidovudine. These include any drug that affects the bone marrow, such as anticancer drugs, and drugs that interfere with the breakdown and elimination of zidovudine, such as trimethoprim, sulfamethoxazole, and acetaminophen.

PROLONGED USE

There is an increased risk of serious blood disorders with prolonged use of zidovudine.

Monitoring Regular blood checks are required during treatment.

A – Z OF VITAMINS AND MINERALS

This section on individual vitamins and minerals gives detailed information on the 24 major chemicals that are required by the body for good health – chemicals that are essential, but which the body is unable to manufacture itself. These include the main vitamins – A, C, D, E, K, H (biotin), and the six B vitamins, together with twelve essential minerals.

The section on Vitamins in Part 3 (p.177) describes in general terms the main sources of the major vitamins and minerals, their roles in the body, and their primary uses, while the following profiles discuss each vitamin and mineral in detail.

The following pages may be particularly useful as a guide for those who think their diet lacks sufficient amounts of a certain vitamin or mineral, and for those with disorders of the digestive tract or liver, who may need extra vitamins. If you think that you may be deficient in a particular vitamin or mineral, refer to the table on p.178 to check that your diet includes good sources of each vitamin and mineral.

The vitamin and mineral profiles

For ease of reference the vitamin and mineral profiles are arranged in alphabetical order and give information under standard headings. These include the different names by which each chemical is known; whether it is available over the counter or by prescription only; its role in body maintenance; specific foods in which it can be found; the recommended daily amounts; how to detect a deficiency; how and when to supplement your diet; and the risks of excessive intake of a particular vitamin or mineral.

Normal daily vitamin and mineral requirements are usually based on US recommended daily allowances (RDA). Dosages for treating deficiency are largely based on the recommendations of the AMA Council on Scientific Affairs.

HOW TO UNDERSTAND THE PROFILES

Each vitamin and mineral profile contains information arranged under standard headings to enable you to find the information you need.

Availability
Tells you whether the vitamin or mineral is available over the counter or by prescription only.

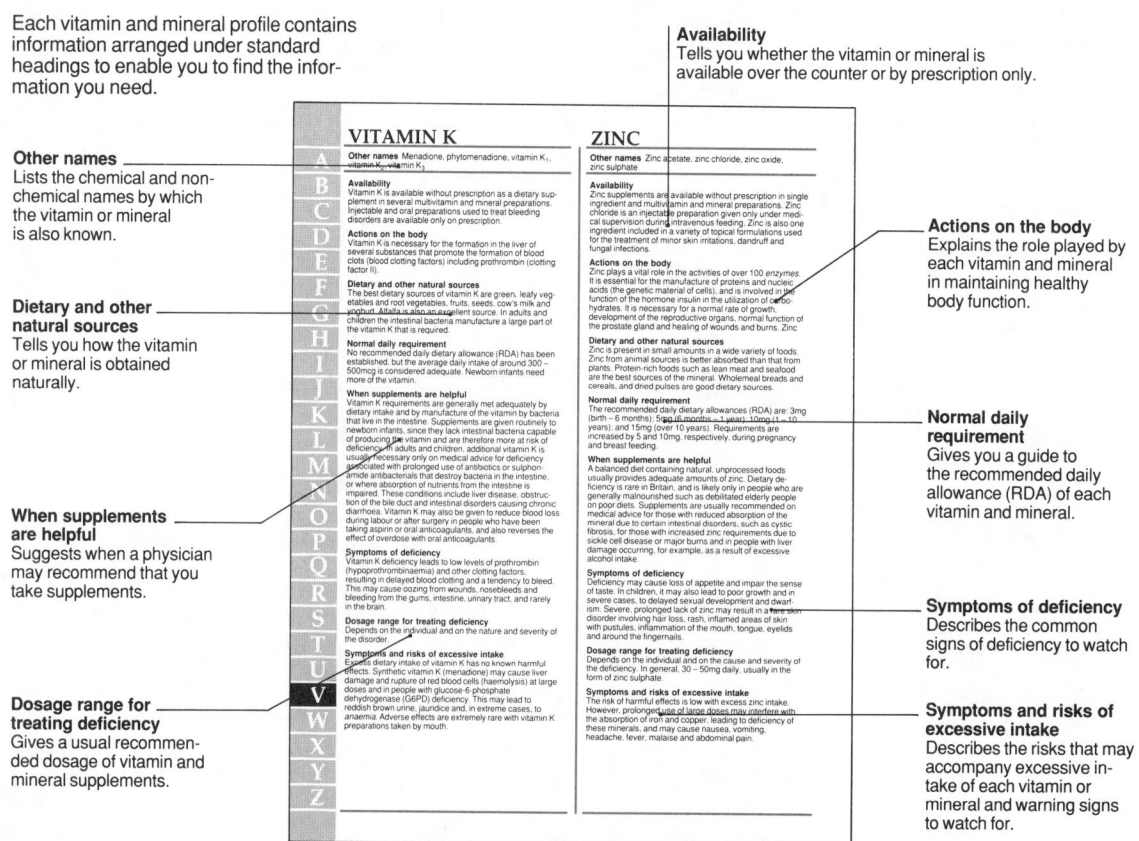

Other names
Lists the chemical and non-chemical names by which the vitamin or mineral is also known.

Dietary and other natural sources
Tells you how the vitamin or mineral is obtained naturally.

When supplements are helpful
Suggests when a physician may recommend that you take supplements.

Dosage range for treating deficiency
Gives a usual recommended dosage of vitamin and mineral supplements.

Actions on the body
Explains the role played by each vitamin and mineral in maintaining healthy body function.

Normal daily requirement
Gives you a guide to the recommended daily allowance (RDA) of each vitamin and mineral.

Symptoms of deficiency
Describes the common signs of deficiency to watch for.

Symptoms and risks of excessive intake
Describes the risks that may accompany excessive intake of each vitamin or mineral and warning signs to watch for.

BIOTIN

Other names Coenzyme R, vitamin H

Availability
Biotin is available without a prescription, alone and in a wide variety of vitamin/mineral preparations.

Actions on the body
Biotin plays a vital role in the activities of several *enzymes*. It is essential for the breakdown of fatty acids and carbohydrates in the diet for conversion into energy, for the manufacture of fats, and for excretion of the products of protein breakdown.

Dietary and other natural sources
Traces of biotin are present in a wide variety of foods. Rich dietary sources include liver, nuts, beans, egg yolks and cauliflower.

Normal daily requirement
A recommended daily allowance (RDA) has not been established, but a daily intake of 100 – 200 micrograms (mcg) meets the body's requirements.

When supplements are helpful
Most diets provide adequate amounts of biotin, and it is also manufactured in relatively large amounts by bacteria that live in the intestine. The need for supplements is rare. However, deficiency can occur with prolonged, excessive consumption of raw egg whites (as in eggnogs), since these contain a protein – avidin – that prevents absorption of the vitamin in the intestine. The risk of deficiency is also increased during long-term treatment with antibiotics or sulfonamide antibacterial drugs, which may destroy the biotin-producing bacteria in the intestine. However, additional biotin is not usually necessary with a balanced diet.

Symptoms of deficiency
Symptoms of biotin deficiency include weakness, tiredness, poor appetite, hair loss, and depression. Severe deficiency may cause eczema of the face and body, and inflammation of the tongue.

Dosage range for treating deficiency
Depends on the individual and on the nature and severity of the disorder. In general, dietary deficiency is treated with 150 – 300 mcg of biotin daily. Deficiency of biotin resulting from a genetic defect that limits use of the vitamin by body cells is treated with doses of 5mg given once or twice daily.

Symptoms and risks of excessive intake
None known.

CALCIUM

Other names Calcium amino acid chelate, calcium carbonate, calcium chloride, calcium citrate, calcium glubionate, calcium gluceptate, calcium gluconate, calcium lactate

Availability
Oral forms are available over the counter. Injectable forms of calcium are available only under medical supervision.

Actions on the body
The most abundant mineral in the body, calcium makes up more than 90 percent of the hard matter in bones and teeth. It is essential for the formation and maintenance of strong bones and healthy teeth, blood clotting, the transmission of nerve impulses, and the contraction of muscle.

Dietary and other natural sources
The main dietary sources of calcium are milk and other dairy products, sardines, dark green, leafy vegetables, dried beans, and nuts. Calcium may also be obtained by drinking water in hard-water areas.

Normal daily requirement
The recommended daily allowances (RDA) of calcium are 360mg (birth – 6 months); 540mg (6 months – 1 year); 800mg (children aged 1 – 10 and adults aged 19 and over); and 1,200mg (adolescents and young adults aged 11 – 18). Daily requirements of calcium are increased by 400mg during pregnancy and breast feeding.

When supplements are helpful
Unless a sufficient amount of dairy products is consumed – a pint of milk contains approximately 600mg – the diet may not contain enough calcium, and supplements may be needed. Women are especially vulnerable to calcium deficiency because pregnancy and breast feeding demand large amounts of calcium, which may be extracted from the skeleton if intake is not adequate. Osteoporosis (fragile bones) has been linked to dietary calcium deficiency in some cases, but may not be helped by supplements in all women. Hormone replacement therapy may also be necessary (see Drugs for bone disorders, p.150).

Symptoms of deficiency
Symptoms of deficiency do not develop because when dietary intake is inadequate, the body obtains the calcium it needs from the skeleton. Long-term lack of calcium can lead to softening of the bones, which in children leads to abnormal bone development (rickets) and in adults to osteoporosis and osteomalacia, causing backache, muscle weakness, bone pain, and fractures of the long bones. Severe deficiency, resulting in low levels of calcium in the blood, causes abnormal stimulation of the nervous system, resulting in cramplike spasms in the hands, feet, and face.

Dosage range for treating deficiency
Oral supplements of up to 800mg daily may be advised for children with rickets, and up to 1,000mg daily may be given for osteoporosis and osteomalacia. Severe deficiency is treated in hospital by intravenous injection of calcium. Vitamin D is usually given together with calcium to increase its absorption from the intestine.

Symptoms and risks of excessive intake
Excessive intake of calcium may reduce the amount of iron and zinc absorbed and also may cause constipation and nausea. There is an increased risk of palpitations and, for susceptible persons, of calcium deposits in the kidneys, leading to kidney stones and kidney damage. These symptoms do not usually develop unless calcium is taken with large amounts of vitamin D.

A
B
C
D
E
F
G
H
I
J
K
L
M
N
O
P
Q
R
S
T
U
V
W
X
Y
Z

CHROMIUM

Other names Chromium amino acid chelate, glucose tolerance factor (GTF)

Availability
Chromium supplements are available without prescription.

Actions on the body
Chromium plays a vital role in the activities of several *enzymes*. It is involved in the breakdown of sugar for conversion into energy and in the manufacture of certain fats. It works together with insulin and is thus essential to the body's ability to use sugar. It may also be involved in the manufacture of proteins in the body.

Dietary and other natural sources
Traces of chromium are present in a wide variety of foods. Meat, dairy products, and whole-grain cereals are good sources of this mineral.

Normal daily requirement
Only minute quantities of chromium are required. A recommended daily dietary allowance (RDA) has not been determined, but 80 –100 micrograms is an average daily adult intake.

When supplements are helpful
Most people who eat a healthy diet containing plenty of fresh or unprocessed foods receive adequate amounts of chromium. However, supplements may be advised in malnourished children and elderly people (who retain less of the mineral). Diabetics and those with diabetes-like symptoms may also benefit from additional chromium. Supplements may also be helpful if symptoms show chromium deficiency.

Symptoms of deficiency
Chromium deficiency is fairly common in the United States, since the soil contains low levels of the mineral. A diet of too many processed foods may contribute to chromium deficiency. Inadequate intake of chromium over a prolonged period may impair the body's ability to use sugar, leading to high blood sugar levels. However, in most cases, this is symptomless. In some people, there may be diabetes-like symptoms such as tiredness, mental confusion, and numbness or tingling of the hands and feet. Deficiency may worsen pre-existing diabetes and may depress growth in children. Chromium deficiency may also contribute to the development of atherosclerosis (narrowing of the arteries).

Dosage range for treating deficiency
Severe chromium deficiency may be treated with daily doses of up to 5 – 10mcg.

Symptoms and risks of excessive intake
Chromium is poisonous in excess. Levels that produce symptoms are usually obtained from exposure to industrial waste in drinking water or the atmosphere, not from excessive dietary intake. Symptoms include inflammation of the skin and, if inhaled, damage to the nose. People who are repeatedly exposed to chromium fumes have a greater-than-average risk of developing lung cancer.

COPPER

Other names Copper amino acid chelate, cupric chloride, copper chloride dihydrate, copper gluconate, copper sulfate

Availability
Copper gluconate, copper sulfate, and copper amino acid chelate are available in oral preparations without a prescription. Cupric chloride is an injectable form and is available only by prescription. Copper chloride dihydrate is part of a multiple-ingredient preparation for hospital use.

Actions on the body
Copper is an essential constituent of several proteins and *enzymes*. It plays an important role in the development of red blood cells, helps to form the dark pigment that colors hair and skin, and helps the body to use vitamin C. It is essential for the formation of collagen and elastin – proteins found in ligaments, blood vessel walls, and the lungs – and for the proper formation and maintenance of strong bones. It is also required for central nervous system activity.

Dietary and other natural sources
Most unprocessed foods contain copper. Liver, shellfish, nuts, mushrooms, whole-grain cereals, and dried peas and beans are particularly rich sources.

Normal daily requirement
The recommended intake is: 0.6mg (birth – 1 year); 1mg (1 – 4 years); and 2mg (adults and children over 4 years).

When supplements are helpful
A diet that regularly includes a selection of the foods mentioned above provides sufficient copper. Supplements are rarely necessary. However, physicians may advise additional copper for malnourished children and infants.

Symptoms of deficiency
Copper deficiency is very rare. The major change is anemia due to failure of production of red blood cells, the main symptoms of which are pallor, fatigue, shortness of breath, and palpitations. In severe cases, abnormal bone changes may occur. An inherited copper deficiency disorder called Menke's syndrome (kinky hair disease) results in brain degeneration, retarded growth, sparse and brittle hair, and weak bones.

Dosage range for treating deficiency
This depends on the individual and on the nature and severity of the disorder.

Symptoms and risks of excessive intake
As little as 10 – 15mg of copper taken by mouth can produce toxic effects. Symptoms of poisoning include nausea, vomiting, abdominal pain, diarrhea, and general aches and pains. Large overdoses of copper may cause destruction of red blood cells (hemolytic anemia), and liver and kidney damage. Copper poisoning can occur in people who drink homemade alcohol distilled through copper tubing.

FLUORIDE

Other names Calcium fluoride, sodium fluoride, sodium monofluorophosphate, stannous fluoride

Availability
Sodium fluoride is added to drinking water and is available by prescription in single or multiple ingredient preparations. Fluoride mouth rinses and toothpastes containing sodium fluoride, stannous fluoride, or sodium monofluorophosphate are available over the counter. Calcium fluoride is the naturally occurring form of the mineral.

Actions on the body
Fluoride helps to prevent tooth decay and contributes to the strength of bones. It is thought to work on the teeth by strengthening the mineral composition of the tooth enamel, making it more resistant to attack by acid in the mouth. Fluoride is most effective when taken during the formation of teeth in childhood, since it is then incorporated into the tooth itself. It may also strengthen developing bones.

Dietary and other natural sources
Fluoride has been added to drinking water in many states, and water is therefore a prime source of this mineral (fluoride levels in water vary among states, and untreated water also contains a small amount of fluoride). Foods and beverages grown or prepared in areas with fluoride-treated water may also contribute fluoride.

Normal daily requirement
The daily requirement is around 1.5mg (in adults); 0.1 – 1.0mg (infants up to 2 years old); and 0.5 – 2.5mg (children aged 2 – 14 years). A recommended daily allowance (RDA) has not been established.

When supplements are helpful
Most diets typically provide 0.9 – 2.6mg of fluoride per day, depending on whether or not the water supply contains fluoride. Drinking water containing fluoride at 1 part per million (the recommended level is 0.7 – 1.2 ppm) provides an additional 1.4 – 1.8mg per day for adults and 0.4 – 0.8mg per day for young children. If the level is inadequate, children may be given fluoride drops or tablets. The use of supplements is currently under investigation for the prevention and treatment of osteoporosis (fragile bones).

Symptoms of deficiency
Fluoride deficiency increases the risk of tooth decay, especially in children.

Dosage range for treating deficiency
Dietary supplements may be given to children when the concentration of fluoride in the water supply is less than 0.7 ppm. When fluoride is present at less than 0.3 ppm, the recommended daily dose is: 0.25 mg (birth – 2 years); 0.5mcg (2 – 3 years); and 1mg (3 – 13 years). When the fluoride concentration is 0.3 – 0.7ppm, supplements are not recommended for infants under 2, and the recommended daily dose for older children is 0.25mcg (2 – 3 years) and 0.5mcg (3 – 13 years).

Symptoms and risks of excessive intake
In large quantities, fluoride may cause slow poisoning – called fluorosis. Prolonged intake of water containing more than 2 parts per million may lead to mottled or brown discoloration of the enamel in developing teeth. Very high levels (over 8 ppm) may also lead to bone disorders and degenerative changes in the kidneys, liver, adrenal glands, heart, central nervous system, and reproductive organs. Suggestions of a link between fluoridation of the water supply and cancer are without foundation. A child who has taken a number of fluoride tablets may vomit and lose consciousness. Give milk if the child is conscious, and seek immediate medical help.

FOLIC ACID

Other names Folacin, vitamin M, folate sodium, leucovorin calcium (folinate calcium, citrovorum factor), folates

Availability
Folic acid is available without prescription, alone and in a variety of vitamin/mineral preparations. Strengths of 1mg and over are available only by prescription.

Actions on the body
Folic acid is essential for the activities of several *enzymes*. It is required for the manufacture of nucleic acids – the genetic material of cells – and thus for the processes of growth and reproduction. It is vital for the formation of red blood cells by the bone marrow and the development and proper function of the central nervous system.

Dietary and other natural sources
The best sources are green, leafy vegetables, mushrooms, and liver. Root vegetables, oranges, nuts, dried beans and peas, and egg yolks are also rich sources.

Normal daily requirement
The recommended daily allowances (RDA) of folic acid in micrograms (mcg) are: 30mcg (birth – 6 months); 45mcg (6 months – 1 year); 100mcg (1 – 3 years); 200mcg (4 – 6 years); 300mcg (7 – 10 years); and 400mcg (ages 11 and over). In pregnancy and breast feeding, requirements are increased by 400 and 100mcg, respectively.

When supplements are helpful
A varied diet containing fresh fruit and vegetables usually provides adequate amounts. However, minor deficiency is fairly common, and can be corrected by the addition of one uncooked fruit or vegetable or a glass of fruit juice daily. Supplements are given routinely during pregnancy and breast feeding, and may also be needed in premature or low birth-weight infants and those fed on goat's milk (breast and cow's milk contain adequate amounts of the vitamin). Doctors may recommend additional folic acid for people on hemodialysis, or those who have certain blood disorders or psoriasis. It is given for certain conditions in which absorption of nutrients from the intestine is impaired, severe alcoholism, and liver disease. Supplements may be helpful if you are a heavy drinker or if you are taking certain drugs that deplete folic acid, including anticonvulsants, antimalarial drugs, estrogen-containing contraceptives, certain analgesics, corticosteroids, and sulfonamide antibacterial drugs.

Symptoms of deficiency
Folic acid deficiency leads to abnormally low numbers of red blood cells (anemia). The main symptoms include fatigue, loss of appetite, nausea, diarrhea, and hair loss. Mouth sores are common and the tongue is often sore. Deficiency may also cause poor growth in infants and children.

Dosage range for treating deficiency
Symptoms of anemia are usually treated with 1,000mcg of folic acid daily, together with vitamin B_{12}. Occasionally, doses of up to 1mg daily may be given if absorption of folic acid from the intestine is impaired. A lower maintenance dose of 100 – 400mcg daily may be substituted after symptoms have subsided.

Symptoms and risks of excessive intake
Excessive folic acid is not toxic. However, it may worsen the symptoms of a coexisting vitamin B_{12} deficiency and should never be taken to treat anemia without a full medical investigation of the cause of the anemia.

IODINE

Other names Calcium iodide, potassium iodide, sodium iodide

Availability
Iodine supplements are available without prescription as kelp tablets and in several vitamin/mineral preparations. Iodine skin preparations are also available without a prescription for antiseptic use. Treatments for thyroid suppression and expectorant cough medicines containing iodine are available only by prescription.

Actions on the body
Iodine is essential for the formation of thyroid hormone, which regulates the body's energy production, promotes growth and development, and helps burn excess fat.

Dietary and other natural sources
Seafood is the best source of iodine, but bread and dairy products are the main sources of this mineral in most diets. Iodized table salt is also a good source. Iodine may be inhaled from the atmosphere in coastal regions or from pollution produced by automobile exhaust fumes.

Normal daily requirement
The recommended daily allowances (RDA) of iodine in micrograms are: 40mcg (birth – 6 months); 50mcg (6 months – 1 year); 70mcg (1 – 3 years); 90mcg (4 – 6 years); 120mcg (7 – 10 years); and 150mcg (11 years and over). Requirements are increased during pregnancy and breast feeding by 25mcg and 50mcg, respectively.

When supplements are helpful
Most diets contain adequate amounts of iodine, and use of iodized table salt can usually make up for any lack. Supplements are rarely necessary except on medical advice. However, excessive intake of raw cabbage or nuts may reduce uptake of iodine into the thyroid gland and lead to deficiency if iodine intake is otherwise low. Kelp supplements may be helpful.

People exposed to radiation from radioactive iodine released into the environment may be given sodium iodide at 10 – 100mg per day (adults and children over 1 year) or 15mg per day (children under 1 year) for 3 – 10 days.

Symptoms of deficiency
Deficiency may result in a goiter (enlargement of the thyroid gland) and hypothyroidism (deficiency of thyroid hormone). Symptoms of hypothyroidism include tiredness, physical and mental slowness, weight gain, facial puffiness, and constipation. Babies born to iodine-deficient women are lethargic and difficult to feed. Left untreated, they develop cretinism, with poor growth and mental retardation.

Dosage range for treating deficiency
Deficiency may be treated with doses of 150mcg of iodine daily, often as iodized table salt (4g or 1teaspoon daily).

Symptoms and risks of excessive intake
Iodine that occurs naturally in food is non-toxic, but iodine taken as a drug can be harmful in excess. Large overdoses of iodine may cause abdominal pain, vomiting, bloody diarrhea, and swelling of the thyroid and salivary glands. Prolonged use of 6mg or more daily may suppress the activity of the thyroid gland.

IRON

Other names Ferrous fumarate, ferrous gluconate, ferrous sulfate, iron dextran, iron-polysaccharide complex

Availability
Ferrous sulfate, ferrous fumarate, ferrous gluconate, and iron-polysaccharide complex are available without prescription, alone and in vitamin/mineral preparations. Iron dextran, an injectable form, is available only by prescription.

Actions on the body
Iron has an important role in the formation of red blood cells and is a vital component of the oxygen-carrying pigment hemoglobin. It is involved in the formation of myoglobin, a pigment that stores oxygen in muscles for use during exercise. It is also an essential component of several *enzymes*, and is involved in the uptake of oxygen by the cells and the conversion of blood sugar to energy.

Dietary and other natural sources
Liver is the best dietary source of iron. Meat (especially organ meat), eggs, chicken, fish, green, leafy vegetables, dried fruit, enriched or whole-grain cereals, breads or pastas, nuts, and dried beans are also rich sources. Iron in meat, eggs, chicken, and fish is better absorbed than that in vegetables.

Normal daily requirement
The recommended daily allowances (RDA) of iron are: 10mg (birth – 6 months); 15mg (6 months – 3 years); 10mg (4 – 10 years); 18mg (males aged 11 – 18 and females aged 11 – 50); 10mg (males aged 19 and over and females over 51). Requirements are increased during pregnancy and for two to three months after childbirth.

When supplements are helpful
Most average diets supply adequate amounts of iron. However, larger amounts are necessary during pregnancy. Supplements are therefore given throughout pregnancy and for two to three months after childbirth to maintain and replenish adequate iron stores in the mother. Premature babies may be prescribed supplements soon after birth (breast fed) or after 6 months of age (formula fed) to prevent deficiency. Supplements may be helpful in young vegetarians, women with heavy menstrual periods, and people with chronic blood loss due to disease (for example, peptic ulcer).

Symptoms of deficiency
Iron deficiency causes *anemia*, symptoms of which are pallor, fatigue, shortness of breath, and palpitations. Apathy, irritability, and lowered resistance of the body to infection may also occur.

Dosage range for treating deficiency
Depends on the individual and the nature and severity of the condition. In adults, iron deficiency anemia is usually treated with 30 – 100mg of iron two or three times daily. In children the dose is reduced according to age and weight. Iron supplements of 30 – 60mg daily are prescribed throughout pregnancy.

Symptoms and risks of excessive intake
Iron poisoning is extremely dangerous. Abdominal pain, nausea, and vomiting may be followed by fever, abdominal bloating, dehydration, and dangerously lowered blood pressure. Immediate medical attention is vital.

Excessive intake, especially when taken with large amounts of vitamin C, may cause iron to accumulate in organs, causing congestive heart failure, cirrhosis of the liver, and diabetes mellitus.

MAGNESIUM

Other names Magnesium amino acid chelate, magnesium gluconate, magnesium oxide, magnesium oxide dolomite, magnesium sulfate

Availability
Magnesium is available without prescription in a variety of vitamin/mineral preparations. Magnesium is also an ingredient of numerous over-the-counter antacid and laxative preparations, but it is not absorbed well from these sources.

Actions on the body
About 70 percent of the body's magnesium is found in bones and teeth. It is essential for the formation of healthy bones and teeth, the transmission of nerve impulses, and the contraction of muscles. It activates several *enzymes*, and is important in the conversion of blood sugar into energy. It also helps to regulate body temperature.

Dietary and other natural sources
The best dietary sources of magnesium are leafy, green vegetables. Nuts, whole grains, soybeans, and seafood are also rich in magnesium. Drinking water in hard-water areas may also be a source of this mineral.

Normal daily requirement
The recommended daily allowances (RDA) of magnesium are: 50mg (birth – 6 months); 70mg (6 months – 1 year); 150mg (1 – 3 years); 200mg (4 – 6 years); 250mg (7 – 10 years); 300mg (females over age 11); 350mg (males aged 11 – 14 and over 19); and 400mg (males aged 15 – 18). Requirements are increased by 150mg, both in pregnancy and in breast feeding.

When supplements are helpful
A varied diet provides adequate amounts of magnesium, particularly in hard-water areas. Supplements are usually necessary only on medical advice for magnesium deficiency associated with certain conditions in which absorption from the intestine is impaired, which occurs in repeated vomiting or diarrhea, advanced kidney disease, severe alcoholism, or prolonged treatment with certain diuretic drugs.
   Estrogens and estrogen-containing oral contraceptives may reduce blood magnesium levels, but women on adequate diets do not need supplements.

Symptoms of deficiency
Symptoms include anxiety, restlessness, tremors, confusion, palpitations, depression, irritability, and disorientation. Severe magnesium deficiency causes marked overstimulation of the nervous system, resulting in cramp-like spasms of the hands and feet and seizures. Inadequate intake may be a possible factor in the development of coronary heart disease, and may also lead to calcium deposits in the kidneys, resulting in kidney stones.

Dosage range for treating deficiency
This depends on the individual and on the nature and severity of the disorder. Severe deficiency is usually treated in the hospital by injection of magnesium sulfate.

Symptoms and risks of excessive intake
Magnesium toxicity (hypermagnesemia) is rare but can occur in people with impaired kidney function after prolonged intake of large amounts (more than 3,000mg daily) found in antacid or laxative preparations. Symptoms include nausea, vomiting, dizziness (due to a drop in blood pressure), and muscle weakness. Very large increases in magnesium in the blood may cause fatal respiratory failure or heart arrest.

NIACIN

Other names Niacinamide, nicotinamide, nicotinic acid, nicotinyl alcohol tartrate, vitamin B$_3$

Availability
Niacin is available without prescription in a wide variety of single-ingredient and vitamin/mineral preparations. Nicotinyl alcohol tartrate is available only by prescription.

Actions on the body
Niacin plays a vital role in the activities of many *enzymes*. It is important in the production of energy from blood sugar and in the manufacture of fats. Niacin is essential for the proper functioning of the nervous system, for a healthy skin and digestive system, and for the manufacture of sex hormones (estrogens, progesterone, and testosterone).

Dietary and other natural sources
Liver, lean meat, poultry, fish, whole-grain products, nuts, and dried beans are the best dietary sources of niacin.

Normal daily requirement
The recommended daily allowances (RDA) of niacin are: 6mg (birth – 6 months); 8mg (6 months – 1 year); 9mg (1 – 3 years); 11mg (4 – 6 years); 16mg (7 – 10 years); 18mg (males aged 11 – 18 and aged 23 – 50); 19mg (males aged 19 – 22); 16 mg (males over 51); 15mg (females aged 11 – 14); 14mg (females aged 15 – 22); 13mg (females over 23). Requirements are increased by 2 and 5mg, respectively, during pregnancy and breast feeding.

When supplements are helpful
Most North American diets provide adequate amounts of niacin, and dietary deficiency is rare, except in areas where corn is the staple diet. Supplements are required for niacin deficiency associated with bowel disorders in which absorption from the intestine is impaired, and with liver disease and severe alcoholism. Large doses of niacin (up to 9g daily) lower the levels of certain fats in the blood, including cholesterol, and are used in the treatment of hyperlipidemia (raised blood fat levels). There is no convincing medical evidence that niacin helps psychiatric disorders (except those associated with pellagra) or that it has a beneficial effect in peripheral vascular disease.

Symptoms of deficiency
Severe niacin deficiency causes pellagra (literally, rough skin). Symptoms include sore, red, cracked skin in areas exposed to sun, friction or pressure, inflammation of the mouth and tongue, abdominal pain and distension, nausea, diarrhea, and mental disturbances such as the anxiety, depression, and dementia that accompany pellagra.

Dosage range for treating deficiency
For severe pellagra, adults are usually treated with 100 – 500mg niacinamide daily by mouth, and children are usually given 100 – 300mg daily. For less severe deficiency, doses of 25 –50mg are given.

Symptoms and risks of excessive intake
At doses of over 50mg, niacin (nicotinic acid) may cause transient itching, flushing, tingling, or headache. The synthetic form of niacin, niacinamide (nicotinamide), is free of these effects. Large doses of niacin may cause nausea and may aggravate a peptic ulcer. This can be prevented by taking the drug on a full stomach. At doses of over 2g daily (which have been used to treat hyperlipidemia), there is a risk of gout, liver damage, and high blood sugar levels, which lead to nervousness and extreme thirst.

PANTOTHENIC ACID

PANTOTHENIC ACID

Other names Calcium pantothenate, panthenol, vitamin B$_5$

Availability
Pantothenic acid, calcium pantothenate, and panthenol are available without prescription in a variety of vitamin/mineral preparations. Pantothenic acid is available alone in lower tablet strengths (of up to 200mg) without a prescription; 1,000mg tablets are available only by prescription.

Actions on the body
Pantothenic acid plays a vital role in the activities of many *enzymes*. It is essential for the production of energy from sugars and fats, for the manufacture of fats, cortico-steroids and sex hormones, for the utilization of other vitamins, for the proper function of the nervous system and the adrenal glands, and for normal growth and development.

Dietary and other natural sources
Pantothenic acid is present in almost all vegetables, cereals, and animal foods. Liver, kidney, heart, fish, and egg yolks are good dietary sources. Brewer's yeast, wheat-germ, and royal jelly (the substance on which queen bees feed) are also rich in the vitamin.

Normal daily requirement
A recommended daily allowance (RDA) has not been established, but requirements are met by 4 – 7mg daily.

When supplements are helpful
Most diets provide adequate amounts of pantothenic acid. Any deficiency is likely to occur together with other B vitamin deficiency diseases such as pellagra (see niacin), beriberi (see thiamine), or in alcoholism, and is treated with B complex supplements. There is no firm evidence that large doses help, as some believe, in the prevention of graying hair, nerve disorders in diabetes, or psychiatric illness. As with other B vitamins, the need for pantothenic acid is increased by injury, surgery, severe illness, and psychological stress.

Symptoms of deficiency
Pantothenic acid deficiency may cause low blood sugar levels, duodenal ulcers, respiratory infections, and general ill-health. Symptoms include fatigue, headache, nausea, abdominal pain, numbness and tingling in the limbs, muscle cramps, faintness, confusion, and lack of coordination.

Dosage range for treating deficiency
Usually 5 – 20mg per day.

Symptoms and risks of excessive intake
In tests, doses of 1,000mg or more of pantothenic acid have not caused toxic effects. The risk of toxicity is con-sidered to be very low, since pantothenic acid is a water-soluble vitamin that does not accumulate in the tissues. Any excess is eliminated rapidly in the urine. Very high intakes of 10 – 20g can cause diarrhea.

POTASSIUM

Other names Potassium acetate, potassium amino acid, potassium chloride, potassium citrate, potassium gluconate

Availability
Potassium chloride, potassium gluconate, and potassium amino acid complex are available without prescription in a number of single-ingredient and vitamin/mineral supplements. Potassium chloride and gluconate are also widely available in sodium-free salt. Potassium citrate and acetate supplements are given by prescription only.

Actions on the body
Potassium works together with sodium in controlling the body's water balance, conduction of nerve impulses, contraction of muscle, and maintenance of a normal heart rhythm. It is essential for storage of carbohydrate and its breakdown for energy.

Dietary and other natural sources
The best dietary sources of potassium are green, leafy vegetables, oranges, potatoes, and bananas. Lean meat, beans, and milk are also rich in the mineral. Many methods of food processing may lower potassium levels found in fresh food.

Normal daily requirement
A recommended daily allowance (RDA) has not been established, but many authorities suggest a daily intake of 2 – 6g.

When supplements are helpful
Most diets contain adequate amounts of potassium, and supplements are rarely required in normal circumstances. However, people who drink large amounts of coffee or alcohol or eat lots of salty foods may become marginally deficient. Diabetics may also be deficient in potassium. Supplements are usually advised only when symptoms suggest deficiency or for people at particular risk. Prolonged treatment with certain diuretics is the most common cause of deficiency; long-term use of corticosteroids may also deplete the body's potassium. People with certain types of kidney disease and those who abuse laxatives may also become deficient in potassium. Prolonged vomiting and diarrhea may also deplete potassium.

Symptoms of deficiency
Early symptoms of potassium deficiency may include muscle weakness, fatigue, dizziness, and mental con-fusion. Impairment of nerve and muscle function may progress to cause disturbances of the heart rhythm, paralysis of the skeletal muscles, and paralysis of the bowel, leading to constipation.

Dosage range for treating deficiency
Depends on the preparation, the individual, and the cause and severity of deficiency. In general, daily doses equivalent to 4 – 6g of potassium chloride are given to prevent deficiency (for example, in people treated with diuretics that deplete potassium). Doses equivalent to 3.0 – 7.2g of potassium chloride daily are used to treat deficiency.

Symptoms and risks of excessive intake
Blood potassium levels are normally regulated by the kidneys, and any excess is rapidly eliminated in the urine. Doses of over 18g may cause serious disturbances of the heart rhythm and muscular paralysis. In people with impaired kidney function, excess potassium may accumulate, increasing the risk of potassium poisoning. People on hemodialysis treatment should stay on a carefully controlled low-potassium diet.

PYRIDOXINE

Other names Pyridoxine hydrochloride, vitamin B$_6$

Availability
Pyridoxine and pyridoxine hydrochloride are available without prescription in a variety of single-ingredient and vitamin/mineral preparations.

Actions on the body
Pyridoxine plays a vital role in the activities of many *enzymes*. It is essential for the breakdown and utilization of proteins, carbohydrates, and fats from food; for the release of carbohydrates stored in the liver and muscles for energy; and for the manufacture of niacin (vitamin B$_3$). It is needed for the production of red blood cells and *antibodies*, for healthy skin, and for healthy digestion. It is also important for normal function of the central nervous system and the action of several hormones.

Dietary and other natural sources
Liver, chicken, fish, whole-grain cereals, wheat germ, and eggs are rich in this vitamin. Bananas, avocados, and potatoes are also good sources.

Normal daily requirement
The recommended daily allowances (RDA) of pyridoxine are: 0.3 mg (birth – 6 months); 0.6mg (6 months – 1 year); 0.9mg (1 – 3 years); 1.3mg (4 – 6 years); 1.6mg (7 – 10 years); 1.8mg (11 – 14 years); 2.0mg (females over 15 and young males aged 15 – 18); and 2.2mg (males aged 19 and over). Daily requirements are increased by 0.6mg and 0.5mg in pregnancy and breast feeding, respectively.

When supplements are helpful
Most balanced diets contain adequate amounts of pyridoxine, and it is also manufactured in small amounts by bacteria that live in the intestine. However, breast-fed infants may require additional pyridoxine. Elderly adults may also require supplements. Supplements may be given on medical advice together with other B vitamins to people with certain conditions in which absorption from the intestine is impaired. Supplements may also be recommended to prevent or treat deficiency caused by alcoholism and treatment with drugs such as penicillamine and hydralazine. Supplements may also help relieve depression caused by a deficiency of the vitamin in women taking estrogen-containing oral contraceptives, and may help prevent morning sickness in pregnancy. Supplements may help relieve premenstrual depression, irritability, and breast tenderness.

Symptoms of deficiency
Pyridoxine deficiency may cause weakness, irritability, nervousness, depression, skin disorders, inflammation of the mouth and tongue, and cracked lips. In adults, it may cause anemia (abnormally low levels of red blood cells). Seizures may occur in infants.

Dosage range for treating deficiency
Depends on the individual and the nature and severity of the disorder. In general, deficiency is treated with 5 – 25mg daily for three weeks followed by 1.5 – 2.5mg daily in a multivitamin preparation. Deficiency resulting from genetic defects that prevent use of the vitamin is treated with doses of 2 – 15mg daily in infants and 10 – 250mg daily in adults and children. Daily doses of 50mg given with other B vitamins from day 10 of a menstrual cycle to day 3 of the following cycle may help relieve premenstrual syndrome.

Symptoms and risks of excessive intake
Daily doses of over 500mg taken over a prolonged period may damage the nervous system, resulting in unsteadiness, numbness, and awkwardness of the hands.

RIBOFLAVIN

Other names Vitamin B$_2$, vitamin G

Availability
Riboflavin is available without a prescription, alone and in a wide variety of vitamin/mineral preparations.

Actions on the body
Riboflavin plays a vital role in the activities of several *enzymes*. It is involved in the breakdown and utilization of carbohydrates, fats, and proteins and in the production of energy in cells using oxygen. It is needed for utilization of other B vitamins and for production of hormones by the adrenal glands.

Dietary and other natural sources
Riboflavin is found in most foods. Good dietary sources are liver, milk, cheese, eggs, leafy green vegetables, whole grains, and beans. Brewer's yeast is also a rich source of the vitamin.

Normal daily requirement
The recommended daily allowances (RDA) are: 0.4mg (birth – 6 months); 0.6mg (6 months – 1 year); 0.8mg (1 – 3 years); 1.0mg (4 – 6 years); 1.4mg (7 – 10 years); 1.6mg (males aged 11 – 14); 1.7mg (males aged 15 – 22); 1.6mg (males aged 23 – 50); 1.4 mg (males over 51); 1.3mg (females aged 11 – 22); and 1.2mg (females over 23 years). Requirements of the vitamin are increased by 0.3mg in pregnancy and by 0.6mg in breast feeding.

When supplements are helpful
A balanced diet generally provides adequate amounts of riboflavin. Supplements may be beneficial in people on very low calorie diets. Requirements may also be increased by prolonged use of phenothiazine antipsychotics, tricyclic antidepressants, and estrogen-containing oral contraceptives. Supplements are required for riboflavin deficiency associated with certain conditions in which absorption of nutrients from the intestine is impaired. Riboflavin deficiency is also common among alcoholics. As with other B vitamins, the need for riboflavin is increased by injury, surgery, severe illness, and psychological stress. In all cases, treatment with supplements works best in a complete B-complex formulation.

Symptoms of deficiency
Prolonged deficiency may lead to chapped lips, cracks and sores in the corners of the mouth, and a red, sore tongue. The eyes may itch, burn, and may become unusually sensitive to light. Twitching of the eyelids and blurred vision may also occur.

Dosage range for treating deficiency
Usually treated with 5 – 25mg daily in combination with other B vitamins.

Symptoms and risks of excessive intake
Excessive intake does not appear to have harmful effects. However, prolonged use of large doses of riboflavin alone may deplete other B vitamins; it is therefore best taken with other B vitamins.

SELENIUM

Other names Selenious acid, sodium selenite, selenium sulfide, selenium yeast

Availability
Selenium is available without a prescription in single-ingredient tablets (50 and 200mcg) and in capsules in combination with vitamin E. It is also available by prescription in a number of vitamin/mineral preparations. Selenium sulfide is the active ingredient of several antidandruff shampoos.

Actions on the body
Selenium works in association with vitamin E to preserve elasticity in the tissues, thus slowing down the processes of aging. It also increases endurance by improving the supply of oxygen to the heart muscle. It is necessary for the formation of a group of substances called prosta-glandins, which give protection against high blood pressure, help to prevent the abnormal blood clotting in arteries that may lead to a stroke or heart attack, and stimulate contractions of the uterus in labor.

Dietary and other natural sources
Meat, fish, whole grains, and dairy products are good sources. The amount of selenium found in vegetables depends on the content of the mineral in the soil where they were grown.

Normal daily requirement
Only minute quantities are required. A recommended daily allowance (RDA) has not been determined, but the average intake is around 60 – 150 mcg.

When supplements are helpful
Most normal diets provide adequate amounts of selenium, and supplements are, therefore, rarely necessary. At present, there is no conclusive medical evidence in support of some claims that selenium may provide protection against cancer or that it prolongs life. A daily intake of more than 150mcg is not recommended except on the advice of a physician.

Symptoms of deficiency
Long-term lack of selenium may result in loss of stamina and reduced elasticity of tissues, leading to premature aging. Severe deficiency may cause muscle pain and tenderness, and can eventually lead to a fatal form of heart disease in children in areas where selenium levels in the diet are very low.

Dosage range for treating deficiency
Depends on the individual and on the nature and severity of the disorder. Severe selenium deficiency may be treated with doses of up to 200mcg daily.

Symptoms and risks of excessive intake
Selenium is the most poisonous of dietary minerals. Excessive intake may cause baldness, loss of nails and teeth, fatigue, nausea, vomiting, and sour-milk breath. A massive overdose of this mineral may be fatal.

SODIUM

Other names Sodium acetate, sodium bicarbonate, sodium chloride, sodium phosphate

Availability
Sodium is widely available in the form of common table salt (sodium chloride). Sodium acetate is a prescription-only drug used in intravenous feeding. Sodium phosphate is a laxative available only by prescription.

Actions on the body
Sodium works with potassium in controlling the water balance in the body, transmission of nerve impulses, contraction of muscle, and maintenance of a normal heart rhythm.

Dietary and other natural sources
Sodium is present in almost all foods as a natural ingredient, or as an extra ingredient added during processing. The main sources are table salt, processed foods, cheese, breads and cereals, and smoked, pickled or cured meats and fish. High concentrations are found in pickles and snack foods, including potato chips and olives. Sodium is also present in water that has been treated with water softeners.

Normal daily requirement
There is no official recommended daily allowance (RDA) for sodium, but the National Research Council suggests an intake between 1 – 3g. Approximately 2g of sodium is obtained from one teaspoon of sodium chloride.

When supplements are helpful
Most North American diets contain amounts of sodium far exceeding requirements. The average consumption of sodium is 3 – 7g daily. The need for supplementation is rare in temperate climates, even with low-salt diets. In tropical climates, however, sodium supplements may help prevent heat stroke from occurring as a result of sodium loss caused by excessive perspiration during heavy work. Supplements may be given on medical advice to replace salt lost due to prolonged diarrhea and vomiting, particularly in infants, and to prevent or treat deficiency due to certain kidney disorders, cystic fibrosis, adrenal gland insufficiency, use of diuretics, or severe bleeding.

Symptoms of deficiency
Dietary sodium deficiency is rare. Most deficiency usually results from conditions that increase loss of sodium from the body, such as diarrhea, vomiting, and excessive perspiration. Early symptoms include lethargy, muscle cramps, and dizziness. In severe cases, there may be a marked drop in blood pressure leading to confusion, fainting, and palpitations.

Dosage range for treating deficiency
Depends on the individual and on the nature and severity of symptoms. In extreme cases, intravenous sodium chloride may be required.

Symptoms and risks of excessive intake
Excessive sodium intake is thought to contribute to the development of high blood pressure. In people whose blood pressure is already raised, it may increase the risk of heart disease, stroke, and kidney damage. Other adverse effects include abnormal fluid retention leading to dizziness and swelling of the legs and face. Large overdoses, even of table salt, may cause seizures or coma and can be fatal.

THIAMINE

Other names Thiamine hydrochloride, thiamine mononitrate, vitamin B$_1$

Availability
Thiamine is available without prescription in a variety of vitamin/mineral preparations and as single-ingredient tablets.

Actions on the body
Thiamine plays a vital role in the activities of many *enzymes*. It is essential for the breakdown and utilization of carbohydrates. It is important for a healthy nervous system, healthy muscles, and normal heart function.

Dietary and other natural sources
Thiamine is present in all unrefined food. Good dietary sources include pork, whole-grain or enriched cereals and breads, brown rice, pasta, liver, kidneys, meat, fish, beans, nuts, eggs, and most vegetables. Wheat germ and bran are excellent sources.

Normal daily requirement
The recommended daily allowances (RDA) of thiamine are: 0.3mg (birth – 6 months); 0.5 mg (6 months –1 year); 0.7mg (1 – 3 years); 0.9mg (4 – 6 years); 1.2mg (7 – 10 years); 1.4mg (males aged 11 – 18); 1.5mg (males aged 19 – 22); 1.4mg (males aged 23 – 50); 1.2mg (males over 51); 1.1mg (females aged 11 – 22); 1.0mg (females over 23). Requirements are increased by 0.4 and 0.5mg in pregnancy and breast feeding, respectively.

When supplements are helpful
A balanced diet generally provides adequate amounts of thiamine. However, supplements may be helpful in elderly people and in those with high energy requirements caused, for example, by overactivity of the thyroid or heavy manual work. As with other B vitamins, requirements of thiamine are increased during severe illness, surgery, serious injury, and prolonged psychological stress. Additional thiamine is usually necessary on medical advice for deficiency associated with conditions in which absorption of nutrients from the intestine is impaired, and for prolonged liver disease or severe alcoholism.

Symptoms of deficiency
Mild deficiency may cause fatigue, irritability, loss of appetite, and disturbed sleep. Severe deficiency may cause confusion, loss of memory, depression, abdominal pain, constipation, and beriberi, a disorder that affects the nerves, brain and heart. Symptoms of beriberi include tingling or burning sensations in the legs, cramps and tenderness in the calf muscles, incoordination, palpitations, mental disturbances, and heart failure. In infants, beriberi can cause seizures, vomiting, and heart failure. In chronic alcoholics with malnutrition, vitamin B$_1$ deficiency may lead to a characteristic deterioration of central nervous system function known as Wernicke's syndrome, which results eventually in paralysis of the eye muscles, severe memory loss, and dementia, for which urgent treatment is needed.

Dosage range for treating deficiency
Depends on the individual and on the nature and severity of the disorder. In general, 5 – 25mg is given three times daily by mouth. Injections of the vitamin are sometimes given when deficiency is very severe or when symptoms have appeared suddenly.

Symptoms and risks of excessive intake
The risk of adverse effects is very low, since any excess is rapidly eliminated in the urine. However, prolonged use of large doses of thiamine may deplete other B vitamins; it should therefore be taken in a vitamin B complex formulation. Allergic reactions have occurred in rare cases after intravenous injection of large doses of this vitamin.

VITAMIN A

Other names Beta-carotene, retinol, retinol palmitate

Availability
Retinol, retinol palmitate, and beta-carotene are available without prescription in various single-ingredient and vitamin/mineral preparations. Etretinate, tretinoin, and isotretinoin are related to vitamin A and are available only by prescription for skin disorders such as acne and psoriasis.

Actions on the body
Vitamin A is essential for normal growth and strong bones and teeth in children. It is necessary for normal vision and healthy cell structure. It helps keep skin healthy and protects the linings of the mouth, nose, throat, lungs, and digestive and urinary tracts against infection. Vitamin A is also necessary for fertility in both sexes.

Dietary and other natural sources
Liver, fish liver oils, eggs, dairy products, orange and yellow vegetables and fruits (carrots, squash, apricots and peaches), and dark green, leafy vegetables (spinach, kale and broccoli) are good dietary sources. Vitamin A is also added to margarine.

Normal daily requirement
Vitamin A requirements are expressed in international units (IU) and retinol equivalents (RE). Recommended daily allowances (RDA) are: 420 RE (2,100 IU) birth – 6 months; 400 RE (2,000 IU) 6 months – 3 years; 500 RE (2,500 IU) age 4 – 6; 700 RE (3,500 IU) age 7 – 10; and over 11 years, 1,000 RE (5,000 IU) for males and 800 RE (4,000 IU) for females. Requirements are increased by 200 RE in pregnancy and 400 RE in breast feeding.

When supplements are helpful
Most diets provide adequate amounts of vitamin A. However, diets exceptionally low in fat or protein can lead to deficiency. Supplements may be necessary for people with certain intestinal disorders, cystic fibrosis, obstruction of the bile ducts, diabetes mellitus, and overactivity of the thyroid gland, and for people on long-term treatment with lipid-lowering drugs, since these reduce absorption of the vitamin from the intestine.

Symptoms of deficiency
Night blindness (difficulty in seeing in dim light) is the earliest symptom of deficiency. Other symptoms include dry, rough skin, loss of appetite, and diarrhea. Resistance to infection is decreased. Eyes may become dry and inflamed. Severe deficiency may lead to corneal ulcers and weak bones and teeth.

Dosage range for treating deficiency
Severe deficiency in adults and children over age 8 is treated with 1,000 – 9,000 RE (5,000 – 30,000 IU) until the amount of vitamin in the blood returns to normal.

Symptoms and risks of excessive intake
Prolonged excessive intake of 2,000 RE (10,000 IU) in children and 7,500 RE (25,000 IU) in adults can cause headache, nausea, diarrhea, dry, itchy skin, hair loss, and loss of appetite. Fatigue and irregular menstruation are also common. In extreme cases, bone pain and enlargement of the liver and spleen may occur. High doses of beta-carotene may turn the skin orange but are not dangerous. Excessive intake of vitamin A in pregnancy may lead to birth defects.

A B C D E F G H I J K L M N O P Q R S T U **V** W X Y Z

A B C D E F G H I J K L M N O P Q R S T U V W X Y Z

VITAMIN B$_{12}$

Other names Cobalamin, cyanocobalamin, cobalamins, hydroxycobalamin

Availability
Vitamin B$_{12}$ is available without prescription in a wide variety of preparations. Hydroxycobalamin is given only by injection under medical supervision.

Actions on the body
Vitamin B$_{12}$ plays a vital role in the activities of several *enzymes*. It is essential for the manufacture of the genetic material of cells and thus for growth and development. The formation of red blood cells by the bone marrow is particularly dependent on this vitamin. It is also involved in the utilization of folic acid and carbohydrates in the diet, and is necessary for maintaining a healthy nervous system.

Dietary and other natural sources
Liver is the best dietary source of vitamin B$_{12}$. Kidney, lean meats, fish, chicken, eggs, and dairy products are also rich in the vitamin.

Normal daily requirement
Only minute quantities of vitamin B$_{12}$ are required. Recommended daily allowances (RDA) of the vitamin in micrograms are: 0.5mcg (birth – 6 months); 1.5mcg (6 months – 1 year); 2.0mcg (1 – 3 years); 2.5mcg (4 – 6 years); 3.0mcg (over 7 years). Requirements are increased by 1.0mcg during pregnancy and breast feeding.

When supplements are helpful
A balanced diet usually provides more than adequate amounts of the vitamin, and deficiency is generally due to impaired absorption from the intestine rather than a low dietary intake. However, a strict vegetarian or vegan diet lacking in eggs or dairy products is likely to be deficient in vitamin B$_{12}$, and supplements are usually needed. The most common cause of deficiency is pernicious anemia, in which absorption of the vitamin is impaired due to inability of the stomach to secrete a special substance – intrinsic factor – that normally combines with the vitamin so that it can be taken up in the intestine. Supplements are also prescribed on medical advice in certain bowel disorders such as celiac disease and steatorrhea, after surgery to the stomach or intestine, and in tapeworm infestation.

Symptoms of deficiency
Vitamin B$_{12}$ deficiency usually develops over months or years – the liver can store up to 6 years' supply. It leads to *anemia*. The mouth and tongue often become sore. Deficiency of the vitamin also affects the brain and spinal cord, leading to numbness and tingling of the limbs, memory loss, and depression.

Dosage range for treating deficiency
Depends on the individual and on the type and severity of deficiency. Pernicious anemia (deficiency due to impaired absorption of B$_{12}$) is treated in adults with 1,000mcg twice during the first week, followed by 100 – 200mcg monthly by injection until anemia disappears. Higher doses of up to 1,000mcg of B$_{12}$, together with folic acid, may be given if deficiency is severe. Children are treated with doses of 30 – 50mcg daily. Dietary deficiency is usually treated with oral supplements of 6mcg daily (2 – 3mcg in infants). Deficiency resulting from a genetic defect that prevents use of the vitamin is treated with 250mcg every three weeks throughout life.

Symptoms and risks of excessive intake
Harmful effects from high doses of vitamin B$_{12}$ are unknown. Allergic reactions may in rare cases occur with impure preparations given by injection.

VITAMIN C

Other names Ascorbic acid, ascorbate calcium, ascorbate sodium

Availability
Vitamin C is available without prescription in a wide variety of single-ingredient and vitamin/mineral preparations. Ascorbate sodium is given only by injection under medical supervision.

Actions on the body
Vitamin C plays an essential role in the activities of several *enzymes*. It is vital for the growth and maintenance of healthy bones, teeth, gums, ligaments, and blood vessels and is an important component of all body organs. It is important for the manufacture of certain *neurotransmitters* and adrenal hormones. It is also required for the utilization of folic acid and absorption of iron. Vitamin C is also necessary for normal immune responses to infection and for wound healing.

Dietary and other natural sources
Vitamin C is found in most fresh fruits and vegetables. Citrus fruits, tomatoes, potatoes, and green, leafy vegetables are good dietary sources. Strawberries and cantaloupe are also rich in the vitamin.

Normal daily requirement
Recommended daily allowances (RDA) are: 35mg (birth – 1 year); 45mg (1 – 10 years); 50mg (11 – 14 years); and 60mg (ages 15 and over). Requirements are increased by 20mg in pregnancy and by 40mg in breast feeding.

When supplements are helpful
A healthy diet generally contains sufficient quantities of vitamin C. However, it is used up more rapidly after a serious injury, major surgery, burns, and in extremes of temperature. Because inhalation of carbon monoxide destroys the vitamin, city dwellers need more than people who live in the country, and smokers are likely to be deficient. Supplements may be necessary to prevent or treat deficiency in the elderly and chronically sick, and in severe alcoholism; women taking estrogen-containing contraceptives may also require supplements. There is no convincing evidence that vitamin C in large doses prevents colds, although it may reduce the severity of symptoms.

Symptoms of deficiency
Mild deficiency may cause weakness, aches, pains, swollen gums, and nosebleeds. Severe deficiency results in scurvy, the symptoms of which include inflamed, bleeding gums, excessive bruising, and internal bleeding. In adults, bones fracture easily and teeth become loose. In children there is abnormal bone and tooth development. Wounds fail to heal and become infected. Deficiency often leads to anemia (abnormally low levels of red blood cells), symptoms of which are pallor, fatigue, shortness of breath, and palpitations. Untreated scurvy may cause seizures, coma, and death.

Dosage range for treating deficiency
For scurvy, 300mg of vitamin C is given daily for several weeks. Adding a daily source of vitamin C, such as a glass of orange juice, is also recommended.

Symptoms and risks of excessive intake
The risk of harmful effects is low, as excess vitamin C is excreted in the urine. However, doses of over 1g daily may cause diarrhea, nausea, and stomach cramps. Kidney stones may occasionally develop.

VITAMIN D

Other names Alfacalcidol, calcefediol, calciferol, calcitriol, cholecalciferol, ergocalciferol, vitamin D_2, vitamin D_3

Availability
Vitamin D is available without prescription in various single-ingredient and vitamin/mineral preparations. Injections are given only under medical supervision.

Actions on the body
Vitamin D (with parathyroid hormone) helps regulate the balance of calcium and phosphate in the body. It aids the absorption of calcium from the intestinal tract, and is essential for strong bones and teeth.

Dietary and other natural sources
Fortified milk is the best dietary source of vitamin D. Oily fish (sardines, herring, salmon, and tuna), liver, dairy products and egg yolks are good, but not reliable, sources of this vitamin. It is also formed by the action of ultraviolet rays in sunlight on chemicals naturally present in the skin.

Normal daily requirement
Recommended daily allowances (RDA), expressed in micrograms (mcg) of cholecalciferol and international units (IU) of vitamin D are: 10mcg (400 IU) up to age 18; 7.5mcg (300 IU) ages 19 – 22; and 5mcg (200 IU) over 23 years. Requirements are increased by 5mcg (200 IU) in pregnancy and breast feeding.

When supplements are helpful
Vitamin D requirements are small and usually adequately met by dietary sources and normal exposure to sunlight. However, a poor diet and inadequate sunlight may lead to deficiency; dark-skinned people (particularly those living in smoggy urban areas) and night shift workers are more at risk. In areas of moderate sunshine, supplements may be given to infants. Premature infants, strict vegetarians, and the elderly may benefit from supplements. Supplements are usually necessary on medical advice to prevent and treat vitamin D deficiency-related bone disorders, and for conditions in which absorption from the intestine is impaired, deficiency due to liver disease, certain kidney disorders, prolonged use of certain drugs, and genetic defects. It is also used in treatment of hypoparathyroidism.

Symptoms of deficiency
Long-term deficiency leads to low blood levels of calcium and phosphate, which results in softening of the bones. In children, this causes abnormal bone development (rickets), and in adults, osteomalacia, causing backache, muscle weakness, bone pain, and fractures.

Dosage range for treating deficiency
In general, rickets caused by dietary deficiency is treated initially with 5,000 – 10,000 IU of vitamin D daily, followed by a maintenance dose of 400 IU. Osteomalacia caused by vitamin D deficiency is treated initially with 3,000 – 50,000 IU daily, followed by a daily maintenance dose of 400 IU. Deficiency caused by impaired intestinal absorption is treated with doses of 10,000 – 50,000 IU daily (adults) and 10,000 – 25,000 IU daily (children).

Symptoms and risks of excessive intake
Doses of over 400 IU of vitamin D daily are not beneficial to most people and may increase the risk of adverse effects such as weakness, unusual thirst, increased urination, gastrointestinal disturbances, and depression. Prolonged, excessive use disrupts the balance of calcium and phosphate in the body and may lead to abnormal calcium deposits in the soft tissues, blood vessel walls, and kidneys and retarded growth in children. Daily doses of over 25mcg (1,000 IU) in infants and 1.25mg (50,000 IU) in adults and children are considered excessive.

VITAMIN E

Other names Alpha-tocopherol acetate, tocopherol, tocopherols

Availability
Vitamin E is available without prescription in many single-ingredient and vitamin/mineral preparations. It is also included in skin creams. Alpha-tocopherol is the most powerful form.

Actions on the body
Vitamin E is vital for healthy cell structure, for slowing the effects of the aging process on cells and for maintaining the activities of certain *enzymes*. Vitamin E protects the lungs and other tissues from damage by pollutants, and protects red blood cells against destruction by poisons in the bloodstream. It also helps to form red blood cells, and is involved in the production of energy in the heart and muscles.

Dietary and other natural sources
Vegetable oils are good sources. Other sources rich in this vitamin include green, leafy vegetables, whole-grain cereals, and wheat germ.

Normal daily requirements
Vitamin E requirements are expressed in alpha-tocopherol equivalents (alpha-TE) and international units (IU). The recommended daily allowances (RDA) are: 3mg alpha-TE (4.5 IU) from birth – 6 months; 4mg alpha-TE (6 IU) at 6 months – 1 year; 5mg alpha-TE (7.5 IU) from 1 – 3 years; 6mg alpha-TE (9 IU) from 4 – 6 years; 7mg alpha-TE (10.5 IU) from 7 – 10 years; 8mg alpha-TE (12 IU) males aged 1 – 14 and females aged 11 and over; and 10mg alpha-TE (15 IU) for males over 15. Requirements are increased by 2 and 3mg alpha-TE (3 and 4.5 IU) in pregnancy and breast feeding, respectively.

When supplements are helpful
A normal diet supplies adequate amounts of vitamin E, and supplements are rarely necessary. However, people consuming large amounts of polyunsaturated fats in vegetable oils, especially if used in cooking at high temperatures, may need supplements, as may people with impaired intestinal absorption, liver disease, or cystic fibrosis. Supplements of vitamin E are also recommended for premature infants.

Symptoms of deficiency
Vitamin E deficiency leads to destruction of red blood cells (hemolysis) and eventually anemia (abnormally low levels of red blood cells), symptoms of which are pallor, fatigue, shortness of breath, and palpitations. In infants, deficiency causes irritability and fluid retention.

Dosage range for treating deficiency
Doses are generally four to five times the recommended daily allowance (RDA) in adults and children.

Symptoms and risks of excessive intake
Harmful effects are rare, but prolonged use of over 250mg daily may lead to nausea, abdominal pain, vomiting, and diarrhea. Large doses may also reduce the amounts of vitamin A, D, and K absorbed from the intestines.

VITAMIN K

Other names Menadione, phytonadione, vitamin K_1, vitamin K_2, vitamin K_3

Availability
Vitamin K is available without prescription as a dietary supplement on its own and in several vitamin/mineral preparations. Injectable and oral preparations used to treat bleeding disorders are available only by prescription.

Actions on the body
Vitamin K is necessary for the formation in the liver of several substances that promote the formation of blood clots (blood clotting factors) including prothrombin (clotting factor II).

Dietary and other natural sources
The best dietary sources of vitamin K are green, leafy vegetables and root vegetables, fruits, seeds, cow's milk, and yogurt. Alfalfa is also an excellent source. In adults and children the intestinal bacteria manufacture a large part of the vitamin K that is required.

Normal daily requirement
No recommended daily allowance (RDA) has been established, but the average daily intake of around 300 – 500mcg is considered adequate. Newborn infants need more of the vitamin.

When supplements are helpful
Vitamin K requirements are generally met adequately by dietary intake and by manufacture of the vitamin by bacteria that live in the intestine. Supplements are given routinely to newborn infants, since they lack intestinal bacteria capable of producing the vitamin and are therefore more at risk of deficiency. In adults and children, additional vitamin K is usually necessary only on medical advice for deficiency associated with prolonged use of antibiotics or sulfonamide antibacterials that destroy bacteria in the intestine, or when absorption of nutrients from the intestine is impaired. These conditions include liver disease, obstruction of the bile duct, and intestinal disorders causing chronic diarrhea. Vitamin K may also be given to reduce blood loss during labor or after surgery in people who have been taking aspirin or oral anticoagulants; it also reverses the effect of an overdose of oral anticoagulants.

Symptoms of deficiency
Vitamin K deficiency leads to low levels of prothrombin (hypoprothrombinemia) and other clotting factors, resulting in delayed blood clotting and a tendency to bleed. This may cause oozing from wounds, nosebleeds, and bleeding from the gums, intestine, urinary tract, and, rarely, in the brain.

Dosage range for treating deficiency
Depends on the individual and on the nature and severity of the disorder.

Symptoms and risks of excessive intake
Excess dietary intake of vitamin K has no known harmful effects. Synthetic vitamin K (menadione) may cause liver damage or rupture of red blood cells (hemolysis) at large doses and in people with glucose-6-phosphate dehydrogenase (G6PD) deficiency. This may lead to reddish-brown urine, jaundice and, in extreme cases, *anemia*. Adverse effects are extremely rare with vitamin K preparations taken by mouth.

ZINC

Other names Zinc amino acid chelate, zinc chloride, zinc sulfate, zinc gluconate

Availability
Zinc supplements are available without prescription in single-ingredient and vitamin/mineral preparations. Zinc chloride is an injectable preparation given only under medical supervision during intravenous feeding. Zinc is also one ingredient included in a variety of topical formulations used for the treatment of minor skin irritations, dandruff, and fungal infections.

Actions on the body
Zinc plays a vital role in the activities of over 100 *enzymes*. It is essential for the manufacture of proteins and nucleic acids (the genetic material of cells), and is involved in the function of the hormone insulin in the utilization of carbohydrates. It is necessary for a normal rate of growth, development of the reproductive organs, normal function of the prostate gland, and healing of wounds and burns.

Dietary and other natural sources
Zinc is present in small amounts in a wide variety of foods. Zinc from animal sources is better absorbed than that from plants. Protein-rich foods such as lean meat and seafood are the best sources of the mineral. Whole-grain breads and cereals and dried beans are good dietary sources.

Normal daily requirements
The recommended daily allowances (RDA) are: 3mg (birth – 6 months); 5mg (6 months – 1 year); 10mg (1 – 10 years); and 15mg (over 10 years). Requirements are increased by 5 and 10mg, respectively, during pregnancy and breast feeding.

When supplements are helpful
A balanced diet containing natural, unprocessed foods usually provides adequate amounts of zinc. Dietary deficiency is rare in the United States and is likely only in people who are generally malnourished, such as debilitated elderly people on poor diets. Supplements are usually recommended on medical advice for those with reduced absorption of the mineral due to certain intestinal disorders, such as cystic fibrosis, for those with increased zinc requirements due to sickle cell disease or major burns, and for people with liver damage (e.g., as a result of excessive alcohol intake).

Symptoms of deficiency
Deficiency may cause loss of appetite and impair the sense of taste. In children, it may also lead to poor growth and, in severe cases, to delayed sexual development and dwarfism. Severe, prolonged lack of zinc may result in a rare skin disorder involving hair loss, rash, inflamed areas of skin with pustules, and inflammation of the mouth, tongue, eyelids, and around the fingernails.

Dosage range for treating deficiency
Depends on the individual and on the cause and severity of the deficiency. In general, 30 – 50mg daily, usually in the form of zinc sulfate.

Symptoms and risks of excessive intake
The risk of harmful effects is low with excess zinc intake. However, prolonged use of large doses may interfere with the absorption of iron and copper, leading to deficiency of these minerals, and may cause nausea, vomiting, headache, fever, malaise, and abdominal pain.

DRUGS OF ABUSE

The purpose of these pages is to clarify the medical facts concerning certain drugs (or classes of drugs) that are most commonly abused in the United States. Their physical and mental effects, sometimes including a dangerous habit-forming potential, have led to their use outside a medical context. Some of the drugs listed here are illegal; others have legitimate medical uses (for example, sleeping drugs and anti-anxiety drugs) and are also discussed elsewhere in the book. Alcohol, nicotine, and solvents, although not medical drugs, are all substances with drug-like effects and high abuse potential. They are also listed for the sake of completeness.

The individual profiles are designed to instruct and inform the reader so that he or she may become more aware of the hazards of drug abuse and be able to recognize signs of abuse in others. Since a large proportion of drug abusers are young people, the following pages may serve as a useful source of reference for parents and teachers concerned that young people in their charge may be taking drugs.

The drugs of abuse profiles

The profiles are arranged in alphabetical order under their medical names, with street names, drug categories, and cross-references to other sections of the book where appropriate. Each profile contains information on that drug under standard headings. Topics covered include the various ways it is taken, its habit-forming potential, its legitimate medical uses, effects, and risks, the signs of abuse, and interactions with other drugs.

HOW TO UNDERSTAND THE ENTRIES

Each drug of abuse profile contains standard headings under which you will find information covering important aspects of the drug.

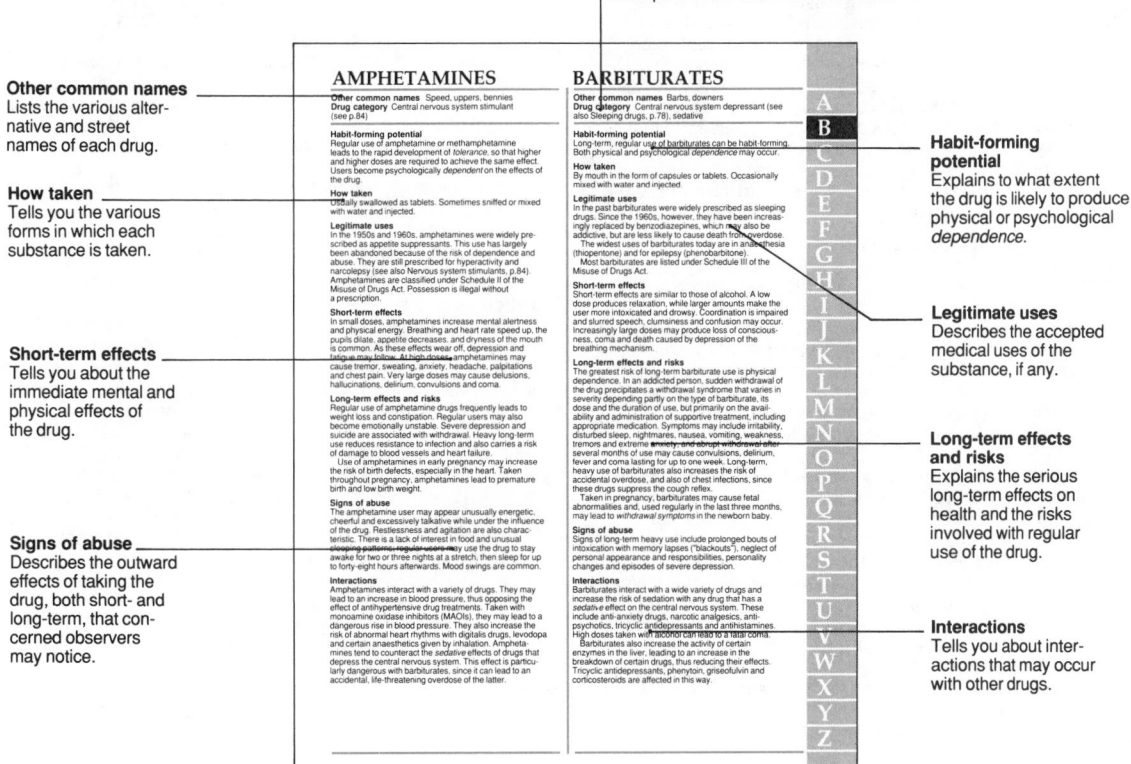

Drug category
Categorizes the drug according to its principal effects on the body, with cross-references to other parts of the book where relevant.

Other common names
Lists the various alternative and street names of each drug.

How taken
Tells you the various forms in which each substance is taken.

Short-term effects
Tells you about the immediate mental and physical effects of the drug.

Signs of abuse
Describes the outward effects of taking the drug, both short- and long-term, that concerned observers may notice.

Habit-forming potential
Explains to what extent the drug is likely to produce physical or psychological *dependence*.

Legitimate uses
Describes the accepted medical uses of the substance, if any.

Long-term effects and risks
Explains the serious long-term effects on health and the risks involved with regular use of the drug.

Interactions
Tells you about interactions that may occur with other drugs.

AMPHETAMINES

Other common names Speed, uppers, bennies
Drug category Central nervous system stimulant (see p.84)

Habit-forming potential
Regular use of amphetamine or methamphetamine leads to the rapid development of *tolerance*, so that higher and higher doses are required to achieve the same effect. Users become psychologically *dependent* on the effects of the drug.

How taken
Usually swallowed as tablets. Sometimes sniffed or mixed with water and injected.

Legitimate uses
In the 1950s and 1960s, amphetamines were widely prescribed as appetite suppressants. This use has largely been abandoned because of the risk of dependence and abuse. They are still prescribed for hyperactivity and narcolepsy (see also Nervous system stimulants, p.84). Amphetamines are classified under Schedule II of the Misuse of Drugs Act. Possession is illegal without a prescription.

Short-term effects
In small doses, amphetamines increase mental alertness and physical energy. Breathing and heart rate speed up, the pupils dilate, appetite decreases, and dryness of the mouth is common. As these effects wear off, depression and fatigue may follow. At high doses, amphetamines may cause tremor, sweating, anxiety, headache, palpitations and chest pain. Very large doses may cause delusions, hallucinations, delirium, convulsions and coma.

Long-term effects and risks
Regular use of amphetamine drugs frequently leads to weight loss and constipation. Regular users may also become emotionally unstable. Severe depression and suicide are associated with withdrawal. Heavy long-term use reduces resistance to infection and also carries a risk of damage to blood vessels and the heart.
Use of amphetamines in early pregnancy may increase the risk of birth defects, especially in the heart. Taken throughout pregnancy, amphetamines lead to premature birth and low birth weight.

Signs of abuse
The amphetamine user may appear unusually energetic, cheerful and excessively talkative while under the influence of the drug. Restlessness and agitation are also characteristic. There is a lack of interest in food and unusual sleeping patterns; regular users may use the drug to stay awake for two or three nights at a stretch, then sleep for up to forty-eight hours afterwards. Mood swings are common.

Interactions
Amphetamines interact with a variety of drugs. They may lead to an increase in blood pressure, thus opposing the effect of antihypertensive drug treatments. Taken with monoamine oxidase inhibitors (MAOIs), they may lead to a dangerous rise in blood pressure. They also increase the risk of abnormal heart rhythms with digitalis drugs, levodopa and certain anaesthetics given by inhalation. Amphetamines tend to counteract the *sedative* effects of drugs that depress the central nervous system. This effect is particularly dangerous with barbiturates, since it can lead to an accidental, life-threatening overdose of the latter.

BARBITURATES

Other common names Barbs, downers
Drug category Central nervous system depressant (see also Sleeping drugs, p.78), sedative

Habit-forming potential
Long-term, regular use of barbiturates can be habit-forming. Both physical and psychological *dependence* may occur.

How taken
By mouth in the form of capsules or tablets. Occasionally mixed with water and injected.

Legitimate uses
In the past barbiturates were widely prescribed as sleeping drugs. Since the 1960s, however, they have been increasingly replaced by benzodiazepines, which may also be addictive, but are less likely to cause death from overdose.
The widest uses of barbiturates today are in anaesthesia (thiopentone) and for epilepsy (phenobarbitone).
Most barbiturates are listed under Schedule III of the Misuse of Drugs Act.

Short-term effects
Short-term effects are similar to those of alcohol. A low dose produces relaxation, while larger amounts make the user more intoxicated and drowsy. Coordination is impaired and slurred speech, clumsiness and confusion may occur. Increasingly large doses may produce loss of consciousness, coma and death caused by depression of the breathing mechanism.

Long-term effects and risks
The greatest risk of long-term barbiturate use is physical dependence. In an addicted person, sudden withdrawal of the drug precipitates a withdrawal syndrome that varies in severity depending partly on the type of barbiturate, its dose and the duration of use, but primarily on the availability and administration of supportive treatment, including appropriate medication. Symptoms may include irritability, disturbed sleep, nightmares, nausea, vomiting, weakness, tremors and extreme anxiety; and abrupt withdrawal after several months of use may cause convulsions, delirium, fever and coma lasting for up to one week. Long-term, heavy use of barbiturates also increases the risk of accidental overdose, and also of chest infections, since these drugs suppress the cough reflex.
Taken in pregnancy, barbiturates may cause fetal abnormalities and, used regularly in the last three months, may lead to *withdrawal* symptoms in the newborn baby.

Signs of abuse
Signs of long-term heavy use include prolonged bouts of intoxication with memory lapses ("blackouts"), neglect of personal appearance and responsibilities, personality changes and episodes of severe depression.

Interactions
Barbiturates interact with a wide variety of drugs and increase the risk of sedation with any drug that has a *sedative* effect on the central nervous system. These include anti-anxiety drugs, narcotic analgesics, antipsychotics, tricyclic antidepressants and antihistamines. High doses taken with alcohol can lead to a fatal coma.
Barbiturates also increase the activity of certain enzymes in the liver, leading to an increase in the breakdown of certain drugs, thus reducing their effects. Tricyclic antidepressants, phenytoin, griseofulvin and corticosteroids are affected in this way.

ALCOHOL

Other common names Liquor, drink, booze, sauce, hooch
Drug category Central nervous system depressant; sedative

Habit-forming potential
Because individual responses vary so widely, it is difficult to measure the habit-forming potential of alcohol. But there is certainly a disease called alcoholism, characterized by a person's inability to control intake. Regular drinking and heavy drinking do not cause alcoholism so much as indicate that it may be present. Alcoholism involves psychological and physical *dependence*, evidenced by large daily consumption, heavy weekend drinking, or long episodic binges.

How taken
By mouth, usually in the form of wines, beers and a variety of liquors.

Legitimate uses
Alcoholic beverages are generally available throughout the US although there are restrictions on sale and consumption. Sale of alcohol is generally restricted to people 21 or older.

Medically, rubbing alcohol (which is isopropyl, or denatured ethyl alcohol) is widely used as an *antiseptic* before injections to minimize the risk of infection. It is also used to harden the skin and thus prevent pressure sores in bedridden people, and foot sores in hikers or runners.

Short-term effects
Alcohol acts as a central nervous system depressant, thus reducing anxiety, tension, and inhibitions. In moderate quantities, it gives the drinker a feeling of relaxation and confidence and increases sociability and talkativeness. Moderate amounts also dilate small blood vessels, particularly those in the skin, leading to flushing and a feeling of warmth. With increasing amounts, concentration and judgment are progressively impaired and the body's reactions are increasingly slowed. Accidents, particularly driving accidents, are more likely. As blood alcohol levels rise, violent or aggressive behavior is possible. Speech is slurred, and the person becomes unsteady, staggers, and may experience double vision and loss of balance. Nausea and vomiting are frequent; urinary incontinence may occur. Loss of consciousness may follow if blood alcohol levels continue to rise, and there is a risk of death from inhalation of vomit or cessation of breathing.

Long-term effects and risks
A large number of heavy drinkers develop liver diseases, including alcoholic hepatitis, cirrhosis, liver cancer, or fatty liver (excess fat deposits that may lead to cirrhosis). Coronary heart disease, high blood pressure, and strokes are also possible consequences of heavy drinking. Inflammation of the stomach (gastritis) and peptic ulcers are also more common. Alcoholics have an above average risk of developing dementia (irreversible mental deterioration).

Long-term heavy drinking is usually associated with physical dependence. An alcoholic may appear to be sober, even after heavy drinking, because of built-up *tolerance*. But a reverse-tolerance effect is often seen in long-time alcoholics, in whom relatively little alcohol causes signs of overt intoxication. In addition to health problems, alcohol dependence is associated with a range of personal and social problems. Alcoholic-dependent persons may suffer from anxiety and depression, and since they often eat poorly, they are at risk of nutritional deficiency diseases, particularly thiamine deficiency (see p.543).

Drinking during pregnancy can cause fetal abnormalities and poor physical and mental development in infants; even taking moderate amounts of alcohol can lead to miscarriage, low birth weight, and mental retardation.

Signs of abuse
Signs that alcohol consumption is getting out of control include any or all of the following: changes in drinking pattern (for example, early morning drinking or a switch from beer to vodka); changes in drinking habits (such as drinking alone or having a drink before an appointment or interview); personality changes; neglect of personal appearance; poor eating habits; furtive behavior; increasingly frequent or prolonged bouts of intoxication with memory lapses ("blackouts") about events that occurred during drinking episodes. Physical symptoms may include nausea, vomiting, or shaking in the morning, abdominal pain, cramps, weakness in the legs and hands, redness and enlarged blood vessels in the face, unsteadiness, poor memory, and incontinence. Sudden discontinuation of heavy drinking, if untreated, can lead to delirium tremens (severe shaking, hallucinations, and, occasionally, fatal convulsions) beginning after two to four days of abstinence and lasting for up to three days.

Interactions
Alcohol interacts with a wide variety of drugs. In particular, it increases the risk of sedation with any drug that has a *sedative* effect on the central nervous system. These include anti-anxiety drugs, sleeping drugs, general anesthetics, narcotic analgesics, antipsychotics, tricyclic antidepressants, antihistamines, and certain antihypertensive drugs (methyldopa and clonidine). Taking alcohol with other depressant drugs of abuse, particularly narcotics, barbiturates, or solvents, can lead to coma and may be fatal.

Taken with aspirin and similar analgesics, alcohol increases the risk of bleeding from the stomach, particularly in people who have had peptic ulcers.

People on a regimen of disulfiram (Antabuse), a drug used to help people stay in an alcohol-free state, will experience highly unpleasant reactions if they then take even a small amount of alcohol. The results include flushing of the face, throbbing headache, palpitations, nausea, and vomiting.

Alcohol may inhibit the breakdown of some oral antidiabetic drugs and oral anticoagulants, and thus increase their effects.

Taken with monoamine oxidase inhibitors (MAOIs), alcohol, particularly in the form of red wine, may cause a dangerous rise in blood pressure.

Practical points
If you drink, know what your limits are. They vary from person to person, and capacity depends a good deal on body weight, age, experience, and mental and emotional state. If you are a woman and are pregnant, or are planning to have a baby soon, the safest course is abstinence. If you are planning to drive, don't drink. If you find that you are having trouble controlling your drinking, seek help and advice from your physician or from one of the treatment programs available in most parts of the country. And even if you don't have a control problem, don't drink heavily – remember that alcohol can have harmful effects on many parts of your body, including your brain.

AMPHETAMINES

Other common names Speed, uppers, bennies
Drug category Central nervous system stimulant
(see p.116)

Habit-forming potential
Regular use of amphetamines and methamphetamine
leads to the rapid development of *tolerance*, so that higher
and higher doses are required to achieve the same effect.
Users become psychologically dependent on the effects of
the drug.

How taken
Usually swallowed as tablets. Sometimes sniffed or mixed
with water and injected.

Legitimate uses
In the 1950s and 1960s, amphetamines were widely prescribed as appetite suppressants. This use has largely
been abandoned because of the risk of *dependence* and
abuse. They are still prescribed for hyperactivity and
narcolepsy (see also Nervous system stimulants, p.116).
Amphetamines are classified under Schedule II drugs of the
Controlled Substances Act. Possession is illegal without
a prescription.

Short-term effects
In small doses, amphetamines increase mental alertness
and physical energy. Breathing and heart rate speed up, the
pupils dilate, appetite decreases, and dryness of the mouth
is common. As these effects wear off, depression and
fatigue may follow. At high doses, amphetamines may
cause tremor, sweating, anxiety, headache, palpitations,
and severe chest pain. Very large doses may cause
delusions, hallucinations, delirium, seizures, and coma.

Long-term effects and risks
Regular use of amphetamine drugs frequently leads to
weight loss and constipation. Regular users may also
become emotionally unstable. Severe depression and
suicide are associated with withdrawal. Heavy long-term
use reduces resistance to infection and also carries a risk
of damage to blood vessels and heart failure.

Use of amphetamines in early pregnancy may increase
the risk of birth defects, especially in the heart. Taken
throughout pregnancy, amphetamines lead to premature
birth and low birth weight.

Signs of abuse
The amphetamine user may appear unusually energetic,
cheerful, and excessively talkative while under the
influence of the drug. Restlessness and agitation are also
characteristic. There is a lack of interest in food and
unusual sleeping patterns; regular users may use the drug
to stay awake for two or three nights at a stretch, then
sleep for up to forty-eight hours afterwards. Mood swings
are common.

Interactions
Amphetamines interact with a variety of drugs. They may
lead to an increase in blood pressure, thus opposing the
effect of antihypertensive drug treatments. Taken with
monoamine oxidase inhibitors (MAOIs), they may lead to a
dangerous rise in blood pressure. They also increase the
risk of abnormal heart rhythms with digitalis drugs, levodopa,
and certain anesthetics given by inhalation. Amphetamines
tend to counteract the *sedative* effects of drugs that
depress the central nervous system. This effect is particularly dangerous with barbiturates, since it can lead to an
accidental, life-threatening overdose of the latter.

BARBITURATES

Other common names Downers, goofballs
Drug category Central nervous system depressant (see
also Sleeping drugs, p.110), sedative

Habit-forming potential
Long-term, regular use of barbiturates can be habit-forming.
Both physical and psychological *dependence* may occur.

How taken
By mouth in the form of capsules or tablets. Occasionally
mixed with water and injected.

Legitimate uses
In the past, barbiturates were widely prescribed as sleeping
drugs. Since the 1960s, however, they have been increasingly replaced by benzodiazepines, which may also be
addictive but are less likely to cause death from overdose.

The widest uses of barbiturates today are in anesthesia
and for epilepsy (phenobarbital).

Most barbiturates are listed under Schedule II of the
Controlled Substances Act.

Short-term effects
Short-term effects are similar to those of alcohol. A low
dose produces relaxation, while larger amounts make the
user more intoxicated and drowsy. Coordination is impaired
and slurred speech, clumsiness, and confusion may occur.
Increasingly large doses may produce loss of consciousness, coma, and death caused by depression of the
breathing mechanism.

Long-term effects and risks
The greatest risk of long-term barbiturate use is physical
dependence. In an addicted person, sudden withdrawal of
the drug precipitates a withdrawal syndrome that varies in
severity, depending partly on the type of barbiturate, its
dose, and the duration of use, but primarily on the availability and administration of supportive treatment, including
appropriate medication. Symptoms may include irritability,
disturbed sleep, nightmares, nausea, vomiting, weakness,
tremors, and extreme anxiety; abrupt withdrawal after
several months of use may cause seizures, delirium, fever,
and coma lasting for up to one week. Long-term, heavy use
of barbiturates increases the risk of accidental overdose,
and also of chest infections, since these drugs suppress
the cough reflex.

Taken in pregnancy, barbiturates may cause fetal
abnormalities and, used regularly in the last three months,
may lead to withdrawal symptoms in the newborn baby.

Signs of abuse
Signs of long-term heavy use include prolonged bouts of
intoxication with memory lapses ("blackouts"), neglect of
personal appearance and responsibilities, personality
changes, and episodes of severe depression.

Interactions
Barbiturates interact with a wide variety of drugs and
increase the risk of sedation with any drug that has a
sedative effect on the central nervous system. These
include anti-anxiety drugs, narcotic analgesics, antipsychotics, tricyclic antidepressants, and antihistamines.
High doses taken with alcohol can lead to a fatal coma.

Barbiturates also increase the activity of certain
enzymes in the liver, leading to an increase in the
breakdown of certain drugs, thus reducing their effects.
Tricyclic antidepressants, phenytoin, griseofulvin, and
corticosteroids are affected in this way.

BENZODIAZEPINES

Other common names Tranquilizers
Drug category Central nervous system depressants
(see Sleeping drugs, p.110, and Anti-anxiety drugs, p.111)

Habit-forming potential
The addictive potential of benzodiazepines is much lower
than that of some other central nervous system depressants such as barbiturates. However, regular long-term use
of these drugs can lead to psychological and physical
dependence on their sedative effects.

How taken
By mouth as tablets or capsules.

Legitimate uses
Benzodiazepines are among the most commonly prescribed
drugs. They are used mainly for short-term treatment of
anxiety and stress and for relief of sleeplessness. They are
also used in anesthesia both as *premedication* and for
induction of general anesthesia. Other medical uses include
the management of alcohol withdrawal, control of seizures,
and relief of muscle spasms. Benzodiazepines are
classified as Schedule IV drugs under the Controlled
Substances Act.

Short-term effects
Benzodiazepines can reduce mental activity along with
anxiety. In moderate doses, they may also cause
unsteadiness, reduce alertness and slow the body's
reactions, thus impairing driving ability and increasing the
risk of accidents. Any benzodiazepine in a high enough
dose induces sleep. Very large overdoses may cause
depression of the breathing mechanism.

Long-term effects and risks
Benzodiazepines tend to lose their *sedative* effect with long-
term use. This may lead the user to increase the dose
progressively, a manifestation of tolerance and physical
dependence. Older people may become apathetic or
confused when taking these drugs. On stopping the drug,
the chronic user may develop *withdrawal symptoms* that
may include anxiety, panic attacks, palpitations, shaking,
insomnia, headaches, dizziness, aches and pains, nausea,
loss of appetite, and clumsiness. Symptoms can last for
days or weeks. Babies born to women who use
benzodiazepines regularly may suffer withdrawal symptoms
during the first week of life.

Signs of abuse
Abuse can occur, but it is uncommon. The typical abuser
is a middle-aged or elderly person who may have been
taking these drugs by prescription for months or years. He
or she is usually unaware of the problem, and may freely
admit to taking "nerve pills" in large quantities. As long as
moderate drug intake continues, general health is not
noticeably affected.

Interactions
Benzodiazepines increase the risk of sedation with any
drug that has a sedative effect on the central nervous
system. These include other anti-anxiety and sleeping
drugs, alcohol, narcotic analgesics, antipsychotics,
tricyclic antidepressants, and antihistamines.

Practical points
Benzodiazepines should normally be used for courses of
two weeks duration or less. If these drugs have been taken
for longer than two weeks, it is usually best to reduce the
dose gradually to reduce the risk of withdrawal symptoms. If
you have been taking benzodiazepines for many months or
years, it is best to consult your doctor to work out a dose
reduction program. If possible, it will help to tell your family
and friends and enlist their support.

COCAINE

Other common names Coke, crack, nose candy, snow
Drug category Central nervous system stimulant and
local anesthetic

Habit-forming potential
Taken regularly, cocaine is habit-forming. Users may become psychologically dependent on its physical and mental
effects, and may step up their intake to maintain or increase
these effects or to prevent the feelings of severe fatigue
and depression that may occur after the drug is stopped.
The risk of *dependence* is especially pronounced with the
form of cocaine known as "freebase" or "crack" (see below).

How taken
Smoked, sniffed, or occasionally injected.

Legitimate uses
Cocaine was once widely used as a local anesthetic. It is
still sometimes given for *topical* anesthesia in the mouth
and throat prior to minor surgery or other procedures.
Because of its side effects and potential for abuse, cocaine
has now largely been replaced by safer local anesthetic
drugs. Cocaine is classified under Schedule II of the
Controlled Substances Act.

Short-term effects
Cocaine is a central nervous system stimulant. In moderate
doses it overcomes fatigue and produces feelings of well-
being and elation. Appetite is reduced. Physical effects
include an increase in heart rate and blood pressure,
dilation of the pupils, tremor and increased sweating. Large
doses can lead to agitation, anxiety, paranoia, and hallucinations. Paranoia may cause violent behavior. Very large
doses may cause seizures and death due to heart attack or
heart failure.

Long-term effects and risks
Heavy, regular use of cocaine can cause restlessness,
anxiety, hyperexcitability, nausea, insomnia, and weight
loss. Continued use may lead to increasing paranoia and
psychosis. Repeated sniffing also damages the membranes
lining the nose and may eventually lead to the destruction of
the septum, the structure separating the nostrils.
   People with heart disease, high blood pressure, or an
overactive thyroid gland run the risk of heart problems.

Signs of abuse
The cocaine user may appear unusually energetic and
exuberant under the influence of the drug and show little
interest in food. Heavy, regular use may lead to disturbed
eating and sleeping patterns. Agitation, mood swings,
aggressive behavior, and suspiciousness of other people
may also be signs of a heavy user.

Interactions
Cocaine can increase blood pressure, thus opposing the
effect of antihypertensive drugs. Taken with monoamine
oxidase inhibitors (MAOIs), it can cause a dangerous rise in
blood pressure. It also increases the risk of adverse effects
on the heart when taken with certain general anesthetics.

CRACK
This potent form of cocaine is taken in the form of crystals that are smoked. Highly addictive, it has more
intense effects than other forms of cocaine and there is
an increased risk of abnormal heart rhythms, high blood
pressure, stroke, and death. Long-term consequences
include coughing of black phlegm, wheezing, irreversible
lung damage, hoarseness, and parched lips, tongue and
throat from inhaling the hot fumes. Mental deterioration,
personality changes, social withdrawal, paranoia or
violent behavior, and suicide attempts may occur.

LSD

Other common names Lysergic acid, acid, haze
Drug category Hallucinogen

Habit-forming potential
Although it is not physically addictive, LSD may cause psychological *dependence*. After several days of regular use, a person develops a resistance to its actions. A waiting period must pass before resumption of the drug will produce the original effects.

How taken
By mouth, as tiny colored tablets, or absorbed onto small squares of paper (known as "microdots"), gelatin sheets, or sugar cubes.

Legitimate uses
None. Early interest of the medical profession in LSD focused on its possible use in psychotherapy, but additional studies suggested that it could lead to psychosis in susceptible people. Strict legal controls were introduced in 1966. It is listed under Schedule I of the Controlled Substances Act.

Short-term effects
The effects of usual doses of LSD last for about 12 hours, beginning almost immediately after taking the drug. Initial effects include restlessness, dizziness, a feeling of coldness with shivering, and an uncontrollable desire to laugh. Subsequent effects include distortions in perception of sound and vision; true hallucinations are rare. Introspection is often increased and mystical, pseudo-religious experiences may occur. Unpleasant or terrifying hallucinations, loss of emotional control, and overwhelming feelings of anxiety, despair, or panic may occur, particularly if the user is suffering from underlying anxiety or depression. Suicide may be attempted. Driving and other hazardous tasks are extremely dangerous. Some people under the influence of this drug have fallen off high buildings, mistakenly believing they could fly.

Long-term effects and risks
Long-term LSD use increases the risk of mental distur-bances, including severe depression. In those with existing psychological difficulties, it can lead to lasting mental problems. In addition, some frequent users experience brief but vivid recurrences of LSD's effects ("flashbacks") for months or years after last taking the drug, causing anxiety and disorientation. There is no evidence of lasting physical ill effects from LSD use.

Signs of abuse
A person under the influence of LSD may feel strange but rarely shows outward signs of intoxication. Occasionally, a user drugged with LSD may seem overexcited, or appear withdrawn or confused.

Interactions
None known.

MARIJUANA

Other common names Cannabis, grass, pot, dope, weed, hash
Drug category Central nervous system depressant, hallucinogen, anti-emetic

Habit-forming potential
There is evidence that regular users of marijuana can become physically and psychologically dependent on its effects.

How taken
Usually smoked. May be eaten, often in cakes or cookies, or brewed like tea and drunk.

Legitimate uses
Preparations of the leaves and resin of the cannabis plant (marijuana) have been in medical use for over two thousand years. Introduced into Western medicine in the mid-19th century, marijuana was once taken for a wide variety of complaints, including anxiety, insomnia, rheumatic disorders, migraine, painful menstruation, strychnine poisoning, and opiate withdrawal. Today, marijuana derivatives can be prescribed with certain restrictions in the United States for the treatment of glaucoma and the relief of nausea and vomiting caused by treatment with anticancer drugs. Marijuana itself is listed under Schedule I of the Controlled Substances Act, but the derivative dronabinol (an anti-emetic) is listed under Schedule II.

Short-term effects
These partly depend on the effects expected by the user as well as on the amount and strength of the preparation used. Marijuana available today is arguably more potent than that of a few years ago. In small doses, it promotes a feeling of relaxation and well being, enhances auditory and visual perception, and increases talkativeness. Appetite is usually increased. In some individuals the drug may have little or no effect.

Under the influence of the drug, short-term memory may be impaired and driving ability and coordination are dis-rupted. Loss of the sense of time, confusion, and emotional distress can result. Hallucinations may occur in rare cases. The effects last for one to three hours after smoking marijuana and for up to twelve hours or longer after it is eaten. Death from overdose is unknown.

Long-term effects and risks
Marijuana smoking, like tobacco smoking, probably increases the risk of bronchitis and other pulmonary disorders. Regular users may become apathetic and lethargic, and neglect their work or studies and personal appearance. In susceptible people, heavy use may trigger a temporary psychiatric disturbance. Marijuana is thought by some physicians to increase the likelihood of experimentation with other drugs.

Since marijuana may lower blood pressure and increase the heart rate, people with heart disorders may be at risk from adverse effects of this drug. Regular use of marijuana may reduce fertility in both men and women and, during pregnancy, may contribute to premature birth.

Signs of abuse
The marijuana user may appear unusually talkative or drunk under the influence of the drug. Appetite is increased.

Marijuana smoke has a distinct herbal smell that may linger in the hair and clothes of those who use it.

Interactions
Marijuana may increase the risk of sedation with any drugs that have a *sedative* effect on the central nervous system. These include anti-anxiety drugs, sleeping drugs, general anesthetics, narcotic analgesics, antipsychotics, tricyclic antidepressants, antihistamines, and alcohol.

A
B
C
D
E
F
G
H
I
J
K
L
M
N
O
P
Q
R
S
T
U
V
W
X
Y
Z

MESCALINE

Other common names Peyote, cactus buttons, big chief
Drug category Hallucinogen

Habit-forming potential
Mescaline has a low habit-forming potential; it does not cause physical *dependence* and does not usually lead to psychological dependence. After several days of taking mescaline, the user is resistant to further doses of the drug, which discourages daily use.

How taken
By mouth as capsules or in the form of peyote cactus buttons, eaten fresh or dried, drunk as tea, or ground up and smoked with marijuana.

Legitimate uses
The peyote cactus has been used by Mexican Indians for over 2,000 years, both as a religious sacrament and as a herbal remedy for various ailments ranging from wounds and bronchitis to failing vision. It is still used legally in the Native American Church in North America, which was set up for North American Indians in 1918. Outside this organization, mescaline and peyote are illegal, and mescaline is classified under Schedule I of the Controlled Substances Act.

Short-term effects
Mescaline alters visual and auditory perception, although true hallucinations are rare. Appetite is reduced under the influence of this drug. There is also a risk of unpleasant mental effects, particularly in people who are anxious or depressed.

Peyote may have additional effects caused by several other active substances (beside mescaline) in the plant. Strychnine-like chemicals may cause nausea, vomiting, and, occasionally, tremors and sweating, which usually precede the perceptual effects of mescaline by up to two hours.

Long-term effects and risks
The long-term effects of mescaline have not been well studied. It may increase the risk of mental disturbances, particularly in people with existing psychological problems. Studies have shown that after taking mescaline, most of the drug concentrates in the liver rather than in the brain, and it may therefore have special risks for people with impaired liver function.

Signs of abuse
Signs of mescaline or peyote abuse may not be obvious. Users might sometimes appear withdrawn, disoriented, or confused.

Interactions
The combination of alcohol and peyote is recognized to be dangerous. There is a risk of temporary derangement, leading to disorientation, panic, and violent behavior. Vomiting is likely to occur.

NARCOTICS (HEROIN)

Other common names Horse, junk, smack, scag, H
Drug category Central nervous system depressant

Habit-forming potential
Narcotic analgesics include not only drugs that are derived from the opium poppy (opium, morphine) but also synthetic drugs whose medical actions are similar to those of morphine (meperdine, methadone, propoxyphene). Their frequent use leads to tolerance, and all have a potential for dependence. Among them, heroin is the most potent, widely abused, and dangerous.

After only a few weeks of use *withdrawal symptoms* may occur when the drug is stopped; fear of such withdrawal effects may be a strong inducement to go on using the drug. In heavy users, the drug habit is often coupled with a lifestyle revolving around its use.

How taken
A white or speckled brown powder, heroin is either sniffed or injected. Other narcotics may be taken by mouth.

Legitimate uses
Heroin has no accepted medical use in the US and is listed under Schedule I of the Controlled Substances Act. Other narcotics, listed under Schedule II, are used for the relief of moderate to severe pain. Mild narcotics such as codeine are also sometimes included in cough suppressant and antidiarrheal medications and are listed under Schedule V.

Short-term effects
Strong narcotics induce a feeling of well-being and contentment. Pain is dulled and the activity of the nervous system is depressed; breathing and heart rate are slowed and the cough reflex is inhibited. First-time users often feel nauseated and vomit. With higher doses, there is increasing drowsiness, sometimes leading to coma and, in rare cases, death from respiratory arrest.

Long-term effects and risks
Long-term regular use of narcotics leads to constipation, reduced sexual drive, disruption of menstrual periods, and poor eating habits. Poor nutrition and personal neglect may lead to general ill-health.

Street drugs are often mixed ("cut") with other substances, such as caffeine, quinine, talcum powder and flour, that can damage blood vessels and clog the lungs. There is also a risk of abscesses at the injection site. Dangerous infections, such as hepatitis, syphilis and AIDS, may be transmitted via unclean or shared needles.

After several weeks of regular use, sudden withdrawal of narcotics produces a flu-like withdrawal syndrome beginning 6 – 24 hours after the last dose. Symptoms may include runny nose and eyes, hot and cold sweats, sleeplessness, aches, tremor, anxiety, nausea, vomiting, diarrhea, muscle spasms, and abdominal cramps. These effects are at their worst 48 – 72 hours after withdrawal and fade after 7 – 10 days.

Signs of abuse
Signs of abuse include apathy, neglect of personal appearance and hygiene, loss of appetite and weight, loss of interest in former hobbies and social activities, personality changes, and furtive behavior. Signs of intoxication include pinpoint pupils and a drowsy or drunken appearance.

Interactions
Narcotics dangerously increase the risk of sedation with any drug that has a sedative effect on the central nervous system, including barbiturates and alcohol.

NICOTINE

Other common names None
Drug category Central nervous system stimulant

Habit-forming potential
The nicotine in tobacco is largely responsible for tobacco *addiction* in up to 52 million American cigarette smokers. Most are also probably psychologically *dependent* on the process of smoking. Most people who start to smoke go on to do so regularly and most become physically dependent on nicotine. Stopping can produce temporary *withdrawal symptoms* that include nausea, headache, diarrhea, hunger, drowsiness, fatigue, insomnia, irritability, inability to concentrate, depression, and craving for cigarettes.

How taken
Usually smoked in the form of cigarettes, cigars, and pipe tobacco. Sometimes chewed (chewing tobacco), sniffed (tobacco snuff), or held between cheek and gum and sucked (snuff dipping). Nicotine is also available in chewing gum.

Legitimate uses
There are no legal restrictions on tobacco use. Its sale, however, may be restricted to those over the age of 16 or 18. Nicotine chewing gum is sometimes prescribed on a temporary basis along with behavior modification therapy to help people who want to give up smoking.

Short-term effects
Nicotine stimulates the sympathetic nervous system (see p.107). In regular tobacco users, it increases concentration, relieves tension and fatigue, and counters boredom and monotony. These effects are short-lived, thus encouraging frequent use. Physical effects include narrowing of blood vessels, increase in heart rate and blood pressure, and reduction in urine output. First-time users often feel dizzy and nauseated, and may vomit.

Long-term effects and risks
Nicotine taken regularly may cause a rise in fatty acids in the bloodstream. This effect, combined with the effects of the drug on heart rhythm and blood vessel size, increases the risk of diseases of the heart and circulation, including angina, high blood pressure, peripheral vascular disease, stroke, and coronary thrombosis. In addition, its stimulatory effects may lead to excess production of stomach acid, thereby increasing the risk of peptic ulcers.

Other well-known risks of tobacco smoking, such as chronic lung diseases, adverse effects on pregnancy, and cancers of the lung, mouth, and throat, are likely to be due to other harmful ingredients in tobacco smoke, principally tar and carbon monoxide.

Signs of abuse
Regular smokers often have yellow, tobacco-stained fingers and teeth, and bad breath. The smell of tobacco may linger on hair and clothes. A smoker's cough or shortness of breath are early signs of lung damage or heart disease.

Interactions
Cigarette smoking reduces the blood levels of a variety of drugs and reduces their effects. Such drugs include theophylline, propranolol, heparin, tricyclic antidepressants, phenothiazine antipsychotics, benzodiazepines, and caffeine. Diabetics may require larger doses of insulin. The health risks involved in taking oral contraceptives are increased by smoking.

Practical points
▼ Don't start smoking; nicotine is highly addictive.
▼ If you smoke already, give up now even if you have not yet suffered adverse effects.
▼ Ask your physician for advice and support.
▼ Inquire about self-help groups for people trying to give up smoking.

NITRITES

Other common names Amyl nitrite, butyl nitrite, poppers, snappers
Drug category Vasodilators (see also p.126)

Habit-forming potential
Nitrites do not seem to cause physical *dependence*; major *withdrawal symptoms* have never been reported. However, users may become psychologically dependent on the stimulant effect of these drugs.

How taken
By inhalation, usually from small bottles with screw or plug tops or from small glass ampules that are broken.

Legitimate uses
Amyl nitrite was originally introduced as a treatment for angina but has now largely been replaced by safer, longer-acting drugs. It is still used as an *antidote* for cyanide poisoning. Because of its potential for abuse, it was restricted to *prescription*-only status in 1969. Butyl and isobutyl nitrites are not used medically.

Short-term effects
Nitrites increase the flow of blood by relaxing blood vessel walls. They give the user a rapid high, felt as a strong rush of energy. Less pleasant effects include an increase in heart rate, intense flushing, dizziness, pounding headache, nausea, and coughing. High doses may cause fainting, and regular use may produce a blue discoloration of the skin due to alteration of hemoglobin in the red blood cells.

Long-term effects and risks
Nitrites are very quick-acting drugs. Their effects start within thirty seconds of inhalation and last for about five minutes. Regular users may become tolerant to these drugs, thus requiring higher doses to achieve the desired effects. Lasting physical damage, including cardiac problems, can result from chronic use of these drugs, and deaths have occurred.

The risk of *toxic* effects is increased in those with low blood pressure. Nitrites may also precipitate the onset of glaucoma in susceptible people, by increasing pressure inside the eye.

Signs of abuse
Nitrites have a pungent, fruity odor. They evaporate quickly; the contents of a small bottle left uncapped in a room usually disappear within two hours. Unless someone is actually taking the drug or is suffering from an overdose, the only sign of abuse is a bluish skin discoloration.

Interactions
The blood pressure-lowering effects of these drugs may be increased by alcohol, beta blockers, calcium channel blockers, and tricyclic antidepressants, thus increasing the risk of dizziness and fainting.

A B C D E F G H I J K L M N O P Q R S T U V W X Y Z

PHENCYCLIDINE

Other common names PCP, angel dust, crystal, hog, monkey, tranq, goon, DOA, ozone, cyclone, T
Drug category General anesthetic, hallucinogen

Habit-forming potential
There is little evidence that phencyclidine causes physical *dependence*. Some users become psychologically dependent on this drug and tolerant to its effects.

How taken
May be sniffed, used in smoking mixtures (in the form of angel dust), eaten (as tablets) or, rarely, injected.

Legitimate uses
Although it was once infrequently given as an anesthetic, it no longer has any medical use. Its only legal use now is in veterinary medicine. It is the substance in the darts fired by animal tranquilizing guns.

Short-term effects
Phencyclidine taken in small amounts generally produces a "high" but sometimes leads to anxiety or depression. Coordination of speech and movement deteriorates and thinking and concentration are impaired. Hallucinations and violent behavior may occur. Other effects include increase in blood pressure and heart rate, dilation of the pupils, dryness of the mouth, tremor, and numbness and reduced sensitivity to pain, which may make it difficult to restrain a person who has become violent under the influence of the drug. Shivering, vomiting, muscle weakness, and rigidity may occur. Higher doses lead to coma or stupor. The recovery period is often prolonged, with alternate periods of sleep and waking, usually followed by memory blackout of the whole episode.

Long-term effects and risks
Repeated phencyclidine use may lead to paranoia, auditory hallucinations, violent behavior, anxiety, and severe depression. While depressed, the user may attempt suicide by overdosing on the drug. Heavy users may also develop brain damage, causing memory blackouts, disorientation, visual disturbances, and speech difficulties.

    Deaths due to prolonged seizures, cardiac or respiratory arrest and ruptured blood vessels in the brain have been reported. After high doses or prolonged coma, there is also a risk of mental derangement, which may be permanent.

Signs of abuse
The phencyclidine user may appear drunk while under the influence of the drug. Hostile or violent behavior, and mood swings with bouts of depression, may be more common with heavy use.

Interactions
May inhibit effects of *anticholinergic* drugs, as well as beta blockers and antihypertensive drugs.

SOLVENTS

Other common names Inhalants, glue
Drug category Central nervous system depressant

Habit-forming potential
There is a low risk of physical *dependence* with solvent abuse, but regular users may become psychologically dependent. Young people with family and personality problems are particularly at risk of becoming habitual users.

How taken
By breathing in the fumes, usually from a plastic bag placed over the nose and/or mouth or from a cloth or handkerchief soaked in the solvent.

Legitimate uses
Solvents are used in a wide variety of industrial, domestic, and cosmetic products. They function as aerosol propellants for spray paints, hair lacquer, lighter fuel, and deodorants. They are used in adhesives, paints, paint stripper, lacquers, gasoline, kerosene, and cleaning fluids. There are no legal restrictions on the sale of solvents.

Short-term effects
The short-term effects of solvents include lightheadedness, dizziness, confusion, and progressive drowsiness and loss of coordination with increasing doses. Accidents of all types are more likely. Large doses can lead to disorientation, hallucinations, and loss of consciousness. Nausea, vomiting, and headaches may also occur.

Long-term effects and risks
One of the greatest risks of solvent abuse is accidental death or injury while intoxicated. Some products, particularly aerosol gases, butane gas, and cleaning fluids, may seriously disrupt heart rhythm or cause heart failure and sometimes death. Aerosols and butane gas can also cause suffocation by sudden cooling of the airways and are particularly dangerous if squirted into the mouth. Butane gas has been known to ignite in the mouth. Aerosol products such as deodorant and paint may suffocate the user by coating the lungs. People have also suffocated while sniffing solvents from plastic bags placed over their heads. There is also a risk of death from inhalation of vomit and depression of the breathing mechanism.

    Long-term misuse of solvent-based cleaning fluids can cause permanent liver or kidney damage, while long-term exposure to benzene (found in plastic cements, lacquers, paint remover, gasoline, and cleaning fluid) may lead to blood and liver disorders. Hexane-based adhesives may cause nerve damage leading to numbness and tremor. Repeated sniffing of leaded gasoline may cause lead poisoning.

    Regular daily use of solvents can lead to pallor, fatigue, and forgetfulness. Heavy use may affect school performance and lead to weight loss, depression, and general deterioration of health.

Signs of abuse
The majority of abusers are adolescents between the ages of 12 and 17, although the average age for this type of drug abuse is thought to be falling.

    Obvious signs of solvent abuse include a chemical smell on the breath and traces of glue or solvents on the body or clothes. Other signs include furtive behavior, uncharacteristic moodiness, unusual soreness or redness around the mouth, nose, or eyes, and a persistent cough.

Interactions
Sniffing solvents increases the risk of sedation with any drug that has a *sedative* effect on the central nervous system. Such drugs include anti-anxiety drugs, sleeping drugs, narcotics, antipsychotics, tricyclic antidepressants, and alcohol.

FOOD ADDITIVES

Almost all of us consume a number of processed, packaged, or other types of convenience foods every day. These include canned, dried, and frozen foods, breads, candy, and preserves. In addition to their basic food ingredients, most of these products contain a number of additional substances – chemicals that are supposed to enhance the appearance, flavor, texture, or freshness of the food.

All chemicals added to foods for sale in the United States are subject to rigorous scrutiny; only after they have been certified as safe are they approved for use by the Food and Drug Administration. Like other chemicals, food additives can be harmful if consumed in large quantities. But the amounts of additives allowed in foods have been regulated to prevent this possibility. Except in the small number of people with sensitivity to certain additives, adverse effects are not common. For most people, the benefits of food additives outweigh any risks. Besides enhancing the appeal of food, these chemicals often act as safeguards by preventing production of poisons from spoilage and by inhibiting growth of disease-producing bacteria, molds, and other organisms. Nevertheless, increasing concern about the effects of chemicals taken in the form of medication is paralleled by a growing interest in the chemicals that are added to our diet. People want to know the purpose and possible effects of the often mysterious-sounding substances included in the list of ingredients on the labels of food products.

This page contains descriptions of the major types of food additives, explaining why they are used. The most common food additives are described individually and listed alphabetically on the following pages.

MAJOR TYPES OF ADDITIVES

Anticaking agents
These help powdered food or food particles, such as confectioner's sugar and dried milk, to flow freely, preventing lumps from forming. They do this by absorbing moisture, thereby preventing it from entering the food particles.

Humectants
Humectants have a function opposite to that of anticaking agents – they attract moisture from the atmosphere, not from the food. They pass it on to the food and thus prevent it from drying out or becoming brittle.

Chemical preservatives
Chemical preservatives prevent foods from spoiling and increase their shelf life. They fall into two groups – anti-oxidants and antimicrobials. Anti-oxidants prevent certain fats (and to a lesser extent, the vitamins) in food from deteriorating when they combine with oxygen. Without anti-oxidants, oxygen in the air reacts with chemicals in food (a process called oxidation), to produce substances that taint the food and make it taste or smell unpleasant, or even make it harmful. Vegetable oils contain varying amounts of vitamin E (tocopherol, which is a natural anti-oxidant), but it is often lost during processing. It can be replaced by the addition of synthetic anti-oxidants such as BHA (butylated hydroxyanisole) or BHT (butylated hydroxytoluene). Because of increasing public concern about the safety of synthetic anti-oxidants, many manufacturers are replacing them with ascorbic acid (vitamin C) in moist foods such as meat, bakery products, and beer, and with vitamin E in foods with a high fat content.

Antimicrobials prevent the multiplication of microorganisms that cause foods to decay. Sulfur dioxide and benzoic acid act as antibacterials; sorbic acid is an antifungal agent and is more effective against molds and yeasts; propionic acid is a fatty acid produced by bacteria and is also an antifungal agent. Antimicrobials include nitrates and nitrites, which prevent the growth in meats of *Clostridium botulinum*, the bacterium responsible for botulism, a sometimes fatal disorder.

Emulsifying agents
Emulsifiers are substances that help to form a stable mixture between two substances that do not normally mix. In food, this is usually fat and water. As an example, when egg yolk is used to make mayonnaise, the lecithin in the egg yolk works as an emulsifier. Emulsifiers also reduce the amount of fat that is needed in foods to which emulsifiers are added.

Sequestrants
Traces of metal, especially copper and iron, present in some foods, can speed the oxidation of fats and oils. By making those metals chemically inactive, sequestrants prevent foodstuffs from spoiling.

Flavorings
Flavorings are a very complex group; any one natural flavor can be a mixture of up to several hundred chemical substances.

Flavorings may be natural substances obtained from fruits, nuts, vegetables, herbs, or spices. They may also be factory-made chemical copies of the original, or synthetic flavors developed in a laboratory. Synthetic flavors form the largest group. Manufacturers generally prefer synthetics because they are less likely to break down under the rigorous extremes of food processing and are less costly than their natural or nature-identical counterparts.

Most flavorings are safe, although some are only safe in limited use. A few have harmful effects.

Flavor enhancers
Flavor enhancers are included in foods to heighten the taste of the ingredients. Monosodium glutamate is a particularly interesting flavor enhancer that occurs naturally in some soups when a meat-bone or fish stock is combined with vegetable ingredients to create a unique taste. MSG added to processed foods can bring out the sometimes weak flavor of a natural ingredient or intensify that of small amounts of artificial flavors.

Stabilizers
Stabilizers may have the same basic function as emulsifiers, or they may thicken the fat or, more usually, the watery part of the emulsion. They may also make the emulsion stickier and prevent its components from separating, or curdling. Stabilizers therefore have a second function as jelling, thickening, or suspending agents.

A – Z OF ADDITIVES

ACACIA
Also known as gum arabic, sudan gum, gum Hashab, or Kordofan gum

Use Emulsifier, stabilizer, and thickening agent.
Found in Candies, jellies, glazes, puddings, gelatin desserts, ice cream, salad dressing, sodas, beer, wine, and appetite-reducing pills.
Adverse effects or risks Acacia slightly reduces the level of cholesterol in the blood. A few people have allergic reactions to it, either after eating it or inhaling it.

ACETATES
Also known as acetic acid. Includes allyl phenoxyacetate and allyl phenyl-acetate

Use Flavoring to give foods a variety of different flavors from liquor, nut, coffee, vanilla, and cheese to honey or pine-apple flavor.
Found in Beverages, ice creams, sherbets, cakes, cookies, pastries, and candy.
Adverse effects or risks None with normal use. May be irritating to the stomach if consumed in large quantities.

AGAR-AGAR
Also known as agar or Japanese isinglass

Use Thickener, stabilizer, and jelling agent.
Found in Ice cream, sherbet, baked goods, icings, and beverages.
Adverse effects or risks None in normal use. Excessive consumption could have a laxative effect and produce temporary distension of the abdomen and/or flatulence.

ALLYL ISOTHIOCYANATE
Also known as volatile oil of mustard, redskin, and allyl isosulfocyanate

Use Meat and spice flavoring.
Found in Mustard, horseradish, and onion (occurs naturally), beverages, ice creams, sherbets, candy, relishes, sauces, meats, and pickles.
Adverse effects or risks Negligible in the amounts used in food.

ANTHRANILATES
Also known as ethylanthranilate

Use Synthetic flavoring that gives a citrus, aniseed, licorice, vanilla, or rum flavor.
Found in Beverages, ice creams, sherbets, cakes, cookies, pastries, and candy.
Adverse effects or risks None.

ASCORBIC ACID
Also known as vitamin C

Use Anti-oxidant preservative. Prevents browning of cut fruit and fixes meat color in sausages.
Found in Frozen fruit, beer and ale, apple juice, candy, frankfurters, and cured or pickled meats.
Adverse effects or risks Although ascorbic acid is essential for healthy growth and iron absorption, excessively large amounts can cause diarrhea and some other disorders (see p.544).

BENZOIC ACID
Includes sodium benzoate

Use Antifungal and antibacterial preservatives.
Found in Margarine and a wide variety of acid-based foods and drinks, including purees, syrups, pickles, preserves, and alcoholic and non-alcoholic beverages.
Adverse effects or risks May have a numbing effect on the mouth and may trigger an asthma attack in asthma sufferers. People sensitive to aspirin may find that benzoic acid causes allergic symptoms, such as breathlessness and watering eyes. It may also cause skin rashes.

BUTYLATED HYDROXYANISOLE
Also known as BHA

Use Anti-oxidant preservative.
Found in Many packaged foods, shortening, dry breakfast cereals, potatoes, ice creams, baked goods, candies, and beverages. It is the most widely used of the anti-oxidants.
Adverse effects or risks Safe at normal levels of intake.

BUTYLATED HYDROXYTOLUENE
Also known as BHT

Use Anti-oxidant preservative.
Found in Packaged convenience foods and snack foods, dry breakfast cereals, enriched rice, shortening, and chewing gum.
Adverse effects or risks Can cause skin rashes in certain people, who are often also sensitive to aspirin.

BUTYRATES
Includes butyraldehyde, 2-ethyl-butyraldehyde, 2-ethylbutyric acid, isobutyl butyrate, alpha-alpha dimethyl-phenylbutyrate, isopropyl butyrate, and many more

Use Butter, butterscotch, caramel, chocolate, and fruit flavorings.
Found in Coffee and strawberries (occurs naturally), sodas and alcoholic beverages, ice creams and sherbets, candy, baked goods, puddings, and icings.
Adverse effects or risks None known in food use, but may cause skin irritation in factory workers.

CAFFEINE
Also known as methyltheothrombine, guaranine, or theine

Use Flavoring.
Found in Coffee, cola, cocoa, root beer, and tea (occurs naturally).
Adverse effects or risks Stimulates the central nervous system, the heartbeat, and respiration rate, and acts as a diuretic (see p.127). An excess may cause insomnia, nervousness, irregular heartbeat, and diarrhea.

CALCIUM ALGINATE
Includes sodium alginate and potassium alginate

Use Stabilizer, thickener, suspending and jelling agent. Also a solvent and vehicle for flavorings. Sodium alginate is by far the most common of the three.
Found in Ice cream, popsicles, soft and cottage cheeses, cheese snacks, dressings and spreads, fruit drinks, beverages, and instant desserts.
Adverse effects or risks None known.

CARAMEL
Also known as plain (spirit) caramel, caustic sulfite caramel, ammonia caramel, and sulfite ammonia caramel

Use Brown coloring. It is the most widely used food coloring.
Found in Beverages, especially cola and a wide range of candy, chocolates, cakes and pastries, ice cream, and soya products.
Adverse effects or risks Its safety has been questioned for some time, especially when taken in large quantities. Sulfite ammonia caramel tested on humans produced soft to liquid stools and increased the frequency of bowel movements.

CARNAUBA WAX

Use Glazing and polishing agent for candy.
Found in Chocolates and candy.
Adverse effects or risks Occasional reports of skin irritation from skin contact with this substance.

CARRAGEENAN

Also known as Irish moss and Chondrus extract

Use Stabilizer, emulsifier, thickener, and suspending and jelling agent, especially in dairy products.
Found in Evaporated, condensed, and chocolate milks; milk shakes; sterilized, sour, and aerosol cream; and milk-based alcoholic beverages, pudding and custard mixes, ice cream, yogurt, cheese spreads, and salad dressing.
Adverse effects or risks Evidence suggests that carrageenan is safe.

CITRIC ACID

Use Sequestrant (especially in wine). Also used to prevent browning of cut fruit, to firm vegetables, add flavor, set jam, assist brewing, and cure meat.
Found in Canned and frozen fruit and vegetables, beer, wine, and cider, breakfast cereals, cheese, and cream.
Adverse effects or risks None likely in normal use.

ERYTHORBIC ACID

Also known as isoascorbic acid. Includes sodium erythorbate

Use Anti-oxidant preservative, color fixative in meat.
Found in Cured meat products, baked goods, beverages, and pickled products.
Adverse effects or risks None.

ETHYLENEDIAMINE TETRA-ACETIC ACID (EDTA)

Includes calcium disodium salt of EDTA and disodium dihydrogen salt of EDTA

Use Sequestrant.
Found in Canned foods, including crab, lobster, clams, shrimp, potato salad, mayonnaise, sandwich spreads, soda, beer, and malt whisky.
Adverse effects or risks None likely in food use.

ETHYL VANILLIN

Also known as ethovan

Use Flavoring.

Found in Ice creams, beverages, cakes, pastries, and other desserts.
Adverse effects or risks Appears to be safe in quantities used in foods.

FD & C RED No. 3

Also known as erythrosine

Use Red coloring.
Found in Cherries in canned fruit salads, maraschino and glacé cherries, and cherry pie mixes.
Adverse effects or risks Contains iodine and has been shown to affect the thyroid glands of laboratory animals, but not of humans. Children who eat huge amounts of artificially colored cherries could be at risk.

GLYCERIN

Use Humectant, sweetening agent, solvent.
Found in Candy, beverages, baked goods, chewing gum, and in edible coatings for meat and cheese.
Adverse effects or risks Safe in normal amounts.

GUAR GUM

Also known as guar flour, jaguar gum, and cluster bean gum

Use Stabilizer and suspending agent, thickener, dietary bulking agent, and firming and binding agent.
Found in Bottled sauces and salad dressings, carbonated beverages, meats, candies, baked goods, cream cheese, cheese spread, ice cream, yogurt, frozen fruit, and fruit drinks.
Adverse effects or risks In excessive amounts may cause nausea, flatulence, or abdominal cramps.

LECITHIN

Use Emulsifier, anti-oxidant, defoaming agent in yeast and sugar beet processing, cocoa substitute in chocolate. Increases volume in bread, protects vitamin A in margarine, and keeps the water content in food products.
Found in Chocolate and bakery products, breakfast cereals, frozen desserts, powdered milk, and popcorn.
Adverse effects or risks None.

MAGNESIUM CARBONATE

Also known as magnesite

Use Anticaking agent, alkali, acidity regulator, anti-bleaching agent.
Found in Table salt, flour, blue cheese,

sour cream, and ice cream.
Adverse effects or risks None likely in the small amounts present in food.

METHYLCELLULOSE

Also known as methocel and cologel

Use Thickener, emulsifier, stabilizer, bulking and binding agent, and clarifier to form edible films for food products.
Found in Vinegar, beverages, and imitation jellies or jams. Used in foods for people on low calorie diets.
Adverse effects or risks In large amounts may cause flatulence, distension of the abdomen, or intestinal obstruction; may also affect the absorption of minerals or other drugs.

METHYL PARABEN

Also known as methyl p-hydroxy-benzoate. Includes propyl p-hydroxy-benzoate and propyl paraben

Use Antimicrobial preservative.
Found in Beer, soda and fruit drinks, flavoring syrups, dessert sauces, fruit pulp and pie fillings, baked goods, candy, artificially sweetened jellies and preserves, and pickles.
Adverse effects or risks Asthmatics and people who are sensitive to aspirin may be sensitive to the parabens and develop skin rashes or irritation of the lining of the mouth.

MONOGLYCERIDES

Includes diglycerides, mono- and diglycerides of fatty acids, glyceryl monostearate, distearate, and mono-sodium glycerides of edible fats and oils

Use Emulsifiers.
Found in Baked goods, margarines and shortenings, beverages, ice cream, ice milk, whipped toppings, and chocolate.
Adverse effects or risks None recorded.

MONOSODIUM GLUTAMATE

Also known as MSG

Use Flavor enhancer.
Found in A variety of savory canned and packaged foods, candy, baked goods, condiments, and pickles. Used extensively in Chinese cooking.
Adverse effects or risks MSG has been implicated in the "Chinese restaurant syndrome"(which includes facial flushing and headaches), but links with this condition have recently been shown to be tenuous.

A – Z OF ADDITIVES continued

MYRISTIC ACID
Also known as myristicin

Use Natural flavorings.
Found in Coconut, mace, palm seed, and sperm whale oils; most animal and vegetable fats (occurs naturally); butterscotch, cocoa and fruit flavorings for beverages; and candy, ice cream, butter, and desserts.
Adverse effects or risks In the amounts used in foods it is not harmful.

OILS
Includes almond oil, bergamot oil, sandalwood oil, and many others

Use Natural flavorings.
Found in Beverages, ice cream, cakes, cookies, pastries, candy, chewing gum, soups, syrups, sauces and relishes, liqueurs, pickles, and meats.
Adverse effects or risks Some oils increase the levels of cholesterol and triglycerides in the blood.

PAPAIN
Also known as carica papaya, benase, and tomasin

Use Meat tenderizer and clarifying agent for beverages.
Found in Meat and meat products, beverages, and enriched farina.
Adverse effects or risks None known in normal food use. Most known cases of allergic reactions to papain have occurred in factory workers who have inhaled the powder, which caused asthma and urticaria (hives).

PECTIN
Includes sodium pectinate and low-methoxyl pectins

Use Stabilizer, jelling and thickening agent.
Found in Jams, jellies, marmalades, puddings and desserts, ice cream and sherbet, beverages, and syrups.
Adverse effects or risks Pectin is sometimes prescribed for diarrhea but has also been used as a bulk laxative (see Laxatives p.139). It may cause distension or flatulence.

POLYSORBATE 60
Also known as polyoxyethylene (20) sorbitan monostearate

Use Emulsifier, stabilizer, wetting and dispersing agent for powdered processed foods, and a foaming agent for beverage mixes. It is added to chocolate coatings to prevent cocoa butter substitutes from tasting greasy.
Found in Frozen and gelatin desserts, cakes, cake mixes, doughnuts and artificial chocolate coatings, nondairy whipped cream and creamers, powdered convenience foods, salad dressings made without egg yolks, and vitamin supplements.
Adverse effects or risks None in normal food use.

POLYSORBATE 80
Also known as polyoxyethylene (20) sorbitan mono-oleate

Use Emulsifier, stabilizer, and humectant. Prevents oil from separating in nondairy whipped cream and helps nondairy coffee whiteners to dissolve.
Found in Baked goods, nondairy whipped cream, coffee whiteners, ice cream, frozen custard, shortenings, and in vitamin and mineral supplements.
Adverse effects or risks None in normal use.

PROPIONIC ACID
Includes calcium propionate and sodium propionate

Use Antifungal preservative, especially against the mold known as "rope" that affects bread. Also used as a flavoring.
Found in Baked goods such as bread and rolls, dairy products, pizzas, and processed cheeses. Propionic acid is also used in butter, fruit flavoring for beverages, ice creams, and candy. Calcium propionate is also used in poultry stuffing, chocolate products, cakes, and cupcakes.
Adverse effect or risks May cause migraine in migraine sufferers and contact with chemical may cause skin irritations in bakery workers.

PROPYLENE GLYCOL
Use Humectant, solvent, and inhibitor of mold growth.
Found in Cakes, cookies, pastries, candy, breads and bread products, ice cream, icings and toppings, shredded coconut, beverages, emulsifiers, and meat products.
Adverse effects or risks None in normal use.

PROPYL GALLATE
Also known as propyl 3,4,5 trihydroxybenzoate

Use Anti-oxidant preservative, on its own or combined with butylated hydroxyanisole or butylated hydroxy-toluene. Also used as a flavoring.
Found in Margarines, oils and shortenings; packaged snack foods such as popcorn, soup bases, potato flakes, dehydrated mashed potatoes and mayonnaise. Propyl gallate provides citrus or spice flavors to beverages, ice cream, candy, and baked goods.
Adverse effects or risks Can cause stomach or skin irritation, especially in people who suffer from asthma or are sensitive to aspirin.

SODIUM CARBOXYMETHYL-CELLULOSE
Also known as carboxymethylcellulose sodium salt, and cellulose gum

Use Stabilizer, thickener, jelling agent, and non-nutritive bulking aid. Used to prevent water loss, make food opaque, and to enhance the texture of food.
Found in Cakes, cookies, pastries, candy, bread and bread products, cake mixes, powdered beverages, pie fillings, dips and spreads, salad dressings, ice cream, whipped toppings, whipped cream, batter coatings, and processed and cottage cheeses.
Adverse effects or risks Could cause digestive disturbances.

SODIUM CITRATE
Includes monosodium citrate and disodium citrate

Use Adds acidity to food. Also used as a sequestrant.
Found in Candy, ice cream, processed cheeses, fruit juices, and carbonated beverages.
Adverse effects or risks None known.

SODIUM HEXAMETA-PHOSPHATE
Also known as sodium polymeta-phosphate. Includes calcium hexa-metaphosphate

Use Emulsifier, texturizing agent used to cure hams, sequestrant, and used in bottled drinking water to prevent corrosion and buildup of scale.
Found in Bottled beer, water, and other beverages; processed cheese; breakfast cereals, angel food cake, ice cream, reconstituted lemon juice, and preserves.
Adverse effects or risks Phosphorus is an essential nutrient taken in balance with other minerals in the diet, such as calcium and magnesium. Too much phosphorus in the form of phosphates can upset the balance.

SODIUM NITRATE

Includes potassium nitrate (saltpeter), sodium nitrite, and potassium nitrite

Use Color fixatives.
Found in Processed meat and fish products.
Adverse effects or risks May cause dizziness, headaches, or difficulty in breathing, especially in children. There is some danger of nitrites (and converted nitrates) forming carcinogenic substances (nitrosamines), resulting in stomach cancer. The risk may be reduced by taking additional amounts of vitamins C and E.

SODIUM SULFITE

Also known as sodium and potassium hydrogen sulfite, disodium, and potassium pyrosulfite. Includes sodium and potassium bisulfites and meta-bisulfites

Use Antimicrobial preservatives, anti-oxidants, anti-browning agents.
Found in An extensive range of foods and beverages, including beer, wine, cider, fruit juices, syrups and purees, peeled potatoes, and cut, dried or frozen fruit.
Adverse effects or risks Foods and drinks containing sulfites may release sulfur dioxide. If this is inhaled by people who suffer from asthma it can trigger an asthmatic attack. Sulfites are known to cause stomach irritation, nausea, diarrhea, skin rash, or swelling in sulfite-sensitive people. People whose kidneys or livers are impaired may not be able to produce the *enzymes* that break down sulfites in the body. Sulfites may destroy thiamine and consequently are not added to foods that are sources of this vitamin.

SORBIC ACID

Includes potassium sorbate, calcium sorbate, and sodium sorbate

Use Preservatives against yeasts, molds, and bacteria in acid foods.
Found in Yogurts, processed cheeses, pickles and sauces, fruit pies, cordials, juices, jams, and jellies.
Adverse effects or risks None known in food use, although sorbic acid applied to the skin is irritating.

SORBITOL

Also known as D-glucitol and L-glucitol

Use Sweetening agent, especially in diabetic foods, humectant, sequestrant, stabilizer, and texturizer. Reduces the tendency of sugar to form crystals. It is also a dilutant for food colors, masks the bitter aftertaste of saccharin, and helps to maintain the texture of chewy candy.
Found in A variety of chocolate, cakes, cookies, pastries, candy, ice cream, vegetable oils, bacon, and sausages.
Adverse effects or risks In small amounts, sorbitol presents no problems. Large amounts (2oz for adults, 1oz for children) may have a laxative effect or cause distension of the abdomen or flatulence.

SULFUR DIOXIDE

Use Preservative. Used to prevent oxidation and browning.
Found in Wine, beverages, fruit pulp, juice and flavors, dehydrated fruit and vegetables, corn and table syrup, soups, sauces, and relishes.
Adverse effects or risks Only residual amounts should be present in or on the food, but even small amounts may provoke asthma in susceptible people. Sulfur dioxide may destroy thiamine and so is not added to foods containing this vitamin.

TARTARIC ACID

Includes sodium tartrate and sodium potassium tartrate (Rochelle salts)

Use Sequestrant (especially in wine), emulsifier, and acid dilutant for food colors, constituent of grape and artificial sour- or tart-tasting products.
Found in Grapes (occurs naturally), wine, canned sodas and colas, candy, preserves, baked goods, dried egg white, lemon meringue pie mix, pasteurized processed cheese, cheese food and cheese spread, and some types of baking powder.
Adverse effects or risks Large amounts may have a laxative effect.

TRIBASIC CALCIUM PHOSPHATE

Also known as tricalcium diortho-phosphate and tricalcium phosphate

Use Anticaking agent, calcium supplement in grain products.
Found in Packaged cake mixes, candy, baked goods, gelatin desserts, powdered beverage mixes, seasoning mixes, soup mixes, and sugar.
Adverse effects or risks Too much phosphorus in the form of phosphates from processed food can upset the body's mineral balance.

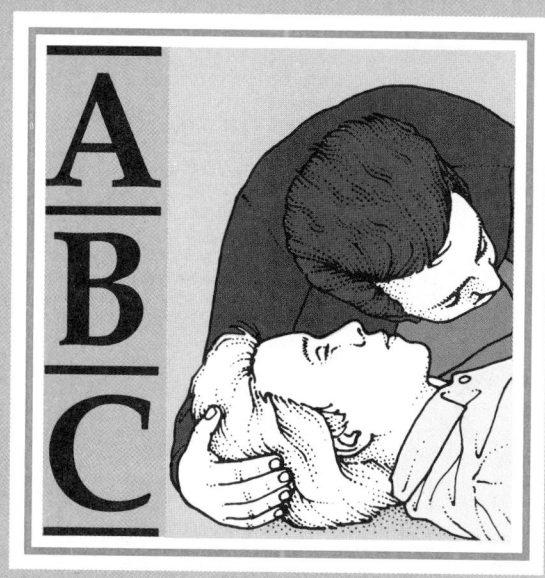

GLOSSARY

The following pages contain definitions of drug-related terms whose technical meanings are not explained in detail elsewhere in the book, or for which an easily located, precise explanation may be helpful. These are words that may not be familiar to the general reader or that have a slightly different meaning in a medical context than in ordinary use. Some of the terms included refer to particular drug actions or effects; others describe methods of drug administration. A few medical conditions that may occur as a result of drug use are also defined. All words printed in italics within the main text are included as entries in this glossary.

The glossary is arranged in alphabetical order. Each entry has a bold heading. In order to avoid unnecessary repetition, where relevant, entries include cross-references to further information on that topic in sections elsewhere in the book, or to another glossary term.

A

Addiction
An imprecise term that can cover any-thing from intense, habitual cravings for coffee, tea, or tobacco, to physical and psychological dependence on more potent agents such as narcotics. See also *Dependence*.

Adjuvant
A drug that enhances the therapeutic effect of another, but that does not necessarily have a beneficial effect alone. An example is aluminum added to certain vaccines to enhance the protection given by the vaccine.

Adrenergic
See *Sympathomimetic*.

Adverse reaction
An unexpected or unpredictable reaction to a drug that is unrelated to the drug's usual effects. The cause may some-times be an allergic reaction or a genetic disorder such as the lack of an enzyme that normally inactivates the drug. See also The effects of drugs (p.15).

Agonist
A term meaning to have a positive, stimulating effect. An agonist drug is one that binds to a *receptor*, thereby triggering or increasing a particular activity in that cell.

Amebicide
A drug that kills amebas (single celled microorganisms). See also Antiproto-zoal drugs (p.164).

Analeptic
A drug given in the hospital to stimulate breathing. See also Respiratory stimu-lants (p.116).

Analgesia
Relief of pain, usually by administration of drugs. See also Analgesics (p.108).

Anaphylaxis
A severe hypersensitive reaction to an allergen, such as a bee sting or a drug (see Allergy, p.151). Symptoms may include rash, swelling, breathing difficulty and collapse. See also Dealing with anaphylactic shock (p.592).

Anemia
A condition in which the concentration of the oxygen-carrying pigment of the blood, hemoglobin, is below normal. Many different disorders may cause anemia, and it may sometimes occur as a result of drug treatment. Severe anemia may cause fatigue, pallor and, occasionally, breathing difficulty.

Anesthetic, general
A drug or drug combination given to produce unconsciousness prior to and during surgery or potentially painful investigative procedures. General anesthesia is usually induced initially by injection of a barbiturate drug, such as thiopental, and maintained by inhalation of a volatile liquid, such as halothane, or a gas, such as nitrous oxide mixed with oxygen. See also *Premedication*.

Anesthetic, local
A drug applied topically or injected to numb sensation in a small area. See also Local anesthetics (p.108).

Antagonist
A term meaning to have a negative effect. An antagonist drug (often called a "blocker") is one that binds to a *receptor* without stimulating cell activity and prevents any other substance from occupying that receptor.

Antibody
A protein manufactured by lymphocytes (a type of white blood cell) to neutralize an antigen (foreign protein) in the body. The formation of antibodies against an invading microorganism is part of the body's natural defense against infec-tion. Immunization carried out to increase the body's resistance to a specific disease involves either injection of specific antibodies or administration of a vaccine that stimulates antibody production. See also Vaccines and immunization (p.162).

Anticholinergic
A drug that blocks the action of acetyl-choline, or a term that refers to the *parasympathomimetic* effects of such a drug. Acetylcholine is a *neurotransmitter* secreted by the endings of nerve cells that allows certain nerve impulses to be transmitted, including those that relax some involuntary muscles, tighten others, and affect the release of saliva. Anticholinergic drugs are used to treat urinary incontinence because they relax the bladder's squeezing muscles while tightening those of the sphincter. Anticholinergic drugs also relax the muscles of the intestinal wall, helping to relieve irritable bowel syndrome (p.138). See also Autonomic nervous system (p.107).

Antidote
A substance that neutralizes or counter-acts the effects of a poison. Very few poisons have a specific antidote.

Antineoplastic
An anticancer drug (p.182).

Antiperspirant
A substance applied to the skin to reduce excess sweating. Antiperspir-ants work by reducing the activity of the sweat glands or by blocking the ducts that carry sweat to the skin surface.

Antipyretic
A drug that reduces fever. The most commonly used antipyretic drugs are aspirin and acetaminophen.

Antiseptic
A chemical that, when applied to the skin, destroys bacteria and prevents infection from spreading. See Anti-infective skin preparations (p.203).

Antispasmodic
A drug that reduces spasm (abnormally strong or inappropriate contraction) of the muscles of the gastrointestinal tract, airways, and blood vessels. Antispas-modic drugs are most commonly prescribed to relieve irritable bowel syndrome (p.138).

Antitussive
A drug that prevents or relieves a cough. See also Drugs to treat coughs (p.122).

Aperient
A mild laxative. See Laxatives (p.139).

Astringent
A substance that causes tissue to dry and shrink by reducing its ability to absorb water. Astringents are used in a number of antiperspirants and skin tonics because they remove excessive moisture from the skin surface. They are also used in ear drops for outer-ear inflammation because they promote healing of the inflamed tissue.

B

Bactericidal
A term used to describe a drug that kills bacteria. See also Antibiotics (p.156) and Antibacterial drugs (p.159).

Bacteriostatic
A term used to describe a drug that stops the growth or multiplication of bacteria. See also Antibiotics (p.156) and Antibacterial drugs (p.159).

Balm
A soothing or healing preparation applied to the skin.

Bioavailability
The amount of a drug that enters the bloodstream and thus reaches tissues throughout the body, usually expressed as a percentage of the dose given. The injection of a drug directly into a vein produces 100 percent bioavailability. Drugs given by mouth generally have a much lower bioavailability because only a proportion of the drug can usually be absorbed through the digestive system. Also, some of the drug may be broken down in the liver before reaching the general circulation.

Body salts
Also known as electrolytes, these are compounds of various minerals that are present in such body fluids as blood, urine, and sweat, and within cells. These salts play an important role in regulating water balance, acidity of the blood, conduction of nerve impulses, and muscle contraction. The balance between the various salts can be upset by such conditions as diarrhea and vomiting. The balance may also be altered by the action of drugs such as diuretics (p.127).

Brand name
See *Generic drug*.

Bronchoconstrictor
A substance that causes the airways in the lungs to narrow, or constrict. An attack of asthma may be caused by the release of bronchoconstrictor substances such as histamine or certain prostaglandins.

Bronchodilator
A drug that widens the airways. See Bronchodilators (p.120).

C

Cathartic
A drug that stimulates bowel action to produce a soft or liquid bowel movement. See also Laxatives (p.139).

Chelating agent
A chemical used in the treatment of poisoning by metals such as iron, lead, arsenic, and mercury. It acts by combining with the metal to form a less poisonous substance and in some cases increases excretion in the urine. Penicillamine is a commonly used chelating agent.

Chemotherapy
The treatment of cancer or infections by drugs. *Cytotoxic* drugs (p.182) and antibiotics (p.156) are examples of drugs used in chemotherapy.

Cholinergic
A drug, also known as *parasympathomimetic*, that stimulates the parasympathetic nervous system. See also Autonomic nervous system (p.107).

Coma
A state of unconsciousness and unresponsiveness to external stimuli such as noise and pain. Coma results from disturbance or damage to part of the brain. Drug overdose is a common cause.

Contraindication
A factor in a person's current condition, medical history, or genetic make-up that may increase the risks of an adverse effect from a particular drug, so that the drug should not normally be prescribed.

Counterirritant
Another term for *rubefacient*.

Cycloplegic
The action of paralyzing the ciliary muscle in the eye. This muscle alters the shape of the lens when it contracts, enabling the eye to focus on objects. A cycloplegic drug prevents this action, and by doing so makes both examination of and surgery on the eye easier. See also Drugs affecting the pupil (p.198).

Cytotoxic
A drug that kills or damages cells, most commonly used to treat cancer. Although they primarily affect abnormal cells, they may kill or damage healthy cells. See also Anticancer drugs (p.182).

D

Dependence
A term that relates to physical or psychological dependence, or both, on a substance. Psychological dependence involves intense mental cravings if a drug is unavailable or withdrawn. Physical dependence produces physical withdrawal symptoms (sweating, shaking, abdominal pain, seizures, etc.) if the substance is not taken. Dependence also implies loss of control over intake. See also Drug dependence (p.23).

Depot injection
Injection into a muscle of a drug that has been specially formulated to provide for a slow, steady absorption of its active ingredients by the surrounding blood vessels. The drug may be mixed with oil or wax. The release period can be made to last up to several weeks, depending on the formulation. See also Methods of administration (p.17).

Designer drugs
A group of unlicensed substances whose only purpose is to duplicate the effects of certain illegal drugs of abuse or to provide even stronger ones. Designer drugs differ chemically in some minor degree from the original drug, enabling the user and supplier to evade prosecution for possession of an illegal drug. They are extremely dangerous because they are often highly potent and may contain impurities. New laws have been introduced in many states to outlaw the use of these drugs.

Double-blind
A type of test commonly used by drug companies to measure the effectiveness of a new drug against an existing medicine or a *placebo*. Neither the patients nor the physicians administering the drug know who is receiving what substance. Only after the test is complete and the patients' responses recorded is the identity of those who received the new drug revealed. Double-blind trials are carried out for almost all new drugs. See also Testing and approving new drugs (p.12).

Drip
A nonmedical term for *intravenous infusion*.

E

Electrolyte
See *Body salts.*

Elixir
A sweetened liquid often containing alcohol that forms a base for many medicines, such as those used to treat coughs.

Embrocation
An ointment rubbed on to the skin to relieve joint pain, muscle cramp, or muscle injury. An embrocation usually contains a *rubefacient.*

Emetic
Any substance that causes a person to vomit. An emetic may work by irritating the lining of the stomach and/or by stimulating the part of the brain that controls vomiting. An emetic, such as ipecac, may be used in the treatment of drug overdose. See also Drug poisoning emergency guide (p.590).

Emollient
A substance that has a soothing, softening effect when applied to the skin. An emollient also has a moisturizing effect on dry skin, preventing loss of water from the skin surface by forming an oily film. See also Bases for skin preparations (p.203).

Emulsion
A combination of two substances that normally do not mix together properly but remain as particles of one suspended in the liquid form of the other. Many lotions are emulsions; they need to be shaken before use in case the constituent substances have separated.

Endorphins
A group of substances that occurs naturally in the brain. Released in response to pain, they bind to specialized *receptors* and reduce perception of pain. Narcotic analgesics such as morphine work by mimicking the action of endorphins. See also Analgesics (p.108).

Enzyme
A protein that controls the rate of one or more chemical reactions in the body. There are thousands of enzymes active in the human body. Each type of body cell produces a specific range of enzymes. Cells in the liver contain enzymes that stimulate the breakdown of nutrients and drugs; cells in the digestive tract release enzymes that help digest food. Some drugs work by altering the activity of enzymes – for example, certain anticancer drugs halt tumor growth by altering enzyme function in cancer cells.

Excitatory
A term meaning having a stimulating or enhancing effect. A chemical released from a nerve ending that causes muscle contraction has an excitatory effect. See also *Inhibitory.*

Expectorant
A type of cough remedy that enhances the production of sputum (phlegm) and is used in the treatment of a productive (sputum-producing) cough. See also Drugs to treat coughs (p.122).

F G

Formula, chemical
A way of expressing the constituents of a chemical in symbols and numbers. Every known chemical substance has a formula. Water, for instance, has the formula H_2O, indicating that it is composed of two hydrogen atoms (H_2) and one oxygen atom (O). Drugs have more complicated formulas.

Formulary
See *Pharmacopoeia.*

Generic drug
The official name for a single, therapeutically active substance. It is distinct from a brand name, a term chosen by a manufacturer for a product containing a generic drug. Example: diazepam is a generic name; Valium is a brand-name product that contains diazepam.

H

Half-life
A term used in pharmacology for the time the body takes to eliminate half of the drug from the bloodstream. Knowledge of the half-life of a drug helps to determine frequency of dosage.

Hallucinogen
A drug that causes hallucinations (unreal perceptions of surroundings and objects). Common hallucinogens include the drugs of abuse LSD and marijuana (p.551). Alcohol taken in large amounts may also have a hallucinogenic effect; hallucinations may also occur during alcohol withdrawal. Certain prescribed drugs may rarely cause hallucinations.

Hormone
A chemical released directly into the bloodstream by a gland or tissue. The body produces numerous hormones, each of which has a specific range of functions such as controlling the *metabolism* of cells, growth, sexual development, and the body's response to stress or illness. Hormone-producing glands make up the endocrine system (see Hormones and endocrine system, p.168); the kidneys, intestine, and brain also release hormones.

I J

Immunization
The process of inducing immunity (resistance to infection) as a preventive measure against the spread of infectious diseases. See Vaccines and immunization (p.162).

Infusion pump
A machine for administering a continuous, controlled amount of a drug or other fluid through a needle inserted into a vein or under the skin. It consists of a small battery-powered pump that controls the flow of fluid from a syringe into the attached needle. The pump is usually strapped to the patient and programmed to deliver the fluid at a constant rate. See also Methods of administration (p.17).

Inhaler
A device used for administering a drug in powder or vapor form. Inhalers are used principally in the treatment of respiratory disorders such as asthma and chronic bronchitis. Among the medications administered in this way are corticosteroids and bronchodilator drugs. See also Methods of administration (p.17).

Inhibitory
A term meaning to have a blocking effect on cell activity. A chemical released from a nerve ending that prevents a muscle from contracting has an inhibitory effect. See also *Antagonist.*

Inoculation
Administration of microorganisms or other biological substances, usually by injection, to produce immunity to disease. See Vaccines and immunization (p.162).

Intramuscular injection
Injection of a drug into a muscle, usually into the upper arm or buttock. The drug is absorbed from the muscle into the bloodstream.

Intravenous infusion
Prolonged, slow injection of fluid (often a solution of a drug) into a vein. The fluid flows at a controlled rate from a bag or bottle through a fine tube inserted into a needle placed in a vein. An intravenous infusion may also be administered via an *infusion pump.*

Intravenous injection
Direct injection of a drug into a vein, which puts the drug immediately into circulation. Because it has a rapid effect, intravenous injection is useful in an emergency.

Investigational
A term used for a drug that is still being tested for efficacy and safety before approval for marketing is granted.

Jaundice
A condition in which the skin and whites of the eyes are yellowed. Jaundice is caused by an accumulation in the blood of the pigment bilirubin. Jaundice is a sign of many disorders of the liver. A drug may cause jaundice as an adverse effect either by damaging the liver or causing an increase in the breakdown of red blood cells in the bloodstream.

L M

Lotion
A liquid preparation that may be applied to large areas of skin. See also Bases for skin preparations (p.203).

Medication
Any substance prescribed to treat illness.

Medicine
A medication or drug that maintains, improves, or restores health.

Metabolism
The term for all chemical processes in the body that involve the formation of new substances or the breakdown of a substance to release energy. Metabolism provides energy required to keep the body functioning at rest – to maintain breathing, heartbeat, and body temperature. It also provides energy needed during exertion. Metabolism produces this energy from the breakdown of digested foods.

Miotic
A drug that constricts (narrows) the pupil. Opiate drugs such as morphine have a miotic effect, and someone who is taking one of these drugs characteristically has pinpoint pupils. The pupil is sometimes deliberately narrowed by other miotic drugs in the treatment of glaucoma. See also Drugs for glaucoma (p.196) and Drugs affecting the pupil (p.198).

Mucolytic
A drug that liquefies mucous secretions in the airways. See also Drugs to treat coughs (p.122).

Mydriatic
A drug that dilates (widens) the pupil. *Anticholinergic* drugs such as belladonna have this effect and may cause *photophobia* as a consequence. Mydriatic drugs may occasionally provoke the onset of glaucoma in susceptible people. See also Drugs affecting the pupil (p.198).

N

Narcotics
Stemming from the Greek word for numbness or stupor and once applied to drugs derived from the opium poppy, the word narcotics no longer has a precise medical meaning. Physicians today use the term narcotic analgesics to refer to opium-derived and synthetic drugs that have pain-relieving properties and other effects similar to those of morphine (see Analgesics, p.108). See also Narcotics (p.552).

Nebulizer
A method of administering a drug to the airways and lungs in aerosol form through a face mask. The apparatus includes an electric or hand-operated pump that sends a stream of air or oxygen through a length of tubing into a small canister containing the drug in liquid form. This inflow of gas causes the drug to be dispersed into a fine mist, which is then carried through another tube into the face mask. Inhalation of this drug mist is much easier than inhaling from a pressurized aerosol (see also *Inhaler*).

Neuroleptic
A drug used to treat psychotic illness. See Antipsychotic drugs (p.113).

Neurotransmitter
A chemical released from a nerve ending after an electrical impulse arrives at the nerve ending. A neurotransmitter may carry a message from the nerve to another nerve so that the electrical impulse passes on, to a muscle to stimulate contraction, or to a gland to stimulate secretion of a hormone. Acetylcholine and norepinephrine are examples of neurotransmitters. See also Brain and nervous system (p.106).

O

Orphan drug
A drug that is effective for a rare condition, but that may not be marketed by a drug manufacturer because of the small sales and profit potential compared with the high cost of development, testing, and production.

OTC
The abbreviation for over-the-counter. Over-the-counter drugs can be bought from the drugstore without a prescription from your physician.

P

Parasympathomimetic
A drug that stimulates the parasympathetic nervous system (see Autonomic nervous system, p.107). Parasympathomimetic (or cholinergic) drugs are used as *miotics* and to stimulate bladder contraction in urinary retention (see Drugs used for urinary disorders, p.194).

Parkinsonism
Neurological symptoms including tremor of the hands, muscle rigidity, and slowness of movements that resemble Parkinson's disease. Parkinsonism may be caused by prolonged treatment with an antipsychotic drug.

Pharmacist
A licensed, trained health professional who is concerned with the preparation and dispensing of drugs. Pharmacists may advise on the correct use of non-prescription drugs and may answer many questions about the use of prescribed medication.

Pharmacokinetics
The term used to describe how the body deals with a drug, including how it is absorbed into the bloodstream, distributed to different tissues, broken down, and finally excreted from the body.

Pharmacologist
A scientist concerned with the study of drugs and their actions. Pharmacologists are responsible for research into new drugs. Clinical pharmacologists often may have an MD degree. They are primarily concerned with the actions of drugs in the treatment of specific disorders and with monitoring their effects on patients in clinical trials and in medical practice.

Pharmacopoeia
A publication that lists and describes drugs used in medicine. This term usually refers to an official national publication such as the United States Pharmacopoeia (USP). Used as a reference book by physicians and pharmacists, a pharmacopoeia describes sources, preparations, doses, and tests that can be used to identify individual drugs and to determine their purity. It may also contain information about mechanisms of action, possible adverse effects,

comments about the relative effectiveness and safety of a drug in treating a particular disorder, and price comparisons between similar drugs. The first official US Pharmacopoeia was published in 1820 and included information on 217 drugs.

Pharmacy
A term used to describe the practice of preparing drugs and making up prescriptions, or a place where these activities are carried out.

Photophobia
Dislike of bright light. Photophobia may be induced by certain drugs.

Placebo
A "medicine," often in tablet or capsule form, that contains no medically active ingredient. Placebos are frequently used in clinical trials of new drugs (see *Double-blind*). A physician may administer a placebo because of the positive emotional or psychological benefit it may give to a patient convinced that his or her condition calls for some form of medication.

Poison
A substance that, in relatively small amounts, disrupts the structure and/or function of cells, causing harmful and sometimes fatal effects. Many drugs are poisonous if taken in overdose.

Premedication
The term applied to drugs given between one and two hours before an operation to prepare a person for surgery. Premedication usually contains a narcotic analgesic to help relieve pain and anxiety and to reduce the dose of anesthetic needed to produce unconsciousness (see also *Anesthetic, general*). An *anticholinergic* drug is sometimes included to reduce secretions in the airways.

Prescription
A written instruction from the physician to the pharmacist, detailing the name of the drug to be dispensed, the dosage, how often it has to be taken, and other instructions as necessary. A prescription is filled and signed by a physician and carries the name and address of the patient for whom the drug is prescribed. The pharmacist keeps a record of all prescriptions dispensed. See also Managing your drug treatment (p.25).

Prophylactic
A drug, procedure, or piece of equipment used to prevent disease. For example, a course of drugs given to a traveler to prevent malarial infection is called malaria prophylaxis.

Proprietary
A term now generally applied to a drug that is sold over the counter, its name being registered to a private manufacturer (i.e. a proprietor). An ethical drug is one that virtually always requires a physician's prescription. Early in this century, ethical drugs were those employed by "ethical" physicians, who had confidence in their safety and effectiveness.

Purgative
A drug that helps eliminate feces from the body. See also *Cathartic*.

R

Receptor
A specific site on the surface of a cell with a characteristic chemical and physical structure. Natural body chemicals such as *neurotransmitters* bind to cell receptors to initiate a response in the cell. Many drugs also have an effect on cells by binding to a receptor. They may promote cell activity or may block it. See also *Agonist* and *Antagonist*.

Replication
The duplication of genetic material (DNA or RNA) within a cell as part of the process of cell division, which enables a tissue to grow or a virus to multiply.

Rubefacient
A preparation, also known as a counter-irritant, that, when applied to an area of skin, causes it to redden by increasing blood flow in vessels in that area. A rubefacient such as methyl salicylate may be included in an *embrocation*.

S

Sedative
A drug that dampens the activity of the central nervous system. Sleeping drugs (p.110) and anti-anxiety drugs (p.111) have a sedative effect, and many other drugs such as antihistamines (p.152) and antidepressants (p.112) can produce sedation as a side effect.

Side effect
A reaction to a drug that can be explained by the established effects of the drug itself. A side effect may be a predictable effect, such as dry mouth caused by an *anticholinergic* drug, or an exaggeration of the normal therapeutic effect, such as bleeding caused by an anticoagulant drug. The term is distinct from *adverse reaction*, which is an unpredictable effect.

Subcutaneous injection
A method of administering a drug by which the drug is injected just beneath the skin. The drug is then slowly absorbed over a few hours into the surrounding blood vessels. Insulin is given in this way. See also Methods of administration (p.17).

Sublingual
A term meaning under the tongue. Some drugs are administered sublingually in tablet form. The drug is then very rapidly absorbed through the lining of the mouth into the bloodstream within a few seconds. Nitrate drugs may be given this way to provide rapid relief of an angina attack. See also Methods of administration (p.17).

Suppository
A bullet-shaped pellet usually containing a drug for insertion into the rectum or vagina. See also Methods of administration (p.17).

Sympatholytic
A term meaning blocking the effect of the sympathetic nervous system. Sympatholytic drugs work either by reducing the release of the stimulatory *neurotransmitter* norepinephrine from nerve endings, or by occupying the *receptors* that the neurotransmitters epinephrine and norepinephrine normally bind to, thereby preventing their normal actions. Beta blockers are examples of sympatholytic drugs. See also Autonomic nervous system (p.107).

Sympathomimetic
Having the same effect as stimulation of the sympathetic nervous system to cause, for example, an increase in the heart rate. A drug with a sympathomimetic action may work by causing the release of the stimulatory *neurotransmitter* norepinephrine from nerve endings or by mimicking the action of stimulatory neurotransmitters. See also Autonomic nervous system (p.107).

Systemic
Having a generalized effect, causing physical or chemical changes in tissues throughout the body. For a drug to have a systemic effect it must be absorbed into the bloodstream, usually via the digestive tract, by injection or by rectal suppository.

T

Tardive dyskinesia
Abnormal, uncontrolled movements, mainly of the face, tongue, mouth, and neck, that may be caused by prolonged treatment with antipsychotic drugs. This condition is distinct from *parkinsonism*, which may also be caused by such drugs. See also Antipsychotic drugs (p.113).

Tolerance
The need to take a higher dosage of a specific drug to maintain the same physical or mental effect. Tolerance may occur during prolonged treatment with narcotic analgesics and benzodiazepines. See also Drug dependence (p.23).

Tonics
A diverse group of remedies prescribed or bought over the counter for relieving vague symptoms such as malaise, lethargy, and loss of appetite for which no obvious cause can be found. Tonics sometimes contain vitamins and minerals, but there is no scientific evidence that such ingredients have anything other than a *placebo* effect. Nevertheless, many individuals feel better after taking a tonic for a few weeks, and this does no harm.

Topical
The term used to decribe the application of a drug to the site where it is intended to have its effect. Disorders of the skin, eye, outer ear, nasal passages, and vagina are often treated with drugs applied topically.

Toxic reaction
Symptoms, which can sometimes be dangerous, caused by a drug as the result of either an overdose or an *adverse reaction*.

Toxin, toxic
A toxin is a poisonous substance such as a harmful chemical released by bacteria or created by a drug interaction. Drugs that are usually safe in normal doses may produce toxic effects when taken in overdose. An *adverse reaction* may also produce a toxin. See The effects of drugs (p.15).

Tranquilizer, major
A drug used to treat psychotic illnesses such as schizophrenia. See Antipsychotic drugs (p.113).

Tranquilizer, minor
A *sedative* drug used to treat anxiety and emotional tension. See Anti-anxiety drugs (p.111).

Transdermal patch
A method of administering a drug in which an adhesive patch impregnated with the drug is placed on the skin. The drug is slowly absorbed through the skin into the underlying blood vessels. Drugs administered in this way include nitrates and estrogens. See also Methods of administration (p.17).

V W

Vaccine
A substance administered to induce active immunity against a specific infectious disease (see Vaccines and immunization, p.162).

Vasoconstrictor
A drug that narrows blood vessels, often prescribed to reduce nasal congestion. See Decongestants (p.121). Vasoconstrictors are also frequently given with injected local anesthetics (p.108). Ephedrine is a commonly prescribed vasoconstrictor.

Vasodilator
A drug that widens blood vessels. See Vasodilators (p.126).

Withdrawal symptom
Any symptom caused by abrupt stopping of a drug. These symptoms occur as a result of physical *dependence* on a drug. Drugs that may cause withdrawal symptoms after prolonged use include narcotics, benzodiazepines, and nicotine. Withdrawal symptoms vary according to each drug, but common examples include sweating, shaking, anxiety, nausea, and abdominal pain. See also Drug dependence (p.23).

GENERAL INDEX

Use this index to look up specific drugs and medications or general topics such as drug groups, diseases, and conditions. In Part 2 there is also a special Index of Generic and Brand-Name Drugs (Index of drugs for short) where further information on individual drugs can be found (see pp.64–103).

Entries for brand-name tablets and capsules that are shown in the Color Identification Guide contain italicized references to the appropriate page and grid letter.

References that consist of a page number followed by the letter "g" indicate terms that are defined in the glossary.

O

DRUG POISONING EMERGENCY GUIDE

The information on the following pages is intended to give practical advice for dealing with a known or suspected drug poisoning emergency. Although many of the first-aid techniques described can be used in a number of different types of emergency, instructions apply only to drug overdose or poisoning.

Emergency action is necessary in any of the following circumstances:

● If a person has taken an overdose of any of the high-danger drugs listed in the box on p.592.
● If a person has taken an overdose of a less dangerous drug, but has one or more of the danger symptoms listed below.
● If a person has taken, or is suspected of having taken, an overdose of an unknown drug.
● If a child has swallowed, or is suspected of having swallowed, any prescription or non-prescription drug.

What to do

If you are faced with a drug poisoning emergency, it is important to carry out first aid and arrange immediate medical help in the right order. The Priority Action Decision Chart, below, will help you to assess the situation and to determine your priorities. The following information should help you to remain calm in an emergency if you ever need to deal with a case of drug poisoning.

DANGER SYMPTOMS

Take emergency action if the person has one or more of the following symptoms:
● Drowsiness or unconsciousness
● Shallow, irregular, or stopped breathing
● Vomiting
● Seizures or convulsions

PRIORITY ACTION DECISION CHART

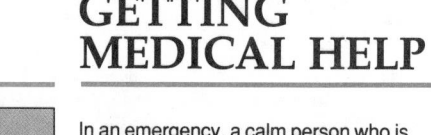

Is the person breathing? — **NO** →
Carry out mouth-to-mouth resuscitation and, if necessary, cardiac compression (facing page).
Then
Get medical help (right).

YES ↓

Is the person conscious? — **NO** →
Clear airway (step one, facing page) and place person in the recovery position (facing page).
Then
Get medical help (right).

YES ↓

Is the person drowsy? — **NO** →
Get medical help (right). Keep the person under observation in case of a change in his or her condition. See also Things to remember (right).

YES ↓

Place in recovery position.
Then
Get medical help (right). Keep the person under observation in case of a change in his or her condition. See also Things to remember (right).

IMPORTANT

Do not give anything by mouth unless specifically instructed to do so by a physician or poison control center. Fluids may hasten absorption of the drug, thereby increasing the danger to the overdose victim.

GETTING MEDICAL HELP

In an emergency, a calm person who is competent in first aid should stay with the victim while others summon help. However, if you have to deal with a drug poisoning emergency on your own, use first aid (see the Priority Action Decision Chart) before getting help.

Call the emergency medical service (911 in many areas) for an ambulance. Then call the poison control center or your physician for advice. If possible, tell what drug has been taken, how much has been taken, and the age of the victim. Follow instructions precisely, especially with regard to vomiting.

THINGS TO REMEMBER

Effective treatment of drug poisoning depends on the physician's making a rapid assessment of the type and amount of drug taken. Collecting evidence that will assist the diagnosis will help. After you have carried out first aid, look for empty or opened medicine containers. Keep any of the drug that is left together with its container (or syringe), and give these to the physician. Save any vomit for analysis.

ESSENTIAL FIRST AID

MOUTH-TO-MOUTH RESUSCITATION

When there is no rise and fall of the chest and you can feel no movement of exhaled air, immediately commence mouth-to-mouth resuscitation.

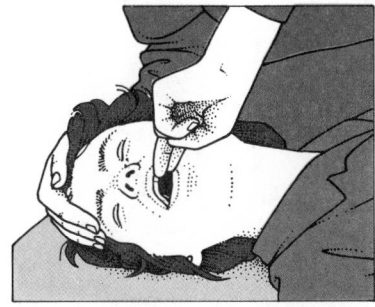

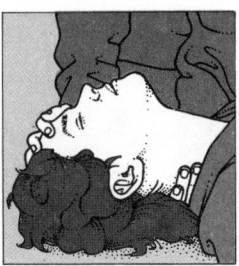

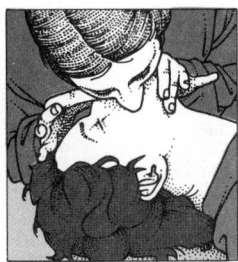

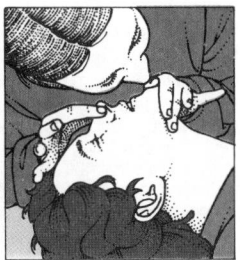

1 Lay the victim on his or her back on a firm surface. Clear the mouth of vomit or any other foreign material that might otherwise block the airways, and remove false teeth.

2 Place one hand under the neck and lift gently to tip the head back and raise the chin, while pressing down on the forehead. This should allow the mouth to drop open.

3 Pinch the victim's nostrils closed with the hand that is placed on the forehead and use the other to grip his or her chin firmly to keep the mouth open. Take a deep breath, seal your mouth over that of the victim, and give two quick breaths. Continue to give further breaths every 5 seconds.

4 After each breath, turn to watch the chest falling while you listen for the sound of air leaving the victim's mouth. Continue until the victim starts to breathe regularly on his or her own, or until medical help arrives.

CARDIAC COMPRESSION

This is a technique used in conjunction with mouth-to-mouth resuscitation to restart a stopped heartbeat. It is a procedure that should normally be undertaken only by someone who has received training.

Cardiac compression involves putting repeated, strong pressure on the center of the chest with the heels of both hands, at a rate of 80 compressions per minute (right). After every 15 compressions, two breaths should be given using mouth-to-mouth resuscitation (above).

CHECKING PULSE

If the victim does not start breathing after two breaths of mouth-to-mouth resuscitation, check the pulse in the neck. If there is no pulse, start cardiac compression if you have been trained in this technique.

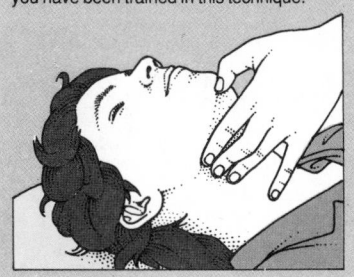

This sequence should be continued until breathing restarts.

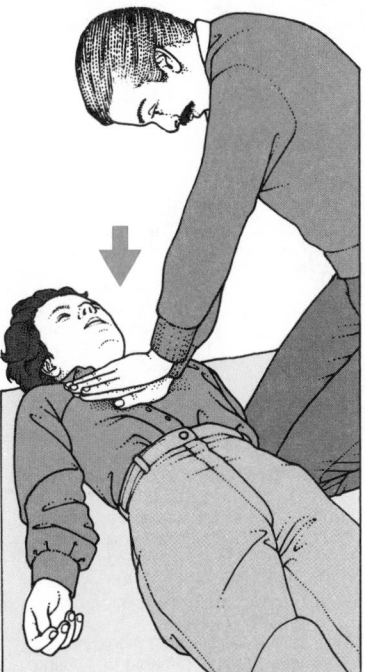

THE RECOVERY POSITION

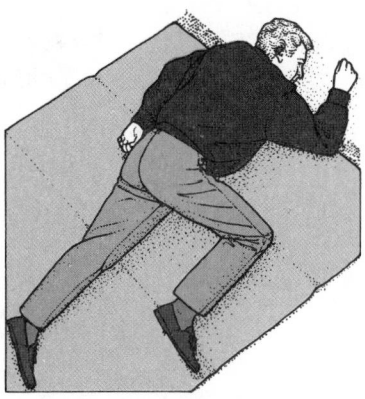

The recovery position is the safest position for an unconscious or drowsy person. It allows the person to breathe easily and will help to prevent choking if vomiting occurs. A victim of drug poisoning should be placed in the recovery position after more urgent first aid, such as mouth-to-mouth resuscitation, has been carried out and when shock (p.592) is not suspected. Place the victim on his or her stomach with one leg bent and the arm on that side raised. Turn the head to the same side. Tilt the head back so that the chin juts forward. Cover the person with a blanket for warmth.

DEALING WITH A SEIZURE

Certain types of drug poisoning may provoke seizures. These may occur whether the person is conscious or not. The victim usually falls to the ground twitching or making uncontrolled movements of limbs and body. If you witness a seizure, remember the following points:

● Do not try to hold the person down.

● Do not put anything into the person's mouth.

● Remove any objects or furniture on which the victim could be injured.

● Once the seizure is over, place the person in the recovery position (p.591).

HIGH-DANGER DRUGS

The following is a list of drugs given a high overdose rating in the drug profiles. If you suspect that someone has taken an overdose of one of these drugs, immediate medical attention must be sought.

Acebutolol
Acetaminophen
Acetohexamide
Alprostadil
Aminophylline
Amitriptyline
Amoxapine
Aspirin

Belladonna

Chloral hydrate
Chloroquine

Chlorpropamide
Codeine
Colchicine
Cyclobenzaprine

Desipramine
Dicumarol
Digitoxin
Digoxin
Disopyramide
Doxepin

Epinephrine
Ergonovine

Glipizide
Glyburide
Guanethidine

Heparin
Hydralazine

Imipramine

Insulin
Interferon
Isocarboxazid
Isoniazid
Isoproterenol

Labetalol
Lithium

Maprotiline
Meperidine
Methotrexate
Metoprolol
Minoxidil
Morphine

Nadolol
Neostigmine

Orphenadrine
Oxtriphylline

Phenelzine

Phenobarbital
Phenylbutazone
Phenylpropanolamine
Primidone
Procyclidine
Propoxyphene
Propranolol
Pseudoephedrine
Pyridostigmine

Quinidine
Quinine

Secobarbital

Theophylline
Timolol
Tolazamide
Tolbutamide

Vasopressin

Warfarin

DEALING WITH ANAPHYLACTIC SHOCK

Anaphylactic shock occurs as the result of a severe allergic reaction to a drug or insect sting or bite. Blood pressure drops dramatically and the airways may become narrowed. The reaction usually occurs within minutes of taking the drug. The main symptoms are:

● Pallor
● Tightness in the chest
● Breathing difficulty
● Rash
● Facial swelling
● Collapse

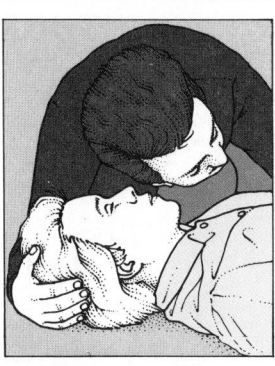

1 First ensure that the person is breathing. If breathing has stopped, immediate mouth-to-mouth resuscitation should be carried out as described on p.591.

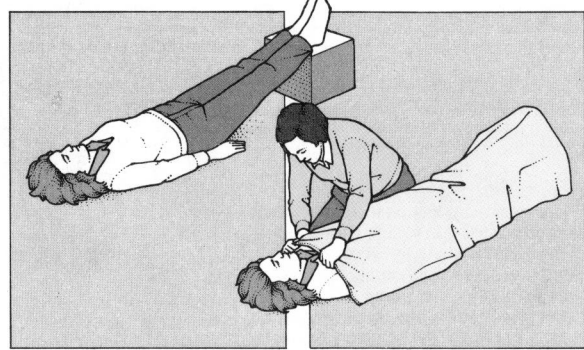

2 If the person is breathing normally, lay him or her down, face-up, with legs raised above the level of the heart to ensure the adequate circulation of the blood. Use a footstool, carton, or a similar item to support the feet.

3 Cover the person with a blanket or articles of clothing and phone for medical help. Do not attempt to administer anything by mouth.

HOW TO INDUCE VOMITING

In certain circumstances you may be advised to make a person vomit in order to expel a drug from the stomach, thus preventing the drug from being absorbed. This should be attempted only when specifically advised, and never when the person is unconscious. The simplest method of inducing vomiting is to give syrup of ipecac, a drug that should be kept among your regular medical supplies. Recommended dosages are 2 teaspoons (children under 18 months); 1 tablespoon (18 months – 12 years); and 2 tablespoons (adults). This normally stimulates vomiting within 20 – 30 minutes. Do not push fingers down the throat. When vomiting occurs, remember the following:

1 Ensure that the victim leans well forward to avoid choking or inhaling vomit.

2 Keep the vomit for later analysis (see Things to remember, p.590).

3 Give water to rinse the mouth. This should be spit out, not swallowed.